Second Edition

A Practical Approach to Occupational and Environmental Medicine

Edited by

Robert J. McCunney, M.D., M.P.H., M.S.

Director, Environmental Medical Service, Medical Department, Massachusetts Institute of Technology, Cambridge; Corporate Medical Director, Cabot Corporation, Boston

Foreword by

Paul W. Brandt-Rauf, Sc.D., M.D., Dr.P.H.

Professor of Environmental Sciences, Columbia University School of Public Health, New York

Little, Brown and Company
Boston   New York   Toronto   London

Library of Congress Cataloging-in-Publication Data
A Practical approach to occupational and environmental medicine /
    edited by Robert J. McCunney ; foreword by Paul W. Brandt-Rauf. —
    2nd ed.
        p.   cm.
    Rev. ed. of: Handbook of occupational medicine. c1988.
    Includes bibliographical references and index.
    ISBN 0-316-55534-7

Third Printing

    1. Medicine, Industrial—Handbooks, manuals, etc.
    2. Environmental health—Handbooks, manuals, etc.
    3. Environmentally induced diseases—Handbooks, manuals, etc.
    I. McCunney, Robert J.   II. Handbook of occupational medicine.
        [DNLM: 1. Occupational Diseases—handbooks.   2. Occupational
    Medicine—handbooks.   WA 39 H2356 1994]
    RC963.H34 1994
    616.9'803—dc20
    DNLM/DLC
    for Library of Congress   94-11269
Printed in the United States of America   CIP
QW/F

Editorial: Nancy Megley, Laurie Anello
Production Editor: Cathleen Cote
Copyeditor: Debra Corman
Indexer: Alexandra Nickerson
Production Supervisor: Michael A. Granger
Cover Designer: Michael A. Granger

Contents

Contributing Authors

Donald Accetta, M.D.
Consultant, Department of Medicine, New England Medical Center, Boston
19. Allergy and Immunology

L. Kristian Arnold, M.D.
Assistant Clinical Professor of Sociomedical Sciences, Boston University School of Medicine; Attending Physician, Emergency Department, Boston City Hospital and Boston University Medical Center Hospital, Boston
47. Emergency Response to Environmental Incidents

Cheryl Barbanel, M.D., M.B.A., M.P.H.
Director, Occupational Medicine, Boston University School of Medicine; Assistant Medical Director, Occupational and Environmental Medicine, Boston University Medical Center Hospital, Boston
Appendix A. Health Effects of Common Substances

Thomas Beck, J.D.
Associate Attorney, Jones, Day, Reavis & Pogue, Washington
2. Legal and Ethical Issues

Jonathan Borak, M.D.
Associate Clinical Professor of Internal Medicine, Yale University School of Medicine; President, Jonathan Borak and Company, Inc., New Haven, Connecticut
46. Environmental Medical Emergencies

Reid T. Boswell, M.D., M.P.H.
Assistant Medical Director, Occupational and Environmental Medicine Unit, Boston University Medical Center Hospital, Boston
12. Musculoskeletal Disorders

Christopher R. Brigham, M.D.
Clinical Instructor of Medicine, University of Vermont College of Medicine, Burlington, Vermont; Director, Division of Occupational Health, Maine Medical Center, Portland, Maine
7. The Disability/Impairment Evaluation

Ron Brookmeyer, Ph.D.

Professor of Biostatistics, School of Hygiene and Public Health, Johns Hopkins University, Baltimore
24. Epidemiology and Biostatistics

William E. Browning, Jr., A.B.

Consultant, Scientific Literature Research, Environmental Health and Safety, P.C., Boston
27. Searching the Occupational Medical Literature

William B. Bunn, M.D., J.D., M.P.H.

Director, International Medical Services, Mobil Corporation, Princeton, New Jersey
42. Environmental Medicine: The Regulatory Issues
49. The Environmental Audit
50. Environmental Risk Assessment

Kenneth H. Chase, M.D.

Clinical Assistant Professor of Medicine, George Washington University School of Medicine and Health Sciences, Washington
26. Risk Assessment

Chang-Ming Chern, M.D.

Fellow in Occupational and Environmental Neurology, Boston University School of Medicine, Boston; Attending Physician, Neurological Center, Veterans General Hospital, Taipei, Taiwan
15. Neurotoxic Disorders

Barry A. Cooper, M.H.A.

Vice President, Occupational Health Strategies, Inc., Arlington, Virginia
36. Computers in Occupational Medical Practice

Alan M. Ducatman, M.D., M.Sc.

Professor of Medicine, West Virginia University School of Medicine; Director, Institute for Occupational and Environmental Health, West Virginia University School of Medicine, Morgantown, West Virginia
43. Clinical Environmental Medicine

Alan L. Engelberg, M.D.

Clinical Associate Professor of Community and Family Medicine, St. Louis University School of Medicine; Medical Director, Monsanto Company and NutraSweet Company, St. Louis
7. The Disability/Impairment Evaluation

Nancy English, Ph.D.

SmithKline Beecham, Philadelphia
Appendix B. Government and Regulatory Agencies

Jack E. Farnham, M.D., M.P.H.

Assistant Professor of Medicine, Occupational Medicine Division, University of Texas Health Center, Tyler, Texas
19. Allergy and Immunology

Robert G. Feldman, M.D.

Professor and Chairman of Neurology, Boston University School of Medicine; Chief of Neurology, Boston University Medical Center and VA Medical Center, Boston
15. Neurotoxic Disorders

Jean Spencer Felton, M.D.

Clinical Professor, Department of Medicine, University of California, Irvine, College of Medicine
Appendix C. A History of the American College of Occupational and Environmental Medicine and the Growth of a Specialty

Howard Frumkin, M.D., Dr.P.H.

Director, Division of Environmental and Occupational Health, Emory School of Public Health; Director, Environmental and Occupational Medicine Program, The Emory Clinic, Atlanta
13. Occupational Cancers
Appendix A. Health Effects of Common Substances

Robert Galvin, M.D.

Clinical Assistant Professor of Internal Medicine, Boston University School of Medicine, Boston; Clinical Coordinator, Inpatient Teaching Service, North Shore Medical Center, Salem, Massachusetts
40. Health Care Management

David H. Garabrant, M.D., M.P.H.

Director of Occupational Health, Department of Environmental and Industrial Health, University of Michigan School of Public Health, Ann Arbor, Michigan
37. Training and Communications

Donald C. Gasaway, M.A.

Hearing Conservation Consultant, Hearing Conservation–ASP, San Antonio, Texas
16. Noise-Induced Hearing Loss

Rose H. Goldman, M.D.

Assistant Professor of Medicine, Harvard Medical School, Boston; Director, Occupational and Environmental Health, Cambridge Hospital, Cambridge, Massachusetts
21. Suspecting Occupational Disease

Douglas C. Gray, Ph.D.

Manager, Corporate Industrial Hygiene, Department of Safety, Health, and Environment, Cabot Corporation, Boston
4. The Establishment of an Occupational Health Program

Ian A. Greaves, M.D.

Associate Professor and Head, Environmental and Occupational Health, School of Public Health, University of Minnesota, Minneapolis
11. Occupational Pulmonary Disease

William W. Greaves, M.D., M.S.P.H.

Associate Professor and Acting
Chairman of Preventive Medicine,
Medical College of Wisconsin;
Chairman, Department of Preventive
Medicine, Froedtert Memorial
Lutheran Hospital, Milwaukee
31. Reproductive Hazards

Tee L. Guidotti, M.D.

Professor of Public Health Sciences,
University of Alberta Faculty of
Medicine, Edmonton, Alberta
41. The Environment and Health

David Mueller Gute, Ph.D., M.P.H.

Interim Director, Center for
Environmental Management, Tufts
University, Medford, Massachusetts
48. Accessing Environmental Data

Nortin M. Hadler, M.D.

Professor of Medicine and
Microbiology/Immunology, University
of North Carolina at Chapel Hill
School of Medicine; Attending
Rheumatologist, Department of
Medicine, UNC Hospitals, Chapel
Hill, North Carolina
20. Arm Pain in the Workplace

Ridgway M. Hall, Jr., LL.B.

Attorney, Crowell & Moring,
Washington, D.C.
49. The Environmental Audit

Philip Harber, M.D., M.P.H.

Associate Professor of Medicine,
University of California, Los Angeles,
UCLA School of Medicine; Attending
Physician, UCLA Medical Center, Los
Angeles
25. Medical Surveillance

Jeffrey S. Harris, M.D.

Assistant Clinical Professor of Family
Medicine, Medical College of
Wisconsin, Milwaukee; National
Practice Leader, Strategic Health
Care Practice, Alexander &
Alexander Consulting Group,
San Francisco
*34. Economics of Occupational
Medicine*
39. Workers' Compensation

Joseph Harzbecker, Jr., M.S.(L.S.)

Reference Librarian, Alumni Medical
Library, Boston University School of
Medicine, Boston
*27. Searching the Occupational
Medical Literature*
*Appendix E. References in
Occupational and Environmental
Medicine*

James A. Hathaway, M.D.

Associate Clinical Professor,
Environmental Sciences, Columbia
University School of Public Health,
New York; Corporate Medical
Director, Rhone-Poulenc, Inc.,
Princeton, New Jersey
3. The Role of Regulatory Agencies

Benjamin Haskell Hoffman, M.D., M.P.H.   Adjunct Assistant Professor of
Medicine, Dartmouth Medical School,
Hanover, New Hampshire; Medical
Director, Business Health
Management, P.C., Exeter, New
Hampshire
*4. The Establishment of an
Occupational Health Program*

Peter J. Holland, M.D.   Clinical Instructor of Psychiatry,
University of Miami School of
Medicine, Miami; President, Boca
Raton Psychiatric Group, Boca Raton,
Florida
*18. Psychiatric Aspects of
Occupational Medicine*

John Howard, M.D., J.D.   Assistant Clinical Professor of
Medicine, University of California,
Irvine, College of Medicine, Irvine
California
*30. Medical Center Occupational
Health*

Craig Karpilow, M.D.   Medical Director, Department of
Occupational Medicine, Clinical
Associates; President, International
Professional Associates, Seattle
38. International Occupational Health

Todd D. Kissam, B.A.   Health Examinetics, Inc.,
Charlottesville, Virginia
*36. Computers in Occupational
Medical Practice*

Frank H. Leone, M.P.H., M.B.A.   Executive Director, National
Association of Occupational Health
Professionals and President, Ryan
Associates, Santa Barbara, California
*8. Working with the Business
Community*

David C. Logan, M.D.   Clinical Toxicologist, Medical
Department, Mobil Corporation,
Princeton, New Jersey
23. Toxicology

Molly J. McCauley, M.P.H., R.N.   Division Manager, Health Promotion,
Health Affairs Organization, AT&T,
Basking Ridge, New Jersey
32. Health Promotion

Roger O. McClellan, D.V.M.   Adjunct Professor of Toxicology,
Department of Community and
Family Medicine, Duke University
School of Medicine, Durham;
President, Chemistry Industry
Institute of Toxicology, Research
Triangle Park, North Carolina
50. Environmental Risk Assessment

James M. McCunney, M.S., C.I.H.   Safety and Health Administrator,
Boeing Company, Seattle
22. Industrial Hygiene

Robert J. McCunney, M.D., M.P.H., M.S.

Director, Environmental Medical Service, Medical Department, Massachusetts Institute of Technology, Cambridge; Corporate Medical Director, Cabot Corporation, Boston
1. Occupational Medical Services
12. Musculoskeletal Disorders
14. Cardiovascular Disorders
25. Medical Surveillance
32. Health Promotion
44. Indoor Air Pollution
Appendix A. Health Effects of Common Substances

Junius C. McElveen, Jr., J.D.

Partner, Jones, Day, Reavis & Pogue, Washington, D.C.
2. Legal and Ethical Issues

Joseph K. McLaughlin, Ph.D., M.P.H.

Deputy Chief, Biostatistics Branch, National Cancer Institute, Bethesda, Maryland
24. Epidemiology and Biostatistics

Robert K. McLellan, M.D.

Medical Director, Center for Occupational and Environmental Health, Exeter Hospital, Exeter, New Hampshire
44. Indoor Air Pollution

Frank L. Mitchell, D.O.

Chief Medical Officer, Agency for Toxic Substances and Disease Registry, Atlanta
45. The Agency for Toxic Substances and Disease Registry

Ira H. Monosson, M.D.

Assistant Clinical Professor of Medicine, University of California, Los Angeles, UCLA School of Medicine; Clinical Faculty, Department of Medicine, UCLA Medical Center, Los Angeles
25. Medical Surveillance

J. Steven Moore, M.D., C.I.H.

Assistant Professor of Preventive Medicine, Medical College of Wisconsin, Milwaukee
28. Ergonomics

Kent W. Peterson, M.D.

Clinical Associate Professor of Environmental Medicine, New York University School of Medicine, New York; President, Occupational Health Strategies, Inc., Charlottesville, Virginia
5. The Americans with Disabilities Act
9. Drug Testing
36. Computers in Occupational Medical Practice

Jack Richman, M.D.

Supervisor Elective of Acupuncture and Alternative Medicine, University of Toronto Faculty of Medicine, Toronto; Affiliate Staff, Department of Family Medicine, Oakville Trafalgar Memorial Hospital, Oakville, Ontario
10. Accreditation of Occupational Health Clinical Centers

Bonnie Rogers, R.N., Dr.P.H., C.O.H.N.

Director and Associate Professor of Occupational Health Nursing, School of Public Health, University of North Carolina at Chapel Hill, Chapel Hill, North Carolina
6. The Role of the Occupational Health Nurse

Victor S. Roth, M.D., M.P.H.

Assistant Professor of Occupational and Environmental Medicine, University of Alabama School of Medicine; Attending Physician, Division of Occupational and Environmental Medicine, Birmingham, Alabama
37. Training and Communications

Stephen M. Schmitz, M.D., M.P.H.

Associate Medical Director, Business Health Management, P.C., Exeter, New Hampshire
14. Cardiovascular Disorders

Dennis Schultz, M.D.

Assistant Professor of Preventive Medicine, Medical College of Wisconsin, Milwaukee
10. Accreditation of Occupational Health Clinical Centers

Steven K. Shama, M.D., M.P.H.

Clinical Instructor in Dermatology, Harvard Medical School; Active Staff, Department of Medicine, New England Deaconess Hospital, Boston
17. Occupational Skin Disorders

Peter G. Shields, M.D.

Senior Clinical Investigator, Laboratory of Human Carcinogenesis, National Cancer Institute, Bethesda, Maryland
29. Molecular Genetics

David J. Tollerud, M.P.H.

Associate Professor of Environmental and Occupational Health, Graduate School of Public Health, University of Pittsburgh; Director, Occupational and Environmental Medicine, University of Pittsburgh Medical Center, Pittsburgh
35. Educational Opportunities

John Whysner, M.D., Ph.D., D.A.B.T.

Executive Secretary, Environmental Health Safety Council, American Health Foundation, Valhalla, New York; Vice President, Washington Occupational Health Associates, Inc., Washington, D.C.
26. Risk Assessment

William E. Wright, M.D. M.S.P.H.

Program Manager, Dyncorp • PRI, Reston, Virginia
33. The Case Report: Discovery of Occupational Disease

Foreword: Occupational Medicine's Expanding Scope

The purpose of a book such as this should be to help all the parties involved in occupational health (including employees, employers, and health care professionals) to achieve the mutual objective of advancing the healthfulness of the workplace. This process includes the identification of health hazards at work and the diagnosis, treatment, and, most important, the *prevention* of health effects from associated hazards. Knowledge of this process can help to empower employees so that they can participate in a more meaningful way in the protection of their own health. It can also serve to orient employers to their responsibilities in this area and to provide guidance for effective ways of fulfilling these responsibilities through the expertise of health care professionals. Most significant, however, this book is designed for health care professionals, particularly physicians, who are primarily responsible for the health of a workplace. For the expert in occupational medicine, this book, based on the successful *Handbook of Occupational Medicine,* will continue to serve as a useful reference. However, because specialists in occupational medicine are few and far between and insufficient by all estimates to meet the nation's needs into the foreseeable future, most occupational medicine in this country will continue to be practiced by physicians trained in other specialties. For this majority of occupational medicine practitioners, *A Practical Approach to Occupational and Environmental Medicine* is an invaluable resource.

The value becomes increasingly apparent as one compares the size and content of the first and second editions. Compared to other medical specialties, occupational medicine has always required a particularly broad scope of knowledge for its effective practice, but this edition demonstrates that the field of occupational medicine is clearly expanding its knowledge base in scope and depth at an extraordinarily rapid pace. It is impossible for the expert in occupational medicine, let alone the nonexpert practitioner, to keep abreast of all relevant areas. This book, however, makes the most important and practical aspects of this knowledge accessible to all practitioners. From the physics and engineering of ergonomics to the legal/ethical intricacies of drug testing and the Americans with Disabilities Act to the role of computers in occupational medicine, we are responsible for knowledge from the micro/molecular to the macro/societal if we are to do the best job of advancing occupational health. And now we have added a whole new dimension to occupational medicine practice— environmental medicine, with 10 chapters devoted entirely to this emerging area of importance.

Because of our knowledge base in occupational medicine, practitioners should take the lead in addressing the *prevention* of adverse health effects due to such environmental problems as air and water pollution, toxic waste, ozone depletion, and global warming. The assessment of these environmental health risks, the balanced communication of these risks to employees, employers, and the general public, and the promotion of preventive strategies are now part of the enlarging responsibilities of occupational medicine practitioners. The astute occupational medicine physician has always known that concern for the health of the employee does not stop at the factory gates. It now clearly extends to the home, the community, and the entire planet. Achieving a healthful environment, inside and outside the workplace, must now be the objective of all responsible occupational medicine physicians.

Paul W. Brandt-Rauf, Sc.D., M.D., Dr.P.H.

Preface

A Practical Approach to Occupational and Environmental Medicine, Second Edition, began as a revision of the *Handbook of Occupational Medicine,* which was published in 1988. Intended as a practical guide, the handbook found wide applicability in various settings. As a result, it seemed appropriate to update the book, especially in light of the numerous changes that have occurred in the regulatory and scientific aspects of occupational medical practice.

Since the *Handbook of Occupational Medicine* was reviewed by the Publications Committee of the American College of Occupational and Environmental Medicine (ACOEM), a draft outline of the second edition was developed for the committee's review in late 1991. This draft included new chapters on topics such as clinical environmental medicine, medical center occupational health, and searching the literature. It was evident that the range of occupational medicine practice had expanded considerably over the intervening six years. Changes in the delivery of occupational health services, wider recognition and regulation of biological hazards, and the growing importance of environmental health issues are but a few of the developments that led to either new or considerably revised chapters. As a result of the more than 50 percent expansion in content, it became clear that the publication was actually a new book, hence the change in title as proposed by the publisher. The book remains practical in focus with sufficient background in each chapter to enable the uninitiated reader to quickly grasp the essentials of a topic. Each chapter includes a "Further Information" section of annotated references to facilitate additional review.

Occupational medicine has continued to become more widely recognized as a specialty with unique capabilities for preventing and treating illnesses and injuries related to work. Federal regulations, in particular, have furthered the expansion of clinical occupational medical services; but, in the process, the purchasers of health care have begun to place a priority on specialized training in occupational medicine. Group practices, hospitals, and private practitioners have continued a trend in adding occupational medicine physicians to their staffs with more regularity than ever before.

Challenges to the occupational physician in the 1990s will likely be broad in scope. This book, with its 50 chapters in 5 sections, addresses the range of activities that can be assumed by the practitioner. It also attempts to provide a framework for incorporating environmental medicine activities into the sphere of occupational medicine practice. Understanding appropriate regulations and the methods to access public data can be as demanding as evaluating the health implications of exposure to a hazardous substance.

Developing this book has been a challenging experience that has proved to be wonderfully educational. I am indebted to the efforts of the contributing authors who persevered through numerous drafts and revisions, all in the attempt to ensure a high-quality book that will help define the range of occupational medical practice.

R. J. M.

Acknowledgments

The following members of the Publications Committee of the American College of Occupational and Environmental Medicine participated in the peer review process of various sections of this book. Their insights and suggestions played a major role in improving the quality of the final effort. All of the reviewers contributed chapters to the text as well.

William B. Bunn, M.D., J.D., M.P.H.
William W. Greaves, M.D., M.S.P.H.
Jeffrey S. Harris, M.D.
Alan L. Engelberg, M.D.
Tee L. Guidotti, M.D.

Royalties from the sale and distribution of this book benefit the Samuel E. Bacon Research and Education Fund of the American College of Occupational and Environmental Medicine.

American College of Occupational and Environmental Medicine Code of Ethical Conduct

This code establishes standards of professional ethical conduct with which each member of the American College of Occupational and Environmental Medicine (ACOEM) is expected to comply. These standards are intended to guide occupational and environmental medicine physicians in their relationships with: the individuals they serve; with employers and workers' representatives; with colleagues in the health professions; with the public and with all levels of government, including the judiciary.

Physicians should:

1. accord the highest priority to the health and safety of individuals in both the workplace and the environment;
2. practice on a scientific basis with integrity and strive to acquire and maintain adequate knowledge and expertise upon which to render professional service;
3. relate honestly and ethically in all professional relationships;
4. strive to expand and disseminate medical knowledge and participate in ethical research efforts as appropriate;
5. keep confidential all individual medical information, releasing such information only when required to by law or overriding public health considerations, or to other physicians according to accepted medical practice, or to others at the request of the individual;
6. recognize that employers may be entitled to counsel about an individual's medical work fitness, but not to diagnoses or specific details, except in compliance with the law or other regulations;
7. communicate to individuals and/or groups any significant observations and recommendations concerning their health and/or safety; and
8. recognize those medical impairments in oneself and others, including chemical dependency or abusive personal practices, which interfere with one's ability to follow the above principles, and take appropriate treatment measures.

Occupational Medical Services

Notice

The indications and dosages of all drugs in this book have been recommended in the medical literature and conform to the practices of the general medical community. The medications described do not necessarily have specific approval by the Food and Drug Administration for use in the diseases and dosages for which they are recommended. The package insert for each drug should be consulted for use and dosage as approved by the FDA. Because standards for usage change, it is advisable to keep abreast of revised recommendations, particularly those concerning new drugs.

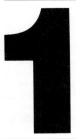

Occupational Medical Services

Robert J. McCunney

The range of services provided by a physician who practices occupational medicine depends largely on the *setting* of the practice. Occupational medicine specialists must work much more closely than many traditional medical specialists with other professionals such as epidemiologists, toxicologists, and industrial hygienists. In fact, a *team* approach to controlling occupational illnesses and injuries is essential. This chapter is designed to provide an introduction to the *range of occupational medical services,* provided by physicians who deliver health care to the working population.

Although occupational medicine has been a distinct discipline within the American Board of Preventive Medicine since 1954, a considerable shortage of well-trained and certified specialists in this field exists. In large part, this shortage is due to a deficiency of post-graduate training positions. The situation is now changing. Over the past 15 years, Educational Resource Centers established by the National Institute for Occupational Safety and Health (NIOSH) and other institutions, such as hospitals [1], have been instrumental in educating physicians in the discipline of occupational medicine. More recently, additional residency programs have been established. As of 1992, 37 institutions sponsored graduate medical education training in occupational medicine. In addition, "mini-residency" programs and other educational opportunities such as those established by the American College of Occupational and Environmental Medicine have furthered the growth and influence of the specialty. Unfortunately, these recent endeavors still fail to provide the number of highly trained physicians necessary for the provision of quality occupational medical services.

The shortage of occupational medicine specialists combined with wider awareness of occupational and environmental hazards creates an opportunity for the primary care physician [2]. One needs only to read a daily newspaper to come into contact with topics such as the Superfund, contamination of the water supply, "right to know" laws, and periodic reports associating certain illnesses with a particular workplace or environmental substance. Educated workers and consumers offer further challenges to the physician to become abreast of these issues and to develop protocols for the evaluation and prevention of occupationally related illnesses [3].

History of Occupational Medicine

The history of occupational medicine can be traced into antiquity. Observations related to increased rates of illnesses and mortality among miners date back to Roman times; however, explanations for this phenomenon were often attributed to the fact that workers were slaves and thus of a more feeble constitution. It was not until the late seventeenth century, when an Italian physician published *Disease and Occupations,* that physicians were formally urged to pay attention to the role of one's work in the development of certain illnesses [4].

Throughout the two centuries after Dr. Ramazzini's book appeared, periodic reports described illnesses associated with a variety of substances [5]. In the first part of the twentieth century, a rising number of employee-directed suits against employers for work-related injuries prompted the development of workers' compensation statutes [6]. The workers' compensation system essentially established a "no fault" insurance program such that any injured worker would be guaranteed compensation for medical bills, time lost from work, and permanent impairment or death. In turn, employers were granted immunity from further legal action by workers for work-related illnesses or injuries.

About this time (1916), the Industrial Medical Association, the forerunner of the American College of Occupational and Environmental Medicine, was formed. This early group was composed primarily of surgeons who had developed a strong interest and expertise in treatment of work-related injuries. Most of the occupational medicine practice at this time was directed primarily toward injury care and management. Little, if any, recognition was given to certain hazardous substances such as silica or asbestos, although the US Public Health Service began to do worksite surveys during this period.

Clinical activities associated with treating work-related injuries were referred to as *industrial* medicine. As physicians became more concerned with *preventing* work-related injuries and illnesses, the medical discipline became known as occupational medicine.

Eventually, the area of knowledge and expertise associated with delivering health care to the working population began to incorporate other disciplines within its sphere. Toxicology, epidemiology, industrial hygiene, ergonomics, and other related disciplines became integral elements of the education of the well-trained occupational physician. In 1946, the American Academy of Occupational Medicine was founded to foster the growth and development of the more formally educated occupational physician; its founding led to occupational medicine becoming a distinct medical specialty in 1954. The American Academy eventually merged with the American Occupational Medical Association to form the American College of Occupational Medicine, which eventually added "Environmental" to its title.

Throughout the first four to five decades since the establishment of the workers' compensation laws, the provision of occupational health services has been primarily in the corporate setting and in some cases from the private physician's office. Larger corporations with a sufficient number of employees could economically justify on-site facilities, especially if the work situations warranted immediate medical care. During this period, however, the needs of small businesses for occupational medical services appeared to have been overlooked. A relatively unknown fact is that over 90% of businesses in the United States *and the world* have 100 or fewer employees. It is rarely economically feasible for these enterprises to provide anything other than meager health care and, in some cases, at best first aid.

To meet the need for providing occupational health services to small businesses, a number of approaches can be effective. An entire medical facility can provide occupational health services to a range of small businesses within a certain geographic area. Alternatively, occupational health services can be delivered from the private physician's office or by the physician making periodic visits to the local business facility.

Occupational Health Services

What does one *do* in occupational medicine? The occupational physician lacks the trademark associated with other specialties, such as the electrocardiogram of the cardiologist, the bronchoscope of the pulmonary specialist, or the scalpel of the surgeon. Occupational health services, in their broadest sense, can include the entire form of health care delivery to the working population. Although any definition is likely to be arbitrary, the description of occupational health services to follow is designed mainly for the primary care physician who may provide such services at a local plant, as part of a private practice or multispecialty group, or at an occupational health center designed for small businesses. Residents and other health care professionals such as physician assistants and nurse practitioners will also find that many of these services are within their realm of expertise. These services should be considered *essential* in primary occupational health care. Clinicians are advised that business professionals responsible for overseeing the delivery of these services will expect knowledge and understanding in these areas. The physician in turn is advised to become familiar with the scientific principles of occupational medicine practice through the educational programs that are widely available (see Chap. 35).

The scope of services provided in an occupational medicine practice setting will vary depending on a variety of factors. To help set a framework of consistency, the American College of Occupational and Environmental Medicine published guidelines regarding essential and elective components (Tables 1-1 and 1-2).

Table 1-1. Occupational and environmental health programs:
Essential components

1. Health evaluation of employees
   A. Preassignment
   B. Medical surveillance
   C. Post illness or injury
2. Diagnosis and treatment of occupational and environmental injuries or illnesses, including rehabilitation
3. Emergency treatment of nonoccupational injury or illness
4. Education of employees and jobs where potential occupational hazards exist
5. Implementation of programs for personal protective equipment
6. Evaluation, inspection, and abatement of workplace hazards
7. Toxicologic assessments, including advice on chemical substances that have not had adequate toxicologic testing
8. Biostatistics and epidemiology assessments
9. Maintenance of occupational medical records
10. Immunization against possible occupational infections
11. Medical interpretation and participation in governmental health and safety regulations
12. Periodic evaluation of the occupational or environmental health program
13. Disaster preparedness: planning for the workplace and community
14. Assistance in rehabilitation of alcohol- and drug-dependent employees or those with emotional disorders

Source: Adapted from Scope of occupational and environmental health programs and practices, report of the Occupational Medical Practice Committee of the American College of Occupational and Environmental Medicine. *J. Occup. Med.* 34:436, 1992.

Table 1-2. Elective components of occupational and environmental health programs

1. Palliative treatment of nonoccupational disorders
2. Repetitive treatment of nonoccupational conditions prescribed and monitored by personal physicians
3. Assistance and control of illness-related job absenteeism
4. Assistance and evaluation of personal health care
5. Immunizations against nonoccupational infectious diseases
6. Health education and counseling
7. Termination and retirement administration
8. Participation in and planning and assessing of the quality of employee health benefits
9. Participation and systematic research

Source: Adapted from Scope of occupational and environmental health programs and practices, report of the Occupational Medical Practice Committee of the American College of Occupational and Environmental Medicine. *J. Occup. Med.* 34:436, 1992.

Clinical Services

Preplacement Evaluation
Preplacement evaluations, formerly known as the preemployment physical, are an essential part of many occupational health programs. The purpose of a preplacement evaluation is to ensure that the person examined does not have any medical condition that may be aggravated by the job duties or that may affect the health and safety of others. Although this category is reasonably broad, the physician should recognize that the primary obligation is to the patient's health and to evaluate such situations accordingly. The critical determinants in this decision-making process are the person's health and the *job* itself. Incumbent on physicians conducting preplacement examinations is a thorough understanding of the job duties and the *work environment* (see Chap. 4 for discussion of the worksite visit).

Preplacement evaluations can also be of value in complying with certain Occupational Safety and Health Administration (OSHA) standards and in serving as a baseline for health improvement programs. For example, the OSHA standard for occupational exposure to asbestos requires that workers undergo a chest film and pulmonary function studies prior to job assignment. Health promotion and wellness programs often include baseline examinations and routine ancillary testing; results are used to screen for certain illnesses, promote more healthful behavior, and serve as a frame of reference to evaluate the effectiveness of certain interventions.

The decision regarding the need for and content of preplacement evaluations depends on the nature of the industry and the particular *job*. In some cases, however, in particular when workers are exposed to substances regulated by OSHA standards, such evaluations are legally mandatory. Other situations that call for mandatory preplacement examinations include the transportation industry, for example, the Interstate Commerce Commission (ICC) and the Federal Aviation Administration (FAA).

The type of testing to be conducted at a preplacement examination depends on the job for which the worker is being considered. For example, in workers who paint with isocyanates, pulmonary function testing prior to assignment can help to assess the person's breathing capacity and capability of safely wearing a respirator. This examination can also serve as a baseline upon which to compare future evaluations that are part of a medical surveillance program.

The physician is urged to exercise restraint, however, in recommending the type of ancillary testing (e.g., laboratory, x-ray) that should be included in a preplacement evaluation. Attention needs to be directed to the effectiveness of the ancillary procedure as a screening tool to uncover unrecognized illness or as a "predictor" of future occupational illness or injury. Indiscriminate testing can divert resources away from programs of potentially greater benefit as well as cause needless alarm and greater expense in evaluating the inevitable false-positive results. Arbitrary use of certain tests can also be considered discriminatory, legally unsound, and of limited medical utility. (Random use of low back films to "predict" future back disorders falls under this category; see Chap. 12.) In light of the Americans with Disabilities Act, physicians are likely to be called on to ensure that testing is job specific and has some pertinence in evaluating a person's fitness for duty.

The physician conducting a preplacement evaluation has an obligation to the business enterprise to report functional limitations and corresponding accommodations that may be necessary to work. The physician should pay heed to *medical confidentiality* on non–work-related illnesses [7]. Although the criteria used to define health conditions that fall under this category may be blurred at times, the physician should strive to be recognized as impartial in these often difficult settings. Ideally, the patient should be advised as to what information will be released to the employer. Similarly, as part of this process, it is advisable that a person undergoing a preplacement evaluation sign an appropriate release form that allows the physician to discuss pertinent medical findings with the business (Fig. 1-1).

To communicate effectively with the business enterprise, it is advisable to have a simple form that notifies a designated person that an examination has taken place and that the person is either medically suitable with or without certain restrictions or not medically suitable (Fig. 1-2). Medical records should be kept on site at the medical facility. Medical records should not be released to the business unless an on-site medical office is maintained and supervised by a registered nurse or physician who can assume responsibility for the ethical maintenance of the medical records.

A protocol to follow-up of abnormalities noted during preplacement evaluations should be developed. During these examinations, people may exhibit abnormalities such as idiopathic hematuria, mild hypertension, and other conditions that will not interfere with work ability [8]. Ideally, these people should be apprised of the abnormal findings and referred to their personal physician for diagnostic and therapeutic care. The occupational health program will most likely need to develop referral patterns, however, because as many as 40% of the workforce have a primary care physician.

Work-Related Injuries

The physician who provides primary occupational health care will likely encounter a variety of minor injuries ranging from cuts and lacerations to strains and burns, treatment of which is well within the expertise of the primary care clinician. According to workers' compensation statutes, the injured worker may have the right to choose the *site and provider of medical care,* although businesses often establish

---

Name: _____   Employer: _____
Address: _____   Occupation: _____
_____   Age: _____ Date of birth: _____
Phone: _____   SS#: _____

Person to contact in case of medical emergency: _____
Relationship to you: _____   Phone number: _____

Are you allergic to any medications?   Yes   No
If *Yes,* what medications are you allergic to: _____
Do you have a family physician?   Yes   No   Do you have health insurance?   Yes   No
Physician's name: _____   Name of insurance: _____
Address _____   Membership #: _____
_____   Subscriber: _____

I authorize this medical facility, its physicians and health care professionals, to provide treatment, examinations, and/or evaluations, etc. as deemed necessary, and in accordance with sound medical procedures.

Signature: _____   Date: _____

Release of Information to Employer

(The section below applies to patients being treated or examined for work-related illness and injury, and for those patients undergoing preplacement, fitness for duty, and return to work evaluations.)

The answers that I give are true to the best of my knowledge. The information shall be used to determine whether: (a) I am capable of performing the job requirements of the position for which I am being considered; or (b) I am able to return to work after an illness or work-related injury. Medical information related to this evaluation will pertain only to my ability to perform essential job functions. Specific diagnostic information will not be released, in accordance with the Code of Ethical Conduct of the American College of Occupational and Environmental Medicine. Medical records will not be released to any party, without my consent, except in the context of workers' compensation, when information related only to a specific injury or illness can be transmitted. Other information will be held strictly confidential.

Signature: _____   Date: _____

Figure 1-1. Sample medical treatment authorization form.

relationships with designated medical facilities or physicians to provide occupational health services. These regulations, however, may have variations among the states.

Principles of *medical confidentiality* regarding *work-related* injuries and illnesses allow the employer to know about the nature of the occupational illness or injury, the type of treatment, and need for continual care. Following a work-related injury, it is advisable for the physician to *inform* an appropriately designated representative at the organization as to the need for further medical evaluations or work-site restrictions. In some cases, such notification may be required by workers' compensation regulations. Similarly, counseling on the potential time away from work secondary to the injury can aid in the proper planning of the worker's medical and occupational rehabilitation. Enhanced *communication* between the business facility and the physician can facilitate better medical care as well. Appropriate forms that outline this information are essential. Uniform reports are also required by most workers' compensation statutes (Fig. 1-3).

The physician is advised to be aware of *recurring* clinical events such as injuries

```
┌─────────────────────────────────────────────────────────────────────┐
│                                      Report of Preplacement Physical Exam │
│                                                                        │
│ Company: _____       ☐ Individual is medically suitable │
│ Name: _____        ☐ Individual is medically suitable with │
│                                          these restrictions:           │
│ Was examined on: _____        _____    │
│ Tests performed: _____        _____    │
│ _____                                        │
│                                        _____    │
│ _____  _____     ☐ Individual is not medically suitable │
│ EXAMINER'S SIGNATURE     DATE             NOTE: All medical records and test │
│                                           results are maintained at this med- │
│                                           ical facility.               │
└─────────────────────────────────────────────────────────────────────┘
```

Figure 1-2. A sample form for reporting results of a preplacement evaluation.

from one type of machinery or certain tasks such as lifting or repetitive motion activities. Businesses are required to record work-related injuries, periodic review of which can stimulate the search for preventive measures (OSHA 200 Log) (see Chap. 2).

Return to Work Evaluation
Following a lengthy absence from work, many businesses request a medical evaluation before the person may resume job duties. Such examinations are conducted on workers who have missed a prescribed amount of *time* as a result of a non–work-related or work-related *disorder.* The respective *time* periods and *disorders* (e.g., lumbar disk disease, coronary artery disease, tendonitis) covered by "return to work" policies are arbitrary and vary among organizations. Sound clinical judgment coupled with an understanding of the needs of both the business and the worker is essential. More time away from work is not always in the best interests of the worker's health.

The purpose of these examinations is to ensure proper placement of the worker to prevent future injury and illness. The physician is advised that the focus of these examinations should be on the patient's health. In turn, the decision related to ability to work is based on whether *health* will be adversely affected by the work duties. In some cases, it may be appropriate to recommend alternative or modified duty assignments for a certain period of time. All decisions regarding work capabilities, however, should be based on a thorough review of the job history. Physicians performing such examinations are advised to request suitable job descriptions and become generally familiar with the worksite. A brief report is recommended.

Periodic Examinations
Certain occupations such as those regulated by the ICC and FAA require periodic medical evaluations for licensing purposes. Other occupations come under the auspices of OSHA, which has established standards for periodic medical evaluations of workers exposed to materials such as asbestos and lead. In some cases, such as the ICC examinations, guidelines are *strict,* and adherence is mandatory. For example, people with insulin-dependent diabetes are not considered qualified for interstate driving, although regulations are periodically reviewed and amended.

Another type of periodic examination is the so-called preventive medicine examination. Over the past few years, the effectiveness of periodic medical evaluations has been evaluated by a variety of professional groups, including the American Cancer Society, American College of Physicians, and Council on Scientific Affairs of the American Medical Association These reviews were in turn assessed by the US Preventive Services Task Force, which published a monograph that evaluated the effectiveness of 169 interventions. The pace and need for developing screening interventions, however, has proceeded unabated with new concern toward the use of prostatic specific antigen for prostatic cancer and use of biomarkers for ovarian cancer. The thrust of the respective reviews is that most "annual physicals" and other periodic medical evaluations include more ancillary services (laboratory and x-ray) than are necessary to ensure good health. Moreover, these reports indicate that more attention should be directed toward lifestyle issues such as diet, exercise, and smoking habits to prevent illness. Physicians asked to provide these types of examinations are encouraged to review the recent guidelines [9].

Health Assessments

Since nearly 40% of the workforce has no primary care physician, it is likely that individuals evaluated for occupational health purposes (i.e., a preplacement evaluation, treatment of a work-related injury) may return for care of routine illnesses. These illnesses are often described as "episodic" and range from influenza to pharyngitis and sunburn. Following initial evaluation and treatment, it is often appropriate for the occupational health center to refer these patients to primary care physicians or appropriate specialists for follow-up care, especially for chronic ailments such as hypertension, asthma, or allergic disorders. In other cases, cooperation between the private physician and the occupational health service can facilitate treatment measures, especially for conditions such as hypertension.

The occupational physician may also be requested to conduct second opinions regarding an individual's work capabilities. Although the factors involved in these decisions are often complicated, the focus should always be on the worker's *health*. Physicians, however, may hear counterbalancing opinions about whether the business wants the person back to the position or whether the person actually wants to return to work. If the physician always focuses on health with attention to the job duties, however, some of the inherent difficulties in making these decisions will be minimized. If the physician believes that a certain job will *more than likely* aggravate the medical condition or impede recovery, an alternative assignment should be recommended if suitable accommodations are not feasible. The ultimate decision regarding placement rests with the organization; the physician's role is to serve as a consultant and to render a *medical* opinion.

The clinician may also be asked to conduct a *disability evaluation* of a worker who does not appear medically able to return to a particular position. In these settings, it is advisable to employ standard guidelines such as the American Medical Association's guidelines to the evaluation of permanent impairment [10]. The physician should appreciate that in most situations the medical opinion concerns *impairment; disability* is far more complex, with medical considerations representing only part of the entire picture, along with educational and vocational factors.

An assessment of *disability* also incorporates a review of social factors, such as level of education and occupational experiences. A person with emphysema, for example, may demonstrate severe pulmonary impairment that disables him from work as a material handler but does not disable him from work as an accountant. The term *impairment* refers to a measurable deficit in physiologic functioning (e.g., decrease in lung function, abnormal hearing, reduced motion of a joint), whereas *disability* refers to how the medical impairment affects work capabilities.

Ancillary Services

Because of wider awareness of the health implications of certain jobs, industries, and materials, occupational physicians are often called on to conduct more detailed evaluations. These reviews necessitate supportive diagnostic information, such as radiographic examinations, laboratory testing, and air sampling. A proper coordination of these efforts can help provide quality care, while preventing illness and injury.

Ancillary services refer to *laboratory* and related procedures conducted as part of clinical evaluations. The type and level of ancillary services depend on the practice setting and the local medical community. In the provision of occupational health services to small businesses, however, the following items are considered essential: an audiometric booth and audiometer, a well-functioning and calibrated spirometer, and a vision screener. Optional services include laboratory, x-ray, and physical therapy; however, the appropriateness of including these services will vary. In some cases, it may be suitable to employ referral services.

According to the OSHA Hearing Standard, as many as 10 million Americans may be exposed to sufficient noise at work to damage their hearing. Numerous industries have the potential to produce noise-induced hearing loss. Consequently, physicians

1. Name of injured person: _____ Age: _____ Sex _____
2. Address: No. and St. _____ City or town _____ State _____
3. Name and address of employer: _____
4. Date of accident: _____ Hour _____ M. Date disability began: _____
5. State in patient's own words where and how accident occurred: _____

6. Give accurate description of nature and extent of injury and state your objective findings: _____

7. Will the injury result in (a) permanent defect? _____ If so, what? _____ (b) Facial or head disfigurement? _____

8. Is accident above referred to the only cause of patient's condition? _____ If not, state contributing causes: _____

9. Is patient suffering from any disease of the heart, lungs, brain, kidneys, blood, vascular system, or any other disabling condition not due to this accident? _____ Give particulars: _____

10. Has patient any physical impairment due to previous accident or disease? _____ Give particulars: _____

11. Has normal recovery been delayed for any reason? _____ Give particulars: _____

12. Date of your first treatment: _____ Who engaged your services? _____

13. Describe treatment given by you: _____

14. Were x-rays taken? _____ By whom? _____ When? _____
    (Name and Address)

15. X-ray diagnosis: _____

16. Was patient treated by anyone else? _____ By whom? _____ When? _____
    (Name and Address)

17. Was patient hospitalized? _____ Name and address of hospital: _____

18. Date of admission to the hospital: _____ Date of discharge: _____

19. Is further treatment needed? _____ For how long? _____

20. Patient (was/will be) able to resume regular work on: _____

21. Patient (was/will be) able to resume light work on: _____

22. If death ensued give date: _____

23. Do you recommend vocational rehabilitation services will be: Likely _____ Probable _____ Unlikely _____

Remarks: (Give any information of value not included above.) _____

Diagnosis _____

I am a duly licensed physician in the State of _____

I was graduated from _____ Medical school in _____ Year _____

Date of this report: _____ (Signed:) _____

This report must be signed personally by physician. Address: _____ Telephone: _____

Figure 1-3. A first-report form for a work-related injury.

providing occupational health services are urged to have an audiometric booth and audiometer on site or have access to such. Many preplacement evaluations will require an audiometric evaluation prior to job assignment. Strict adherence to the OSHA Hearing Standard is recommended.

A well-functioning spirometer is a critical component of any occupational health program. NIOSH has established guidelines for the proper training of technicians conducting this particular procedure. Many OSHA standards, especially those concerning asbestos and cotton, require periodic pulmonary function testing. Pulmonary function testing is often performed in the context of determining medical suitability for wearing a respirator. There are no specific guidelines for the type of examination to perform, and discretion is left to the examining physician. By convention, however, most occupational physicians administer a questionnaire and pulmonary function testing as a minimum. Other settings, such as hazardous waste work, may warrant detailed evaluations that include an exercise electrocardiogram, usually as a result of the need to wear bulky, cumbersome protective equipment in potentially hot environments that pose a risk of heat stress. The level of pulmonary function below which a person should not be advised to wear a respirator is subject to opinion. In general, however, results below 70% (FEV_1) warrant a careful review. The types of spirometers that are commercially available have been reviewed [11].

Since people rarely undergo routine eye examinations, a properly functioning vision testing machine is strongly recommended (as opposed to the standard Snellen chart). Many periodic examinations such as ICC and FAA examinations require vision screening and adherence to strict guidelines. The importance of good vision in an effective safety program should not be overlooked. As a result of eye fatigue and strain among video display (VD) operators, periodic vision screening has been recommended in some settings. A directive in the European Community requires periodic eye examinations of those who use VD terminals for designated periods of time.

Optional services include laboratory, x-ray, and physical therapy. Customarily, it is not practical, even for an occupational health center, to have complete on-site laboratory services. The decision to employ laboratory services depends on many factors, including the type of specimen to be analyzed, as well as volume of testing and cost effectiveness. The physician who provides occupational health services, however, should be aware that some medical monitoring and toxicologic analyses for substances such as mercury, trichloroethanol, and lead are not routinely performed at most hospitals. Thus, the physician needs to ensure that the laboratory chosen to provide such services is appropriately qualified. Quality control, proficiency, and pricing can vary widely. For measurement of blood lead levels, however, the Centers for Disease Control periodically evaluate laboratories according to defined criteria. With the increased interest demonstrated in the value of biomarkers in the diagnosis of occupational illness, a quality reference laboratory becomes an important service in the delivery of occupational medical services.

For occupational health programs that treat work-related injuries, it is essential to have access to radiology facilities. Often it is worthwhile to have x-ray facilities on site for proper assessment of injuries, illnesses, or medical monitoring examinations. If on-site facilities are not available, provisions should be made for local referral.

Physical therapy can play an instrumental role in promoting prompt and efficient recovery from work-related injuries. A physical therapy unit can also be helpful to the occupational physician in other ways, such as playing an educational role in instructing workers in lifting techniques and proper back care and in conducting strength testing. Strength testing of back musculature has been heralded as offering potential benefit in predicting back injuries. With the advent of the Americans with Disabilities Act (ADA), strength testing will play a role in assessing a person's ability to handle certain job duties. Although routine use of dynamic strength testing is sporadic, the evaluation of back functioning prior to certain job assignments is becoming more common. The effectiveness of this procedure in predicting future back injuries, however, remains to be clarified. A physical therapy unit can also assess work capabilities. (For example, a worker considered for a material handling position in a delivery firm presented with amputated second through fifth fingers at the middle phalanx. Since the position required frequent lifting of up to 70 pounds, his work capabilities were assessed by the physical therapy unit, which offered a reasonably objective approach.)

Nonclinical Activities

Educational activities are an essential component of an occupational health service. The physician will likely be asked to give presentations on a variety of health-related topics to both manager and worker groups. The physician is encouraged to recognize his or her own role in educating the workforce and management on matters of health related to the occupational environment. For example, a discussion on causes, prevention, and treatment of back pain can help managers understand why injured workers need sufficient *time* away from the job for effective treatment and that modified assignments may be needed on return to work. Other topics of interest include occupational risks associated with acquired immunodeficiency syndrome (AIDS), urinary screening for abused drugs, and the role of smoking policies. The physician may also be asked to discuss with worker groups the value of medical surveillance examinations or how to interpret health-related information on material safety data sheets (see Chap. 2 on Hazard Communication Standard).

The physician providing occupational health care is often viewed as *health consultant* to the business. Thus, the physician may be asked to recommend first-aid protocols, hazard control programs, or back education seminars. It is not realistic to expect the physician to be even remotely involved in all of these activities; however, he or she is encouraged to become aware of available resources and to assist in review of programs. Working together with and supervising the efforts of other health care professionals such as nurses, physician assistants, and physical therapists can help expand the physician's role. As corporations become more aware and accountable for the health and welfare of their employees, occupational physicians are being called on to address many of the nonclinical health issues associated with operating a business. Serving as an advisor on epidemiology, toxicology, or health policy is a notable example.

Worksite policies related to health issues, such as annual examinations, cigarette smoking, or health promotion programs, may need to be developed. In some cases, however, a local business facility may be part of a larger corporation that has established guidelines for specific occupational health issues. In other cases, unions associated with particular occupations have issued guidelines and prepared information that may be of assistance to the clinician.

Health Promotion Activities

The definition of health promotion is considerably broad and includes virtually any type of preventive medicine activity designed to *educate people regarding the role of lifestyle* in promoting health and to facilitate behavior change. Typically considered under this heading are smoking cessation, weight reduction, stress management, fitness, and hypertension and cancer screening. Because of rising health care costs and greater awareness of the public regarding the role of prevention, the clinician is likely to be faced with questions such as whether the local business facility should institute a health promotion program and may be asked to design its components (see Chap. 32). It is unrealistic to expect the physician to be involved in the administration and planning of these activities; however, an advisory role to ensure that all activities are conducted in accordance with current medical standards is recommended.

Referral Patterns

The provision of primary occupational health services requires occasional referrals to a certified occupational medicine physician; other medical specialists, such as orthopedic surgeons and neurologists; and other occupational health professionals, such as industrial hygienists.

Occupational Medicine Physician

Although fewer than 1000 practicing physicians are board certified in occupational medicine [12], it is wise for the clinician to investigate within the local community whether such a physician may be available as a consultant. Information related to occupational physicians can be obtained through the directory of the American College of Occupational and Environmental Medicine. The clinician is urged to be aware of the complicated nature of many occupational medical problems and is advised to seek appropriate advice on medical monitoring of substances not covered by OSHA standards and in evaluating the work-relatedness of certain illnesses. For some substances, such as asbestos or lead, OSHA has established standards that define medical guidelines on the *type of testing* to be performed and measures to be followed based on the results. In other cases, however, especially in work settings where exposure may occur to untested substances or to materials with unusual health risks, further consultation is suggested. These settings may require more intense worksite monitoring, including air level measurements in addition to toxicology testing, before appropriate advice can be given.

Because of wider awareness of occupational illnesses in the general population, a clinician will likely encounter patients concerned as to whether a particular health condition may be due to exposure to an occupational or environmental substance. At times, these decisions can be straightforward, such as evaluating lead intoxication in a pistol shooter or pleural abnormalities in a sheet metal worker who spent 30 years working in the vicinity of asbestos. In other cases, the decision can be considerably complicated by either insufficient medical information regarding the toxicity of a substance or inadequate information regarding working conditions. Most occupational illnesses, however, are originally recognized by astute clinicians. When an unusual occupational illness is suspected, appropriate consultation with a trained and experienced occupational physician is suggested (see Chap. 33 on the case report).

Local Medical Specialists

The clinician is advised to be active in the local medical community. Specific needs for specialists include orthopedic surgeons, general surgeons, otolaryngologists (particularly as part of the OSHA hearing standard), pulmonary specialists, neurologists (to conduct nerve conduction studies and neuropsychiatric testing), and psychiatrists or psychotherapists. In provision of occupational health services, these specialists are likely to be called on routinely. Consequently, it is strongly advised that a good working professional relationship be established to enhance communication between the clinician and the specialist. It is important that the specialist be sensitive to the need for prompt scheduling and a complete and timely report. Unfortunately, not all physicians are willing to meet these specific needs of an occupational health service.

Other Professionals

The occupational physician will occasionally require the services of other professionals such as industrial hygienists, audiologists, or physical therapists. Professional ties with these professionals can help the clinician provide quality occupational health care.

A wide array of government agencies such as NIOSH and OSHA provide educational information related to the workplace and environmental substances. Other professional organizations such as the American College of Occupational and Environmental Medicine, American Conference of Governmental Industrial Hygienists, and other professional societies publish material related to occupational health that may be of benefit to the physician.

The Delivery of Occupational Medical Services

Today, occupational medical services are delivered from a variety of perspectives, most commonly by the primary care clinician, although hospitals have become more assertive in the past few years. Most recently, however, occupational health centers have been developed to provide health services to a range of small businesses in the immediate geographic area of the facility. In some cases, freestanding health centers have incorporated occupational medical services as part of their program. Unions and corporations have also sponsored health care clinics.

Determining the Need for Occupational Medical Services

The goals of an occupational health service include the following:

1. To protect people at work from health and safety hazards
2. To protect the local environment

3. To facilitate safe placement of workers according to their physical, mental, and emotional capacities
4. To assure adequate medical care and rehabilitation of the occupationally ill and injured
5. To assist in measures related to personal health maintenance

In deciding the economic feasibility of an occupational health center, a number of factors need to be considered (Table 1-3). The type and diversity of the business community should be reviewed, since some types of industries require more health care than others. Business groups should be categorized by the number of workers, respective location to the medical facility, and type of industry. It is also worthwhile to review who else may be providing occupational health services in the geographic region under consideration for the occupational health program. Based on this review, one can determine the *type* of medical services that may be required, such as preplacement evaluations, treatment of injuries, or more complicated occupational medical consultations. The expectations of the business and labor community should also be considered. Finally, after careful evaluation of the market area and costs involved in equipment and staff, a decision can be made.

In the establishment of an occupational health service, professionals knowledgeable in marketing, accounting, and management will be valuable aids to the success of the venture. The quality of the medical staff, however, is crucial, especially regarding training and experience in occupational medicine. Careful attention should be directed toward the *type* of staff that is employed, including the cost effectiveness of medical care providers, such as physician assistants and nurse practitioners [13]. Organizations or physicians considering establishing an occupational health program should be aware of the code of ethical conduct of the American College of Occupational and Environmental Medicine.

Once a decision is made to develop an occupational health service, one should have realistic expectations in terms of when the facility can become self-supporting. Appropriate business counseling regarding fee schedules, equipment, and staffing costs is advisable. Policies and procedures need to be implemented. In addition, appropriate forms for preplacement evaluations and treatment of work-related injuries need to be developed. Attention to medical confidentiality is essential. Guidelines for referrals to local physicians are essential.

A well-run program depends on *effective communication* between the business facility and the physician. In providing occupational health services, the physician is advised that the primary responsibility is always to the patient and that the physician should not be confused as an advocate of the company but instead should be viewed as an *impartial* professional concerned primarily with the worker's health. Proper communication, however, requires strict attention to medical confidentiality. (See Chap. 2 for further discussion on this complex issue.)

Once an occupational health center has been established or a physician has decided to incorporate occupational medical services into his or her practice, *a visit to the business is essential*. Such a visit can enable the physician to become acquainted with the nature of the enterprise and with respective work responsibilities. This knowledge will enhance the physician's ability to make effective determinations as

Table 1-3. Factors in establishing need for occupational medical services for small businesses

Determine:
1. The number of *businesses* in the service area and categorize by
   a. Number of employees
   b. Geographic concentration
   c. Type of industry (SIC* code may be helpful)
2. Level of local *competition,* i.e., presence of other group practices or occupational health programs providing occupational health care
3. *Types* of occupational medical services in *demand* by the local business community (i.e., workers' compensation, preplacement examinations, treatment of work-related injuries)
4. Cost analysis, including marketing, equipment, staff, and operating expenses

*Standard Industrial Classification.

to whether someone can handle a job duty in light of existing health or whether worksite modifications are necessary. During this visit, the physician can also be apprised of the expectations of the organization. One should realize, however, that one visit is hardly adequate to become familiar with the intricacies of many jobs. (Chapter 4 describes issues the physician should consider in holding discussions during a plant visit.)

An occupational health center ideally should provide fundamental clinical services, such as preplacement evaluations and treatment of work-related injuries. Other types of services, such as health promotion, educational seminars, and screening programs, will likely be requested as the business gains confidence in the capabilities of the physician and/or organization providing basic care.

The considerations described refer to an occupational health center or physicians who provide occupational health services as part of their practice. These physicians are encouraged to become aware of other types of occupational health care delivery, such as corporate and union settings and hospitals.

Corporate-Sponsored Health Care Delivery

Corporations assumed a role in providing occupational health services shortly after the institution of the workers' compensation statutes. Sears, Roebuck, for example, and some insurance companies were some of the first to institute "preemployment" examinations, as they were known at that time. Because some corporate or business settings employed a large group of people, it was economically feasible to deliver health care on site. Episodic illnesses and minor injuries, for example, could be more promptly and accurately treated. Similarly, in the event of a more serious injury, prompt medical treatment was close at hand. Corporate-sponsored health care delivery later evolved into more comprehensive programs that also included treatment of non–work-related illnesses. Most recently, however, corporations have tended to reduce their commitment to *on-site* programs and in turn have looked toward local physicians for provision of these services. Staffing and medical equipment used at an on-site corporate facility will parallel that necessary at an occupational health center. The trend for businesses to contract occupational health services continued through the late 1980s, but has begun to stabilize. In some settings, for example, it is cost effective to deliver services on site [14]. Nonetheless, this decline in corporate-sponsored services was reflected in a study of positions available in corporate occupational medicine [15].

Many corporations employ professionals skilled in fields related to occupational medicine, including epidemiology, toxicology, and industrial hygiene. The clinician is urged to contact the parent corporation when providing occupational health services for a subsidiary plant or division. Valuable information and policy guidelines can often be obtained from corporate staff.

Union-Sponsored Occupational Health Care

Although few medical facilities sponsored by unions actually deliver health care, unions have been active in various aspects of occupational health. Other union efforts related to occupational health have been directed toward the collective bargaining process, lobbying local legislators, and preparation of educational material for their members.

With respect to occupational health, labor has identified three main goals [16]: (1) to prevent disease by ensuring a safe work environment, (2) to notify and treat workers when prevention has failed, and (3) to compensate workers and families when disease takes its toll. In evaluating individual patients, the physician should be aware that some unions have implemented educational programs directed toward preventing occupational illness. The patient may be able to obtain valuable information that can be of assistance to the physician in evaluating an illness. Union groups may also have access to medical information related to products used at a particular business. Unfortunately, because of the adversarial nature of many labor and management dealings, the physician may be inadvertently thrust into a conflict. To enhance effectiveness, however, it is critical that the physician *maintain neutrality* and make decisions based on *health*. Table 1-4 outlines questions that a physician might ask either management or the union regarding occupational health care.

Table 1-4. Local union health and safety involvement

1. Does a joint union/management *health and safety committee* exist at the plant?
2. Is there a shop floor committee with health and safety interests?
3. Does the union conduct *training* for its members in health and safety, and if it does, are materials available for the health care providers?
4. Are there *grievance procedures* for health and safety?
5. Do *collective bargaining agreements* pertain to health and safety issues?
6. How does the union help its members in handling *compensation claims*?
7. How does the union handle its relationship with the Occupational Safety and Health Administration?
8. Does the union have a working relationship with a local clinic for occupational health programs?
9. What is the local union's involvement in substance abuse, rehabilitation, and/or employee assistance programs?
10. Do joint union/company health screening programs exist for non–work-related problems, such as blood pressure, cholesterol, diabetes, and glaucoma detection?
11. Some unions have educational arragements with local physicians to educate members on general health topics. Does such exist in your area?
12. Does the local union have available medical consultants through their international affiliation?

Hospital-Based Occupational Health Programs

Although most hospitals have had some type of employee health service for many years, hospitals have been marketing occupational health services to the local business community with vigor since the mid to late 1980s. These types of programs have varied considerably from provision of services through the emergency department or through a separate department within the hospital [6], or by a group of hospital staff physicians who individually provide some type of clinical occupational health services. Some hospitals have developed independent subsidiaries *off site* to provide health care to the small business community. Guidelines presented for the establishment of an independent occupational health center are applicable to hospital programs as well.

University-Based Teaching Centers

Few university-based residency training centers for occupational medicine exist in the United States (at last count, fewer than 40) [1]. Some hospitals, however, have developed sections of occupational medicine within departments of internal or community medicine, or at a school of public health.

These centers often can be of value to the clinician as a source to refer people with more complex occupational medical problems. In addition, some occupational medical sections at universities are Educational Resource Centers (ERCs) funded by the National Institute for Occupational Safety and Health for graduate training in occupational medicine. These ERCs also provide educational programs related to occupational medicine for physicians and other health professionals (see Chap. 35).

Because of the need for well-trained occupational physicians, the clinician who provides occupational medical services can be instrumental in the educational process. University programs may sponsor students or house staff at appropriate health care centers, where the student of occupational medicine can gain valuable practical experience.

The university-based center can channel a patient to the appropriate specialist, such as physicians skilled in occupational lung disease, dermatology, or neurology. University programs also have access to consultants in toxicology, audiology, and industrial hygiene. Since research activities are a major emphasis of university programs, opportunities may exist for an occupational health program to coparticipate in certain ventures.

References

1. McCunney, R. J., and Couturier, A. C. Where do occupational medicine residency programs fit in the institution? *J. Occup. Med.* 35:889, 1993.
2. Warshaw, L. J. Toward the year 2000: Challenges to the occupational physician. *J. Occup. Med.* 32:524, 1990.
3. Walsh, D. C. The vanguard and the rearguard. Occupational medicine revisits its future. *J. Occup. Med.* 30:124, 1988.
4. Ramazzini, B. Diseases of Workers. Translated by W. C. Wright. From *DeMorbis Artificum. Diatriba,* 1713. New York: Hafner, 1964.
   The classic text by the so-called father of occupational medicine.
5. Raffle, P. A. B., et al. *Hunter's Diseases of Occupations* (2nd ed.). Boston: Little, Brown, 1988.
   A comprehensive review of occupational illnesses and injuries with attention to historical aspects of occupational medicine.
6. Felton, J. S. 200 years of occupational medicine in the U.S. *J.O.M.* 18:809, 1976.
   A good summary of the history of occupational medicine.
7. McCunney, R. J. Medical records and confidentiality. *J.O.M.* 26:790, 1984.
   An overview of the multifaceted aspects of medical confidentiality in providing occupational health services.
8. McCunney, R. J. A hospital based occupational health program. *J. Occup. Med.* 26:375, 1984.
9. US Preventive Services Task Force. *Guide to Clinical Preventive Services: An assessment of the effectiveness of 169 interventions.* Baltimore: Williams and Wilkins, 1989.
10. American Medical Association (AMA). *Guidelines to the Evaluation of Permanent Impairment* (3rd ed.). Chicago: AMA, 1991.
    A uniform approach to evaluating disabilities of a variety of organ systems.
11. Gardner, R. M., Hankinson, J. L., and West, B. J. Evaluating commercially available spirometers. *Am. Rev. Respir. Dis.* 121:73, 1980.
    Although a bit dated, this article offers practical advice in selecting a spirometer. The practitioner may find it of value to select a device with digital printouts to ensure uniformity in interpreting results.
12. Pransky, G. Occupational medical specialists in the United States—a survey. *J. Occup. Med.* 32:985, 1990.
13. Baxter, P. Management of a multi-client occupational health clinic. *Occup. Health Nurs.* 32:151, 1984.
14. Anstadt, G., et al. The business planning process applied to an in-house corporate occupational medicine unit. *J. Occup. Med.* 33:354, 1991.
15. Ducatman, A. M. Career options of occupational physicians. *J. Occup. Med.* 30:776, 1988.
16. Parsons, M. *Seminars in Occupational Medicine—The Role of Occupational Medicine: Prospectives from Labor.* Vol. 1, No. 1, March 1986.

Further Information

Felton, J. S. *Occupational Medicine Management.* Boston: Little, Brown, 1989.
Written by a renowned occupational physician, this book addresses many of the operational and managerial aspects of running an occupational and environmental health program.

Guidotti, T. L., Cowell, J. W. F., and Jamleson, G. G. *Occupational Health Services. A Practical Approach.* Chicago: American Medical Association, 1989.
An excellent overview of the type of occupational health services that may be appropriate for a variety of settings.

Levy, B., and Wegman, D. *Occupational Health: Recognizing and Preventing Work-Related Disease* (2nd ed.). Boston: Little, Brown, 1988.
A handy text and reference in paperback.

Moser, R. *Effective Management of Occupational and Environmental Health and Safety Programs. A Practical Guide.* Boston: OEM Press, 1992.
A practical guide to managing an occupational health service.

National Institute for Occupational Safety and Health (NIOSH). *Occupational Diseases: A Guide to their Recognition.* Washington, DC: US Government Printing Office, 1977.
An ideal reference. Includes an overview of the toxicity of the major substances used in commerce today.

The Occupational and Environmental Medicine Report. Available from OEM Health Information, 55 Tozer Rd, Beverly, MA 01915 (508-921-7300)
This monthly report, published since 1987, includes critical reviews of articles pertinent to occupational medicine practice by a board of directors from hospitals, corporations, academia, and government.

Rom, W. N. *Environmental and Occupational Medicine* (2nd ed.). Boston: Little, Brown, 1992.
The most comprehensive text in the field. This edition includes 129 chapters that address specific toxins in detail. The text is especially strong in occupational pulmonary disorders.

Rom, W. N., et al. *Environmental and Occupational Medicine.* Boston: Little, Brown, 1983.
The most definitive and comprehensive text in the field. Essential reference for occupational physicians and those who provide a broad scope of occupational medical services.

Scope of occupational and environmental health programs and practice. Report of the Occupational Medical Practice Committee of the American College of Occupational and Environmental Medicine. *J. Occup. Med.* 34:436, 1992.

Zenz, C., Dickerson, O. B., and Horvath, E. *Occupational Medicine: Principles and Practical Applications* (3rd ed.). St. Louis: Mosby, 1994.
A comprehensive text on occupational medicine that makes a valuable contribution to any medical library.

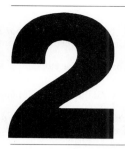

Legal and Ethical Issues

Junius C. McElveen, Jr.,
and Thomas Beck

The practice of occupational medicine is likely to present the practitioner with legal, ethical, and regulatory issues, not customarily a part of clinical medicine. It is necessary, however, for the clinician to develop a working knowledge of topics such as workers' compensation, medical record confidentiality, the Hazard Communication Standard, the Americans with Disabilities Act, toxic torts, and drug testing in order to practice effectively. This chapter is designed to present the essentials of these issues along with practical guidelines to enhance the delivery of occupational health care.

Workers' Compensation Law

Until the early years of the twentieth century, if employees were injured in their place of employment, the only remedy against the employer was a suit at common law. In that lawsuit, the only way in which damages could be recovered would be for the employee to prove the employer had failed to act as a reasonable person would have (i.e., had been negligent) and that negligence had resulted in injury to the employee. No one liked that system. Employers objected to the costliness of the lawsuits. Employees did not like the fact that certain defenses the employers could raise might bar their recovery completely. For example, if a jury found the employee's lack of care had contributed to the injury (contributory negligence), the employee, by law, was not entitled to recover any damages at all. Similarly, if the jury determined the employee had knowingly and voluntarily assumed the risk of the kind of work that resulted in the injury (assumption of the risk), the employee was barred from any recovery. Finally, if the employee was injured by a co-employee (the co-employee doctrine), the employee could not get damages.

Therefore, in the early twentieth century, employers and employees in the various states began to make a deal. That deal was known as workers' compensation. The workers' compensation statutes varied a bit from state to state (each state has its own workers' compensation law), but each is composed of several compromises:

1. Employees gave up their right to sue employers at common law and agreed to accept a certain sum of money per week for their inability to work as a result of work-related injuries. They agreed to accept this compensation as their *exclusive remedy* against the employer.
2. Employers give up their right to assert the defenses of contributory negligence, assumption of the risk, and the co-employee doctrine and agreed to give injured employees a certain sum of money per week, if they were unable to work as a result of work-related injuries. Thus, payment would be made, *regardless of fault.*
3. Payment would be automatic unless disputes arose. The disputes over issues of work-relatedness, amounts of entitlement, timeliness of claim, etc., would (generally) be decided by *administrative bodies,* rather than courts.
4. Payments would only be made for disability (i.e., inability to work).[1] There would be no damages recoverable for pain and suffering. No damages would be allowed as a punishment for the employer (punitive damages).

[1]Most state laws did contain scheduled awards, in which a certain percentage of impairment resulted in a certain payment of compensation, even though the employee continued to work. Thus, loss of a finger or partial loss of vision or hearing might result in payment of a number of weeks of compensation, even though it did not affect ability to work.

Thus, although the monetary recovery for employees (usually 66⅔% of their weekly wage) would generally not be as much as they *might* recover at common law, the recovery would be substantially more certain, since who was at fault was no longer an issue. Moreover, since matters were determined administratively, recovery would presumably be quicker.

At first, most of the state workers' compensation systems covered only work-related accidents. Illness and disease coverage were added later. When disease coverage was added, it was generally grafted onto statutory schemes designed to compensate for accidents. Therefore, a disease or illness would be considered work related if it satisfied the prerequisites for accident coverage, that is, it "arose out of and in the course of employment." However, unlike accidents, diseases do not generally manifest themselves immediately after exposure. Many have extremely long latency periods. By the time a disease occurred, the employee might have had a large number of different jobs and exposures. He or she might not even be working. Furthermore, the period of time during which a claim would be filed, known as the "statute of limitations," was generally only 1 or 2 years, depending on the state, and often was held to run from the date on which the last exposure occurred. For a disease with a long latent period, such as cancer, a worker might be barred from even filing a claim. In some states, statutes even forbade the filing of a claim after 5 years from the last exposure. Therefore, states have been obliged to create ways to determine if a disease is work related and create more workable statutes of limitation for disease.

Some states developed statutory schedules of occupational diseases [1]. Those diseases listed in the statute were presumed to be employment related. Those not listed were not compensable. The unfairness of this concept soon became apparent, and most states developed more *general concepts of compensability*.

Two lines of authority developed. The first held that a disease was compensable if a work-related "accident" aggravated or accelerated the underlying disease [2]. Thus, if a myocardial infarction occurred at work and the employee could show that some work-related stress contributed to precipitate the myocardial infarction, the employee's disability was compensable, even though the underlying disease process—coronary artery disease—was not work related. Gradually, courts have abolished the requirement that a special stress occur. Now, in many states, if a doctor is prepared to testify that *ordinary working conditions aggravated a non–work-related condition,* disability produced by the disease will be *compensable*.

The second line of authority postulated that a disease would be compensable if the employee's occupation put him or her at a greater risk of getting the disease than the general public had. Thus, diseases caused by hazardous substances at the workplace, to which the employee had greater exposure than the general public, were compensable, but so-called ordinary diseases of life, to which everyone ran the same risk, were not compensable. As one court said, "Such [occupational] disease is not the equivalent of a disease resulting from the general risks and hazards common to every individual regardless of the employment in which he is engaged" [3]. Thus, early decisions identified lead colic or lead poisoning in painters, ear trouble in telephone operators, and phosphorus poisoning in fireworks manufacturing employees as ". . . injuries or diseases common to workers in those particular trades" [4]. However, state boards were loath to extend coverage to most infectious diseases and cancers, which are "ordinary diseases of life" in the sense that both workers and nonworkers get them.

However, in recent years, that barrier has also fallen in most states. The first incursion into "ordinary diseases of life" was a line of cases in which those "ordinary" diseases were found compensable if they occurred under "unusual circumstances." Thus, for example, an employee on a ship who contracted meningitis after being required to work with numerous passengers who had meningitis was compensated through the workers' compensation system [5]. This exception has now evolved to the extent that, in some jurisdictions, a disease may be considered occupationally related if epidemiologic studies demonstrate a significantly elevated risk of contracting certain illnesses secondary to particular workplace conditions, when compared to the general population [6].

Other chronic diseases, most notably, psychological or psychiatric problems arising from work "stress" and cumulative trauma disorders (CTDs) may also be included in this exception.

Just as courts found heart attacks and strokes (even those not occurring on the job) to be covered by workers' compensation if it could be shown that workplace stress or exertion materially contributed to the progression of cardiovascular disease [7], courts recently have awarded workers' compensation for mental stress and anguish, if triggered by a significant employment incident. The Supreme Court of Texas held that workers' compensation was the only available remedy to a woman who suffered mental anguish as a result of the stillbirth of a child after an accident at work. The employee had not been physically injured, but the court viewed the stillbirth and concomitant emotional distress as part and parcel of the accident [8].

However, courts have not gone so far as to award compensation for mental stress or simple upset attributable to the general work environment. Some specific precipitating incident must have occurred, and the claimed mental problem must be clearly causally related to the incident [9]. Moreover, some states have legislatively excluded from coverage minor mental upset without any accompanying injury [10], and disorders stemming from an employer's bona fide disciplinary or termination decisions [11].

Cumulative trauma disorders are conditions, such as carpal tunnel syndrome, tendinitis, and bursitis, that are due to excessively forceful and repetitious movements over time. The view that CTDs occur frequently in the general population and should be classified as "ordinary diseases of life" has been approached by most jurisdictions in the manner taken by the Missouri Court of Appeals, that is, finding a disorder compensable if the employee has had an exposure at work greater than or different from that of the general public, and if there is a recognizable link between the disorder and some distinctive feature of the employee's job that is common to all jobs of that type [12]. Essentially, if some excessively forceful and repetitious motion is a requirement of the job, and if medical evidence attributes the disorder to that motion to a reasonable degree of medical probability, the disorder is compensable.

With regard to statutes of limitation, most states have adopted the *discovery rule*. A claim is timely if it is filed within a certain number of years after the claimant becomes aware of the disease *and* its potential work-relatedness. Almost all states have eliminated the requirement that a claim be filed within a certain number of years after exposure. However, as noted, workers' compensation law is state law, and occupational health professionals must be familiar with the law of the state in which they practice.

Determining When a Disorder Is Occupational

A doctor who determines that an injury or illness is occupational must report that fact to some state workers' compensation agencies, and unless the worker requires only first aid, the business must make an entry on an Occupational Safety and Health Administration (OSHA) Log 200 form, a special form that is required by OSHA. As has been noted, many jurisdictions consider *aggravation* of a non–work-related disorder by workplace agents or conditions to be occupational in origin and thus compensable. Some states may consider an illness occupationally related if epidemiologic studies show the disorder occurs with a statistically significantly greater incidence in the work population than in the general population. However, as other chapters of this book indicate, some diseases have long latency periods, and others produce nonspecific symptoms, so that it is extremely difficult to determine if a particular problem is occupationally related.

Promulgated OSHA guidelines [13] set out some of the inquiries a physician should make in determining whether a condition is work related. These inquiries include

1. A comparison of the *date of onset of symptoms* with [a carefully and thoroughly taken] occupational history
2. Evaluation of the results of any past biologic or medical monitoring and previous physical examinations [and symptomatology]
3. Evaluation of various laboratory tests for suspected disease agents
4. Review of the literature, including relevant Material Safety Data Sheets, to ascertain what the health effects of particular substances in the employee's workplace are, and whether the levels (of these substances) to which the employee was exposed could have produced the ill effects (See Chaps. 21 and 33 for a thorough discussion on evaluating whether a medical disorder is occupationally related.)

Information regarding the chemical substances to which the employee has been exposed will be easier to obtain now than has been the case in the past. In recent years, many states and OSHA have enacted rules mandating that employees be provided with information about the chemical exposures they are receiving in the workplace and how those exposures may affect their health. OSHA's rule is known as the Hazard Communication Standard (HCS) [14]. The HCS originally covered only entities in the manufacturing sector and importers of chemicals; however, several recent cases made it quite clear that although the HCS preempts any state or local laws that attempt to regulate employer obligations to their employees in the manufacturing workplace, it does not preempt state laws imposing obligations on the nonmanufacturing sector. Because of the potential for conflicting regulations, OSHA expanded the coverage of the HCS to all employers covered by the OSH Act. However, the federal HCS, even as expanded, does not preempt state laws that regulate the conduct of any employer as to *environmental* (as opposed to workplace) hazards [15].

Generally, the HCS requires that

1. Containers in the workplace that contain hazardous chemicals[2] must be labeled with the chemical's identity, appropriate hazard warnings, and the identity of the manufacturer.
2. Employees must be *trained* about the hazards of chemicals to which they are or may be exposed.
3. *Material Safety Data Sheets* (MSDS), which set out in considerable detail the hazards of specific chemicals, must be made available to employees who may be exposed to those chemicals.

In taking a complete occupational history, it will be very useful to find out from the patient what type of information was conveyed in the training program and what warnings are on containers of materials with which the employee frequently works. However, the most valuable information to the practicing physician may be that contained on an MSDS. Although the MSDS contains an enormous amount of information (Table 2-1), some may be incomplete. Thus, the physician may find it necessary to conduct a separate toxicologic review. Employees are entitled to review the MSDS on the materials with which they work, and physicians would be well advised to elicit this information from their patients in those types of jobs when a diagnosis is in question. In addition, under the 1986 amendments reauthorizing the "Superfund" Act (SARA Amendments), MSDSs or a list of the chemicals for which the company has MSDSs must be supplied to local emergency planning committees, state emergency planning committees, fire departments, and state emergency response commissions. In addition, inventories on hazardous chemicals must be submitted to these state and local agencies. Any citizen who requests that information from the state or local authorities is entitled to receive it with certain trade secret exceptions [16].

The HCS provides protections for information about chemical identities that are alleged by the manufacturer to be *trade secrets.* However, under certain circumstances, treating physicians and other health professionals can obtain that information, as follows: (1) If a treating physician determines a *medical emergency* exists and the chemical identity of a trade secret-protected hazardous chemical is necessary for proper treatment, the physician can obtain that information immediately from the manufacturer, importer, or employer who asserts the trade secret (telephone numbers, for example, are listed on the MSDS). However, the manufacturer or other party asserting the trade secret may obtain a statement of need and a confidentiality agreement as soon as circumstances permit. (2) In *nonemergency situations,* physicians, industrial hygienists, toxicologists, or epidemiologists providing medical or other occupational health services to employees may obtain trade secret information, if certain prerequisites are met, if a need for the actual chemical identity is shown to be necessary, and if a guarantee of confidentiality is set out [17].

---

[2]*"Hazardous" chemicals* are defined in the HCS as being those chemicals that present one of several *physical hazards* (e.g., flammability, reactivity, or explosiveness) or a *health hazard.* Health hazards include carcinogens, mutagens, teratogens, and toxins to any of the body's organ systems. 29 CFR 1910.1200(c), (d). A determination as to what constitutes a hazard *must be made by the manufacturer or importer,* but downstream users may also make that determination. 29 CFR 1910.1200(d)(1), (2).

Table 2-1. Information provided on Material Safety Data Sheets (MSDS)

1. The *label identity* of the chemical
2. The *chemical and common names* including synonyms
3. If the substance is a *mixture* that has been tested as a whole to determine its hazards, the chemical and common names of the ingredients that contribute to the known hazards
4. If the substance is a mixture that has *not* been tested as a whole, the chemical and common names of all ingredients that have been determined to be health hazards and that constitute 1% or more of the mixture (or *0.1% or more, if the hazard is a carcinogen)*
5. The chemical and common names of all ingredients that have been determined to present a *physical hazard*
6. The physical and chemical characteristics of the chemical
7. The physical hazards of the chemical
8. The *health hazards of the chemical,* including signs and symptoms of exposure, and any medical conditions that can be aggravated by exposure to the chemical
9. The primary routes of exposure
10. The *OSHA Permissible Exposure Limit,* the American Conference of Governmental Industrial Hygienists (ACGIH) Threshold Limit Value, or any other recommended exposure limit
11. Whether the substance is listed on the National Toxicology Program's "Annual List of Carcinogens" or has been found to be a potential carcinogen by the International Agency for Research on Cancer or OSHA
12. Known precautions for safe handling and use
13. Applicable control measures
14. The date of preparation of the latest MSDS or its latest change
15. The name, address, and telephone number of the manufacturer, importer, employer, or other responsible party preparing or distributing the MSDS, who can provide additional information on the hazardous chemical and appropriate emergency procedures

Note: See Chaps. 13 and 50 for information on how various organizations determine whether a substance is a carcinogen.

Exceptions to the Exclusivity of Workers' Compensation

In recent years, some courts have created rather significant exceptions to the rule that the *exclusive remedy* of an employee for workplace injuries and illnesses is workers' compensation. The reasons for these exceptions are quite complex, but physicians should be aware of their potential liability even when performing services in the context of a work-related injury or disease.

The Intentional Tort Exception

A number of states have long had one major exception to the "exclusive" remedy doctrine. Workers' compensation is not the employee's exclusive remedy *if the injury was caused by a deliberate and intentional act of the employer* (the so-called intentional tort exception). For many years, this exception to the *exclusivity* rule was narrowly construed; only situations in which an employer actually assaulted an employee were customarily included. In recent years, however, the exception has been interpreted more broadly, particularly in cases alleging occupational disease.[3] In 1980, for example, the California Supreme Court held that an employee could sue the employer at common law for *aggravation* of an occupational disease if the employee could prove that the employer knew of the presence of the disease, and failed to tell the employee, and that the disease was exacerbated as a result [18].

[3]On the other hand, courts of some states have taken the restrained position that workers' compensation truly is the exclusive remedy for any work-related disease or injury, absent express exceptions articulated by the legislature, e.g., *Abbott v. Gould, Inc.,* 443 N.W.2d 591 (Neb. 1989) (despite employees' allegations of intentional misconduct of employer, such as misrepresenting the safety of the work environment where lead was smelted, workers' compensation law provided absolute relief from tort actions for any diseases "arising out of" and "in the course of" employment).

In the California case, the employee had asbestosis. The court held that the employee could not sue for asbestosis because that disorder was covered under workers' compensation—even if the infliction of the disorder was intentional.[4] However, once the employer knew of the employee's asbestosis, the employer had a responsibility to inform the affected worker. Intentional failure to meet this obligation allowed the employee to file a suit under common law. The California Supreme Court also put the burden of proof on the employer to differentiate impairment caused by the disease and that caused by aggravation of the disease. To the extent the employer could not do so, it would be liable for the whole disease.

The New Jersey Supreme Court has recently followed the California Rule, with an additional twist. It also held that damages for *aggravation* of an occupational disease could be recovered at common law, saying [19]:

> An employer's fraudulent concealment of diseases already developed is *not* one of the risks an employee should have to assume. Such intentionally deceitful action goes beyond the bargain struck by the Compensation Act.

However, in the New Jersey case, the court also permitted the plaintiffs to sue physicians who allegedly knew of the presence of the disease and fraudulently concealed that fact from the employees.[5] As the court pointed out, though, the problems of proving such allegations could be substantial. Nonetheless, a physician is advised of the importance, both medically and ethically, of advising the patient of abnormal findings noted during an evaluation.

An additional problem in this area of the law is that some courts seem to be willing to let an employee sue an employer at common law, based on the intentional tort exception, for conduct that is not intentional. For example, the Ohio Supreme Court held that allegations that a company knew of dangerous chemicals, knew their employees might get sick from exposure to the chemicals, and failed to tell the employees of the dangers constituted sufficient allegations to go to trial on the theory that the employer's conduct was "intentional" and thus outside the workers' compensation system.[6] A later decision by the Ohio Supreme Court held that allegations that dangerous conditions existed and that the employer knew the dangerous conditions existed but failed to warn employees of the conditions or correct the conditions constituted sufficient allegations for an intentional tort suit [20].

> A defendant who fails to warn of a known defect or hazard which poses a grave threat of injury may reasonably be considered to have acted despite a belief that harm is substantially certain to occur [20].

This standard is substantially lower than the standard articulated in the vast majority of jurisdictions, including New Jersey and California.[7]

There has also been a notable, if not yet widespread, expansion of the exceptions to workers' compensation as an exclusive remedy, to allow civil action against employers for egregious workplace conduct resulting in emotional distress. For instance, a Pennsylvania decision recently allowed an employee to pursue a claim against his employer for alleged emotional distress caused by racial harassment by co-workers. Such a claim was found not to be preempted by the Pennsylvania Workers' Compensation Act [21].

Similarly, the California Supreme Court held that an employer's conduct in allegedly accusing its employee of gross misconduct before finally firing him so "exceeded the normal risks of the employment relationship" that it was not

---

[4]The court noted that the California Code contains a provision that if an employer's intentional misconduct results in a workplace injury or illness, the employer must pay 150% of the ordinarily payable compensation.

[5]In the California case, the employee had also sued two doctors who treated him for his illness. However, that part of the case was not considered by the California Supreme Court.

[6]*Blankenship v. Cincinnati Milacron Chemicals, Inc.*, 433 N.E.2d 572 (Ohio 1982). Although the majority in that case purported to focus only on the issue of whether an employee in Ohio could seek common law damages for an intentional tort, several members of the court spoke of workers who were "intentionally chemically poisoned on-the-job." 433 N.E.2d 572 at 578. However, the facts of this case, even as set out in the plaintiff's allegations, could as easily refer to any workplace at any time. As one of the justices in this case said, "'The mere knowledge and appreciation of a risk, short of substantial certainty [of harm], is not the equivalent of intent.' Appellants have not clearly alleged any degree of certainty." 433 N.E.2d 572 at 581 (Locher, concurring in part and dissenting in part).

[7]State legislatures have limited some of these exceptions to the workers' compensation exclusivity rule.

entitled to insulation from civil liability. The court allowed the employee's claim for severe emotional distress, but carefully noted that emotional distress caused by everyday management decisions (hiring, firing, demotion, criticism) would be covered exclusively by workers' compensation [22].

The Dual Capacity Doctrine
A few states permit actions against corporations or co-employees, such as medical personnel, for violation of a concept called the *dual capacity* doctrine. This doctrine provides that an employee may sue at common law if the employee is injured as a result of some action of the employer that occurs when the employer and employee stand in some relationship other than the employer-employee relationship. For example, in a California case, a chiropractor's receptionist sought treatment from the chiropractor for a back disorder. The chiropractor's treatment was allegedly negligent because it made the employee's back worse. The California Supreme Court held that the injury (to the employee) arose as a result of the doctor-patient relationship, not the employer-employee relationship. Because the injury arose in this context, the employee could sue the chiropractor [23].

Similarly, an Ohio court held that an allegation that a company physician's *failure to inform* an employee that he had silicosis was a case that could proceed at common law because of the dual capacity doctrine. The court stated that once the employer got into the medical examination business, it took on obligations to the employee over and above those duties it had as the employer [24].

Obligations of the Occupational Physician

The *potential for liability* is another reason, in addition to good medical and ethical practice, *for being completely candid with the employee* regarding a suspected occupational disorder. If further testing is necessary, the employer should be consulted, as that testing may be covered under workers' compensation rather than other insurance. As soon as an occupational condition is identified, the employer and the appropriate state workers' compensation agency should be notified [25].

Health care professionals have been sued for malpractice or negligence in a number of states by individuals who have either been employees of the same employer (i.e., co-employees) or employees of a company for which the health care professional was doing contract work. The allegations of malpractice and negligence have covered a wide range of conduct. In some states, courts have held that the exclusive remedy provisions of the state's workers' compensation law bar a lawsuit against the health care professional. Here, the employee's exclusive remedy is workers' compensation benefits [26]. Other courts have held, in a variety of circumstances, that health care professionals can be sued outside the compensation system.

In a landmark case, the New Jersey Supreme Court held that company physicians could be sued outside the compensation system based on employee allegations that the physicians knew the employees had an occupational disease, and did not tell the employees about the disease [27]. In that case the employees alleged that the employer's physicians had diagnosed asbestosis, based on chest x-ray findings, but had fraudulently failed to tell the employees.

Similarly, some courts have said that when a physical examination or some type of testing, such as drug or alcohol testing, is a condition of future or continued employment, that examination creates a physician-patient relationship between the examiner and the employee. That relationship imposes a duty to conduct the required test and diagnose the results thereof in a nonnegligent manner. However, it should be noted that courts have not held any testing laboratories liable if their sole function is to obtain samples, test them, and report the results, if the work was done nonnegligently.

Occupational Safety and Health and Other Record-Keeping and Reporting Requirements

To the extent a condition is identified as occupationally related, certain statutory reporting, disclosure, and record retention requirements are triggered. It is incumbent upon the physician to be familiar with those requirements, in part to ensure compliance with his or her obligations and in part to avoid even the appearance of impropriety. These requirements can be divided into two categories. The *first* group of requirements are those mandated by the Occupational Safety and Health Act and its regulations. The *second* group are those mandated under the workers' compensation laws of the jurisdiction in which the work-related injury or illness occurred.

Record-Keeping Requirements

OSHA Requirements

Regulations promulgated under the Occupational Safety and Health Act of 1970 require that occupational injuries and illnesses be recorded and reported [28]. Although the obligation to generate these records is restricted to *employers of 11 or more employees* in certain Standard Industrial Classification (SIC) Codes [29], physicians should always be aware of the requirements because they may be called on to determine if a condition is work related and how it should be recorded or reported. That determination must be made within 6 workdays after the employer receives information that an injury or illness has occurred. Basically, all injuries (except extremely minor ones treated only with first aid) and all deaths and illnesses that result from a work-related accident or from an exposure in the work environment must be recorded.

There are two OSHA forms that have been developed for record-keeping purposes, the OSHA Form 200, Log and Summary of Occupational Injuries and Illnesses, and the OSHA Form 101, Supplementary Record of Occupational Injuries and Illnesses. The first of these, the OSHA 200 Log, is used to record the occurrence and extent of occupational injuries and illnesses, and at the end of the year, it is used to summarize the injuries and illnesses that occurred during the year. Each injury or illness must be classified as either (1) a death case, (2) a case involving lost workdays (which includes days of *restricted work activity* as well as days off work), or (3) a case not involving lost workdays. In addition, for occupational illnesses, the log must record whether the illness was a skin disorder, a dust disease of the lungs, a respiratory condition caused by a toxic agent, systemic poisoning, a disorder due to repeated trauma or physical agents, or another type of occupational illness. New entries should not be made on the OSHA 200 Log if the employee is merely experiencing a recurrence of symptoms from an earlier injury or illness.

An OSHA Form 101 must be completed for every injury or illness entered on the Form 200. This supplementary record provides *details* of the occurrence and nature of the illness or injury. Other forms, such as workers' compensation forms, may be used instead of the Form 101 if they contain the same information.

The OSHA Forms 200 and 101 must be maintained for *5 calendar years* following the year to which they relate. In addition to OSHA inspectors and various other officials listed in the regulations, employees, former employees, and their representatives may inspect the OSHA 200 Log. Employee access to the OSHA 200 Log is limited to the logs for the establishment where the employee worked or formerly worked. However, *all relevant logs must be made available for inspection,* by OSHA representatives and access must be within a reasonable time and in a reasonable manner.

All employers *must report to OSHA, within 48 hours,* accidents that result in one or more *deaths* or in the *hospitalization* of five or more employees. The report must describe the circumstances surrounding the occurrence, the number of fatalities, and/or the number of those who were hospitalized [30]. Other OSHA standards or state or federal regulations may set out other reporting requirements, but those requirements are beyond the scope of this chapter.

Workers' Compensation Law Requirements

Each state's workers' compensation statute imposes certain reporting requirements for all physicians who treat occupational injuries and illnesses. It is imperative that all physicians be familiar with the reporting requirements of the workers' compensation laws of the state in which they practice. In some jurisdictions, the time during which an employee is obliged to file a claim for a work-related condition (the statute of limitations period) does not begin to run until the employer files a report of accident. What the employer actually knows, however, often depends on what is related by the treating physician. In the case of work-related injuries and illnesses, the physician is entitled to be paid by the employer or the employer's workers' compensation insurance plan. However, in some states, *failure to file an attending physician's report within a certain period of time may excuse the employer's obligation to pay the bill.*

Medical Record Access

The physician may be asked to provide the medical records of an employee who has been treated. There are two types of considerations in a request of this sort: the *confidentiality* expectations of the patient and the *rights,* guaranteed by statute or otherwise, of the employer to have the records examined. There are also two types of laws to consider, federal and state. The *federal* law is OSHA's Access to Employee Exposure and Medical Records Standard, and the state laws are those statutory or case law pronouncements regarding who can examine medical records and under what circumstances.

OSHA's Exposure and Medical Record Access Standard

WHO IS COVERED. By its terms, OSHA's Record Access Standard "applies to all employee exposure and medical records, and analyses thereof, made or maintained in any manner, including on an in-house or contractual (fee-for-service) basis" [31]. Therefore any patient seen at an employer's medical facility or seen, at the employer's request, by any physician has records covered by this standard.

WHAT CONSTITUTES A MEDICAL RECORD. The first decision that must be made is what constitutes "medical records." OSHA's Record Access Standard defines medical records to include, but not necessarily be limited to, medical and employment questionnaires or histories; results of all medical examinations, laboratory tests, and biologic monitoring; medical opinions, diagnoses, progress notes, and recommendations; descriptions of treatments and prescriptions; and employee medical complaints. Health insurance records are also covered, if they are accessible to the employer by employee name, social security number, or "other personal identifier."

There are three specific *exemptions* from coverage. *First,* physical specimens, such as blood or urine, which are routinely discarded, are not required to be kept (although the written results of such tests are). *Second,* health insurance records to the extent they are not accessible by personal identifier are not part of the medical records. *Finally,* records regarding employee alcohol, drug abuse, or personal counseling programs are *not* covered if they are maintained separate and apart from the employee's medical program and its records [32]. Given the highly sensitive nature of some of these last records and the high public visibility these cases may receive, it is prudent to keep records related to alcohol and substance abuse *separate.* Failure to do so may result in an unsuspected lawsuit.

WHO IS ENTITLED TO REVIEW THE RECORDS AND UNDER WHAT CIRCUMSTANCES. Under the Record Access Standard, any employer who has employees exposed to "toxic substances" or "harmful physical agents" must provide the employee (or his or her authorized representative) access to his or her medical record *within 15 days of a request.* The employer must provide to the requesting employee, or his or her designated representative, either (1) a copy of the employee's medical record, *at the employer's expense;* (2) the necessary copying facilities, supplied at the employer's expense, so the employee can make copies of the record; or (3) temporary custody of the record, so that the employee can make copies. This provision applies to *all present and former employees* exposed to toxic substances or harmful physical agents. *Employers must advise all employees of their rights under the standard when they are hired and at least annually thereafter.* All medical records must be retained for the duration of the employee's employment plus 30 years, and all analyses using medical records must be retained for 30 years (unless another OSHA standard directs otherwise). The length of this retention period is justified, according to OSHA, because of the extremely long latency periods of some occupational diseases.

Under the Record Access Standard, the employee can also utilize a "designated representative" to obtain medical record information. That "representative" may be a collective bargaining representative, physician, attorney, family member, fellow employee, or anyone else.

To obtain access to medical records, any of these designated representatives *must have the written consent of the employee.* That written consent need not be in any particular form, but it must contain the following [33]:

1. The name and signature of the employee authorizing the release of medical information

2. The date of the authorization (*because any authorizations expire after 1 year*)
3. The name of the organization or individual authorized to release the information
4. The name of the designated representative to whom the information is authorized to be released
5. A general description of the purpose for the release of the medical information
6. The date or condition on which the release will expire, if less than a year

It is quite likely that a large number of employees will be entitled to see medical records because of the broad definition given to "toxic substances" and "harmful physical agents."

THE DEFINITION OF "TOXIC SUBSTANCE." A "toxic substance," under the Record Access Standard, includes chemical substances, biologic agents, and physical stress (noise, heat, cold, vibration, repetitive motion, ionizing and nonionizing radiation, hypo- and hyperbaric pressure).

The Record Access Standard covers substances and agents that

1. Are regulated by any federal law or rule due to a hazard to health
2. Are listed in the latest edition of the National Institute for Occupational Safety and Health (NIOSH) Registry of Toxic Effects of Chemical Substances
3. Have yielded evidence of an *acute or chronic health hazard* in human, animal, or other biologic testing conducted by, or known to, the employer
4. Have an MSDS available to the employer indicating that the material may pose a hazard to human health

When medical records are provided, employers may delete trade secret information from medical (and exposure) records, to the extent they disclose manufacturing processes or the percentage of chemical substances in mixtures. However, the employee must be notified the deletions have been made, and the employer must provide effective alternative information about when and where the exposure occurred. In addition, the employer may *not* withhold chemical names or levels of exposure, although it may obtain a confidentiality agreement [34].

REFUSAL TO PERMIT ACCESS TO EMPLOYEE MEDICAL RECORDS. There is one circumstance under which a physician for the employer may prohibit an employee from seeing his or her medical record. If the physician believes that direct employee access to records concerning a terminal illness or a psychiatric condition of that employee could be detrimental to the employee's health, the employer may refuse to show these records to the employee. However, the records must be shown to the employee's authorized representative.

EXPOSURE RECORDS. The Record Access Standard also provides that an employee or an authorized representative can obtain access to records of *exposure monitoring* to hazardous substances. This portion of the Access Standard is applicable to *current and former employees*.

Exposure records are broadly defined as "records containing exposure information concerning the employee's workplace or working conditions" and "exposure records pertaining to workplaces or working conditions to which the employee is being assigned or transferred." Exposure records include (1) *environmental* (workplace) *monitoring* or measuring, including personal, area, grab, wipe, or other forms of sampling, including collection and analytic methodologies, calculations, and other background data relevant to interpretation; (2) *biologic monitoring* results that directly assess the absorption of a substance or agent by a body system; and (3) Material Safety Data Sheets. Since exposure records may not be available for all employees, the standard provides that an employee can review other "exposure records [of employees] . . . with past or present job duties or working conditions related to or similar to those of the employee." Similarly, a request for records of exposures made in particular worksites, but not tied to any specific employee, would also be obtainable.

Employers must also advise employees of their exposure record access rights upon commencement of employment and at least annually thereafter. *Exposure records must be maintained for 30 years.*

Exposure records may also be obtained by designated representatives. However, with regard to exposure records, a collective bargaining representative of the employee is automatically deemed to be a "designated representative," and, without written employee authorization, is entitled to review exposure records [35].

ANALYSES USING EMPLOYEE EXPOSURE OR MEDICAL RECORDS. Employees and their designated representatives are also entitled, by the Record Access Standard, to review any *analysis* using employee exposure or medical records. This term *analysis* is defined as

> Any compilation of data, . . . research . . . [or] statistical . . . study based . . . in part on information collected from . . . employee exposure or medical records; [and] information . . . from health insurance records, . . . [if] the analysis has been reported to the employer. . . .

This portion of the rule also permits collective bargaining representatives to examine analyses without obtaining specific employee written consent. However, if the analyses contain any information by which individual employees can be identified, the employer must remove that information before it is turned over [36].

State Laws Governing Access to Medical Records

State laws regarding the availability of medical records are basically of two types. The *first* is statute or case law that sets out a physician's obligations to disclose medical record information. All physicians should familiarize themselves with any pertinent state law regarding who can obtain medical records and when they may be obtained. These, in the main, are designed for purposes of setting out the conditions under which patients themselves may obtain their records.

The other type of state law is that found in the workers' compensation statutes. Generally, those laws provide that if an employee has made his or her physical condition an issue in a workers' compensation proceeding, that employee's medical records are discoverable by the parties to that proceeding. However, to be on the safe side, physicians should (1) make sure they know what the law of their particular state provides and (2) in a compensation proceeding, insist on a *subpoena* setting out the style of the case and precisely the types of records requested.

Confidentiality

OSHA's Record Access Standard and certain state laws provide that, under certain specified circumstances, patients, their representatives, and opposing parties in litigation can get medical records. Two other situations in which the physician might be asked for medical information should be addressed.

The *first* situation is when records are requested by an agency such as NIOSH, investigating worker health or attempting, in some way, to cope with a public health problem. In a recent United States Supreme Court case, for example, the court upheld the right of New York State to require that a copy of any prescription for a narcotic drug be sent to the state health department. The court held that public health concerns outweighed privacy considerations [37]. State court rulings may interpret state agency rights in the various jurisdictions. Physicians should familiarize themselves with these decisions. Insofar as federal agencies are concerned, the most commonly litigated issue has been the request by NIOSH for employee medical information to conduct studies regarding potential health hazards in the workplace. Courts have routinely permitted NIOSH to obtain this information pursuant to a subpoena [38]. However, one court of appeals has held that, to prevent unwanted invasions of privacy, *NIOSH should notify employees* that their records will be examined after a certain period of time has elapsed, unless the employee requests that the record not be reviewed [39].

The *second* situation occurs when an employer wants information about an employee's medical condition. An employer's request for information may arise in several contexts. The first is in conjunction with a preplacement or periodic physical examination, the second is in connection with workers' compensation, and the third is not, to the physician's knowledge, in conjunction with anything in particular.

With regard to preplacement or periodic examinations, physicians should be aware of the Code of Ethical Conduct of the American College of Occupational and Environmental Medicine, originally adopted in 1976 and updated in 1994:

> . . . Employers are entitled to counsel about the medical fitness of individuals in relation to work, but are not entitled to diagnoses or details of a specific nature.

Thus, under this section and without a release from the patient, physicians may advise employers, for example, that an employee should not work in high places because of possible dizziness but would not convey information about the etiology of the dizziness if the dizziness is not work related. As to non–work-related conditions that would have no effect on the ability to do the job, the physician should not convey those to the employer at all. If the employee wants the employer's insurance to pay the medical bill, however, as a practical matter, a release will be required by the employer or insurance company to process appropriate payments.

As to work-related disorders, the situation is a bit different. State workers' compensation statutes *mandate* reporting of work-related disorders, and the *employer is obliged to know* what the employee's condition is, so as to protect him or her from further exposure and not violate any necessary restrictions. Again, as a practical matter, the information contained on most state workers' compensation "Attending Physician Reports" will suffice to provide the employer with the necessary information.

Finally, an employer may request information on a patient's health status *for no apparent reason*. OSHA's rule making on the Record Access Standard revealed that management access to employee medical records might be much more extensive than the ACOEM Code of Ethical Conduct permits. OSHA, however, specifically declined to issue specific rules limiting management access to records [40]. However, a physician who provides such information may be open to a malpractice suit by the patient whose records are so disclosed. In the absence of one of the permissible situations outlined above, the physician is advised not to release medical information without the patient's consent.

The Americans with Disabilities Act

Now more than ever, practitioners of occupational medicine will have to concern themselves with the legal ramifications of disabilities in the workplace. This is because, in 1990, Congress passed the Americans with Disabilities Act (ADA), which comprehensively regulates how employers treat the disabled. (See Chap. 5 for a comprehensive discussion of the ADA.)

The ADA is intentionally worded very broadly, and even the Equal Employment Opportunity Commission (EEOC), charged with issuing regulations and enforcing the Act, has yet to give detailed guidelines as to the requirements of some of the Act's provisions. The EEOC and others have acknowledged that explication of the ADA's specific requirements will only come as courts interpret the Act on a case-by-case basis. At this time, we can only look to the language of the Act itself, and some of EEOC's regulations and interpretations, for enlightenment [41].

Under the ADA a "disability" is (1) a physical or mental impairment that substantially limits one or more of the major life activities of an individual, (2) a record of such an impairment, or (3) a situation in which an individual is regarded as having such an impairment. The thrust of the ADA (relevant to employers) is that employees or job applicants with such disabilities may not be discriminated against in any aspect of the employment relationship if that employee or applicant is "qualified" for the job. A disabled person is "qualified" if, with "reasonable accommodation" he or she can perform the "essential functions" of the job as well as one who is not disabled. Obviously, many questions arise in the face of such vague terms as "major life activity" and "reasonable accommodation."

A "major life activity" is exemplified in the EEOC rules by such things as caring for oneself, seeing, hearing, speaking, walking, learning, and working [42]. A major life activity is "substantially limited" if, due to disability, the person cannot perform that activity, or cannot perform it as well as or as easily as the average person in the general population [43].

Notably, a person is disabled, even if not presently impaired, if he or she "has a record of such impairment" or "is regarded as having" a disability. The first phrase covers those who have been misclassified as having a disability, or who were impaired but have at least temporarily recovered [44]. The second phrase covers those who are not actually impaired in the major life activities, but are nevertheless viewed and treated by others as being impaired [45].

No doubt much of the inevitable ADA-spawned litigation will center on what are and are not "essential functions" of jobs. A lawyer could hardly imagine a more fact-specific, case-by-case issue. The EEOC sets out three factors, to which others may be added, to aid in the analysis. The function may be essential if (1) the position exists specifically to perform that function, (2) only a limited number of employees can perform the function, and/or (3) the function is highly specialized and the person is hired specifically for his or her expertise in performing that function [46].

Evidence considered in assessing whether a job function is essential includes, among other things, (1) the employer's judgment as to what is essential, (2) the amount of time spent on the particular function, (3) written job descriptions, and (4) the consequences of not requiring the employee to perform the function [47].

Once the essential functions are determined, the employees or applicants may not be treated differently due to their disability, if any "reasonable accommodation" will enable them to do the job. An accommodation is necessarily reasonable if it does not impose on the employer an "undue hardship." An accommodation must be effective, but it need not be the best available accommodation [48]. Reasonable accommodations include making work facilities physically accessible, and acquiring or modifying equipment. It might even require steps such as hiring readers for blind employees or interpreters for deaf employees [49].

An "undue hardship" is "action requiring significant difficulty or expense." The EEOC elaborates by explaining an undue hardship as an accommodation that would (1) be unduly costly, (2) be extensive, (3) be substantial, (4) be disruptive, or (5) fundamentally alter the nature or operation of the business [50]. In analyzing the financial burden of an accommodation, the cost of accommodation is not compared to the value of the position being accommodated (i.e., employee's salary) but is analyzed in light of the employer's entire financial resources [51].

Of special note to medical practitioners is the ADA's impact on employment-related medical examinations. The ADA prohibits such examinations before an offer of employment is made. Examinations are allowed only after an offer is made, and the offer may be conditioned on passing the examination. However, the same examination must be given to all entering employees in the same job classification, and the information derived therefrom may not be used to discriminate against the disabled applicant.

The practitioner may also be called on to assess whether an applicant should be rejected as posing a "direct threat" to others "that cannot be eliminated by reasonable accommodation." This will be an issue in situations in which the disability is, or is related to, an infectious disease. The regulations emphasize that the "direct threat" determination must be an individualized assessment, relying on the most current medical knowledge and the best available objective evidence [52]. The risk must be evaluated in terms of its duration, and the likelihood, imminence, and severity of the potential harm [53].

Toxic Torts

The "toxic tort" is another possible concern for the practitioner of occupational medicine. Toxic tort suits are suits at common law, brought by those who claim that exposure to the toxic substance caused them some injury or disorder. Normally, but not always (see the exception to workers' compensation exclusivity for intentional torts), workers' compensation will be the sole remedy for employees harmed by exposure to toxic substances at the workplace that are being manufactured by their own employer. However, workers can always sue third-party suppliers of materials to their employers (e.g., asbestos). Consumers of products (e.g., pharmaceuticals such as diethylstilbestrol) or those exposed to allegedly toxic waste in the environment (e.g., a Superfund site) can also bring a civil suit.

Toxic tort lawsuits can be brought under many different legal theories, including (1) negligence (lack of reasonable care by defendant), (2) strict liability (defendant liable for his or her abnormally dangerous activity or defective and unreasonably dangerous product), (3) breach of express or implied warranty, and even (4) intentional misconduct (defendant knew that injury was substantially certain to flow from his or her act or omission).

Most peculiar to toxic tort suits are the types of damages that are recoverable by plaintiffs. In addition to the usual damages for medical expenses, lost earning capacity, and pain and suffering, plaintiffs who claim exposure to toxins may, in some states, seek damages for future risk of illness, fear of future illness, or the cost of medical surveillance.

Plaintiffs who claim future risk of injury are arguing that their exposure to a toxin has increased their risk of a particular illness or illnesses associated with such exposure. It is very difficult to prove that a future illness will probably occur absent some present injury or symptoms. Thus, most courts allow recovery for increased risk only if there is some present manifestation of the deleterious effects of the exposure. Even if such is the case, plaintiffs still must prove, usually with expert testimony, that the possible future illness is produced by exposure to the toxin, and that the illness is likely to occur some time in the future.

Closely related to increased risk of future illness is fear of future illness. Here, as in a claim for infliction of emotional distress, the claimant is claiming psychic injury—damages for worry and anxiety [54]. Courts that allow such a claim require that the fear be "reasonable." This requirement is sometimes met when there is a sufficiently rational causal relationship between the toxin and the disease. In a number of cases, courts have held that the chance of contracting the disease need not be greater than 50% to justify a reasonable fear. Thus, even where a plaintiff's claim for increased risk fails, he or she might still recover for fear. Even here, in the great majority of cases that have permitted this cause of action, some physical injury or some physical manifestation of the fear must be shown in order to prove the genuineness of the fear [55]. However, courts have, on occasion, allowed corroborative medical and psychological testimony to substitute for actual injury. A few courts have found a reasonable fear based only on *proof of exposure* to the toxin [56].

Injured plaintiffs always seek damages for medical expenses incurred in treating injuries. Sometimes, after exposure to a toxic substance, expenses for medical surveillance, rather than treatment, are incurred. Medical surveillance involves regular examination and testing designed to monitor the patient's health, with an eye toward early detection and treatment of a future illness stemming from exposure. Most courts will allow such expenses if there is a reasonable probability of the plaintiff contracting the disease. Of course, this is proved by expert testimony. As would be expected, damages for medical surveillance are more easily obtained if the plaintiff already shows symptoms or some related injury. If no injury is present, the trend in the courts that have considered and approved this element of damages is to allow the costs as long as enough of a concern about future illness exists to justify medical intervention.

Fetal Protection Programs

Practitioners of occupational medicine need no longer concern themselves with monitoring or enforcing fetal protection programs, since the Supreme Court recently found such programs to be unlawfully discriminatory [57]. Fetal protection programs directed solely at women, solely for the protection of fetuses, are not legitimate employer policies.

In that case the employer excluded fertile women from battery production jobs that exposed them to lead. The fear was that in utero, or even preconception, exposure might interfere with proper fetal development. The Court found the policy to be facially discriminatory in targeting women only. While facial discrimination is permitted if based on a bona fide occupational qualification (BFOQ), the Supreme Court held that these policies were not BFOQs.

Drug Testing

Substance abuse is a problem that must be confronted by occupational medicine practitioners in today's workplace. Of particular significance is the issue of whether and how to test employees for substance abuse. Given the fact that drug use by employees (both on and off the job) visits enormous costs on employers in the form of increased absenteeism, lower productivity, increased chance of accidents, and increased health care costs [58], and given that testing based solely on suspicion of abuse is only slightly effective at best [59], more employers every year are implementing random drug testing procedures.

This is an area where knowledge of applicable state law and precedent is a necessity. In the private sector, random drug testing is a question of state law, although the evolution of state law will likely be influenced by federal decisions.

In 1989, the United States Supreme Court decided two major cases involving challenges to drug testing conducted or required by the federal government [60].

These cases involved testing of railroad employees in safety-sensitive positions, and Customs Service employees whose jobs were "sensitive," in that the employees interdicted narcotics, carried weapons, or had access to classified information.

Since the "tester" in these situations was the government, the Fourth Amendment prohibition to unreasonable searches was implicated. The Supreme Court essentially found that a government employer's right to conduct employee drug testing is far from absolute, and must be weighed against an employee's reasonable expectation of privacy. In both cases, the testing procedures were upheld, given the limited expectations of privacy in such sensitive jobs, and the government's compelling interest in maintaining safety on the rail lines, and in maintaining the fitness and integrity of front-line Customs personnel. Subsequently, courts have approved government-mandated drug testing of air traffic controllers [61] and workers on natural gas pipelines [62].

Most state constitutions have a provision similar to that of the Fourth Amendment preventing unreasonable searches and seizures. Some state constitutions go further, having express protections of privacy as such [63]. Normally, such constitutional provisions apply only to governmental conduct, and so do not impact the private employment relationship [64]. Accordingly, drug testing by private employers will typically be limited (if at all) by state privacy statutes [65], and a state's common law on privacy.

Most challenges to private employer drug testing have been based on common-law privacy interests. Most of these cases have involved testing of employees in safety-sensitive jobs and, predictably, testing has been upheld [66]. As in the federal Fourth Amendment cases, the courts usually have reached their conclusions by balancing employee privacy expectations against employer interest in safety.

The propriety of testing is most uncertain where employers wish to test employees in nonsensitive positions. In one California case, the court ruled that the constitutional privacy guarantee was applicable even to strictly private sector employment, and that random drug testing is justified only by an employer's compelling interest [67]. On the other hand, a Texas court seemed to say that any drug testing by private employers would be legal. The court recognized a right to privacy under Texas law, but reasoned that an employee who did not wish to submit to an intrusive drug test could vindicate this privacy right by simply quitting his or her job [68].

Informed by trends in both federal and state law, it is likely that drug testing of employees in sensitive jobs will normally be upheld. Testing of employees in nonsensitive jobs is a much riskier proposition, and some jurisdictions will find it to be an unwarranted invasion of employee privacy (see Chap. 9).

References

1. 1920 N.Y. Laws Ch. 538 [codified as amended at N.Y. Workmen's Comp. Law § 3(2)] (McKinney 1965 and Supp. 1982).
2. *Southern Shipping Co. v. Lawson,* 5 F. Supp. 321 (S.D. Fla. 1933) (heavy labor resulted in rupture of preexisting aortic aneurysm; death held to be compensable).
3. *Chausse v. Lowe,* 35 F. Supp. 1011, 1014 (E.D.N.Y. 1938) [(quoting *Goldberg v. 954 Marcy Corp.,* 276 N.Y. 313, 12 N.E.2d 311 (1938)].
4. *Ivancik v. Wright Aeronautical Corp.,* 68 F. Supp. 270, 273 (D.N.J. 1946) [(quoting *Bollinger v. Wagaraw Building Supply Co.,* 122 N.J.L. 12, 6 A.2d 396 (1939)].
5. *Todd Dry Docks, Inc. v. Marshall,* 61 F.2d 671 (9th Cir. 1932).
6. *Dower v. General Dynamics Corp.,* 14 Ben. Rev. Bd. Serv. (MB) 342 (1981) (rectal cancer allegedly potentiated by asbestos exposure); *Compton v. Pennsylvania Avenue Gulf Service Center,* 14 Ben. Rev. Bd. Serv. (MB) 472 (1981) (leukemia allegedly caused by exposure to benzene).
7. *Ryan v. Connor,* 503 N.E.2d 1379 (Ohio 1986).
8. *Witty v. American General Capital Distributors, Inc.,* 727 S.W.2d 503 (Tex. 1987).
9. *Sparks v. Tulane Medical Center Hospital and Clinic,* 546 So. 2d 138 (La. 1989); *Barnes v. City of Cincinnati,* 590 N.E.2d 294 (Ohio App. 1990).
10. Fla. Stat. Ann. 440.02(1).
11. Maine Rev. Stat., Ann., Title 39, Section 51(3).
12. *Prater v. Thorngate Ltd.,* 761 S.W.2d 226 (Mo. App. 1988).
13. Occupational Safety and Health Administration. *A Brief Guide to Recordkeeping Requirements for Occupational Injuries and Illnesses* (OMB No. 1220-0029), April 1986. Chapter IV.

14. 29 CFR §§ 1910.1200.
15. *New Jersey State Chamber of Commerce v. Hughey,* 774 F.2d 587 (3rd Cir. 1985); *Manufacturers Association of Tri-County v. Knepper,* 801 F.2d 130 (3rd Cir. 1986); *cert. denied* 108 S. Ct. 66 (1987); *Ohio Manufacturers' Association v. City of Akron,* 801 F.2d 824 (6th Cir. 1986); *cert. denied* 108 S. Ct. 44 (1987).
16. Superfund Amendments and Reauthorization Act of 1986, "Emergency Planning and Community Right-to-Know Act" (EPCRA) (Public Law 99-499) §§ 311-312; see also, 52 FR 38344.
17. 29 CFR § 1910.1200(i); see also, 3 part trade secret test proposed by EPA under EPCRA, 52 FR 38312 (Oct. 15, 1987).
18. *Johns-Manville Product Corporation v. Contra Costa Superior Court,* 165 Cal. Rptr. 858; 612 P.2d 948 (1980).
19. *Millison v. E.I. duPont de Nemours and Co.,* 501 A.2d 505, 516 (N.J. 1985).
20. *Jones v. VIP Development Co.,* 472 N.E.2d 1046, at 1052 (Ohio 1984).
21. *Price v. Philadelphia Electric Co.,* 1992 W.L. 99227 (Ed. Pa. 1992).
22. *Levitsanos v. Superior Court,* 2 Cal. 4th 744 (1992).
23. *Duprey v. Shane,* 39 Cal. 2d 781, 249 P.2d 8 (1952).
24. *Delamotte v. Unit Cast Division of Midland Ross Corp.,* 411 N.E.2d 814, 818 (Ohio App. 1978).
25. Billauer, B. F. The legal liability of the occupational health professional. *J.O.M.* 27:185, 1985.
26. *Abbott v. Gould, Inc.,* 443 N.W.2d 591 (Neb. 1989).
27. *Millison v. E.I. DuPont de Nemours and Co.,* 5 A.2d 505 (N.J. 1985).
28. 29 USC 651 et seq. and 29 CFR Part 1904.
29. Occupational Safety and Health Administration. *A Brief Guide to Recordkeeping Requirements for Occupational Injuries and Illnesses* (OMB No. 1220-0029), April 1986. Chapter I.
30. Occupational Safety and Health Administration. *A Brief Guide to Recordkeeping Requirements for Occupational Injuries and Illnesses* (OMB No. 1220-0029), April 1986. Chapters IV-VII.
31. 29 CFR § 1910.20(b), (c), (e), and (f).
32. 29 CFR § 1910.20(b) and (c).
33. 29 CFR § 1910.20(c) and (e).
34. 29 CFR § 1910.20(c) and (f).
35. 29 CFR § 1910.20(c) and (e).
36. 29 CFR § 1910.20(c)(2).
37. *Whalen v. Roe,* 429 U.S. 589 (1977).
38. *General Motors Corporation v. Director,* NIOSH, 9 OSHC (BNA) 1139 (6th Cr. 1980).
39. *Westinghouse v. United States,* 8 OSHC (BNA) 2131 (3rd Cir. 1980).
40. 45 FR 35243 (1980).
41. 56 Fed. Reg. 35725 (July 26, 1991) ("Regulations"); *EEOC Technical Assistance Manual* (1992) ("TAM").
42. Regulations, Section 1630.2(i).
43. Regulations, Section 1630.2(j)(1).
44. Regulations, Section 1630.2(k).
45. Regulations, Section 1630.2(1).
46. Regulations, Section 1630.2(n)(2).
47. Regulations, Section 1360.2(n)(3).
48. TAM III-3-5.
49. Regulations, Section 1630.2(o)(2).
50. Appendix to Regulations, 56 Fed. Reg. 35744.
51. TAM III-15.
52. Regulations, Section 1630.2(r).
53. *Id.*
54. *Jackson v. Johns-Manville,* 781 F.2d 394 (5th Cir.), *cert. denied,* 478 U.S. 1022 (1986).
55. *E.g., Payton v. Abbott Laboratories,* 437 N.E.2d 171 (Mass. 1982).
56. *In re Moorenovich,* 634 F. Supp. 634 (D. Me. 1986).
57. *International Union, United Automobile, Aerospace and Agricultural Implement Workers of America, UAW v. Johnson Controls, Inc.,* 111 S. Ct. 1196, 113 L. Ed. 2d 158, 59 U.S.L.W. 4209 (1991).
58. *Potomac Electric Power Company v. International Brotherhood of Electrical Workers, Local Union 1900,* AAA Case No. 16 30 0016 5 865 (Stone, May 8, 1987).
59. *Brotherhood of Maintenance of Way Employees, Lodge 16 v. Burlington Northern R.R.,* 802 F.2d 1016 (8th Cir. 1986).

60. *Skinner v. Railway Labor Executives Association,* 489 U.S. 602 (1989); *National Treasury Employees Union v. Von Raab,* 489 U.S. 656 (1989).
61. *Bluestein v. Department of Transportation,* 908 F.2d 451 (9th Cir. 1990), *cert. denied,* 111 S. Ct. 954 (1991).
62. *I.B.E.W. v. Department of Transportation,* 913 F.2d 1454 (9th Cir. 1990).
63. Wests Ann. Cal. Const. Art. I, Sec. 1 (1983); S.H.A. Ill. Const. Art. I, Sec. 6 and 7 (1971).
64. *But see Wilkinson v. Times Mirror Corp.,* 264 Cal. Rptr. 194 (1st Dist. 1989) (concluding after review of legislative history and case law that privacy provision applies to private employer drug testing programs).
65. Mass. Gen. L. Ann. Ch. 214 Sec. 1B (West 1989); Ga. Code Sec. 26-3002.
66. *Horne v. J.W. Gibson Well Service Co.,* 894 F.2d 1194 (10th Cir. 1990); *Grace Drilling Company v. Director of Labor,* 790 S.W.2d 907 (1990); *DiTomaso v. Electronic Data Systems,* 3 Indiv. Empl. Rts. Cas. (BNA) 1700 (E.D. Mich. 1988).
67. *Luck v. Southern Pacific Transportation Co.,* 267 Cal. Rptr. 618 (1st Dist.), *cert. denied,* 111 S. Ct. 344 (1990).
68. *Jennings v. Minco Technology Labs, Inc.,* 765 S.W.2d 497 (Tex. Ct. App. 1989).

Further Information

Ashford, N. A., and Andrews R. A. Workers' Compensation. In W. Rom (ed.), *Environmental and Occupational Medicine.* Boston: Little, Brown, 1983. Pp. 907-912.

Billauer, B. F. The legal liability of the occupational health professional. *J.O.M.* 27:185, 1985.

Boden, L. I. Workers' Compensation. In B. S. Levy and D. H. Wegman (eds.), *Occupational Health: Recognizing and Preventing Work Related Diseases.* Boston: Little, Brown, 1983. Pp. 439-452.

29 CFR § 1910.20.

Letter to the Editor by M. A. Silverstein, and Author's Response by R. J. McCunney *J.O.M.* 27(1):5-7, 1985.

Lieberman, M. Confidentiality of Medical Records: Legal Precedents and Issues. In J. S. Lee and W. N. Rom (eds.), *Legal and Ethical Dilemmas in Occupational Health.* Ann Arbor, MI: Ann Arbor Science, 1982. Pp. 235-242.

Loomis, L. *Drug Testing: A Workplace Guide to Designing Practical Policies and Winning Arbitrations.* Washington, DC: BNA, 1990.

McElveen, J. C. Expert Witnesses. In J. T. O'Reilly (ed.), *Toxic Torts: Practice Guide,* Colorado Springs, CO: Shepards/McGraw Hill, 1992. Pp. 16-1–16-25.

McElveen, J. C., and Postol, L. P. Compensating occupational disease victims under the Longshoremen's and Harbor Workers' Compensation Act. *Am. Univ. Law Rev.* 32(3):717, 1983.
General overviews of the development of workers' compensation laws.

NIOSH Registry of the Toxic Effects of Chemical Substances. Washington, D.C.: U.S. Government Printing Office, 1992.
The latest edition can be purchased from the Superintendent of Documents, U.S. Government Printing Office, Washington, D.C. 20402.

Occupational Safety and Health Administration. *A Brief Guide to Recordkeeping Requirements for Occupational Injuries and Illnesses* (OMB No. 1220-0029), April 1986.

Swotinsky, R. B. *The Medical Review Officer's Guide to Drug Testing.* New York: Van Nostrand Rheinhold, 1992.

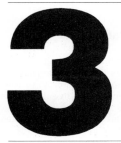

The Role of Regulatory Agencies

James A. Hathaway

The practice of medicine has become increasingly affected by governmental activity, as evidenced by diagnostic-related groups (DRGs), prospective budgeting for hospitals, and limitations on fees. Virtually all medical specialties, including occupational medicine, have been affected by the public sector regarding the cost and delivery of medical care. Additional changes are anticipated from proposed health care reform legislation.

The delivery of occupational health services, however, has a unique background with respect to governmental activity. Not only do issues such as workers' compensation statutes affect the practitioner, but also regulations established by federal and state agencies have a direct effect on the practice of occupational medicine. In particular, the Occupational Safety and Health Administration (OSHA), the National Institute for Occupational Safety and Health (NIOSH), and the Environmental Protection Agency (EPA) all carry out activities that directly affect the practice of occupational medicine in some capacity. OSHA standards, NIOSH research activities, and certain EPA regulations should become familiar topics for physicians who provide occupational health care. This chapter provides an overview of the activities of these and other agencies that have the most significant impact on practitioners providing occupational and environmental health services.

It is not the purpose of this chapter to review the history of the regulatory agencies or to discuss in detail the philosophy behind their stated lofty objectives. Whether the agencies are accomplishing their goals or doing so efficiently and effectively will also not be covered even though this is often a topic of debate. Interested individuals are referred to textbooks that have chapters on these topics [1, 2]. How these agencies affect the day-to-day practice of occupational medicine in either a clinical or administrative setting and what a practitioner should know are the focus of this chapter.

Agencies that focus mainly on worker health and safety and those that have primarily an environmental focus are discussed. Government agencies seem to be particularly fond of acronyms and an occupational medicine practitioner would be wise to develop at least a passing knowledge of this alphabet soup (Table 3-1).

Table 3-1. Federal agencies with rules that affect the practice of occupational and environmental medicine

Occupational Safety and Health Administration (OSHA)
National Institute for Occupational Safety and Health (NIOSH)
Mine Safety and Health Administration (MSHA)
Nuclear Regulatory Commission (NRC)
Department of Transportation (DOT)
    Federal Aviation Administration (FAA)
    Federal Railroad Administration (FRA)
    Federal Highway Administration (FHA)
Equal Employment Opportunity Commission (EEOC)
Environmental Protection Agency (EPA)
Agency for Toxic Substances and Disease Registry (ATSDR)

Occupational Safety and Health Administration

The Occupational Safety and Health Administration is mandated to assure safe and healthful working conditions for employees. OSHA has legislative authority to accomplish this mission by setting health and safety standards, enforcing these standards through workplace inspections, and assisting employers in solving worksite problems by offering consultation. Of all the regulatory agencies that affect the practice of occupational medicine, OSHA has the greatest impact. Some states have taken advantage of an option in the Occupational Safety and Health (OSH) Act to establish and administer their own state OSHA plan. Standards promulgated by these states are usually identical to the federal OSHA standards but in some cases may be more stringent. The OSH Act does not cover federal, state, or local municipal employees. However, executive branches of the federal government are expected to have equivalent regulations and most state-run programs cover state and local municipal employees.

The OSHA standards that have the greatest potential impact on physicians who provide occupational health services are listed in Tables 3-2 and 3-3. The numerical reference in the tables refers to the specific section(s) of Title 29 of the Code of Federal Regulations (CFR), which provide more detailed information.

Occupational Injuries and Illnesses

Recording of occupational injuries and illnesses is the responsibility of the employer. In some cases, determining whether an injury is work related, and therefore recordable, is difficult. With illnesses, the determination of work-relatedness is even more problematic. Physicians are frequently asked to assist with this determination. Dermatitis and cumulative trauma disorders are examples of conditions that are often controversial regarding work-relatedness. Physicians can assist by making a definitive diagnosis and then weighing the probable impact of workplace and other exposure factors to make a decision as to whether or not the condition is work related.

Injuries and illnesses are recorded on an *OSHA form 200* by the employer. The threshold of recordability is different depending on whether the case is an injury or illness. These terms are defined differently by OSHA than they have been traditionally defined in medicine. OSHA's definition of an injury is something that is caused by an instantaneous exposure, for example in the snap of the fingers. An illness is anything caused by a longer exposure even if it is as short as a couple of seconds. Because of this definition, *the same physical condition might be classified as an illness or injury depending on the nature of the exposure.* For example, a drop of acid falling on a worker's hand and causing a minor first-degree burn would be classified as an *injury*. A weaker solution of acid that was in contact with a worker's hand for several minutes that results in an identical first-degree burn would be classified as

Table 3-2. OSHA standards that impact occupational medicine

Section title	Section no.[a]
Log and Summary of Occupational Injuries and Illnesses	1904.2
Access to Employee Exposure and Medical Records	1910.20
Occupational Noise Exposure	1910.95
Hazardous Waste Operations and Emergency Response	1910.120
Respiratory Protection	1910.134
Medical Services and First Aid	1910.151
Fire Brigades	1910.156
Commercial Diving Operations	1910.401–1910.441
Air Contaminants and Chemical Specific Standards[b]	1910.1000 and following
Bloodborne Pathogens	1910.1030
Hazard Communication	1910.1200
Occupational Exposure to Hazardous Chemicals in Laboratories	1910.1450

[a]From Title 29 of the Code of Federal Regulations.
[b]See Table 3-3 for details.

Table 3-3. OSHA chemical specific standards

Section no.*	Chemical
1910.1001	Asbestos
1910.1003	4-Nitrobiphenyl
1910.1004	alpha-Naphthylamine
1910.1006	Methyl chlormethyl ether
1910.1007	3,3'-Dichlorobenzidine (and its salts)
1910.1008	bis-Chloromethyl ether
1910.1009	beta-Naphylamine
1910.1010	Benzidine
1910.1011	4-Aminodiphenyl
1910.1012	Ethyleneimine
1910.1013	beta-Propiolactone
1910.1014	2-Acetylaminofluorene
1910.1015	2-Dimethylaminoazobenzene
1910.1016	N-Nitrosodimethylamine
1910.1017	Vinyl chloride
1910.1018	Inorganic arsenic
1910.1025	Lead
1910.1027	Cadmium
1910.1028	Benzene
1910.1029	Coke oven emissions
1910.1043	Cotton dust
1910.1044	1,2 dibromo 3-chloropropane
1910.1045	Acrylonitrile
1910.1047	Ethylene oxide
1910.1048	Formaldehyde
1910.1050	Methylene dianiline

*From Title 29 of the Code of Federal Regulations.

an *illness*. This distinction is generally considered unimportant to the treating physician but it is of great interest to the employer. *An injury that requires only first-aid care as opposed to medical treatment is not recordable.* In contrast, all illnesses are recordable regardless of how trivial they may be. Employers greatly appreciate injuries being given first aid rather than medical treatment whenever this level of care is sufficient. OSHA also has definitions of what is first aid and what is medical treatment. For example, use of over-the-counter medication is first aid, use of prescription medication is medical treatment. Likewise, use of a Band-Aid is first aid, whereas use of a steristrip is considered medical treatment. For minor injuries, the selection of treatment can determine OSHA recordability. Physicians can gain the appreciation of employers by selecting modalities that are considered by OSHA as first aid whenever this will not adversely affect the outcome of the case. Occupational physicians should be aware of one exception: OSHA has defined all work-related back problems as injuries even though, with the exception of direct trauma, most authorities consider these problems to occur over time [3].

Access to Employee Medical Records

Physicians practicing occupational medicine may expect to be asked to maintain medical records for their employer or client. These records must be maintained for the duration of a person's employment plus 30 years. This time period is much longer than that typically required for non–work-related inactive patient files. OSHA also requires that medical records be released to designated representatives, including the employee, on presentation of signed consent. Compliance with such requests is required within 15 working days [4].

Occupational Noise Exposure

This OSHA standard requires annual examinations for employees exposed to noise of 85 dBA or higher on a daily time-weighted average (TWA) basis. The hearing level thresholds are compared each year to the baseline audiogram. Audiograms that show a standard threshold shift (STS), which is defined as an age-adjusted decrease of 10 dB or greater in either ear averaged for the frequencies of 2000, 3000, and 4000 Hz, must be evaluated by an audiologist or physician to determine the need for further evaluation. Employers frequently expect physicians practicing occupational medicine to perform these evaluations and provide medical direction for their hearing conservation program. One controversial area is recordability of work-related hearing loss. Based on current OSHA field directives, a work-related change in hearing of 25 dBA averaged over the frequencies of 2000, 3000, and 4000 Hz must be recorded on the OSHA form 200 as a disorder due to repeated trauma. (See Chap. 16 for more details.)

Physical Fitness Evaluations

Several OSHA standards, including Hazardous Waste Operations and Emergency Response, Respiratory Protection, and some Chemical Specific Standards, require the employee to have a medical examination to determine physical fitness to perform certain jobs, or to wear specific personal protective equipment (e.g., respirators). Two other standards, fire brigades and commercial diving operations, do *not* require examinations unless the employee has a specific medical condition; however, the need for examinations is implied due to the strenuous physical activities.

None of these standards specify *details* of the medical examination, which are left to the discretion of the examining physician. Employers may specify requirements, and additional guidance can be found in Chap. 25. Physicians should request authorization for additional tests from employers if the tests are clinically appropriate.

In general, the OSHA standards require the physician to furnish the employer a *written opinion* on whether the employee has any medical conditions that would place the employee at increased risk of impairment from the work or use of protective equipment. The physician must provide in writing any limitations on the employee's assigned work. The employee should be informed of any conditions that require further examination or treatment and be referred to private physicians, as necessary.

Medical Services and First Aid

This standard requires employers to ensure ready availability of medical personnel for advice and consultation on matters of plant health. It is common practice for employers to develop agreements with physicians or clinics to obtain this advice and to have a resource for treatment of injuries or illnesses and for medical examinations.

The standard also requires that a physician approve first-aid supplies for the worksite. Many employers have the physician visit the site annually and sign the list of approved first-aid supplies.

Chemical Specific Standards

There are detailed individual standards for 26 chemicals. Each of these standards includes a section on medical surveillance. In all standards, medical examinations are required if certain conditions are met. These conditions typically refer to airborne exposure levels above a designated concentration (usually 50% of the permissible exposure limits [PEL]) or dermal exposure to material containing the substance at a level above 0.1% or 1.0% by weight or volume. (See Chap. 25 for a detailed description on the methods used to determine the need for medical examinations.)

With the exception of the Carcinogen Standards (1910.1003–1910.1016), most OSHA regulations include detailed requirements for specific examinations and tests. The Asbestos Standard (1910.1001) even includes a required medical history form. All the standards include a provision that additional tests can be performed at the option of the examining physician. More recent standards include an appendix on medical surveillance that provides additional information in determining the type of additional tests that may be useful in specific situations.

In addition to the specified requirements of OSHA standards, several administrative procedures affect the physician performing the examinations. For example, the employer must furnish the physician with a copy of the standard, a description of the employee's duties as they relate to exposure, information on the employee's level of exposure, a description of personal protective equipment used, and information from previous medical examinations. After completion of the medical surveillance examination, the physician must furnish a *written opinion* as to whether the employee has any detected condition that would put him/her at increased risk of material health impairment. Also required is a statement that the employee is fit to wear a respirator or other protective equipment or whether there are limitations in using such equipment.

Some of the more recent standards also include provisions for *medical removal protection* and multiple physician review (e.g., lead [1910.1025] and methylene dianiline [1910.1050]). In some cases, the criteria for medical removal may be straightforward. In lead exposure, for example, temporary removal from exposure is required if the average of the last three blood tests for lead is greater than 50 µg/100 g whole blood and the last test is over 40 µg/100 g whole blood. In other cases, greater discretion is given the physician. An abnormal liver function test in someone exposed to methylene dianiline (MDA) requires medical removal if the abnormal results are believed due to MDA or if the abnormal results are not due to MDA but the physician believes MDA exposure may exacerbate the condition. Methylene dianiline causes choleostasis, which results in elevated alkaline phosphatase and bilirubin levels. Usually no hepatocellular damage occurs. In contrast nonoccupational conditions such as viral infections or alcohol abuse cause hepatocellular damage with elevated levels of alanine aminotransferase (ALT, SGPT) and aspartate aminotransferase (AST, SGOT). There is no experimental evidence or clinical experience to know whether MDA exposure would exacerbate viral or alcoholic hepatitis. One can therefore imagine that physicians may have differences of opinion regarding the risk of MDA exacerbating hepatocellular damage, which could trigger the multiple physician review provisions of the standard. Future standards will likely incorporate medical removal protection and multiple physician review.

In addition to the 26 Chemical Specific Standards, over 600 other chemicals have an OSHA-specified permissible exposure level (PEL). In 1989, OSHA revised downward the airborne exposure limit for many of these chemicals. In 1992, a circuit court of appeals invalidated those revisions. At the time this chapter was written, there was no requirement for medical surveillance for these other chemicals. However, OSHA is considering a standard on generic medical surveillance. If such a standard is adopted in the future, it will probably require medical examinations if exposure is above an action level (most likely 50% of the PEL).

Bloodborne Pathogens

OSHA's standard on bloodborne pathogens is directed primarily at the health care industry, but also affects blood processing and research activities using human blood or other bodily fluids, as well as any employer that has designated first-aid responders. Physicians who practice occupational medicine may be asked to assist employers in drafting written exposure control plans, in conducting training, and particularly in reviewing exposure incidents and providing counseling and advice. (See Chap. 30 for a detailed description of this standard.)

Hazard Communication

The Hazard Communication Standard requires manufacturers and distributors of chemicals to draft *Material Safety Data Sheets* (MSDS) that include detailed information on the product. Of particular interest to the physician are sections on health hazards and first aid. In addition, many companies also include a section on notes to physicians. The MSDS can be a very useful reference to determine the ingredients of a chemical mixture and to learn summary information on toxicity and expected effects of overexposure. First-aid recommendations and, in some cases, specific medical treatment information, are also available. The MSDS includes a phone number for the manufacturer/distributor who can be a source of more detailed information. In some cases, because of trade secret concerns, the identity of all ingredients may not be listed on the MSDS. In an emergency, a treating physician or nurse can request immediate disclosures of the chemical identity of the ingredients. The health care professional can and probably will be required to sign a confidentiality agreement as soon as possible after such a request. In nonemergency situations, similar information can be requested in writing if a legitimate health concern is stated. A signed confidentiality agreement may be required from the manufacturer/distributor.

Occupational Exposure to Hazardous Chemicals in Laboratories

This standard requires employers to furnish medical examinations if employees develop signs or symptoms related to exposure to chemicals in the laboratory, or if they have routine exposures above the action level of a regulated chemical (see Chemical Specific Standards) or following an accidental overexposure from a spill, leak, explosion, or similar occurrence. The content of the examination is left to the discretion of the physician but should be based on the known toxic effects of the chemical(s) of concern. There are similar administrative requirements for written opinions, and related functions as found in chemical specific standards.

National Institute for Occupational Safety and Health

The National Institute for Occupational Safety and Health is the research agency created by the OSH Act. In 1973, under the auspices of the former Department of Health, Education and Welfare (now Health and Human Services), NIOSH became part of the Centers for Disease Control (CDC). In addition to its Atlanta headquarters, it has regional offices in Boston, Massachusetts, and Denver, Colorado, and research facilities in Morgantown, West Virginia, and Cincinnati, Ohio. The institute is mandated to protect the health and safety of workers by conducting research on workplace hazards. In addition to its responsibilities designated under the OSH Act, NIOSH has responsibilities legislated by the Federal Mine Safety and Health Act, the Public Health Service Act, the Toxic Substance Control Act, the Clean Air Act, and the Superfund legislation.

NIOSH plays an important role in providing information pertinent to the development of OSHA standards. Before making specific recommendations, NIOSH performs research and conducts a literature review of human and animal literature and other test systems. This information is assembled into a "criteria document" that OSHA often uses as a basis for its standards. This document contains information on hazards, material use, and control measures. The NIOSH paper on labeling hazardous chemicals, for example, formed the basis of the Hazard Communication Standard promulgated by OSHA in October 1985.

Health Hazard Evaluations

At either employee or employer request, NIOSH may conduct a Health Hazard Evaluation (HHE), which includes an industrial hygiene study and appropriate medical evaluation of an occupational health problem.

Training and Publications

The majority of the training and educational services provided by NIOSH are conducted at 15 Education Resource Centers (ERCs), which were established in 1977 because of the shortage of occupational health professionals. A variety of programs are offered, including occupational medicine residencies and graduate school training in occupational nursing, industrial hygiene, and safety. Physicians who desire training in occupational disease epidemiology may enroll in a 2-year program administered by NIOSH in conjunction with the CDC in the Epidemic Intelligence Service.

NIOSH publishes its findings in a variety of scientific journals and government publications including the CDC's *Morbidity and Mortality Weekly Report*. It also maintains a library, several databases, and a publication office to respond to inquiries about occupational safety and health concerns.

The physician can use several NIOSH publications when evaluating a patient who may have been exposed to a hazardous substance. Additional sources of information include the Criteria Documents and Current Intelligence Bulletins (CIBs), which describe new scientific information about occupational hazards. A CIB may discuss a previously unrecognized hazard or report that a known hazard is more or less dangerous than previously considered.

Although NIOSH makes its own publications available to the public, it will **not** perform literature reviews for inquiring health personnel.

Mine Safety and Health Administration

The Mine Safety and Health Administration (MSHA) was established by the Federal Mine Safety and Health Act of 1977. Its purpose is similar to that of OSHA except it covers only workers in the mining industry. Rules issued by MSHA are found in Title 30 of the CFR. Many of the standards promulgated by MSHA are similar to those issued by OSHA. In addition there are regulations specific to the mining industry. For example, *health and safety training* is mandated for all new miners and refresher teaching is required annually. All underground mines are inspected four times a year and all surface mines twice a year. NIOSH develops health standards for MSHA, but only *advises* OSHA concerning health standards. In general, health standards under MSHA place requirements on physicians regarding medical examinations that are similar to OSHA standards.

Nuclear Regulatory Commission

The Nuclear Regulatory Commission (NRC) has primary responsibility for regulating hazards from ionizing radiation, including x-rays, gamma rays, and radioactive material that can be taken into the body. Regulations issued by the NRC are found in Title 10 of the CFR. Part 20 covers radiation protection programs and occupational dose limits. Section 20.1703 requires that a physician determine a worker's ability to wear a respirator every 12 months. This is in contrast to OSHA's standard, in which an annual review is suggested but longer time intervals are acceptable.

Enforcement of NRC regulations is usually delegated to state departments of health. Medical examination requirements are typically included in the facility's operating license. Physicians providing services to employers with an NRC license should follow appropriate requirements. In addition, they should review potential exposures to radionucleotides. Specific biologic monitoring may be possible using whole body counting or assaying urine samples for radioactivity. External radiation hazards are monitored with personal dosimeters. The results of such monitoring should be reviewed by the physician and explained to the employee.

Department of Transportation

Several Department of Transportation (DOT) agencies have issued regulations of potential interest to the physician practicing occupational medicine. These agencies include the Federal Aviation Administration (FAA), the Federal Railroad Administration (FRA), and the Federal Highway Administration (FHA). All of these agencies have issued regulations dealing with drug and alcohol testing (see Chap. 9).

Federal Aviation Administration

Title 14 of the CFR, part 67, includes the medical standards and certification requirements of the FAA. These standards are very detailed regarding medical or physical conditions that disqualify airmen and pilots. The standards also include qualifications regarding who can perform medical examinations. A physician who wants to examine pilots under these standards must become an aviation medical examiner approved by the FAA.

Federal Railroad Administration

Medical fitness requirements for railroad locomotive engineers are found in Title 49 of the CFR, section 240.119 related to substance abuse disorders, and section 240.121 covering vision and hearing acuity. Section 240.119 details specific conditions and time periods for return to service following alcohol or drug abuse. Section 240.121 details visual acuity and hearing threshold levels required for one to be certified as a locomotive engineer. After an appropriate medical evaluation, a physician may conclude that someone can safely operate a locomotive despite not meeting the visual and hearing thresholds and may condition that certification on special instructions.

Federal Highway Administration

Truck drivers in interstate commerce must meet the physical qualifications required by the FHA. Sections 391.41 to 391.49 of Title 49, CFR, detail the specific examinations and criteria required to be used when examining interstate truck drivers. These rules must be carefully followed by physicians performing these examinations.

Equal Employment Opportunity Commission

The Equal Employment Opportunity Commission (EEOC) is charged with enforcing the *Americans with Disabilities Act*. This act and the EEOC regulations in Title 29 of the CFR, Part 1630, affect the practice of occupational medicine in three major areas. These regulations establish federal laws regarding the confidentiality of occupational medical records. They limit mandatory examinations and tests of employees to those that are job related. They also require "reasonable" accommodation of applicants or employees with medical impairments. Physicians who practice occupational medicine must have knowledge of employees' work assignments and the physical requirements of essential job functions to properly advise employers regarding the placement of persons with impairments (see Chap. 5).

Environmental Protection Agency

The EPA was established by presidential order in 1970. It is responsible for implementation of numerous acts of Congress promulgated to protect the environment. Although these laws should be of general interest to physicians in occupational medicine, most do not have a significant impact on the day-to-day activities of most physicians in the field. However, it is worth noting that standards related to the quality of air and water are increasingly being based on *health effects* rather than engineering technology. Cleanup criteria at hazardous waste sites are also based on potential health effects in addition to technical feasibility. Some physicians in occupational medicine may serve as consultants to government agencies or to private companies in coordinating and/or evaluating risk assessments related to proposed ambient air and water standards or cleanup criteria. Other physicians practicing clinical occupational medicine may be asked questions concerning such standards by their patients or by citizens in their community. While it is not necessary for most occupational physicians to have detailed knowledge of the specifics of environmental laws and regulations, it is desirable for them to become more knowledgeable concerning the concepts and process of *risk assessment* (see Chap. 26, 50).

Physicians who practice occupational medicine should become familiar with two provisions of one of the environmental laws, the *Toxic Substance Control Act (TSCA)*. Section 8(c) of this act requires manufacturers or users of a specific chemical to keep a record of any allegation of a heretofore unknown adverse health effect. The purpose of these records is similar to that of adverse reaction reports for pharmaceuticals. If a company sees several similar reports, further investigation is warranted. Physicians practicing occupational medicine will often be the first to learn of a purported relationship between exposure to a substance and an adverse health effect. If it is a previously unknown effect, they should notify the manufacturer or user of the chemical or encourage the patient to do so.

Section 8(e) of TSCA requires manufacturers, producers, and users of chemicals to report to the EPA new information that reasonably supports the conclusion that the chemical or mixture presents a substantial risk of injury to health or the environment. Such information is often discovered during toxicity testing but may also be developed from investigations of 8(c) allegations. Occasionally, clinical information from a single case may be strong enough to warrant reporting. Information reported under section 8(e) becomes more widely known so that other users of the same substance can take action to prevent adverse health effects. Early recognition of unrecognized health effects is an important role of the physician. Physicians learning of such effects should be encouraged to report new information to companies so that the TSCA 8(c) and 8(e) provisions work effectively (see Chap. 42).

Agency for Toxic Substances and Disease Registry

The Agency for Toxic Substances and Disease Registry (ATSDR) is a Public Health Service Agency created in 1980 under the Superfund legislation to implement the health-related activities of the Comprehensive Environmental Response, Compensation, and Liability Act (CERCLA). ATSDR is primarily concerned with the potential adverse health effects associated with environmental exposure to toxic substances. ATSDR's mission is to support activities designed to protect the public from the adverse health consequences of toxic chemical exposure. Specific responsibilities include health consultations at Resource Conservation Recovery Act sites and at hazardous chemical spills, such as an overturned railway car filled with toxic gases. Part of its mission is to conduct research about the health effects of toxic materials identified at these locations.

ATSDR is mandated to establish a disease and exposure registry to provide an information base of health effects of toxic substances. It also provides continuing education training for physicians through case studies in environmental medicine. In addition, it has developed medical management guidelines for treatment of some chemical overexposures. (See Chap. 45 for more details.)

References

1. Felton, J. S. *Occupational Medical Management*. Boston: Little, Brown, 1990.
2. Rom, W. N., et al. *Environmental and Occupational Medicine* (2nd ed.). Boston: Little, Brown, 1992.
3. US Department of Labor, Bureau of Labor Statistics. *Recordkeeping Guidelines for Occupational Injuries and Illnesses* (OMB No. 1220-0029). September 1986.
4. Doyle, J. R. Access to medical record standard. *Occup. Env. Med. Rep.* 3:53, 1989.

Further Information

See the federal regulation that pertains to the agency of interest. The title and part or section is referenced in the text as the agency is discussed.

Morbidity and Mortality Weekly Report, published by the Massachusetts Medical Society, PO Box 9120, Waltham, MA 02254-9120.

Appendix to Chapter 3: An Overview of OSHA Regulations

B. Hoffman

The OSHA regulations are contained in Title 29 of the Code of Federal Regulations, part 1910 (29 CFR 1910). This part is divided into subparts A–Z, sections 1–1500.

Subpart A contains sections 1–7 under the title "General." It cites the references and applicability of the regulations, and defines the procedures established to appeal or amend them. This subpart has had one major change since its promulgation, which is the addition of 29 CFR 1910.7, titled "Definition and Requirements for a Nationally Recognized Testing Laboratory" (NRTL). It allows the establishment of privately owned NRTLs to test and certify OSH equipment of various kinds, similar to the way Underwriters Laboratory tests and certifies electrical equipment.

Subpart B contains sections 11–19 under the title "Adoption and Extension of Established Federal Standards." It deals with the construction and maritime trades. **Subpart C,** section 20, is titled "Access to Employee Exposure and Medical Records," and is very important to occupational physicians and industrial hygienists. **Subpart D** contains sections 21–32 under the heading "Walking and Working Surfaces." It deals with ladder safety, floor and wall openings, scaffolding, and fall protection. None of these three subparts have been the subject of major revisions.

Subpart E contains sections 35–40 under the title "Means of Egress." Major changes have been proposed for this subpart in the form of a new Confined Spaces regulation working its way through the process.

Subpart F, sections 66–70, deals with "Powered Platforms, Manlifts, and Vehicle-mounted Work Platforms." **Subpart G** contains sections 94–100, titled "Occupational Health and Environmental Control." It includes ventilation, noise exposures, and ionizing and nonionizing radiation exposures. No major changes in these subparts.

Subpart H, sections 101–120, deals with "Hazardous Materials." It gives specific instructions for the use and handling of specific materials, such as acetylene, hydrogen, oxygen, nitrous oxide, flammable and combustible materials, explosives, anhydrous ammonia, and hazardous waste operations and emergency response (HAZOPs and ER). This last regulation, 29 CFR 1910.120, HAZOPs and ER, is a major addition to the OSHA regulations, and is of concern to every industry or individual whose activities are affected by these regulations. It sets requirements for training of individuals involved in HAZOPs and in ER, and sets minimum requirements for safe operations of these activities. This subpart also contains section 29 CFR 1910.119, "Process Safety Management of Highly Hazardous Chemicals." This section defines a list of chemicals for which greatly extended written procedures and risk analysis documentations are required, and is a major addition to the OSHA regulations. This section's provisions are still being challenged in the courts.

Subpart I, sections 132–140, deals with "Personal Protective Equipment." It covers general requirements, and eye and face, respiratory, head, foot, and electrical protective devices and measures. There have been several changes in this subpart, all relatively minor, clarifying and extending the original regulations.

Subpart J, containing sections 141–150, is titled "General Environmental Controls." It deals with sanitation, temporary labor camps, non–water carriage disposal problems, safety color codes for marking physical hazards, specifications for accident prevention signs and tags, and lock-out/tag-out regulations for energy sources. This last section, 29 CFR 1910.147, lock-out/tag-out, is a major revision, and is still being challenged in the courts.

Subpart K, sections 151–153, deals with "Medical Services and First Aid," and is of concern to occupational physicians. **Subpart L,** containing sections 155–165, deals with "Fire Protections." **Subpart M,** sections 166–171, is titled "Compressed Gas and Compressed Air Equipment." **Subpart N,** sections 176–190, deals with "Materials Handling and Storage." It covers servicing of wheel rims, powered industrial truck operations, crane operations, crawler locomotive operations, derricks, helicopters, and slings. These subparts have had fairly frequent changes, but no major revisions.

Subpart O contains sections 211–222 under the title "Machinery and Machine Guarding." **Subpart P,** sections 241–247, is titled "Hand and Portable Power Tools and Other Hand-held Equipment." **Subpart Q** holds sections 251–257 under the heading "Welding, Cutting and Brazing." **Subpart R** contains sections 261–275, and is titled "Special Industries." It contains regulations of operations in selected industries, including pulp, paper, pulpwood logging, agricultural operations, telecommunications, and grain handling facilities. No major changes in any of these subparts.

Subpart S contains sections 301–399, under the heading "Electrical." It has had continual small changes since its promulgation, but no major changes. **Subpart T,** sections 401–441, is titled "Commercial Diving Operations." It is a special case, and has little application to most occupational health specialists. No major changes.

Subparts U to Y are not used. These subparts are set aside for future regulations.

Subpart Z, sections 1000–1500, are titled "Toxic and Hazardous Substances." These are the sections in which all of the specific permissible exposure limits (PELs) and specific procedures for selected toxic materials are listed. This subpart has been the site for most of the changes in OSHA regulations, and includes one former and three recent major revisions. The oldest major revision is 29 CFR 1910.1200, the OSHA Hazard Communication standard. When it was first promulgated, it was subjected to lengthy court challenges before finally being accepted. The first recent revision in subpart Z was the PEL update, in which OSHA attempted to change over 600 PEL values at one time. Previous PEL changes had been tackled one by one, and numbered only about 24 in the first 20 years of OSHA's existence. The PEL Update was successfully challenged in court, and OSHA has appealed the action. This issue is still in doubt, but OSHA has vowed to pursue the changes it desires in order to keep up with the pace of change. If the court appeal is not successful, OSHA may petition Congress for additional authority granted by a new federal law.

The second recent revision was 29 CFR 1910.1450, titled "Occupational Exposure to Hazardous Chemicals in Laboratories." This section did not face major court challenges, since it supersedes existing provisions of the Hazard Communication regulations for laboratories, and is thus really a modification of OSHA's previous regulations. The final recent major change is section 29 CFR 1910.1030, titled "Bloodborne Pathogens." This section applies to every person or organization in which any person might be occupationally exposed to human blood or body fluids, such as emergency response teams, first-aid workers, and medical aid personnel. This section has been, and is currently, under challenge in the courts.

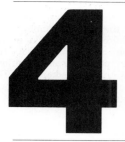

The Establishment of an Occupational Health Program

Benjamin Haskell Hoffman
and Douglas C. Gray

Most businesses have occupational health needs. The ever-increasing federal and state regulation of workplace health and safety, environmental compliance, spiraling workers' compensation premiums, and the many diverse hazards encountered in the modern workplace have given increasing importance to the role of the occupational and environmental health professional. Even with the financial pressures encountered by business during recessionary times, budgets to manage these problems have increased steadily.

Occupational health programs are as varied as the organizations they serve. They are influenced by a multitude of factors, including the business itself (its products or services), corporate philosophy, and the economy. An occupational medical program can be conducted on site or through contract facilities. The key player in the development of an occupational health program is the occupational and environmental medicine (OEM) physician.

In whatever organization he or she chooses to practice, the OEM physician has become an integral component of senior management within many business communities. Whether he or she practices within industry as the company physician, directs a freestanding or hospital-based occupational health clinic, or serves in the government/academic medical community, the OEM physician plays a pivotal role in the spectrum of occupational health services critical to the operation of a business. Essential to the OEM physician's skills is an understanding of the basic tenets of business, legal, and regulatory requirements in occupational health. Often, the OEM physician is the "jack-of-all-trades" and must have a "global perspective" on health issues. Consultation with other medical specialists, industrial hygiene and safety specialists, attorneys, and engineers is frequently necessary when the mastery of a specific subject is required.

Because of their professional interests and training and the specific health needs of a business, OEM physicians may be involved in a variety of ways. This involvement may include assessment, development, and/or operation of occupational health programs. All OEM physicians, regardless of the setting in which they practice, need to be familiar with the universe of programs and services that are the essential ingredients of the field.

Assessment

The type of occupational health programs needed by any business is directly dependent on the goals, activities, and operations of that organization. Regardless of who provides the services, whether it be a company physician or off-site facility, an understanding of the activities of the organization is critical to the development of a quality program. When a physician, hospital, or medical clinic is asked by a business to "set up a program," a variety of motivations may have led to this decision, including concern for the health of employees, legislation, or increasing health costs, among others. The basic approach to the initial assessment includes conducting a *walk-through* of the facility regardless of the setting, whether it be an office or factory. The formal process of the walk-through is described later in this chapter.

A successful relationship between an OEM physician and an organization requires that the physician become familiar with the operations. Review of the workplace is necessary to understand and evaluate the working conditions of the employees. A checklist of items to review is included in Table 4-1. These reviews are preferably made with an industrial hygienist, safety engineer, and other persons familiar with

Table 4-1. Guidelines for the physician conducting a facility walk-through

1. Are there substances used in the workplace for which established OSHA standards exist?
2. Are carcinogenic substances used?
3. Are corporate policies in effect for certain issues such as alcohol or drug abuse?
4. Are rehabilitative or modified duty assignments available?
5. Are collective bargaining agreements in place that may affect delivery of medical care?
6. Are Material Safety Data Sheets available?
7. What is the level of existing first-aid services?
8. Is a disaster plan in place?
9. What is the nature of control measures (e.g., engineering devices, personal protective equipment)?
10. What staff members are responsible for health and safety measures?
11. What training procedures are in place (regarding Hazard Communication Standard, respiratory use, etc.)?
12. Review current facilities, especially storage of medical records.

the operations. During the walk-through, various types of jobs should be noted. In particular, the physician should be concerned with whether there is potential and actual exposure to chemical, physical, and/or biologic hazards and whether appropriate control measures such as engineering devices or personal protective equipment are available. A tour of the facility to become familiar with the operations and the general environment will enable the physician to understand specific job requirements and make more informed decisions. (The latter part of this chapter includes a description of a facility walk-through, written from the perspective of an industrial hygienist.)

Following the walk-through, a meeting can enhance a discussion of the specific needs of the organization. Initially, the physician is advised to discuss specific expectations for the occupational health services with the representative who solicited the meeting. At that time, representatives of the enterprise can express their particular needs regarding occupational health programs for the facility. Where feasible, additional perspectives can be gained from key employees such as members of the safety and health committees. The OEM physician, in turn, can address his or her own capabilities for providing occupational health services. If an outside occupational and environmental medicine clinic is selected to provide services, the clinic should identify a contact person both at the business and at the clinic to enhance communication regarding the occupational and medical services.

The OEM physician must realize that a balanced perspective is necessary for the effective practice of occupational and environmental medicine because the field often has strong political crosscurrents. Clearly, each situation needs to be approached differently, but it is strongly advised that the physician be recognized as a fair and impartial health professional.

Development and Operation

The field of occupational and environmental medicine has undergone substantial changes in the last decade. The delivery of occupational medical care has expanded from the industrial in-plant clinic to hospital-based clinics, multispecialty groups, and occupational medicine programs within academic settings. Some companies have moved away from the traditional on-site medical dispensary and have contracted with occupational health programs in their community. Other companies have moved toward maintaining on-site services, but through the hiring of contractors.

In many business settings, there is a stronger emphasis on *preventive* interventions than on medical treatment alone. The practice of occupational and environmental medicine is at its core a field within preventive medicine. The OEM physician often directs care to *groups* of workers, in contrast to the routine practice of clinical medicine. While clinicians may offer expertise concerning particular aspects of care (cardiologists for cardiovascular evaluation and pathologists for tissue diagnosis), the OEM physician integrates the information from diverse clinical perspectives into a group analysis to provide occupational medical services.

Prevention has particular value in the design and operation of programs since all occupational medical problems are potentially preventable. Public health professionals use the principles of prevention in their daily development of programs. Prevention has three components: primary, secondary, and tertiary. *Primary prevention* is any intervention that addresses a risk factor for a disease or injury. Examples include immunization against infectious diseases and reduction in blood cholesterol levels to reduce the risk of heart disease and stroke. *Secondary prevention* refers to early detection of disease and intervention before symptoms appear. The goal is to reverse, halt, or retard the progression of a disorder. Examples include the use of mammography in the early detection of breast cancer and periodic cytologic testing of the uterine cervix (Papanicolaou smear) in screening for cervical cancer. *Tertiary prevention* refers to minimizing the effects of disease and disability by reducing complications and premature deterioration. Examples include the care of pressure points and bladder function in bedridden individuals. Traditionally, occupational health programs (both company based and contract services) limited their role to tertiary prevention—the management of occupational injury and illness. Recently, there has been a much greater emphasis on programs addressing primary and secondary prevention. With the increasing costs of workers' compensation, these programs should have a greater emphasis.

One of the cornerstones of a productive and healthy workforce is an effective occupational health program. Once a business's needs have been assessed, the OEM physician should focus on the types of programs that are likely to prevent occupational injury and illness, contain health care costs, and reduce liability. Adopting the tenets of preventive medicine is useful in designing such a program.

Primary Prevention Programs

The goal of primary prevention in the workplace is to reduce the rate of occupational injury and illness through three types of programs.

Properly Designed Workplace

Historically, the vast majority of industrial machinery was not manufactured with the worker's health, safety, and comfort in mind. If and when these factors were considered, equipment was designed for the traditional 25- to 55-year-old white man of average height and weight [1]. However, population demographics in the workplace have changed considerably in the past three decades. Women and a wide variety of nonwhite ethnic groups now comprise a large percentage of workers in the manufacturing sector of the United States. Their physical characteristics bear little resemblance to those of the predominant employee of the 1930s. Although engineering experts have attempted to make industrial equipment more user-friendly, poor equipment design remains a major problem in many industries.

The development of an ergonomics team is an essential ingredient in a primary prevention program. The team should analyze jobs routinely to assess potential problems. Team members should represent a cross section of engineering, production, medicine, and rehabilitation/biomechanics expertise and be provided with adequate training in ergonomics to exercise their duties. Such training programs are provided on a regular basis through the Occupational Safety and Health Administration (OSHA) and numerous academic centers. Additional invaluable resources are mechanic and electrical engineers. A specialized discipline within electrical engineering, the field of rehabilitation engineering is primarily involved in engineering the workplace to meet the physical capabilities of workers (see Chap. 28, Ergonomics).

Matching Workers to the Job

Many workers may not be able to perform the job for which they were hired [2]. When applicants are tested for specific job tasks, testing protocols rarely take into account factors that may affect job performance.

The first step in establishing whether prospective employees are capable of performing the job for which they may be placed is to establish the job task that they are to perform. This approach necessitates the development of a *functional job description* that outlines the job requirements, including exposures to biologic, chemical, and physical hazards. The data are then converted into testing protocols to assess the physical and/or psychological capabilities of the prospective employee. An example of a functional job description is given in Fig. 4-1.

INITIALING INFORMATION

Corporation: _____ Job Title: _____
Department: _____ Grade: _____ Date: _____
Hours/Day: _____ Days/Week: _____ DOT#: _____

NARRATIVE JOB DESCRIPTION **TOOLS**

KEY

| O | Occasional ≤ 33% of day | F | Frequently 34-66% of day | C | Continuous 100% of day | E | Essential | OVH FW WC | Overhead Floor to Waist Waist to Chest |

FUNCTION LIST

TASK	O	F	C	E
Crawling				
Sitting				
Standing				
Walking				
Stair Climbing				
Ladder Climbing				
Balancing				
Squatting				
Reaching				
Reaching	Near	Far	OVH	
Sustained Bending				

HAND/ARM

TASK	O	F	C	E	Right	Left
Pinch						
Grip						
Fine Manipulation						
Finger Press						
Keyboard						
Keypad						
Hand/Arm Vibration						
Required Force	Light	Mod	Hvy			

LIFT & CARRY

TASK	R	O	F	C	E	Force/Wt.
Zone						
F-W						
W-C						
C-OVH						
Two-hand Carry						
One-hand Carry						
Pushing						
Pulling						
Twisting						
Handles						

Exposures
☐ Noise ≥ 85 db ☐ Dampness ☐ Cold ≥ 47° F ☐ ≤ 75° F ☐ Height < 4'
☐ Dust ☐ Chemicals

Protective Equipment
☐ Shoes ☐ Helmet ☐ Glasses ☐ Mask ☐ Respirator
☐ Other

Sensory Functional
☐ Light Touch ☐ Seeing ☐ Color ☐ Vision ☐ Speaking
☐ Depth Percep ☐ Hearing ☐ Remembering ☐ Reading ☐ Problem Solving
☐ Work ϖ others ☐ Work Independently

Restrictive Duty
☐ LBP ☐ Hand/Arm ☐ Wheelchair ☐ Crutches ☐ Blind
☐ Deaf ☐ Heart ☐ Stroke ☐ Arthritis ☐ Hip/Knee/Foot
☐ Diabetes ☐ ALS/MS ☐ Other

Figure 4-1. Elemental job analysis.

Testing protocols are critical to avoid unnecessary injuries or illness because of worker–job task mismatch. In the same way that a company would not hire a person who could not type a specific number of words per minute to be a typist, it is not appropriate to hire someone who is incapable of performing forceful repetitive motion, heavy lifting, or similar job tasks if that is what the position requires. Not only does this level of analysis make sense, but this approach will be necessary under the requirements of the Americans with Disabilities Act (see Chap. 5).

The development of functional job description often requires a team approach, combining the efforts of employees familiar with the job tasks and occupational health professionals. Appropriate testing protocols may be performed by a variety of professionals, including physical therapists, occupational therapists, kinesiologists, or physicians experienced in physical medicine and occupational health.

Worker Training

It is essential for workers to be properly trained, even if they *are* matched to their jobs. The *majority* of injuries occur in recently hired people [3]. Severe injuries in particular tend to occur among employees who are *not* properly trained to use the equipment they are operating. Similarly, inadequate training in hazardous material handling accounts for a large percentage of accidental overexposures. Training in hazard communication, lock-out/tag-out, forklift, and driver safety are examples of programs that can help reduce occupational injuries and illness. Training is not a "one-shot deal," however, and should be repeated at routine intervals (see Chap. 37).

Industrial Hygiene

Industrial hygiene involves the recognition, evaluation, and control of industrial hazards that may cause illness among workers. Industrial hazards frequently encountered by workers include chemicals, physical energy (such as electromagnetic and ionizing radiation), noise, vibration, repetitive motion, temperature extremes, and microorganisms (such as fungi, bacteria, and viruses) [4].

In the United States, the primary source of industrial hygiene regulations is the Occupational Safety and Health Act of 1970 (OSH Act). The Congressional act established the National Institute for Occupational Safety and Health (NIOSH) to recommend new or changed regulations, OSHA to promulgate and enforce regulations, and the Occupational Safety and Health (OSH) Review Board to review appeals of OSHA regulations or actions under the OSH Act. NIOSH is under the Centers for Disease Control (CDC) in the Department of Health and Human Services, whereas OSHA and the OSH Review Board are in the Department of Labor.

Initially, OSHA was charged by the OSH Act to promulgate existing federal and consensus health and safety standards as its initial regulations. After that, regulations could only be changed by an elaborate process involving public hearings, NIOSH recommendations, and publication in the *Federal Register*. Major standards promulgated via this route have been limited to about two dozen. The OSHA regulations are contained in Title 29 of the Code of Federal Regulations, part 1910 (see the Appendix to Chapter 3).

The industry hygienist routinely evaluates the work environment and reports findings to the medical, engineering, and operational components of the company. Although OSHA standards mandate routine industrial hygiene practices in specified situations (such as in the development of a new process, change in the process, or situations in which air levels of chemicals are above specified thresholds), it is highly advisable to conduct regular industrial hygiene evaluations of certain workplaces, even if it is anticipated that the regulatory requirements will be satisfied. A well-run industrial hygiene program will enhance employee confidence in the company's ability to maintain a safe work environment. Routine industrial hygiene data may also be instrumental in defending workers' compensation claims, reducing liability, and performing epidemiologic surveys.

Industrial hygienists, like OEM physicians, work in a variety of different settings. Depending on the size and needs of a business, an industrial hygienist may be hired as a contract worker or as an employee. Many OEM physicians hire a consulting industrial hygienist and encourage his or her involvement as a member of the health and safety team.

Secondary Prevention Programs

Secondary prevention in the workplace involves detecting occupational health problems at an early stage, before a worker develops symptoms of an illness or injury. The goal of secondary prevention is to address problems before they become more advanced. Secondary prevention has far-reaching implications for any occupational health program and includes two major types of programs, medical surveillance and employee assistance programs.

Medical Surveillance

Medical surveillance is the systematic evaluation of employee health to monitor for the early occurrence of disease. Medical surveillance may be applied to workers with four major types of workplace exposures: hazardous substances, repetitive motion, manual lifting, and physical hazards.

HAZARDOUS SUBSTANCES. Medical surveillance of workers exposed to hazardous substances has become routine practice in occupational health for many types of work settings. Although OSHA has established medical surveillance standards for only 26 substances, it is in the process of developing a "generic medical surveillance standard" to cover *all* hazardous chemicals.

Numerous changes have occurred in medical surveillance over the last 10 years. Traditional programs have been slanted toward organ system dysfunction. This approach, however, is relatively insensitive and nonspecific. Abnormal findings tend to occur late in the disease process beyond the time when treatment would be curative. Examples include the use of chest x-rays to determine asbestos-related lung disease and liver function tests to assess chemical-induced hepatitis. Therefore, in recent years, other methods (including biologic monitoring) have become more widely used.

Biologic monitoring is an attempt to assess the internal "dose" of overall worker exposure to chemicals in the workplace through measurement of the appropriate determinant in biologic specimens such as urine, blood, or exhaled air. The American Conference of Governmental Industrial Hygienists (ACGIH) has developed biologic exposure indices (BEIs) that are intended as guidelines for analyzing the results of biologic monitoring [5]. High body fluid levels that suggest overexposure to chemicals should prompt a worksite evaluation by an industrial hygienist. Low levels tend to indicate a healthy working environment, help to establish confidence among workers, and reduce frivolous lawsuits. Although biologic monitoring may or may not be part of a medical surveillance program, it has advantages over air monitoring, including the following:

It takes into account absorption via routes other than inhalation.
The substances measured in body fluids relate more directly to an adverse health effect than any environmental measurement.
Personal hygiene habits (such as hand washing, smoking, etc.) are considered.
Individual variation in physiologic parameters, such as respiratory rate (which may alter the amount of exposure measured by air monitoring), are addressed.
Environmental monitoring is not always feasible.

See Chap. 25, Medical Surveillance, for a more comprehensive discussion of this topic.

A sophisticated medical surveillance program should supplement workplace control measures. These programs can become complex in design, but are relatively simple to operate. Abnormal values must be dealt with in a uniform way and results must be effectively communicated to both the employee and the personal physician. Management needs to be informed of the aggregate findings to evaluate potentially unsafe working conditions. Clear guidelines should be established regarding *medical confidentiality*, with attention to the OSHA Access to Medical and Exposure Records Standard.

REPETITIVE MOTION. Repetitive motion injuries have become more widely recognized of late. Regulatory agencies such as OSHA have developed a strong interest in the prevention of such injuries, so much so that an effective prevention program will likely become an OSHA standard. Unfortunately, many physicians do not fully understand such injuries since they defy the traditional paradigm of injury, that is, they do not occur at one particular time, they develop gradually, and they may not respond to traditional treatment. Moreover, routine diagnostic tests may not help in assessing early symptoms.

Repetitive motion injuries are the result of force, rate, position, and rest factors that tax tissues beyond their ability to fully recover or heal [6]. Secondary modifying variables, such as extremes of temperature, humidity, vibration, surface texture changes, or grip sizes, can increase ergonomic stress and tissue injury. Carpal tunnel syndrome and similar forms of cumulative trauma may be the result of an exposure combined with the active involvement of the worker. The early detection and prevention of cumulative trauma such as carpal tunnel syndrome is a high priority. Toward that end, devices such as the digital vibrometer, which assess sensory thresholds in a similar manner as audiometry, may be useful [7]. These devices are the first attempt to provide objective measurement of sensory changes reflective of early nerve compression in the hand.

MANUAL LIFTING. Today, it is possible to enhance our ability to predict those workers who are most likely to experience a work-related back injury. The technology for this surveillance technique appeared in the early 1980s with the publication of the NIOSH *A Work Practices Guide for Manual Lifting,* which has recently been updated [8]. The scientific underpinnings used in the creation of this text and other more recent advances in human performance measurement systems allow a clinical evaluation to place workers' spinal function on an "injury-risk" ratio scale. This procedure is performed by relating information on spinal function during tests of spinal load capacity while the individual is lifting, and then by analyzing certain physiologic parameters such as muscle strength, trunk strength, and velocity of spinal motion. The data can then be applied to create proper worksite accommodations and generate improvements in employee work technique and overall level of physical conditioning [9].

The outcome of these and other measures may reduce the incidence and cost of back injury while at the same time increasing the worker productivity. Many physical therapists and kinesiologists are familiar with these techniques. With their assistance, testing protocols may be developed that should be consistent with the Americans with Disabilities Act. This legislation does not consider strength testing or other types of agility assessments as medical examinations (the Act takes a similar position with drug testing) and as a result these can be performed *prior to* a job offer.

PHYSICAL HAZARDS. Exposures to physical hazards (radiation, vibration, noise and temperature extremes) may impose undue stress on workers. Recognition and control of hazards are an important part of an industrial hygiene plan. A medical surveillance program must incorporate an effective hearing conservation program (as required by OSHA) and monitor the worker's exposure to noise.

Employee Assistance Program

Stress, emotional problems, and substance abuse can affect work performance and increase the rate of injury and absenteeism. An effective approach to prevent and manage such problems is through an employee assistance program (EAP). EAPs are counseling services designed to help employees and their dependents cope with stressful situations that arise at work and at home. The typical EAP provides confidential and voluntary counseling for psychological or financial problems, alcohol or drug abuse, and family difficulties.

With the increasing role of drug-testing programs in the work setting, EAPs provide resources for assessing and treating employees who test positive for drugs. (The Department of Transportation rules do not require rehabilitation of individuals who test positive. Rather, that follow-up is left to labor management negotiation.) The development of an EAP program usually requires cooperation with the human resources department. Local hospitals and many companies specializing in multisite EAP programs are available.

Employers covered under the federal Department of Transportation (DOT) drug testing rules must provide an EAP program, which shall, as a minimum include

An educational and training component for drivers, supervisory personnel, and company representatives that addresses controlled substances
A written statement, on file and available for inspection, of the motor carrier's principal place of business, outlining that the motor carrier has an EAP
At least 60 minutes of training on the consequences of substance use on health and safety in the work environment along with the manifestations and behavioral changes that may indicate substance use or abuse [10]

Tertiary Prevention Programs

Tertiary prevention involves *clinical management* of people injured or ill and appropriate *rehabilitation* (vocational and physical) to assure a timely return to work. The goal of this form of prevention is to manage the care of the worker from the onset of the injury to the point at which the worker returns to the job, regardless of the time frames. A continuum of health care may be necessary, depending on the severity of the injury or illness. For instance, the medical services required for a worker who herniates a disk and requires surgery vary greatly from those of the worker who merely sustains a minor contusion. In the former case, a broad array of services, ranging from monitoring the hospitalization and surgical intervention to vocational rehabilitation, is necessary. With a minor injury, merely tracking a worker's medical care and assuring a timely return to work are necessary.

The traditional approach to providing medical care to injured or ill workers was via the *on-site medical department,* staffed by health professionals. Because of increasing concerns of cost and quality assurance, many businesses have begun to reduce the amount of general health care services provided, and focus primarily on *occupational health* as opposed to primary care. Currently, a range of options are available to businesses that can provide high-quality and cost-effective occupational health services. These include maintaining an on-site program through the hiring of community-based contractors on a part-time or full-time basis; completely contracting out occupational health services to a local provider, such as a community hospital; or providing a mix of on-site health care professionals (either contractors or company employees, part-time or full-time) and targeting the use of certain occupational health services through community-based resources.

On-site Services

Maintaining an on-site problem can be a cost-effective method of delivering occupational health services for many organizations, depending on the number of employees and the complexity and health risks of the operations. Services can be delivered through hiring of contractors or company employees on a part-time or full-time basis. The staff number is dependent on the facility size, the number of injuries or illnesses that occur, and other organizational priorities, such as wellness, health promotion, and the provision of non–work-related medical care.

In many industries, an occupational health nurse, nurse practitioner, and/or physician assistant provide cost-effective occupational health services. At times, these professionals are also responsible for the assessment and management of workplace health and safety programs and coordinating the off-site services. Responsibilities include tracking injured or ill employees, maintaining the OSHA 200 Log, and delivering a variety of other health- and safety-related prevention programs. If appropriately trained, the professional may also provide supervised clinical care for both work-related and non–work-related medical problems, such as performing preplacement medical surveillance examinations. State regulations vary, however, regarding the degree of autonomy and level of physician supervision that are necessary. In some cases, nurse practitioners and physician assistants may function independently and prescribe medications.

A physician, preferably with certification or training in occupational medicine, is usually necessary. The physician, who may be contracted through a local occupational medicine program, should be present routinely, at an interval that varies depending on a number of factors, including the number of employees, the incidence rate of occupational illnesses and injuries, and related variables. Although a physician may be present for as few as 2 to 3 hours per week, he/she should be available throughout the week to the staff of the occupational medical department. The physician provides medical direction to the staff on the management of work injury and illness, medical surveillance, preplacement, and fitness-for-duty examinations. The physician should be an active member of the team, keep the staff up to date on new regulations, and perform medical review officer–related activities, where appropriate.

On-site physicians are generally hired on an hourly basis with a yearly retainer that guarantees a specified number of hours. If it is elected to contract clinical services with an off-site clinic, fees are negotiable and less than the usual and customary fee arrangement.

The delivery of occupational health care at the workplace can be enhanced by the availability of the rehabilitation staff, including physical therapists and occupational (hand) therapists. These professionals are critical to the treatment of musculoskeletal injuries (such as repetitive motion injuries and back pain) that may affect some employees in manufacturing and service environments. Frequently, a local rehabilitation provider, such as a hospital or private group, is willing to provide these services on site through a contractual arrangement and thereby reducing costs by avoiding the traditional "fee for service" arrangement. Appropriate space needs to be provided, but the equipment needs are minimal and usually worth the investment. If rehabilitation is provided off site, similar contractual relationships may be developed to reduce cost through service "bundling," a concept that hospitals have recently used to attract businesses to use their facilities.

When a business chooses to provide the majority of occupational and medical services on site, adequate space is essential. Ideally, the facility should be in a central area, easily accessed by employees, and kept clean and quiet, especially the hearing booth. Privacy should also be ensured. Good lighting and ventilation are necessary as well as wide doors to allow passage of stretchers and wheelchairs.

To estimate the size needed for the facility, one can use the factor of *1.5 sq ft of floor space for each employee* of the medium to large business. Proportional space needs increase in smaller organizations to meet minimum standards for a waiting room, records room, clerical offices, and exam rooms. A waiting room and reception area plus a room to serve as a patient treatment area are ideal. Space will also be necessary for safe storage of medical records. A bed or reclining couch should be available to allow people to rest who are too ill to work but do not require further medical care. Adequate toilet facilities, hot and cold water, and a shower for flushing the whole body or a part of the body such as the eyes are necessary, as well as dust-free, locked instrument storage cabinets. A reclining first-aid chair, particularly for treating eye injuries, is ideal. Additional office space for the physician or other health care providers is also of help.

Team Management of Cases

The occupational health coordinator or "contact person," occupational physician and nurse, and related personnel work as a team. If any of the team members are not "on site," the occupational health coordinator should be responsible for coordinating their efforts and ensuring that responsibilities are properly met. They should meet at regular intervals to discuss the management of cases and judicious return to work, including alternative assignments. Team members can visit the worksite of an injured employee, assess hazardous exposures, and facilitate necessary job modification. A team promotes consistency in treatment, continuity of care, and appropriate use of resources. In addition, the on-site team has a greater understanding of the employer's concerns, but, nonetheless, can remain as patient advocates.

With a well-functioning team, costs become more controllable. Although most states have statutes that allow workers the right to any health care provider, most workers are pleased with the easy access, lack of billing problems, and coordinated approach to their return to work.

Case Management

Injured employees who do not use the plant medical facilities should have their medical care managed similarly by the company medical staff. Routine visits to the designated occupational medicine department, coupled with effective communication between the company's health professionals and the personal physician(s) of the employee, are essential. Outside medical professionals are usually willing to use the rehabilitation professionals at the worksite, if apprised of their availability.

The goals of the occupational health department should be communicated to local physicians to minimize conflicts. It is paramount to the success of the process that a company select the most reputable health care providers of the highest quality to staff their programs.

The Walk-through Survey[*]

After visiting certain business facilities, the physician will recognize that additional review by an industrial hygienist may be necessary. In some cases, an industrial hygiene audit with air sampling may have been conducted and the results available for review. Where feasible, the physician should review plant operations with the hygienist, who can comment on the hazards present and the adequacy of the respective control measures to protect workers from those hazards.

Use of the term *occupational physician* implies responsibilities for the maintenance, care, and treatment of the health of certain workers and is based on the assumption that the workers' health may be affected by conditions in the workplace. An awareness of those conditions is necessary to correlate them with the potential health effects that may be seen in workers during routine physical examinations, biologic assay or monitoring procedures, or treatment of work-related complaints.

---

[*]This description is from the perspective of an industrial hygienist and details an approach to evaluating a manufacturing or production facility. See Chap. 22 for a detailed description of industrial hygiene and its role in occupational medicine.

The best way to become aware of workplace conditions is to make a walk-through survey.

Initial Recognition of Hazards

The following description is designed to su.nmarize the major avenues whereby toxic substances can enter the body. (Although Chaps. 22 and 23 cover these areas in more detail, some key points deserve emphasis.)

The three primary routes of exposure to hazardous materials are inhalation, ingestion, and skin contact. Materials can be *inhaled* if they are present in the form of a gas, a vapor, or an aerosol. The term *aerosol* refers to dusts (formed from suspending finely divided solids in air), mists (droplet clouds), fumes (formed from the condensation or reaction products of a gas), and combinations of these types, such as smokes. Gases and vapors may be absorbed from the deep lung directly into the bloodstream, may irritate or damage the respiratory tract at any point, or may condense or react with the moisture in the breath to form an aerosol. Aerosols entering the respiratory tract, or produced there, deposit at locations primarily determined by size [11]. The largest tend to deposit in the nose and pharynx. Medium-sized aerosols, below 10 μm in diameter, tend to deposit in the nose, pharynx, trachea, and bronchi. Fine aerosols, below about 5 μm in diameter, deposit throughout the respiratory tract, including the deep lung.

Materials can be *ingested* in the form of aerosols, liquids, or solids. Eating, drinking, or smoking in the work area increases the likelihood of ingestion, as does poor personal hygiene. Good personal hygiene includes frequent washing of exposed skin surfaces; finding an uncontaminated area before eating, drinking, or smoking; and avoiding transfer of materials to the skin, eyes, nose, and mouth from contaminated objects.

Materials can contact the *skin* in any form. Such materials may be inert, cause local irritation but fail to penetrate the skin, penetrate the skin without local effects, or both irritate and penetrate the skin. Some materials can be absorbed through the skin directly into the bloodstream. At least two of these substances, *jojoba oil* and the solvent *dimethyl sulfoxide*, have the hazardous property of carrying with them any dissolved materials. Some materials (e.g., hydrogen fluoride in solution) penetrate deep into the skin and surrounding tissues before damage is detected. Many solvents defat and dry the skin, causing discomfort, chapping, dermatitis, and an increased probability of infection and skin absorption of other chemicals.

Physical agents, such as high and low relative humidities, sound and vibration, high and low temperatures, radiant energies, and ionizing and nonionizing radiations, can affect the body in much the same ways as chemical substances. Many of these agents produce effects similar to those produced by skin contact with material substances. Others, such as ultrasonic and electromagnetic radiation, may penetrate the body to various depths, depending on frequency, and cause damage or heating effects throughout the region of penetration.

The Systematic Approach to a Walk-through Survey

Hazard recognition is best accomplished by a systematic approach.

1. Obtain a list of all starting, intermediate, final, and waste stream materials involved in each process or operation to be reviewed. This tabulation should be done before the actual survey, by contacting appropriate supervisors. A Material Safety Data Sheet (MSDS) should be obtained for each material on the list.

2. This step should be accomplished during the actual survey. The materials list should provide room to fill in information about each item, such as the physical state or states, the conditions of use, and any safety devices or protective equipment used to protect workers from the material. In addition, a notation of the approximate daily exposure duration or work schedule should be made. This information can be obtained by observation and by speaking to workers and supervisors in each work area. Workplace conditions should be observed, including temperature; ventilation; labeling on containers, vessels, and pipes; housekeeping; lighting; protective equipment; and the general appearance of workers in the areas.

3. During or after the survey, prepare a process flow diagram that shows all materials and energies that go into a process; the time of reaction or flow; all changes in

physical state, composition, and energies during the process; and all product and waste streams that come out. This information is usually available from the engineering or maintenance departments.

4. Use the information obtained to prepare a hazard checklist. For example, where any material or agent enters or escapes from a process, the location and type of safety devices or controls used to reduce exposures should be noted. If no controls are provided, some justification for believing none are needed should be noted. Where controls are provided, the frequency and type of maintenance needed and the frequency and types of performance tests used to assure their proper operation should be noted. Where the process produces heat, pressure, or gaseous reaction products, the flow diagram should be amended to show rupture disks, pressure relief valves, dump tanks, and exhaust stacks as appropriate. Process failure modes and precautions or emergency plans to cope with each should be noted.

5. After the survey or as a separate survey, investigate off-production maintenance procedures; rest areas and toilets; wash facilities; cafeterias; food storage and handling areas; drinking water sources; garbage and waste disposal procedures; lockout/tag-out procedures for electrical, mechanical, liquid tanks, and lines; compressed gas line repairs; confined space entry procedures; welding and cutting work permit procedures; contractor and visitor safety procedures; emergency procedures; and protective equipment cleaning, issue, storage, and repair procedures.

6. Organize the observations made before, during, and after the survey into a written report. Items of information not available, issues not resolved, and recommendations to modify factors that might adversely affect the health, comfort, or well-being of one or more workers should be included.

7. Follow up on recommendations made, to see that operating personnel have satisfactorily addressed each item where action was necessary. This step includes paying closer attention to the health of workers in areas where improvements were recommended, to be sure that these areas are not causing obvious health effects. This step may also include initiation of research or epidemiologic studies to answer the physician's concerns if that information is not otherwise available.

Relationship with Industrial Hygienists

Many large companies employ industrial hygienists, who customarily have an undergraduate degree in some basic discipline (e.g., engineering, chemistry, physics, or related biologic sciences), and who by virtue of special studies and training have acquired competence in the field of industrial hygiene. Most industrial hygienists have one or more graduate degrees in industrial hygiene or related areas of study. Industrial hygiene is that science and art devoted to the recognition, evaluation, and control of environmental factors or stresses, arising in or from the workplace, that can cause significant discomfort and inefficiency among workers or among the citizens of the community. When the walk-through survey and the experiences of the occupational physician do not provide enough information to decide whether a health finding is related to workplace conditions, an industrial hygienist is best able to investigate workplace conditions further and make the additional measurements required for that decision. The hygienist can take samples, evaluate health implications of concentrations measured, test control equipment, and estimate worker exposures to hazardous materials or conditions. The hygienist will usually have records that document exposure concentrations to materials of concern over some previous period of time and will be familiar with the process.

For subtle health effects not reported in the literature, the physician and the hygienist may recommend an epidemiologic study to try to assess the relationship between exposure concentrations or conditions to observed symptoms. The hygienist may also recommend specific air sampling methods, bioassay procedures, and biomonitoring methods to obtain the epidemiologic information desired.

The physician should think of the hygienist and use this individual whenever possible as a bridge between the medical and production/engineering departments of the plant. The hygienist may also serve as an expert witness when medical problems are the subject of legal proceedings before courts, hearing boards, or workers' compensation commissions to testify on conditions in the workplace based on industrial hygiene records used to support that testimony.

References

1. Frymoyer. J. W., et al. Epidemiologic studies of low back pain. *Spine* 5:419, 1980.
2. Cady, L. D., et al. Strength and fitness and subsequent back injuries in fire fighters. *J. Occup. Med.* 21:269, 1979.
3. Spangfort, E. V. The lumbar disc herniation. *Acta Orthop. Scand.* 142:(Suppl.)1, 1972.
4. Plog, B. A. *Fundamentals of Industrial Hygiene* (3rd ed.) Chicago: National Safety Council, 1988.
5. *Documentation of the Threshold Limit Values and Biological Exposure Indices* (7th ed.). Cincinnati: American College of Industrial Hygienists, 1991.
6. Silverstein, B. A., Fine, L. J., and Armstrong, T. J. Hand, wrist cumulative trauma disorders in industry. *Br. J. Ind. Med.* 43:779, 1986.
7. Jetzer, T. C. Use of vibration testing in early evaluations of workers with carpal tunnel syndrome. *J. of Occup. Med.* 33-2:117, 1991.
8. NIOSH. *A Work Practices Guide for Manual Lifting.* DHHS (NIOSH) Publication, No. 81-122, Cincinnati, OH, 1981.
9. Pope, M. H., et al. *Occupational Low Back Pain: Assessment, Treatment and Prevention.* St. Louis: Mosby-Yearbook, 1991.
10. *The Federal Register.* 49 CFR Part 40 and the chapter on Drug Testing.
11. Hatch, T. F., and Gross, P. *Pulmonary Deposition and Retention of Aerosols.* New York: Academic, 1964.

Further Information

American Association of Occupational Health Nurses. *A Guide for Establishing an Occupational Health Nursing Service.* New York: American Association of Occupational Health Nurses, 1977.
Available from the American Association of Occupational Health Nurses, Inc., Suite 400, 3500 Piedmont Road, NE, Atlanta, GA 30305.

American Association of Occupational Health Nurses. *A Guide for the Setting Up of a Record System.* New York: American Association of Occupational Health Nurses, 1977.
Available from the American Association of Occupational Health Nurses, Inc.

American Occupational Medical Association Occupational Medical Practice Committee. Scope of occupational health programs and occupational medical practice. *J.O.M.* 34: , 1992.

Breslow, L. Prospects for improving health through reducing risk factors. *Prev. Med.* 7:449, 1978.

Burgess, W. *Recognition of Health Hazards in Industry.* New York: Wiley, 1981.
An overview of the occupational health issues of major industries and industrial processes. Excellent reading to acquaint the practitioner with special concerns for controlling respective health risks.

Cralley, L. V., and Cralley, L. J. *Industrial Hygiene Aspects of Plant Operations.* Vol. 1., *Process Flows.* London: Macmillan, 1982.
A comprehensive presentation of the technical aspects of major types of industrial process.

McCunney, R. J. Providing high quality occupational and medical services. *J. Amb. Health Care Marketing* 4:9, 1990.

McCunney, R. J. (ed.). *A Manager's Guide to Occupational Health Services.* Boston: OEM Press, 1994.

Moser, R. *Effective Management of Occupational and Environmental Health and Safety Programs, Practical Guide.* Boston: OEM Health, 1992.

Newkirk, W. L. (ed.). *Occupational Health Services.* Chicago: American Hospital Association, 1989.

Silver, R. R. *Basic Occupational Medicine: A Guide to Developing Delivery System.* Boston: CRC Press, 1991.

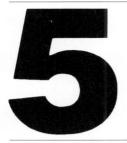

The Americans with Disabilities Act

Kent W. Peterson

In 1990, the United States Congress enacted Public Law 101-336, the most far-reaching civil rights legislation in recent history, with the following words [1]:

> The Congress finds that . . . some 43,000,000 Americans have one or more physical or mental disabilities, and this number is increasing as the population as a whole is growing older; . . . historically, society has tended to isolate and segregate individuals with disabilities, and, despite some improvements, such forms of discrimination against individuals with disabilities continue to be a serious and pervasive social problem; . . . individuals with disabilities are a discrete and insular minority who have been faced with restrictions and limitations, subjected to a history of purposeful unequal treatment, and relegated to a position of political powerlessness in our society, based on characteristics that are beyond the control of such individuals and resulting from stereotypic assumptions not truly indicative of the individual ability of such individuals to participate in, and contribute to, society; . . . the continuing existence of unfair and unnecessary discrimination and prejudice denies people with disabilities the opportunity to compete on an equal basis and to pursue those opportunities for which our free society is justifiably famous, and costs the United States billions of dollars in unnecessary expenses resulting from dependency and nonproductivity.

The Americans with Disabilities Act (ADA) is intended to bring those with physical and mental disabilities into the mainstream of American society. Of these one in six disabled Americans, two thirds are not employed. In 1986, a Louis Harris poll reported that 82% of those with disabilities would give up their government benefits in favor of full-time employment.

The ADA built on many provisions of sections 503 and 504 of the Rehabilitation Act of 1973 [2], which covered government employees and federal contractors. The ADA covers four areas: Title 1, employment, extends protections to applicants and employees of companies with 25 or more employees as of July 26, 1992, and with 15 or more employees as of July 26, 1994. Title II covers access to public services; Title III deals with public accommodations and services operated by private entities, including hospitals and medical clinics; Title IV covers telecommunications.

The Civil Rights Act of 1991 strengthened the ADA by allowing punitive and compensatory damages of up to $300,000 for each infraction.

In preparing for Title I implementation, the Equal Employment Opportunity Commission (EEOC) prepared detailed regulations [3], interpretative guidance, and an extensive technical assistance manual [4]. This chapter focuses on Title I employment provisions as they affect employee health and safety.

The ADA breaks ground in a number of new areas that will have a profound impact on occupational medical practice. These include the need to distinguish between "essential" and "nonessential" job functions and the need for health professionals to share previously confidential medical information with employers, who are charged with making "reasonable accommodations" and determining if individuals represent a "direct threat" to themselves or others. In addition, the ADA prohibits medical examinations in the preemployment phase, allowing them only after a bona fide job offer has been made, and even then, only when all employees within a job category are required to have a medical examination. For current employees, examinations can only be required when mandated by statute (such as by the Occupational Safety and Health Administration) or when job related and consistent with business necessity. They must be limited to determining the ability to perform essential job functions. If conducted on a voluntary basis, blood pressure or cholesterol screening, health risk appraisal, periodic physician's examinations, and other wellness programs are permitted.

Key Concepts, Terms, and Definitions

Terminology is instructive about the evolution of thinking in our society. The term *the handicapped* (allegedly taken from beggars with cap in hand) yielded to *the disabled* (those lacking certain abilities) and, more recently, to *individuals with disabilities*. Speaking of the handicapped or the disabled carries a sense of inherent limitation. The current term emphasizes the person first and only secondly any disability that he or she might have. It also reflects the ADA's strong emphasis on considering each individual situation on a case-by-case basis. Curiously, the shift in terminology has created the cumbersome title of the President's Committee on Employment of People with Disabilities.

Sawisch's [5] distinction between pathology, impairment, functional limitation, and disability is fundamental. *Pathology* is an interruption or interference with normal bodily processes or structures. It occurs at a structural level within cells and tissues. *Impairment* is the loss and/or abnormality of mental, emotional, physiologic, or anatomic structure or function. It includes all losses or abnormalities including pain, not just those attributable to active pathology. It occurs at an organ system level. *Functional limitation* is a restriction or lack of ability to perform an action or activity in the manner or within the range considered normal. Functional limitation results from impairment. It occurs at the level of action or activity performance of the whole person or organism. *Disability* is the inability or limitation in performing socially defined activities and roles expected of individuals within a social and physical environment. It occurs on a societal level, that is, in the performance of tasks within the social and cultural context.

For example, pathology may be a denervated muscle in the arm due to trauma. Impairment is the resultant muscle atrophy. The functional limitation is the inability to pull with the arm. The disability is that the person cannot perform certain job or recreational tasks. An accommodation is to use the other arm to perform the task successfully.

Two important distinctions should be noted. First, *the relationship between impairment, functional limitation, and disability varies enormously from individual to individual*. This is due to biologic, psychological, social, environmental, lifestyle, and cultural factors. Some employees with apparently minimal impairment appear to have severe functional limitations and to be disabled. Conversely, many individuals with major impairments and limitations have minimal disability.

Second, *disability determination is a nonmedical managerial task*. Health professionals make medical technical judgments about pathology, impairment, and functional limitation within a framework of generally accepted medical principles and practice [6]. Established medical diagnostic criteria such as the AMA *Guides to the Evaluation of Permanent Impairment* are intended to bring objectivity and uniformity to the process [7]. The technical medical information must then cross an information interface into the nonmedical realm. The ADA places clear responsibility on management to make appropriate decisions about disability, "direct threat" to the health of the individual or others, and reasonable accommodation, taking into consideration information provided by the applicant/employee, occupational health professionals, personal physicians, rehabilitation specialists, psychologists, and others. It is the employer, not the health professional, who is liable for errors in judgment.

Understanding the precise terminology as defined by the EEOC is critical to understanding and interpreting the ADA. Key ADA definitions are set forth in Table 5-1. The ADA's tripartite definition of disability takes into account not only current actual disability, but also powerful potential for discrimination against those with a past history of impairment (e.g., addiction, back pain, cancer) or those who become inappropriately labeled as disabled (e.g., being treated as if one were positive for human immunodeficiency virus or using illicit drugs).

The ADA's definition of disability differs from others. For example, a person who is disabled under Veteran's Administration, Social Security Administration, Railroad Retirement Board, or state workers' compensation criteria may or may not have a disability under the ADA definition.

Because of the wide individual variation in response to an impairment, disability

Table 5-1. Definitions from the Americans with Disabilities Act

Disability (with respect to an individual)
1. A physical or mental impairment that substantially limits one or more of the major life activities of such individual,
2. A record of such an impairment, or
3. Being regarded as having an impairment

Physical or mental impairment
1. Any physiologic disorder or condition, cosmetic disfigurement, or anatomic loss that affects one or more of the following body systems: neurologic, musculoskeletal, special sense organs, respiratory (including speech organs), cardiovascular, reproductive, digestive, genitourinary, hemic and lymphatic, skin and endocrine; or
2. Any mental or psychological disorder, such as mental retardation, organic brain syndrome, emotional or mental illness, and specific learning disabilities

Major life activities
Functions such as caring for oneself, performing manual tasks, walking, seeing, hearing, speaking, breathing, learning, and working

Substantial limits
1. Unable to perform a major life activity that the average person in the general population can perform, or
2. Significantly restricted as to the condition, manner, or duration under which an individual can perform a particular major life activity as compared to the . . . average person in the general population. . . .

Qualified individual with a disability
An individual with a disability who satisfies the requisite skill, experience, education, and other job-related requirements of the employment position such individual holds or desires, and who, with or without reasonable accommodation, can perform the essential functions of such position

Reasonable accommodation
Modifications or adjustments
1. To a job application process that enable a qualified applicant with a disability to be considered for the position . . . ; or
2. To the work environment, or to the manner or circumstances under which the position held or desired is customarily performed, that enable a qualified individual with a disability to perform the essential functions of that position; . . . or
3. That enable a covered entity's employee with a disability to enjoy equal benefits and privileges of employment as are enjoyed by its other similarly situated employees without disabilities

Direct threat
A significant risk of substantial harm to the health or safety of the individual or others that cannot be eliminated or reduced by reasonable accommodation. The determination that an individual poses a "direct threat" shall be based on an individualized assessment of the individual's present ability to safely perform the essential functions of the job. This assessment shall be based on a reasonable medical judgment that relies on the most current medical knowledge and/or on the best available objective evidence. In determining whether an individual would pose a "direct threat," the factors to be considered include:
1. The duration of the risk,
2. The nature and severity of the potential harm,
3. The likelihood that the potential harm will occur, and
4. The imminence of the potential harm

Source: From *Equal Employment Opportunities for Individuals with Disabilities*. EEOC; Final Rule. *Federal Register* 56(144):35735, July 26, 1991.

is defined in terms of its effects on the person's major life activities. A substantial limitation of a major life activity means that an individual's activities, such as caring for him/herself, performing manual tasks, walking, seeing, hearing, speaking, breathing, learning, working, and participating in community activities, are restricted as to the conditions, manner, or duration that they can be performed as compared to most other people.

The provision of *reasonable accommodation* is central to the ADA (see definition). Reasonable accommodation may include making existing facilities readily accessible, job restructuring through modified work schedules, reassignment to vacant positions, use of equipment or devices, modifying training materials or policies, and provision of qualified readers or interpreters.

Basic ADA Provisions

In essence, the ADA prohibits discrimination on the basis of disability against a qualified individual with a disability. Covered entities include an employer, employment agency, labor organization, or joint labor-management committee. As stated previously, the ADA protects applicants and employees of companies with 25 or more employees as of July 26, 1992, and with 15 or more employees as of July 26, 1994. Although 85% of US employers have fewer than 15 employees, the ADA will cover more than 85% of the US workforce.

Discrimination is prohibited in recruitment, advertising, job application procedures, hiring, upgrading, promotion, transfer, layoff, termination, and return from layoff or rehiring. Discrimination pertains to pay rates or other compensation, job assignments, job classifications, organizational structure, position descriptions, lines of progression, seniority lists, leaves of absence, sick or other leave, fringe benefits, training, and social or recreational programs.

Discrimination means not making a reasonable accommodation to *known* physical or mental limitations of an otherwise qualified individual with a disability. The duty to accommodate must first be initiated by a request from the applicant or employee. The examining health professional can play a significant role in helping to initiate or facilitate this process both with the employer and with appropriate vocational rehabilitation professionals. The Job Accommodation Network is a valuable resource that provides consultation on individual situations (see Further Information).

It is helpful to distinguish between the responsibilities of individuals, of management, and of health professionals in this process. The individual applicant or employee must make the employer aware of a "hidden" disability and request a reasonable accommodation. Management is responsible for making employment decisions and must face the legal consequences. As a result, the health professional becomes an expert advisor, responsible for providing management with sufficient information to make his or her own decision and thus be accountable. A health professional often finds him/herself with multiple roles: as a company agent and member of a management team, as a contract physician or nurse, or as a private treating physician or other health professional. The ADA forces us to sharpen our awareness of these overlapping, sometimes conflicting roles.

The ADA does not override other health and safety requirements established by other federal laws. This allows certain blanket exclusions to remain, for example, Federal Highway Administration driver qualifications. If a standard is required by another law, the employer does not need to show that it is job related or consistent with business necessity. However, the employer still has an obligation to determine whether a reasonable accommodation is possible. When the ADA conflicts with health and safety provisions of state and local laws, the situation is less clear.

Impact of ADA on Occupational Health Practice

The ADA impacts many occupational health procedures and the role of the occupational health professional in general. Table 5-2 highlights some ways in which traditional practices are being affected by the ADA. Fortunately, many employers and occupational health services providers long ago adopted the approach now required under the ADA. Employers operating under sections 503 and 504 of the Rehabilitation Act of 1973 have had to comply with many of these provisions.

Table 5-2. Influence of the ADA on employee medical examinations

	Traditional approach	ADA approach
Employment application	Inquiries into medical conditions/disabilities	Inquiries only regarding ability to perform essential functions
Drug testing	Pre-offer	Pre-offer (not considered a medical test)
Agility or strength testing	Pre-offer	Pre-offer (not considered a medical test)
Applicant medical examination	Pre-offer preemployment; no restrictions	Post-offer preplacement; no restrictions
Job information received by medical examiner	Job title, possibly job description	Essential job functions, likely detailed information on job, environment, etc.
Medical criteria	Blanket restrictions permitted	Individual consideration on case-by-case basis
Medical information reported back	Qualified/not qualified; specific job restrictions	Functional abilities and limitations with/without reasonable accommodation; detailed information re "direct threat"
Confidentiality of medical information	Often kept in personnel files	Separate files, with restricted access
Medical information provided to supervisor	No legal restrictions; guideline is ACOEM Code of Ethical Practices	Work abilities/limitations; recommended reasonable accommodations
Employer medical standards for job eligibility	Employer dependent: For some, all employees must be 100% functional	Employees must perform essential functions with reasonable accommodation
Return to work practices	Employer dependent: For some, no light duty; all employees must be 100% functional	Light duty not required; reasonable accommodation encouraged
Mandated current employee exams	No restrictions	By mandate (e.g., OSHA) or by business necessity but related to essential job functions
Voluntary exams	No restrictions	No restrictions

Key: ACOEM = American College of Occupational and Environmental Medicine.

However, compliance with the ADA requires more sophisticated occupational health services delivery.

Medical examinations are performed for many purposes, including general medical screening, preemployment, preplacement, medical biomonitoring, periodic health evaluation, exposure-related surveillance, symptomatic evaluation, impairment and disability evaluation, and return to work [8].

Fitness for duty must be *individually determined,* taking into consideration the nature of the individual's disability and the nature of the individual's job. Medical fitness and risk evaluation can best be achieved by the examiner having intimate familiarity with the essential job functions, frequency and importance of job tasks/demands, and workplace environment (e.g., exposures, use of personal protective equipment, emergency procedures). This familiarity can be gained through extremely clear written descriptions (Figs. 5-1 through 5-3), walk-through inspections, or videotapes. Although the ADA requires employers to distinguish between essential and marginal job functions, they are not required to have detailed written job descriptions. Furthermore, employment job descriptions often do not specify functional job requirements in a level of detail required for an optimal medical exami-

Job title: _____

1. Description (essential functions):

2. Physical demands (see attached requirements):

   Body part most   Type of stress (force/repetitive/   Priority
   affected   awkward position)

   Environment: noise/heat/cold/vibration

3. Chemical, biologic, psychological hazards:

   Personal protective eqipment:

4. Previous health problems from employees in same/similar jobs:

   Information source: _____WC data _____ employer _____ employee

5. Emergency and unusual situations or risks:

6. Accommodations available/previously made for job:

7. A regulatory standard: ____ Dept. of Transportation

                          ____ Respirator

                          ____ OSHA for noise

                          ____ OSHA for chemical substance _____

                          ____ Other _____

8. Medical examination for this job:

       ____ Basic hx/exam   ____ Back fitness

       ____ Hand/arm fitness   ____ Hearing

       ____ Vision   ____ Respirator

       ____ Aerobic fitness

       ____ Special (test or system) _____

   Information provided by: _____

   Date: _____

Figure 5-1. Information requested from employer. (Adapted from G. S. Pransky, Presentation Materials. In K. W. Peterson and B. A. Cooper (eds.), *Americans with Disabilities Act Handbook*. Arlington Heights, IL: American College of Occupational and Environmental Medicine, 1992.)

Body Part	Effort Level	Continuous Effort Time	Efforts/ Minute	Priority
Neck/ Shoulders	___	___	___	___
Back	___	___	___	___
Arm/Elbow	___	___	___	___
Wrists/hand fingers	___	___	___	___
Legs/knees	___	___	___	___
Ankles/feet	___	___	___	___

KEY:

Effort Categories	Continuous Effort Time Categories	Efforts/Minute Categories
1 = Light	1 = < 6 seconds	1 = < 1/minute
2 = Moderate	2 = 6-20 seconds	2 = 1-5/minute
3 = Heavy	3 = > 20 seconds	3 = > 5/minute

Priority for Change/Relative Risk

Moderate:	123 132 213 222 231 232 312	High:	223 313 321 322	Very High:	323 331 332 333

Figure 5-2. Ergonomic job analysis.

nation. Figure 5-1 outlines the kind of information that occupational health professionals should request from the employer.

Employment Examinations

The ADA prohibits pre-offer, preemployment medical *"inquiries"* (e.g., health histories), medical *examinations,* and other medical information gathering (e.g., workers' compensation claims) until *after* a job offer has been made. In doing so, Congress wanted to prohibit employers from using medical information to discriminate against those who might have a silent disability or be more likely to incur higher health benefit costs, for example, those with diabetes, cancer, heart disease, epilepsy, or mental illness. Further, they wanted applicants to know when they were being rejected for medical reasons. Thus, job application forms may not inquire about current or past medical conditions, limitations, or disabilities; they may only ask about current ability to perform the essential job functions. An employer may condition a job offer on satisfactorily completing a post-offer medical examination as

Please place an "X" in the box that best describes current job activities					
WORK TASKS	**NEVER**	**OCCASIONAL** 0.33%	**FREQUENT** 34-66%	**CONSTANT** 67-100%	**JOB RESPONSIBILITIES**
SITTING					
STANDING					
WALKING					
CLIMBING					
STAIRS					
RAMPS					
LADDERS/ POLES					
BENDING					
SQUATTING					
LIFTING					
VERY LIGHT (<10lb)					
LIGHT (10-19lb)					
MEDIUM (20-49lb)					
HEAVY (50-99lb)					
VERY HEAVY (100lb)					
PUSHING					
PULLING					
TWISTING					
REACHING FORWARD					
REACHING OVERHEAD					
KNEELING					
CRAWLING					
HAND TASKS (BOTH HANDS)					
RIGHT HAND					
LEFT HAND					
TOOLS/ EQUIPMENT					
TEMPERATURE (HOT)					
TEMPERATURE (COLD)					
HIGH NOISE					
VIBRATION					

ARE MODIFICATIONS AVAILABLE? TEMPORARY: ☐ YES   ☐ NO   PERMANENT: ☐ YES;   ☐ NO

Figure 5-3. Physical demand requirements.

long as this is required of all other entering employees in the same job category. However, examinations may be required of all production employees or those performing physical labor, but not of those with clerical or managerial jobs.

Of note, strength testing and agility tests are not considered to be medical procedures, and therefore may be required *before* a job offer. Employers may require applicants to take job-related strength, agility, and other tests, work simulations, or even demonstrations of their ability to perform essential job functions through an actual job trial.

The post-offer, pre-hire medical examination is a unique opportunity for employers, because it is the only time that a comprehensive medical history, physical examination, and battery of tests may be performed without restriction. Questions may be asked about previous illness and injuries and workers' compensation claims. Thus, a complete "baseline" of health information can be collected for future comparison.

Although the scope of the medical examination is not limited to functional assessment of job capabilities, any assessment which concludes that the individual cannot perform essential functions without accommodation will need to be extremely well documented. If the individual is rejected from the job, the employer must be able to demonstrate that the reasons were job related and necessary for the business, and that no reasonable accommodation was possible. Individuals may be disqualified because they pose a *"direct threat"* to themselves or others (see below). If they can currently perform essential job duties, however, they may not be rejected because of speculation that the disability will cause a future injury.

Because all employees within a job category must be treated the same, if one has a medical inquiry, all must have some kind of medical inquiry. If one has a medical examination, all must have some kind of medical examination. However, the inquiries or examinations do not have to be identical. Therefore, screening questions can be used, for example, "Do you or have you ever had any problems with back pain that restricted your activity?" An examiner may go into detail for those who answer affirmatively. Similarly, positive screening tests may be followed by more definitive ones on a case-by-case basis. The ADA restricts employers from requiring all new hires to complete a medical history, with follow-up medical examinations being performed only on those with significantly positive test results.

Examinations of Current Employees

The ADA places severe restrictions on employee medical inquiries and examinations. Unless required by other federal laws, disability-related inquiries or examinations must be job related and necessary for business. This means that the inquiries/examinations must relate to the individual's ability to perform the essential functions of the job or to whether he/she poses a "direct threat" in the position. Employers may conduct examinations for "fitness for duty" for a particular job, or where there is evidence of a job performance or safety problem. Although an early draft of the legislation prohibited voluntary health screening and wellness examinations, these may be performed as part of a voluntary employee health program.

A number of gray areas have yet to be resolved. One is the extent to which medical histories administered to current employees must be tailored to each individual based on his/her particular job. This creates a problem for employers and clinics that use standardized medical history questionnaire forms. Another uncertainty involves medical surveillance. Whereas the Department of Transportation (DOT) mandates pilot, driver, and other examinations, the Occupational Safety and Health Administration (OSHA) only requires medical examinations that are actually to be performed in limited instances, for example, audiometry as part of a hearing conservation program. More often, OSHA requires the employer to offer medical surveillance examinations, but they do not have to be taken. Furthermore, with limited exceptions, OSHA does not specify the detailed content of a medical history done as part of a medical surveillance examination. Thus, EEOC and OSHA very closely overlap and the content of the OSHA medical history and examination may be restricted by the ADA. A third area of uncertainty is the extent to which employers may inquire about personal employee illness, for example, among those who are returning to work after absence.

An "informal discussion" letter reinforces EEOC's intent, but does not resolve these issues [9]. It states:

> Examinations of employees *are* limited in scope/content because they must be job-related and consistent with business necessity, or required by federal law. Fitness-for-duty examinations/inquiries must be tailored to measure an employee's ability to perform the essential functions of his/her job. Therefore, it would be inappropriate for an employer to require broad medical histories in cases where such histories are not job-related and consistent with business necessity or are not federally required. In addition, medical histories taken pursuant to a federally required examination must be required for the examination. In short, an employer may not ask disability-related questions as part of a medical history which are broader than required for the examination.

Confidentiality of Medical Information

The ADA is one of the first federal laws to strongly reinforce confidentiality of medical records. Specifically, it calls for information obtained from medical inquiries or medical examinations to be collected and maintained on separate forms, and to be kept in separate medical files. Confidential medical records are to be maintained by the employer in locked cabinets, separate from personnel files, accessible only to designated persons. Access to this confidential medical information is limited to five situations: (1) informing supervisors and managers about necessary work restrictions and accommodations; (2) informing first-aid and safety personnel, as necessary, if a disability might require emergency treatment (e.g., limited mobility, epilepsy, or diabetes); (3) providing government officials investigating compliance with relevant information on request; (4) providing relevant information to state workers' compensation offices or second-injury funds; and (5) providing relevant information to insurance companies that require a medical examination to provide employee health or life insurance.

The applicant/employee should sign a medical release authorizing the dissemination of certain medical information (see Fig. 1-1). Note that Fig. 5-4 contains a signature line for the individual to confirm knowledge of the information being provided to the employer. Such a safeguard will help protect the physician against charges of inappropriate release of medical information. For risk management purposes, most medical societies now recommend that a physician not release any medical information, even in the presence of a subpoena, without a signed release from the patient.

Under the ADA, sharing of medical information about people with disabilities differs sharply from the traditional view of medical confidentiality, outlined in the Code of Ethical Conduct for Physicians Providing Occupational Medical Services of the American College of Occupational and Environmental Medicine (ACOEM). In the past, it has been customary for physicians to indicate to an employer only that an applicant was "qualified" (meets qualifications based on company standards) or "not qualified" (does not meet qualifications based on company standards). The ADA requires health professionals to share sufficient information for employers to make management decisions about the presence of a disability, a "direct threat" to health or safety, and reasonable accommodation (see ADA Information Flow).

Evaluating Impairment and Fitness for Duty

Because the ADA opens up the employment examination to direct legal scrutiny, occupational health professionals must be prepared to have their recommendations challenged. Yet, as former ACOEM president, Irving R. Tabershaw [10], has written, "The content, scope, tests, procedures, etc. of pre-placement examinations have in the past been arbitrarily adopted by the company or a contract physician without any peer review. Most of the protocols have never been made public and may be open to attack as discriminatory, unfair, biased, incompetent and not pertinent to the job. If litigation develops, they will be made public."

The health professional must consider each case through a rigorous, logical process. First, is the employer or entity covered by the ADA? Second, does the individual in question have a disability as defined by the ADA? Third, does the disability create workplace limitations? Fourth, how do the individual's abilities and limitations relate to the essential job functions? Fifth, would a reasonable accommodation make it possible for the person to perform the essential job functions without causing a "direct threat" to health and safety? And sixth, what information needs to be conveyed to the employer to facilitate an appropriate decision?

The medical examiner should not be lured into making employment decisions or determining whether a reasonable accommodation can be made. The occupational health professional should advise the employer about two things only: (1) an individual's functional abilities and limitations in relation to functional job requirements, that is, can this person currently perform this specific job, with or without an accommodation, and (2) whether the individual meets the employer's overall health and safety requirements, that is, whether the individual can perform the job without posing a "direct threat" to the health or safety of him/herself or others.

The ADA does not permit blanket exclusions from certain categories of jobs (e.g., medical standards that exclude all those with diabetes, epilepsy, hypertension, or a learning disorder). Each individual's situation must be considered on its own merits. For example, a person with epilepsy may not have had a seizure for more than 10 years, or may have a distinct aura that allows adequate time to deal with safety threats. Often, the best predictor of job performance is past job performance.

Direct Threat to Oneself or Others

The ADA allows employers to refuse to hire or to terminate the employment of an individual who constitutes a *"direct threat"* to the health or safety of the individual or others, which cannot be eliminated or reduced by reasonable accommodation (see definition in Table 5-1). The EEOC went beyond Congress' provision for threats only to others; it allows for a direct threat to oneself, but only at a very high level.

The employer must show a *significant risk of substantial harm* (i.e., a high probability). It is not enough to conclude that an individual is at higher risk than others. Raising the specter of safety hazards (e.g., insulin-dependent diabetes out of control) is not sufficient reason to discriminate. Some interpretations conclude that the risk must be "more likely than not" (i.e., >50% chance of harm). Even if a significant risk of substantial harm is verified, the employer must determine whether a reasonable accommodation can reduce the risk to below the level of a "direct threat."

The specific risk must be identified. Four factors must be considered in "direct threat" determinations:

1. The duration of risk; some risks may be quickly reduced through treatment, for example, for an infectious disease
2. The nature and severity of potential harm, taking into consideration the person's past medical and work history and the nature of the job
3. The likelihood that the potential harm will occur
4. The imminence of the potential harm; it must be a current risk, not one that is speculative or remote

The assessment of risk must be based on objective medical or other evidence related to a particular individual. It cannot be based on blanket exclusions or stereotypes about the nature or effect of a disability. The regulations call for reasonable medical judgment that relies on the most current medical knowledge or best available objective advice, or both. Decisions must be made on a case-by-case basis, looking at the specific risk posed by each individual, information provided by the individual, the person's experience in previous similar positions, and opinions of physicians, rehabilitation counselors, physical therapists, and other professionals.

Drug and Alcohol Abuse

Congress took a neutral position with regard to the President's war on drugs. The ADA specifies that employers may ensure that the workplace is free from illegal drug use and the use of alcohol, and they may comply with other federal drug and alcohol laws. Employers may require employees not to be under the influence of drugs or alcohol at work, prohibit the use of illegal drugs and alcohol in the workplace, require employees to submit to drug testing, discharge or deny employment to current users of illegal drugs, and hold illegal drug users and alcoholics to the same performance standards as other employees.

Testing for illegal drugs is specifically excluded as being a "medical test." The schedule of drugs is broader than those covered by the Department of Health and Human Services (DHHS) drug testing regulations, and includes any drug that is unlawful under the five schedules of the Controlled Substance Act. Therefore, tests for illicit drugs may be conducted before a job offer. However, an interesting gray area still exists. The EEOC had not considered that, in the case of a positive laboratory test, medical review officers (see Chap. 9) must inquire about legitimate explanations. The DOT considers the medical review officer's function to be an integral part of drug testing, thus excluded from coverage under the ADA [11]. The EEOC has recommended informally that employers arrange drug testing so that any associated medical inquiry is conducted after a conditional job offer has been made. It is also not clear whether alcohol testing, which will be required by DOT regulations, will also be excluded as a medical test (see Chap. 9).

The ADA provides limited protection to alcoholics and former drug users who have the disability of addiction. The critical distinction for illegal drug users is between current and former use. Current drug use is defined as "use recently enough to justify an employer's reasonable belief that involvement with drugs is an ongoing problem." The time is not limited by days or weeks, but must be determined on a case-by-case basis. Former users of illegal drugs are protected if they have completed a supervised rehabilitation program, which can include self-help programs such as Narcotics Anonymous; are participating in a drug rehabilitation program and are not currently using drugs illegally; or were erroneously regarded as using illegal drugs.

Alcoholics, while having a disability and being entitled to a reasonable accommodation, may be disciplined or discharged where alcohol use adversely affects job performance or conduct to the extent that the person is no longer "qualified" for the job. However, the same performance standard must be applied to other employees in the same position. Employers are not required to provide alcohol/drug rehabilitation as a reasonable accommodation.

The law is silent with regard to prescription drugs. Thus, there is a large gap in coverage regarding misuse of and addiction to drugs not included in the Controlled Substances Act and use of prescription drugs that can affect performance and the safety of the individual and others.

Emotional and Mental Disabilities

The highly stigmatized area of mental health was scrutinized very carefully by Congress in passing the ADA. One proposed amendment would have excluded mental illness from coverage under the ADA. Mental illnesses were carefully reviewed; nowhere else were symptoms or diagnoses included or excluded with the same degree of specificity. Kleptomania, pyromania, compulsive gambling, transvestism, homosexuality, bisexuality, pedophilia, and other disorders were specifically excluded from protection by the ADA.

Conditions found to be impairments under section 504 of the Rehabilitation Act of 1973 include autism, cerebral palsy, chronic fatigue, dyslexia, learning disabilities, and mental retardation. Borderline cerebral palsy and acrophobia without an effect on work performance were among the conditions that were excluded.

The ADA's definition of "any mental or psychological disorder" is very broad, especially given the prevalence of psychological problems in the general population. Repeated studies cite 20 to 25% of the population showing significant emotional symptoms [12]. Depression is astonishingly prevalent. Further, an estimated 10 to 15% of the workforce is alcohol or drug dependent or impaired, and an even greater number have used illegal substances regularly in the past.

Unfortunately, assessment techniques are not very good in terms of their ability to predict successful employment. An extensive literature review by Anthony and Jansen [13] showed that for severely psychiatrically impaired individuals, symptoms, diagnosis, intelligence, aptitude, and personality tests are all poor predictors of future work performance. There is no correlation between symptoms and functional skills. The best demographic predictor is prior employment history; the best clinical predictors are ratings of adjustment in sheltered job sites or workshops. A significant predictor is ability to "get along" or function socially with others. The best paper and pencil test predictors are ego strength or self-concept in the role as worker.

These findings help to validate the ADA's philosophy of considering every individual on a case-by-case basis. The EEOC's ADA technical assistance manual provides some helpful guidance. For example, common personality traits such as poor judgment, quick temper, or irresponsible behavior (e.g., "being a jerk") are not protected unless they are symptoms of a mental disorder.

Stress and depression may or may not be considered impairments, depending on whether these conditions result from a documented psychological or mental disorder. If a psychiatrist diagnoses a stress disorder, the individual would have an impairment that might or might not be considered a disability.

Functional job descriptions can include a number of attributes in the psychological and social realm. These include the ability to:

Maintain concentration over time
Screen out external stimuli
Manage time effectively
Relate to others beyond giving and receiving simple instructions
Handle intense interpersonal contacts
Influence people, for example, negotiate
Accept and respond appropriately to negative feedback
Comprehend and follow instructions
Perform simple and repetitive tasks
Perform complex or varied tasks

Handle multiple simultaneous tasks
Make decisions without immediate supervision
Evaluate and make appropriate generalizations
Maintain work pace appropriate to workload
Accept and carry out responsibility for direction, planning, control over others

Many reasonable accommodations can address mental health issues. Examples in five categories are contained in Table 5-3.

Communicable Diseases

Specific communicable diseases, such as tuberculosis or human immunodeficiency virus (HIV) infection, were defined by Congressional statute as disabilities. An employer can limit the activities of such individuals only if it can demonstrate that the contagious disease constitutes a significant risk to the health or safety of others that cannot be eliminated by reasonable accommodation.

The ADA allows food service industry employers to remove an individual with a contagious disease or infection from a food-handling position if the disease can be spread from this position and the employer cannot take other measures (e.g., use of gloves or masks) to prevent the problem. The DHHS published a list, which is updated annually [14].

Voluntary Health Examinations and Wellness Programs

The initial legislation would have severely restricted all medical inquiries and examinations for current employees. Fortunately, this was amended to allow *voluntary* examinations that are part of an employer's program, as long as they do not discriminate against those with disabilities.

Health Insurance Benefits

The 1991 EEOC regulations provided a limited exemption that allowed a covered entity to sponsor a benefit plan based on underwriting risks, as long as risks were

Table 5-3. Examples of reasonable accommodations to emotional and mental disabilities

---

1. Modification of the supervisory process
   Put work requests in writing
   Train supervisors to give positive feedback, as well as criticism, especially in light of the sensitive emotional antennae of those with mental illness
   Allow worker to appraise own performance before getting criticism
   Written agreement between worker and supervisor of how crises will be handled (e.g., if worker becomes insensitive, manic, alienates others, or work performance slips)
   Individualized job training (for those with anxiety or learning disabilities)
2. Job modification
   Work at home
   Eliminate marginal job functions that cause problems, e.g., greeting perople or handling switchboard during lunch
   Modified work schedule (e.g., to attend therapy sessions)
   Job sharing or part-time work
   Use of sick leave for emotional or cognitive reasons (mental health days)
3. Changing policies
   Advance unpaid sick leave during treatment
   Allow water or soda to be used by cashier with dry mouth
4. Physical environment changes
   Reduce stimuli, e.g., noise, light, vibration, activity
   Enclose an office
5. Human assistance
   Use of a job coach
   Peer counselor/advocate as needed
   Supervisor available to meet with employee

---

classified or administered in accordance with state law. Interpretative guidance indicated that the purpose was to permit development of plans in accordance with accepted principles of risk assessment. The ADA provisions were not intended to disrupt the current nature of insurance underwriting or practices. However, a qualified applicant or employee with a disability cannot be denied *access* to the insurance process or given different terms or conditions of insurance based on disability alone, if the disability does not pose increased risks. One practical limitation is that many employers have instituted surcharges or longer periods of exclusion from insurance coverage for preexisting conditions. The insurance provisions include arrangements with insurance companies, health maintenance organizations, third-party administrators, or stop-loss carriers.

Interim Enforcement Guidelines released in June 1993 [15] identify four basic ADA requirements: (1) Disability-based insurance distinctions are permitted only if the employer-provided health insurance plan is bona fide and if the distinctions are not being used as a subterfuge for purposes of evading the Act; (2) decisions about the employment of an individual with a disability cannot be motivated by concerns about the impact of the individual's disability on the employer's health plan; (3) employees with disabilities must be accorded equal access to whatever health insurance the employer provides to employees without disabilities; and (4) an employer cannot make an employment decision about any person, whether or not that person has a disability, because of concerns about the impact on the health plan of the disability of someone with whom that person has a relationship.

A gray area is the extent to which the ADA may limit risk-rated benefit and other financial health incentive programs, such as programs that offer reduced deductibles or copayments to those who voluntarily participate in health programs or who have healthier risk factors, such as blood pressure, cholesterol, weight, or cardiovascular fitness.

ADA Information Flow

Another useful way to review the ADA is in terms of the flow of information among the various participants. First, information needs to be obtained about the applicant or employee, the job, and the work environment. Ideally, this includes job title, job description broken down into essential and nonessential functions, job assessment, job analysis, physical job demands, environmental demands, psychological and social requirements, information about the work environment, and even the availability of emergency and other medical services. This information can be conveyed in writing (see Fig. 5-1) or through discussion with supervisor/employer, workplace walk-through inspections, videotaping of the workplace, job analysis, or sophisticated ergonomic analyses.

Second, information emerges from the medical examination: the medical history inquiry, general physical examination, laboratory and other tests, individualized assessment tests or procedures, and specialized information from personal physicians, occupational therapists, rehabilitation specialists, or other providers. Third is the medical assessment of impairment (not disability), what the individual can or cannot do, increased risk that might impose a "direct threat" to oneself or others, and recommended accommodations.

The fourth step is communication from the health professional to the employer. Information sharing can range from being quite restricted to full disclosure. For example, the health professional can limit information provided to (1) whether the applicant/employee is able to perform key functions, (2) the identification of work restrictions, (3) recommended accommodations, or (4) notification of potential "direct threat." This reflects the attitude of sharing with the employer on a need-to-know basis. An example of a suitable communication form is contained in Fig. 5-4. Additional information is often best shared through an iterative dialogue between management and medical advisor, a process that is encouraged by the ADA.

At the level of "full disclosure," the health professional may need to release medical history, diagnoses, and/or all medical information (e.g., to support a "direct threat" decision or workers' compensation hearing). It may also be necessary to document that a medical opinion reflects "the most current available medical knowledge," a standard to which the ADA explicitly holds the employer for "direct threat" exclusions. The health professional can also reinforce that information must be kept confidential and used on a need-to-know basis (e.g., by first-aid personnel). The full

---

Employee name _____ Date _____

Employer _____

Job title _____

My evaluation of this employee indicates:

_____ 1. No medical contraindication to performing this job without accommodation.

_____ 2. No medical contraindication to performing this job, with the following recommended accommodations, or job training:

_____

_____

_____ 3. Based upon probability of substantial harm, this employee could pose a *direct threat* to self or others. Please refer to the attached information on the extent of the threat and accommodations that may significantly decrease the threat.

_____ 4. Further testing is required to fully evaluate ability or risk.

_____ 5. Medical hold: waiting for additional data. Reevaluate on ____ / ____ / ____ .

Comments: _____

_____

If 2, 3, or 4 is checked, please call me to discuss this further, including recommendations for other information that may aid in accommodations or clarification of risk.

Any attached information on medical conditions should be treated as confidential medical information, in accordance with the Americans with Disabilities Act, with distribution only as needed.

_____   _____
Employee signature   Physician signature

Figure 5-4. Report of pre-placement medical evaluation. (Adapted from G. S. Pransky, Presentation Materials. In K. A. Peterson and B. A. Cooper (eds.), *Americans with Disabilities Act Handbook*. Arlington Heights, IL: ACOEM, 1992.)

ramifications of medical confidentiality and information sharing under the ADA are not clear at this time.

Finally, the ADA offers the occupational health professional the challenge and the opportunity of serving as internal or external consultants to employers. Clinicians can evaluate particular cases and advise the employer accordingly. An even more valuable role is helping the employer to interpret physician reports and knowing what to do with the information. The ADA is deceptively complex in its nuances for the employer to administer; occupational health professionals can play an invaluable educational role.

ADA's Impact: Two Views

Because the final outcome of the ADA will be determined through arbitration hearings and courtroom decisions about individual cases, much is still unclear. Thus, the ADA has been described in dramatically different contexts by disability rights advocates and those who fear its consequences. Both sides are summarized in this section.

ADA: A Costly Burden

On the negative side, the ADA has been described as a well-intentioned but poorly designed law, a financial disaster, and a litigator's delight. Proponents of this view complain that the definition of who is covered is extremely broad. In some sense, almost everyone has or could claim an abnormality or impairment that substantially limits one or more major life activities (e.g., working). When employers subject employees to stringent performance standards, many will claim to have a disability. Second, because medical examinations cannot be performed until after a conditional job offer has been made, a subsequent rejection will attract unprecedented legal scrutiny into the medical evaluation process. Thus, it will be hard to use medical information to exclude employment, although this information can be used to identify increased risks and to suggest job alternatives. Some employers will perceive the legal liabilities of preplacement medical examinations to be too great and will discontinue them. Third, defining "essential functions" will be difficult, with few guidelines available to help. Regarding safety, Congress did not consider a worker's own risk of accident or injury. The EEOC corrected this problem by defining the "direct threat" provision to include a threat to oneself, although this has not yet been tested in court. The phrase "significant risk of substantial harm" may be interpreted as an employee "more likely than not" will injure him or herself. However, requiring an employee's risk of harm to be greater than 50% probability is not good preventive medicine and will halt further developments in risk appraisal and risk assessment.

ADA: A Beneficial Opportunity

On the positive side, the ADA is perceived as long overdue for bringing the disabled into the mainstream of the American workforce, and a financial boon for the nation and for employers facing shortages of qualified workers [16]. The ADA will require employers and occupational health professionals to implement far more rigorous and effective occupational health programs. For example, the ADA will strongly encourage development of clear, functional job descriptions that define physical, emotional, and other job requirements. In turn, preplacement examinations will become more focused on the applicant or employee's specific job requirements and his/her ability to perform the essential job functions. Medical criteria and standards will be encouraged to help meet this challenge. Strong impetus will be given to advancing the science of functional capacity assessment and tailoring specific jobs to individual needs. Because of the complexities, job-related medical examinations will need to be performed by competent, well-trained health professionals. Physical medicine and rehabilitation, once used only in the final workers' compensation ritual, will be engaged more frequently and more appropriately. Employers will be encouraged to create healthy work environments where no one is placed at increased risk. The distinction between work-related and non–work-related disability will become blurred, and employers will need to focus on providing appropriate job accommodation to those with short-term as well as long-term disabilities.

Which parts of these two scenarios will prove true has not yet been determined. The ADA book has not yet been written. In the end, the success of the ADA will depend not only on applicants, employees, attorneys, and courts, but on actions by employers and their health advisers. As health professionals we can play a major role in assuring the most positive possible outcome.

References

1. Findings and Purposes, section 2, 42 US Code 12101, The Americans with Disabilities Act of 1990, as amended. In Appendix A, *A Technical Assistance Manual on the Employment Provisions (Title I) of the Americans with Disabilities Act.* Washington, DC: Equal Employment Opportunity Commission, January 1992.
2. Rehabilitation Act of 1973, Public Law 93-112, amended by Public Law 93-516 in 1974.
3. Equal Employment Opportunities for Individuals with Disabilities. Equal Employment Opportunity Commission; Final Rule. *Federal Register* 56(144):35726, July 26, 1991.
4. *A Technical Assistance Manual on the Employment Provisions (Title I) of the Americans with Disabilities Act.* Washington, DC: Equal Employment Opportunity Commission, January 1992. Appendix B contains the Interpretive Guidance published earlier by EEOC.

5. Sawisch, L. P. Americans with Disabilities Act: An Historical Overview of Discrimination and Legislation. In K. W. Peterson and B. A. Cooper (eds.), *Americans with Disabilities Act Handbook*. Arlington Heights, IL: American College of Occupational and Environmental Medicine, 1992.
6. Smith, G. M. The Role of the Occupational Medicine Physician in the Management of Industrial Injury. In T. G. Mayer and R. J. Gatchel (eds.), *Contemporary Conservative Care for Painful Spinal Disorders*. Philadelphia: Lea & Febiger, 1991. Pp. 191–201.
7. Engelberg, A. L. (ed.) *Guides to the Evaluation of Permanent Impairment* (3rd ed.). Chicago: American Medical Association, 1987.
8. Himmelstein, J. S. Worker Fitness and Risk Evaluations in Context. In J. S. Himmelstein and G. S. Pransky (eds.), Worker Fitness and Risk Evaluations. *Occupational Medicine State of the Art Reviews* 3:169, April–June, 1988.
9. June 17, 1993, letter to Elizabeth E. Gresch, MD, President, ACOEM, from Elizabeth M. Thornton, Deputy Legal Counsel, EEOC, in response to a May 18, 1993, letter from Dr. Gresch to Ms. Thornton.
10. Tabershaw, I. R., letter to L. A. Shaptini MD, President, ACOEM, 1991.
11. Smith, D. R. Office of the Secretary, US Department of Transportation, personal communication, June 1993.
12. Robbins, D. B. Psychiatric Conditions in Worker Fitness and Risk Evaluation. In J. S. Himmelstein and G. S. Pransky, (eds.), Worker Fitness and Risk Evaluations. *Occupational Medicine State of the Art Reviews* 3:309, April–June, 1988.
13. Anthony, W. A., and Jansen, M. A. Predicting the vocational capacity of the chronically mentally ill; research and policy implications. *Am. J. Psychol.* 39:537, 1984.
14. Centers for Disease Control, Department of Health and Human Services. Diseases Transmitted Through the Food Supply. *Federal Register* 56(159):40397, August 16, 1991. This material is contained in Appendix C of the EEOC's ADA *Technical Assistance Manual*, referenced above. (#1)
15. Interim Enforcement Guidance on the Application of the ADA to Disability-Based Distinctions in Employer Provided Health Insurance. EEOC Notice no. N-915.002, June 8, 1993.
16. Johnston, W. B., and Packer, A. E. *Workforce 2000: Work and Workers for the Twenty-first Century*. Indianapolis, IN: Hudson Institute, Inc. Herman Kahn Center, June 1987.

Further Information

EEOC. Equal Employment Opportunities for Individuals with Disabilities. Equal Employment Opportunity Commission; Final Rule. *Federal Register* 56(144):35726, July 26, 1991.
This contains the basic EEOC Title I Regulations and Interpretive Guidance in 27 pages. This material is reprinted as Appendix B of the ADA Technical Assistance Manual, *cited below.*

EEOC. *A Technical Assistance Manual on the Employment Provisions (Title I) of the Americans with Disabilities Act*. Washington, DC: Equal Employment Opportunity Commission, (800-669-EEOC voice; 800-800-3302 TDD), January 1992.
Detailed but highly readable manual provides an excellent overview, filled with illustrative case study examples. See Chaps. VI, Medical Examinations and Inquiries; VIII, Drug and Alcohol Testing; and IX, Workers' Compensation and Work-Related Injury. Appendix B contains the EEOC Title I Regulations and Interpretive Guidance, cited above. A Resource Directory (second volume) describes and provides contact information for hundreds of federal agency and national nongovernmental technical assistance resources, as well as regional and state locations of federal programs.

Fasman, Z. D. *What Business Must Know About the ADA: 1993 Compliance Guide*. Washington, DC: US Chamber of Commerce (800-638-6582), 88 pages.
This little guide provides a concise, readable summary of provisions under Title I employment and Title III public accommodations and services operated by private entities. Intended for employers, it includes case examples and "helpful hints."

Job Accommodation Network, PO Box 6123, 809 Allen Hall, Morgantown, WV 26506-6123. (800-526-7234 provides accommodation assistance for out-of-state voice/TDD; 800-526-4698 provides accommodation assistance for in-state voice/TDD; 800-

ADA-WORK provides ADA information for voice/TDD; 800-DIAL-JAN provides ADA information for computer modem.)
Provides free consultant service, funded by the President's Committee on Employment of People with Disabilities, to individuals, health professionals, and employers on customized job and worksite accommodations. Provides individualized searches for workplace accommodations based on the job's functional requirements, the individual's functional limitations, and environmental and other factors.

Peterson, K. W., and Cooper, B. A. (eds.). *Americans with Disabilities Act Handbook.* Arlington Heights, IL: American College of Occupational and Environmental Medicine (ACOEM), 55 W. Seegers Rd. 60005 (708-228-6850).
Originally assembled for ACOEM's ADA 2-day courses, this loose-leaf binder is available to individuals for $100. It contains the entire EEOC Technical Assistance Manual, cited above, plus an equal amount of information on a framework for looking at disability, historical events leading to the ADA, medical versus management responsibilities, job descriptions, job analysis, reasonable accommodation, medical fitness and risk evaluation examinations, workers' compensation and other disability benefits, substance abuse and mental disabilities under the ADA, an ADA planner, and company programs.

Pimentel, R. K., et al. *The Workers' Compensation–ADA Connection.* Chatsworth, CA: Milt Wright & Associates, 1993.
Subtitled "Supervisory Tools for Workers' Compensation Cost Containment that Reduce ADA Liability," this concise guide includes a section on management communication with physicians, identifying "red flag" ADA workers' compensation issues, and fraud and the malingerer. It also explores the often overlapping relationship between obligations for workers' compensation and ADA compliance.

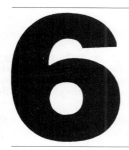

The Role of the Occupational Health Nurse

Bonnie Rogers

The practice of occupational medicine, unlike many medical disciplines, requires a team approach to include a variety of professional disciplines, including nursing, industrial hygiene, toxicology, business management, and epidemiology, among others. Occupational health nurses in particular have played a major role in the delivery of health services at the worksite. Over the past few years, the role of the nurse has expanded considerably and ranges from clinical care to administration to case management to education and research. The actual responsibilities assumed by an occupational health nurse vary and depend on the nurse's educational background and training, unique challenges of the worksite, availability of medical support, and supervision, as well as business culture and legal restraints. The purpose of this chapter is to describe the scope of occupational health nursing as currently practiced in the United States, as well as the specific roles that can be assumed by a nurse at the worksite. It is hoped that this chapter will emphasize how a well-trained occupational health nurse can participate in the team approach, which is so essential in the prevention, treatment, and rehabilitation of work-related ailments.

The breadth of occupational health nursing has expanded significantly in recent decades to support the growth of occupational health. In addition to the provision of direct supervised care of occupational illnesses/injuries in most areas of the country, support roles in health promotion and wellness education, disease and injury prevention, and service administration and research have become challenges for the future [1, 2]. When examining the contemporary domains of occupational health nursing, an historical perspective is helpful in providing the context for the practice framework.

Historical Perspectives

Historically, nursing care to worker populations, then referred to as industrial nursing, began in the late nineteenth century. In 1888, a group of coal miners employed Betty Moulder, a graduate of Blockley Hospital School of Nursing in Philadelphia, to care for ailing miners and their families [3–6]. However, little else is known about this individual or the services rendered.

Ada Mayo Stewart, hired in 1895 by the Vermont Marble Company in Rutland, Vermont, is often credited as being the first industrial nurse [4, 7]. Miss Stewart, whose primary mode of transportation was a bicycle, visited sick employees in their homes, provided emergency care, taught habits for healthy living, and taught mothers about child care. She learned much about the customs and methods of caring for the sick in the native countries of the workers and their families. Miss Stewart also gave talks on health and hygiene to schoolchildren, initially at the request of the schoolteacher, a personal friend, but also because child health care was considered extremely important by the company's president [7, 8].

In the early 1900s, employee health services proliferated rapidly throughout the United States as awareness grew that the provision of health services at the worksite resulted in a more productive workforce, decreased illnesses and injuries, and reduced absenteeism. At that time, working conditions in many factories were deplorable in the face of an industrial ethic that placed property rights above human rights. The proponents of this ethic maintained that industrial accidents were inevitable and were simply the cost of progress [9]. This type of attitude was not supported by the public; thus, safeguards for workers were encouraged, resulting in the institution of the workers' compensation system.

During the first half of the twentieth century, interest in industrial nursing expanded, state professional societies were established, and educational courses in occupational health nursing were instituted. With the advent of World War II, industries grew and the demand for nursing services increased dramatically with a reported 4000 industrial nurses employed [10]. With a sufficient number of nurses to support a national association, the American Association of Industrial Nursing (AAIN) was established in 1942 to improve industrial nursing practice and education and increase interdisciplinary collaborative efforts [3].

In the late 1960s and early 1970s, several laws designed to protect worker health and safeties were enacted (e.g., Federal Mine Safety and Health Act, 1969; Occupational Safety and Health Act, 1970). This legislation resulted in an increased need for occupational health nurses at the worksite. The passage of the Occupational Safety and Health (OSH) Act of 1970 provided a major stimulus to prepare occupational health professionals for the demands of many new legislated occupational health services.

As the nurse's role in industry expanded and evolved, the AAIN changed its name to the American Association of Occupational Health Nurses in 1977 to better reflect the broad scope of service delivery of the occupational health nurse. The 1980s witnessed a concomitant expansion of the role of the occupational health nurse, with more involvement in clinical management and health promotion, administration and policy development, cost containment, research, and regulatory monitoring.

Role of the Occupational Health Nurse

In light of population growth and these historical trends, economic demands, and regulatory mandates, more emphasis will likely be placed on primary care delivery at the worksite, case management, disability management, and possibly extended care to families. Occupational health nurses will need to enhance their skills in these direct support services as well as become even more active team participants to identify health problems and hazards as the means for health improvement and enhancement within the worksite. The nurse collaborates with specialists in other disciplines to help the employer recognize the economic and human benefits of occupational health programs, such as increased worker productivity by cost-effective health promotion [11].

Most nurses employed by industry must assume a generalist approach to their position, and others function in direct patient care, in administration or in a consultative role. In contrast, a multi-nurse unit involves responsibilities that are usually more clearly differentiated. The occupational health nurse may be hired specifically for direct patient care, as a health services manager, or health promotion specialist.

Five major functional roles of the occupational health nurse have been identified: clinician, administrator, educator, researcher, and consultant [12]. The clinician practitioner is primarily responsible for delivering supervised direct care to employees in the management of illnesses and injuries and in the promotion of health. The administrator provides functional direction to accomplish the goals and objectives of the occupational health service by the use of human and operational resources. When the nurse teaches individuals or groups of workers, the functional role is as an educator. As a research team member, the occupational health nurse may conduct or participate in scientific investigations. As consultant, the nurse provides advice and recommendations related to occupational health nursing. Each of these roles is discussed in more depth below.

The occupational health nurse *clinician/practitioner* applies the nursing process (i.e., assessment, diagnosis, planning, implementation, and evaluation) in providing nursing care for occupational and nonoccupational health problems. In this functional role, the nursing process is applied to health promotion, and other prevention programs based on worker needs and health hazards. Depending on individual knowledge, training, and experience, as well as the legal scope of the licensing authority, the occupational health nurse clinician/practitioner may perform the following major activities:

Assess the work environment for actual and/or potential health hazards

Collect data about the health status of the worker, through an occupational health history, physical assessment, and appropriate laboratory measurements

Develop a nursing diagnosis to formulate a plan of nursing care in collaboration with the employee and other health care professionals, as appropriate

Record health data and maintain accurate employee health records

Provide counseling for worker health problems, health promotion, and disease prevention interventions (e.g., immunization, respiratory protection, hypertension screening, hearing conservation programs)

Develop liaison relationships with community health care providers and organizations for worker health enhancement (e.g., referral to private providers and nonprofit and governmental agencies)

The occupational health nurse *administrator* provides direction for the planning, implementation, and evaluation of occupational health nursing services. To accomplish this task, the administrator must collaborate with others and facilitate interpersonal relationships for the smooth running of the organizational unit. The occupational health nurse administrator performs the following major activities:

Assesses the health needs of the workforce to help plan and develop cost-effective health services

Defines goals and objectives for the occupational health nursing service

Determines resources, such as facilities, staff, and operating expenses, necessary to accomplish unit goals; develops an appropriate, realistic budget; and policies and procedures aimed to foster goal attainment and work performance

Provides nursing leadership in the management and evaluation of human and operational resources, such as opportunities for enhancement of professional growth and quality management.

The functional role of the occupational health nurse *educator,* while usually described in relation to formal and continuing education within academic institutions, is less distinct in the occupational health setting, where the educator role is usually coupled with the role of the clinician/practitioner. Health education is often provided during a nursing health assessment, a visit to the occupational health unit, or at informal group meetings (e.g., lunch) or more formal training sessions. As a worksite health educator, the occupational health nurse performs the following major activities:

Assesses the needs of the workforce with respect to health information and educational interventions

Develops, implements, and evaluates health promotion and education programs and materials

Acts as a liaison to community agencies in establishing networks for health education and promotion resources

Provides current information to all workers regarding health issues, trends, and factors that influence health behaviors and impact on health outcomes

The occupational health nurse *researcher* works to increase the knowledge in occupational health nursing to improve the health of the workforce and the working conditions [13]. In the occupational health setting, the nurse may function in several capacities, ranging from identification of trends in illness and injury that may stimulate a research investigation or participation in data collection activities, to the actual design and implementation of a nursing research study. The breadth and depth of the role the occupational health nurse plays in research will depend on the individual knowledge and skills that the nurse can contribute to the research effort. Collaboration with others involved in research will be a key to a successful research project. The occupational health nurse who functions in a nursing research role may engage in the following major activities:

Identify issues to be considered through an occupational health and safety research effort

Participate with others in the conduct of research

Disseminate research findings

Incorporate research findings into the delivery of occupational health nursing services

The occupational health nurse *consultant* serves as a resource to management and members of the occupational health and safety team. Often, this functional role is performed by a nurse not employed by the organization; however, a corporate or regional occupational health nurse who works within the organizational structure may provide consultation to nurses and other health care professionals within the company. A nurse consultant may provide services such as suggesting policies and procedures, record systems, and job descriptions. In the consultant role, the occupational health nurse may perform the following major activities:

Provide advice about the scope and development of occupational health services and programs, considering regulatory and other trends in health care
Serve as a resource to management on occupational health nursing issues
Serve as a resource for information and professional networking.

In addition to these five functional roles, an occupational health nurse may function in such diverse roles as an academician, policy maker in governmental agencies, disability/claims specialist, or lobbyist.

Scope of Occupational Health Nursing

The definition of occupational health nursing has evolved over time to reflect the changing role of the occupational health nurse within the occupational health team, such as autonomous decision-making under medical directives. The practice of occupational health nursing is defined by the American Association of Occupational Health Nurses as "the application of nursing principles in conserving the health of workers in all occupations. It emphasizes prevention, recognition, and treatment of illnesses and injuries, and requires special skills and knowledge in the fields of health education and counseling, environmental health, rehabilitation, and human relations" [14]. The ultimate goal of the nurse in the occupational health setting is to improve, maintain, and restore the health of the worker. Many factors affect this goal, including external and internal or work-setting influences [2].

Factors *external to the organization* play a major role in the type and methods of nursing care delivered. How the organization reacts to and handles these factors will have a significant impact on health-related costs, programs, and outcomes. External factors or influences include

Economic constraints (e.g., decreased profits), more costly health care delivery methods, and costs related to health insurance premiums and workers' compensation claims
Demographics of the population, reflected in the workforce (e.g., aging workforce, more women and minority workers), changes in benefits packages, and job restructuring
Legislation requiring implementation of regulations for workplace health and safety resulting in increased costs for programs, controls, resources, and administrative practices (e.g., Americans with Disabilities Act)
Advances in technology requiring acquisition of more professional/technical knowledge and skills, and equipment

Internal factors or those within the work setting itself play a major role in nursing support for health and safety programs, the type and degree of exposure to health hazards in the environment, and the overall view of health and safety at the worksite. These factors affect trends in illness and injury at work and the health of the worker population. Internal influences include the following:

Workforce size, composition and demographics, health status, and projected needs
Corporate culture through the mission and philosophy of workforce health and workplace hazard control
Human and capital *resource allocation* to accomplish occupational health and safety goals
Collaborative *interdisciplinary functioning* necessary to conduct occupational health and safety programs, assessments, surveillance activities, and research

Prevention is the cornerstone of occupational health nursing [15, 16]. In the framework of prevention, the primary goals of occupational health nursing are to

Protect the worker from hazards that may occur as a result of the work experience
Promote, maintain, and restore the physical and psychosocial well-being of the worker in order to enhance optimal functioning

Encourage and participate in a company culture supportive of health
Collaborate as a team member with workers, management, and other disciplines
  and health care professionals to ensure a safe and healthful work environment [8]

Primary prevention is aimed at health promotion and protection, secondary prevention focuses on early diagnosis and detection, and tertiary prevention is aimed at disability limitation through treatment and rehabilitation [17]. The occupational health nurse contributes at all levels of prevention, including an emphasis on cost containment that preserves and improves quality health services [8, 18] (see Table 6-1).

The scope of activities addressed by occupational health nursing is broad and is directed toward achievement of cost-effective health promotion and protection goals.

1. *Health hazard assessment and surveillance.* To determine worker health status, the occupational health nurse may perform assessments and monitoring and surveillance activities such as initial occupational health histories. Hazard detection and surveillance of the workplace are critical to identify hazards harmful to worker health. Familiarity with the work and work processes, including personal protective equipment, is critical to accurate hazard detection. Multidisciplinary collaboration is essential to a successful hazard detection, surveillance, and control program (see Chap. 4 for a discussion on points to address in conducting a workplace walkthrough assessment).

2. *Primary health care and counseling.* Basic initial health care and counseling are provided to workers for work-related illnesses or injuries and for episodic nonoccupational illnesses and injuries. Nursing primary care for nonoccupational health conditions usually includes assessment of emergencies and minor and chronic health problems such as upper-respiratory infections or blood pressure monitoring, as well as appropriate medical referral and follow-up evaluation. Counseling is an integral component of the nurse's practice and one in which the nurse is particularly trained. Counseling about physical and psychosocial health-related problems, family dynamics, parenting, coping, and grief associated with a loss are but a few examples of counseling interventions. The type of care provided must be guided by nursing protocols or guidelines in accordance with state legal requirements.

3. *Health promotion/protection.* These activities aim to increase worker awareness and knowledge about occupational toxic exposures, lifestyle risk factors associated with health and illness (e.g., smoking, nutrition), attitudes and behaviors to improve health, and self-responsibility for health. Supporting a philosophy of illness prevention is important to health enhancement and improvement. In addition to activities described above, program planning and management of health promotion and special health programs include regulatory programs (e.g., hearing conservation, respiratory protection), screening programs for early detection (e.g., hypertension, mammography), rehabilitation and disability management programs including return to work, and employee assistance programs for workers' mental health needs and for performance-related problems.

4. *Administration, management, and quality assurance.* Administration of the occupational health service involves policy development, planning, and budgeting. The occupational health nurse is often responsible for the effective and efficient management of the occupational health service, regardless of the resources available. Establishment of criteria to measure goal achievement is a necessary component.

Table 6-1. Examples of occupational health nursing practice activities within a prevention framework

Primary	Secondary	Tertiary
Immunizations	Health assessment and surveillance	Work hardening
Wellness programs	Preplacement/periodic examinations	Rehabilitation
Nutrition education	Screening programs, i.e., high blood pressure, mammography	Disability management
Exercise/fitness programs		

Quality assurance, including record audits and attention to quality process activities (e.g., identifying quality indicators and barriers), are important to improving the functioning of the occupational health nursing service.

5. *Research.* The foundation for occupational health nursing is based on soundly conducted research. The occupational health nurse is in a key position to contribute to the examination of relationships between exposures, the work environment, and the health or illness of the worker. Once data are collected and analyzed, results can be used to improve current nursing practice or develop new techniques and methods, such as counseling and health education strategies to reduce risk and improve worker health.

6. *Community orientation.* The occupational health nurse should collaborate with community groups and organizations to develop a network of resources. For example, agencies such as the American Heart Association, American Lung Association, or American Cancer Association can offer valuable materials, information, and expertise to help with health programs or referrals, or both. In addition, working with health departments and hospitals in relation to employee return to work can be mutually beneficial to the company and worker.

7. *Legal-ethical practice.* The occupational health nurse must be familiar with the laws that govern the occupational health and safety of workers (e.g., OSH Act, Hazard Communication Standard, Americans with Disabilities Act) and the laws regarding proper physician supervision, and must be able to recommend or develop programs to meet requirements. The occupational health nurse must be cognizant of the state nurse practice acts, standards for occupational health nursing practice, and ethical practice parameters. The Code of Ethics from the American Association of Occupational Health Nurses provides guidance for ethical decision-making and addresses the following areas:

Provision of nondiscriminatory health care in the work environment with regard for human dignity
Collaboration with other health professionals/agencies to meet the needs of the workforce
Protection of the employee's right to privacy and protection of confidential information
Provision of quality care and monitoring of unethical/illegal actions
Acceptance of accountability for health care actions
Maintenance of individual competence
Participation in knowledge-building activities such as research

While many occupational health nurses practice in traditional manufacturing industry settings, many others provide services to workers in hospitals, government, construction sites, and university settings. The types of services and programs provided will be dependent on such factors as the composition and size of the workforce, potential and actual workplace hazards, and a recognized need for occupational health and safety. Thus, the number and mix of occupational health nurses at a given worksite will be determined not only by the size of the workforce but also the relative type and severity of potential workplace hazards, trends in occupational illness and injuries, regulatory mandated programs, availability of physician services, and provision of nonoccupational health services and health promotion and screening programs.

Organizational needs should determine the type of nurse recruited for an occupational health nursing position; that is, the nurse's skills, knowledge, and training should be commensurate with the job requirements. However, prospective employers have reported difficulties in locating qualified occupational health nurses for employment [19]. Resources such as the *AAOHN Newsletter,* state and local professional occupational health nursing constituent groups, occupational health nursing consultants, and academic institutions that offer occupational health nursing programs may be potential contact sources for employers.

Conclusion

The occupational health nurse is an integral part of the occupational health and safety team and is often the lead health care provider at the worksite with physician oversight. The nurse often functions in a variety of roles depending on the needs of the workforce and resources available to expand services and programs.

The role of the occupational health nurse has expanded considerably in recent decades, with greater emphasis on advanced clinical, management, and cost containment skills, and regulatory monitoring. The occupational health nurse will continue to assume a major role in the management of occupational health services, with increased emphasis on policy making and expansion of research skills to better identify and define occupational health problems in order to improve worker health.

References

1. Cox, A. Planning for the future of occupational health nursing. *AAOHN J*. 37:356, 1989.
2. Rogers, B. Occupational health nursing practice, education and research: Challenges for the future. *AAOHN J*. 38:536, 1990.
3. American Association of Industrial Nurses. *The Nurse in Industry*. New York: The American Association of Industrial Nurses, 1976.
4. Markolf, A. S. Industrial nursing begins in Vermont. *Public Health Nursing* 37:125, 1945.
5. McGrath, B. J. Fifty years of industrial nursing. *Public Health Nursing* 37:119, 1945.
6. Wright, F. S. *Industrial Nursing*. New York: Macmillan, 1919.
7. Felton, J. The genesis of American occupational health nursing. Part I. *Occup. Health Nurs*. 33:615, 1985.
8. Rogers, B. *Occupational Health Nursing: Concepts and Practice*. New York: Saunders. In press.
9. LaDou, J. *Occupational Health Law*. New York: Marcel Dekker, 1981.
10. Brown, M. L. *Occupational Health Nursing*. New York: Macmillan, 1981.
11. Harper, A. *The Health of Populations*. New York: Springer Publishers, 1986.
12. Randolph, S. A. Occupational health nursing: A commitment to excellence. *AAOHN J*. 36:166, 1988.
13. Rogers, B. Establishing research priorities in occupational health nursing. *AAOHN J*. 37:493, 1989.
14. American Association of Occupational Health Nurses. *A Guide to Establishing a Comprehensive Occupational Health Service*. Atlanta: AAOHN J, 1987.
15. Babbitz, M. The practice of occupational health nursing in the U.S. *Occup. Health Nurs*. 31:23, 1983.
16. Rogers, B. Perspectives in occupational health nursing. *AAOHN J*. 36:151, 1988.
17. Last J. M., and Wallace, R. B. (eds.). *Public Health and Preventive Medicine* (13th ed.). Norwalk, CT: Appleton & Lange, 1992.
18. Wachs, J., and Parker-Conrad, J. Occupational health nursing in 1990 and the coming decade. *Appl. Occup. Environ. Hygiene* 5:200, 1990.
19. McCunney, R. Personal communication, 1992.

Further Information

American Association of Occupational Health Nurses. 50 Lenox Pointe, Atlanta, GA, 30324.
This national organization, which includes local chapters in the US, sponsors a variety of educational activities, including a national meeting each spring. It will provide guidance in selecting an occupational health nurse, as well as information for obtaining certification in occupational health nursing.

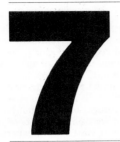

The Disability/Impairment Evaluation

Christopher R. Brigham
Alan L. Engelberg

The evaluation of work-related injury and illness requires clarification of physical, behavioral, psychosocial, vocational, and legal issues [1, 2]. Occupational medicine physicians must therefore be knowledgeable about the terminology and systems involved [3, 4]. Physicians participate in this arena through clinical care, case consultation, and performance of independent medical evaluations (IMEs). This chapter discusses the role and context of IMEs in the provision of occupational medicine services.

IMEs are examinations performed by a physician not involved in the person's care for the purpose of clarifying medical and job issues. Key issues associated with an IME differ from clinical consultations in role and focus (Table 7-1). Occupational medicine physicians are often the most appropriate specialists to evaluate work-related injuries and other disability cases to determine whether worksite accommodations may be necessary for certain medical disorders.

IMEs are performed to provide information for case management and for evidence in hearings and other legal proceedings [5]. IMEs are a component of all workers' compensation statutes, although the specifics vary by state. IMEs also are used in clarifying liability (personal injury) and disability. Insurers, third-party administrators, employers, and attorneys usually request IMEs. A survey by the Alliance of American Insurers found that 100% of workers' compensation carriers use IMEs, and they rated the technique as of primary importance 68% of the time, higher than any other technique. States may impose limitations on the number of examinations an injured person may have, and may specify requirements for evaluating physicians. IMEs may also have different roles, dependent on the context of the evaluation. For example, in some states, examinations performed by an agreed upon examiner or requested directly by the court or commission may be given particular credence.

The physician who performs the IME is not involved in a treating capacity. No clinical management is provided and the fee is paid by the party requesting the examination. The information obtained is presented to the client in a written report. The physician must be impartial and unbiased in performing the assessment. Ethics and moral character must be without question.

Assessments are often requested because of a lack of medical information or conflict on specific matters, especially regarding the cause of the condition and a person's ability to work. The physician makes a careful assessment and addresses the issues raised by the referring sources. The assessment process must be precise and detailed, and assure that conclusions are valid, reliable, defensible, and useful. Many assessments undergo legal scrutiny, and the physician must be able to support the conclusions in deposition or testimony.

Table 7-1. Key issues in an IME

Diagnoses
Causal relationship
Prognosis
Maximum medical improvement
Permanent impairment
Work capacity
Disability
Appropriateness of care
Recommendations

The examinee is not necessarily a willing participant, and may present with more dysfunctional behavior than is usually encountered in a typical treatment setting. The assessments, therefore, are more challenging and require greater patience. A thorough assessment of chronic pain associated with a musculoskeletal disorder may require 2 to 3 hours of physician time. The use of other staff, structured assessment protocols, and software will reduce the time needed to conduct a thorough evaluation.

The performance of these assessments requires specific skills in addition to clinical acumen. The physician must not only have a strong clinical background, but also have an appreciation of the biomedical, emotional, and vocational aspects of injury and illness. Credentials should be solid; this is not an arena for an inexperienced physician or someone who is unable to support conclusions if challenged.

IMEs are a valuable component of case assessment and management. Unfortunately, many IMEs are inadequate, superficial, and biased, and do not address specific questions. A physician who provides a thorough, detailed IME, however, delivers a valued, needed service. The performance of these assessments is challenging because of the intense effort involved and the complexity of the workers' compensation and legal systems.

Depending on the complexity of the case and the tools used in the process, a comprehensive IME may require 1 to 4 hours of physician time. It is best to schedule an IME at a time separate from other clinical visits. Because of the challenges involved, it is difficult to devote all one's effort to performing IMEs; they are best approached as one component of a practice in occupational medicine. Physicians with some clinical, consulting, or teaching involvement are considered to be more credible than those who only perform IMEs.

Challenges in Independent Medical Evaluations

It is imperative to learn the specific elements to be addressed in a report (see Table 7-1). In conducting IMEs, challenges relate to diagnoses, causal relationship, prognosis, maximum medical improvement, permanent impairment, work capacity, and appropriateness of care. The occupational physician should recognize the importance of addressing these items in both the performance of an IME and the preparation of a report.

Diagnoses

Clinical impressions include not only the primary illness or injury, but also other conditions that need further evaluation. It is useful to prepare a problem list of clinical diagnoses, particularly other pertinent conditions that contribute to the patient's functional status. It is helpful to present the problem list in relative order of significance, and to number each problem. Standard classification of diagnoses is useful, such as the *International Classification of Diseases (ICD-9)* [6] and, for psychiatric illness, the *Diagnostic and Statistical Manual of Mental Disorders* [7].

Pain, pathology, impairment, residual functional capacity, and disability are separate concepts. *Pain,* especially chronic pain, may not be associated with significant physical pathology [8, 9]. *Pathology* may be present without symptoms or dysfunction. *Impairment* is a measurable decrement in some physiologic function, whereas *disability* considers not only the physical or mental impairment but also the social, psychological, or vocational factors associated with a person's ability to work [10–12]. Functional limitations are manifestations of impairment [13]. Factors relating to each of these issues should be identified in the problem list.

The significance of medical problems should be discussed, such as the relationship between the extent of symptoms (subjective complaints) and signs (objective findings). It is necessary to identify which problems are acute and which are chronic or degenerative in nature. Problems that predated an injury and may relate to current dysfunction directly or indirectly must be determined, since this information is used in assessing causal relationship. Psychosocial problems, health behaviors, and the examinee's perceptions/values are often more predictive of the future than is the physical condition.

Chronic pain, the most common problem seen in the performance of IMEs, may be not a symptom of an underlying acute somatic injury but a multidimensional bio-psycho-social phenomenon [14–16]. A multi-axial assessment of biomedical, psychosocial, and behavioral-functional issues is necessary [17–20].

Causal Relationship

Causation is a critical issue in work-related and liability cases. A work-related problem is defined as one that "arose out of and during the course of employment." [21] With an acute injury such as a fracture, this determination may be simple. In many workers' compensation cases, however, the process is far more complex, particularly with preexisting, chronic conditions and environmental exposures.

The physician must establish *causation* to a reasonable degree of medical *probability,* which implies that it is more probable than not (i.e., there is more than a 50% probability) that a certain condition arose out of or in the course of work duties. *Possibility* implies less than 50% likelihood. Stating that a problem is work related implies that, based on the available information, to a reasonable degree of medical certainty, work activities caused the problem. States may vary in the definition of causation, particularly for cumulative trauma disorders and preexisting conditions.

Apportionment refers to the extent to which a problem is caused by various factors. For example, a worker may have sustained an injury with one employer, then returned to work and sustained a similar injury with another employer. In reviewing the case, it may be necessary to apportion current dysfunction between the two parties. It also may be necessary to apportion responsibility between work- and non–work-related conditions. This process depends largely on judgment, since the science supporting apportionment is in its infancy.

Different definitions of causation may exist for physical and mental conditions; for example, a mental condition may be attributed to work activities only if the factors associated with the illness were unique. A condition may be the result of one or more factors, or may be due to multiple factors. These factors may occur in a sequence of events. Causation can be ultimate or proximate [22]. Ultimate causation refers to the initial factor that leads to the effect. Proximate cause is the factor that immediately or closely precedes the effect. Unique causation occurs when a condition is due to a specific cause, for example, asbestosis. Multifactorial causation, where there are several possible causes, is more common.

Work activities may influence underlying problems. An *aggravation* implies a long-standing effect due to an event, resulting in a worsening, hastening, or deterioration of the condition. An *exacerbation* is a temporary increase in symptoms from the condition. Thus, an aggravation has an ongoing substantial impact on the physical condition, whereas an exacerbation results in a *flare* of symptoms.

The evaluator needs to scrutinize the specifics of the case and compare this information to the known pathogenesis of a condition. This analytical process requires careful assessment of the diagnoses, mechanism of injury, preexisting status, and clinical history.

The following case examples illustrate some complexities of causation analysis.

Case 1

Mr. B. is a 51-year-old man who sustains a low back injury as a result of a lifting episode. He developed an acute onset of radicular pain and is found to have a herniated nucleus pulposus. His physician treats him with prolonged bed rest and high-dose steroids, and eventually he undergoes a diskectomy. Later he complains of hip pain, and aseptic necrosis of the hip is diagnosed. He undergoes a total hip replacement, and during the associated hospitalization a pulmonary embolism develops.

Each event would be causally related to the injury at work, since each situation either directly or indirectly resulted in the next one. If there were a break in the chain of events, causation would not be present. For example, if the avascular necrosis had not been caused by the steroids but by alcoholism, the complications would not be causally related, unless it was shown that the alcohol consumption resulted from his injury.

Case 2

A 40-year-old obese woman with hypothyroidism develops a right carpal tunnel syndrome. Her treating physician believes that this disorder is associated with her work as a cashier. Nerve conduction studies are positive on the right, and she undergoes a carpal tunnel release. One year later, similar problems develop on the left, and her treating physician states that these problems must be due to the fact that she now uses her left arm rather than her right.

Careful assessment revealed that this patient did not make significant use of the left hand, and analysis of her previous job as a cashier showed that her work was in a convenience store, with only occasional use of the cash register. It is more probable that her carpal tunnel syndrome was due *not* to her work activities but to her risk factors of obesity and hypothyroidism. The evaluator therefore concluded that her left carpal tunnel problem was not related to work activities.

Case 3

A 50-year-old woman diagnosed as having "overuse syndrome" is seen for further assessment, which reveals that she has upper and lower body complaints that are symmetric. She has 12 of 18 possible painful tender points, consistent with a diagnosis of fibromyalgia.

The evaluator finds that although the work activities resulted in temporary exacerbation of her symptoms, there is inadequate evidence to conclude that fibromyalgia was caused by these activities.

Case 4

A 41-year-old man sustains a low back muscular strain while lifting. Magnetic resonance imaging (MRI) reveals degenerative disk disease with bulging. There is no evidence, however, that his episode of low back pain is related to the degenerative disease. He improves and returns to usual work activities. One year later, while lifting at home, he has another episode of acute back pain, this time with a radicular component. A herniated nucleus pulposus is diagnosed.

The initial work-related injury was muscular in origin. The degenerative disk disease predated the injury, although this was not known until the imaging study was performed. There is no evidence that the soft-tissue injury aggravated the degenerative disk disease. The herniation a year later was unrelated to the muscle injury a year earlier. It was concluded, to a reasonable degree of medical probability, that the subsequent problems were not causally related to the work-related lifting injury.

Prognosis

The physician may need to identify the outlook for a problem, that is, the predicted time of recovery. This opinion is based on a careful clinical assessment that compares the results with the natural history of the problem. Influencing factors are also identified. This information is used in case management to establish the case's financial reserves, which are the predicted expenses for medical care and lost wages. Analysis is influenced largely by concurrent problems. The relative role of each of these factors in determining the clinical prognosis should be identified.

Case 5

A 41-year-old physician falls on the ice and sustains comminuted scapular and thoracic fractures. She is in excellent health, motivated, and unable to afford any work absence.

Although the injury itself is significant, her motivation and the sedentary nature of her job suggest that the prognosis for full recovery and employability is good.

Case 6

A 31-year-old, obese deconditioned woman with a history of prolonged disability associated with carpal tunnel syndrome and a postural disturbance develops a myofascial pain syndrome involving her trapezius. She left school in eighth grade, did not receive a graduate equivalency diploma, and has a disabled spouse. She is dissatisfied with her work and supervisor, and angry with her employer about being injured.

The prognosis for the physical problem alone would be good; however, the prognosis for full employability is grim.

Maximum Medical Improvement

Maximal medical improvement is a phrase used to indicate when further recovery and restoration of function can no longer be anticipated to a reasonable degree of medical probability. This assessment implies that a condition is permanent and static. Considerations include whether the current or proposed treatment will result in functional improvement, if surgery has occurred recently, and whether enough time has passed for the process to be stable.

Permanent Impairment

Often a physician is asked to conduct an *impairment evaluation* as part of the assessment. To physicians who are not independent medical evaluators, an impairment evaluation and an independent assessment are synonymous, but they are not [23]. The basic philosophies that have been detailed in the American Medical Association's *Guides to the Evaluation of Permanent Impairment* [24] define an *impairment* evaluation, which should be distinguished from a *disability* evaluation. The definitions according to the *Guides* are the following: *Impairment* is "the loss of, the loss of use of, or a derangement of any body part, system or function." *Disability* is "the limiting loss of the capacity to meet personal, social or occupational demands, or to meet statutory or regulatory requirements."

Impairment is a measurable decrement in health status evaluated by medical means; disability is the gap between what a person can do and what he or she needs to do, partly because of a diminished health status. Disability is assessed by the consideration of nonmedical issues, such as the person's educational and vocational skills, experience, age, and, in workers' compensation cases, potential for future loss of wages. Assessing education, vocation, and potential for future loss of wages is *not* a skill most physicians possess, and, thus, the medical role usually is limited to evaluating impairment, not disability [25].

What does impairment reflect? An erroneous impression is to think that an evaluation of impairment is indicative of a person's ability or inability to do a task or set of tasks relating to work. Rather, an impairment evaluation is based on activities of daily living (Table 7-2). Note that specific tasks of employment are not considered activities of daily living for the purposes of an impairment evaluation.

Independent medical evaluators, because of the nature of their current role and experience, may feel more comfortable in assessing the impact of nonmedical aspects of disability on the functioning of the people they evaluate. This extra role, however, should be delineated from the impairment evaluation itself. A difference exists between the *evaluation* of impairment and the *rating* of impairment. The former includes the latter, but also much more. For example, an impairment evaluation must consider all pertinent clinical and laboratory reports, and attempts at management and rehabilitation. This information should be used with the evaluator's own examination to form a conclusion about the patient's impairment, and should be included in the final report. Following the conducting of an independent evalu-

Table 7-2. Activities of daily living

Self-care and personal hygiene	Urinating, defecating, brushing teeth, combing hair, bathing, dressing oneself, eating
Communications	Writing, typing, seeing, hearing, speaking
Normal living postures	Sitting, lying down, standing
Ambulation	Walking, climbing stairs
Travel	Driving, riding, flying
Nonspecialized hand activities	Grasping, lifting, tactile discrimination
Sexual function	Having normal sexual function and participating in usual sexual activity
Sleep	Restful nocturnal sleep pattern
Social and recreational activities	Ability to participate in group activities

Source: Adapted from American Medical Association, *Guides to the Evaluation of Permanent Impairment* Chicago: American Medical Association, copyright June 1993.

ation, a report is usually necessary. The wise occupational physician will inquire as to whether time restraints are associated with the preparation of the report. A report should address, in particular, those items raised in the context of the impairment evaluation (Table 7-3).

The physician who reviews medical records for an impairment evaluation may need to contact a treating physician (as any physician would do outside of the workers' compensation process) to gain a better understanding of the health of a patient, or to arrive at some agreement. These two physicians can also agree if specialty referral is warranted.

In some workers' compensation jurisdictions, either by law, regulation, or administrative practice, a formula is used, whereby the impairment rating becomes the primary piece of information on which a compensation level is established. This situation is unfortunate, because an impairment evaluation can only document a

---

Table 7-3. Steps in impairment rating

1. Medical evaluation in accordance with the protocols of the AMA *Guides* include
    A. A *narrative history* of the medical condition(s) with specific reference to onset and course of the condition, findings on previous examinations, treatments, and responses to treatment
    B. *Results* of the most recent clinical evaluation, including (if obtained): physical examination findings, laboratory test results, electrocardiogram, radiographic studies, rehabilitation evaluation, mental status and psychological tests, and other specific tests or diagnostic procedures
    C. Assessment of *current clinical status,* and statement of plans for future treatment, rehabilitation, and reevaluation
    D. *Diagnosis* and clinical impressions
    E. Estimate of the expected *date of full or partial recovery*
2. Analysis of findings, which includes explanation of
    A. The *impact* of the medical condition(s) on life's activities
    B. The medical basis for any conclusion that the *medical condition has, or has not, become static or well stabilized*
    C. The medical basis for a conclusion that the person *is, or is not, likely to suffer sudden or subtle incapacitation* as a result of the medical condition
    D. The medical basis for any conclusion that the person *is, or is not, likely to suffer injury or harm or further impairment* by engaging in activities of daily living or any other activity necessary to meet personal, social, and occupational demands
    E. Any conclusion that *restrictions or accommodations*[a] are warranted for daily activities or activities required to meet personal, social, and occupational demands, if restrictions or accommodations are necessary, their value should be delineated
3. Comparison of the results of the analysis with the impairment criteria in the *Guides,* which include
    A. A description of *specific clinical findings* related to each impairment, with reference to how the findings *relate to the criteria* described in the respective chapter; reference to the absence of, or to the examiner's inability to obtain, pertinent data is essential
    B. *Comparison* of specific clinical findings to the specific criteria that pertain to the particular body system, as they are listed in the *Guides*
    C. *Explanation of each percent of impairment rating,* with reference to the applicable criteria
    D. Summary list of all impairment ratings
4. Rating of impairment of the whole person[b]
    An explanation of how ratings of body parts are combined to obtain impairment rating of the whole person.

---

[a]Accommodations are a central feature of complying with the Americans with Disabilities Act (see Chap. 5).
[b]This step may or may not be required, depending on the nature of the impairment(s) and the requirements of the disability system in which the evaluation is to be used.
Source: Adapted from American Medical Association, *Guides to the Evaluation of Permanent Impairment.* Chicago: American Medical Association, copyright June 1993.

person's health status at a point in time, and not the impact on functioning in society or employability. The impairment evaluation does not determine if a person may meet "personal, social or occupational demands."

For most organ systems, the impairment rating guidance is broad. For example, with the skin, each category of impairment spreads across 10 percentage points; for the pulmonary system, each category spreads across 15 percentage points. Even for those organ systems, such as the musculoskeletal system, where the rating guidance is more precise, the *Guides* allow for rounding of impairment rating results to the nearest 5%. These are clear indications that impairment ratings reflect the innate variability in human biologic systems; they were never intended to be the major factor in determining compensation for permanent impairment.

Assessment of impairment in patients with chronic pain is particularly challenging [26]. There are presently no completely objective means for measuring pain or impairment or for determining resultant disability [27, 28]. Controversy occurs due to the multifaceted concept of pain, and the fact that pain cannot be measured objectively. There is no exact relationship among degree of pain, extent of pathologic change, or extent of impairment. In most chronic pain syndromes, two kinds of impairments can be identified: a primary impairment due to a documented pathologic condition affecting an organic system, and a secondary impairment due to the consequences of a painful experience, such as inactivity, disuse, drug misuse, and learned helplessness [29]. Pain is usually considered in determining impairment only if substantiated by objective findings affecting both organic systems and function [30]. The *Guides* state: "Since chronic pain by definition is primarily a perceptual, maladaptive behavioral problem, since pain per se cannot be validated objectively or quantitated, and since the underlying substrate of somatic pathology is minimal or nonexistent, it follows that *little, if any, impairment exists in most instances of the chronic pain syndrome.*"

Work Capacity

Work capacity is a primary issue in IMEs. Judgments of work capability and *direct threat* are important aspects of addressing the Americans with Disabilities Act. Opinions are formed by the patient's report, clinical condition, and measurements of functional performance. Individuals may provide information on their capabilities, particularly if symptom magnification is absent. Certain clinical conditions suggest specific restrictions. For example, in a patient with low back pain, the amount of lifting, bending, sitting, and certain body postures may need to be altered. Cumulative trauma disorders suggest low-repetition, low-force tasks and an ergonomic assessment.

Functional performance assessments are more accurate determinations of ability, if the assessment is valid and reliable and relates to particular jobs. Caution should be exercised because various methodologies are available. A structured protocol is essential. It is customary to express work capacity following parameters in the *Dictionary of Occupational Titles,* United States Department of Labor, which are based primarily on lifting requirements (Table 7-4).

The examining physician should estimate capacities as carefully as possible, including the number of hours of work per day, based on endurance and tolerance for sitting, standing, and walking. Estimates of lifting and carrying capabilities are noted for specific frequencies. Guidelines should be provided for the *frequency and duration of tasks* such as bending, crouching, squatting, pushing/pulling, climbing

Table 7-4. *Dictionary of Occupational Titles* work demands

Category	Lifting occasionally	Lifting frequently
Sedentary	10 lb	5 lb
Light	20 lb	10 lb
Moderate	50 lb	25 lb
Heavy	100 lb	50 lb
Very heavy	150 lb	75 lb

Source: US Department of Labor. *Dictionary of Occupational Titles* (4th ed.). 1991.

stairs, climbing ladders, reaching above shoulder level, lifting above shoulder level, balancing, and working on uneven ground or at heights.

These capacities are compared with the functional requirements of the job, obtained from job descriptions, videotapes, or direct observations. The physician must advise in consideration of the Americans with Disabilities Act, and avoid arbitrary restrictions that do not meet the criteria of a direct threat (see Chap. 5). Specific assessments of work capacity based only on a clinical evaluation may be difficult. As a result, a functional performance assessment may be incorporated into the IME or be used as a separate recommendation.

Appropriateness of Care

Many IMEs call for a review of the appropriateness of clinical management, which should be based on the specifics of the case and not be reflective of bias against a certain discipline or approach. This process includes issues of unnecessary and/or omitted diagnostic evaluation, and inappropriate, excessive, and/or omitted treatment. The need for repeated imaging studies should be assessed. Areas of possible inappropriate treatment may include, for example, use of prolonged bed rest and immobilization, protracted passive physical therapy or manipulation, repeated surgery, and use of narcotic analgesics. A beneficial approach that is sometimes neglected includes the physician's involvement in functional restoration that addresses behavioral issues and focus on return to work. The details of the evaluation should be compared to the accepted standards of care for the problem. For example, manipulative therapy can be compared against standards set forth by the Rand Expert Panel [31], the Mercy Center Consensus Conference [32], and the North American Spine Society's Ad Hoc Committee on Diagnostic and Therapeutic Procedures [33].

Specific recommendations on further diagnostic studies, treatment, or other aspects of the case may be sought. If further testing or treatment is not needed, the physician should so state. It may be appropriate to recommend obtaining missing records.

Conducting an Evaluation and Preparing a Report

The IME process should address the issues posed by the referral source. The assessment consists of three phases: preevaluation, evaluation, and postevaluation. The use of structured questionnaires and inventories, workbooks, and software for report generation facilitates this procedure. The physician may want to include ancillary staff members in this process to make the most efficient use of time.

Preevaluation

A request for an IME should specify issues to be addressed and background demographic, clinical, and claims information. The referral source (or your office) needs to identify the party responsible for notifying the person to be examined. Often this responsibility is assumed by the requesting party, often by certified letter. The client should forward records before the examination. Since records may be poorly organized and incomplete, a clerical staff member can organize the records in advance; medical records should be separated from other information in the file and be organized chronologically. Reports of consultants and results of laboratory tests and surgical procedures can be tagged. It is important to review the medical records before the evaluation and to read correspondence from the client, so that the evaluation can be structured to answer specific questions. The examinee may be asked to complete a questionnaire before the evaluation, to facilitate the interview. Pain and functional inventories are particularly helpful in identifying behavioral and psychological components related to an illness or injury.

Evaluation

At the beginning of the visit, the physician should explain the nature of the evaluation and that an independent evaluation will be conducted, but that no treatment will be performed. There is no patient-physician relationship, and a report will be sent to the requesting client. The person should sign a release, stating, for example:

I understand that the purpose of the examination is for an evaluation only, and that no treatment will be provided. I further understand that the client requesting and paying for the assessment will receive a report. I realize that no physician-patient relationship is established during the course of this assessment.*

Key Components of the Evaluation

HISTORY. The history, organized in sections (Table 7-5), usually commences with a detailed review of the *injury* or illness, including the reported mechanism, symptoms at the time, and events immediately thereafter. These comments are compared to other medical records for consistency. The mechanism of injury is important in deciding causal relationship.

The history includes relevant *preexisting conditions* and prior injuries. The patient's baseline is established to determine the framework for examining the effect of the referenced condition. For example, in a patient with a preexisting low back problem, a subsequent event may result in an exacerbation or an aggravation of the condition. If records are available, they should be reviewed to determine the accuracy of the history. Other work- or liability-related incidents should be determined. This information may be particularly significant from a behavioral standpoint. For example, a history of multiple claims or claims associated with significant disability or large monetary settlement may warrant concern.

The *chronology* of events from the time of injury through the present is examined. The pattern of the condition is determined, and the specifics of providers, opinions of other consultants, results of diagnostic studies, and treatment approaches are reviewed. It should be determined whether the complaints are consistent over time, if the symptoms are supported by objective findings, and if the clinical management has been appropriate. The results of various diagnostic studies are examined to clarify the diagnoses and determine whether the evaluations were appropriate. The treatment and corresponding results are detailed and compared with the customary

Table 7-5. Preparation of the IME report

Background
History
  Preexisting status
  Injury
  Clinical history
    Chronology
    Providers
    Studies
    Treatment
  Current status
    Complaints
    Functional reports
    Perceptions
  Occupational history
  Psychosocial history
  Past medical history
  Review of systems
  Family history
Pain Inventories
Examination
  Behavioral
  Structural
  Regional
Conclusions
  Diagnosis
  Prognosis
  Recommendations
  Work status

*See Chap. 1 for a sample medical release form that the individual should sign before undergoing an evaluation.

therapeutic approach. Failure of the patient to have any response to multiple treatment modalities suggests a chronic pain syndrome.

The *current status* is explored in detail, with attention directed to the examinee's primary concern. Most often the complaint is pain, and therefore the location, pattern, and nature of the pain, as well as aggravating/relieving factors, are defined. Associated symptoms such as numbness, tingling, weakness, morning stiffness, and other physiologic difficulties are assessed. It is important to identify not only positives but negatives as well. Anxiety, discouragement, depression, and sleep disturbance are referenced.

The person's perceived *functional status* is documented to clarify both work capacity and behavioral issues. Tolerances for sitting, standing, walking, lifting, and carrying, and the ability to carry out a variety of tasks associated with activities of daily living, are noted. In a patient with symptom magnification, inconsistencies may be present.

The examinee's *perceptions* are useful in understanding the personal experience with the medical problem. Several questions can be asked to clarify these issues. For example, "What do you think is causing your problem?" "What do you think will happen in the future?" "How satisfied are you with your medical care, employer, insurer, and the workers' compensation system?" "What is your primary goal?"

A thorough *occupational history* begins with a detailed description of the job at the time of injury, and includes not only physical characteristics but also issues of job satisfaction. For toxicology cases, a detailed review of exposures at the current and previous jobs is required. The events from the injury to the present, relative to disability, are explored. If the patient is not working, the involvement of vocational rehabilitation, possibilities for work in the future, and the patient's plans for the future are defined. If the patient is working, the details of this position are explored. It should be identified whether work restrictions have been imposed, along with their rationale. It should be determined if there has been a functional performance assessment; if so, the results should be scrutinized. The patient's previous work experiences, educational background, and future work plans should be defined.

A *psychosocial history* should be directed to the family unit, activities on a usual day, recreational activities, and changes in the household since the injury. Smoking, alcohol use, and use of recreational drugs are documented. One should attempt to clarify reinforcements for disability, such as changes in roles of other family members.

The complete medical history concludes with a traditional past medical history that notes medical and surgical procedures, medications and allergies, review of systems, and family history.

EXAMINATION. The meticulous history is followed by a physical examination, including a behavioral assessment and a detailed examination of the involved area(s). The behavioral assessment commences when the patient is greeted. Pain behavior and inconsistencies should be documented. A structural examination focuses on posture, body position, and body movements.

Regional examinations should ensure reliability and ideally reproducibility of positive, negative, and nonphysiologic findings [34, 35]. For example, in a patient with low back pain, the examination should note gait, structure of the back (lordotic curves, pelvic symmetry, surgical scars), palpatory findings (localized tenderness, spasm, trigger points), and range of motion, among others. Range of motion of the spine should be determined using an inclinometer that measures cervical, thoracic, and lumbosacral angles. A neurologic examination includes, among others, sensory assessment, motor evaluation (strength and atrophy), and straight-leg raising both sitting and supine. Specific maneuvers also should be performed, for example, to determine sacroiliac problems, piriformis syndrome, somatic dysfunction syndrome, and problems that may be masquerading as low back pain. The assessment also should look for nonphysiologic (Waddell) findings of symptom magnification (see Chap. 12, Musculoskeletal Disorders).

PAIN AND DISABILITY INVENTORIES. Psychological and behavioral factors must be considered in a disability assessment [36]. A number of self-report, interview, and behavioral measures have been developed to assess pain and disability [37]. Numerous self-report instruments have been developed, using both comprehensive and brief formats. It is useful to include these in an IME to assess the behavioral and psychosocial aspects.

The self-report instruments have been developed to assess disability in patients with chronic pain. The Multidimensional Pain Inventory (MPI) was designed specifically for patients with chronic pain [38]. Another comprehensive measure of disability is the Sickness Impact Profile (SIP), which was designed as a generic measure of disability associated with any chronic illness [39]. The Oswestry Disability Questionnaire [40] and the Roland Disability Questionnaire [41] were developed to assess changes in functional limitations associated with treatment for back pain. Another brief instrument is the Pain Disability Index [42], which measures changes in role functions associated with chronic pain. The Functional Assessment Screening Questionnaire [43] and the Functional Interference Estimate Scale [44] assess both functional limitations and role interference associated with chronic pain. Several interview measures have also been developed, but these have not been researched as intensively as the self-report measures. The Mensana Pain Inventory is a useful screening test designed to assist in the diagnosis of patients with chronic pain complaints and to clarify the extent of exaggerating pain behavior [45]. Pain drawings have been widely used to assess pain distribution and symptom magnification [46, 47].

Distress and disability are associated; factors include personality, emotion, cognition, education, and attention/concentration deficits. The Minnesota Multiphasic Personality Inventory (MMPI) assesses personality factors and disability in individuals with chronic pain [48]. Depression is common in chronic pain syndromes [49]. Several scales have been used to rate depression, including the Center for Epidemiologic Studies–Depressed Mood Scale (CES-D), Zung Depressive Inventory, and Beck Depressive Inventory. Coping responses and attitudes/beliefs affect perception of disability. Attitudes (feelings about a subject) and beliefs (information about a subject) should be clarified when evaluating a patient with chronic pain. The concept of illness behavior refers to the different ways individuals perceive, evaluate, and respond to their symptoms. These have been studied in terms of the overt behaviors that patients use to communicate pain and pain behaviors.

The use of these inventories will assist the evaluator in identifying the behavioral and psychosocial issues. The selection of inventories requires assessment of their intended use, appropriateness for the population being evaluated, validity and reliability of the instruments, and feasibility of administration and scoring. An appropriate battery of inventories may include, for example, the MPI, the Pain Disability Index, and the CES-D. The use of a standardized assessment such as the Short Form–36 (SF-36) is helpful in objectifying medical outcomes [50].

Referral sources, as well as many physicians, may be unfamiliar with the utility of these tools and therefore may not request them in an assessment. Since these inventories require little time to administer and score and provide such useful information, it is suggested that they be included in the IME of a patient with chronic pain.

DIAGNOSTIC STUDIES. Radiographic films brought by the examinee (or supplied by the client) are reviewed at the visit. The findings are compared with those of the reviewing radiologist. Additional studies may be recommended to the referring source; however, they should not be obtained without approval from the referral source to avoid conflicts regarding fiscal responsibilities for the testing.

At the conclusion of the evaluation, it may be appropriate to discuss findings with the examinee, although some referral sources prefer that the examiner withhold certain opinions until the completion of the report.

Postevaluation

The evaluation should address the issues requested by the referring source. The physician may need to support the findings in a legal setting, such as in a deposition or in testimony. As a result, unsupported conclusions, emotional statements, or comments that may suggest libel of the examinee or involved doctors should be avoided.

IMEs are usually performed during a single visit, although the examinee may be seen at a future date, often 1 or 2 years later. The follow-up examination may be called by the client because of the availability of medical information missing at the time of the visit or a change in medical status or working conditions.

Reports

Reports should be organized and detailed, and present the information obtained during the evaluation. The available medical records, the patient's behavior and quality as a historian, individuals accompanying the examinee, and the context of the assessment should be described. The history, physical examination findings, results of pain inventories, and interpretation of radiographic studies follow. (The Chapter appendix includes a sample computer-generated report that uses an integrated system of a questionnaire and clinical protocol workbook.)

Although the appendix includes an example of a report that is a thorough, detailed analysis that may be required in certain settings, occupational physicians are also called on to prepare brief reports related to fitness for duty, focused second opinions, or back-to-work evaluations. In these settings brevity is essential, as long as key information is presented. For example, a party requesting such an evaluation may be primarily interested in a person's ability to work or the need for additional medical care. Too often, physicians do not understand medical confidentiality in the context of workers' compensation and, as a result, employers may not receive adequate information to which they are entitled.

A brief report in these settings should address the following:

1. Chief complaint
2. History of illness or injury
   A. Precipitating event
   B. Follow-up activities, including diagnostic studies and treatment
   C. Condition at time of evaluation
3. Past medical history of direct pertinence to the condition
4. Examination results
5. Laboratory result interpretation
6. Diagnosis
7. Prognosis
8. Recommendations
9. Return to work status

References

1. Aronoff, G. M. Chronic pain and the disability epidemic. *Clin. J. Pain* 7:330, 1991.
2. Turk, D. C., Rudy T. E., and Steig R. L. The disability determination dilemma: Toward a multi-axial solution. *Pain* 3:217, 1988.
3. Brigham, C. R. Independent medical evaluations and disability assessment. *O.E.M. Rep.* 6:5, 1992.
4. Brigham, C. R. Medical analysis of workers' compensation claims. *Workers' Comp. Monthly* 11:1, 18, 1990.
5. Tompkins, N. Independent medical examinations: The how, when, and why of this useful process. *OSHA Compl. Adv.* 215:7, 1992.
6. World Health Organization. *International Classification of Diseases* (9th revision [*ICD-9*]). Hyattsville: World Health Organization Collaborating Center, 1991.
7. American Psychiatric Association. *Diagnostic and Statistical Manual of Mental Disorders*. Washington, DC: American Psychiatric Association, 1987.
8. Loesser, J. D. What is chronic pain? *Theor. Med.* 12:213, 1991.
9. Spektor, S. Chronic pain and pain-related disabilities. *J Disabil.* 1:98, 1990.
10. Ryley, J. F., Ahern, D. K., and Follick, M. J. Chronic pain and functional impairment: Assessing beliefs about their relationship. *Arch. Phys. Med. Rehab.* 69:579, 1988.
11. Brena, S. F., and Spektor, S. Systematic assessment of impairment and residual functional capacity in pain-impaired patients. *J. Back Musculoskel. Rehabil.* 3:6, 1993.
12. Vasudevan, S. V. The relationship between pain and disability: An overview of the problem. *J Disabil.* 2:44, 1991.
13. Vasudevan S. V. Impairment, Disability, and Functional Capacity Assessment. In D. C. Turk and R. Melzack, *Handbook of Pain Assessment*. New York: Guilford Press, 1992.
14. American Medical Association. Pain and Impairment. Appendix B in AMA *Guides to the Evaluation of Permanent Impairment* (3rd ed. revised). Chicago: American Medical Association, 1991.
15. Loesser, J. D. What is chronic pain? *Theor. Med.* 12:213, 1991.
16. Melzack, R. *Pain Measurement and Assessment*. New York: Raven Press, 1983.
17. Turk, D. C. Evaluation of pain and disability. *J. Disability* 2:24, 1991.

18. Turk, D. C., Rudy T. E., and Steig, R. L. The disability determination dilemma: Toward a multi-axial solution. *Pain* 3:217, 1988.
19. Turk, D. C., and Melzack, R. *Handbook of Pain Assessment.* New York: Guilford Press, 1992.
20. Turk, D. C. *Multiaxial Assessment of the Injured Worker.* Presentation at the American Occupational Health Conference, Atlanta, Georgia, April 28, 1993.
21. Larson, A. *The Law of Workmen's Compensation.* New York: Matthew Bender, 1982.
22. Balsam, A. Evaluation of Disability Under Workers' Compensation. In A. Balsam and A. P. Zabin, *Disability Handbook.* New York: Shepard's/McGraw-Hill, 1990. Chapter 15.
23. Frymoyer, J. W., Haldeman, S. and Andersson, G. B. J. Impairment Rating—the United States perspective. In M. H. Pope et al., *Occupational Low Back Pain: Assessment, Treatment and Prevention.* St. Louis: Mosby Year Book, 1991. Chapter 16.
24. American Medical Association. *Guides to the Evaluation of Permanent Impairment,* (4th ed.). Chicago: American Medical Association, 1993.
25. Babitsky, S., and Sewall, H. D. *Understanding the AMA Guides in Workers' Compensation.* Colorado Springs: Wiley Law Publications, 1992.
26. Ryley, J. F., Ahern, D. K., and Follick, M. J. Chronic pain and functional impairment. *Arch. Phys. Med. Rehabil.* 69:579–82, 1988.
27. Andersson G. B. J. Impairment Evaluation Issues and the Disability System. In T. G. Mayer, V. Mooney, and R. J. Gatchel, *Contemporary Conservative Care for Painful Spinal Disorders.* Philadelphia: Lea & Febiger, 1991.
28. Vasudevan, S. V., and Monsein, M. Evaluation of Function and Disability in the Patient with Chronic Pain. In P. P. Raj (ed.), *Practical Management of Pain (2nd ed.).* St. Louis: Mosby Year Book, 1992.
29. Brena, S. F. and Koch, D. L. A pain estimate model for quantification and classification of chronic pain status. *Anesthesia Review* 3:28, 1975.
30. Brena, S. F., and Turk, D. C. Chronic pain and disability: An overview for legal professionals. *Def. Counsel J.* 122, 1987.
31. Shekelle, P. G., et al. The appropriateness of spinal manipulation for low back pain. Santa Monica, CA: Rand Corporation, 1992.
32. Mercy Center Consensus Conference. Rockville, MD: Aspen, 1992.
33. North American Spine Society's Ad Hoc Committee on Diagnostic and Therapeutic Procedures. Common diagnostic and therapeutic procedures of the lumbosacral spine. *Spine* 16(10): 1991.
34. Waddell, G., et al. Objective clinical evaluation of physical impairment in chronic low back pain. *Spine* 17:617, 1992.
35. Harris, J. S., and Brigham, C. R. Low back pain: Impact, causes, work relatedness, diagnosis and therapy. *O.E.M. Rep.* 4:84, 1990.
36. Institute of Medicine Committee on Pain, Disability and Chronic Illness Behavior; Osterweis, M., Kleinman, A., and Mechanic, D. (eds.). *Pain and Disability: Clinical, Behavioral, and Public Policy Perspectives.* Washington, DC: National Academy Press, 1987.
37. Tait, R. C. Psychological factors in the assessment of disability among patients with chronic pain. *J. Back Musculoskel. Rehabil.* 3:20, 1993.
38. Kerns, R. D., Turk, D. C., and Rudy, T. E. The West Haven–Yale Multidimensional Pain Inventory (WHYMPI). *Pain* 23:345, 1985.
39. Bergner, M., et al. The Sickness Impact Profile: Development and final revision of a health status measure. *Med. Care* 19:787, 1981.
40. Fairbanks, J. C., et al. The Oswestry low back pain disability questionnaire. *Physiotherapy* 66:271, 1980.
41. Roland, M., and Morris, R. A study of the natural history of back pain. Part I: Development of a reliable and sensitive measure of disability in low-back pain. *Spine* 8:141, 1983.
42. Pollard, C. A. Preliminary validity study of the Pain Disability Index. *Percept. Mot. Skills.* 59:974, 1984.
43. Millard R. W. The Functional Assessment Screening Questionnaire: Application for evaluating pain-related disability. *Arch. Phys. Med. Rehabil.* 70:303, 1989.
44. Toomey, T. C., et al. Assessment of functional impairment in chronic pain patients: Description of a scale and relation to other pain measures. Proceedings of the VIth World Congress on Pain, Adelaide, Australia, April 1990.
45. Hendler, N., et al. A preoperative screening test for chronic back pain patients. *Psychosomatics* 20:801, 1979.

46. Ransford, A. O., Carson, D. C., and Mooney, V. The pain drawing as an aid to the psychologic evaluation of patients with low-back pain. *Spine* 1:127, 1976.
47. McNeill, T. W., Sinkora, G., and Leavitt, F. Psychological classification of low-back pain patients: A prognostic tool. *Spine* 11:955, 1986.
48. Love, A. W., and Peck C. L. The MMPI and psychological factors in chronic low back pain: A review. *Pain* 28:1, 1987.
49. Romano, J. M., and Turner, J. A. Chronic pain and depression: Does the evidence support a relationship? *Psychol. Bull.* 97:18, 1985.
50. Ware, J. E., and Sherbourne, C. D. The MOS 36-Item Short Form Health Survey (SF-36). *Med. Care* 30:473, 1992.

Further Information

American Medical Association. *Guides to the Evaluation of Permanent Impairment* (4th ed. revised). Chicago: American Medical Association, 1993.
The standard guidelines to the evaluation of permanent impairment, required by most states.

Aronoff, G. M. Chronic pain and the disability epidemic. *Clin. J. Pain* 7:330, 1991.
Insightful article on the issues associated with chronic pain and disability.

Babitsky, S., and Sewall, H. D. *Understanding the AMA Guides in Workers' Compensation.* Colorado Springs: Wiley Law Publications, 1992.
Text written for attorneys on the AMA Guides; also very useful for physicians.

Turk, D. C., and Melzack, R. *Handbook of Pain Assessment.* New York, Guilford Press 1992.
Superb resource for understanding the complex process of assessing patients with pain. This text includes works by the leaders in this field.

Training in the performance of independent medical evaluations is provided by several organizations, including:
American Academy of Disability Evaluating Physicians (2045 S. Arlington Heights Rd., Suite 304, Arlington Heights, IL 60005-4151)
American College of Occupational and Environmental Medicine (55 West Seegers Rd., Arlington Heights, IL 60005)
Occupational Health Excellence (Foreside Place, US Route One, Falmouth, ME 04105)

Appendix to Chapter 7: Independent Medical Evaluation*

Examinee	James Sample III
Date of birth	December 27, 1950
Date of evaluation	January 4, 1993
Date of injury	October 1, 1991
Referral organization	Unified Mutual
Referral individual	Marge Smith
Referral reference no.	WC112-456-1
Examining physician	George Wood, MD, FACOEM, FAADEP
Location of examination	Orono, Maine
Type of examination	Workers' compensation

Background

This 42-year-old, right-handed man was referred for an independent medical evaluation by the above client. The IME process was explained to the examinee, and he understands that no patient–treating physician relationship exists and that a report will be sent to the requesting client. History was provided by the examinee, who was a cooperative, fair historian. He arrived on time for the appointment and was driven by his wife, who often answered for him and reinforced statements of dis-

---

*OHX Evaluation, copyright 1993. All rights reserved. The names and situations given in this evaluation are fictitious.

ability. Approximately 1½ hours were spent directly with the examinee, with an additional 45 minutes in review of clinical information and preparation of the report. OHX systems, including questionnaire, clinical workbook, and software, were used in this assessment and in preparing this report (Occupational Health Excellence, Inc., Foreside Place, US Route 1, Falmouth, ME 04105).

The referral source provided limited clinical records of Chris Smart, MD, and Fred Cutter, MD. No records prior to December 1, 1991, or subsequent to September 10, 1992, were available for review. Significant missing records included the most recent clinical visits, emergency room records, and records of Debbie Fixer, DC. A detailed list of the records reviewed is available upon request.

To verify accuracy, the clinical synopsis was dictated in the presence of the examinee. The issues requested in the referral are addressed in the Conclusions. The examinee is represented by William Settle, Esq.

History

Preexisting Status
Mr. Sample denies any prior similar injury or problems. He had a previous work-related injury to the left shoulder while employed by Smith Trucker. He was out of work for 2 months and was treated with a sling.

Mr. Sample had complete resolution. There was no settlement. He denies any symptoms or dysfunction immediately prior to this injury.

Injury
Mr. Sample reports that on October 1, 1991, while unloading a tractor trailer, "I lifted up on a heavy box [estimated weight 100 lb.], and twisted and got pain in my back. Later that day it went down my right leg." He lifted the box from floor level and twisted to the left. The pain was in the right low back.

Initial Clinical Encounter
On October 2, 1991, one day after the injury, Mr. Sample saw the emergency room physician at Eastern Maine Medical Center with a complaint of back pain. The assessment was a back strain. He was advised to rest and take pain pills. These records are not available for review.

Clinical Synopsis
Mr. Sample sought chiropractic care with Debbie Fixer, DC, within a week of the injury and was manipulated for approximately 6 weeks without improvement. Dr. Fixer obtained an orthopedic consultation with Dr. Smart 2 months after the injury. He ordered a magnetic resonance imaging (MRI), which revealed a herniated disk at L4–5 with compression to the right. On December 10, 1991, the examinee was seen by neurosurgeon Fred Cutter, MD, who believed it was appropriate to proceed with surgery. On December 24, 1991, the patient underwent a lumbar diskectomy at L4–5, with findings of a herniated nucleus pulposus compressing the right L5 nerve root. The operation was uncomplicated. Since surgery, his primary treatment has been passive physical therapy and analgesics. He performed exercises for 2 weeks in August 1992, but these were discontinued because of pain. As discussed under Occupational History, he has been out of work since his injury.

Clinical Management Summary
HEALTH CARE PROVIDERS. Fred Cutter, MD, a neurosurgeon, is identified as the primary treating doctor. The last appointment was on December 11, 1992, and the next is scheduled for December 1993. His primary care physician is Dr. Smith. He has also seen Chris Smart, MD, and Debbie Fixer, DC.

CONSULTANT REPORTS. Chris Smart, MD, orthopedics, December 3, 1991: "History and clinical examination suggestive of a herniated disk with a right L5 radiculopathy."

Fred Cutter, MD, neurosurgeon, December 10, 1991: "The MRI scan was quite positive for a herniated nucleus pulposus at the L4–L5 disk level with compression on the right, which correlates with my clinical examination. I feel that surgery is required."

EVALUATION SUMMARY. X-ray, lumbosacral (LS) spine, October 10, 1991: The report is not available; films were reviewed and are apparently within normal limits, although they are of poor quality.

X-ray, LS spine, December 1, 1992: normal; the films are not available for review.

MRI scan, lumbar, December 3, 1992: "1. L4–5 disk herniation, centrally and to the left resulting in encroachment upon the right L5 nerve root. 2. Minor disk bulging at L3–4 and L5–S1 levels."

No myelogram, electromyography (EMG)/nerve conduction studies, or psychological testing have been performed.

TREATMENT SUMMARY.

Physical therapy	Currently none; previously ultrasound and electrostimulation (beneficial) and flexibility/strengthening (patient discontinued after 2 weeks because of pain; last 8/92); no trial of conditioning, swim program, or education
Exercise	Currently independent flexibility and strengthening, equivocal benefit
Manipulation	Currently none; previously chiropractic adjustment, equivocal benefit; no trial of osteopathic manipulation
Injections	Previous spinal injection; doubtful benefit
Medications	Currently propoxyphene dapsylate and acetaminophen (Darvocet), 2–4/day, as well as nonnarcotic analgesics, both helpful; previously also nonsteroidal antiinflammatory medication (doubtful benefit) and muscle relaxant (not helpful); no trial of tricyclic antidepressant
Surgery	December 24, 1991, lumbar diskectomy, L4–5, with equivocal result
Other	Currently none; previously splint/brace, doubtful benefit; no trial of counseling or pain program
Planned	None that the examinee is aware of or identified in the records

Current Status

The examinee's major concern is that his "back hurts and I can't lift." He reports that since the injury he has remained the same. The pain is located primarily in the right low back, and is described as nagging. It radiates down the right leg posterior to the knee.

AGGRAVATING FACTORS. Mr. Sample's condition is significantly worsened by forceful use, movement, lifting, cold or damp weather, and sitting, and somewhat by exercise, coughing or sneezing, standing, walking, and "driving my car."

RELIEVING FACTORS. Rest, ice, and heat provide some relief. The pain is constant. On a scale from 0 (no pain) to 10 (excruciating pain), initially it was a 10. During the past month it averaged a 7, with a low of 4 and a high of 10. Today the pain is a 7.

Mr. Sample has numbness on the outside of the right leg to the knee, and rare tingling. He reports weakness of the back and right leg, and morning stiffness that lasts an hour or so. He admits feeling discouraged at times and depressed, although he denies suicidal thoughts. His sleep is disturbed, with primary and secondary insomnia due to pain. He mentions as another problem that "my neck is occasionally stiff."

Functional Status

He feels he can sit for half an hour, stand for one hour, walk for half an hour, and lift up to 10 lb occasionally. He reports being unable to lift heavy weights, and has major difficulty lifting a heavy bag of groceries, bending, lifting from floor to waist or waist to shoulder, lifting above shoulder level, climbing stairs, or driving. He indicates minor problems lifting a light bag of groceries, reaching above shoulder level, pulling, pushing, sweeping or vacuuming, and moving the neck. He is unsure of his ability to climb ladders. His most difficult task is "driving my car over bumpy roads."

Perceptions

Mr. Sample believes the pain is the result of a "busted disk," and blames his employer for the injury. He does not know what will happen in the future, and is not sure if any other treatment would help. He has been satisfied with his medical care, but not with his employer, who has not contacted him since the injury. He is not sure how he feels about the insurer, but states that he has occasionally received checks late. His primary goal is "a new back." When asked, "If you had three wishes for anything in the world, what would you wish for?," the examinee responds, "Get rid of the pain, win the lottery, [and] go on vacation." He is unsure whether any legal action is upcoming on this case.

Occupational History

The examinee was employed by Jones Trucking since August 1, 1989. At the time of the injury he was working full-time as a truck driver. According to the description provided by the examinee, this involved long-haul driving of a tractor trailer and helping with loading and unloading. The physical demands included sitting for 3 hours at a time, standing for 2 hours at a time, walking for 1 hour at a time, and frequent lifting. The heaviest object he usually had to lift was a box weighing 100 lb. The examinee reports enjoying the job but having only a fair relationship with his direct supervisor, who was not friendly to him. He rates his employers as only fair, stating that they were not sympathetic.

From 1982 to 1989, Mr. Sample worked at Smith Trucking, leaving for more money. He belongs to a labor union and is a high school graduate. He has a driver's license. He is currently receiving workers' compensation and disability loan payments. He has no specific long-term occupational plans.

The examinee has been out of work for over 2 years, since the date of his injury. He is not currently receiving vocational rehabilitation counseling, but previously worked with Jane Smith in evaluation and job search. Records of this are not available. There is no projected return to work date, and the examinee does not expect to return to work in the near future. He hopes to be retrained. He does not know what work is available.

He reports that in December 1992, Dr. Cutter imposed work restrictions of 4 hours per day, 5 days per week, with no frequent bending and no lifting over 10 lb. A functional capacity evaluation has not been performed. A functional job description is not available; however, I am familiar with its demands from having viewed similar jobs.

Lifestyle/Contributory History

The examinee has been married for 4 years (twice), and lives in a two-story house in Old Town with his wife and 17-year-old child. His wife works outside the home. He reports that another person in his family has been disabled. During the day he rests, watches TV, reads, does light chores, and visits friends or family. He denies being able to do heavy chores, clean house, or work. He describes his average day as: "Get up at 7, have breakfast, walk my dog, visit friends, get coffee, get lunch, watch soap, eat dinner, watch TV, go to bed at 11." Before the injury his recreation consisted of fishing, hunting, and bowling, but he reports only fishing a little now. He is not involved in any community or religious activities. He states that "I can't do anything—my wife and daughter have to do all the chores."

Mr. Sample has smoked one pack of cigarettes a day for 20 years, and has three or four alcoholic drinks a week. He reports that on rare occasions he uses alcohol to help with the pain, and that there is a family history of alcoholism. He consumes six caffeinated beverages per day, but denies the use of recreational drugs.

Medical History

Surgery	Hernia
Medical	Noncontributory
Allergies	Penicillin
Medications	None
Review of systems	Positive for fatigue, recent weight gain, overweight; occasional cough; hypertension in the past, not now. Negative for eye-ear-nose-throat (EENT) problems; chest pain, heart disease; stomach problems, ulcers, liver disease; abdominal pain, bowel problems; urinary problems; rashes, skin problems; seizure, other neurologic problems; arthritis; thyroid disease, diabetes, endocrine problems; and psychiatric or emotional problems.
Family history	Positive for heart disease; denies similar problems, disability, arthritis, hypertension, and diabetes. Both parents are alive and in good health.

Pain Status Inventories

Pain Drawing

The examinee completed a pain drawing using symbols to describe sensations. This drawing received a score of 8, suggesting poor psychometrics.

Pain Disability Index

The Pain Disability Index uses rating scales to measure the extent of perceived disability in seven areas of life. The results are as follows:

Area	Perceived disability
Family/home responsibilities	90%
Recreation	90%
Social activity	90%
Occupation	100%
Sexual activity	80%
Self-care	60%
Life support activities	70%

The overall score is 58 out of 70, for a high level of perceived disability (83%).

McGill Pain Questionnaire

The patient completed the McGill Pain Questionnaire (Short Form), rating 15 pain descriptors on a scale from 0 (none) to 3 (severe). The sum of 11 sensory descriptors was 25, averaging 2.3. The sum of four affective descriptors was 11, averaging 2.75. The total of all descriptors was 36 (an elevated score). The descriptors were primary affective, suggesting exaggerated pain. The descriptors rated as severe were stabbing, hot-burning, aching, tender, splitting, tiring-exhausting, sickening, and punishing-cruel. The overall pain intensity was rated at 4 (horrible) on a scale of 0 to 5.

Multidimensional Pain Inventory

The patient completed the University of Pittsburgh School of Medicine Multidimensional Pain Inventory. The examinee rated the impact of the pain in several areas on a 0 to 6 scale. The first page reports the scores and statistical analysis, and the second page gives a graphic representation of the results compared with those of a control group.

The profile is that of a dysfunctional individual. Compared with the control group, these individuals report a higher severity of pain, greater interference with their lives, a higher degree of psychological distress, a lower perceived ability to control their lives, and lower activity levels. They are labeled dysfunctional because the pain has affected a broad range of their functioning.

Center for Epidemiologic Studies Depressed Mood Scale

The Center for Epidemiologic Studies Depressed Mood Scale (CES-D) was administered. The examinee scored 34, suggestive of a depressed mood.

Oswestry Function Test

Mr. Sample's score on the Oswestry Function Test was 27 out of a possible 50 (54th percentile), indicating a perception of severe disability.

Physical Examination

General

The examinee appeared healthy and had no callus on the hands. He was overweight, with a protuberant abdomen. He reported his weight as 204 lb and his height at 5 ft 9 in. His resting pulse rate was 72, and it remained at 72 when reporting pain.

Behavioral Examination

The examinee was cooperative and attentive, although somewhat irritable. His affect was normal and he maintained eye contact. He appeared comfortable during the interview, sitting continuously for 45 minutes. However, he appeared uncomfortable during the examination, displaying guarding, bracing and grimacing. He displayed more pain behavior during the examination than at other times. Nonphysiologic findings were present and are detailed in the examination.

Structural Examination

In the standing neutral position, cervical and thoracic curves were well maintained. No loss of lower cervical lordosis or exaggeration of upper thoracic kyphosis was seen, but lumbar hypolordosis was present. The examinee had no scoliosis or protraction of the shoulders. The upper and lower extremities appeared grossly normal. The pelvis appeared symmetric. Gait was normal, with no antalgia. There was normal gluteal participation in weight-bearing and leg-clearing phases. There was no tendency to asymmetric external rotation at the hips. Heel and toe walking were intact.

No focal tender points were identified. Examination focused on the low back region.

Low Back Examination

Surgical scars were present. There was generalized tenderness over the low back, but no paraspinal muscle tenderness or spasm. There was no vertebral, sciatic, sacroiliac, or coccygeal tenderness. Active trigger points were identified in the right gluteus medius.

Lumbar motion (degrees)	Normal	Angle
Flexion forward	60	6–17
Extension backward	25	7–18
Left lateral flexion	25	13–25
Right lateral flexion	25	5–29

Range-of-motion measurements were made with an inclinometer and were not reproducible. They were inconsistent with straight-leg raising. Sacroiliac tests were negative for pain bilaterally.

LOWER-EXTREMITY NEUROLOGIC EXAMINATION. Patellar reflexes were +¼L, +¼R; Achilles were +¼L, +¼R.

The examinee had normal strength symmetrically of hip flexion, knee flexion and extension, ankle dorsi- and plantar flexion, and great-toe plantar flexion. There was mild weakness of great-toe extension on the right. No muscle atrophy was present. Midthigh circumferences 15 cm above the patella were 51 cm L and 51 cm R. Midcalf circumferences in extension were 32 cm L and 32 cm R.

Sensation was diminished to light touch and pinprick on the right, in a distribution consistent with the L5 dermatome. Straight-leg raising (SLR) while sitting was negative bilaterally, limited to 80° L and 80° R by hamstring tautness. Straight-leg raising supine was positive for back pain at 40° L and 30° R.

NONPHYSIOLOGIC FINDINGS. Numerous nonphysiologic findings were present: Light pressure on the skull caused complaints of increased back pain, rotation of the trunk as a unit resulted in complaints of increased pain, superficial touch caused severe pain, superficial pressure resulted in radicular pain complaints, range of motion measurements were inconsistent, range of motion was inconsistent with straight-leg raising, and SLR supine measurements were inconsistent with SLR sitting.

Conclusions

Diagnoses*

1. Chronic pain syndrome (307.8)
   1.1. Symptom magnification (316)
2. Depressive disorder (311)
3. Lumbar or lumbosacral disk degeneration (722.52)
   3.1. Lumbar disk with radiculopathy (722.73)
   3.2. Lumbar postlaminectomy (722.83)
4. Myofascial pain syndrome (728.89)
5. Obesity (278.0)
6. Deconditioning (728.2)
7. Tobacco use (305.1)
8. Shoulder and upper-arm sprain, history of (840.9)
9. Drug allergy (995.2)

Mr. Sample does have underlying physical pathology; however, his far more significant barrier to returning to work is his chronic pain behavior and depression. Symptom magnification behavior is suggested by the clinical history, abnormal pain inventories, pain behavior, and nonphysiologic findings on examination.

EXPLANATIONS. Chronic pain (*ICD-9* 309) is a useless, malevolent, and destructive process that can be long-lived and progressive. Pain perception is markedly enhanced, and pain behavior becomes maladaptive and counterproductive. Both pain

*Classification numbers according to *ICD-9* [6].

perception and pain behavior are grossly disproportionate to any underlying noxious tissue. Tissue damage generally has healed and no longer serves as an underlying generator of pain. Chronic pain is often improperly diagnosed and inadequately treated, resulting in deteriorating coping mechanisms and pacing skills, and progressive limitations in functional capacity, which contribute to the evolution of the syndrome. Chronic pain syndrome is a biopsychosocial phenomenon of maladaptive behavior. The presence of two or more of the following characteristics, "the six Ds," is considered sufficient to establish the diagnosis of chronic pain syndrome: *duration* (although classically 6 months, this can be recognized far earlier), *dramatization* (use of emotionally charged words; exaggerated, histrionic deportment; or physical presentation), overuse or abuse of *drugs, despair* (emotional upheaval, dysphoric manifestations, impairment of pacing and coping mechanisms), *disuse* (physical deconditioning, further aggravating and perpetuating the chronic pain cycle), and *dysfunction.*

The diagnosis of symptom magnification syndrome is not intended to discredit entirely the subjective complaint of pain, its possible basis in organic pathology, or the existence of a certain degree of objective disability. However, this individual reports symptoms that are essentially nonnegotiable, which serve to control his environment, and which result in significant amplification of his perceived and expressed functional limitations. This should not be interpreted to suggest an intentional misrepresentation of pain and disability, but more likely represents a learned pattern of illness behavior. There may be significant behavioral barriers to full functional recovery, and these may need to be addressed aggressively in the management of this individual's represented disability.

Causation
Based upon the available information, to a reasonable degree of medical certainty, there is a probable causal relationship between the current complaint and the occupational injury reported.

Prognosis
Mr. Sample's prognosis is poor, based primarily on length of time out of work and chronic pain behavior.

Maximum Medical Improvement
Maximum medical improvement is defined as the date after which further recovery and restoration of function can no longer be anticipated, based on reasonable medical probability. MMI is equivocal. Mr. Sample may benefit from changes in his treatment program, although he appears unlikely to seek such treatment. It is estimated that he achieved MMI on December 24, 1992, one year after surgery.

Permanent Impairment
The American Medical Association *Guides to the Evaluation of Permanent Impairment* (4th ed.), was used for the impairment rating. The presence of objective evidence of radiculopathy (sensory deficit in the anatomic distribution of L5 nerve root) qualifies for Diagnosis-related Estimates Model lumbosacral category III, 10% total body impairment. No additional impairment is given for neurological deficit, loss of range of motion, or chronic pain. Neither the surgical treatment nor the results of treatment affect the rating.

Disability
The Americans with Disabilities Act, Title I, defines an individual with disability as having "physical or mental impairment that substantially limits one or more of the individual's major life activities; a record of such an impairment; and regarded as having such an impairment." Specific definitions of these terms are provided in the Act and in the technical assistance manual prepared by the Equal Employment Opportunity Commission.

Based on a review of this case, it is my professional opinion that this examinee would be considered an individual with a disability.

Work Capacity
This examinee has at least a light work capacity as defined in the *Dictionary of Occupational Titles,* US Department of Labor. Light work is defined as exerting up to 20 lb force occasionally and/or up to 10 lb force frequently and/or a negligible amount of force constantly to move objects. Physical demands are in excess of those for sedentary work. Light work usually requires a substantial amount of walking

or standing. However, if the worker sits most of the time but the use of arm and/or leg controls requires exertion of forces greater than those for sedentary work, the job is rated as light work.

He can work full-time. The return to work process may be facilitated by starting with less than a full day and slowly increasing the number of hours per day. He should alternate between sitting and standing based on comfort. He can lift up to 25 lb occasionally and up to 10 lb frequently, depending on the circumstances. Factors include the height of the lift, the distance from the body, and the bulk. He may have greater capabilities, particularly with conditioning. He can occasionally bend and twist. If the examinee has no pain into the legs, there are no restrictions on operating foot controls. Prolonged whole body vibrations should be avoided.

The above restrictions should remain in effect until performance of a functional capacity assessment. His current work status is indicated on the enclosed Functional Capacities Evaluation form. The recommendations are based on the examinee's own report and on my clinical assessment. A formal functional capacities evaluation by a physical therapist skilled in these assessments is recommended. This would best be performed utilizing a standardized, validated protocol such as the Key Functional Assessment. He is capable of performing other work within the above guidelines.

I would be pleased to review any written functional job descriptions or videotapes of jobs, to make arrangements to view work being considered, and/or to discuss any issues concerning work capability or the return to work process.

Appropriateness of Care
Mr. Sample has not been involved in needed treatment. A functional restoration approach should have been applied postoperatively.

Recommendations
DIAGNOSTIC. No further diagnostic testing is indicated. A chronic pain assessment is recommended.

THERAPEUTIC. It is recommended that Mr. Sample undergo a conditioning/work hardening program for 4 to 6 weeks, followed by an independent exercise program. He should increase his physical activity, lose weight, stop smoking, and stop the use of addictive drugs. A trial of nonsteroidal antiinflammatory medication and tricyclic agents is recommended. The focus should be on returning to work, with consideration of medical management and vocational rehabilitation.

CASE ANALYSIS. The missing clinical records should be obtained and reviewed.

The above analysis is based upon the subjective complaints, the history given by the examinee, the medical records and tests provided, the results of pain status inventories, and the physical findings. It is assumed that the material provided is correct. If more information becomes available at a later date, an additional report may be requested. Such information may or may not change the opinions rendered in this evaluation.

The examiner's opinions are based upon reasonable medical probability and are totally independent of the requesting agent. Medicine is both an art and a science, and although an individual may appear to be fit for return to duty, there is no guarantee that the person will not be reinjured or suffer additional injury. If applicable, employers should follow the process established in the Americans with Disabilities Act, Title I. Comments on appropriateness of care are professional opinions based upon the specifics of this case, and should not be generalized to the involved providers or disciplines. The opinions expressed do not constitute a recommendation that specific claims or administrative functions be made or enforced.

Thank you for asking me to see this examinee in consultation. If you have any further questions, please do not hesitate to contact me.

Respectfully submitted,

George Wood, MD, FACOEM, FAADEP
Enclosures: Functional Capacities Evaluation form
                Pain drawing
                Multidimensional Pain Inventory
                Body diagram
                Inclinometer measurements (Fig. 83, Lumbar range of motion)
cc: Fred Cutter, MD

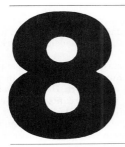

Working with the Business Community

Frank H. Leone

Overview—The 1990s: A Decade of Change

In the practice of occupational medicine, the physician has traditionally worked within an organization, primarily as an employee at an on-site occupational health service. Over the past decade, however, corporate-sponsored delivery of occupational health services has declined in frequency, although this decline seems to have stabilized [1]. In contrast to the decline of corporate-sponsored services, there has been a substantial increase in interest in the provision of occupational health services to small businesses. In the United States, as well as in most other countries, the average manufacturing or business site has fewer than 100 employees. These organizations must fulfill the same regulatory and ethical responsibilities toward the health of their employees as larger organizations. As a result, significant opportunities exist for physicians and other health care providers to deliver occupational medical services to the small-business community [2].

A major theme of this chapter is change. This change has occurred not only within the field of occupational medicine and the delivery of its services, but also within the business community itself. For example, businesses have been charged with the responsibility of understanding more about occupational health and safety in terms of their effect on business [3]. Deficiencies still exist, however, in graduate schools of business with respect to education of students and knowledge of faculty in occupational health principles and practices as they pertain to operating an organization. Nonetheless, improvements are occurring. In addition, some occupational health analyses emphasize the importance of understanding the business perspective [4].

The point of this chapter is to highlight some of the changes in the business community that may affect the delivery of occupational medical services in the next decade and to describe opportunities for physicians in providing health services to the business community.

Opportunities for physicians to work closely with the business community are virtually limitless in the 1990s. Challenges range from affiliations with hospital-based occupational health programs to roles as private consultants. Physicians are finding that occupational medicine is an evolving specialty with a captive audience—millions of working Americans whose health, safety, and livelihoods are at stake. In an era with increasing emphasis on primary care, employers are becoming the leading gatekeepers of the nation's health care system; partnerships and networking are replacing the traditional private practice concept of medicine.

Many large professional associations and industry groups consider occupational health and safety to be central to strategic planning in the 1990s. The Chemical Manufacturers Association, for example, has developed a responsible care initiative for its employee health and safety code [5]. Chemical manufacturing companies must adhere to the code to maintain membership in the organization. In another example, Giant Food, Safeway, and the Local 400 of the Food and Commercial Workers Union recently signed a 4-year labor contract that includes a rehabilitation program for employees and their dependents for cardiovascular or cerebrovascular accidents, closed head or spinal cord injuries, and neurologic disorders [6].

Close associations with employers are becoming a paramount positioning strategy for both physicians and medical centers as the private sector assumes greater influence in health care funding and medical service delivery. Well-conceived occupational health programs and delivery systems represent extraordinary opportunities for physicians, clinics, and hospitals who can position themselves accordingly.

The emerging provider-employer partnership is not limited to contracting and government mandate. As the US becomes oriented toward the prevention of deleterious health and safety habits that result in injuries and illnesses, the workplace is the optimal setting for training, health monitoring, and management of some acute and chronic conditions.

Several characteristics of the 1990s are worthy of attention:

Health care delivery is moving toward managed competition, with greater emphasis on employer responsibility.

Reform of the Occupational Safety and Health Act and state and local regulatory activity in occupational health will result in a vastly different atmosphere in which to practice medicine.

The Occupational Safety and Health Administration (OSHA) and the Environmental Protection Agency (EPA) promise to be more aggressive in promulgating and enforcing federal standards.

Environmental health issues of business will attract more attention of business and medicine and demand additional expertise of health care providers [7].

The Changing Occupational Health Environment

Today occupational health professionals are focusing more effort on the provision of health-related consultations to businesses and other organizations. This "information-brokering" approach, which is not typical of traditional clinical care, involves providing assistance to employers, especially smaller ones, on regulatory, policy, and medical areas [8].

Several significant changes have occurred in the regulatory environment that affect occupational medical practice. The deregulatory fervor of the 1980s has been overshadowed by public health regulation, especially enforcement activities. Recent initiatives include the Americans with Disabilities Act, the Drug-Free Workplace Act, and the OSHA Bloodborne Pathogens Standard. As regulatory reforms continue in both scope and enforcement, employers need even more counsel by qualified occupational medicine practitioners. In fact, recent changes in state occupational health and safety law and proposed federal reforms emphasize workplace prevention efforts that stress planning, education, and collaboration between management and labor. In the area of prevention, opportunities for the creative occupational medicine practitioner are likely to abound. Meanwhile, employers are becoming more sophisticated in understanding occupational medicine and in their expectations of quality service. As financial pressures increase, they become more selective and tend to rely on professionals with specialty training, as opposed to general physicians.

Health care cost control is a major motivator for employers to establish partnerships with providers, especially physicians, the essential ingredients for addressing the complex occupational and environmental health issues facing business today. (See Chap. 40, Health Care Management, for a discussion of innovative roles assumed by some occupational health physicians in managing health care costs.) Growing awareness, sensitivity, and liability related to environmental issues are other driving factors in many corporate decisions. Continued pressure from the public to address environmental exposures and health issues at the workplace is likely to continue.

Perhaps the most profound change in the practice of medicine is the decline of fee-for-service reimbursement in favor of a variety of managed care arrangements, such as those used by many health maintenance organizations. The workers' compensation system, under enormous financial and political pressure in some states, is easing away from the fee-for-service means of funding health care toward preferred provider organizations and related arrangements between employers and providers.

Reimbursement for workers' compensation–related medical care is becoming more tightly controlled through the use of nurse managers and other "gatekeepers" who encourage return to work and scrutinize the need for additional diagnostic testing. Workers' compensation reform will ultimately force both providers and employers to become more prevention oriented.

The Changing Role of the Physician

The practice of medicine in the United States appears poised for a significant change in which physicians are evaluated on both their ability to address broad community health care concerns and their clinical skills. Accordingly, prevention is likely to assume a more pronounced role, both in reducing workplace risk factors and in using the workplace as a forum for health education. At its best, occupational medicine is a preventive discipline, as evidenced by its specialty oversight by the American Board of Preventive Medicine.

The successful occupational physician of the 1990s will be adept at organizational dynamics, consumer education, entrepreneurship, and marketing, along with the clinical practice of medicine. Occupational medicine necessitates the ability to work as part of a team, deal with multiple constituencies (e.g., employers, workers, insurance carriers), and show leadership.

Occupational medicine physicians need to strive for objectivity and consistency in a field in which political crosscurrents abound. They must practice medicine while appreciating the pressures under which organizations operate without compromising patient care or ethical principles [9]. Frequently, a physician faces labor/management conflicts in some aspect of delivering occupational medical services. Ideally, a balanced perspective that addresses the legitimate rights of each party will be perceived as fair and ultimately effective. A review of the Code of Ethical Conduct of the American College of Occupational and Environmental Medicine may be helpful in sorting out the competing pressures in the practice of occupational medicine [10].

The traditional physician-hospital relationship is also changing. Some version of the community care concept is likely to be developed in response to competitive pressures or political mandates during this decade. Physicians are becoming hospital employees in increasing numbers; hospital and medical groups are forming joint ventures and both groups are recognizing that collaborative arrangements may be the best way to address the broad opportunities in ambulatory care. One example of a collaborative venture is the Physician-Hospital Organization, an entrepreneurial company dedicated to marketing and developing the hospital and its medical staff. Hospitals and physicians who work as partners can be significant players in a competitive market [11].

Opportunities

A board-certified occupational physician can work in academia, government, or private industry, or from the health care perspective [11A]. It is the latter setting, from the position of a hospital, a multispecialty clinic, or a freestanding facility, that offers some of the more interesting, challenging, and wide-open opportunities [12]. This chapter focuses on positions at hospitals, multispecialty groups, or freestanding occupational health clinics.

The trained occupational medicine physician has the option of selecting from a variety of practice settings, each of which offers unique advantages and opportunities. To be effective, the occupational health physician, in practicing in one of these settings, should emphasize the following to prospective clients:

"One-Stop Shopping." Programs with a broad range of services that can be provided in one setting, especially by a single physician, have great appeal.
The partnership concept. Employers in partnership with health care providers are part of the future of medical care in the United States. The physician, in particular, should be seen as a partner in preventing occupational injuries and illnesses.
Training. The value of specialized training in occupational medicine is more recognized today. The physician should emphasize certification in occupational medicine or appropriate related disciplines such as toxicology.

Hospital-Based or -Affiliated Programs

The recent growth of hospital-based or -affiliated occupational health programs has been dramatic. In the late 1980s, with the advent of the prospective payment system, many hospitals recognized occupational health as a prudent diversification strategy and entered the market in large numbers. In the past, injury care and other occupational health–related services were loosely provided out of hospital emergency departments. Today, injury care is "bundled" with other health-related services to create a defined "product" line.

In 1990, an estimated 1000 or more hospitals of approximately 7000 in the United States had dedicated programs that provided occupational medical services for employers. Although some programs are still based in emergency departments, freestanding clinics within the hospital or at other ambulatory sites are developing. Of 118 respondents to a 1989 survey of provider-based occupational health programs conducted by RYAN Associates (101 East Victoria St., Santa Barbara, CA 93101) and Occupational Health Research, 35.6% were hospital emergency department based, 33.1% were based elsewhere in hospitals, and 31.4% were freestanding. In 1992, when the survey was refielded, of 119 survey respondents, 25.2% of programs were emergency department based, 24.4% were hospital based, and 28.6% were hospital based/freestanding [13].

Furthermore, hospital-affiliated programs have matured and are expanding services to include screening, education, and rehabilitation services along with injury management and other core services. A hospital base provides several competitive advantages:

Hospitals possess a breadth of services to offer a comprehensive approach in one setting.

Hospitals typically have the financial resources to withstand a development period that may last 12 to 18 months.

Hospitals can profit from existing personnel in management, finance, and marketing to offer immediate support for a program.

The physician/medical director is a critical part of the hospital-affiliated program team. Given the chronic undersupply of trained occupational medicine physicians, compensation and negotiation leverage is favorable for the physician. Compensation for medical directors is becoming more creative and ranges from direct salary, to salary plus incentive, to salary plus fee for service. A hospital setting is especially attractive for the physician who thrives in a team atmosphere and is interested in environmental as well as clinical challenges.

Freestanding Occupational Health Clinics

Freestanding occupational health clinics with no formal ties to a hospital are also growing rapidly. Such clinics can include ambulatory care in addition to occupational medicine. Many successful clinics are large and multispecialty while others may involve only a few physicians or a single practitioner.

The freestanding occupational health clinic is likely to provide the physician with greater autonomy; it also gives employers an impression of greater efficiency, easier access and less cost than services provided by hospitals. Many primary care physicians have sought to increase their patient base by offering occupational medicine services as an adjunct to an existing primary care practice.

As employers become more prudent users of occupational health services, physicians will need to broaden their services and become better acquainted with the workplace. The era of the freestanding injury care mill that lacked an appreciation of the gamut of occupational health responsibilities is beginning to slip away.

Consulting

The shortage of physicians with training in occupational medicine provides yet a third practice option: that of a consultant. The well-trained occupational medicine physician can provide consultative services to employers, labor groups, attorneys, and professional associations [14]. Physicians may be part-time employees or consultants under contract. Compensation ranges from a specified hourly rate to fee for service or a retainer to cover an agreed upon amount of services.

Numerous hospitals and clinics are actively seeking physicians to develop an occupational health program or to serve as a part-time medical director, or both. The occupational medicine physician with administrative and managerial expertise has appealing opportunities in many settings, and is especially attractive to institutions such as hospitals and medical centers. Likewise, opportunities to work directly with employers are considerable, including more than one employer on a part-time basis. The more compelling opportunity, however, may be to develop a relatively narrow niche of expertise and provide replicable services to large numbers of organizations. Examples of services include advice related to medical surveillance, training, health policy, program development, and regulatory compliance. Cost-containment activities such as workers' compensation loss control [15] and managed care are increasingly discussed with occupational medicine consultants.

The physician serving as a consultant must know how to package and market the services. Methods include:

1. Maintain and publicize a narrow scope of services. A highly specialized consultant in virtually any field is invariably better positioned than the generalist. The physician consultant should define the service (or series of services) to be provided rather than appear as the consultant for all causes.
2. Evaluate each discrete issue in terms of the overall health and safety of the workplace in order to deal effectively with the business community and other organizations, including labor groups.
3. Publicize services in terms of benefits. High-quality services coupled with sensitivity to cost and awareness of the implications on normal operations will demonstrate the benefit.
4. Put it in writing. Although formal contracts between physicians who provide episodic services and employers are rare and in most instances unnecessary, a letter of agreement is highly recommended. The simpler the letter the better; it should simply reiterate the scope of services, fees as applicable, and any special agreements between the physician and employer.

What the Astute Physician Can Do Now

In a dynamic field replete with opportunity, a physician may wonder where to start. There are seven key elements to developing a profile that will allow the physician to succeed and be instrumental when working with the business community to prevent and manage work-related ailments.

1. *Gain a basic foundation in occupational medicine.* Many physicians offer little more than basic work injury care under the guise of occupational medicine. The discipline is far too complex for such a narrow approach. Physicians must establish a strong foundation in the field, ideally through formal training in an occupational medicine residency or short courses or other educational opportunities, and through the use of a plethora of texts and journals that cover the field. For physicians in practice, it is usually not feasible to enroll in a formal residency program. Nonetheless, programs such as the core curriculum of the American College of Occupational and Environmental Medicine can be invaluable in providing a framework for advanced education. In addition, accredited academic course work can be conducted through off-site computer programs. The Medical College of Wisconsin's Department of Preventive Medicine is a notable example. (See Chap. 35 for educational opportunities for the physician entering the field of occupational medicine.)
2. *Address the range of occupational medicine.* To work optimally with other organizations, especially the business community, the physician must embrace the entire occupational medicine continuum, including prevention and policy as well as acute injury treatment and the return to work process. Prevention should be incorporated into routine services and extend directly to the workplace to develop a safe environment and a more trusting relationship between management and labor. The physician needs to visit workplaces, communicate by telephone frequently with appropriate parties, and view injury and disease in terms of cause as well as cure. Prevention includes formal health education at the workplace, counseling during screening examinations, and treatment for injuries or illnesses.
3. *Remain abreast of regulatory measures.* As regulations governing occupational health and safety evolve, so will the role of occupational medicine specialists, who must keep abreast of the changes and implement the regulations into routine practice. In fact, the astute occupational health professional will recognize the entrepreneurial opportunities in helping organizations meet their regulatory responsibilities.
4. *Address interventions in terms of health care cost containment.* The evolving partnership between occupational medicine physicians and the business community is

contingent upon the awareness of *cost control* associated with preventive and clinical services. This daunting task can be tackled by developing systems for tracking costs and quantifying cost-containment efforts, especially the effect of case management on reducing days lost due to injuries and illnesses. Several basic parameters such as changes in lost work days associated with workplace injuries, employee absenteeism, group health, and workers' compensation premiums provide objective data. Computer software programs have been developed specifically to address these matters, among others. (See Chap 36, Computers in Occupational Medicine Practice.) Softer assessments of employee morale, job satisfaction, and productivity can also add valuable information regarding cost-containment efforts.

5. *Be an educator.* Inadequate training and education contribute to most workplace health and safety problems. Moreover, the failure of organizations to meet their responsibilities for training is a consistent reason for the issuance of OSHA citations. In addition, the successful occupational medicine practitioner recognizes the value of educating employers, workers, and professional colleagues. Giving presentations to local medical staff, for example, can raise awareness of occupational medicine and promote benefits to both physicians and patients. An effective educator is also a good listener. To practice effectively, the occupational medicine physician must heed the concerns of both employers and workers.

6. *Be prepared to play multiple roles.* The modern occupational medicine physician is at once an educator, clinician, consultant, and visionary. Although this disparate array of skills may seem daunting, many physicians find these requirements invigorating.

7. *Commit to professional and aggressive marketing.* Success in either product or service delivery is invariably contingent upon developing a product/service appropriate to its market and then effectively educating the market about its availability. Frequently, an occupational health service program is strong on quality but woefully weak in promoting the product to its public. The effective marketing of occupational health services usually involves two components: an aggressive, targeted *sales effort* and the ability to focus on *program benefits* (e.g., cost containment, health status) rather than features (e.g., extended hours, training, and experience). An aggressive effort usually involves retaining the services of at least one full-time salesperson, providing appropriate financial incentives for that person, and targeting employers who are most in need of the services.

The Occupational Medicine Physician of the Future

Change in the nation's health care system and the role of its practitioners is inevitable. In this author's view, the occupational medicine physician will be in the mainstream of the practice of medicine by the 21st century. The employer-provider interface is the centerpiece of this evolution. This relationship addresses two central issues: control of runaway health care costs and the need to continually improve productivity for American business to maintain a competitive edge in an increasingly global economy.

The emergence of the employer as a key figure in health care reform and as a gatekeeper and financial supporter of the health care system presents an extraordinary opportunity to the physician with training and expertise in occupational medicine. Opportunities abound in provider-based and corporate-based programs, and, increasingly, in private consulting. The supply of physicians with specialty training continues to fall short of demand; given the magnitude of this shortfall, it is unlikely to abate in the foreseeable future.

There is much to motivate the physician to join the ranks of a growing and highly evolutionary specialty that places a premium on prevention by recognizing the workplace as a perfect venue to address the nation's health through the reduction of workplace health and safety hazards and the practice of genuine preventive medicine. Occupational medicine appears poised to become a key medical specialty.

References

1. Ducatman, A. M., et al. Occupational physician staffing in large US corporations. *J. Occup. Med.* 33:613, 1991.

2. Chapman-Walsh, D. The vanguard and the rearguard: Occupational medicine revisits its future. *J. Occup. Med.* 30:124, 1988.
3. Waters, C. F., and Heath, E. D. The Minerva Program: New kid on the occupational safety and health block. *J. Occup. Med.* 31:925, 1989.
4. Snyder, T. B., et al. Business analysis in occupational health and safety consultations. *J. Occup. Med.* 33:1040, 1991.
5. Chemical Manufacturers Association. *Employee Health and Safety Resource Guide.* Washington, D.C.: CMA, 1992.
6. *Developments in Industrial Relations,* Monthly Labor Review, US Department of Labor, Bureau of Labor Statistics; Dec. 1992. P. 54.
7. McCunney, R. J., Boswell, R., and Harzbecker, J. Environmental health in the journals. *Environ. Res.* 59:114, 1992.
8. LaDou, J. Occupational medicine consultant. *Am. J. Ind. Med.* 19:257, 1991.
9. McCunney, R. J., and Brandt-Rduf P. Ethical issues in the private practice of occupational medicine. *J. Occup. Med.* 33:80, 1991.
10. Code of Ethical Conduct. American College of Occupational and Environmental Medicine. *J. Occup. Med.* 36:28, 1994.
11. Reece, R. and Coombes, D., Clinical corner. *Visions* 3:14, 1993.
11A. American College of Occupational and Environmental Medicine. Careers in Occupational and Environmental Medicine. *J. Occup. Med.* 35:628, 1993.
12. McCunney, R. J. Providing high quality occupational medical services. *J. Amb. Care Marketing* 4:9, 1990.
13. Newkirk, W., and Leone, F. H. Occupational Health Research, Skowhegan, ME/ RYAN Associates, Santa Barbara, CA. *Survey of Occupational Health Programs: 1989 and 1992.* (Available from RYAN Associates, 101 East Victoria St., Santa Barbara, CA 93101.)
14. McCunney, R. J. The Academic Occupational Physician as a Consultant: A Ten-Year Perspective. *J. Occup. Med.* vol. 36, 1994.
15. McCunney, R. J., and Barbanel, C. S. Controlling Workers Compensation Costs: The Role of an Audit. *Occup. Health Saf.* 62(10):75, 1993.

Further Information

Chapman-Walsh, D./Corporate Physicians. *Between Medicine and Management.* New Haven: Yale University Press, 1987.
This now classic work describes some of the dilemmas and their solutions for occupational physicians as they strive to balance the competing interests of labor and management in providing quality medical care.

Guidotti, T. et al. *Occupational Health Services: A Practical Approach.* Chicago: American Medical Association, 1989.

LaDou, J. (ed.). *Occupational Medicine.* Norwalk, CT: Appleton & Lange, 1990.

Leone, F. H. *Marketing Health Care Services to Employers.* Binghamton, NY: Haworth Press, 1994.

Levy, B., and Wegman, D. (eds.). *Occupational Health.* Boston: Little, Brown, 1994.

Mack, K. E., and Newbold, P. *Health Care Sales.* San Francisco: J.E. Bass Publishers, 1991.

Moser, R. *Effective Management of Occupational and Environmental Health and Safety Programs.* Boston: OEM Press, 1992.
An excellent primer on management responsibilities that many occupational health professionals must address in overseeing various programs.

Newkirk, W., and Jones, L. *Providing Hospital Occupational Health Services to Business* (2nd ed.). Chicago: American Hospital Association, 1993.

The Occupational and Environmental Medicine Report. OEM Health Information, 24 Spice St., Boston, MA 02129.
This monthly publication includes summaries and critical commentaries of articles related to occupational medicine that were originally published in various professional

journals. Since 1987, this compact newsletter has been helpful in keeping practitioners up to date on the medical issues that affect the practice of occupational medicine.

Occupational Safety and Health Reporter. Washington, DC: Bureau of National Affairs.
This weekly publication addresses regulatory issues associated with the practice of occupational medicine. It is essential for quality programs to aid in keeping abreast of the numerous rules, standards, and other guidelines that affect the practice.

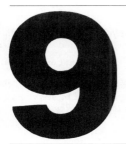

Drug Testing

Kent W. Peterson

Employee drug testing has grown dramatically during the last decade. In 1980, drug testing was confined to the military, nuclear power industry, and a few other employers. Now, almost every Fortune 500 company prohibits illegal drug use on or off the job, and requires preemployment drug tests. Approximately 7 million Americans are subject to federal drug testing requirements; this number is expected to reach 10 million by 1995.

This chapter reviews the growth of workplace drug testing; the nature and magnitude of the drug problem in the United States; types of drug tests; regulated versus unregulated testing models; components of a drug-free workplace program; urine collection procedures; laboratory analysis; review, interpretation, and reporting of laboratory results by medical review officers (MROs); new federal alcohol testing regulations in the transportation industry; and current technical and legal issues.

Two basic forms of drug testing reflect two different purposes. Federally mandated drug testing was initiated to deter workers from using illicit drugs, as one component of the federal Drug-Free Workplace Program. Other components include a written policy restricting possession and use of illicit drugs and alcohol, employee education, supervisor training, rehabilitation, and employee assistance. Fitness-for-duty programs, such as that in the nuclear power industry, are quite different.

Growth of Drug Testing

The extraordinary growth of drug testing is due to many factors. Most essential was the technological breakthrough of simple, inexpensive immunoassay urine screening tests in the 1960s. Sensitive immunoassay tests produce many false positives, however, because of cross reactivity with other substances. Testing using this method alone adversely affected some of those tested, with consequent litigation. A two-test standard has evolved, with a more specific test—gas chromatography/mass spectrometry (GC/MS)—used to confirm positive screening test results. GC/MS has become the "gold standard" for forensic drug testing and is required in all federally mandated programs.

In the 1970s, the US military successfully reduced the prevalence of drug use by introducing a random testing program with witnessed urine collections. In the 1980s, large corporate employers began drug testing. In response, the American College of Occupational and Environmental Medicine (ACOEM) offered guidance to private employers and occupational health professionals by issuing *Drug Screening in the Workplace: Ethical Guidelines* in 1986, later updated in 1991 (see Chapter Appendix) [1, 2]. These guidelines have become a standard of practice among private employers.

Drug testing of public sector employees was shaped by Executive Order 12564 and Public Law 100-71, which commissioned the Department of Health and Human Services (DHHS) to develop technical procedures for drug testing. These were published as the April 1988 *Mandatory Guidelines for Federal Workplace Drug Testing Programs* [3]. These mandatory guidelines outlined the framework for regulations published by the Department of Transportation (DOT) [4], Department of Defense (DOD), Department of Energy (DOE), and other federal agencies. Landmark decisions by the US Supreme Court validated that properly conducted drug testing programs, including random testing, were lawful for private and public sector employees working in security and safety-sensitive positions [5].

The Bureau of Labor Statistics (BLS) and The Conference Board have studied the growth of drug programs in industry. For example, BLS reported that in 1990 companies with more than 250 employees were much more likely to have written policies (74 vs. 12%), sponsor employee assistance programs (79 vs. 9%), and conduct drug testing (46 vs. 3%) than those with fewer than 50 employees [6].

What is the "Drug Problem" Being Addressed?

Substance abuse in the US includes unauthorized or inappropriate use of controlled substances, prescription drugs, alcohol, and tobacco. To date, drug testing has focused largely on illicit drugs. In 1991, 12.6 million Americans aged 12 and over used one or more illicit drugs during the previous month, a decrease of 45% from 1985. Of the 19.5 million people who in 1991 used marijuana at least once during the past year, 5.3 million used it once a week or more, and 3.1 million used it daily or almost daily. In 1991, 1.9 million people reported having used cocaine in the last month [7]. Although the prevalence of illicit drug use in 1991 was markedly reduced compared to 1989, these figures are still high. However, prevalence has remained constant among frequent cocaine users. Recidivism after rehabilitation for illicit drug abuse is high compared to those treated for alcoholism.

Drugs in the workplace are a concern because 66.5% of current illicit drug users are employed, 51.7% full-time and 14.8% part-time. Illicit drug use is higher among men than women. Among employees 18 years or older, 7% of men and 4.8% of women were current illicit drug users in 1991. Even more dramatic is the variation by age, as shown in Table 9-1. Illicit drug use is heavily concentrated among those aged 18 to 34. Based on 1991 surveys, 9.7% of full-time employees aged 18 to 34 use illicit drugs, largely marijuana (7.9%) and cocaine (1.8%). This percentage is considerably higher than the usual rates of positive urine drug screens among this age group. Reasons for this gap include urine substitution or adulteration and the fact that recreational users abstain from drug use before scheduled drug tests. Illicit drug use crosses all industries, but is highest in construction, wholesale, and retail trades (15.4, 13.6, and 12.2%, respectively, of full-time employees aged 18–34). Interestingly, the transportation industry clusters in the middle of other industries.

Illicit drug use among employees is associated with higher rates of absenteeism, accidental injury, involuntary separation, medical care usage, and health care costs. For example, in a study of US Postal Service applicants, those who screened positive for drugs had 66% higher absenteeism, 77% greater likelihood of being fired, 143% more employee assistance program referrals, and 26% higher medical claims over a 3.3-year period than those who screened negative [8]. Even though supervisors did not know the results of employment drug tests, disciplinary action for problems of attendance, performance, and conduct was almost twice as high for those with positive tests. In a study of Georgia Power employees, hours of absenteeism for those testing positive for drugs was 165, compared to 91 for those treated for drug abuse, 73 for those treated for alcoholism, and 41 for the average worker [9]. Annual general medical benefit costs were $1314 for those testing positive for drugs, $1347 for those treated for drugs, and $842 for those treated for alcohol, in contrast to $590 for the average worker.

Table 9-1. Current illicit drug use among full-time US employees by age and sex, 1991

Age	Male	Female
35+	4.2%	2.7%
26–34	9.7%	6.1%
18–25	15%	10.8%
All ages (18+)	7%	4.8%

Source: Adapted from NIDA capsules, *Population Estimates of Lifetime and Current Drug Use, 1991; National Household Survey of Drug Abuse.* Rockville, MD: National Institute on Drug Abuse, December 1991.

Types of Worksite Drug Testing

There are six major situations in which drug testing is performed at the worksite.

Preemployment/Preplacement

This is the most prevalent form of drug testing. For federal employees, it is limited to those in safety-sensitive positions and all military personnel. However, many private employers require preemployment drug tests of all those entering the workplace. Preplacement testing can include employees who are transferred and/or promoted to covered positions and those who are returning to work after extended absences. Although the Americans with Disabilities Act (ADA) prohibits preoffer/preemployment medical examinations, it specifically allows drug testing before a job offer is made.

Periodic

Employers may require drug testing as part of fitness-for-duty or other examinations. Because those examinations are scheduled in advance, recreational users can abstain from drug use before testing and positive rates tend to be low. Scheduled drug tests are not included in the new DOT alcohol and drug testing regulations (see p. 125).

Postaccident/Incident

Testing may be required after an accident, incident, and/or safety violation. Each employer must define specific conditions under which postaccident testing is required. The DOT regulations define conditions that trigger postaccident testing. Postaccident specimens must be collected quickly, often after-hours and away from the usual collection site. In anticipation of this testing, the employer should explore available collection options. Proper urine collection, chain-of-custody techniques, and consent procedures must be observed in the emergency department or other clinical setting. A number of employers have been successful in invoking the "voluntary intoxication defense" in order to avoid paying workers' compensation claims for injuries when the employee tested positive [10].

Reasonable Cause/Reasonable Suspicion

This testing is performed when there is reason to believe that the employee has used drugs in violation of company policy or agency rules. A supervisor must document the behavior and usually obtain the approval of a second supervisor prior to testing. Indications for testing can include unsafe practices, violating operating rules, changes in personality, or aberrant behavior.

Return to Duty and Follow-up

An employee who has refused or previously failed a drug test may be required to provide drug-free urine before returning to work. Frequently, employees who complete a rehabilitation program are subject to unannounced follow-up testing for 6 months to 2 years.

Random

Unannounced random drug testing provides the highest deterrent against drug use. Usually, names of employees in specific safety-sensitive jobs (e.g., pilots, drivers, or security personnel) are included in a pool, from which individuals are selected based on randomly generated numbers. Tests are conducted on short notice, for example, within 1 to 3 hours. To maintain the deterrent effect, employees who have already tested negative remain within the pool, subject to retesting. It is crucial that information about the dates of random testing, locations of testing, and employees to be tested be kept confidential.

Random testing also raises the greatest concerns of civil liberties, invasion of privacy, and unreasonable search and seizure. Proposed random testing among private companies of *all employees* regardless of job category has led to employee relations concerns and legal challenges. Employers are urged to adopt policies that are reasonable, as well as legally defensible, which recognize that the vast majority of employees are not illicit drug users, and which presume innocence rather than guilt.

Regulated Versus Nonregulated Drug Testing Models

Currently, there are two divergent worlds of drug testing. In the unregulated private sector, a wide spectrum of approaches is found. For example, urine may be tested for 2 to 20 different drugs; custody and control forms may include the employee's name and list prescription drugs taken within the last 2 weeks. Urine may be analyzed at any laboratory, laboratory cutoff levels may be specified by the employer, and results may go directly to the employer, without physician review. Because of concerns about the quality and appropriateness of some company drug testing programs, Congress is considering legislation that would establish a federal standard for all workplace drug testing in the US.

The other world of drug testing is proscribed by detailed government regulations from the DHHS, DOT, DOD, DOE, and other agencies. DOT regulations are particularly important, because they currently affect over 4 million Americans in five transportation modes: aviation, commercial marine, interstate trucking, pipelines, and railroads. Federal regulations contain detailed procedures for urine collection, completion of custody and control forms, analysis by laboratories certified by the National Institute on Drug Abuse (NIDA) *for only five specified illicit drugs* (amphetamines, cocaine, marijuana, opiates, and phencyclidine—the "NIDA-5"), and mandatory reporting of all results to an MRO for review and interpretation before reporting to the employer.

The NIDA-DOT regulations have clearly emerged as the standard of practice, that is, a gold standard. The remainder of this chapter summarizes these detailed federal drug testing procedures. Those conducting urine collection and medical review are urged to carefully review federal regulations and participate in training offered by federal agencies or by professional societies such as ACOEM.

Frequently, there is confusion about the relationship of DOT drug testing to the DOT physical examination required of certain transportation workers, for example, pilots and truck drivers [11]. A few years ago, drug testing was included as part of scheduled periodic examinations. DOT medical forms and operator's certificates made reference to both physical examinations and drug testing. The advent of random drug testing within most transportation sectors has separated it from scheduled periodic medical examinations. Reference to drug testing has been removed from the DOT physical examination card.

Nuclear Regulatory Commission (NRC) drug testing provisions differ from those of other federal agencies in that they represent a fitness-for-duty rather than a deterrent program. The NRC permits on-site screening; if an individual tests positive, he/she is removed from safety-sensitive duties until confirmation results are received. Screening cutoff levels may be lower for marijuana and cocaine, testing for other drugs is allowed, and alcohol testing is required [12].

Department of Defense contractors are required to have a Drug Free Workplace Program, but drug testing is not mandated. While employee assistance programs (EAPs) are mandated for federal agencies, they are not required to be offered to private sector employers or defense contractors covered by drug testing regulations. Instead, the regulations require that individuals be informed about any available counseling, rehabilitation, and employee assistance programs.

Urine Collection

Drug testing can be broken down into three steps: collection of the specimen and completion of custody and control forms, laboratory analysis for screening and confirmation of positive tests, and review, verification, and reporting to the employer of test results.

Urine collection is particularly crucial because so many errors occur here. It is vitally important that the urine collection process treat each person with respect and allow the maximum reasonable privacy, while minimizing the opportunity to substitute or adulterate urine specimens. Attention to detail in completing paperwork is also essential. Most positive drug tests that are invalidated are due to improper urine collection or documentation. The DHHS *Mandatory Guidelines* and DOT rules [13] provide excellent urine collection procedures, summarized in Table 9-2.

There are three ways to conduct urine collection. In private collection, the donor provides a specimen in a separate room with complete privacy. In monitored collection, the urine collection is conducted in a public restroom or other facility that offers partial privacy, for example, inside a stall with partitions that block direct view. A licensed health professional of either gender may monitor urine collection; a nonmedically licensed collector must be the same gender as the donor. The third form of collection is under direct observation of the urine exiting the urinary meatus—so-called witnessed collection. Collection site personnel must be the same gender as the donor when a collection is conducted under direct supervision.

Following collection, the collector and the donor should keep the sample in constant view until it is sealed and labeled. The collector places a tamper-proof seal on the specimen bottle's cap and down the sides of the bottle, together with an identification label showing the date and specimen identification number. The tested individual must initial the label to certify that it is the specimen collected from him or her.

If an employer has requested both a federally mandated drug test for the NIDA-5 and a test for additional drugs, *separate specimens must be collected* (separate urine voids into separate containers) for the federally mandated test and for the additional drugs. It is unacceptable to pour any remaining urine from the void for the federally mandated test into another container for additional drug testing. Separate custody and control forms must be used for each specimen.

Split Samples

An employer may authorize or require a split specimen to be collected. Proposed DOT regulations will require split specimens for all DOT urine collections. A split specimen is obtained from a single void into one collection receptacle; 30 to 60 ml is then poured into the first (primary) specimen container. The remainder (up to 60 ml) is kept or poured into a second specimen container. The split specimen may be retained by the urine collection facility or sent to the primary laboratory or to a secondary laboratory. The split specimen is tested only if the primary specimen tests positive and the employee or MRO requests reanalysis of the split. The reanalysis is performed by GC/MS only for the analyte that was positive initially at the laboratory's lower limits of detection. If the split-specimen analysis is negative, the overall test should be reported as negative.

Completion of Custody and Control Forms

All urine collection requires a use of a custody and control form. The DOT form has six paper copies (7 copies if a split specimen is collected). The copies that go to the laboratory may not contain the name of the donor, only the social security or other identification number. Although forms currently have varied widely from laboratory to laboratory, DOT will soon require mandatory use of a standard form.

There is often confusion about completing the chain of custody blocks. A minimum of four entries (date, 2 actual signatures, and courier) must appear in the chain of custody block of the DOT-type form. The first line should register that the specimen was provided by "Donor," usually preprinted on the form. The donor's actual name should not be written. On the same line, the name and signature of the collector should be written, along with the date. On the second line, the collector's name and signature should appear a second time as being released either to another attendant in the collection facility or to the "Courier." The actual name of the delivery person need not appear because the specimen and forms are sealed in boxes before courier pickup.

Table 9-2. Specimen collection procedures

Employers must designate specimen collection sites that have
1. An enclosure for urinating in private
2. A toilet or receptacle large enough to contain a complete void
3. A source for washing hands
4. A suitable surface for writing

The collection site must be secure to prevent unauthorized access during the collection process.

The specimen must be kept in sight of the donor and collection site person until sealed and ready for shipment.

Employees are required to have individual privacy when providing a specimen except when
1. The employee presents a specimen that is outside the accepted temperature range and he/she refuses to have an oral body temperature measurement, or the body temperature measurement varies more than 1°C from the specimen temperature
2. The collector observes the employee attempting to adulterate or substitute the specimen
3. The employee's last provided specimen was determined to be diluted
4. The employee has previously had a verified positive test

In 1 and 2 above, the employee must provide a specimen under direct observation. In 3 and 4, the employer may require a direct observation collection.

Specific procedures must be followed during collection of the specimen, including
1. Positive identification of the donor
2. Removing of outer garments only; employees should not undress or wear a hospital gown or other examination gown
3. Washing hands before collection of specimen
4. Securing water sources in the collection site enclosures
5. Adding bluing agent to toilet tank and bowl
6. Collector remains outside the enclosure
7. Donor may flush toilet only after releasing specimen to collector
8. The specimen should contain at least 60 ml urine

If donor cannot provide a sufficient volume of urine, he/she should remain at the collection site and be provided fluids to drink.

The collector must measure the temperature of the specimen within 4 minutes after collection, and inspect the specimen for color and unusual signs of contamination.

Collector and donor must complete the collection process together, including
1. Sealing and labeling of specimen bottle
2. Donor initialing label or seal
3. Signing and dating of custody and control form

Collector must prepare specimen for shipment, including and dating a seal on shipping container.

An employer may authorize collection of a split specimen. A split specimen is obtained when urine from a single void is divided into two specimen containers. The first (primary specimen) must contain at least 60 ml urine; the second (split specimen) contains the remainder of the urine up to 60 ml.

All procedures and documentation must be carried out for the split specimen. The split specimen is only tested at the request of the employee when the primary specimen has been reported positive to the MRO.

The split specimen, if tested, is only tested by GC/MS to confirm the presence of the drugs found in the primary specimen.

Disciplinary action against the employee does not have to be deferred while awaiting the result of the split-specimen analysis.

Source: Adapted from US Department of Transportation, Employer's Guide to 49 CFR Part 40: Procedures for Transportation Workplace Drug Testing Programs, October 1990. P. 19.

Laboratory Analysis

Federally regulated drug tests must be analyzed in NIDA-certified laboratories. Almost 100 laboratory sites have been NIDA certified as of 1993. Since most laboratories have NIDA and non-NIDA sections, it is important to specify whether a drug specimen should be analyzed under NIDA provisions. Because of rigorous internal open and blind quality control and external blind proficiency testing checks, prices for NIDA-certified drug testing are usually higher.

Laboratories use internal chain of custody documents to track specimens in-house. From the accessioning area where specimens are logged in and stored, small aliquots are removed and sent for screening or confirmation tests. Screening is first performed using one of several approved immunoassay methods. Screening tests are recorded as either positive or negative. If the screen is positive, then another aliquot is taken from the specimen for confirmation testing for the identified drug. GC/MS confirmation provides quantitative results, but under DOT provisions, laboratories may report routinely quantitative results only for opiates. However, quantitative levels may be requested on a case-by-case basis for any drug specimen.

When the laboratory identifies a specimen as negative, it is discarded. *Positive specimens are frozen and retained at the laboratory for at least one full year in case the analysis is questioned and retests must be performed.* The laboratory must retain all specimen records for a minimum of 2 years. Laboratories must also send to each employer a monthly statistical report of all testing conducted, but this report does not contain individual results.

Occupational physicians can help employers meet their obligations to submit quality control specimens. DOT requires that employers submit three quality control specimens to their laboratory for every 100 employee specimens tested. These "external blind proficiency tests" should not be known to the laboratory; hence, ID numbers, signatures on labels, and other information should appear just as if they were typical specimens. Blind specimens can be known negatives, purchased specimens that are positive at a given cutoff level, or split specimens obtained from employees who are not subject to drug testing. If a specimen is reported as falsely negative or positive, the laboratory should be notified and an attempt made to investigate the error. Because of its significance, any false-positive test should also be communicated immediately to the DOT or other federal agency for immediate investigation. *If verified, a single false-positive test could result in the laboratory's certification being suspended.*

Although only a few milliliters are required for each analysis, separate GC/MS confirmation of several different positive screens can add up to more than 30 ml. DOT now requires collection of a 60-ml specimen, but has considered reducing the requirement to 30 ml once split-specimen requirements are in place.

The laboratory certifying scientist must review the test results and sign for any positive specimens. Medical review officers may request laboratory reanalysis of specimens when there is some question as to the validity of findings or on the donor's request.

The Department of Transportation has issued guidance to laboratories regarding "fatal flaws" that constitute grounds for rejecting a specimen [14]; these are outlined in Table 9-3. Some flaws (nos. 3, 4, 10) may be corrected by a signed statement from the appropriate individual. Because affidavits can permit an otherwise unacceptable sample to be tested, laboratories have been requested to retain specimens not suitable for testing for a minimum of 5 working days.

The cutoff levels issued by NIDA for both screening and confirmation tests are shown in Table 9-4. The screening level for marijuana of 100 ng/ml represents a variety of metabolites; the confirmation cutoff level of 15 ng/ml represents one specific metabolite—delta-9-tetrahydrocannabinol-9-carboxylic acid. DHHS has proposed lowering the screening level to 50 ng/ml, but not changing the confirmation cutoff level [20]. The cocaine screening level of 300 ng/ml is also for various metabolites, whereas the confirmation cutoff level of 150 ng/ml is for benzoylecgonine. For opiates and phencyclidine (PCP), the screening and confirmation levels are identical. Screening levels for amphetamines of 1000 ng/ml are paralleled by confirmation cutoff levels of 500 ng/ml each for amphetamine and/or methamphetamine.

When repeat analysis is requested or when split samples are tested, only GC/MS confirmation is performed. Under these circumstances, cutoff levels do not apply;

Table 9-3. "Fatal flaws" to DOT-mandated drug testing programs

Specimens presented to laboratories should be rejected for testing when any of the following procedural errors occur.
1.   Specimen ID number on specimen bottle and custody and control form do not match.
2.   Specimen ID number is omitted on specimen bottle.
3.* Collector's signature is omitted from certification statement.
4.* Chain of custody block is incomplete (minimum: 2 signatures; shipping entry; date).
5.   Donor Social Security or ID number is omitted on custody and control form unless "refusal of donor to provide" is stated in remarks section.
6.   Specimen volume is less than 30 ml; if on arrival at the laboratory, specimen volume is slightly below the 30-ml minimum (within 10%), the specimen may be accepted if the laboratory can ensure that sufficient volume will be available for storage and any necessary reanalyses for quality control or reconfirmation of results.
     Note: This provision does not change the DOT requirement for the donor to provide 60 ml urine. The provision is meant to apply to situations such as leakage.
7.   Specimen bottle seal is broken or shows evidence of tampering.
8.   Specimen shows obvious adulteration (i.e., color, foreign objects, unusual odor).
     Positive specimen results reviewed by the medical review officer should be canceled when the following procedural errors occur:
9.   Donor's signature is omitted from the certification statement unless "donor refusal to sign" is stated in the remarks section.
10. Certifying scientist's signature is omitted on laboratory copy of the drug testing custody and control form.

*Correctable by signed affidavit.
Source: From R. Knisely, *Operating Guidance for DOT Mandated Drug Testing Programs*. US Department of Transportation, Office of the Secretary, June 1, 1992.

Table 9-4. DHHS cutoff levels for drugs of abuse

Drugs	Initial screening (ng/ml)	Confirmatory (GC/MS)
Marijuana metabolites	100	15[a]
Cocaine metabolites	300	150[b]
Opiate metabolites	300	
Morphine		300
Codeine		300
Phencyclidine	25	25
Amphetamines	1000	
Amphetamine		500
Methamphetamine		500

[a]As delta-9-tetrahydrocannabinol-9-carboxylic acid.
[b]As benzoylecgonine.
Source: From DHHS, Alcohol, Drug Abuse, and Mental Health Administration, Mandatory guidelines for Federal Workplace Drug Testing Programs; Final guidelines. *Fed. Register* 53(69):11979, April 11, 1988.

the analyte is tested at the laboratory's lowest limit of detection. The cutoff is removed because over time, analytes often degrade or adhere to the sides of the specimen container.

Results from the laboratory are reported in federally regulated testing to a medical review officer; in unregulated testing, results may go directly to the employer. Results may be communicated electronically by facsimile, teleprinter, or modem, but a written copy of the custody and control form must also be provided. Results may not be communicated by telephone.

Review of Test Results by a Medical Review Officer

The MRO designation and role emerged from federal regulations, which referenced a "medical review official." For example, the 1988 DHHS guidelines governing drug testing under the federal Drug-Free Workplace Program described the MRO as "a licensed physician . . . who has knowledge of substance abuse disorders and has appropriate medical training to interpret and evaluate an individual's positive test result together with his/her medical history and any other relevant biomedical information" [3].

By *receiving, reviewing, interpreting, verifying, and reporting* drug test results, the MRO plays a vital role in protecting individuals from being inappropriately labeled as drug users, with adverse consequences. Approximately 5000 MROs have received 2-day training from organizations such as the ACOEM, American Society of Addiction Medicine, Federal Aviation Administration, DOT, and others. MRO manuals have been published by NIDA, DOT, professional societies, and seasoned MROs. [15–18]. DHHS and DOT regulations that enumerate specific duties of MROs are summarized below [3, 4].

The MRO *receives* negative and confirmed positive results from the laboratory, including a certified copy of the custody and control form. Under federally regulated testing, all results must come directly to the MRO. Although DOT considered allowing negative results to be reported directly to the employer, this approach was rejected because of concerns that employers would label as drug users those whose test results were verified as "negative" from the MRO.

The MRO must perform an administrative *review* of the custody and control form for each negative specimen to assure it was completed in conformance with the employer's policy and procedures. Negative laboratory results with a flawed chain of custody section must be reported as a *canceled test,* rather than negative, unless corrected by signed affidavit.

The MRO must understand the urine collection, forms completion, and analytic procedures. Deviance from procedures may lead the MRO to negate apparently positive results, while knowledge that prescribed procedures were carefully followed permits the MRO to discount statements from an applicant/employee that a collection site person or laboratory adulterated the sample.

The most critical MRO function is to *interpret and verify positive test results.* The MRO must allow individuals with positive tests the opportunity to provide a legitimate medical explanation. The MRO should follow the procedure outlined in Table 9-5. Figure 9-1 contains an example of an MRO verification work sheet.

Staff under an MRO's supervision may contact individuals, discuss positive results, and request verification of medical prescriptions. However, before reporting verified positives an MRO must personally speak with individuals who have positive results unless the individual refuses to talk with the MRO or if an employer representative has notified the donor to contact the MRO and 5 days have elapsed.

The MRO may ask the laboratory for the concentration of the detected drug. The MRO may authorize reanalysis of the original sample. Consultation with the toxicologist or laboratory certifying scientist can also be helpful.

Many prescription and over-the-counter (OTC) drugs can cause positive test results. Verification of legitimate medical explanations for positive tests often requires clinical judgment. For example, tetrahydrocannabinol, the active ingredient of marijuana, is used as an antinausea agent for cancer patients under the prescription name Marinol. Although inhalation of sidestream marijuana smoke is offered as an explanation for a positive test result, toxicology studies have not confirmed this explanation as feasible. Cocaine is used in ear-nose-throat (ENT), ophthalmology, and surgical procedures, such as injection of TAC (tetracaine, adrenaline, and co-

Table 9-5. DOT guidelines: MRO/employee interview checklist

1. Identify yourself as a physician serving as the MRO for the specific employer, with the duty of receiving and reviewing drug test results.
2. Establish the identity of the applicant or employee (i.e., full name, social security or employee ID number, date of birth).
3. Inform the employee that medical information discussed during the interview is confidential, and may only be disclosed under special circumstances (e.g., impact on fitness for duty) as required by law.
4. If the employee holds a medical certificate under a DOT agency (e.g., airline pilot or train engineer), advise the employee that information regarding drug test results and information supplied by the employee will be provided to the DOT agency as required.
5. Tell the employee you are calling about the specific drug test he/she underwent on the specific date and at the specific location. Inform the employee for what drug the specimen tested positive.
6. If the employee requests the quantitative levels of the confirmed results, provide him/her with it, if available. If quantitative levels are not available, the MRO should request them from the laboratory. However, pending quantitative levels should not delay verification decisions.
7. Ask for recent medical history, when appropriate, regarding use of prescription medication, over-the-counter drugs, dental, ear-nose-throat, ophthalmologic, or other medical procedures, and food ingestion if pertinent (e.g., poppy seeds if positive test for opiates).
8. Request that the employee provide medical records or documentation of prescription for controlled substance when appropriate. Set a specific deadline for receipt of the medical records.
9. Request the employee to undergo a medical evaluation, when appropriate (e.g., to provide clinical confirmation of opiate abuse). Make arrangements for medical evaluation.
10. Notify the employee that he/she may request a re-test of the original specimen and, if appropriate, provide information about payment for re-test in accordance with employer's policy. Tell the employee that a re-test will not delay verification of the initial test result. Similarly, if a split specimen was collected, notify the employee of the procedures under which it may be analyzed.
11. When the verification process is complete, inform the employee that the appropriate official of the employer will be notified.
12. If the test result was verified positive, inform the employee of any employee assistance program made available by the employer, as appropriate.
13. Offer to answer any further questions.
14. Give your name and telephone number in case the employee has any further questions or wishes to provide further information.

Source: Adapted from guidelines prepared by the DOT, Office of the Secretary, Office of Drug Enforcement and Program Compliance, 202-366-3784, 1992.

caine) for suturing skin lacerations. Because extremely high doses of ephedrine or l-methamphetamine (e.g., Vicks Inhaler) can cause a positive immunoassay screening, the MRO should request d- and l-isomer isolation on confirmed methamphetamine specimens with a level over 10,000 ng/ml. Ingestion of poppy seeds can cause high levels of urine opiates. The federal regulations require that verification of an opiate test as positive requires clinical confirmation of opiate abuse, or the identification of the heroin metabolite monoacetylmorphine (6-MAM). Clinical signs include medical history, physical findings, or behavior fitting DSM-III (Diagnostic and Statistical Manual of Mental Disorders, 3rd ed.) definitions of opiate abuse ascertained by a trained medical professional [19]. Medical review officers must determine whether quantitative levels are compatible with prescription drug use.

Another issue in MRO judgment involves the use of medication prescribed for one's spouse, child, or other relative or acquaintance. DOT recommends that these be verified as positive, that is, representing unauthorized use of controlled substances. Unless this issue is specifically addressed in company policy, consideration of whether spousal use is legitimate or unauthorized drug use remains an MRO

Employee name: _____
                    Last   First   Middle

Date of collection: _____

Employee SS or ID #: _____

Date positive result received: _____ Time: _____

Date of initial contact with employee: _____

Initial contact made by: _____

_____ Employee refused to discuss test result, declined interview with MRO

_____ Medical records are forthcoming. Date records to be available: _____

_____ Date MRO interview conducted: _____ Time: _____

_____ Date medical examination conducted (if applicable): _____

        Examining physician name: _____

_____ Address: _____ Phone #: _____

_____ Date re-test ordered (if applicable): _____

        Result and date received _____

_____ Date split analysis ordered (if applicable): _____

        Result and date received: _____

Comments/attempts to contact employee/Interview details: _____

_____

_____

_____

_____

Date employee notified of verified result: _____ Time: _____

Date employer notified of verified result: _____ Time: _____

Employer contact: _____

Date DOT agency notified of verified result

(if applicable): _____ Time: _____

Name of DOT agency and contact: _____

General comments: _____

_____

Verification Decision:

_____ Positive _____ Negative _____ Test canceled

Drug: _____

_____

Reason for test cancellation: _____

_____

_____   _____
MRO signature   Date

Figure 9-1. MRO Verification Work Sheet. (From guidelines prepared by the US DOT, Office of the Secretary, Office of Drug Enforcement and Program Compliance, 202-366-3784, 1992.)

judgment. It is best to resolve this issue in advance through consultation with the employer. This is also true regarding use of a dated prescription issued to the individual tested. It is important for the MRO to document evidence provided as substantiation of authorized drug use.

Once the tests have been verified as positive, negative, or canceled because of errors, the MRO must *report the results* to the employer. Verified positives may also be reported to designated EAP contacts or a federal management official with the power to recommend or take administrative action. Reporting should be in writing, with safeguards to protect confidentiality. Under federal programs, employers are not routinely entitled to quantitative results, but must be told the specific drug for which test results were positive. The completed custody and control forms should not be used for reporting results to the employer, because many forms will show laboratory positives that, because of legitimate medical use, were verified as negative.

DOT Alcohol Breath Testing

In the Omnibus Transportation Employee Testing Act of 1991, Congress mandated testing for misuse of alcohol as well as controlled substances in preemployment, random, reasonable suspicion, postaccident, and posttreatment testing in most transportation sectors. It also provided legislative authority for drug and alcohol testing for Mass Transit vehicle operators, controllers, and maintenance workers. The February 15, 1994 final rules require those subject to urine drug testing to also undergo alcohol breath testing [20]. In effect, these regulations broaden the previous deterrent program into a fitness-for-duty program. Individuals in qualified safety-sensitive functions will not be able to work (1) with breath alcohol concentrations of 0.04% or greater, (2) while their behavior or appearance indicates intoxication or impairment, (3) while using alcohol, or (4) within 4–8 hours after using alcohol. Employees involved in an accident will not be able to use alcohol until they have been tested or 8 hours have passed.

Employment alcohol tests may be conducted any time between the preplacement examination and initiation of the safety-sensitive functions. Postaccident testing will be required for employees whose performance could have contributed to an accident as soon as possible, preferably within 2 hours. Random tests may be given just before, during, or just after performing safety-sensitive functions. Reasonable suspicion testing will be based on the observations of a supervisor trained in recognizing signs of alcohol misuse. *For those returning to duty after evaluation and/or necessary rehabilitation, at least six tests will be required in the first 12 months.*

Tests must be conducted using evidential grade breath testing devices approved by the National Highway Transportation Safety Administration (NHTSA). Confirmation tests must provide a permanent record of results and identification of the individual tested (e.g., a printed result of sequentially numbered tests), be capable of testing blank air samples, and discriminate between alcohol and acetone, which can be produced by diabetics in ketoacidosis. Both initial screening and confirmation tests will be required, with a 15-minute wait between tests. The lower of the two results determines the consequence. Testing must be conducted by a trained, certified breath alcohol technician (BAT) who has demonstrated proficiency in a NHTSA-approved course. The DOT has also proposed that blood alcohol testing be permitted for postaccident and reasonable-suspicion testing when approved breath testing devices are not available.

Employees with alcohol concentrations of 0.04 or greater will be removed from *safety-sensitive duty.* Return to work will be permitted only after evaluation and rehabilitation, if indicated, as well as follow-up testing. The regulations call for removal from safety-sensitive duty if the alcohol concentration is between 0.02% and 0.04% for 8 hours or until the tested alcohol concentration falls below 0.02%. While cumbersome to implement, this two-tier provision underscores the DOT's concern that even low levels of alcohol are inconsistent with safety. Although correlated with blood alcohol levels, the breath alcohol results will stand on their own merit.

The new rules will affect a vastly expanded population of employees. Current DOT regulations require drug testing of an estimated 4.2 million Americans; the new rules will require both drug and alcohol testing of approximately 7.5 million people. Most significant is expansion to include all intrastate vehicle operators who hold a commercial driver's license, including school bus drivers and motor coach drivers. This program will be effective on January 1, 1995 for those with 50 or more safety-sensitive employees and on January 1, 1996 for smaller employers. Once alcohol testing is required of some employers, many others are also likely to begin testing.

Current Issues

Individual Privacy Versus Public Health and Safety

Drug testing programs must balance carefully the individual right to privacy and personal freedom versus public health and safety needs. The federal drug testing regulations seek to protect the individual against false accusation of illicit drug use and, in the collection process, to balance the right to privacy against unreasonable search and seizure. For this reason, directly witnessed specimen collection is permitted only in instances of likely specimen adulteration or substitution. Drug testing is also restricted to those in safety-sensitive jobs.

Although private sector drug testing is not restricted to those in safety-sensitive positions, health professionals are urged to be sensitive to privacy issues, to recognize that the vast majority of those tested are not illicit drug users, and to ensure each individual confidentiality and respect.

Specimen Dilution and Adulteration

A quarrelsome issue for MROs has been interpretation of dilute specimens. By water loading, a donor can reduce the specific gravity of urine to 1.002 or below and the creatinine to below 0.15 mg/ml. However, when a laboratory reports specimen as being both dilute and negative, DOT guidelines require that it be verified as a negative, rather than as a canceled test. In response to commercial urine specimen adulterants such as UrinAid and Mary Jane Superclean 13, laboratories are developing sophisticated adulteration panels. The DOT has issued guidance to all NIDA-certified laboratories urging reporting in three categories: Specific gravity < 1.003 and creatinine < 0.2 g/liter; Specimen not suitable; or Specimen adulterated for XYZ substance [20A]. If a specimen is not suitable for testing, MROs are encouraged to talk with the laboratory forensic toxicologist and with the donor. If a suitable explanation is not identified (e.g., use of nonsteroidal antiinflammatory agents), the MRO should report to the employer that another specimen should be collected under direct observation. If a specimen is reported adulterated, the MRO should report this to the employer along with the guidance that the laboratory finding constitutes a "refusal to be tested," requiring removal from safety-sensitive functions.

MRO Credentialing

Because of concerns about quality of MRO services, federal officials urged establishment of voluntary MRO credentialing and certification within the private sectors. Although MRO certification is not required by current federal regulations, physicians seeking to demonstrate their competence in a competitive marketplace and a litigious environment have shown strong interest in MRO credentialing. The Medical Review Officer Certification Council (MROCC) was established in 1992 by ACOEM; it has been joined by the American Medical Association, the American Academy of Family Practice, the College of American Pathologists, the American Society of Clinical Toxicologists, and other medical specialty societies. MROCC eligibility requires at least 12 hours of approved MRO training, followed by a rigorous certifying examination [21]. Certificates are valid for 5 years.

Evidence of Drug Testing Effectiveness

Many studies have shown a strong association between illicit drug use and increased absenteeism, accidents, injuries, disciplinary measures, and health care costs [8, 9, 22]. NIDA surveys indicate that the prevalence of drug use among high school seniors and employees dropped significantly from 1985 to 1991 [7]. The former is believed due to health education, the latter to a broad-based deterrent program, which includes education and drug testing. To date, few studies have looked at the ability of drug testing programs to reduce either the prevalence of drug use or consequent effects [23, 24]. The Federal Railroad Administration has noted a significant decrease in the number of accidents, accompanied by a steady drop in the rate of positive drug tests in postaccident testing [25]. Successful corporate case studies are reported by the Institute for a Drug-Free Workplace [26].

Americans with Disabilities Act

ADA excludes testing for controlled substances as a medical test, thus permitting drug testing at any time, including prior to an employment offer. Additionally, ADA distinguishes current and former drug users. Those who test positive are excluded from protection under ADA, but former drug users are protected. Employers may require periodic, unscheduled testing for a reasonable period of time to assure that former users are successfully rehabilitated. However, a positive test automatically voids ADA protection. Users of alcohol and drugs may also be held to the same performance standards in the workplace as all other employees, including attendance, productivity, and conduct.

On-site Testing

Although on-site testing is permitted under the NRC fitness-for-duty program, it is not allowed under other federal agency regulations. However, on-site screening can be valuable for highly safety-sensitive jobs in the unregulated private sector. Employees testing positive can immediately be removed from duty pending results of confirmation tests.

Choice of Drug Panel

Even when testing only for the NIDA-5, considerable MRO dialogue is required with those testing positive. However, employers often seek to reduce accidents, injuries, absenteeism, and increased medical costs caused by inappropriate use of other controlled substances and prescription drugs not covered by current federal regulations. Quality medical review becomes essential when testing for more commonly used drugs such as barbiturates and benzodiazepines.

Screening Cutoff Levels

A 1989 NIDA consensus conference recommended reducing screening levels for marijuana from 100 to 50 ng/ml and cocaine from 300 to 150 ng/ml [27]. NIDA has subsequently proposed adoption of the 50 ng/ml marijuana cutoff level [28]. Estimated impact of cutting the marijuana screening level in half is a 10% increase of marijuana positives. Preliminary results of toxicology studies to determine the impact of lower screening levels on those exposed to sidestream crack cocaine smoke show little likelihood of detection, even at lower cutoff levels.

Hair Analysis

Most toxicologists do not believe that this technology has been sufficiently validated to replace urinalysis. Issues that hold back this technology include challenges of standardization; blind specimen quality control; uncertain impact of shampoos, permanents, and other adulterants and secondary exposure on results; and the fact that many collection techniques require pulling hairs from their roots, hardly a noninvasive procedure.

Conclusions

This chapter has briefly reviewed the wide-ranging area of drug and alcohol testing, laboratory analyses, and medical review of results. Because drug testing programs cannot assure a drug-free workplace, the importance of EAPs cannot be overemphasized. Well-trained MROs should be an integral part of any drug testing program.

As drug testing expands among employees, litigation will increase, placing the urine collection facility, laboratory, and MRO at growing risk.

A positive drug test identifies an individual to be at high risk of impaired work performance. However, a positive test means only the presence of a drug above the cutoff level at the time of testing. It does not mean that the individual was under the influence, impaired, addicted, or an abuser of substances. Furthermore, the quantitative test result cannot distinguish between the recreational user and the drug addict. Occupational health professionals need to help employers understand these limitations.

Alcohol and drug abuse often reflect dissatisfaction with one's life, be it personal or at work. Employers must seek ways to foster healthier work environments filled with challenge, support, creativity, and human concern—in short, high-level wellness. Addressing these issues will help solve the "drug problem" our society faces.

References

1. ACOEM Committee Report. Drug screening in the workplace: Ethical guidelines. *J. Occup. Med.* 33: 651, 1991.
2. Peterson, K. Employee drug screening: Issues to be resolved in implementing a program. *Clin. Chem.* 33:54B, 1987.
3. Department of Health and Human Services; Alcohol, Drug Abuse, and Mental Health Administration. Mandatory guidelines for Federal Workplace Drug Testing Programs; Final guidelines. *Fed. Register* 53(69):11979, April 11, 1988.
4. US Department of Transportation, Office of the Secretary. Procedures for Transportation Workplace Drug Testing Programs; Final rule. *Fed. Register* 54(230):49854, December 1, 1989. See also Interim final rule. Federal Highway Administration. *Fed. Register* 55(22):3546, February 1, 1990.
5. *Skinner v. Railway Labor Executives Association,* 109th Supreme Court, 1989.
6. US Department of Labor, Bureau of Labor Statistics. *Survey of Employer Anti-drug Programs.* Washington, DC, Report 760, 1989.
7. NIDA Capsules. *Population Estimates of Lifetime and Current Drug Use, 1991; 1991 National Household Survey of Drug Abuse.* Rockville, MD: National Institute on Drug Abuse, December 1991.
8. Zwerling, C., Ryan, J., and Orav, E. J. The efficacy of preemployment drug screening for marijuana and cocaine in predicting employment outcome. *J.A.M.A.* 264:2639, 1990.
9. Sheridan, J. R., and Winkler, H. An Evaluation of Drug Testing in the Workplace. In S. W. Gust and J. M. Walsh (eds.), *Drugs in the Workplace: Research and Evaluation Data.* NIDA Research Monograph 91. US Department of Health and Human Services; Alcohol, Drug Abuse, and Mental Health Administration; National Institute on Drug Abuse, 1989. Pp. 195–216.
10. Judge, W. J. *"Outside the Circle": The Impact of Drug Testing on Workers' Compensation.* Tort and Insurance Practice Section, American Bar Association, 1991.
11. US Department of Transportation, Federal Highway Administration. 49 CFR 391.41-391.49. Subpart E: Physical Qualifications and Examinations, and subpart F: Files and Records.
12. US Nuclear Regulatory Commission. Fitness-for-duty programs; final rule and statement of policy. *Fed. Register* 54(108):24468, June 7, 1989.
13. See *Specimen Collection Workbook.* US Department of Transportation, Office of the Secretary, Washington, DC, May 1992. See also *Employer's Guide to 49 CFR Part 40: Procedures for Transportation Workplace Drug Testing Programs.* US Department of Transportation, October 1990.
14. Knisely, R. *Operating Guidance for DOT Mandated Drug Testing Programs.* US Department of Transportation, Office of the Secretary, June 1, 1992.
15. DHHS. *Medical Review Officer Manual: A Guide to Evaluating Urine Drug Analysis.* Washington, DC: US Department of Health and Human Services, National Institute on Drug Abuse, September 1988. *This is now outdated, but an updated version is being prepared.*
16. DOT. *Medical Review Officer Guide.* Washington, DC: US Department of Transportation, Office of the Secretary, October 1990.
17. Peterson, K. W. *Medical Review Officer Information Handbook.* Arlington Heights, IL: American College of Occupational and Environmental Medicine, 1990 (updated 1993).

18. Swotinsky, R. *The Medical Review Officer's Guide to Drug Testing.* New York: Van Nostrand Reinhold, 1992.
19. *Diagnostic Criteria from DSM-III.* Washington, DC: American Psychiatric Association, 1982.
20. Department of Transportation. Drug and Alcohol Testing Programs; Final Rules. *Fed. Register* 59(31):7302–7625, February 15, 1994.
20A. Smith, Donna R. US Department of Transportation, Office of the Secretary. *Certified Drug Testing Laboratories and Medical Review Officers* (memorandum to the Department of Health and Human Services). December 9, 1993.
21. Medical Review Officer Certification Council, 55 W. Seegers Rd., Arlington Heights, IL 60005, 708-228-6850.
22. Crouch, D. J., et al. A Critical Evaluation of the Utah Power and Light Company's Substance Abuse Management Program: Absenteeism, Accidents and Costs. In S. W. Gust and J. M. Walsh (eds.), *Drugs in the Workplace: Research and Evaluation Data.* NIDA Research Monograph 91, US Department of Health and Human Services; Alcohol, Drug Abuse and Mental Health Administration, 1989. Pp. 169–193.
23. Zwerling, C., and Ryan, J. Pre-employment drug screening: The epidemiologic issues. *J. Occup. Med.* 34:595, 1992.
24. Upfal, M., and Peterson, K. W. Pre-employment drug screening: The epidemiological issues (letter to the editor, with response by the authors). *J. Occup. Med.* 35:8, 1993.
25. Federal Railroad Administration, Office of Safety. Reducing Substance Abuse in the Railroad Industry—A Success Story (unpublished). Presented to the 71st Annual Meeting of the Transportation Research Board, 1992.
26. Current, W. F. *Does Drug Testing Work?* Institute for a Drug-Free Workplace, 1301 K St., NW, Washington, DC 20005, 1993.
27. *Consensus Report: Technical, Scientific and Procedural Issues of Employee Drug Testing.* DHHS Publication (ADM) 90-1684, 1990.
28. Department of Health and Human Services, Substance Abuse and Mental Health Services Administration. Mandatory guidelines for federal workplace drug testing programs: Notice of proposed revisions. *Fed. Register* 58(14):6063, January 25, 1993.

Further Information

The National Institute on Drug Abuse has funded many valuable research studies, sponsored research conferences, and published many results. Research findings are reported in the NIDA Research Monograph Series. Of note are no.73, *Urine Testing for Drugs of Abuse* (1986); no.91, *Drugs in the Workplace: Research and Evaluation Data* (1989); no.92, *Testing for Abuse Liability of Drugs in Humans* (1989); no.94, *Pharmacology and Toxicology of Amphetamine and Related Designer Drugs* (1989); no.100 *Drugs in the Workplace: Research and Evaluation Data,* vol. II (1990); no.101, *Residual Effects of Abused Drugs on Behavior* (1990); no.106, *Improving Drug Abuse Treatment* (1991); and no.123, *Acute Cocaine Intoxication: Current Methods of Treatment* (1992).

NIDA Capsules. Published by the Press Office of NIDA, 5600 Fischer's Lane, Rockville, MD 20857.
These contain current information on drug use, for example, summaries of NIDA's National Household Surveys on Drug Abuse, National High School Senior Survey, Drug Abuse Warning Network, and National Drug Abuse Treatment Survey.

NIDA's toll-free *Workplace Helpline* (1-800-843-4971).
The Helpline provides consultation to health professionals, employers, and labor representatives on developing drug-free workplace policies and programs. It is linked to the National Clearinghouse for Alcohol and Drug Information (1-800-729-6686), which provides model policies, available publications, and even literature searches, and lends videotapes on drugs in the workplace.

Peterson, K. W. (ed.). *The Medical Review Officer Information Handbook.* Published by the American College of Occupational and Environmental Medicine, 55 W. Seegers Rd., Arlington Heights, IL 60005.
This is an expanded syllabus for ACOEM's ongoing Urine Drug Testing and MRO Training course. The Handbook is updated every 6 months to contain the latest available information in this rapidly evolving field.

Swotinsky, R. B. (ed.). *The Medical Review Officer's Guide to Drug Testing.* New York: Van Nostrand Reinhold, 1992.
Contains chapters on drug abuse in the workplace, drug testing, drug testing collection procedures, forensic laboratory drug testing, the MRO function, risk management, employee assistance programs, monitoring laboratory performance, case studies, and several key federal regulations.

Appendix to Chapter 9: ACOEM Drug Screening in the Workplace: Ethical Guidelines*

Drug and alcohol abuse constitute a significant problem in the workplace, contributing to impaired productivity and job performance, increased accidents and injuries, violations of security, theft of company property, and diminished employee morale. The federal government and many companies have adopted policies regarding the use of drugs, as well as instituting a variety of drug screening, control, and rehabilitation programs.

Appropriate constraints must be observed in order to ethically screen employees and prospective employees for the presence in their bodies of drugs, including alcohol, that might affect ability to perform work in a safe manner.

The following guidelines deal only with ethical issues involved in drug screening in the workplace. Other important considerations that must be addressed in the design and implementation of a drug screening program include biologic factors concerning rates of absorption and elimination of drugs, technical factors relating to specificity and accuracy of analyses, legal safeguards, regulatory requirements, and employee relations concerns.

ACOEM recommends strongly that employers obtain expert legal, medical, and employee relations advice before making a decision to require screening of employees or applicants for drugs. Such experts also should be involved in the actual structuring and implementation of any program of screening of employees and applicants for drugs.

These guidelines are pertinent to drug testing done under the following circumstances: preplacement assessment; job transfer evaluation; periodic mandatory medical surveillance; postincident/accident, for-reasonable-cause, and random testing of those in safety and security-sensitive positions; special work fitness examinations; and monitoring of employees who are under treatment for drug abuse, including alcohol, as a condition of continuing employment. . . .

The following features should be included in any program for the screening of employees and prospective employees for drugs:

1. A written company policy and procedure concerning drug use and screening for the presence of drugs should exist and be applied impartially.
2. The reason for any requirement for screening for drugs should be clearly documented. Such reasons might involve safety for the individual, other employees, or the public; security needs; or requirements related to job performance.
3. Affected employees and applicants should be informed in advance about the company's policy concerning drug use and screening. They should be made aware of their right to refuse such screening and the consequences of such refusal to their employment.
4. Where special safety or security needs justify testing for drugs on an unannounced and possibly random basis, employees should be made aware in advance that this will be done from time to time. Care should be taken to assure that such tests are done in a uniform and impartial manner for all employees in the affected group(s).
5. Written consent for screening and for communication of results to the employer should be obtained from each individual prior to screening.
6. Collection, transportation, and analysis of the specimens and the reporting of the results should meet stringent legal, technical, and ethical requirements. The process should be under the supervision of a licensed physician.
7. A licensed physician who is qualified as a medical review officer should eval-

*From ACOEM Committee Report. Drug screening in the workplace: Ethical guidelines. *J. Occup. Med.* 33:651, 1991.

uate positive results before a report is made to the employer. This may require the obtaining of supplemental information from the employee or applicant in order to ensure that a positive test result does not represent appropriate use of prescription drugs, over-the-counter medication, or other substances that could cause a positive test. Training of the medical review officer should include the pharmacology of substance abuse, laboratory testing methodology and quality control, forensic toxicology, pertinent federal regulations, legal and ethical requirements, chemical dependency illness, employee assistance programs, and rehabilitation.

8. The affected employee or applicant should be advised of positive results by the physician and have the opportunity for explanation and discussion prior to the reporting of results to the employer, if feasible. The mechanism for accomplishing this should be clearly defined.

9. The employee or applicant having indication of a drug abuse problem should be advised concerning appropriate treatment resources.

10. Any report to the employer should provide only the information needed for work placement purposes or as required by government regulations. Identification to the employer of the particular drug(s) found and quantitative levels is not necessary, unless required by law. Reports to the employer should be made by a physician sensitive to the various considerations involved.

The use of a drug screen as part of a voluntary periodic examination program can be acceptable ethically if adequate safeguards as to confidentiality can be assured. It seems probable at present that inclusion of a drug screen as part of a voluntary periodic examination program may lead to a significant reduction in participation, with consequent loss to the nonparticipants, of the benefits of the examination. Potential health benefits should be carefully weighed against potential losses to health before a decision is reached on this matter.

If carefully designed and carried out, programs for the screening of employees and applicants for drugs, including alcohol, serve to protect and improve employee health and safety in an ethically acceptable manner.

American College of Occupational and Environmental Medicine
Approved by Board of Directors
February 9, 1991

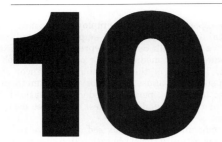

Accreditation of Occupational Health Clinical Centers

Dennis Schultz and
Jack Richman

Accreditation is a process often used to certify that an organization meets certain criteria. The accreditation body must have a defined *set of standards* that represent value or excellence, and a *defined process* by which the organization's performance is judged against these standards. Usually the organization applying for accreditation begins its preparation with a program of evaluation and improvement. It obtains the standard and performs a comprehensive self-assessment, reviewing its policies, procedures, and practices. The organization identifies deficiencies, improves these areas, and repeats its evaluation to assure improvement. Once this process is completed, the organization requests that the accrediting body evaluate its program. Usually the accrediting body conducts an on-site survey with independent auditors.

Medical organizations may pursue accreditation for a variety of reasons. In some cases, the sole motivation may be to improve operations and quality of care. Here, the value of accreditation will depend on several elements: first, the relevance of the standards to the specific medical organization; second, the emphasis of the standards on assuring and improving quality of care; third, the amount of consultative assistance provided by the accreditation organization in the process of performing the audit. In other cases, the organization's primary goal may be financial: assuring reimbursement, expanding market shares, or reducing insurance premiums. Here, the value of accreditation depends on the credibility and prestige of the accrediting body, specifically whether accreditation assures payment or financial gain. Based on experience with hospitals, accreditation only becomes widespread when it is linked to reimbursement. Ideally, accreditation meets the needs of all organizations by enhancing the quality of care and by providing certification useful in improving the organization's financial situation. Financial gain may be the motivating factor to pursue accreditation but improvement in mission is the final result.

The American College of Occupational and Environmental Medicine (ACOEM) has considered the issues surrounding accreditation and has concluded that it is an important element in improving the quality and effectiveness of patient care. Specifically, ACOEM supports the development of standards of practice, the achievement of these standards through self-evaluation, and the participation in accreditation to demonstrate that the standards have been met. These statements are included in ACOEM's *Policy Manual* [1]. The organization has pursued matters further. After reviewing existing accreditation programs, ACOEM chose in 1987 to become a member of the Accreditation Association for Ambulatory Health Care (AAAHC). This decision formally recognized AAAHC as the accrediting body for occupational health services. Together, ACOEM and AAAHC developed standards specifically for occupational health services. The quality of these standards further increases the value of accreditation. Currently, ACOEM has two representatives on AAAHC's Board of Directors. These individuals are active in the executive, accreditation, and standards and policy committees [2].

Other organizations provide accreditation for ambulatory services or guidance in establishing occupational health services. Interested readers are referred to Yodaiken and Zeitz's article on accreditation [3], the comments by ACOEM's occupational medicine practice committee on resources in quality assurance [4], or the publication of the American Association of Occupational Health Nurses on establishing occupational health services [5]. The exclusive focus of this chapter is AAAHC's accreditation process and standards as they relate to the delivery of occupational health services.

The Accreditation Association for Ambulatory Health Care

AAAHC is a nonprofit corporation whose goal is to assist ambulatory health care organizations in providing high-quality care in the most efficient and economically sound manner possible. AAAHC achieves its goal through a voluntary, peer-based accreditation program that is focused on education and counseling.

The organization was founded in 1979, though its charter members had been involved in accreditation issues since the mid-1960s. The development of AAAHC was prompted by a reorganization of the Joint Commission for the Accreditation of Hospitals (now the Joint Commission on Accreditation of Healthcare Organizations). The reorganization eliminated the Council for Ambulatory Health Care and replaced it with technical and consulting services. Believing that this was inadequate, several organizations that were involved with the Joint Commission joined together to form AAAHC. The charter members included the American Group Practice Association, the Group Health Association of America, the Medical Group Management Association, the Freestanding Ambulatory Surgical Association, the American College Health Association, and the National Association of Community Health Care Centers.

Currently, 12 organizations comprise AAAHC, with several others endorsing AAAHC accreditation for their members. ACOEM became a member in 1987. In 1989, AAAHC developed a formal affiliation with the California Medical Association to conduct ambulatory care accreditation.

During its relatively brief tenure, AAAHC has become a leader in ambulatory accreditation. Its certification has been recognized and accepted by a variety of third-party payers who require such credentialing. Examples include Blue Cross and Blue Shield plans, commercial carriers, health maintenance organizations, and governmental agencies. In addition, some major professional liability carriers discount premiums to organizations accredited by AAAHC.

Accreditation Under AAAHC

Criteria used by AAAHCs are published in their *Accreditation Handbook for Ambulatory Health Care 1992–1993 Edition.* This booklet represents the efforts of thousands of experts in the delivery of ambulatory health care. The current edition, written in 1991, is the sixth major revision since 1979. (All comments in this chapter relate to the 1992–93 edition.)

The standards comprise about half of this 70-page document. Background information, appendices, and self-directed questionnaires constitute the remainder of the booklet. Unlike the Occupational Safety and Health Administration (OSHA) or other federal standards, those of AAAHC are brief, simple, and clearly written. The format, which is the same for each standard, begins with one or two opening sentences defining and setting goals for the service or entity. Next it lists a series of "characteristics of accreditable organizations," which delineate specific objectives. Most of the standards are written in general terms, unless there are limited ways of achieving compliance, in which case specific guidelines are noted.

There are 22 individual standards, which are divided into two groups: core and adjunct. *Core* standards apply to *all* organizations and address issues common to ambulatory health care delivery, such as administration, facilities, and records. *Adjunct* standards address specific services or activities and only apply if the organization is active in these areas. One of the adjunct standards is occupational health services. This arrangement of core and adjunct standards provides consistency between ambulatory health care organizations and specific guidance for organizations offering specialized services. The standards can be applied to any occupational health program, whether in-plant, solo, or group practice or hospital based.

Survey Eligibility

AAAHC's goal is to provide quality accreditation services to a wide variety of ambulatory health care organizations. This goal is reflected in the eligibility requirements for accreditation surveys, which are summarized as follows: The organization's primary activity must be provision of health services and it must have been in operation for at least 6 months. Either the organization or its parent organization must be a formally organized, legal entity. If required, the organization must be licensed to provide services and be in compliance with appropriate regulations. For occupational health services, medical care must be under the direction or supervision of a physician(s). The health care organization must also share facilities, equipment, and patient care records among its members providing patient care.

Survey Process

Preparation for the survey starts with a review of the *Self-Assessment Manual* produced by AAAHC. This 100-page book serves as a blueprint to assess an organization's current status and to guide the effort to achieve the standards. Much of the *Manual* consists of AAAHC standards subdivided into component parts. The organization completes a checklist that rates its current level of compliance on a five-point scale for each component. The *Manual* also provides work sheets to guide the organization in assessing and improving performance. Although AAAHC standards do not require these specific steps to achieve compliance, the outline in the *Manual* provides a reasonable approach for most organizations.

The *first step* of the self-assessment process is creation of a committee or team. Collectively, the members of this team should be knowledgeable about all aspects of the organization's operations, be capable of implementing change, and be committed to the process of self-assessment and accreditation. Once the committee is formed, it identifies a chairperson and divides primary responsibilities for the standards among its members. These individuals enlist the support of other organization members, begin the process of assessment, and plan for needed changes. One of the goals at this step of the process is to involve as much of the organization as possible. Ultimately, everyone will be affected by the accreditation process. Through regular meetings, the team creates a timetable for the project and monitors progress.

The self-assessment process may take months to years depending on the status of the organization. Certain of AAAHC standards require that programs be in place long enough to demonstrate effectiveness. In fact, it may take a year to gather sufficient information to demonstrate that it is actually effective, especially if the organization has not been involved in any quality assurance activities. AAAHC also provides consulting services to help organizations identify and correct areas of deficiencies. Once the self-assessment is completed, the organization obtains, completes, and submits the *Presurvey Questionnaire,* a 49-page document published by AAAHC. Responses to these questions form the basis for AAAHC recommendations about the structure and timing of the survey.

The survey consists of an extensive on-site evaluation of the organization's policies, procedures and operations. The process relies heavily on the abilities of AAAHC surveyors, who are volunteers, chosen and trained by AAAHC. Surveyors may be practicing administrators or health care providers, selected based on their knowledge and experience. AAAHC training focuses on using the surveyors' experience to evaluate the organization and to apply the standards fairly. The specific surveyors are selected based on characteristics of the organization to be reviewed. Therefore, occupational health professionals, knowledgeable and experienced in the field, are used for occupational health site visits.

The duration of the review and the number of surveyors are determined by the characteristics of the organization. The manner in which the survey is performed is determined by the AAAHC in consultation with the organization. Organizations with multiple service sites may have all or a representative sample of locations surveyed. The Association strives to minimize the impact of the survey on the organization's day-to-day operation.

A *primary goal* of the surveyors is to determine if the organization is in compliance with the intent of the standards. The surveyors use a variety of information to assess the extent of compliance, such as written documentation of policy and procedure manuals, patient chart reviews, internal audit information, and answers to detailed questions concerning implementation. Surveyors also use information from interviews, observations from the on-site visit, and public comment. The organization must demonstrate that it understands and has implemented the standards. It must also show that its day-to-day operations are consistent with its internal policies and procedures. Compliance with the standard must be evident in both policy and action.

A second goal of the surveyors is to educate and provide consultation to the organization. The surveyors have a formal meeting with representatives of the organization at the end of the site visit. At the meeting, they discuss their findings, answer questions, and make suggestions for improvement. The surveyors' written report and conclusions are submitted to the Accreditation Committee of the Board of Directors of AAAHC, who determine whether the organization is accredited.

Accreditation can be granted for either 1 or 3 years. AAAHC can also decide to defer accreditation if there are deficiencies that are likely to be corrected within 6 months. A third option is to register the survey as a consultation, which occurs if AAAHC finds that the standards are not appropriate for the facility. Lastly, AAAHC may deny accreditation. There is a formal policy for appeals and the organization can apply for reevaluation immediately. The organization receives a *Survey Report Form,* which outlines the survey findings, as well as a *Survey Evaluation Form,* which it uses to critique the accreditation process. The cost of the survey depends on the number of surveyors and the days required to complete on-site activities.

AAAHC Standards

Core Standards

The following eight topics constitute AAAHC's core standards. All organizations must be in compliance with these standards.

Patient Rights
The first of the core standards addresses patients' rights, specifically the obligations of the organization to the patient. It requires that the organization protect the patient's dignity and confidentiality, provide the patient with proper information about his or her medical condition, encourage patient participation in medical decisions, and inform the patient of respective rights and responsibilities. Specific examples include the organization's policy concerning payment, provision of after-hour care, and the accuracy of its advertising. The patient must be informed of the right to change physicians and to refuse treatment.

Governance
The second standard addresses governance, the organization, and activities of the facility's governing body. It delineates the basic responsibilities of a governing body, such as setting the missions, goals, and objectives for the organization, assuring adequate facilities and personnel, determining organizational structure, and adopting policies and procedures. Other areas of responsibility are physician appointments and credentialing, risk assessment, bloodborne pathogens policy, and staff improvement. The governing body must also provide for full disclosure of ownership.

Administration
The third core standard notes that the organization must be administered in a manner that assures quality health care and is consistent with its mission, goals, and objectives. Many topics in this standard are similar to those in governance; however, the focus is on *executing* the policies and procedures. Issues addressed include the *enforcement* of policies, steps taken to comply with applicable laws, and the method of evaluating performance. The standard also requires assessment of patient satisfaction.

Quality of Care
The fourth core standard requires that the organization provide high-quality, cost-conscious health care. The majority of the standard addresses medical management issues such as accuracy of diagnosis, appropriateness of treatment and referrals, and duplication of services. Generally, these types of questions are addressed through patient chart audits. The standard also addresses training and credentialing of health care providers and mandates that the organization provide translators when needed.

Quality Assurance
The fifth core standard is titled *Quality Assurance Program.* Like the previous standard, it addresses quality of care issues; however, the standard is much more comprehensive. It mandates that the organization have an active, organized, peer-based program dedicated to improving professional practice, administrative practice,

and patient outcomes. The standard requires collection and evaluation of data concerning important aspects of the care as well as the development of criteria by which providers judge their performance. It also delineates characteristics of quality assurance activities and provides a questionnaire to guide quality assurance program analysis.

Clinical Records
The sixth core standard addresses all aspects of medical records from legibility to confidentiality. The standard notes the type of information that should be included for any clinical encounter, that telephone contacts be documented, and that records be managed properly. The *Handbook* includes a clinical record work sheet to guide the assessment of clinical care and medical records.

Professional Improvement
The seventh core standard discusses professional improvement. The organization must strive to improve the competence and skills of its members. Issues include continuing education, support for library services, and credentialing.

Facilities and Environment
The last of the core standards addresses the adequacy of the organization's own facilities and its safety procedures. Included in this standard are accommodations for individuals with disabilities, parking issues, smoking policy, appropriate design of patient areas and examination rooms, the organization's hazardous material program, and facilities maintenance.

Adjunct Standards

AAAHC has 14 adjunct standards, each addressing a different clinical activity or service. The individual standard is only applied if it pertains to an activity of the organization. Following are summaries of several of these standards, beginning with the one on occupational health services.

Occupational Health Services
The most pertinent of the adjunct standards is occupational health services. This set of criteria was developed by ACOEM and adopted by AAAHC. The opening statement sets the goals of occupational health services as assuring a safe and healthy workplace through the recognition, evaluation, and control of illness and injury in or from the workplace. The organization must also meet the needs of the employees.

The standard itself contains 12 points, which are summarized below.

1. Services must be in compliance with all pertinent regulations including the Occupational Safety and Health Act and workers' compensation laws. This point was written before the enactment of the Americans with Disabilities Act, which should also be addressed.
2. Individuals providing services must be appropriately trained, have necessary skills, and be knowledgeable about the work environment and the specific risks for the individual patient.
3. Individuals must have access to reference materials and an occupational health physician.
4. Continuing education in occupational health is specifically required.
5. Medical management includes consideration of the relationship of the patient's condition to work, the effect of the condition on fitness for duty, and consideration of disability status.
6. Medical care should strive to minimize disability and restore function as soon as possible.
7. If the patient is off work, the health care provider should consider issues regarding his or her safe return to work. This assessment includes the prognosis for functional improvement, the potential hazards that may interfere with a return to work, and ways to reduce these hazards.
8. Preplacement examinations must consider both the patient's medical status and the work demands. Therefore, both the employee and health provider must know the essential job functions and workplace conditions. All findings and recommendations should be reviewed with the employee; the employer should be informed of the recommendations.

9. Medical surveillance examinations should be appropriately timed to identify adverse health effects of workplace exposures. Employees should be informed of findings and the relationship of these to work. The employers should be advised of any adverse health effects from work exposures and any recommendations regarding risk reduction. In addition, the services should educate the employee about the potential hazards of their workplace and about methods to reduce the risk. This role includes consideration of lifestyle habits, if the habits may affect the risk of workplace exposures.

10. Information that does not relate to the employee's ability to safely perform the job must be handled as confidential and only be released with proper consent, and only if there is a need to know.

11. The organization's records management system must be able to report health surveillance data and any other statutory requirements.

12. If the occupational medicine (OM) service is a subunit within a larger organization, the organization's management must demonstrate that it understands and supports the services provided.

Immediate/Urgent Care Services

A second adjunct standard is applied if the organization provides urgent or immediate medical care. This standard requires that the organization be accurate in describing its services, that it only sees patients who can be appropriately treated in an urgent care setting, and that it has appropriate staff and facilities.

Testing: Diagnostic Imaging and Laboratory Services

AAAHC has two different adjunct standards covering diagnostic testing. The first addresses imaging, such as radiographs, and the second pathology and laboratory testing. The basic issues in both standards are the same. They consider professional staffing, facilities, and administrative policies covering operations, safety, record management, and quality assurance.

Other Professional and Technical Services

Services such as occupational therapy, physical therapy, psychological services, health education, and audiology are covered by an adjunct standard titled Other Professional and Technical Services. The standard is general and brief. It notes that services must be appropriate to the needs of the patient, there must be appropriate staffing and facilities, and evaluation of the services must be consistent with the AAAHC standards.

Other Standards

There are nine other adjunct standards. Some of these may also apply to organizations that provide occupational health services. Individual standards cover emergency, pharmaceutical, surgical, and anesthesia services; teaching and publication activities; research activities; and others.

Problem Areas in Achieving Accreditation

If organizations encounter problems in accreditation, it is usually in one of three areas: clinical records, quality assurance, or occupational health services.

Clinical Records

Deficiencies in medical records are among the most common problems seen in surveys. The clinical record work sheet in the *Handbook* provides 16 specific areas that are used to judge care and medical records. The standard indicates that records must be legible, accurate, current, and accessible, and have a common format. All information, including test reports, dictated notes, and hospitalization records, must be reviewed. In addition, the chart must clearly note allergies. Problems can arise in any of these areas, but *a common problem is failing to adequately document the patient encounter.*

The medical record is the most common source of information about patient care. It is used by all accrediting bodies including the AAAHC. In order to evaluate care, the medical records must provide sufficient detail so that an outside reviewer can (1) determine the patient's primary complaint, (2) independently confirm the patient's diagnosis based on reported findings, (3) confirm that the treatment was appropriate and necessary, and (4) confirm that the patient's care was appropriate over time. Records must be complete and legible.

The specific solutions for charting deficiencies vary from one practice setting to the next. Practitioners must be convinced that documentation is important. In addition, they usually need to be reminded of its importance. Charts and forms can be designed in ways to facilitate documentation. Dictation equipment can reduce the inconvenience of writing lengthy notes. Both measures have been employed to improve documentation. Fortunately, deficiencies in documentation are easy to identify and can usually be solved with a minimum of effort. Unfortunately, organizations generally have to institute an ongoing program to assure that the improvement is maintained.

Quality Assurance

A second common area of noncompliance is quality assurance. The primary reason for this shortcoming is that the standard is demanding. It mandates that organizations continuously evaluate their performance and strive to improve the quality, effectiveness, and efficiency of care. They further require that this be done through an organized, peer-based quality assurance program and that the program be an integral part of the administrative and medical practice. AAAHC does not dictate the structure of the program, but carefully documents the characteristics of acceptable programs.

Structure

Successful programs require commitment and participation from the entire organization, starting with the governing body, which must assume ultimate responsibility for the program. The basis for the program must be a written statement adopted by the organization, which should delineate the program's content, structure, and function. Important points include identifying who is responsible, how often the program reports to the governing body, and how program recommendations are translated into improvements in operations. Because the program is based on peer review, at least two physicians must be involved. The standard includes a provision that there is adequate staff to support the program's function.

The actual structure of the programs will vary substantially. Larger organizations may have a several-tiered program with a single committee monitoring all activities; topic subcommittees addressing utilization management, departmental issues, or ongoing monitoring programs; and study groups addressing specific questions. Small organizations may have several individuals who discuss and manage all concerns.

Content Areas

The nature of successful quality assurance programs is that they are comprehensive in approach, content, and participation. All staff must be involved including professional and administrative. All aspects of the organization's operations must be considered: clinical, administrative, and cost of care. Moreover, there must be provisions for addressing all types of concerns or potential concerns.

The organization must institute ongoing monitoring for important aspects of care, for example, medical records, adverse outcomes, and satisfaction surveys. This responsibility requires ongoing collection and analysis of data to identify trends. Judging patient care activities also requires that practitioners develop criteria to evaluate the effectiveness of treatment. These documents represent ongoing projects because they are continuously discussed and modified, based on research and the data collected.

Quality Assurance Studies

Central to the process of quality assurance is the Quality Assurance Study. These studies apply research principles to analyze a problem, management principles to implement a corrective change, and surveillance principles to assure that the measure is effective. In many cases, repeat assessments are done to assure that the effect is lasting. The initial step in these studies is defining and quantifying the issue in measurable terms. Effectiveness of an influenza immunization program may be measured in lost workdays of immunized versus nonimmunized employees. Effectiveness of a new medical record protocol may be a decrease in the number of charts returned to records without a signature. Next, an intervention is implemented to correct the problem. The situation is reevaluated to assure that the change has been effective. If a problem persists, the process is repeated. Finally, the results must be documented and reported.

Many organizations find it difficult to perform adequate quality assurance studies. The key for success is to be broad in considering areas for improvement and solutions, but narrow in the scope of the study itself. The simpler the study and more easily defined the outcome, the higher the likelihood of success. Multiple studies implementing small changes are generally more effective than a large study with multiple interventions and outcomes. An organization's first quality assurance study is always the most difficult. Once the organization sets precedent by completing its first sound study, additional studies become much easier.

Practice Guidelines

Standards of care are important elements of quality assurance programs; however, some physicians are reluctant to participate in any program that may develop such standards. The rationale for their concern varies. In some cases, physicians believe that guidelines will substitute "cookbook" medicine for clinical judgment. Alternatively they may be concerned that the process is attempting to identify individuals for punitive measures. Neither is true. Practice guidelines attempt to create a template for the best quality care for patients. Clinical judgment is required in developing the guidelines, which may need to be modified and applied to specific patients.

Developing guidelines relies on aggregate data that summarize the experience with many patients. They do not rely on data from a single physician. Furthermore, guideline development focuses on *processes,* not on individuals. An example may clarify these points. An initial quality assurance study notes wide variations in physical therapy utilization from one satellite facility to the next. An additional study shows that the prime determinant of these differences is physician prescribing patterns. This concern initiates meetings of physicians and therapists to discuss the effectiveness and role of physical therapy treatment. After a literature review and further discussion, the practitioners develop a draft criteria for prescribing therapy and a standardized method for monitoring patient progress. Additional information is gathered and the practitioners review the results to determine the effectiveness of treatment. The criteria are modified and evolve. In the process, physicians learn more about physical therapy and both physicians and therapists develop a better working relationship. As knowledge increases, variations in practice patterns decrease and the physicians' understanding of quality, cost-effective treatment improves. Eventually the criteria become an internal practice guideline that continues to be discussed and modified periodically.

Occupational Health Services

Prevention

Another problem area is the occupational health standard itself. The focus of this standard is prevention, whereas the focus of all other standards is treatment. This difference, combined with an emphasis on workplace hazards, demands a different approach to assessing occupational health services. If clinics fail to identify the difference, they will not comply with this standard. The goal of occupational health service is to assure a safe and healthy workplace, which requires identification, evaluation, and reduction of workplace hazards. The only way of accomplishing this task is through understanding of the workplace and the potential hazards. Thus, the standard requires education in occupational health and knowledge of the patient's specific work environment, which must be applied to all aspects of patient care.

For example, job titles usually do not provide enough information for preplacement examinations to be performed. One "fork lift operator" may never lift weights in excess of 10 lb and work in a dust-free environment. Another "fork lift operator" may routinely lift 50 lb while wearing a respirator. "Foundry work" can run the spectrum from high physical demands under harsh and hazardous work conditions to light physical demands under nonhazardous conditions. In order to make meaningful suggestions regarding placement, health care providers must understand the worker's job and the workplace environment.

If practitioners perform surveillance examinations, they must be knowledgeable about the type of work performed and the potential exposure. If the surveillance examination is prompted by exposure to lead, the practitioner should understand the significance of blood lead levels, and be able to interpret values in light of the patient and the work. A blood level of 30 μg/100 ml may represent cause for alarm or celebration depending on the specifics of the situation. Factors such as the patient's ambient lead exposure, previous lead levels, use of protective equipment, history of past exposure, age, gender, and current medical conditions all play a role. While the standard does not necessitate expertise in occupational medicine, it does require that the practitioner be knowledgeable and have access to reference material and to occupational health physicians.

Treatment
Providers must also be knowledgeable about the work environment in delivering care to injured workers, a responsibility that is critical in making recommendations regarding job placement. The primary goal of treatment is to restore function and reduce disability. Encouraging the individual to return to normal home and work activities as soon as feasible is part of the treatment strategy. In order to make meaningful recommendations for work placement, the practitioner must understand the demands of the various jobs and the effects of the individual's medical condition on performance. Using this information, the practitioner can judge when the patient is able to safely return to work, assist the employer in temporary job placement while the patient is recovering, and provide guidance in implementing reasonable accommodations.

Regulations
Other differences between occupational health and primary care services are the applicable rules and regulations. Practitioners should be knowledgeable about occupational safety and health standards, workers' compensation statutes, the Americans with Disabilities Act, and any other regulations that affect the provision of services. Compliance with these regulations should be reflected in the organization's practice policy and procedures.

Integration with Other Standards
Finally, the specific goals of the occupational health services standard should be reflected in all other relevant AAAHC standards. Documentation must include the preventive activities, knowledge of the workplace, and compliance with all applicable rules and regulations. The organization must be able to demonstrate that the preventive services are characterized by quality, efficiency, effectiveness, and continuous improvement.

Rationale for Accreditation

There are a number of reasons why organizations providing occupational health services should pursue AAAHC accreditation. In many cases, there are immediate financial incentives. Accreditation is becoming increasingly important among third-party payers. The trends toward workers' compensation provider networks and mandated managed care programs will continue. As a result, incentives to become accredited will likely increase. Business is becoming more involved in monitoring and purchasing health care. Accreditation and the quality assurance initiatives required under AAAHC are valuable marketing tools. More importantly, the quality of health care improves as an organization moves toward accreditation. AAAHC's standards represent a blueprint for the achievement of excellence. Any organization that seriously attempts to meet these standards will improve patient care, especially for occupational health services. The standards emphasize prevention and workplace assessment, areas commonly ignored in primary care settings.

Every organization that provides occupational health services should consider pursuing accreditation. Just as health care professionals should pursue board certification, health care organizations should pursue accreditation. Accreditation and AAAHC's accreditation process are formally supported by ACOEM. Accreditation is in the best interest of organizations providing occupational health services and it is in the best interest of occupational medicine, but most importantly it is in the best interest of the organization's patients.

References

1. ACOEM. *Policy Manual.* Arlington Heights, IL: American College of Occupational and Environmental Medicine, 1991.
2. ACOM. *Executive Manual.* Arlington Heights, IL: American College of Occupational Medicine (now the American College of Occupational and Environmental Medicine), 1987, D-54.
3. Yodaiken, R. E., and Zeitz, P. S. Accreditation policies in occupational health care. *J.O.M.* 35:562, 1993.
4. Committee on Occupational Medical Practice, ACOEM. Ambulatory occupational health settings. *J.O.M.* 31:644, 1989.
5. Travers, P. *A Comprehensive Guide for Establishing an Occupational Health Service.* Atlanta: American Association of Occupational Health Nurses, 1987.

Further Information

AAAHC. *Accreditation Handbook for Ambulatory Health Care 1992–1993 Edition.* Skokie, IL: Accreditation Association for Ambulatory Health Care, Inc., 1991.
This document provides all AAAHC's accreditation standards. It contains several questionnaire appendices addressing risk management, analysis of quality assurance programs, and clinical chart reviews. The standards are revised periodically.

AAAHC. *Presurvey Questionnaire: 1992–1993 Edition.* Skokie, IL: Accreditation Association for Ambulatory Health Care, Inc., 1991.
This questionnaire provides background information about an organization and its operation. The questionnaire must be submitted to AAAHC and reviewed prior to a site visit.

AAAHC. *Self-Assessment Manual.* Skokie, IL: Accreditation Association for Ambulatory Health Care, Inc., 1991.
This manual is intended to be used in conjunction with the 1992–1993 AAAHC Accreditation Handbook. It uses a series of checklists and work forms to guide an organization through its efforts to assure compliance with the standards.

Felton, J. *Occupational Medical Management.* Boston: Little, Brown, 1990.
This single-author text provides a compendium of information about the structure and function of in-plant occupational health services. It is useful in gaining insight into the possible configurations and activities of corporate occupational health programs.

Harris, J. S., Belk, D. H., and Wood, L. W. *Managing Employee Health Care Costs: Assuring Quality and Value.* Boston: OEM; 1992.
This collection of articles comes from two issues of the Journal of Occupational Medicine, *December 1990 and March 1991. The articles are loosely woven about the theme of quality and value in health care.*

Houston, T. *Occupational Medicine Services: A Practical Approach.* Chicago: AMA, 1989.
This is a concise handbook for providing occupational medicine services. It has several useful appendices including one outlining quality assurance activities.

JCAHC. *1994 Accreditation Manual for Ambulatory Health Care.* Oak Terrace, IL: Joint Commission on Accreditation of Healthcare Organizations, 1993.
JCAHC provides accreditation services to ambulatory health care facilities. This reference contains their criteria, support material, and presurvey questionnaire. The basic approach and organization of the document is similar to AAAHC, though there is no specific Occupational Health Services standard.

NCQA. *1994 Standards for Accreditation of Managed Care Organizations.* New York: National Committee for Quality Assurance, 1994.
NCQA is the primary accrediting body for managed care organizations. Their standards emphasize administrative issues critical to managed care.

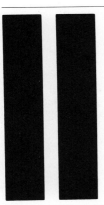

Occupationally
Related Illnesses

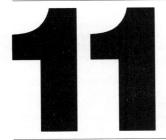

Occupational Pulmonary Disease

Ian A. Greaves

Many of the occupational lung disorders that affect workers today have been known for centuries. Silicosis, for example, has been recognized since antiquity as a disease of stonecutters and quarry workers, and coal workers' pneumoconiosis has been known since miners first dug coal to fire the steam boilers of the industrial revolution. The pioneering Italian physician, Bernadino Ramazzini, in the early eighteenth century noted a long list of occupations that were associated with adverse respiratory effects. Simple awareness of these problems has not eliminated them, however, and work-related pulmonary diseases rank among the top 10 causes of occupational disability and death in the United States and in most other countries.

An occupational lung disorder can be defined as an acute or chronic lung condition that arises, at least partly, from the inhalation of an airborne agent in the workplace. This definition includes lung diseases that are caused solely by workplace exposures, as well as conditions such as asthma that may predate workplace exposures but are exacerbated by them. Broadly speaking, occupational lung disorders fall into four major categories: the pneumoconioses or "dust-related" diseases, irritant reactions, asthmatic responses, and hypersensitivity reactions.

The rates of occurrence of these occupational lung disorders are poorly documented. Data based on workers' compensation claims underestimate the true incidence of many of these disorders; in some cases fewer than 5% of chronic occupational lung diseases are identified as work related, while occupational asthma is probably recognized even less frequently.

Diagnosis

The accurate diagnosis of an occupational cause for lung disease is important for three main reasons.

First, reduction in an individual's exposure to a particular agent may lead to clinical improvement or to arrest of the disease process. Cessation of exposure is most likely to benefit patients with potentially reversible diseases (such as those due to irritant agents, asthma, or other hypersensitivity reactions); reduction or elimination of exposures may not help individuals with one of the pneumoconioses because these disorders are chronic and irreversible, and can progress after cessation of exposure. Second, an accurate diagnosis of the work-relatedness of disease is important for just and fair financial compensation to the patient for his or her disability (see Chap. 2, Legal and Ethical Issues). Finally, an accurate diagnosis may lead to the recognition and prevention of disease among other workers exposed to the same agent.

Patient Evaluation

A physician of first contact is the most likely person to have the opportunity to make the diagnosis of many occupational lung diseases, but such a diagnosis can only be made if a physician is in the habit of asking a patient about his or her work. The most important reason for not diagnosing a work-related illness is failing to consider the individual's occupation.

History
Some knowledge is obviously needed concerning the individual's work. The process of taking an occupational history is described in Chap. 21, Suspecting Occupational Disease. Of particular relevance to establishing a work-related cause for lung disease

is the *temporal relationship of symptoms to work.* For diseases that cause chronic progressive disability (such as advanced silicosis, asbestosis, or coal worker's pneumoconiosis) generally there is a history of at least 10 years of exposure to the relevant dust; even with 10 years of exposure, it may be 20 or more years from first exposure before evidence of a pneumoconiosis appears.

Whenever an occupational lung disease is suspected, the patient should be questioned carefully about *all* jobs (even those as far back as high school) and any relevant hobbies that may be associated with hazardous exposures (such as arts and crafts in which toxic pigments are used; pigeon raising and exposure to avian proteins). *Parental occupation* may be relevant also; the families of asbestos workers, for example, have developed asbestos-related diseases from the asbestos dust brought home on work clothes.

More acute disorders, such as irritant or hypersensitivity reactions, are more likely to be related to workplace exposures at the time symptoms first appear. With these conditions it is important to note whether symptoms are better away from work, whether symptoms are worse on any particular day of the week (e.g., byssinosis), and whether symptoms are associated with certain jobs or assignments. Sometimes the temporal relationships may be misleading, particularly in some patients with occupational asthma whose symptoms of cough and wheezing may actually be most marked at night or in the early hours of the morning.

Another type of *delayed reaction,* and one that is very important to consider in the emergency room, is the inflammatory response that occurs in the airways and alveoli following acute inhalation of highly toxic agents such as chlorine, phosgene, and other potent lung irritants. Up to 48 hours after such an acute inhalation, patients may experience *acute lung edema* with breathlessness, chest tightness, and wheezing. The clinical picture may resemble that of acute asthma or pulmonary edema.

Irritant reactions to airborne agents are generally dose dependent and often affect a relatively large proportion of exposed people. Symptoms usually occur within minutes of first exposure. Depending on the water solubility of the agent, lower-respiratory symptoms will be accompanied by eye, nose, and throat irritation; agents with low water solubility have a greater tendency to affect the deeper lung architecture. Upper-respiratory symptoms (allergic rhinitis) may be prominent in patients with occupational asthma.

Information that other workers in the same area or doing similar jobs were affected similarly is supportive of a work-related etiology. Other workers will more likely be affected when the condition is dose dependent (such as an irritant effect or one of the pneumoconioses) than when a degree of hypersensitivity is required (such as for asthma, hypersensitivity pneumonitis, or chronic beryllium disease).

Physical Examination

The findings on physical examination of occupational lung diseases are similar to those of corresponding nonoccupational disorders. Several of the pneumoconioses, notably "simple" silicosis or coal worker's pneumoconiosis, may have no abnormal features on examination of the respiratory system. On the other hand, the earliest, and sometimes only, clinical finding in mild asbestosis may be fine inspiratory rales at the lung bases. Also, inspiratory rales or rhonchi may be the only abnormal findings following an acute toxic inhalation, and these observations should alert the physician to the possibility of acute lung edema.

No examination of the respiratory system is complete without inspection of the upper airways. Mucosal inflammation is frequently present in the nose, throat, and conjunctivae of workers exposed to irritant gases and fumes, and similar responses can be seen in hypersensitivity reactions. There are no features of these responses, however, to point exclusively to an occupational etiology.

Laboratory Evaluation

A chest radiograph and simple spirometry are *essential* to any assessment of occupational lung disease, and both tests should be obtained by the physician of first contact.

Chest X-ray

The chest film is the cornerstone in the diagnosis and evaluation of the pneumoconioses (asbestosis, silicosis, coal worker's pneumoconiosis) and beryllium disease, and has been widely used to screen workers exposed to asbestos, silica, coal dust, and beryllium for evidence of lung disease. The chest x-ray is also useful in the diagnosis of hypersensitivity pneumonitides (such as farmer's lung, bird fancier's lung), but of relatively little value in the assessment of occupational asthma.

A standard, clinical interpretation of chest films by a qualified radiologist is adequate for most clinical purposes. When any of the pneumoconioses, asbestos-related pleural disease, or beryllium disease is suspected, however, the chest films should be read according to the classification that has been developed by the International Labor Office (ILO) of the World Health Organization [1]. Only certain radiologists and physicians are certified to read films according to this classification. These special readers are termed *B-readers;* they have undertaken a period of training and passed an examination supervised by the National Institute for Occupational Safety and Health (NIOSH) and by the American College of Radiology.

The standard technique that B-readers use to evaluate chest x-rays is a semiquantitative method for determining *the nature, size, and extent of radiographic opacities* observed in the lung fields. Recent additions to the ILO criteria allow grading of pleural shadows also. An important feature of the ILO system is the provision of a standard series of graded x-rays against which a B-reader judges the degree of abnormality present. This approach to grading x-ray changes can be used to classify x-rays at a single point in time, or can be used to quantify changes that occur over time. One of the major applications of the ILO system has been in epidemiologic studies of the pneumoconioses.

The intra- and interobserver variability of B-readers in reading x-ray films has been assessed in recent years [2, 3]. When presented with the same x-ray films on separate occasions, most B-readers show high agreement in their reading of x-rays at different times; greatest intraobserver variability is seen with mild abnormalities, particularly with respect to pleural changes and small, irregular parenchymal densities. When the same chest x-rays are read by different B-readers, it is apparent that the experts can disagree substantially. As might be expected, interobserver variability is also greatest for x-rays that show minimal parenchymal or mild pleural changes.

Although chest radiographs can demonstrate radiodense opacities in the lungs, such opacities may not indicate appreciable impairment of lung function or disability of the patient. "Simple" forms of silicosis or coal worker's pneumoconiosis typically have scattered, small, rounded opacities visible on the chest x-ray, but lung function is usually well preserved. Also, some inhaled agents (such as particles of iron oxide or barium salts) can produce striking radiographic opacities in the lung fields, but these are simply depositional changes caused by the retention of radiodense materials in the lungs, and they do not reflect lung fibrosis or impairment of function.

Lung Function Tests

All patients suspected of having an occupational lung disease should, as a minimum investigation, perform ventilatory function tests. Spirometers are now readily available in physicians' offices and hospital clinics, while any well-equipped company medical clinic should have a high-quality machine that at least meets the performance standards proposed by the US National Institute for Occupational Safety and Health and which has been incorporated into several workplace standards of the US Occupational Safety and Health Administration (OSHA). All spirometers should provide an adequate written record of forced expiratory volumes. An alternative instrument to the standard spirometer is a pneumotachograph, which measures flow in relation to time; by electronically integrating flow over time, this instrument creates a volume-time curve similar to the output of a conventional spirometer. Another way of graphing volume-time information is the flow-volume curve, in which flow is plotted against lung volume and flows are reported at 25, 50, and 75% of the forced vital capacity (Fig. 11-1).

Measurements of the forced expiratory volume in one second (FEV$_1$) and of the forced vital capacity (FVC) are within the capabilities of any physician, nurse practitioner, or nurse. Care is required, however, in obtaining efforts from the subject that are technically satisfactory. A manual [4] for performing spirometry has been prepared by NIOSH to meet the requirements of the OSHA Cotton Dust Standard, and many laboratories offer spirometry training that has been approved by NIOSH. Another excellent account of spirometry requirements appears in the American Thoracic Society's (ATS) Epidemiology Standardization Project [5].

An important feature of spirometry is *repeatability* of the test in a given individual.

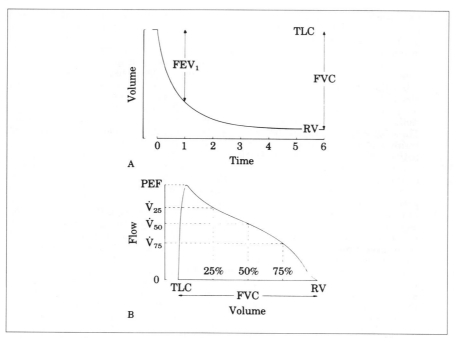

Figure 11-1. Volume-time (A) and flow-volume (B) curves depicting a maximum forced expiratory maneuver. Total lung capacity (TLC) and residual volume (RV) are the beginning and end points, respectively, of a forced vital capacity (FVC). The volume of gas exhaled in one second (FEV_1) can be expressed as a ratio (percentage) of the FVC to yield the forced expiratory ratio (FEV_1/FVC%). Peak expiratory flow (PEF) and flows (V) at 25%, 50%, and 75% of the FVC are often derived to describe the relationship of flow to lung volume. Units: volume (liters), time (seconds), flow (liters per second).

In more than 95% of people without lung disease, the two largest values for FEV_1 agree within 200 ml or 5% of the maximum value, and the two largest values for FVC agree similarly. This 200-ml or 5% criterion (whichever is the larger volume) has been used as a test for the validity of the data; tests that fall outside this range might represent submaximal efforts and be of doubtful value. Patients with respiratory impairment, however, can have difficulty repeating their tests satisfactorily and some judgment is required to assess whether the results in such cases are valid. The opinion of a pulmonary specialist and additional lung function tests that are less effort dependent may resolve whether the spirometry data are accurate and whether significant respiratory impairment is present.

Respiratory impairment is assigned primarily in terms of abnormal spirometry. By convention, ventilatory abnormalities are described either as being *obstructive* (defined as an abnormally decreased FEV_1 and decreased FEV_1/FVC ratio) or *restrictive* (an abnormally decreased FVC, with well preserved FEV_1/FVC ratio). These are purely descriptive terms to imply, respectively, abnormal limitation of airflow from the lungs or a decrease in the number of functioning lung units. Confusion arises, however, when the FEV_1 and FVC are both decreased in a particular patient. In severe asthma, for example, the FEV_1 and FVC are each decreased and the FEV_1/FVC ratio may be mildly decreased. The tendency to describe this as a "combined obstructive-restrictive disorder" should be discouraged; the decrease in FVC in this case is due primarily to airway closure, and is thus part of the overall obstructive disorder. In some diseases, such as conglomerate silicosis, there may indeed be extensive lung fibrosis and airway disease that results in a true, mixed obstructive-restrictive disorder, and the term has a sensible meaning in such cases. The term *restrictive disorder* should be reserved for conditions in which there is an acute or chronic loss of functioning alveoli resulting from a parenchymal lung disease (e.g., pneumonitis, lung fibrosis).

Important features of evaluating spirometry are appropriate prediction equations for *normal values*. An excellent account of normal ventilatory function, and the selection of appropriate normal values for assessing an individual's tests, has been published recently by the ATS [6]. Typically, predicted values for FEV_1 and FVC are obtained from a reference group (usually nonsmoking healthy subjects from the general population). There have been several excellent studies of healthy subjects in the United States [5]. Perhaps the most representative of these studies involved 8432 adults from six major cities in the US [7]; findings from this group are very similar to the earlier equations of Knudson and associates [8] that have been used widely for many years. The American Medical Association [9] has recommended the prediction equations of Crapo and colleagues [10], but these equations yield predicted values that are systematically greater than values obtained from other US population studies, probably because Crapo's measurements were obtained at an altitude of 1400 meters [6]. The prediction equations of Crapo thus overestimate the abnormality of lung function in many patients.

Most prediction equations for lung function relate to whites only. Studies among blacks have been few and have all suffered from small numbers. In practice, predicted values for blacks have been obtained by multiplying the respective predicted value for whites by a value between 0.85 and 0.88. For workers, a correction factor for blacks of 0.87 seems appropriate for most purposes [6, 7].

The evaluation of individuals' lung function has been reviewed critically by the ATS [6]. The most common method for expressing lung function relative to the predicted value is as a percentage. Convention dictates that a value of 80% predicted is the cutoff for an abnormal result. Population studies confirm that the standard deviations around the mean predicted values for FEV_1 and FVC are each about 9 to 10% of predicted, so that 80% of predicted is approximately the lower 95% confidence interval for the percent-predicted values. Other lung function tests—including flows at specific lung volumes and the diffusing capacity for carbon monoxide—generally have larger standard deviations, and therefore the use of 80% of predicted as their lower 95% confidence level is not justified. For example, measurements of the carbon monoxide diffusing capacity (gas transfer factor) have a lower 95% confidence interval of approximately 60% of the mean predicted value.

The practice of using "percent-predicted" as a way of assessing impairment is so entrenched clinically that it is unlikely to change quickly. This approach can be shown, however, to overestimate lung function abnormality in older and short people, and to underestimate abnormality in younger and tall people [5 ,6]. There are sound statistical reasons for considering the absolute difference between observed and predicted values [6], or the number of standard deviations an individual lies from his or her respective mean predicted value [5].

Airway Challenge Testing

Bronchial provocation tests are particularly useful when assessing patients with possible occupational asthma. *Nonspecific airway challenge tests* determine whether an individual's airways are unusually "reactive" to a nonspecific bronchoconstrictor stimulus. The most frequently used nonspecific stimuli are either pharmacologic agents (e.g., methacholine, histamine) administered by nebulized aerosol, eucapneic hyperventilation of subfreezing dry air (cold air challenge), or submaximal exercise for 6 to 8 minutes. There is fairly close agreement between these various tests of airway reactivity within a given subject.

In occupational settings, a dose-response curve to inhaled methacholine has been used most commonly to assess nonspecific airway reactivity. The results of methacholine challenge are expressed as the inhaled concentration that provokes a 20% decrease in FEV_1 from the baseline level (PC_{20}). The other tests of airway reactivity are less well standardized but have been used in clinical and epidemiologic studies.

Specific airway provocation tests involve exposure of the subject to the agent(s) thought to cause asthma. These tests can be performed in the laboratory or at the worksite. The relative merits of where the tests are performed are discussed further in the section on occupational asthma. Specific provocation tests are time consuming and expensive to perform, and should be undertaken by experienced personnel who have adequate resuscitation equipment immediately on hand. Since many industrial agents have "late" asthmatic effects, usually occurring 5 to 8 hours (and up to 24 hours) after exposure, it is important to observe the subject's lung function over at least a 24-hour period.

The value of nonspecific tests of airway reactivity lies in the detection of airway hyperreactivity in someone who has normal lung function, or who has mildly abnormal function with little response to a bronchodilator. The demonstration of airway hyperreactivity in such a person suggests an underlying asthmatic disorder, especially when considered in conjunction with a history of episodic cough, wheezing, chest tightness, or progressive breathlessness, especially in relation to exposure to a known allergen. Specific airway challenge tests are used to determine the etiologic agent(s) for occupational asthma, and to confirm the diagnosis for medicolegal purposes.

Bronchoscopy and Bronchoalveolar Lavage

Fiberoptic bronchoscopy and brushings are established tools for diagnosing malignancy and suspected infections [11]. In occupational settings, diseases classified as "extrinsic allergic alveolitis" have been investigated similarly in an effort to recover fungi or spores and to confirm an etiologic diagnosis. This practice has had limited success and is probably no better than examination of sputum.

Transbronchial biopsy, another procedure applicable to fiberoptic bronchoscopy, is a means to obtain a small fragment of lung tissue for microscopy [11]. While diagnosis of malignant lung disease is reasonable using such fiberoptic biopsy methods, a transbronchial biopsy specimen is usually too small to make a confident diagnosis of nonmalignant disease, and is subject to substantial sampling error. Occasionally a transbronchial biopsy will include a granuloma, thus confirming a type of interstitial lung disease. For the most part, however, transbronchial biopsy is of limited value in assessing occupational lung diseases.

Bronchoalveolar lavage (BAL), with recovery of cells from the airways and alveoli, is an investigative tool that has gained increasing popularity over the last 20 years. Although some problems are associated with using this approach for diagnostic purposes, the technique is now well standardized and has general acceptance [11]. One problem with BAL is the nonspecific nature of many findings in terms of cell counts, protein levels, and enzymes present in lavage fluid. Nevertheless, two occupational settings do seem to have relatively specific BAL findings: chronic beryllium disease and extrinsic allergic alveolitis. In chronic beryllium disease, lymphocytes obtained by BAL can be stimulated in vitro by beryllium salts; in extrinsic allergic alveolitis, BAL shows a high proportion of suppressor T lymphocytes that seems to be characteristic of this disorder.

Immunologic Tests

Immune-mediated occupational lung disorders fall into two main categories: those that cause asthma and those that cause "extrinsic allergic alveolitis." The presence of specific immunoglobulin (IgE) has been demonstrated for several causes of occupational asthma, and these antibodies are usually detected by the radioallergosorbent test (RAST) performed on a sample of blood. The sensitivity and specificity of circulating antibodies are highly variable for predicting the allergic reactions occurring in the lung. Not surprisingly, there are patients who have circulating IgE to a particular allergen and who experience no asthma, whereas there are others who clearly have asthma attributable to a particular agent, but no detectable IgE antibodies to the agent itself or to haptens formed from it.

Similarly, the measurement of circulating IgG precipitins in patients exposed to agents that cause extrinsic allergic alveolitis suffers from the same low sensitivity and specificity in predicting who has disease. Conversely, the absence of precipitins does not exclude the diagnosis of allergic alveolitis. Recent evidence suggests that T cells have a substantial role in the pathogenesis of several forms of "extrinsic allergic alveolitis." As a result, the conventional notion of these disorders being caused by distinct immune complexes may need to be modified. If a substantial component of the "extrinsic allergic alveolitides" were mediated by T cells, this could explain why circulating antibodies are poor indicators and predictors of disease.

The condition in which immune testing seems to have the greatest predictive value, and aids in establishing a diagnosis, is chronic beryllium disease. Lymphocytes in the peripheral blood, or obtained by BAL, from sensitized individuals undergo blastic transformation when exposed in vitro to salts of beryllium.

Finally, a rare complication of several pneumoconioses (chiefly silicosis and coal worker's pneumoconiosis, and perhaps asbestosis) occurs in conjunction with rheumatoid arthritis or in the presence of high titers of circulating rheumatoid factor.

Large necrobiotic nodules develop in the lungs and frequently cavitate to form abscesses. This disorder is termed *Caplan's syndrome.* There is no convincing evidence to suggest that rheumatoid factor, antinuclear factor, or other autoantibodies play a role in the pathogenesis of other occupational lung diseases.

Formulating a Diagnosis

The diagnosis of a work-related lung disease depends first and foremost on the physician considering the possibility and asking the patient about his or her work. Important clues in the history will come from temporal relationships between work and symptoms. Physical examination may contribute some signs of lung disease, which will not be specific for occupational disease; evidence of other respiratory or skin involvement may be important in determining an environmental cause for the lung disease. Laboratory examination is necessary for an objective determination of respiratory impairment, and laboratory tests are often needed to establish an etiologic diagnosis (e.g., challenge testing, immunologic changes, BAL).

Putting all this information together and arriving at a probable work-related cause for lung disease is often straightforward for clinical purposes. The medicolegal consequences of such a diagnosis are more problematic, particularly when compensation or tort liability is involved. The attending physician should not be intimidated, however, by the possible legal outcomes of a work-related diagnosis for lung disease. Without an accurate diagnosis, some patients with occupational lung diseases may continue to be exposed to toxic agents and progress to severe respiratory impairment. Furthermore, without an accurate diagnosis the unsafe workplace from which a patient comes may continue to expose others to the same hazards.

Common Occupational Pulmonary Disorders

The Pneumoconioses

The term *pneumoconiosis* (from the Greek: *pneumos,* the lung; *konios,* dust; *osis,* a state of—that is, a condition of the lungs resulting from inhaling dusts) was coined by the German pathologist Zenker in the last century. A more recent definition has been provided by Parkes [12]: ". . . 'pneumoconiosis' is defined as the non-neoplastic reaction of the lungs to inhaled mineral or organic dusts and the resultant alteration in their structure excluding asthma, bronchitis, and emphysema."

Dating from antiquity, the dust diseases of the lungs are among the oldest occupational diseases known. The chief dusts causing lung problems today are silica, coal, and asbestos. In general, a pneumoconiosis resulting from exposure to one of these agents requires at least 10 to 20 years of exposure. For each of these dusts, the likelihood of developing a pneumoconiosis is proportional to both the intensity and the duration of exposure. Thus, the exposure-response curves for these agents show an effect of cumulative exposure, as well as a latent period before effects appear.

The clearance of silica, coal, and asbestos from the lungs occurs very slowly (over months to years) after these agents are deposited in the lung parenchyma. Autopsy studies have shown large amounts of these dusts retained in the lungs of workers who ceased being exposed many years before their death. Thus, it is not surprising that the major dust-related diseases frequently progress in severity after cessation of exposure because a substantial dose of dust remains in the lungs to cause further pathologic changes.

Another group of agents, termed *inert dusts,* deposit in the lungs and give rise to mild cellular responses. These deposits sometimes cause striking radiographic changes but are accompanied by little impairment of lung function or disability.

A brief clinical review of the classical pneumoconioses follows. The reader is encouraged to consult more comprehensive accounts in the specific texts and review articles listed in the bibliography.

Silicosis

Silicosis is the most common pneumoconiosis worldwide. Silica exposures occur in a wide variety of jobs. One of the most common sources of silica is the soil. Granite and sandstone are two important geologic sources, and people who work in mines or are involved in blasting and drilling operations are at risk of exposure to silica. Other high-risk groups include sandblasters, and foundry workers who grind the surface of iron moldings to remove sand that has been used to make the molds and as a parting agent during the molding process.

Deposition of crystalline silica (SiO_2) in the lung parenchyma and airways causes an intense cellular reaction, with infiltration of macrophages, neutrophils, and lymphocytes. Free silica is toxic to macrophages and thus is cleared relatively slowly from the lungs. Nevertheless, over time, substantial amounts of silica can be found in the hilar lymph nodes of exposed workers as well as in the lung parenchyma.

The characteristic histologic lesion in the lungs and regional lymph nodes is a *granuloma* that has a central, amorphous, hyaline area surrounded by a zone of fibrosis and inflammatory cells. This lesion is termed a *silicotic nodule* and varies in size from less than a millimeter to a centimeter or more in diameter. Silicotic nodules gradually grow in size over time and as cumulative exposure increases.

Nodules 1 to 2 mm in diameter are usually sufficiently radiodense to appear on a chest x-ray. Typically, these small rounded opacities are more prominent in the upper- and midlung zones, but over time the distribution of nodules becomes more generalized throughout the lungs. Nodules may increase rapidly in size or progress very slowly. Presumably the size and number of nodules in the lung reflect the accumulation of silica at particular sites over time, and this in turn depends on the rates of deposition and clearance. Undefined host factors are probably important also in determining the cellular and fibrotic responses to a given dose.

When silicotic nodules are discrete, the condition is termed *simple silicosis*. This condition can be diagnosed readily from the chest x-ray and typically occurs after at least 10 years of exposure to silica dust. Of more concern is progression of the disease to a stage of *conglomerate silicosis* (previously called "progressive massive fibrosis" or PMF). The latter stage results from conglomeration of individual silicotic nodules into increasingly larger fibrotic masses. These masses are usually bilateral, occur mainly in the upper and mid zones of the lungs, and are several centimeters in diameter. Advanced conglomerate silicosis produces a butterfly-shaped opacity in the upper-lung zones.

Lung function is typically well preserved in workers with simple silicosis. Mild abnormalities in forced expiratory flows have been reported, but these have been insufficient to cause disability. Once conglomeration occurs, however, lung function is frequently impaired, and functional deterioration may be rapid. A severe restrictive and obstructive disorder can result from the conglomerate lesions, and respiratory failure with cor pulmonale is seen in severely affected workers.

Other pulmonary effects attributable to silica exposure include inflammation and thickening of the pleura (particularly over the lung apices), a definite increase in risk of pulmonary tuberculosis, and possibly an increased risk of lung cancer. Before the development of effective treatment for tuberculosis, many silica-exposed workers with a simple pneumoconiosis developed tuberculosis and died before a more disabling form of silicosis could develop. The physician today must still be aware of the possibility of tuberculosis in silicotic workers, particularly when the chest x-ray shows a recent change at one of the apices or the abrupt appearance of an opacity elsewhere.

Chronic cough and phlegm (chronic bronchitis) are common symptoms among workers with heavy silica exposure and those who have silicosis. Phlegm production generally increases in advanced stages of silicosis; recurrent bacterial infections are common. Cavitation and chronic infection occur occasionally in conglomerate lesions, and these infections may be tuberculous or due to anaerobic bacteria. A rare variant of silicosis occurs in patients who have rheumatoid arthritis or circulating rheumatoid factor; these people can develop necrobiotic nodules several centimeters in diameter that frequently cavitate and become infected (Caplan's syndrome).

Finally, silicosis has been reported to cause acute lung disease when individuals are exposed to very high concentrations. Silica flower, a very fine silica dust of high purity, still causes this disorder [13]. Acute silicosis resembles alveolar proteinosis, but is more fulminant than the latter and can be rapidly fatal.

With improved dust controls, advanced silicosis should now be a rare disease. Unfortunately, poorly controlled or unmonitored operations persist, and individuals continue to be exposed and become disabled.

Coal Worker's Pneumoconiosis

Coal dust, which is chiefly carbon, produces a relatively mild pulmonary cellular reaction compared with silica. Unlike silica, the characteristic lesion of coal is a pinhead-sized collection of macrophages laden with black coal dust. Typically, these collections are in the vicinity of alveolar ducts and contain increased amounts of reticulin fibers. These characteristic lesions (*macules*) are initially 1 to 2 mm in diameter, but they too may grow in size and number.

Conglomerate lesions also occur with exposure to coal dust, with an outcome similar to that seen with conglomerate silicosis. Advanced coal worker's pneumoconiosis (CWP) with conglomerate lesions is accompanied in most cases by major impairment of lung function and disability attributable to the pneumoconiosis. The factors that promote the sudden development of conglomerate CWP in some coal workers are unknown. Unlike silicosis, which usually shows an orderly progression through increasingly severe degrees of simple silicosis before conglomeration occurs, CWP may progress rapidly from a relatively minor degree of simple pneumoconiosis to the advanced form. The aggressive nature of CWP in some coal workers is surprising because coal is generally less fibrogenic than silica or asbestos. Immune-mediated changes have been proposed to explain the unusual susceptibility of some coal workers to conglomerate CWP, but studies have failed to confirm specific immune features in such workers.

Recent epidemiologic studies of autopsy data have shown an increased risk of centrilobular emphysema associated with increasing grades of CWP [14]. For many years an increased risk of emphysema among coal workers was attributed to cigarette smoking. It is now apparent that coal alone or in combination with smoking can cause emphysema in workers with moderate to severe CWP. Because emphysema leads to airflow obstruction, an obstructive abnormality on lung function testing would be expected in workers with CWP. It is unclear, however, whether mild or minimal CWP is associated with emphysema. The presence of an obstructive pattern of lung function tests in a worker with mild CWP will therefore present some difficulty for the physician who wishes to determine the work-relatedness of that individual's condition.

Coal workers frequently have a cough and phlegm, which are often accompanied by mild reductions in forced expiratory flows; these features are sometimes referred to as an "industrial bronchitis." The reductions in expiratory flow are thought to reflect either involvement of the alveolar ducts and other small airways in the lungs, or the development of centrilobular emphysema. Not all coal workers with cough and phlegm show these mild impairments of lung function, and not all who have some impairment of ventilatory function have cough and phlegm. Cough and phlegm have no causal role in the production of airflow obstruction, but the symptoms of bronchitis and the function changes may be distinct features associated with cumulative exposure to coal dust. For this reason, it is probably wise to avoid the misleading term "industrial bronchitis" when referring to respiratory impairment in coal workers.

As with silicosis, the presence of rheumatoid arthritis or positive circulating rheumatoid factor in association with CWP can result in large necrobiotic nodules (Caplan's syndrome). Low titers of autoantibodies may be found in many patients with CWP; the significance of these titers is unknown.

Asbestosis

Asbestosis is a form of lung fibrosis of the "usual interstitial type" that results from inhalation of asbestos fibers. The term *asbestosis* refers only to this type of parenchymal lung disease and excludes pleural thickening or fibrosis that may accompany the parenchymal lesions. An isolated finding of pleural thickening or fibrosis does not justify the diagnosis of "pleural asbestosis," a term that has no pathologic meaning and has caused confusion.

The interstitial fibrosis accompanying asbestos exposure is indistinguishable histologically from other forms of diffuse lung fibrosis such as idiopathic pulmonary fibrosis. The only feature that is unique to asbestosis is the presence of *asbestos bodies* in the lung tissue. Asbestos bodies comprise an asbestos fiber that has been subjected to attack by alveolar macrophages with the resulting deposition of proteinaceous materials and iron (derived from digestion of hemoglobin by the macrophage) on the surface of the fiber. Asbestos bodies thus stain positively with Prussian blue and other iron stains, and are often referred to as *ferruginous bodies*. Finding an asbestos body in histologic sections can be difficult, but the diagnosis is established if one can be found.

To produce interstitial fibrosis, there needs to have been exposure to substantial air concentration (on the order of 2 fibers per ml or higher) for at least 10 years, and usually for more than 20 years. Asbestosis is a dose-related disease with a long latent period. Asbestos exposures have occurred in many occupations, including asbestos miners and millers, pipe coverers, asbestos textile workers, various construction trades, and shipyard workers. Some relatives of these workers have developed asbestosis and other asbestos-related diseases from dust brought home on the worker's clothing.

Diagnosis of asbestosis is not as simple as that for silicosis or CWP. Unlike the other two disorders, mild or "early" asbestosis is relatively more difficult to detect with a chest x-ray. The first changes are usually irregular linear densities that are seen initially at the lung bases but increase in number, coarseness, and extent as the disease progresses. Lung function changes may precede the radiographic changes, with the most prominent "early" effects being a decrease in FVC and a decrease in the diffusing capacity for carbon monoxide. When other findings are normal, an important clue to possible interstitial disease is the presence of inspiratory rales at the lung bases. Although the presence of inspiratory rales is not pathognomonic of interstitial fibrosis, rales in an asbestos-exposed worker should alert the physician to the possibility of asbestosis and the need to monitor this individual's lung function and to obtain a chest x-ray periodically.

Other Pneumoconioses

A large number of other dusts can cause pulmonary abnormalities, including various minerals that contain different forms of silicates, and some metals and their salts. Examples of *silicates* include kaolin and talc, which can both cause nodular fibrosis in the lungs of exposed workers; each can produce conglomerate lesions similar to those found in advanced silicosis. Several forms of amorphous silica, such as diatomaceous earth and fibrous glass, can also cause problems. *Diatomaceous earth* is a relatively nontoxic material. The principal health concerns about this agent relate to its transformation by calcining into crystalline silica, which causes silicosis in exposed workers. Apart from being a cheap source of silica that can be used as a filler in paints and plastics, diatomaceous earth has been used as a filtering material for wine and beer.

Fibrous glass has been used for many purposes, chiefly as insulation material and as a replacement for asbestos. Some epidemiologic studies have indicated a relationship between exposure to this agent and mild radiographic abnormalities. Human exposures have been associated mainly with irritation of the skin and mucous membranes of the respiratory tract. Animal data suggest that fibrous glass can cause lung and pleural fibrosis. Exposure to fibrous glass may also be associated with an increased risk of bronchogenic carcinoma, but a clear relationship has yet to be demonstrated. Data to date are conflicting regarding the human effects of fibrous glass, but a disturbing trend in industry has been to manufacture glass fibers of fine dimensions similar to asbestos fibers. Depending on the durability in the lung of inhaled fibers, this could result in greater risks of lung fibrosis or malignancies from exposures to fibrous glass.

Various *metals* and some of their salts have been shown to cause abnormalities on the chest x-ray. Tin, barium, antimony, and titanium, all cause radiodense nodules that are collections of dust-filled macrophages with no fibrotic reaction. These dusts are among a group of agents that have been termed *inert dusts* because they deposit in the lungs but elicit little fibrosis reaction.

Irritant Lung Reactions

Many gases, fumes, and aerosols are directly toxic to the respiratory tract by causing acute inflammation of the respiratory mucosa and lung parenchyma. The principal sites in the respiratory tract where different agents have the greatest effect are determined by their water solubility and particle size. Highly soluble agents dissolve readily in the secretions of the eyes, upper respiratory tract (nose, pharynx) and airways; less soluble agents exert their main effects in the peripheral, small airways and in the lung parenchyma. Particles greater than 10μ tend to settle out in the upper-respiratory tract, those 3μ to 10μ settle mainly in the airways, and those less than 3μ deposit mainly in the lung parenchyma and small airways. It is important to note, however, that the "scrubbing" of inspired air by the upper-respiratory tract to remove water-soluble agents and larger particles can be overwhelmed by high air concentrations; when lung ventilation increases (as during exercise or heavy work), greater effects are seen in the lower respiratory tract.

Examples of agents that cause nonspecific irritant effects are shown in Table 11-1. Highly water-soluble gases or aerosols, such as sulfur dioxide or hydrogen chloride, characteristically produce irritant effects in the eyes, nasopharynx, and large airways. Predictably, individuals exposed to these agents may develop sore and watering eyes, sneezing, nasal discharge, coughing, phlegm, and perhaps wheezing. Airflow obstruction can occur as a result of reflex bronchoconstriction. The neural reflex pathways involve afferent nerve fibers in the vagal and glossopharyngeal nerves, and cholinergic efferent fibers in the vagal nerve. Bronchoconstriction from exposure to airway irritants is seen most commonly in asthmatics, who respond at lower air concentrations than do nonasthmatics. The effects of upper-respiratory and airway irritants are usually transient and related to the period of exposure; the irritant effects usually resolve promptly on removal from exposure. Among workers, these symptoms tend to improve over weekends or during vacations.

Chronic exposure to an agent such as sulfur dioxide can lead to persistent symptoms of cough and phlegm that may take many weeks to resolve after cessation of exposure. Such persistent symptoms probably reflect adaptive responses, including hypertrophy and hyperplasia of mucous glands and goblet cells, that follow chronic inflammation of the airway mucosa. Another important effect of airway irritants is an increased permeability of the airway mucosa to other inhaled agents, such as fine particles; airway irritants also cause a transient increase in nonspecific airway reactivity even in workers who are not asthmatic. The importance of increases in airway permeability and airway reactivity is unknown, but these appear to be mechanisms whereby exposure to irritant agents and to other agents toxic to the lungs may result in effects greater than the sum of each agent separately; in other words these may be mechanisms by which synergy could occur between irritant agents and other toxic exposures.

Exposures to high air concentrations of water-soluble agents cause extensive inflammatory changes throughout the respiratory tract. In severe cases, this amounts to a chemical burn of the respiratory mucosa from the nasopharynx to the

Table 11-1. Characteristics of some common irritant gases and fumes

Agent	Industrial sources and uses	Solubility in water
Ammonia	Production of fertilizers, explosives, various chemicals	High
Cadmium oxide	Jewelry making, silver soldering and brazing, smelting, art pigments	High
Hydrogen chloride	Pickling operations, chemical manufacture, electroplating	High
Hydrogen fluoride	Etching and polishing glass, plastics manufacture, insecticide	High
Sulfur dioxide	Paper and pulp manufacture, smelting operations, chemical production, combustion of coal	High
Chlorine	Wide use in chemical industry, water purification, bleaching	Moderate
Vanadium pentoxide	Boiler scaling, chemical industry	Moderate
Mercury vapor	Gold extraction, mercury lamps	Low
Oxides of nitrogen	Chemical and fertilizer manufacture, metal processing, silage, welding, manufacture of explosives	Low
Ozone	Disinfectant, bleaching, oxidizing agent	Low
Phosgene	Production of plastics, pesticides, combustion product of chlorinated hydrocarbons	Low

alveoli, and is a medical emergency. The two principal problems encountered from acute irritant toxicity are laryngeal edema (with the possibility of airway obstruction, which may require a tracheotomy) and severe lung edema, which may necessitate assisted ventilation and oxygen. These serious sequelae of toxic irritants are not always apparent at the time of exposure. Indeed, it is well recognized that these potentially life-threatening outcomes of exposure may be delayed up to 24 to 48 hours after exposure. Quite commonly, individuals will present to an emergency room shortly after exposure to high levels of an irritant and be discharged reasonably well, only to return within 24 hours severely breathless and in need of urgent treatment.

Emergency room management of overexposure to irritant agents is shown in Table 11-2. It is stressed that a careful and prudent policy is to admit to the hospital for 24 to 48 hours of observation those people who appear to be healthy but have been exposed to high levels of an irritant gas, fume, or aerosol, *and* either have evidence of mucosal inflammation in the upper-respiratory tract and conjunctivae, or have rales or rhonchi on auscultation of the chest (regardless of whether there appears to be another plausible explanation for these signs). These comments apply equally to smoke inhalation that combines exposures to toxic gases, fumes, and particles with the additional problem of thermal burns to the respiratory tract.

Irritant agents that are relatively insoluble in water, such as ozone, phosgene, or the oxides of nitrogen, cause slightly different effects. These agents produce few upper-respiratory or airway symptoms, and manifest themselves more insidiously. Following acute severe exposures, the first symptoms are usually a headache and a cough that is triggered by taking a deep breath. A sensation of "chest tightness" may also be present. The major symptom from these agents, however, is progressive breathlessness attributable to toxic pneumonitis with lung edema. The fulminant condition resembles adult respiratory distress syndrome and carries a similar high mortality. Treatment is supportive and recovery occurs slowly. Long-term sequelae of toxic edema include lung fibrosis and occasionally bronchiolitis obliterans. The latter causes chronic irreversible airway obstruction.

Table 11-2. Principles for the management of acute pulmonary effects from inhaling irritant gases, fumes, and aerosols

1. Immediately obtain arterial blood gas measurements and commence oxygen therapy if the patient has any evidence of respiratory impairment.
2. Take a history of likely toxic exposures from the patient or another informed person from the site of exposure. Pay particular attention to whether carbon monoxide (CO), hydrogen sulfide, or hydrogen cyanide exposures could have occurred. Measure the blood carboxyhemoglobin level if there is any suspicion of CO exposure. (Commence treatment for hydrogen sulfide or hydrogen cyanide poisoning if there is any suspicion of exposure.)
3. Examine the eyes, nose, and pharynx for evidence of chemical or thermal burns.
4. Carefully auscultate the lungs for the presence of rhonchi or rales. Listen over the larynx and trachea for an inspiratory stridor, which is best heard when the subject makes a rapid inspiratory effort.
5. Measure baseline spirometry if the subject is capable of performing the test.
6. Obtain an electrocardiograph if the carboxyhemoglobin level exceeds 10% and in anyone who is over the age of 40 years or who has a history of cardiovascular disease.
7. Obtain a baseline chest x-ray in anybody who may have been exposed to possibly toxic levels. Although frequently normal, the chest x-ray is invaluable if the patient's condition deteriorates and early lung edema is suspected.
8. *Admit to the hospital* (if only for 24–48 hours of observation) anyone who has evidence of an acute toxic effect from inhalation of an irritant agent. This includes patients with overt abnormalities on testing and those with positive signs on clinical examination of the upper- or lower-respiratory tract. If in any doubt about discharging the patient, hold him or her for further observation. Those who are discharged after initial evaluation should be advised carefully to return if they feel unwell, and particularly if a cough, wheeze, or breathlessness develops.

Another important sequel of acute exposures to lung irritants is a condition termed *reactive airways dysfunction syndrome* (RADS) [15]. Following an acute exposure to agents such as toluene diisocyanate, welding fumes, or other potent respiratory irritants, individuals may experience the onset of asthma attacks or the return of asthma after many years. Airway reactivity is increased in these patients, presumably as a result of the acute toxic insult. Persistent asthma may occur and it appears that RADS is a variant of occupational asthma. A recent report [16] of 56 people exposed to a formaldehyde spill showed that RADS developed in 3 of 14 (21%) with high exposures. This high rate suggests that the condition is not rare and needs to be considered whenever someone is exposed to high air levels of a respiratory irritant.

Chronic exposures to low levels of poorly soluble irritants such as ozone have also been associated with adverse respiratory effects, notably chronic airflow obstruction and exacerbation of underlying chronic lung conditions. Both ozone and oxides of nitrogen are prominent components of urban air pollution, and exposures also occur in specific work settings. Epidemiologic studies suggest that the workplace hazards of intermittent exposures to high air concentrations of these agents may be more relevant than chronic low-level exposures in the production of respiratory impairment.

Occupational Asthma

Occupational asthma has been defined as "variable airway narrowing causally related to exposure in the working environment to airborne dusts, gases, vapors or fumes" [17]. Considerable differences of opinion exist, however, in the interpretation of this apparently straightforward definition. A very restrictive definition has been developed in Britain by the Industrial Injuries Advisory Council, which defines occupational asthma as a condition "which occurs after a variable period of symptomless exposure to a sensitizing agent at work." It has become clear, however, that chronic airway inflammation may be induced or aggravated by irritant exposures, beyond the individual's hypersensitivity response. Other definitions have included agents that produce bronchoconstriction by mechanisms other than immune sensitization. Some occupational exposures that are known to cause asthma are shown in Table 11-3, which also provides findings for skin testing and circulating IgE for these various exposures. As we develop greater understanding of the different pathogenic mechanisms in occupational asthma, it becomes increasingly clear that non-immune mechanisms are important, particularly for highly reactive chemicals of low molecular weight, such as the isocyanates, formaldehyde, and azodicarbonamide (Table 11-3).

Estimates of the prevalence of asthma resulting from exposures in the workplace vary from about 5 to 50% of individuals, depending on the particular agent. A large proportion of patients who develop asthma as adults, and many workers who experience worsening of long-standing asthma, actually have an occupational cause for their symptoms.

Several clinical features of occupational asthma need to be stressed. First, although many patients experience typical recurrent episodes of wheezing and breathlessness, in some the onset of symptoms may develop more insidiously and may not show typical acute episodic attacks. Individuals can present with steadily increasing exertional breathlessness with evidence of an obstructive defect on spirometry that often responds incompletely (at least initially) to a bronchodilator. Second, symptoms may not be obviously work related: A sizable fraction of workers with occupational asthma experience their symptoms mainly in the evenings or at night. Also, following exposures to some occupational causes of asthma (e.g., western red cedar, toluene diisocyanate), the recovery period may take several days or weeks. As a result, improvement away from work may be seen only over weekends or at times of vacation. Unless the physician is aware of these diverse patterns, an occupational cause of asthma will be overlooked.

Once occupational asthma is suspected, the diagnosis involves two steps. First, it is necessary to show that the individual has asthma. The diagnosis can be confirmed either by measuring variations in lung spirometry that occur spontaneously or with treatment, or, if baseline lung function is normal, by showing that the individual has nonspecific airway hyperreactivity (see above). Second, a causal link needs to be established between workplace exposures and alterations in lung function. Sometimes there is only the patient's history to support the work-related nature of his or her symptoms. Whenever possible, however, direct confirmation should be obtained.

Table 11-3. Agents that cause occupational asthma

Agent	Industries and occupations	Skin test	Specific IgE antibodies
Vegetable dusts and woods			
Grain	Grain handlers	+	−
Flour (wheat/rye)	Millers, bakers	+	+
Coffee beans	Planters, processors	+	+
Castor beans	Oil producers		+
Tea dust	Teaworkers	+	
Tobacco	Tobacco workers	+	+
Western red cedar	Sawmillers, carpenters,	+	+
California redwood	cabinetmakers, other	−	
Oak	woodworkers, construction		−
Mahogany	workers	−	
Colophony (pine resin)	Electronics workers		+
Gum acacia	Printers	+	
Animals, birds, shellfish			
Rats		+	
Mice	Animal handlers, laboratory	+	
Guinea pigs	workers, veterinarians	+	+
Rabbits		+	
Pigeons	Pigeon breeders	+	
Chickens	Poultry workers	+	+
Turkeys	Poultry workers	+	+
Crabs	Crab processors	+	
Prawns	Prawn processors	+	+
Oysters	Oyster farmers	+	+
Enzymes			
Subtilisins	Detergent manufacture	+	+
Papain	Meat packaging	+	+
Trypsin	Pharmaceutical workers	+	+
Pepsin	Pharmaceutical workers	+	+
Metals			
Platinum and salts	Platinum refining and plating	+	
Chromium salts	Tanning of leather	±	+
Nickel	Metal plating	+	±
Cobalt	Manufacture of hard metals	+	
Vanadium	Manufacture of hard metals		
Miscellaneous chemicals			
Toluene diisocyanate (TDI)	Manufacture of polyurethane, foam, painters, plastics manufacture	±	±
Diphenylmethane diisocyanate (MDI)	Core makers in foundries, painters	−	+
Phthallic anhydride	Epoxy resins, plastics	+	+
Trimellitic anhydride	Epoxy resins, plastics	+	+
Formaldehyde	Hospital workers, laboratory technicians, chemical workers	−	−
Azodicarbonamide	Plastics and rubber workers	−	
Ethanolamines	Solderers, spray painters, metal machining	−	

Key: + = positive skin test or specific IgE has been reported in affected workers, but not necessarily in all of those affected; − = no reports of a positive skin test or specific IgE antibodies among those who were tested, although for many of these agents, only small numbers of affected individuals have been examined; ± = conflicting data: some researchers have found a positive skin test or specific IgE, but other investigators did not.
Source: Data derived from M. Chan-Yeung and S. Lam, Occupational asthma (state of art). *Am. Rev. Respir. Dis.* 133:686, 1986.

Skin tests to the suspected agent(s) and the demonstration of circulating specific IgE provide evidence of sensitization to the agent(s) being tested, but the sensitivity and specificity of these tests for detecting respiratory sensitization vary greatly for different agents. Furthermore, not all agents causing occupational asthma exert their effects through IgE-mediated mechanisms.

More direct methods for showing causal relationships involve bronchial challenge with the agent(s) of interest. These challenges can be conducted in the laboratory (where the level and nature of the exposures can be better controlled) or in the workplace (where the offending exposures actually occur). Lung spirometry is obtained before and after a period of exposure, and these tests should be repeated periodically over the next 24 hours to determine whether a "late" asthmatic response is induced (generally maximal at 5 to 8 hours after exposure). Customarily, a decrease in FEV_1 by 15% or greater of the baseline (prechallenge) value is considered a "positive" result. Specific bronchial provocation tests are best performed by experienced personnel in a laboratory where the nature of the exposure can be controlled and where urgent treatment can be administered promptly for an acute severe reaction.

Some careful thought needs to be given to testing an individual's response to the suspected agent(s) in the workplace. The investigator must be sure that the patient is being exposed to the agent(s) of interest, and that the testing protocol is suitable. One approach has been to perform measurements of ventilatory function before and after a work shift. This is an appropriate method when the timing of exposures and responses during the work period are unknown, and it is useful for screening large groups of workers to identify possible "responders," but it is inappropriate for monitoring closely an individual patient with suspected hypersensitivity. Serious reactions to industrial agents have been reported, and some agents (e.g., toluene diisocyanate) can produce severe asthma attacks in sensitized individuals at air concentrations as low as 1 part per billion. If a diagnostic challenge is performed at the worksite, measurements of airway function should be obtained frequently within the first 60 minutes of exposure, and thereafter at regular intervals for at least 24 hours, or as determined by the patient's response.

A mini-Wright peak flow meter is a convenient instrument for measuring a worker's lung function; measurements of maximum expiratory flow can be obtained at frequent intervals without taking a worker off the job. Self-testing and self-recording of the peak flow measurements can be continued at home to take into account possible late reactions that may occur away from work. Although convenient to use, mini-Wright peak flow measurements may be inaccurate and should only be used to consider *relative changes in lung function* over short time periods; they should not be used as a substitute for regular spirometry in assessing whether an individual's ventilatory function is "normal." In general, a decrease in peak flow of 20%, or a decrease in FEV_1 of 10% or greater (see OSHA's *Cotton Dust Standard,* 29 CFR 1910.1000), over a working period is considered an abnormal finding and suggests work-related airflow obstruction. (See Chap. 19, Allergy and Immunology, for a thorough description of the use of peak flow meters in diagnosing occupational asthma.)

Whether in the laboratory or at the worksite, provocative challenge testing must be aborted and bronchodilator therapy given if the subject becomes acutely distressed, or if the peak flow or FEV_1 drops by 50% or more of the baseline value.

Once a diagnosis of occupational asthma is established, prompt job transfer is necessary to an area of no exposure. Because asthma may be precipitated in some cases by minute levels of the responsible agent(s), the sensitized worker must not work near or even pass through an area where exposure may occur. To keep a sensitized individual in an exposed job by using either intensive medication or a respirator cannot be justified on medical grounds, and these practices could subject that worker to a potential life-threatening situation.

Recent data indicate that some workers with occupational asthma do not recover completely after removal from exposure; some will continue to experience episodes of asthma and have persistent hyperreactive airways. Airways that become sensitized initially to an occupational exposure may then develop sensitivities to nonoccupational agents. The probability of recovery is greatest for those who had the least duration and intensity of exposure, and who subsequently have no further exposure to the agent [18]. In general, if a patient with occupational asthma has ongoing or recurrent asthma after removal from the workplace, and the asthma can be attributed to initial airway sensitization by a workplace exposure (that is, to the "occupational phase" of the disease), then the current asthma can be regarded as work-related for workers' compensation purposes even though that person is no longer exposed to the original sensitizing agent.

A condition that resembles occupational asthma in many aspects is *byssinosis,* a disease of cotton textile workers and others who inhale cotton dust, flax, or soft hemp. Byssinosis has a characteristic clinical picture of cough and chest tightness occurring on the first day of a working week, but not on other days of the week. As the disease progresses, symptoms may extend further into the week, until eventually the worker has a chronic cough and breathlessness. Occasionally, the condition develops more insidiously; the typical "Monday cough and tightness" are absent and the patient presents with exertional breathlessness. Accompanying the acute Monday symptoms are impairment of ventilatory function, which shows an obstructive defect.

The etiologic agent in cotton dust is unknown. An allergic reaction is not responsible, and the most likely causes are either a pharmacologic reaction to a compound in cotton bracts, or a reaction to endotoxin that originates from bacterial and fungal contaminants of the cotton. Whichever agent is primarily responsible for the acute symptoms and lung function changes, it is established that the agent is water soluble and heat labile because exposure of byssinotic workers to *steamed raw cotton eliminates their respiratory responses.*

Hypersensitivity Pneumonitis (Extrinsic Allergic Alveolitis)

The prototype of this group of disorders is *farmer's lung,* a condition that resembles recurrent pneumonia. Fungi that grow in wet hay cause this disorder. Exposures occur when farmers come to use the moldy hay and in the process generate enormous air concentrations of the bacteria *Micropolyspora faeni* and various fungi, such as *Thermophilic actinomyces* species. Patients typically present with recurring episodes of fever, cough, headache, breathlessness, and general malaise that mimic acute infectious disease. Examination reveals an acutely ill patient with few physical signs in the chest (occasional, scattered inspiratory rales may be present). The chest x-ray may be normal, but more commonly shows focal or diffuse infiltrates that may occur anywhere in the lung fields, although the upper zones appear to be affected most often. During the acute illness, the white cell count is elevated and generally shows a left shift; the sedimentation rate and serum immunoglobulins are also increased.

Episodic attacks usually resolve spontaneously within several days on removal of the patient from exposure to the offending agents. With repeated acute episodes, however, there may be progression to lung fibrosis with a restrictive ventilatory defect and a decreased diffusing capacity for carbon monoxide. When fibrosis is present these changes are irreversible, but progression does not usually occur unless there are further acute episodes. Respiratory failure has occurred as a result of severe lung fibrosis.

Although acute episodes of pneumonic illness are common in this disorder, some patients will present with a subacute picture that manifests as slowly progressive shortness of breath. A clinical diagnosis of interstitial fibrosis of undetermined cause has usually been made. The correct diagnosis of an allergic alveolitis can be made by first considering the possibility of an environmental agent; second, by taking a careful history of possible exposures; and third, by finding serum precipitins to the offending agent. The finding of precipitins does not necessarily prove a causal relationship between exposure and disease, but is presumptive evidence for such a diagnosis in the absence of contrary findings.

Since the initial description of farmer's lung, many other sources (Table 11-4) have been identified as capable of causing the same acute and chronic clinical picture. In rare cases of indoor air pollution, hypersensitivity pneumonitis has also occurred among susceptible people, presumably as a result of fungal spores contaminating air handling equipment. Culturing air handling systems, however, can be problematic. Thus, careful clinical assessments in these situations are essential (see Chap. 44, Indoor Air Pollution, for further discussion).

The pathogenesis of this group of disorders is traditionally thought to involve a type III (immune complex) response to inhaled antigens. A high preponderance of T lymphocytes (mainly suppressor cells) is found in lung tissue as well as epithelioid granulomas. The latter suggest the additional possibility of a type IV (cell-mediated) immune response. Experimental studies in a mouse model have shown that farmer's lung can be transferred to naive mice by T cells from sensitized animals, but cannot

Table 11-4. Some causes of extrinsic allergic alveolitis

Condition	Responsible agent(s)	Nature of antigen
Farmer's lung	Moldy hay, grain, straw	*Micropolyspora faeni, Thermoactinomyces vulgaris*
Bird fancier's lung	Feathers and droppings	Avian proteins
Humidifier fever (air-conditioner disease)	Humidifier aerosols	*Thermophilic actinomyces,* amebas *(Acanthameba, Naegleria gruberi)*
Sauna-taker's disease	Contaminated steam	*Aureobasidium pullulans*
Bagassosis	Moldy sugar cane	*Thermoactinomyces sacchari*
Mushroom worker's lung	Compost dust	Mushroom spores, *Thermophilic actinomyces*
Malt worker's lung	Moldy barley	*Aspergillus clavatus*
Animal handler's lung	Dusts, dander, dried urine, rats, gerbils	Urine and serum animal proteins
Diisocyanate alveolitis	Polyurethane foam production, paints, adhesives	Toluene diisocyanate
Pyrethrin alveolitis	Insecticide aerosols	Pyrethrins

be transferred by immunoglobulins from sensitized animals. This suggests a central role for sensitized T cells in the pathogenesis of the disease.

Serum precipitins (IgG) to fungal and other suspected causal agents have been demonstrated in individuals with allergic alveolitis, but similar precipitins can also be found in exposed individuals with no evidence of lung disease; thus, serum precipitins are simply thought to reflect exposures to these agents. Bronchoalveolar lavage may have a place in the diagnosis and management of extrinsic allergic alveolitis, because a prominent lymphocytosis (chiefly suppressor T cells) is a characteristic finding in the active phase of the disease. A provocative challenge with the suspected allergen should not be used routinely: These agents will make a sensitized individual acutely ill and may precipitate a severe, acute pneumonitis. Moreover, the long-term sequelae of repeated exposures is unclear, and a provocative challenge may conceivably initiate or exacerbate lung fibrosis.

The outlook for most patients with one of these forms of extrinsic allergic alveolitis is good if they present before lung fibrosis is extensive and if they cease being exposed to the offending agent(s). Corticosteroid therapy may help accelerate recovery during the acute episodes, but corticosteroids have no obvious therapeutic effect once fibrosis has developed. The prophylactic use of steroids to prevent attacks has reduced the frequency and severity of acute symptoms, but it probably does not protect against lung fibrosis.

Prevention

The prevention of diseases caused by airborne agents falls into three broad approaches.

1. The use of engineering controls, ventilation systems, enclosure of hazardous operations, substitution of highly toxic agents with less toxic agents, and other measures to reduce toxic air levels
2. The use of personal protective devices (respirators) to reduce the inhaled dose of air contaminants to the lungs
3. The use of administrative measures to remove from areas of exposure those individuals who are affected or at increased risk

Of these three measures, the most satisfactory is the first because it focuses on the source of the problem. Many industries have employed engineering controls to reduce exposures. Notable examples include coal mining and cotton textile mills. Substitution of highly toxic with less toxic materials has also been effective in reducing risks to workers, and an example of substitution is the extensive use of fibrous glass to replace asbestos for many insulation purposes.

As preventive measures, personal respiratory protection (respirators) are less satisfactory than reductions in air concentrations because the performance and use of respirators is not always optimal and individuals may receive substantial exposures to toxic agents even while wearing them. A wide range of respirators exist, from simple disposable dust masks to supplied air, full-face respirators. One of the chief reasons respirators fail is that the respirator is inappropriate for the type of exposure. A list of respirators suitable for a wide range of workplace exposures is published and updated regularly in the *NIOSH Certified Equipment List,* which is available from NIOSH or the US National Technical Information Service (NTIS). Even when respirators appropriate for the particular exposure are used, problems still arise from poor fitting of the respirator on the worker, from incorrect use by the worker, and most importantly from the fact that respirators are often extremely uncomfortable to wear for prolonged periods—some people simply cannot wear certain respirators because they feel claustrophobic.

Merely giving a respirator to a worker does not constitute adequate respiratory protection. Employers are obligated to conduct a respirator program that includes the provision of a respirator appropriate for the exposures encountered, individual fit-testing of the respirator on the worker, a training program, and frequent checking and repair of respirators.

Before any employee is issued a respirator or assigned to a task that may require a respirator, that worker must have a medical examination to determine whether he or she is capable of performing the work and using the respirator (Code of Federal Regulations, part 29, section 1910.134). Unfortunately, much of the information needed to establish medical guidelines for physicians making these decisions is lacking. As a general rule, however, anyone with documented respiratory impairment of moderate to severe degree (FEV_1 or FVC $< 70\%$ of predicted) should not be required to wear a respirator. Asthmatics with normal or mildly impaired lung function should be evaluated based on the job requirements, but should probably be excluded if they require regular medications for asthma or have had an acute asthmatic episode recently. For making medical decisions regarding respirator use, one needs to heed the *Americans with Disabilities Act,* especially if wearing a respirator is considered an essential job function.

If a respirator program is to succeed, there should be a means of assessing its effectiveness among exposed workers. A medical monitoring program may be needed to detect adverse respiratory effects from exposures and to assess whether protection is inadequate in light of the respirator program.

Administrative controls are generally the least effective methods to reduce adverse health effects from airborne toxic hazards. Medical monitoring of exposed workers and removal of those with "early" effects is obviously unsatisfactory as a preventive measure because, by definition, the individual is affected by the exposure and there is no guarantee that an "early" effect will always be reversible or will not progress to more serious disease. Another form of administrative control that is practiced frequently is exclusion of a worker from entering an area of exposure because that individual may be at increased risk. An example of such a policy is to exclude workers with a history of asthma (whether or not it is present currently) or simply atopy alone from being exposed to potent sensitizing agents such as toluene diisocyanate (TDI), a sensible approach because people with asthma usually respond more severely to potent irritants.

All of these approaches to preventing occupational pulmonary diseases have been incorporated in various standards promulgated by OSHA. Exposures to coke oven emissions (which produce lung cancer), asbestos, and cotton dust are the most completely regulated in terms of prevention (Table 11-5). These standards mandate an upper permissible air concentration (permissible exposure level, or PEL) for each of these agents, provide details of the minimum requirements for medical monitoring and industrial hygiene measurements, require respirator programs, and in some cases recommend administrative measures to be taken for affected workers.

One of the consequences of these standards has been the application by industry of new technologies for controlling air levels of toxic agents. Other industries have not needed the impetus of federal regulations to undertake similar retrofitting of old plants and incorporating engineering controls into new plants. If prevention of

Table 11-5. OSHA standards for occupational respiratory hazards

Agent	Frequency of examinations[a]	Industrial hygiene	Chest x-ray	Spirometry tests	Other	Reference
Asbestos	Preplacement Annual Termination of employment	Yes	Yes	Yes		29 CFR 1910.1001 29 CFR 1926.58 40 CFR 763
Coke oven emissions	Preplacement Annual or semiannual[b]	Yes	Yes	Yes	Sputum cytology	29 CFR 1910.1029
Cotton dust	Initial Annual or semiannual[b,c,d]	Yes	No	Yes	Standard questionnaire	29 CFR 1910.1043 29 CFR 1910.1000

[a]All examinations include a history and physical examination.
[b]Semiannual examinations are required when the worker is 45 years of age or older.
[c]Semiannual examinations are also required if FEV$_1$ decreases by 5% or 200 ml between Monday morning and afternoon; or if the FEV$_1$ is < 80% of the predicted value; or if there is any significant change in questionnaire findings, pulmonary function, or other diagnostic tests.
[d]If FEV$_1$ is < 60% of the predicted value, the worker must be referred to an expert physician for an opinion.

disease is to succeed, however, it requires the cooperation of workers and management at all levels. Potential toxic exposures are inevitable in some industries, and although many of these hazards can be avoided others cannot. Many industries are using novel materials and processes that present unknown hazards. A well-informed workforce and an attentive physician can go a long way toward anticipating potential airborne hazards and recognizing any "early" respiratory effects.

References

1. International Labor Office. *International Classification of Radiology of Pneumoconioses (revised)*. Occupational Safety and Health Science, no. 22 (revised 1980). Geneva: ILO, 1980.
2. Borbeau, J. and Ernst, P. Between- and within-reader variability in the assessment of pleural abnormality using the ILO 1980 International Classification of Pneumoconioses. *Am. J. Ind. Med.* 14:537, 1988.
3. Ducatman, A. M. Variability in interpretations of radiographs for asbestosis abnormalities: Problems and solutions. *Ann. N.Y. Acad. Sci.* 643:108, 1991.
4. Horvath, E. P. (ed.). *Manual of Spirometry in Occupational Medicine*. Washington, DC: US Dept of Health and Human Services, November 1981.
5. Ferris, B. G. (principal investigator). Epidemiology Standardization Project. *Am. Rev. Respir. Dis.* 118: 1978.
6. American Thoracic Society. Lung function testing: Selection of reference values and interpretative strategies. *Am. Rev. Respir. Dis.* 144:1202, 1991.
7. Dockery, D. W., et al. Distribution of forced expiratory volume in one second and forced vital capacity in healthy, white, adult never-smokers in six U.S. cities. *Am. Rev. Respir. Dis.* 131:511, 1985.
8. Knudson, R. J., et al. The maximal expiratory flowvolume curve. *Am. Rev. Respir. Dis.* 113:587, 1976.
9. American Medical Association. The Respiratory System. In *Guides to the Evaluation of Permanent Impairment* (3rd ed., revised). Illinois: AMA, 1990. Pp. 115–126.
10. Crapo, R. O., Morris, A. H., and Gardner, R. M. Reference spirometric values using techniques and equipment that meet the ATS recommendations. *Am. Rev. Respir. Dis.* 123:659, 1981.
11. Zavala, D. C. Diagnostic Procedures in Pulmonary Diseases. In G. L. Baum and E. Wolinsky (eds.), *Textbook of Pulmonary Diseases*. (4th ed.) Boston: Little, Brown, 1989. Pp. 330–331.
12. Parkes, W. R. *Occupational Lung Disorders,* (2nd ed.). London: Butterworth, 1982.
13. Banks, D. E., et al. Silicosis in silica flour workers. *Am. Rev. Respir. Dis.* 124:445, 1981.
14. Soutar, C. A. Update on lung disease in coalminers (editorial). *Br. J. Ind. Med.* 44:145, 1987.
15. Brooks, S. M., Weiss, M. A., and Bernstein, R. L. Reactive airways dysfunction syndrome (RADS). *Chest* 88:376, 1985.
16. Kern, D. G. Outbreak of the reactive airways dysfunction syndrome after a spill of glacial acetic acid. *Am. Rev. Respir. Dis.* 144:1058, 1991.
17. Newman Taylor, A. J. Occupational asthma. *Thorax* 35:241, 1980.
18. Chan-Yeung, M., Lam, S. Occupational asthma (state of art). *Am. Rev. Respir. Dis.* 133:686, 1986.

Further Information

Baum, G. L., and Wolinsky, E. (eds.). *Textbook of Pulmonary Diseases*. (4th ed.). Boston: Little, Brown, 1989.
An excellent text for the diagnosis, investigation, and treatment of pulmonary diseases in general.

Becklake, M. R. Asbestos-related diseases of the lung and other organs (state of art). *Am. Rev. Respir. Dis.* 114:187, 1976; and Becklake, M. R. Asbestos-related diseases of the lung and pleura (editorial). *Am. Rev. Respir. Dis.* 126:187, 1982.
Classic summaries of the malignant and nonmalignant effects of asbestos.

Chan-Yeung, M., and Lam, S. Occupational asthma. *Am. Rev. Respir. Dis.* 133:686, 1986; and Yeung, M., and Grzybowski, S. Prognosis in occupational asthma (editorial). *Thorax* 40:241, 1985.
Excellent reviews of occupational asthma by a foremost authority and experienced clinical investigator.

Ferris, B. G. (principal investigator). Epidemiology Standardization Project. *Am. Rev. Respir. Dis.* 118: 1978.
A concerted effort by senior respiratory epidemiologists and clinicians to standardize methods for the collection of respiratory health effects data. Includes details for respiratory questionnaires, spirometry and other lung function tests, and radiology of the lung.

Morgan, W. K. C., and Seaton, A. *Occupationl Lung Diseases.* Philadelphia: Saunders, 1984.
Another comprehensive text on occupational diseases and rivals Parkes' text for clarity and detail of presentation. Some sections are particularly good, notably the account of coal worker's pneumoconiosis, and the focus is oriented to a North American audience.

Parkes, W. R. *Occupational Lung Disorders,* (2nd ed.). London: Butterworth, 1982.
The premier text on occupational lung diseases. Despite its age, it remains an excellent and detailed account of the major and uncommon occupational lung disorders. It includes clear descriptions of the clinical presentations and pathology of the lung. (A new edition is expected to release in late 1994.)

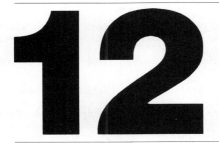

Musculoskeletal Disorders

Robert J. McCunney and
Reid T. Boswell

The diagnosis, treatment, and rehabilitation of musculoskeletal disorders constitute a large portion of clinical occupational medical practice. The physician who provides occupational medical services is likely to encounter sprains, especially to the neck, back, and shoulder; repetitive motion injuries, such as tendonitis and carpal tunnel syndrome; and soft-tissue injuries, such as lacerations and contusions. Although some occupational settings are associated with particular types of musculoskeletal disorders, such as decreased urate clearance in lead nephropathy (saturnine gout), fluorosis associated with exposure to fluorine compounds, and autoimmune dysfunction secondary to silicosis, this chapter does not attempt to discuss these rare conditions. Rather it is intended to review *common* musculoskeletal disorders, including an update on the diagnosis, treatment, and indications for referral by the primary care physician to an appropriate consultant. Because of space limitations, the gamut of musculoskeletal disorders that can be caused or aggravated by work cannot be covered.

Rates of Occupational Injuries

Musculoskeletal injuries constitute the vast majority of all occupational injuries and illnesses. The Bureau of Labor Statistics (BLS) conducts annual surveys of occupational injuries and illnesses based on a sample of various industries' Occupational Safety and Health Administration (OSHA) 200 Log. In addition, the Supplementary Data System (SDS), established under the 1970 Occupational Health and Safety Act, provides information on compensation claims in the 29 states that participate in the SDS. In 1985, occupational injuries accounted for 93% of workers' compensation claims. Of these claims, 45% were sprains and strains [1].

Occupational back injuries are the most common musculoskeletal injury in the workplace, with an estimated incidence rate of 3.5 per 100 workers. Because of the enormous importance of back disorders that limit occupational functioning, particular attention will be directed toward these conditions.

Back Disorders

Acute Back Injuries

Low back problems constitute the most expensive work-related health care problem for people in the 30 to 50 age group [2]. Total direct costs for low back disorders, excluding wage replacement, were estimated to be approximately $24 billion in 1990 [3]. Indirect costs, such as lost productivity and replacement training costs, are difficult to calculate accurately. In an evaluation of over 900 back injuries, 10% accounted for nearly 80% of total costs for all back injuries and for over 30% of all musculoskeletal injuries [2]. Thus, control of costs related to occupational back disorders depends in large part on managing the small percentage of serious disabling conditions.

Risk factors for low back injuries that result in disability include heavy repetitive lifting and pushing and pulling, as well as exposure to industrial and vehicular vibration [3]. In addition, other psychosocial characteristics have been identified as significant risk factors for disabling back injury. These include previous back injury claims; job dissatisfaction; poor ratings from supervisors; repetitive, boring tasks;

younger age and shorter duration of employment; smoking; and a history of *non–back* injury claims [3, 4].

Prolapsed intervertebral disks are most common among persons aged 25 to 45. Major risk factors for prolapsed disk include frequent lifting of objects more than 25 lb, exposure to whole body vibration, cigarette smoking, and narrow lumbar vertebral canals [5]. *Possible* associations with prolapsed disk include lifting and twisting, sedentary occupations, jobs that require prolonged static positions, lack of flexibility or physical fitness, and pregnancy [5].

Table 12-1 lists prevalence of back injury claims among various occupations.

The Diagnosis of Low Back Pain

Most low back problems related to work are diagnosed and treated by primary care physicians. The clinical approach to evaluating such disorders includes an appropriate history, physical examination, and diagnostic imaging or laboratory testing when necessary [6].

The causes of low back pain include: (1) musculo ligamentous injuries; (2) vertebral fractures, including compression fractures; (3) degenerative changes; (4) spinal stenosis; (5) anatomic anomalies, such as spondylolisthesis; (6) herniated intervertebral disks with nerve root compression; (7) systemic diseases, such as cancer, spinal infections, and ankylosing spondylitis; and (8) visceral diseases unrelated to the spine [7]. It should be noted, however, that a definitive diagnosis cannot be reached in up to 85% of patients with low back pain [7].

History

Usually, a worker who experiences back pain is likely to describe a precipitating event associated with the discomfort. It is not uncommon, however, for a person to be unable to relate the onset of back discomfort to a particular incident. Because of certain requirements of the workers' compensation system that encourage the reporting of an *injurious event,* people tend to relate the discomfort to some specific workplace activity. In the absence thereof, workers' compensation benefits may be denied. In the nonoccupational setting, however, only about one third of back problems are associated with a specific event [8].

Elements of a good clinical history are of value in evaluating back pain. An inquiry should be directed to the *onset* of pain, its character, duration, radiation, and measures that relieve the discomfort. Questions regarding neurologic symptoms such as pain radiation, especially down the posterior aspect of the leg; numbness or paresthesias in the feet; or weakness can help determine whether nerve route irritation secondary to a herniated disk is present.

Although pain radiation from the back down the posterior aspect of either leg is strongly associated with nerve irritation secondary to an injured disk, such radicular symptoms are not uncommon in acute non–disk-related back disorders. Pain radiation in the "non-disk" back disorder commonly extends to the buttocks and posterior aspect of the upper leg. This is referred pain based on the common embryologic origin of structures that eventually form the low back and muscles, tendon, and ligaments in the posterior thigh. Pain radiation *beyond the knee* is a more ominous finding and is rare in acute back injuries without associated disk herniation.

Patients will often point to the low back region in a circular manner in the vicinity

Table 12-1. Back compensation claims by occupation

Occupation	Claims/100 workers
Miscellaneous laborers	12.3
Garbage collectors	11.1
Warehouse workers	9.3
Miscellaneous mechanics	5.6
Nursing aides	3.6

Source: Abstracted from B. P. Klein, R. C. Jensen, and I. M. Sanderson. Assessment of workers' compensation claims for back strains/sprains. *J.O.M.* 26:443, 1984; based on 1979 data of the Supplementary Data System (SDS).

of the sacroiliac joints as the source of their discomfort. Rarely, one particular "trigger point" or local area of tenderness can be elicited. The pain is usually relieved by rest and heat applied to the lower back.

In the course of the medical history, it is helpful to inquire about the *nature of the work* that the person performs, including the availability of mechanical lifting devices and the weight of the material that is expected to be lifted. The National Institute for Occupational Safety and Health (NIOSH) has issued guidelines on safe lifting practices [9], which have been updated (see Chap. 28, Ergonomics). Many organizations also restrict the amount of material that can be lifted by the unaided worker.

It is also wise to review whether the person has had a previous back injury, since back injuries have a high rate of recurrence. In fact, most clinical evaluations suggest that subsequent back injuries usually are more uncomfortable for the person and require a longer period of time for resolution of the symptoms.

Although nearly all back injuries will respond to conservative measures, it is critically important during the history for the physician to evaluate the possibility of an emergency surgical disorder, the cauda equina syndrome. This disorder, secondary to a *centrally herniated* disk, usually results in pain radiation down *both legs,* saddle anesthesia, bowel incontinence, or urinary retention. The predictive value of a negative history of urinary retention is estimated to be 0.9999 [7]. Anal sphincter tone is reduced in 60 to 80% of cases [7]. Immediate diagnosis and treatment for this condition are imperative. Otherwise, even in the presence of a herniated disk, initial treatment consists of conservative measures.

Physical Examination

The physical examination of the patient with low back pain is comprehensive and aimed at identifying specific pathology. The history and detailed physical examination will rule out disorders that require further testing 85 to 90% of the time. Initially, the patient is observed walking. The gait should be symmetric, and the extent of ankle dorsiflexion and plantar flexion should be noted. This helps verify motor strength. Overall alignment of the spine is then assessed. Patients with spinal stenosis will frequently maintain a *flexed posture* to increase the area of the spinal canal. Similarly, facet joint disease is usually made more comfortable by mild flexion. Conversely, patients with a herniated disk will frequently maintain a position of *extension.* Next, the range of motion of the lumbar spine should be recorded. Paraspinal muscle spasm should be noted, as should any change in spasm with position.

Testing should always then be performed for pain elicited by the straight-leg raising (SLR) test and Patrick's test (Fig. 12-1). The SLR maneuver produces stretch on the sciatic nerve and in the presence of nerve compression should exacerbate pain. The examination is first done with the patient sitting and then in the supine position. *Results should be identical.* A positive test is noted when SLR causes leg discomfort from 0 to 70 degrees. If only back pain is produced, the examination is negative. Dorsiflexing the foot usually exaggerates the leg pain caused by SLR in the presence of a herniated disk. In contrast, *plantar flexion should not lead to an increase in pain;* when it does, a nonorganic etiology of pain is suggested. Many observers find the *contralateral SLR* test to be very helpful in the diagnosis of a herniated disk; elevation of the nonsymptomatic leg causes sciatic-type pain in the symptomatic leg, which is kept still.

A detailed neurologic examination is then performed. Sensation to light touch, pressure, and vibration is tested in dermatomal distributions L1-S4. The muscle strength of the hip flexors (L1-L3), knee flexors (L2-L4), ankle dorsiflexors (L4), long toe extensors (L5), ankle evertors (L5, S1), and ankle plantar flexors (S1, S2), is sequentially examined and graded. Reflexes are tested for intensity and duration of response. Attempts are then made to elicit ankle clonus and the Babinski reflex.

Finally, a general physical examination should be done, checking for abdominal disorders associated with back discomfort. This approach includes a rectal and, when necessary, a pelvic examination.

Although not exhaustive, the preceding examination will aid the physician in determining the etiology of low back pain.

Diagnostic Imaging

Plain films of the lumbosacral spine are of limited value in the diagnosis of acute back pain, unless there is clinical suspicion of vertebral fracture, primary or metastatic cancer, or infection (osteomyelitis). Magnetic resonance imaging (MRI) is rapidly becoming the procedure of choice in the diagnosis of herniated intervertebral

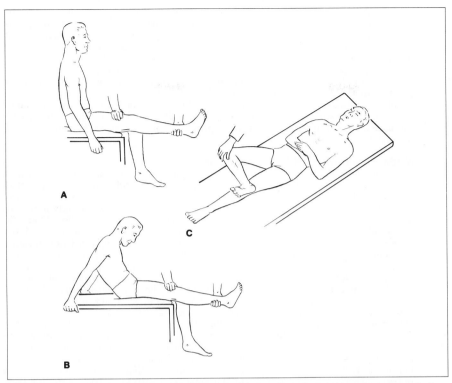

Figure 12-1. A and B. Straight-leg raising test. In A there is no evidence of sciatic irritation. In B the test is positive for sciatic or nerve root irritation. Results should be identical in the sitting and supine positions. A *positive* test elicits *pain radiation* down the
posterior aspect of the leg at 0 to 70 degrees. The production of back pain only is not
considered a *positive* sign. C. Patrick's test. Positive when pain is elicited in the hip joint
or in the sacroiliac joint region as the heel is placed on the opposite knee and leg and the
flexed knee is forced to the table.

disk and spinal stenosis [10]. Indications for obtaining an MRI of the lumbosacral
spine include persistent pain or numbness in a dermatomal distribution; presence
of neurologic abnormalities, such as loss of ankle jerk or muscle strength; and
presence of neurogenic claudication (pain or neurologic deficits after walking or
prolonged standing) [6].

It is important to keep in mind that anatomic evidence of a damaged disk may be
found in 20 to 30% of *normal persons* [6]. Therefore, results of MRI or other imaging
techniques *must* be interpreted in light of clinical findings.

Acute Management of Low Back Pain

The cornerstones of treatment for low back pain arising from a work-related episode
are rest and symptomatic relief of the discomfort. Although the precise amount of
bed rest that is necessary to promote relief of low back pain is debatable, a recent
study suggests no difference in outcome (period of recovery) between the *recommendation* of 2 or 7 days of bed rest [11]. To motivate people to follow suggestions for
bed rest, it is sometimes helpful to point out that bed rest is the only position that
truly rests muscles that may be injured in an acute back disorder. Any other position,
including sitting, standing, or walking, requires the use of the lower back and
associated muscles and ligaments for posture and support.

Within the first 24 hours of acute pain, ice applied to the area of discomfort can
be helpful. An example of an effective technique is an *ice lollie,* a small paper cup
filled with water and then frozen. The person then peels the top of the paper off the

cup; the frozen cup can then be used as a handle by another person to massage the painful area. Deep muscle spasms and associated pain are often relieved by this simple measure. After the *acute phase* of the injury however, locally applied heat through the use of heating pads, whirlpool, or hot baths is usually effective in providing immediate but temporary relief.

In many cases of acute back pain, muscle spasm occurs, for which the administration of a muscle relaxant can afford relief. The use of nonsteroidal antiinflammatory agents can also aid in symptomatic relief [12].

Following treatment, the physician must file an appropriate report in accordance with the state's workers' compensation statutes. Prompt filing of reports will assist the patient in obtaining income replacement benefits guaranteed by workers' compensation.

Medical Follow-Up of Low Back Injury

Because fear and anxiety are often associated with low back pain, it is important for the physician to counsel such patients appropriately. Advising the patient that low back injuries do not generally heal in a few days can help the person respond better to the treatment process. Failing to advise the patient accordingly may lead to frustration in the otherwise healthy younger person (usually between 20 and 50 years old) not accustomed to the limitations in activity that are often associated with back pain. In turn, the person may seek other opinions by practitioners, such as acupuncturists, chiropractors, and others whose diagnostic acumen may be limited. Unfortunately, so much medical uncertainty is associated with back disorders (in terms of cause, source of pain, and treatment) that these differences of opinions may lead the person to become more confused than helped. Consequently, frequent follow-up evaluations, especially in the early phase of an injury, are advisable. In this period, patients often voice their greatest concerns.

During these follow-up evaluations, the physician can inquire about (1) the presence of *symptoms* noted during the initial evaluation, especially those related to nerve route irritation; (2) the *response to treatment;* and (3) how the discomfort has affected activities of daily living. After the initial phase of treatment (3-5 days), it is frequently helpful to refer the patient to a physical therapist who is experienced in treating occupational injuries. The therapist can institute passive treatment, such as thermal modalities and ultrasound, and begin range of motion exercises and patient education.

When the patient's condition begins to improve, one should institute *gentle exercises,* preceded by a hot pack. For stretching, Williams' exercises are appropriate for the patient recovering from the acute phase of a low back injury. The exercises are *not* intended to produce muscle strength but to *stretch* the large paravertebral muscles and the smaller muscles beneath them. The more these muscles receive gentle stretching, the quicker the resolution of deep muscle spasm. Flexion and extension exercises, however, should *not* be done to the point of pain, but gradually so that the individual regains full use of the previously injured area (Fig. 12-2).

Since the recovery process from an acute back injury can be prolonged, physicians will find it of value to be diligent and attentive to detail in note taking during follow-up evaluations. Because of the protracted nature of recovery from many back injuries, subtle improvements may not be easily recognized by the patient. Thus, with proper documentation, the physician can demonstrate that improvements have occurred and in turn encourage the patient toward recovery. The frequency of follow-up evaluations varies considerably and depends on the nature of the disorder, age of the person, history of previous back disorders, underlying medical conditions, and the type of job to which the person will be returning. Ideally, patients should be evaluated at least weekly.

During the follow-up period, the physician is advised to take an active role in facilitating a return to work in either a full or a modified-duty capacity. Early return to work (if sufficient improvement has occurred) can be therapeutic from a number of perspectives. Although modified-duty policies may exist at some places of employment, specific recommendations are essential. General terms such as "light duty" should be discouraged in favor of more specific guidelines. For example, the use of *long-handled objects* such as brooms and rakes can aggravate low back discomfort in many people. A supervisor unaware of this potential problem may inadvertently assign an injured worker to such a task with the assumption that such work is light duty, especially in contrast to a material-handling position. Any back discomfort that develops as a result of these activities is likely not only to frustrate the worker

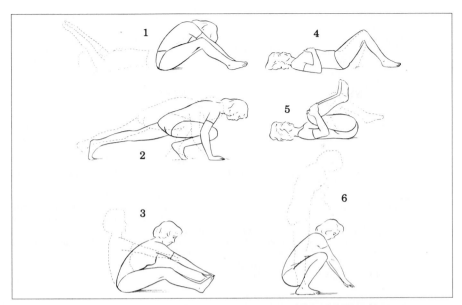

Figure 12-2. Therapeutic exercises helpful in promoting recovery from a back injury.

Exercise 1 is directed toward developing the abdominal muscles. By varying the distance of the heels from the buttocks, it can usually be accomplished without foot anchorage.

Exercise 2 is aimed primarily at stretching the fascia latae and the iliofemoral ligament, as well as hip flexor muscles. This exercise is frequently not indicated in those individuals who present loose joints and a relaxed attitude. The foot of the extended extremity should be dorsiflexed so that the weight is borne on the ball of the foot and rotated internally so that tension is applied principally to the anterolateral aspect of the thigh. The knee of the extended extremity should remain rigidly fixed in the extended position during the exercise.

Exercise 3 is aimed at restoring lumbosacral flexion and stretching shortened hamstring muscles. It should not be used in those experiencing acute radiating pain into the extremities until these symptoms have been relieved.

Exercise 4 is aimed at developing the gluteus maximus. The pelvis is rotated forward by actively contracting these muscles. The buttocks are lifted off the floor, but the abdomen should remain down and the spine should not be lifted from the floor above the waist line.

Exercise 5 is aimed at stretching the contractures of the erector spinae and all structures posterior to the upright center of gravity at this level. The knees should be pulled to the axillae rather than over the shoulders.

Exercise 6 is directed at restoring flexion of the lumbosacral spine and actively developing the gluteus maximus and the femoral quadriceps. The success of a postural program depends to a large extent on the strength of these two muscles, since the lumbosacral spine can be controlled only by those who have the ability to squat up or down with ease, thus avoiding raising the trunk with the erector spinae muscles. The principle involved in this one exercise would avoid most low back disability if rigidly employed in our daily activities. The weight should be borne on the heels, and the entire spine should remain flexed at all times during the course of the exercise.

but also to interfere with the treatment process and affect the trust and credibility of the physician. Consequently, specific instructions, such as no lifting greater than 20 lb or no frequent bending, lifting, or twisting, are preferable. Frequent changes in position to avoid prolonged standing or sitting are also advisable. Fortunately, well over 90% of acute back injuries respond to conservative therapy, and people are able to return to their original line of work [13].

Useful definitions of levels of work could be as follows [14]:

Very heavy work involves lifting objects weighing more than 100 lb at a time, with frequent lifting or carrying of objects weighing 50 lb or more.

Heavy work involves lifting of no more than 100 lb at a time, with frequent lifting or carrying of objects weighing up to 50 lb.

Medium work is defined as involving the lifting of no more than 50 lb at a time, with frequent lifting or carrying of objects weighing up to 25 lb. Workers with 5% or less back-related permanent partial physical impairment can qualify in this category, but those with higher rates cannot.

Light work is described as involving lifting of no more than 20 lb at a time, with frequent lifting or carrying of objects weighing up to 10 lb. Applicants with between 10 and 15% permanent partial physical impairment because of a low back problem should be able to do this type of work.

Sedentary work is described as that involving no more than the lifting of 10 lb at a time and occasional lifting or carrying of articles such as docket files, ledgers, or small tools. Applicants with 20 or 25% permanent partial physical impairment should be capable of this type of work.

Chronic Back Disorders

Chronic back disorders usually refer to back pain that has been present for over 6 weeks and that has not responded to conservative measures. The physician is likely to be asked to evaluate the persistence of a back disorder that has interfered with work capabilities. In this setting, a detailed history and additional laboratory and ancillary procedures are usually necessary to evaluate the possibility of other causes of back pain (Table 12-2).

History

Questions should be directed to the *character* of the pain. For example, morning stiffness can be associated with underlying inflammatory disorders such as ankylosing spondylitis. Pain in the legs precipitated by walking (pseudoclaudication) relieved by rest, especially by flexion of the hip, may be associated with spinal stenosis. Pain that is steady and aggravated by palpation can be due to tumors or multiple myeloma.

A review of medical records, including results of diagnostic tests and treatment measures, is necessary. In some cases, people have been advised merely to "rest" for upward of 3 to 4 weeks. In these settings, the cause of the discomfort may be muscle stiffness and tightness, which can be readily relieved with therapeutic exercises. The physician may also encounter a person who demonstrates a psychological disturbance or fear and anxiety that interfere with the recovery process and ability to return to work.

In the assessment of a chronic back disorder, it is wise to consider the role of psychological and emotional factors that may interfere with recovery. In one study of 111 patients with chronic low back disorders, nearly half were considered disabled primarily "on a psychiatric basis" [15]. In another report, about 20% of patients admitted to a chronic pain rehabilitation program were "overtly or covertly fraudulent, i.e., seeking by their own volition to maximize monetary gain . . ." [16].

Although true malingering (factitious symptoms) is rare, emotional issues often interfere with recovery and return to work. Table 12-3 displays some of the nonorganic physical signs in low back pain [17]. Figure 12-3 indicates aspects of the physical examination that suggest embellishment of symptoms.

Laboratory Testing

Depending on the history and physical examination, appropriate blood testing, especially an erythrocyte sedimentation rate (ESR), may be of value. This nonspecific parameter, if highly elevated, can prompt a search for other disorders such as ankylosing spondylitis, tumors, or infections. Further testing might include an HLA-B27 antigen for ankylosing spondylitis or an alkaline phosphatase for Paget's dis-

Table 12-2. Causes of low back pain

Causes	Examples
Mechanical	
Trauma	Lumbosacral strain and sprain
	Sacroiliac sprain
	Vertebral fractures
Congenital	Spondylolisthesis and spondylolysis
	Transitional vertebra
	Facet tropism
Acquired	Herniated disk
	Spinal stenosis
	Facet syndrome
	Obesity
Nonmechanical	
Rheumatologic disorders	Ankylosing spondylitis
	Reiter's syndrome
	Psoriatic arthritis
	Enteropathic arthritis
	Rheumatoid arthritis
	Vertebral osteochondritis
	Polymyalgia rheumatica
	Fibrositis
Infections	Vertebral osteomyelitis
	Intervertebral disk space infection
	Pyogenic sacroiliitis
	Herpes zoster
Tumors and infiltrative lesions	Osteoid ostema
	Osteoblastoma
	Osteochondroma
	Giant-cell tumor
	Hemangioma
	Eosinophilic granuloma
	Multiple myeloma
	Lymphomas
	Skeletal metastases
	Retroperitoneal tumors
Endocrinologic and metabolic disorders	Osteoporosis
	Osteomalacia
	Parathyroid disease
	Ochronosis
	Pituitary disease
	Paget's disease of bone
Hematologic disorders	Hemoglobinopathies
	Myelofibrosis
Referred pain	Vertebral sarcoidosis
	Retroperitoneal fibrosis
	Abdominal aortic aneurysm

ease. Alterations in serum calcium, phosphorus, and acid phosphatase can also occur in other disorders that are associated with back pain (Table 12-4). A bone scan may be of value, if a tumor, infection, or fracture is suspected.

Electromyography/Nerve Conduction Velocity (EMG/NCV)
Electrodiagnostic techniques can help in the diagnosis of nerve route irritation secondary to a herniated disk. A negative electromyographic study, however, does not exclude neural involvement, because early changes secondary to nerve compression from a herniated disk may not be detected within the first few weeks of the disorder. Properly conducted and analyzed studies can confirm clinical findings of abnormal motor or sensory function. In conjunction with other studies such as MRI [10], EMG/NCV assessment can aid in determining the severity of the disorder.

Table 12-3. Nonorganic physical signs in low back pain

Category	Test	Comments
Tenderness	Superficial palpation	Inordinate, widespread sensitivity to light touch over lumbar spine suggests *amplified symptoms*
Simulation (to assess patient cooperation and reliability)	Axial loading	Light pressure to skull should *not* significantly increase symptoms
	Rotation	Physician should rotate patient's shoulders, which does not move lumbar spine and should not increase pain
Distraction	Straight-leg raising	Physician asks seated patient to straighten knee; patients with true sciatic tension will arch backward and complain; these results should match those of the traditional, recumbent straight-leg test
Regional		Diffuse motor weakness or bizarre sensory deficits suggest functional disturbances if they involve multiple muscle groups and cannot be explained by neuroanatomic principles
Overreaction		Excessive and inappropriate grimacing

In addition, if conducted at periodic intervals, EMG/NVC studies can indicate areas of improvement.

Treatment
The essential element in treating chronic back disorders without a primary cause is patient *education*. People should be thoroughly instructed in activities of daily living that may relieve or aggravate back discomfort. If a referral to a physical therapy unit has not already been initiated, patients with chronic back pain should be evaluated by an experienced physiotherapist. Physiotherapy has been shown to decrease severity of pain complaints compared to continued medical treatment alone [18]. While chiropractic manipulation may also reduce back pain, the long-term efficacy of manipulation therapy has not been conclusively demonstrated [19]. Furthermore, chiropractic is no more effective than physical therapy, which is a far less expensive treatment option [18].

Transcutaneous electrical nerve stimulators (TENS units) have been used for patients with chronic back pain. However, a controlled clinical trial showed *no* benefit of TENS units versus placebo for chronic back pain [20]. The use of steroid injections has been another option in the treatment of chronic back pain. In a double-blind, randomized trial of steroid injections versus placebo in patients with chronic mechanical low back pain, no significant difference was seen in reported improvement in pain over 6 months [21].

Referrals to a neurosurgeon or an orthopedic surgeon should only be considered when surgery is a *reasonable option* for treatment of low back pain. Present indications for operation include cauda equina syndrome, spinal stenosis, and herniated intervertebral disk associated with nerve root impingement and nonresponse to conservative treatment, or progressive neurologic deficits. It should be noted that chronic back pain and radiculopathy resulting from a herniated intervertebral disk frequently respond to conservative treatment alone [22]. Where evidence of depression exists, especially in long-standing disorders, the administration of tricyclic antidepressants may be effective. Clinicians are advised, however, of the importance of referring such individuals to an appropriate therapist.

Rehabilitation and Return to Work Status
Determining a person's ability to return to a job after a back injury can be problematic. In most cases, people with back injuries are able to return to their original type of work without any restrictions. In other cases, however, especially in those rare

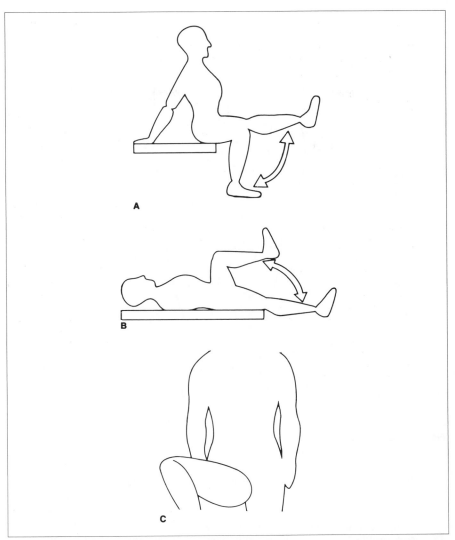

Figure 12-3. Confusion tests in evaluating chronic back pain and determining validity of physical complaints. A. Confusion test 1, knee extension while sitting. If the supine patient has limitation of straight-leg raising, the limitation should be reproducible while the patient is in the sitting position. B. Confusion test 2, hip flexion. Patients with lumbar complaints should *not* experience increased pain when the hip is passively flexed (knee kept in flexion). C. Confusion test 3, Faber's test. Patients with lumbar complaints should *not* experience increased pain when the hip is flexed, abducted, and externally rotated (knee kept in flexion). D. Confusion test 4, skin hypersensitivity to touch in the lumbar area. Patients with lumbar complaints should *not* experience increased pain when the overlying skin is lightly touched. E. Confusion test 5, stocking-type numbness in the lower extremities. Patients with lumbar complaints should *not* have hypesthesia in a stocking-type distribution. (Adapted from William F. Kennedy, MD, Neenah, Wisconsin.)

(continued)

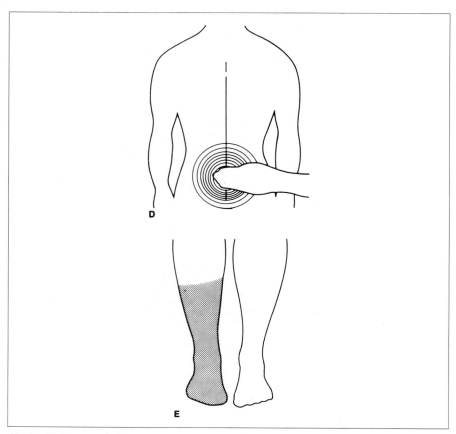

Figure 12-3 (continued)

Table 12-4. Laboratory tests of potential value in assessing chronic back pain

Test	Result
Complete blood count	Elevated in systemic disease
Erythrocyte sedimentation rate	Elevated in infection, tumor, ankylosing spondylitis
Calcium	Elevated in hyperparathyroidism, metastatic tumor; low in advanced osteomalacia
Alkaline phosphatase	Elevated in infiltrative bone disease (tumor), infection (osteomyelitis, diskitis); may be mildly elevated with recent fracture or Paget's disease; a normal glutamyl transpeptidase or 5′-nucleotidase will confirm bone origin
Phosphorus	Increased in renal osteodystrophy, occasionally decreased in osteomalacia
Acid phosphatase	Increased in most cases of metastatic prostate carcinoma
Urinalysis	Abnormal with genitourinary infection of neoplasm
HLA-B27 antigen	Occasionally useful in suspected ankylosing spondylitis with negative or equivocal radiographic changes
Uric acid	Gout
Urine—Bence-Jones protein	Myeloma

disorders that require surgery, considerable alterations may be necessary. Where repeated episodes of back injury have occurred, it may be worthwhile to refer the person to a physical therapy unit for a work hardening program. These types of programs are designed to educate people in proper lifting techniques and gradually to build up their endurance to handle physically demanding jobs. Particular attention to body mechanics, posture, and physical exercise can be instrumental in reducing the risk of future injury.

Prevention of Back Injuries

Because of the prevalence of back problems in the occupational setting, numerous measures have been attempted to prevent, control, and reduce the rate of these disabling ailments. No one preventive approach has proved effective in all situations, and no one specific intervention in itself has been sufficient to reduce the impact of back disorders [23]. An effective preventive program depends on the coordination of a number of efforts, including proper selection and placement, appropriate job design, and maintenance of health through education and physical fitness. Coupled with early recognition and prompt and efficient treatment of back injuries, these preventive measures can reduce the rate of back disorders, which result in the second leading cause of absences from work. (Upper-respiratory infections, such as colds and influenza, lead the list.)

Proper Selection and Placement

Ideally, people at risk of suffering from back injuries could be identified based on a review of individual characteristics and job requirements. Unfortunately, no specific set of criteria applies to all situations. During the preplacement evaluation, attention can be directed toward previous job responsibilities and episodes of back injuries, since the *best predictor* for future back injuries is past history of a back injury [24]. Once a history regarding previous injuries has been obtained, physical examination is unlikely to add any useful information regarding a prospective employee's risk for future back injury [25].

A review of proposed job duties during the examination is essential. The physician should inquire as to the *frequency* that materials might be lifted, their respective weight, and the availability of lifting devices. Proper placement in a material-handling position of a person with a history of back injuries but no current symptoms and a normal examination can be complicated. Many factors will affect whether another back injury occurs, including level of motivation, physical fitness, and circumstances beyond control.

An abnormality that may be noted during a physical examination is leg length inequality. Population studies, however, have demonstrated that leg length discrepancies of up to 4 cm are *not* associated with an increased incidence of low back pain. For people with greater than a 2.5-cm congenital shortening, the use of a small lift in the shoe may increase physical comfort.

It has been suggested that certain personality "types" may be at greater risk of back injuries; however, evidence supporting such claims is lacking. On the other hand, psychological testing has been shown to predict an individual's response to treatment [26]. In fact, one study of 200 workers' compensation cases suggested that psychological factors play a major role in back injuries that occur in workers' compensation settings. The study employed the use of the Minnesota Multiphase Personality Index (MMPI) to measure psychological function [27] and showed that one third of the workers' compensation cases referred for psychological evaluation were back disorders. The authors suggested that psychological disability may profoundly affect an existing physical impairment. The results indicate that a referral to an appropriate therapist may be of value in assessing the many factors involved in long-term disability.

LUMBOSACRAL SPINE FILMS. Lumbosacral spine films have been used since the 1920s in an attempt to identify conditions of the lower back that might predispose one to future injury [28]. Such efforts, however, have failed to meet their promise and are strongly discouraged for routine use [29, 30]. One particular abnormality, however, of the sacrohorizontal angle (i.e., the relationship between the superior border or S1 and a horizontal plane) has been associated with an increased incidence of low back pain only if the angle exceeds 70 degrees. Another abnormality, spondylolisthesis, however, occurs in 2 to 10% of the population [24] and does not appear to increase the risk of back injuries.

Another common condition, narrow disk space, for example, is not associated with an increased rate of low back pain. The rate of disk degeneration varies, and a strong genetic component to its development appears to exist. In rare cases, severe disk generation that occurs at an early age may contribute to low back pain in some people.

STRENGTH TESTING. Isometric strength testing conducted in relation to the requirements of the job has been suggested as a means of predicting those at an increased risk of back injury [31–33]. Measurements of physical capacity have also been recommended as a means of predicting those susceptible to injuries. Although both strength and fitness testing have been advocated for their preventive value, the true impact of these interventions on occupational back disorders has yet to be determined.

Maintenance of a Healthy Back

Once a person begins work in a job with a higher risk of back injuries, efforts should be directed to controlling the development of these disabling conditions. The foremost consideration in preventing back injuries is appropriate *job design.* Proper design of material-handling positions has been estimated to reduce up to one third of compensable low back injuries [8]. Ergonomics, the science directed toward fitting the job to the person, is an essential component of efficient job design.

Other techniques that can be used at work to control back injuries include *guidelines* regarding weights that one can lift without overexertion. For example, some transportation industries as well as the US Postal Service limit the amount of weight that can be lifted without mechanical support to 70 lb or less. If the physician learns that a job requires lifting objects more than 100 lb, efforts should be directed to the use of mechanical lifting devices. NIOSH has established guidelines [9] for safe lifting; however, the appropriateness of the biomechanical criteria proposed has recently been challenged [34].

Education in proper lifting techniques has also been helpful in some situations. Most training programs include basic measures that emphasize the following aspects of lifting [8]: (1) Keep the object close to the body; (2) lift slowly, smoothly, and without a jerking, erratic motion; (3) lift without twisting; (4) maintain good physical fitness; and (5) lift with the knees bent.

Physical fitness programs have also been promoted as effective in preventing back injuries [35]. A study of the Los Angeles Fire Department showed a decrease in injuries between 1971 and 1978 that was attributed, in part, to better fitness levels. The rate of injuries dropped from 2134 in 1971 to 1814 in 1977 without an accompanying change in the size of the workforce or job duties [36]. These findings were contradicted, however, in a study of aircraft workers, which showed no correlation between levels of cardiovascular fitness and back injuries [37]. Persons with previous back injuries who participate in formal "back school" prevention programs have shown a reduction in the incidence of new injuries [38] and a reduction in mean absenteeism for back pain complaints [39].

The physician who is asked to recommend a preventive back program for a local organization is advised to consider a number of issues, including (1) medical data related to back injuries, (2) investigations (job review, in particular) related to the accidents at work, (3) job requirements, and (4) an individual's work capacity.

By coordinating the above measures and implementing prompt and efficient treatment that employs the use of therapeutic exercises, the incidence of back pain and the related sequelae can be controlled. Business personnel must be informed about the need for frequent education of both supervisors and workers on proper back care and lifting techniques. Vigilant review of active back injury cases and appropriate reevaluation prior to return to work are essential.

Shoulder Disorders

A variety of shoulder injuries are common in the occupational setting. *Impingement syndrome,* also referred to as rotator cuff tendonitis or subacromial bursitis, develops when the tendons of the rotator cuff are compressed when the shoulder is flexed and elevated. Repeated impingement can lead to inflammation of the tendons, which can extend to the subacromial bursa. Symptoms of pain may be acute or chronic and the patient may have a history of specific overuse, particularly above shoulder level. Strength and range of motion are often normal, but there will be pain on resisted forward shoulder flexion at 90 degrees while the arm is held extended and internally rotated ("impingement sign"). Treatment consists of antiinflammatory medications, ice, and rest, with subsequent physical therapy referral for range of motion and stretching exercises. Steroid injection should be considered if the patient has no initial improvement.

Bicipital tendonitis is similar to impingement syndrome in that the proximal bicipital tendon becomes inflamed from repetitive motion. The patient usually has pain in the bicipital groove and on resisted forearm flexion. Treatment is similar to that for impingement syndrome.

Rotator cuff tears usually result from acute injury, but may be chronic. Examination reveals weakness on arm abduction through 60 degrees. Magnetic resonance imaging is usually required to confirm the diagnosis. Partial or chronic tears can be treated conservatively with strengthening and range of motion exercises. Complete tears should be evaluated by an orthopedic surgeon for consideration of surgical repair.

Recurrent glenohumeral subluxation can occur following acute shoulder dislocation resulting from a torn glenoid labrum (Bankart lesion) or a fracture of the humeral neck ("fracture dislocation"). Anterior instability is diagnosed by "apprehension sign," wherein the patient becomes apprehensive when the shoulder is abducted and externally rotated. The patient may also give a history of a painful feeling of the joint being "out of place." Posterior instability is diagnosed when the patient is apprehensive when the arm is placed in forward flexion to 90 degrees in full internal rotation and some adduction and the arm is directed posteriorly. Conservative treatment, consisting of strengthening exercises, should be undertaken initially. If unsuccessful, or if posterior instability is present, orthopedic referral should be considered.

Acromioclavicular (AC) separation results from direct trauma to the AC joint. There is tenderness over the AC joint and pain on any shoulder motion. X-rays of the affected shoulder, with and without weights, will reveal displacement of the AC joint. First-degree separation is incomplete AC ligament tear without joint subluxation, second degree is some joint subluxation, while third degree is full tear of the AC ligament and coracoclavicular ligament with obvious subluxation. First- and second-degree separation can be treated with an arm sling, ice, and antiinflammatory medications, followed by strengthening exercises 1 to 3 weeks after the injury. Third-degree tears should be referred to an orthopedic surgeon for possible surgical correction.

Other diagnoses to consider when a patient presents with a shoulder injury or pain are glenoid labrum tears, pericapsulitis, osteoarthritis, and "SLAP" tears (superior labrum, anterior, and posterior). SLAP tears require diagnosis by arthroscopy when conservative treatment is unsuccessful.

Knee Injuries

Traumatic injuries to the knee may result either from direct external trauma, hyperextension, or varus or valgus twisting injuries.

Tears of the *medial or lateral meniscus* occur as a result of twisting with the foot planted. Pain is usually immediate followed by swelling, and there may be a history of "giving way," "locking," or "clicking" on ambulation. MacMurray's test is performed with the hip flexed to 90 degrees and knee flexed to 90 degrees. The knee is then rotated either internally (lateral tears) or externally (medial tears), and the hip and the knee are gradually extended. If pain is elicited, the test is positive, but there is a high rate of false negatives. There is often localized joint line tenderness, which may be the only finding on examination. Definitive diagnosis requires MRI or arthroscopy. Initial treatment consists of immobilization for 1 to 3 weeks with ice and antiinflammatory medications, followed by a quadriceps strengthening program. If pain persists, or if the patient has a history of locking or concurrent ligament tears, referral to an orthopedist should be initiated.

Injuries to the *medial and lateral collateral ligaments* occur with a twisting injury or externally applied trauma. The ligament may be stretched or partially torn (sprain) or completely torn. Medial collateral ligament injuries are more common. One should check for collateral ligament instability by stabilizing the femur with the knee held at 0 degrees and then flexed to 20 degrees with slight external rotation. Varus and valgus stress should be applied, making sure that there is good muscular relaxation; comparison should always be made with the unaffected knee. For acute injuries, x-rays should be performed to rule out an associated fracture. Coexistent meniscal or cruciate ligament tears may be present. Sprains can be treated with immobilization and ice for 24 hours; then progressive weight-bearing can be allowed. Orthopedic referral should be made if instability is present or if an associated meniscus tear cannot be ruled out.

Anterior cruciate ligament (ACL) injuries occur when force is applied to a slightly flexed knee or in twisting injuries. Often, a "pop" with immediate swelling may be noted at the time of the injury. The anterior drawer test is performed by applying anterior force to the fibia with the knee flexed at 90 degrees. This test can be performed in the supine position with the foot at 0 degrees, 30 degrees internal rotation, and 30 degrees external rotation with immobilization by sitting on the foot. The test can also be performed in the sitting position without foot immobilization. Muscular relaxation (especially of the hamstrings) is essential. Results should always be compared with the unaffected side. Lockman's test is performed by stabilizing the femur with one hand and applying anterior force to the tibia with the knee flexed at 30 degrees. The pivot-shift test is performed by applying valgus stress to the knee in extension with the tibia internally rotated, and slowly flexing the knee to about 30 degrees. A "pop" with pain suggests ACL laxity. Diagnosis often requires MRI for confirmation. If there is evidence of ligament instability, one should immobilize the knee and refer the patient to an orthopedic surgeon.

Posterior cruciate ligament (PCL) tears are usually associated with a severe injury involving other structures. Isolated PCL tears are uncommon, but can occur with externally applied trauma to the anterior tibia with the knee flexed. The posterior drawer test is performed by applying posterior force to the tibia with the knee flexed at 90 degrees. Frequently the tibia is in a posterior sagging position ("spontaneous posterior drawer") and it may appear that the *anterior* drawer is positive, when in fact the examiner is simply pulling the tibia into the anatomically correct position. One should always check the initial position of the tibia and evaluate if there is a firm anterior "endpoint" when performing the anterior drawer test. Treatment for isolated PCL tears consists of quadriceps strengthening and gradual return to normal activities. When other structures are involved, referral to an orthopedist is advised.

Diagnoses to consider if the patient has no specific history of trauma include *patellofemoral pain syndrome* (chondromalacia patellae), *anserine tendonitis, osteoarthritis,* and *prepatellar or infrapatellar bursitis.*

Cumulative Trauma Disorders

Cumulative trauma disorders, also referred to as repetitive motion injuries, are conditions that are thought to be due to the repetitive performance of a similar task, rather than an injury that results from a single traumatic event [40]. Cumulative trauma disorders (CTDs) primarily affect the upper extremities, especially the wrist, and include such disorders as carpal tunnel syndrome, wrist tendonitis, ulnar nerve entrapment, epicondylitis, shoulder tendonitis, and hand-arm vibration syndrome [40].

While the understanding of the pathophysiologic mechanism for these disorders has remained controversial [41], the reported incidence of CTDs has risen steadily since 1982 [40]. This apparent increase may be attributable, in part, to improved awareness, diagnosis, and reporting of CTDs.

Carpal Tunnel Syndrome

Carpal tunnel syndrome refers to compression of the median nerve as it traverses the carpal tunnel in the wrist. The tightly bound carpal bones form the dorsal, medial, and lateral walls on the carpal tunnel. Anterior and superior to these bones is the transverse carpal ligament, a dense, nonresilient structure. The carpal tunnel, which is beneath this ligament, contains the median nerve, nine flexor tendons, and their tendon sheaths. At this point, the median nerve has motor fibers to a number of muscles in the hand, including the opponens pollicis, abductor pollicis brevis, and the first and second interosseous muscles. The nerve also gives rise to the sensory branches of the midpalm, the palmar aspect of the first 3½ digits, and the dorsal tips of the fingers.

In a study of 652 workers in jobs with specific hand force and repetitive characteristics, the prevalence of carpal tunnel syndrome ranged from 0.6% among workers in low-force, low-repetitive jobs to 5.6% among workers in high-force, high-repetitive jobs. When the authors controlled for potential confounders, the odds ratio for the high-force repetitive jobs was more than 15 (p less than 0.001) compared to the low-force repetitive jobs [42].

The National Institute for Occupational Safety and Health proposed a case definition for work-related carpal tunnel syndrome in 1989 [43]. The NIOSH criteria are: (1) symptoms suggestive of carpal tunnel syndrome (paresthesia, hypoesthesia, or pain in distribution of the median nerve; (2) objective findings, which can include either a positive Tinel's or Phalen's sign, decreased sensation in the distribution of the median nerve, or abnormal electrodiagnostic findings of the median nerve across the carpal tunnel; and (3) evidence of work-relatedness (frequent, repetitive, or forceful hand work on affected side; sustained awkward hand position; use of vibrating tools; prolonged pressure over wrist or palm; or temporal relationship to work). A study examining the validity of this case definition concluded that reliance on physical examination alone for objective evidence resulted in a significant number of false-positive and false-negative results [44].

Controversy over the diagnostic criteria for this disorder has probably led to a significant amount of overdiagnosis of this condition [40].

History

The patient with carpal tunnel syndrome may experience numbness, burning, and tingling in the first 3½ digits. A frequent complaint also noted is coldness and clumsiness of the hand accompanied by weakness and dropping of objects. Some patients awaken from sleep with numbness and tingling in the hand, which they shake to relieve the discomfort.

Virtually any condition that increases the contents of or decreases the size of the carpal tunnel and in turn compresses the median nerve can lead to the problem. Nonoccupational disorders associated with carpal tunnel syndrome include rheumatoid arthritis, diabetes, degenerative arthritis, gout, hypothyroidism, congenital defects such as anomalous muscles, and acute trauma to the wrist. Any condition that results in edema of the hand or wrist, such as trauma, reflex sympathetic dystrophy, or pregnancy, can also cause carpal tunnel syndrome.

Clinical evaluation usually reveals that the little finger (fifth) is *not* involved and that numbness may be precipitated by gripping a steering wheel; holding tools such as pliers, power screwdrivers, and torque wrenches; or using a broom or kitchen utensil. If a person experiences these symptoms, careful attention should be directed to the possibility of carpal tunnel syndrome.

Physical Examination

The physical examination should focus on assessing the wrist for range of motion in flexion, extension, and lateral and medial mobility. Tapping the dorsum of the wrist anterior to the median nerve (Tinel's sign) can induce numbness in affected persons. Phalen's sign is performed by asking the patient to volar flex the wrist and maintain the position for 60 seconds. If tingling develops in the distribution of the median nerve, that is, the thumb, index, middle, and radial aspect of the ring finger, the test is positive. Positive Phalen's and Tinel's signs are strongly suggestive of carpal tunnel syndrome and indicate the need for further diagnostic evaluation.

Proper evaluation of carpal tunnel syndrome includes a review of other conditions that can cause pain and numbness in the wrist such as thoracic outlet syndrome, brachial plexus lesions, peripheral neuropathy, and herniated cervical disks with nerve root compression.

The use of vibratory perception testing (vibrometry) may prove useful as an early detection tool in carpal tunnel syndrome [45].

Electromyography/Nerve Conduction Velocity

The most useful tool in the *diagnosis of carpal tunnel syndrome* is measurement of EMG/NCV. EMG/NCV studies can confirm clinical findings and aid in the determination of the location and degree of nerve entrapment, if present. These studies are strongly suggested before formulating a diagnosis and initiating a referral to an orthopedic or hand surgeon for surgical correction.

Treatment

Initial treatment of carpal tunnel syndrome can be conducted by the primary care physician. A volar splint with the wrist held in mild dorsiflexion applied prior to sleep can often be effective; the same splint can be used in settings associated with discomfort. If the patient has an illness that contributes to carpal tunnel syndrome, it should be treated initially. Nonsteroidal antiinflammatory medications (NSAIDS) can also be effective.

Once carpal tunnel syndrome develops, the condition usually progresses or at best stabilizes. Eventually, clinical management focuses on the need for and value of surgical correction. Ideally, these decisions are best coordinated by the primary care physician and a consultant in orthopedic or hand surgery. Issues such as the presence of motor weakness, the type of job and availability of reassignment, and the needs and interests of the patient should be considered.

Surgical decompression of the carpal tunnel usually relieves a significant amount of pain, although numbness might persist. Whether numbness is a permanent sequela depends, in part, on the duration and severity of the nerve entrapment. Elderly patients and those with long-standing symptoms, especially muscle weakness and thenar atrophy, may continue to experience numbness and weakness, although pain and discomfort are usually relieved by surgery.

Preventive interventions are essential to avoid progression or recurrence of carpal tunnel syndrome. A work station analysis should be performed, and the risk factors should be identified. Work stations should be redesigned to reduce tasks that require prolonged extension or repetitive motion of the wrist.

Wrist Tendonitis

Although traumatic disorders of the tendons of the hand are serious occupationally related injuries, they tend to be relatively uncommon. On the other hand, irritation of the tendon, referred to as tendonitis, is common in jobs that require frequent and repetitive motions, usually of the upper extremity, especially the hand and elbow but also the shoulder. Sites that may contribute to problems include the muscle, tendon, synovium, tendon sheath, and tendon insertion. Irritation of these structures can occur from repetitive motion activities as well as unaccustomed or severe use of the hand.

A common problem is that associated with excessive or forced repetitive motion that results in irritation of the tendon or its sheath. Ultimately, motion of the affected fingers causes pain and crepitations noted on palpation. The disorder is more accurately described as tenosynovitis, which can progress to the point that the tendon sheath thickens. Restricted motion of the joints of the hand can then result.

One particular type of tenosynovitis is de Quervain's syndrome. The sheaths of the *extensor pollicis longus* (short thumb extensor) and *abductor pollicis longus* (long thumb abductor) become thickened. This condition may be traumatic in origin, especially with repeated abduction and extension of the thumb. Diagnosis is made by noting *tenderness to palpation* of the tendons in the first dorsal compartment of the radial aspect of the wrist. Finklestein's sign is another diagnostic sign that may be helpful. In this maneuver, the patient adducts the thumb into the hand, resting on the palm. The physician then applies an ulnar deviation force to the wrist. The test is positive if this maneuver elicits pain in the first dorsal compartment. In de Quervain's syndrome and in other causes of tendonitis not due to systemic or local infectious disease, the hand should be placed at rest by splinting with a thumb spica splint or with an appropriate support. Systemic nonsteroidal antiinflammatory agents and application of local heat can relieve discomfort. In some cases, careful injection of corticosteroids into the first dorsal compartment provides dramatic and longlasting relief.

Hand-Arm Vibration Syndrome

Hand-arm vibration syndrome, formerly known as vibration white finger, is a condition seen in workers who use handheld vibrating tools. Common presenting symptoms are numbness, tingling, or pain in the fingertips and hands that may progress to weakness and loss of fine motor coordination [46]. It has been postulated that the vibration of the tool can lead to two independent pathologic consequences: arterial spasm (similar to Raynaud's phenomenon), which can cause numbness and blanching of the fingers, and muscular fatigue, produced by slowing of nerve conduction velocities as a result of a direct effect of vibration on peripheral nerves [47]. NIOSH has published diagnostic criteria for hand-arm vibration syndrome [48]. The diagnosis is based primarily on the occupational history, and other disorders that can cause hand paresthesias (Raynaud's phenomenon, collagen vascular disorders, or carpal tunnel syndrome) should be ruled out with appropriate laboratory testing [46].

Treatment is aimed at preventing progression of the disease. Careful review of the use of the vibrating tool is essential and consideration of job modification should be made. In some cases, the worker may be unable to use any vibrating equipment. Nonsteroidal antiinflammatory medications may be helpful in reducing pain. Vasodilators or calcium channel blockers hold some promise in treating the underlying vasospastic episodes [46]. If carpal tunnel syndrome is coexistent, wrist splints may be of some benefit.

Epicondylitis

Two relatively common musculoskeletal conditions that occur at work are lateral and medial epicondylitis of the elbow. These disorders result from excessive stress on the muscle groups around the elbow and *forearm*. In *lateral* epicondylitis, the extensor supinator group of muscles is involved, whereas in *medial* epicondylitis, the flexor pronator muscles are affected. Although these conditions, especially lateral epicondylitis, are frequently associated with sporting activities ("tennis elbow"), use of a hammer, screwdriver, or masonry tools can also precipitate the disorder. Generally, no loss of elbow function occurs; however, pain develops in the affected area of the elbow. Distal radiation of the pain is often associated with a firm grip.

Examination usually reveals tenderness on palpation over the lateral epicondyle, the site of the insertion of the extensor and supinator muscles supplying the wrist. Symptoms are usually reproduced by asking the patient to extend the wrist against resistance. Medial epicondylitis follows a similar course as lateral epicondylitis; however, symptoms are usually reproduced by wrist *flexion* against resistance or by firm palpation of the medial humeral epicondyle.

Primary treatment of both of these disorders requires that the person refrain from aggravating activities. The administration of systemic nonsteroidal antiinflammatory agents, limitation of motion of the elbow through splints and supports, and local heat are advisable initially. Prolonged and marked restriction of activities is ill advised because of the potential for developing stiffness and tightness and ultimately a "frozen" joint. Local infiltration of the affected areas, especially over the trigger site, with 1% lidocaine mixed with a solution of corticosteroids may produce immediate resolution of the symptoms. Repeat injections should be avoided. In general, however, these conditions are apt to recur, especially if the person returns to the same job without changes in job design or work practices.

Other Nerve Entrapment Syndromes

Repetitive motion of the upper extremities can also result in entrapment of the median, ulnar, and radial nerves in other locations [40]. *Pronator teres syndrome* involves entrapment of the median nerve in the forearm, while *radial tunnel syndrome* refers to entrapment of the radial nerve by repetitive motion of the extensor muscles of the forearm. *Cubital tunnel syndrome* is when the ulnar nerve becomes entrapped from external pressure over the cubital tunnel at the elbow.

Neck Injuries

Neck injuries involving muscular strain and spasm are common in the occupational setting [49]. For neck injuries in which there is *any* suspicion of subluxation of the cervical vertebra, immediate immobilization and prompt emergency evaluation are essential. Most acute neck strains result in some degree of overstretching of the paracervical musculature and trapezius muscles. *Cervical strain* usually refers to forced flexion and extension of the neck ("whiplash"), resulting in pain that is often delayed by 12 to 24 hours. *Trapezius strains* are caused by sudden twisting of the neck, often associated with shoulder extension or arm abduction. These types of strains are extremely common and usually respond to conservative treatment with

ice or moist heat, NSAIDs, and muscle relaxants [50]. Initial treatment is similar
to that for low back strains. In cases in which the patient has persistent pain,
referral to a physical therapist may be helpful.

Herniations of cervical intervertebral disks are not as common as herniated lumbar disks. However, if the patient has persistent pain or numbness radiating to the
shoulder or arm and persistent or progressive abnormal neurologic findings on
examination, MRI is indicated to rule out impingement of a cervical nerve root.
Nerve conduction studies can be a helpful adjunct in assessing cervical radiculopathies due to a variety of causes. Neurosurgical referral is appropriate if a cervical
nerve root is compromised or if spinal stenosis is present.

Occupational cervicobrachial disorder (or "fibromyalgia") refers to neck and shoulder pain associated with repetitive extension of the arms above shoulder height
either in static postures or with low external loads [30]. This disorder is difficult to
treat and frequently requires complete work station redesign or job transfer. Physical
therapy, antiinflammatory medications, and muscle relaxants may be of some benefit
in initial treatment of this disorder. If trigger points are identified, an injection with
a combination of anesthetic (such as lidocaine) and corticosteroids may provide some
relief.

References

1. Skovran, M. L. Epidemiology of Occupational Injury. In W. N. Rom (ed.), *Environmental and Occupational Medicine,* (2nd ed.). Boston: Little, Brown, 1992. Pp. 725–
731.
2. Spengler, D. M. et al. Back injuries in industry: A retrospective study. I. Overview
and cost analysis. *Spine* 11:241, 1986.
3. Frymoyer, J. W., and Cats-Bavil, W. L. An overview of the costs and incidence of
low back pain. *Orth. Clin. North Am.* 22:263, 1991.
4. Daltroy, L. H., et al. A case-control study of risk factors for industrial low back
injury. Implications for primary and secondary prevention programs. *Am. J. Ind
Med.* 20:505, 1991.
5. Kelsey, J. L., Golden, A. L., and Mundt, D. J. Low back pain/prolapsed intervertebral
disc. *Rheum. Dis. Clin. North America* 16:699, 1990.
6. Quinet, R. J., and Hadler, N. M. Diagnosis and treatment of back ache. *Semin.
Arthritis Rheum.* 9:261, 1979.
7. Deyo, R. A., Rainville, J., and Kent, D. L. What can the history and physical
examination tell us about low back pain. *J.A.M.A* 268:760, 1992.
8. Snook, S. H. The design of manual handling tasks. *Ergonomics* 21:963, 1978.
9. NIOSH Technical Report. *Work Practices Guide for Manual Lifting.* DHHS (NIOSH)
Publication no. 81–122. Washington, DC: US Government Printing Office, March
1981.
10. Modic, M. T., and Ross, J. S. Magnetic resonance imaging in the evaluation of low
back pain. *Orth. Clin. North Am.* 22:283, 1991.
11. Deyo, R. A. Bed rest for low back pain: How much is enough? *N. Engl. J. Med.*
315:1064, 1986.
12. Muckle, D. S. Comparative study of ibuprofen and aspirin in soft tissue injuries.
Rehabilitation (Bonn) 13:141, 1974.
13. Brown, J. R. Factors contributing to the development of low back pain in industrial
workers. *Am. Ind. Hyg. Assoc. J.* 26–31, Jan. 1975.
14. Wiesel, S. W., Ferrer, H. L., and Rothman, R. H. *Industrial Low Back Pain.* Charlottesville, VA: Michie Co., 1985.
15. Aaronoff, G. M. Pain treatment: Is it a right or a privilege? *Clin. J. Pain* 1:187,
1986.
16. Florence, D. W. The chronic pain syndrome. *Postgrad. Med.* 70:217, 1981.
17. Waddell, G., et al. Nonorganic physical signs in low-back pain. *Spine* 5:117, 1980.
18. Koes, B. W., et al. The effectiveness of manual therapy, physiotherapy, and treatment
by the general practitioner for nonspecific back and neck complaints: A randomized
clinical trial. *Spine* 17:28, 1992.
19. Koes, B. W., et al. Spinal manipulation and mobilization for back and neck pain: A
blinded review. *Br. Med. J.* 303:1298,
20. Deyo, R. A., et al. A controlled trial of transcutaneous electrical nerve stimulation
(TENS) and exercise for chronic low back pain. *N. Engl. J. Med.* 322:1627, 1990.

21. Cavette, S., et al. A controlled trial of corticosteroid injections into facet joints for chronic low back pain. *N. Engl. J. Med.* 325:1002, 1991.
22. Saal, J. A., and Saal, J. S. Nonoperative treatment of herniated lumbar intervertebral disc with radiculopathy: An outcome study. *Spine* 14:431, 1989.
23. Troup, J. D. G. Causes, prediction and prevention of back pain at work, *Scand. J. Work Environ. Health* 10:419, 1984.
24. Snook, S. H. Low Back Pain in Industry. *American Academy of Orthopedic Surgeons Symposium on Idiopathic Low Back Pain.* St. Louis: Mosby, 1982.
25. Bigos, S. J., et al. A prospective evaluation of pre-employment screening methods for acute industrial back pain. *Spine* 17:922, 1992.
26. Bigos, S. J., et al. Back injuries in industry: A retrospective study. III. Employee related factors. *Spine* 11:252, 1986.
27. Repko, G. R., and Cooper, R. A study of the average workers compensation case. *J. Clin. Psychol.* 39:287, 1983.
28. Bohart, W. H. Anatomic variations and anomalies of the spine: Relation to prognosis and length of disability. *J.A.M.A.* 92:698, 1928.
29. Present, A. J. Radiography of the lower back in pre-employment physical examinations. Presented at the ACR/NIOSH Conference, Jan. 11–14, 1973. *Radiology* 8:261, 1979.
30. Rowe, M. L. Are routine spine films on workers in industry cost or risk benefit effective? *J.O.M.* 24:41, 1982.
31. Biering-Sorensen, F. Physical measurements as risk indicators for low back trouble during a one year period. *Spine* 9:106, 1984.
32. Keyserling, W. M., Herrin, G. D., and Chaffin, D. B. Isometric strength testing as a means of controlling medical incidents on strenuous jobs. *J.O.M.* 22:332, 1980.
33. Chaffin, D. B., Herrin, G. D., and Keyserling, W. M. Pre-employment strength testing: An updated position. *J.O.M.* 20:403, 1978.
34. Gracovetsky, S. Determination of load. *Br. J. Ind. Med.* 43:120, 1986.
35. Litchfield, M. M., and Freedson, P. S. Physical training programs for public safety personnel. *Clin. Sports Med.* 5:571, 1986.
36. Mealey, M. New fitness for police and firefighters. *Phys. Sport Med.* 7:96, 1979.
37. Battie, M. C., et al. A prospective study of the role for cardiovascular risk factors and fitness in industrial back complaints. *Spine* 14:141, 1989.
38. Brown, K. C., et al. Cost effectiveness of a back school intervention for municipal employees. *Spine* 17:1224, 1992.
39. Versloot, J. M., et al. The cost effectiveness of a back school program in industry: A longitudinal controlled field study. *Spine* 17:22–27, 1992.
40. Rempel, D. M., Harrison, R. J., and Barnhart, S. Work-related cumulative trauma disorders of the upper extremity. *J.A.M.A.* 167:838, 1992.
41. Hadler, N. M. Cumulative trauma disorders: An intragenic concept. *J.O.M.* 32:38, 1990.
42. Silverstein, B. A., Fine, L. J., and Armstrong, T. J. Occupational factors in carpal tunnel syndrome. *Am. J. Ind. Med.* 11:343, 1987.
43. Matte, T. D., Baker, E. L., and Honchar, P. A. The selection and definition of target work-related conditions for surveillance under SENSOR. *Am. J. Public Health* 79 (Suppl.):21, 1989.
44. Katz, J. N., et al. Validation of a surveillance case definition of carpal tunnel syndrome. *Am. J. Public Health* 81:189, 1991.
45. Jetzer, T. C. Use of vibration testing in the early evaluation of workers with carpal tunnel syndrome. *J.O.M.* 33:117, 1991.
46. Pyykko, I. Clinical aspects of hand-arm vibration syndrome: A review. *Scand. J. Work Environ. Health* 12:439, 1986.
47. McCunney, R. J. Recognizing hand disorders caused by vibrating tools. *J. Musculoskel. Med.* 9:91, 1992.
48. *Criteria for a Recommended Standard: Occupational Exposure to Hand-Arm Vibration.* National Institute for Occupational Safety (NIOSH), Department of Health and Human Services Publication no. 89–106. September 1986.
49. Brisson, P. M., Nordin, M., and Zettenberg, C. Neck and Upper Extremity Impairment in W. N. Rom (ed.), *Environmental and Occupational Medicine.* (2nd ed.). Boston: Little, Brown, 1992. Pp. 719–720.
50. Birnbaum, J. S. *The Musculoskeletal Manual* (2nd ed.). Philadelphia: Saunders, 1986. Pp. 31–38.

Further Information

Birnbaum, J. S. *The Musculoskeletal Manual* (2nd ed.). Philadelphia: Saunders, 1986.
A basic guide to diagnosis and management of musculoskeletal problems for the nonorthopedist.

Bureau of Labor Statistics. *What Every Employer Needs to Know About OSHA Recordkeeping.* Report no. 412–413, 1978.
Guidelines to maintenance of records under the Occupational Safety and Health Act of 1970.

Isernhagen, S. J. Principles of prevention for cumulative trauma. *Occupational Medicine: State of the Art Reviews* 7:147, 1992.
A comprehensive review of occupational cumulative trauma problems and methods of prevention.

Keim, H. (ed.). Low back pain. *Ciba Clinical Symposium* 39:1, 1988.
Primer on the treatment of low back injuries.

O'Donoghue, D. H. *Treatment of Injuries to Athletes.* Philadelphia: Saunders, 1984.

Pariapour, M., et al. Environmentally induced disorders of the musculoskeletal system. *Med. Clin. North Am.* 74:347, 1990.
A review of the pathophysiology, epidemiology, diagnosis, and treatment of musculoskeletal injuries, including psychosocial and organizational factors.

Rowe, M. L. *Orthopaedic Problems at Work.* Fairport, NY: Perinton, 1985.
A practical guide to the diagnosis, treatment, and rehabilitation of common work-related musculoskeletal disorders. Written by an orthopedic surgeon with over 20 years' experience in evaluating occupational musculoskeletal problems.

Seeger, L. L. MRI of the musculoskeletal system. *Orthopedics* 15:437, 1992; and Bassett, L. W., and Gold, R. H. Magnetic resonance imaging of the musculoskeletal system. *Clinical Orthopedics and Related Research* 244:17, 1989.
Both articles are good reviews of the principles, indications, and limitations of this diagnostic modality.

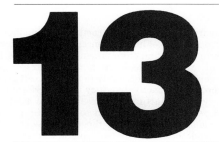

Occupational Cancers

Howard Frumkin

Cancer is one of the most dreaded diseases in our society, and its toll in terms of human suffering and economic costs is enormous. Cancer is second only to cardiovascular disease as a cause of mortality; each year more than a million Americans contract some form of cancer and over half a million die of cancer [1].

With the exception of a few cancer sites, overall progress in cancer treatment during recent decades has been discouraging [2]. Moreover, it is now generally accepted that environmental factors play a major role in causing cancer [3]. For these reasons, the prevention of cancer, both primary and secondary, has assumed great importance. The workplace is an important locus of these preventive activities.

The Process of Carcinogenesis

Cancer encompasses dozens of distinct diseases that share several characteristics: rapid, relatively unrestrained growth by a population of cells; failure of these cells to differentiate and function normally; and survival and propagation of these cells for abnormally long times.

A *carcinogen* is a substance that causes cancer. Carcinogens can be chemicals, physical agents such as ionizing radiation, or biologic agents such as viruses or aflatoxin. In some cases, such as in parts of the rubber industry, elevated rates of cancer have been detected but a specific carcinogen has not been identified.

Carcinogenesis at the Cellular Level

Current knowledge of the mechanisms of carcinogenesis remains incomplete. Based on experimental work with mouse skin in the 1940s, two stages in carcinogenesis were identified, initiation and promotion. *Initiation* was defined as the critical event, when an irreversible change occurred to the cell's genetic material. *Promotion* consisted of one or more subsequent steps, when intra- and extracellular factors allowed the transformed cell to develop into a focal proliferation such as a nodule, then to a malignant tumor, and finally to metastases.

When deoxyribonucleic acid (DNA) was identified as the genetic material of cells, initiation was recognized as an alteration of the DNA, or a *mutation*. In fact, in the 1970s, chemicals began to be tested for mutagenicity in laboratory settings, as a marker for carcinogenicity. Promoters, on the other hand, were viewed not as mutagens, but as *epigenetic* factors that enhanced cell proliferation, interfered with normal control and regulation of cell processes, and/or increased the probability of further genetic damage [4]. Further experimental observations suggested that multiple steps were necessary to induce a neoplasm, leading to *multistep* theories of carcinogenesis [5, 6].

Rapid developments in molecular biology have further clarified the events of carcinogenesis [7]. Early studies of ribonucleic acid (RNA) viruses revealed that some coded for genetic sequences that, when inserted into host genomes, could cause malignant transformation. These were called *oncogenes*. It soon became clear that nascent forms of oncogenes, called *proto-oncogenes*, were common in many human and animal cells, and often played an important role in normal cell function. However, if transformed into oncogenes, their products code for *oncoproteins* that in turn act as growth factors, membrane receptors, or protein kinases, or act in other ways, resulting in rapid cell growth and dedifferentiation. One of the best studied examples is the *ras* oncogene, which was first identified in rat sarcomas. The *ras* oncogene can be activated by polycyclic aromatic hydrocarbons, N-nitroso compounds, and ionizing radiation, and has been found in a wide variety of human cancers including bladder cancer, lung cancer, and others of occupational and environmental importance [8].

A second kind of gene important in carcinogenesis is the *tumor suppressor gene,* or anti-oncogene. Tumor suppressor genes function normally to regulate cell growth and stimulate terminal differentiation. When inactivated, they fail to perform those functions, and increase the probability of neoplastic transformation. The most commonly identified example is the p53 gene, located on chromosome 17 [9]. p53 mutations have been identified in various cancers, including those of the colon, lung, liver, esophagus, breast, and reticuloendothelial and hematopoietic tissues, and in the Li-Fraumeni syndrome of familial multiple cancer susceptibility. Of special interest, carcinogenic exposures such as aflatoxin and hepatitis B virus have been associated with specific mutations on the p53 gene, suggesting that each carcinogen may leave a unique genomic "signature." This gene may have clinical applications, as discussed below.

Carcinogen Metabolism and Individual Susceptibility

Some carcinogens, such as bis(chloromethyl)ether, can damage DNA directly, but most require metabolic activation by enzymes. The enzymes primarily responsible for this activation are those of the cytochrome P450 system [10]. Others include N-acetyltransferase, epoxide hydrolase, and glutathione S-transferase. The primary function of these enzymes is to render xenobiotics more polar and therefore more readily excretable. However, their products are often reactive electrophiles, which can bond with DNA to cause adducts, and result in mutations.

Considerable variation in these metabolic functions has been noted among species and among different people [11]. For example, people vary several thousandfold in their levels of aryl hydrocarbon hydroxylase (AHH), an enzyme of the cytochrome P450 system that helps metabolize polycyclic aromatic hydrocarbons (PAHs). High levels of AHH have been associated with increased risk of lung cancer. These variations reflect genetic factors, but can also result from environmental exposures such as cigarette smoking and diet that induce enzyme activity. Another highly variable factor is the cytochrome P450 enzyme responsible for hydroxylating the antihypertensive drug debrisoquin. So-called extensive hydroxylators have several thousand times more enzyme activity than poor hydroxylators. The extensive hydroxylator phenotype has also been associated with a markedly increased risk of lung cancer.

These insights into gene expression and enzyme activity are important for several reasons. First, the interspecies differences imply that extrapolation from animal evidence to humans must be done with caution. Second, the person-to-person differences imply that some individuals may be at greater risk than others following carcinogenic exposures, because of genetic predisposition and concurrent exposures. Third, understanding the steps in carcinogenesis creates opportunities for clinical testing, including exposure assessment and early detection and diagnosis of cancer. The implications of each of these are discussed below.

Latency

An important issue in carcinogenesis is *latency.* Latency refers to the period of time between the onset of exposure to a carcinogen and the clinical detection of resulting cancers. The latency period for hematologic malignancies is in the range of 4 or 5 years, while the latency period for solid tumors is at least 10 or 20 and possibly as long as 50 years. This period presumably corresponds to the multiple steps of carcinogenesis, from the first DNA mutation or initiation to the ultimate clinical appearance of a malignant tumor. Because of latency considerations, epidemiologic surveillance of workers at risk of cancer should focus on the time *after* latency has elapsed. If surveillance is conducted too soon after the onset of exposure, no increase in risk would be expected. The yield of screening at this stage is likely to be low, the expense is avoidable, and there is a danger that negative results will be falsely reassuring.

Threshold Levels

A *threshold* is a safe level of exposure to a carcinogen, below which carcinogenesis does not occur. Whether thresholds exist has been a controversial question [12].

Since a single mutation in a single cell can theoretically give rise to a malignancy, it has been argued that there is no safe level of exposure. Definitive evidence on this point is elusive, since both epidemiologic and experimental data are inherently uninformative at very low exposure levels. However, several arguments in support of thresholds have been advanced. First, there are known repair mechanisms that correct DNA damage, at least at low levels of exposure. Second, certain carcinogens, such as trace elements and hormones, are ubiquitous and even essential at low doses; it is argued that these substances are carcinogenic only at higher doses. Third, factors that act epigenetically, such as promoters that stimulate cell division, often have reversible effects, implying a threshold phenomenon. Finally, certain empiric data have been interpreted to be consistent with the existence of thresholds. Regulatory approaches have generally made the conservative assumption that carcinogenic thresholds cannot be demonstrated and have not attempted to set safe levels of exposure (see Chap. 26, Risk Assessment).

Interaction

Interaction is another important concept in occupational carcinogenesis. This phenomenon occurs when the joint effect of two or more carcinogens is different than what would have been predicted based on the individual effects. *Synergy,* in which joint effects exceed the combined individual effects, and *antagonism,* in which joint effects are less than combined individual effects, are two examples of interaction. In some cases, interaction may be nothing more than the combined effects of two carcinogens acting through distinct mechanisms, such as an initiator and a promoter. Individually these substances may be predicted to have a certain magnitude of effect, but in sequence they may be far more potent. The statistical and epidemiologic expression of interaction is complex and varies based on whether additive or multiplicative models are selected and other considerations [13].

Clinically, interaction is important when assessing the magnitude of a particular exposure and/or when advising patients about such exposures. Most of the data we have assume individual exposures. However, in practice many exposures occur in tandem, and therefore extra caution may be appropriate. For example, since cigarette smoke and asbestos interact synergistically in causing lung cancer, a worker with past asbestos exposure should be advised especially emphatically to quit smoking. Similarly, a citizen whose drinking water is contaminated by hazardous wastes should be advised that while each component exposure carries some risk, the combined effects are poorly understood and may exceed the individual risks.

Testing and Evaluation of Carcinogens

Several methods have emerged by which carcinogens are identified. These include epidemiologic studies, animal studies, in vitro test systems, and structure-activity relationship analysis.

Epidemiologic studies are potentially the most definitive source of information on human carcinogenicity, since they are based on human exposures in "real-life" situations. However, epidemiologic studies are sometimes difficult to interpret because of confounding, poor exposure data and other problems (see Chap. 24, Epidemiology and Biostatistics). Most of these methodologic limitations of epidemiologic studies bias results toward the null hypothesis, or a finding of no effect. For this reason, great caution is necessary in interpreting their results.

Animal studies usually involve exposing two species of rodents, both male and female, to several dosage levels of a suspected carcinogen. The animals are sacrificed after a prescribed period of time, and the number and sites of tumors are noted. These findings may be extrapolated to humans, on the theory that an animal carcinogen is likely to be a human carcinogen [14]. There are several problems with this extrapolation: Biologic differences between humans and animals may lead to different responses to carcinogens, the high doses that must be given to animals often greatly exceed human exposure levels, and induced animal tumors may be benign or at different sites than in humans, making interpretation difficult.

In vitro testing involves the use of bacterial cultures or human tissue cultures. Suspected carcinogens are added to these systems, and endpoints that reflect DNA damage are monitored. In the best-known in vitro test, the Ames test, mutant strains of *Salmonella typhimurium* are observed for genetic alterations. These tests are obviously less directly applicable to humans than epidemiologic or even animal data, but they have the virtues of rapidity and relatively low cost [15].

Finally, chemical structures can be analyzed with respect to their similarity to known carcinogens. Such structure-activity analysis can direct suspicion to chemicals that may have carcinogenic potential; further testing is generally necessary (see Chap. 23, Toxicology).

Based on these four types of data, regulatory and research agencies have developed standardized ways to classify chemical carcinogenicity. For example, the International Agency for Research on Cancer (IARC) designates three categories [16, 17]. Group 1 includes chemicals and processes established as human carcinogens, based on "sufficient evidence," usually epidemiologic data (Table 13-1). Group 2 includes chemicals and processes that are "probably" (group 2A) or "possibly" (group 2B) carcinogenic to humans. Group 2A (Table 13-2) reflects limited evidence of carcinogenicity in humans and sufficient evidence of carcinogenicity in experimental animals, while group 2B reflects limited evidence in humans without sufficient evidence in animals, or sufficient evidence in animals without any human data. IARC policy has been to recommend treating group 2 chemicals as if they presented a carcinogenic

Table 13-1. Established human occupational carcinogens (IARC group 1)

Industrial processes
Aluminum production
Auramine manufacturing
Boot and shoe manufacturing and repair
Coal gasification
Coke production
Furniture and cabinetmaking
Iron and steel founding
Isopropyl alcohol manufacturing (strong acid process)
Magenta manufacturing
Painting
Rubber industry
Underground hematite mining with radon exposure

Chemicals and mixtures*

Exposures	*Examples of occurrence*
Aflatoxins	Grains, peanuts
4-Aminobiphenyl	Rubber industry
Arsenic and arsenic compounds	Insecticides
Asbestos	Insulation, friction products
Benzene	Chemical industry
Benzidine	Rubber and dye industries
Bis(chloromethyl)ether and chloromethyl methyl ether	Chemical industry
Chromium (VI) compounds	Metal plating, pigments
Coal tar pitches	Coal distillation
Coal tars	Coal distillation
Erionite	Environmental (Turkey)
Mineral oils	Machining, jute processing
Mustard gas	Production, war gas
β-Naphthylamine	Rubber and dye industries
Nickel compounds	Nickel refining and smelting
Radon and its decay products	Indoor environments, mining
Shale oils	Energy production
Soots	Chimneys, furnaces
Talc containing asbestiform fibers	Talc mining, pottery manufacturing
Vinyl chloride	Plastics industry

*Other chemicals and mixtures, including chemotherapeutic agents, tobacco, and others, have been classified in group 1.
Source: From H. Vainio and J. Wilbourn. Identification of carcinogens within the IARC monograph program. *Scand. J. Work Environ. Health* 18 (Suppl.):64, 1992.

Table 13-2. Strongly suspected human occupational carcinogens (IARC group 2A)

Industrial processes
Petroleum refining (certain exposures)
Insecticide application (nonarsenicals)

Chemicals and mixtures*

Exposures	*Examples of occurrence*
Acrylonitrile	Plastics industry
Benz[a]anthracene	Coal distillation
Benzidine-based dyes	Dye industry
Benzo[a]pyrene	Coal and petroleum-derived products
Beryllium and Be compounds	Be extraction, electronics
Cadmium and cadmium compounds	Battery and alloy manufacturing
Creosotes	Wood preservatives
Dibenz[a,h]anthracene	Coal distillation
Diesel engine exhaust	Motor vehicles
Diethyl sulfate	Petrochemical industry
Dimethylcarbamoyl chloride	Dimethylcarbamoyl chloride manufacturing
Dimethyl sulfate	Chemical industry
Epichlorhydrin	Resin manufacturing
Ethylene dibromide	Fumigant, gasoline additive
Ethylene oxide	Sterilizing agent
Formaldehyde	Building materials
4,4′-methylene bis(2-chloroaniline) (MBOCA)	Resin manufacturing
N-nitrosodiethylamine	Solvent
N-nitrosodimethylamine	Solvent
Polychlorinated biphenyls	Electrical equipment
Propylene oxide	Chemical industry
Silica, crystalline	Glass and porcelain manufacturing
Styrene oxide	Chemical industry
Vinyl bromide	Plastics industry

*Other chemicals and mixtures, including chemotherapeutic agents, tobacco, and others, have been classified in group 2A.
Source: From H. Vainio and J. Wilbourn. Identification of carcinogens within the IARC monograph program. *Scand. J. Work Environ. Health* 18 (Suppl.):64, 1992.

risk to humans. Group 3 includes agents that are not classified, and group 4 includes agents that are probably not carcinogenic to humans. Using this classification, IARC has evaluated approximately 750 chemicals, industrial processes, and personal habits. More than 50 have been placed in group 1, and almost 250 have been placed in group 2 (see Appendix D). The American Conference of Governmental Industrial Hygienists (ACGIH), the National Toxicology Program (NTP), and the National Institute of Occupational Safety and Health (NIOSH) have all adopted analogous schemes. In addition, the Generic Carcinogen Policy adopted in 1980 by the Occupational Safety and Health Administration (OSHA), discussed later, incorporates a similar approach.

Molecular Epidemiology of Cancer and Clinical Occupational Medicine

Rapid advances in toxicology and in the molecular biology of cancer have exciting implications for epidemiology and clinical medicine. Many of these will be important in occupational medicine in years to come.

Markers of exposure will be increasingly available, and will play a major role in biomonitoring [18]. For many years carcinogens or their metabolites have been directly measured in biologic media such as blood and urine. For example, benzene exposure can be monitored through expired air and blood benzene levels and through urinary phenol levels; exposure to the aromatic amine 4,4′-methylene bis(2-chloroaniline) (MBOCA) can be monitored through urinary MBOCA levels. More recently assays have measured the level of mutagenicity in urine; the basis for this approach is that carcinogens, when metabolized to active forms and excreted, should be detectable in urine, and should reflect the individual exposure. Perhaps the most direct approach to exposure measurement is to assess the "biologically effective dose" of a carcinogen at the ultimate target, DNA, by measuring DNA adducts [19]. Sensitive methods such as ^{32}P-postlabeling and immunoassay have made this feasible in recent years. As a proxy, RNA adducts and protein adducts may also be studied. This approach has been used to assess exposure among ethylene oxide workers, welders, hazardous waste workers, and others. It has several limitations, including (1) the absence of DNA in the most readily available tissue, red blood cells; (2) the instability and unknown clearance rates of DNA adducts; and (3) the lack of good dose-response data. However, it remains a promising approach to exposure assessment.

Markers of risk may also emerge from molecular biology advances. These fall into at least three general categories: markers of unusually high or low ability to metabolize carcinogens, markers of low ability to repair damaged DNA, and markers of other cancer-prone states. Examples of risky metabolic profiles include high levels of AHH, the extensive debrisoquine hydroxylator phenotype, and the rapid acetylator phenotype, posing increased risks of lung and skin cancer, lung and liver cancer, and bladder cancer, respectively. An example of repair deficiencies is O^6-methyl-transferase deficiency, which increases the risk of liver and intestinal cancers. Finally, examples of other cancer-prone states include the p53 mutations discussed previously. Even when such markers of risk can be reliably identified, their application in occupational medicine will raise profound ethical questions, as "screening out" susceptible workers rather than avoiding carcinogenic exposures may be discriminatory. However, utilizing these data in worker placement may be more acceptable and promising.

Finally, *markers of effect* are increasingly available. These signal that a carcinogen has reached a target tissue and caused changes in genetic material, changes that might predict the development of cancer. Cytogenetic abnormalities such as sister chromatid exchanges and micronuclei have been measured since the 1970s, and have been found to be elevated in many working populations, including those exposed to benzene, epichlorhydrin, styrene, vinyl chloride, asbestos, and ethylene oxide. On the population level these changes correlate with increased cancer risk, but they are not yet adequately standardized or interpretable to be used as clinical tests. The same is true of specific DNA mutations, which can be detected by sensitive techniques such as restriction fragment length polymorphism (RFLP) and polymer chain reaction (PCR) analysis [20]. Finally, the protein products of activated oncogenes can be detected using monoclonal antibodies, an approach with great promise in occupational medicine screening [21]. These techniques are not ready for routine application at present, but in the future they may offer options for sophisticated exposure monitoring and for early detection of precancerous lesions, a sort of molecular Papanicolaou (Pap) smear for workers with carcinogenic exposures.

Regulation of Carcinogens in the Workplace

OSHA's approach to carcinogen regulation was set forth in its Generic Carcinogen Standard, properly called "Identification, Classification, and Regulation of Potential Occupational Carcinogens" [22]. This document prescribes a standardized way of interpreting test data on carcinogenicity and classifying chemicals accordingly. It then provides a framework for the regulation of chemicals found to be carcinogens. In theory, any chemical with sufficient evidence of carcinogenicity is automatically regulated as a carcinogen. However, since its promulgation, the standard has not been utilized by OSHA. Consequently, most known carcinogens that are regulated by OSHA are regulated through earlier consensus standards and not in accordance with the cancer standard.

A major concern in carcinogen regulation is the issue of *potency*. If two substances are both carcinogens but one is much more potent than the other, then some would argue that the two substances should be regulated differently, with more stringent restrictions applied to the more potent carcinogen. The same argument may be advanced when a greater population is exposed to one carcinogen than to another, when one carcinogen is believed to be more essential or irreplaceable than another, or even when control measures for two substances differ in cost. These considerations give rise to cost-benefit analysis in carcinogen regulation, a controversial but increasingly common practice.

Clinical Encounters with Carcinogens

A practitioner of occupational medicine may confront carcinogenic exposures in several ways. The remainder of this chapter poses clinical situations and discusses responses to them.

"Is this Chemical Carcinogenic?"

This question is best answered according to defined criteria, such as those discussed above. The primary animal and epidemiologic data on a chemical may be accessed through standard reference sources, as presented in Chap. 24 and Appendix D. Formal evaluations of carcinogenicity may be found in the *IARC Monographs on the Evaluation of Carcinogenic Risks to Humans* [16], in Annual Reports of the National Toxicology Program, and in NIOSH publications.

"I Am Exposed to a Carcinogen. What Should I Do?"

This query has two components. One pertains to the carcinogenic exposure, and one pertains to the patient.

Ideally, no worker should be exposed to a carcinogen. As discussed previously, safe threshold exposure levels cannot currently be demonstrated. A physician who becomes aware of an ongoing carcinogenic workplace exposure should take appropriate steps to end that exposure. This will often involve contacting responsible individuals at the workplace and/or government agencies. As discussed in Chap. 22, Industrial Hygiene, exposure may be ended through replacement of the carcinogen, enclosure of the process, or, when necessary, personal protective equipment.

The patient who presents following exposure to a carcinogen should be advised to terminate the exposure, to avoid concomitant carcinogenic exposures such as smoking, and to seek appropriate medical follow-up as discussed in the section on medical surveillance.

"Did My Exposure Cause My Cancer?"

Patients with cancer who have been exposed to carcinogens often inquire about the possibility that the exposures were causal. The question sometimes arises in the context of litigation or may simply reflect a patient's psychological need to explain a catastrophic life event. The issue of cancer causation in an individual patient is difficult to address, because it entails the application of epidemiologic and statistical data (which derive from groups) to individuals. The questions that arise are as much philosophic as scientific [23].

Certain requirements must be met before it can be said that an exposure has "causally contributed" to a cancer. There must be evidence that the exposure has indeed occurred. The tumor type in question must be associated with the exposure, based on prior data. Finally, the appropriate temporal relationship must hold; in particular, sufficient latency must have elapsed between the onset of exposure and the diagnosis of cancer.

When these requirements have been met, additional issues should be considered. Suppose that the baseline incidence of lung cancer in unexposed adult men is 80 cases/100,000 men/year. Suppose further that a particular occupational exposure has been associated with a relative risk of lung cancer of 1.8. Therefore, the incidence among exposed men would be 144 cases/100,000 men/year. If an exposed man develops lung cancer and wonders whether his exposure caused his cancer, what should he be told?

The simplest analysis is *qualitative*. Any exposure that markedly increases risk may be considered to contribute to the development of cancer in an exposed individual. A "marked" increase has no firm definition; relative risks as low as 1.3 have been considered in this category. By this analysis, the patient could be told that his exposure contributed to his cancer.

A less simple qualitative approach is to ask whether the patient's cancer would have occurred "but for" the exposure. In the above example, over half the cases of lung cancer in the exposed population would occur even without the exposure. It might then be concluded that any individual case is "more likely than not" to have occurred irrespective of exposure. Similarly, a relative risk of 2.2 would lead to the conclusion in any individual case that cancer would not have occurred "but for" exposure.

This approach is obviously unsatisfactory. It accounts for *no* cancer causation in individual cases when the relative risk is below 2.0, and it accounts for *all* cancer causation in individual cases when the relative risk exceeds 2.0. This violates common sense notions of causation, and it places far too much weight on the precision of the relative risk estimate.

In the *quantitative* approach, causation is allocated to various causes, including occupational exposures. In the above example, the patient might be told that the occupational exposure was "responsible" for 44% (0.8/1.8) of his lung cancer. On the other hand, if he were a smoker, with a consequent 10-fold increase in lung cancer risk, he might be told that smoking accounted for over 80% of his cancer and that the occupational exposure accounted for less than 10%.

This approach has intuitive appeal, since it confronts the multiplicity of exposures and attempts to quantify the relative importance of each. However, the data needed to employ this approach correctly are rarely available. Interaction of multiple exposures, such as synergy, often occurs but is rarely quantitated. Consequently, even if a population's relative risk can be estimated for an occupational exposure, the relative causal contribution of several factors in an individual may be impossible to quantitate.

The two approaches outlined above are often demanded in legal settings, but as noted, they generally have inadequate scientific basis. Until further data or analytic methods are available, the first approach is recommended. It accords with common sense, stays within the confines of available data, and is understandable to patients and their families.

"How Should a Medical Surveillance Program for Cancer be Designed?"

The theory and practice of screening have advanced considerably in recent years (see Chap. 25, Medical Surveillance). With regard to cancer, three goals are sought by screening programs: identifying markers of exposure (biologic monitoring); identifying susceptible or high-risk individuals, presumably before exposure; and identifying early signs of disease (medical surveillance). Some screening tests fall between biologic monitoring and medical surveillance, since they identify physiologic changes related to exposure but of uncertain pathologic significance. Approaches to biologic monitoring and risk detection were discussed previously, and medical surveillance is considered here.

Medical surveillance aims to detect early signs of disease. In general, a successful screening program offers a simple, inexpensive, and accurate test of a population with sufficiently high disease prevalence to confer on the test a high predictive value [24]. Moreover, an intervention should be available for those who test positive that will favorably alter the course of disease. In the occupational setting, conventional principles of medical surveillance may be modified, permitting screening to benefit an exposed population even if no effective treatment can be offered to individual cases and permitting screening programs that might not be cost effective in the community setting [25].

Cancer surveillance in occupational settings has been best explored with regard to bladder and lung cancers. Among workers exposed to beta-naphthylamine, benzidine, and/or benzidine congeners such as *o*-toluidine, two methods have been primarily used: urinalysis for microscopic hematuria and urine cytology. Hematuria is relatively sensitive in detecting both superficial and invasive bladder cancer, but its low specificity results in a high false-positive rate, requiring a large number of invasive studies on healthy individuals. Urine cytology has good sensitivity and specificity for invasive bladder cancer, but no firm evidence demonstrates a survival advantage for patients whose disease is detected through such screening. More advanced techniques such as flow cytometry and quantitative fluorescence image analysis remain unvalidated, but appear to have suboptimal sensitivity and/or specificity. The International Conference on Bladder Cancer Screening in High-Risk

Groups, sponsored by NIOSH in 1989, concluded that urinalysis and cytology might be appropriate, especially following high exposure to known or suspected bladder carcinogens, but that further data were necessary [26]. Ongoing studies of high-risk groups such as the Drake Health Registry [27] should support further recommendations in the near future.

Lung cancer surveillance consists of interval chest radiography or sputum cytology, or both. These approaches were evaluated in a series of trials at the Mayo Clinic, Johns Hopkins University, and the Memorial Sloan-Kettering Cancer Center in the 1970s. The combination of chest x-rays and sputum cytology tests three times a year yielded a significant increase in lung cancer detection and resectability compared to controls (who were merely advised to be tested once a year). However, there was no significant decrease in lung cancer mortality. These results, in combination with other data, have supported the recommendation that no routine surveillance for lung cancer be offered, even to high-risk populations [28, 29].

Other kinds of medical surveillance for occupational cancer are also not recommended. Most approaches carry a high risk of false positives, a low positive predictive value, high cost, worker unacceptability, and/or morbidity. The major exceptions are tests that are generally recommended for the larger population, and that might be easily provided in the workplace setting; these include Pap smears for cervical cancer, stool guaiac testing and sigmoidoscopy for colorectal cancer, physical examination and mammography for breast cancer, and possibly digital examination and prostate-specific antigen for prostate cancer.

"We Have a Cluster of Cancer in Our Plant. How Should We Respond?"

Suspected cancer clusters may be noted by workers or by the company medical department. These situations arouse a great deal of concern, and it is essential that they be handled openly, methodically, and expeditiously [30, 31]. A multidisciplinary approach is necessary, drawing on the experience and knowledge of workers, physicians, epidemiologists, industrial hygienists, and management. The following sequence is suggested.

1. The presence of a cluster should be confirmed or refuted. Each case of cancer should be confirmed, along with tissue type, date of diagnosis, demographic data, and exposure data. The plant population should be enumerated and subdivided by age categories and sex. (If information on retirees is available, it should be included.) Finally, age- and sex-specific state cancer incidence rates should be obtained from the state cancer registry (Table 13-3). With this information, an age-standardized cancer rate can be computed for the plant and compared with the expected rate based on state data. Confidence intervals should be calculated for the plant cancer rate; these will usually be broad because of small numbers. However, even a statistically insignificant elevation in the plant's cancer rate should prompt further evaluation.
2. The tissue types of the cancer cases should be reviewed. An excess of unusual tumors or tumors known to be environmentally induced should prompt further concern [32].
3. The *latency* periods of each cancer case should be reviewed. If many of the patients only began their plant employment shortly before diagnosis, an exposure-related cluster is less plausible.
4. The *occupational histories* of the cases should be reviewed. Detailed personnel histories of each patient may reveal that a particular job title is associated with cancer. It is important that early positions, and not just current ones, be examined.
5. Similarly, an *industrial hygiene review* should be made to determine whether any particular exposures are common among the cases. A variety of job titles may share a common chemical contact, which may help explain the cluster. Again, early exposures must be reconstructed; this may involve interviewing older workers or reviewing production records.
6. The same analysis should be made with regard to worksites. If many of the cases arise from a single building or location, an environmental cause is suggested. Any worksites in question should be subjected to a thorough industrial hygiene evaluation. This should include both the production process and "in-

Table 13-3. How to estimate cancer statistics locally

Community population	Estimated no. who are alive, saved from cancer	Estimated no. of cancer cases under medical care in 1987	Estimated no. who will die of cancer in 1987	Estimated no. of new cases in 1987	Estimated no. who will be saved from cancer in 1987	Estimated no. who will eventually develop cancer	Estimated no. who will die of cancer if present rates continue
1,000	10	5	1	3	1	280	180
2,000	20	11	4	7	3	560	360
3,000	30	16	5	10	4	840	540
4,000	40	21	7	13	5	1,120	720
5,000	50	26	9	16	6	1,400	900
10,000	100	52	18	33	12	2,800	1,800
25,000	250	131	45	79	30	7,000	4,500
50,000	500	262	90	158	59	14,000	9,000
100,000	1,000	525	180	325	122	28,000	18,000
200,000	2,000	1,050	360	650	244	56,000	36,000
500,000	5,000	2,625	900	1,575	590	140,000	90,000

Note: The figures can only be the roughest approximation of actual data for your community and should be used with caution. It is suggested that every effort be made to obtain actual data from a Registry source.
Source: Adapted from Cancer Facts & Figures—1987. *Med. Benefits*, March 31, 1987. Figures are based on data from the National Cancer Institute's SEER program (1981–1983). Nonmelanoma skin cancer and carcinoma in situ have not been included in the statistics. The incidence of nonmelanoma skin cancer is estimated to be over 500,000 cases annually.

cidental" exposures such as the heating, ventilation, and air-conditioning system (HVAC) and the drinking water.

Based on the above analysis, a suspected cancer cluster may be designated as not actually present, present but not consistent with occupational causation, possibly related to occupational exposures, or definitely related to occupational exposures. The results should be carefully and thoroughly communicated to all those concerned. If an occupational cause is implicated, aggressive corrective action should be taken. Whatever the conclusion, careful ongoing surveillance of both the workplace and the workforce should continue.

A physician who undertakes analysis of an apparent cancer cluster may require further assistance. The most appropriate sources are NIOSH or a qualified consultant, such as a university-based occupational health program.

References

1. American Cancer Society, Atlanta, GA. *Cancer Facts and Figures 1993.*
2. Bailar, J. S., and Smith, E. M. Progress against cancer? *N. Engl. J. Med.* 314:1226, 1986.
3. Higginson, J. Importance of occupational and environmental factors in cancer. *J. Toxicol. Environ. Health* 6:941,1980.
4. Drinkwater, N. R. Experimental models and biological mechanisms for tumor promotion. *Cancer Cells* 2:8, 1990.
5. Farber, E. The multistep nature of cancer development. *Cancer Res.* 44:4217, 1984.
6. Fearon, E. R., and Vogelstein, B. A. A genetic model for colorectal tumorigenesis. *Cell* 61:759, 1990.
7. Harris, C. C. Chemical and physical carcinogenesis: Advances and perspectives for the 1990s. *Cancer Res.* 51:(Suppl.) 5023s, 1991.
8. Bishop, J. M. Molecular themes in oncogenesis. *Cell* 64:235, 1991.
9. Hollstein, M., et al. p53 mutations in human cancers. *Science* 1991:253, 1233.
10. Gonzalez, F. J., Crespi, C. L., and Gelboin, H. V. DNA-expressed human cytochrome P450s: A new age of molecular toxicology and human risk assessment. *Mutation Res.* 247:113, 1991.
11. Pelkonen, O. Carcinogen metabolism and individual susceptibility. *Scand. J. Work Environ. Health* 18 (Suppl.):17, 1992.
12. Van Duuren, B. L., and Banerjee, S. Thresholds in chemical carcinogenesis. *J. Am. Coll. Toxicol.* 2:85,1984.
13. Rothman, K. J. Interactions between causes. In *Modern Epidemiology.* Boston: Little, Brown, 1986. Pp. 311–326.
14. Goodman, D. G. Animal testing of carcinogens. *Occup. Med. State of the Art Rev.* 2:47, 1987.
15. Santella R. M. In vitro testing for carcinogens and mutagens. *Occup. Med. State of the Art Rev.* 2:39, 1987.
16. International Agency for Research on Cancer. *IARC Monographs on the Evaluation of Carcinogenic Risks to Humans,* Suppl. 7. Overall Evaluations of Carcinogenicity: An Updating of IARC Monographs Volumes 1 to 42. Lyon, France: IARC, 1987.
17. Vainio, H., and Wilbourn, J. Identification of carcinogens within the IARC monograph program. *Scand. J. Work Environ. Health* 18 (Suppl.): 64, 1992.
18. Wogan, G. N. Markers of exposure to carcinogens. *Environ. Health Perspect.* 81:9, 1989.
19. Perera, F., and Weinstein, I. B. Molecular epidemiology and carcinogen-DNA adduct detection: New approaches to studies of human cancer causation. *J. Chronic Dis.* 35:581, 1982.
20. Hemminki, K. Use of molecular biology techniques in cancer epidemiology. *Scand. J. Work Environ. Health* 18 (Suppl):38, 1992.
21. Brandt-Rauf, P. W. New markers for monitoring occupational cancer: The example of oncogene proteins. *J. Occup. Med.* 30:399, 1988.
22. Occupational Safety and Health Administration. Identification, classification and regulation of potential occupational carcinogens. *Fed. Register* 45:5015, Jan. 15, 1980.
23. Brennan, T., and Carter, R. F. Legal and scientific probability of causation of cancer and other environmental disease in individuals. *Health Polit. Policy Law* 10:33, 1985.

24. Morrison, A. S. *Screening in Chronic Disease.* New York: Oxford University Press, 1985.
25. Halperin, W. E., et al. Medical screening in the workplace: Proposed principles. *J. Occup. Med.* 28:547,1986.
26. Halperin, W., et al. Final discussion: Where do we go from here? *J. Occup. Med.* 32:936, 1990.
27. Marsh, G. M., et al. A protocol for bladder cancer screening and medical surveillance among high-risk groups: The Drake Health Registry experience. *J. Occup. Med.* 32:881, 1990.
28. Eddy, D. M. Screening for lung cancer. *Ann. Intern. Med.* 111:232, 1989.
29. Strauss, G. M., Gleason, R. E., and Sugarbaker, D. J. Screening for lung cancer reexamined. A reinterpretation of the Mayo Lung Project randomized trial on lung cancer screening. *Chest* 103 (Suppl. 4):337S, 1993.
30. Frumkin, H., and Kantrowitz, W. Cancer clusters in the workplace: An approach to investigation. *J. Occup. Med.* 29:949, 1987.
31. Fleming, L. E., Ducatman, A. M., and Shalat, S. L. Disease clusters in occupational medicine: A protocol for their investigation. *Am. J. Ind. Med.* 22:33, 1992.
32. Rutstein, D. D. Sentinel health events (occupational): A basis for physician recognition and public health surveillance. *Am. J. Public Health* 73:1054, 1983.

Further Information

Alderson, M. *Occupational Cancer.* London: Butterworth, 1986.
A general work on occupational carcinogenesis.

Doll, R., and Peto, R. *The Causes of Cancer.* New York: Oxford University Press, 1981.
A focus on the environmental causes of cancer.

Farber, E. Chemical carcinogenesis: A current biological perspective. *Carcinogenesis* 5:1, 1984.
A review on the molecular biology of cancer.

Federal Office of Science and Technology Policy. Chemical carcinogens: A review of the science and its associated principles. *Fed. Register* 50:10372, 1985.
Testing, identification, and regulation of carcinogens.

Maclure, K. M., and MacMahon, B. An epidemiologic perspective of environmental carcinogenesis. *Epidemiol. Rev.* 2:19, 1980.
A thorough but slightly dated review.

Morrison, A. S. *Screening in Chronic Disease.* New York: Oxford University Press, 1985.
The basic principles of cancer screening.

National Institute of Occupational Safety and Health. *J.O.M.* 28:543, 1986, and 28:901, 1986.
The transcript of a NIOSH conference on medical screening and biologic monitoring for carcinogens. The information is up to date and detailed.

Occupational Safety and Health Administration. *Fed. Register* 45:5001, 1980.
OSHA's carcinogen standard.

Schottenfeld, D., and Fraumeni, J. F. (eds.). *Cancer Epidemiology and Prevention.* Philadelphia: Saunders, 1982.
The best general reference on cancer epidemiology.

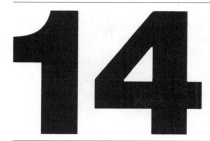

Cardiovascular Disorders

Robert J. McCunney and
Stephen M. Schmitz

Cardiovascular disorders and their ramifications have enormous impact on American society in terms of premature mortality and occupational functioning. Although the range of *cardiovascular* disorders is considerably broad, this chapter is limited to coronary artery disease (CAD), which is also referred to as coronary heart disease (CHD). Attention is directed to the role of the physician in advising preventive programs for the occupational setting, assessing work capabilities of people with CAD, and evaluating whether certain types of cardiovascular disease may be due to exposure to occupational and environmental agents. Since each of these topics could serve as an independent chapter, the material is, of necessity, brief. Coverage of major issues includes appropriate references to facilitate more intensive review of these areas for physicians who provide occupational medical services.

Prevention of Coronary Heart Disease in the Occupational Setting

Although death rates from CHD continue to decline, each year the disorder causes about 1.5 million myocardial infarctions (MI), 500,000 of which are fatal [1] (Tables 14-1 and 14-2). Cost estimates for cardiovascular disease in 1992 are $108.9 billion, which includes the cost of medication, lost productivity, and physician, hospital, and nursing home services [2]. Coronary heart disease refers to narrowing of the coronary vessels due to atherosclerosis, the exact cause of which is unknown, but which is widely acknowledged to be due to the interaction of certain *risk factors*. The principal modifiable risk factors include cigarette smoking, hypertension, elevated serum cholesterol, physical inactivity, and obesity, while increasing age, male gender, and family history are the principal nonmodifiable risk factors [3]. Because of the wide prevalence of CHD in Western societies, numerous preventive measures have been developed. Such efforts have primarily focused on reduction of major risk factors through screening and medical intervention.

The occupational setting has often served as the base from which to provide preventive medical services. Benefits include ready access to large groups of people,

Table 14-1. Estimated prevalence of the major cardiovascular diseases (CVD; United States, 1989 estimate)

CVD type	No. of persons (in millions)
Stroke	3,020,000
Rheumatic heart disease	1,320,000
Coronary heart disease	6,230,000
Hypertensive disease[a]	63,640,000
Total CVD[b]	70,020,000

[a]Hypertensives are defined as persons with a systolic level > 140 and/or a diastolic level > 90 or those who report using antihypertensive medication.
[b]The sum of the individual estimates exceeds 63,400,000 since many persons have more than one cardiovascular disorder.
Source: From National Health and Nutrition Examination Survey II (NHANES II-I: Interview and Examination Data) and the American Heart Association. Data supplied by the American Heart Association ([1], p. 1).

Table 14-2. Estimated economic costs in billions of dollars of cardiovascular diseases by type of expenditure (United States, 1993 estimate)

Expenditure	Estimated cost (in billions)
Physician and nursing services	17.9
Hospital and nursing home services	75.2
Costs of medication	6.7
Lost output due to disability	17.6
Total cost	117.4

Source: From National Health and Nutrition Examination Survey II (NHANES II-I: Interview and Examination Data) and the American Heart Association. Data supplied by the American Heart Association ([1], p. 18).

greater ability to ensure follow-up study of abnormalities noted during screening measures, and financial and administrative support of the organization. All of these considerations can enhance participation and ensure adherence to the behavioral changes necessary to reduce risk factors.

Blood Pressure

Blood pressure control programs in work settings have proved beneficial in controlling the sequelae of hypertension through early recognition, appropriate follow-up study, and greater compliance with treatment regimens [4]. Data from the National Survey of Worksite Health Promotion Activities revealed that blood pressure screening occurred at 55.4% of private sector worksites queried [5]. Such programs have also proved to be cost effective [6]. Successful occupational endeavors include special events, group classes or workshops, and on-site/off-site treatment and follow-up. Optimally, blood pressure screening should be part of a comprehensive health promotion program [7]. Guidelines for the implementation of worksite hypertension control programs are described in Chap. 32. Numerous nonprofit health organizations, such as the American Heart Association, can provide both educational material and staff to implement on-site programs [8].

Cigarette Smoking

Because cigarette smoking is held accountable for nearly one third of MIs (United States Surgeon General's Report, 1984), smoking cessation programs are ideally suited for controlling CHD. Indeed, with the advent of policies that restrict smoking in certain public areas, more organizations are sponsoring these programs. A random sample of a nationwide survey of worksite health promotion activities revealed that smoking cessation programs were offered at 35.6% of all worksites [9]. Many different approaches to encourage people to stop smoking have been attempted; success rates of most efforts are similar. A recent meta-analysis of 20 controlled studies of worksite smoking cessation identified the following factors as those contributing to the highest quit rate: programs that included a group component, programs that were not overly complicated, and programs that shared company and employee time. The worksite appears to be especially effective in assisting heavier smokers in quitting [10]. Interestingly, nearly 90% of people who stop smoking do so on their own, without the benefit of a formal program [11]. Ideally, a few different programs should be offered to enable people to choose the most effective approach for themselves (see Chap. 32).

Cholesterol

The role of cholesterol in the development of CHD has received considerable attention as a result of a National Institute of Health (NIH) National Cholesterol Education Program (NCEP) [12]. The report concluded that cholesterol elevations were *causatively* related to CHD and that the public should be educated accordingly. The report further concluded that levels of serum cholesterol for most Americans are too high and that interventions to reduce these levels should be developed.

The results of the Lipid Research Clinics Coronary Primary Prevention Trial

(LRC-CPPT) indicated that an 8.5% reduction in serum cholesterol in middle-aged hypercholesterolemic men was associated with a 19% reduction in incidence of major coronary events over a 7-year period [13]. A number of other studies have corroborated the association between elevated cholesterol and increased morbidity and mortality from cardiac disease.

Controversy exists, however, as to the most beneficial approach for lowering serum cholesterol levels [14]. Ileal bypass surgery is clearly the most effective approach, although this procedure is not beneficial to most patients. At the NIH conference, a review of 19 diet/drug trials of 36,000 people suggested that interventions designed to lower serum cholesterol reduced coronary events and mortality, but that overall mortality in the study group was not affected (due to increase in noncardiac mortality). Controlled clinical trials in which diets low in saturated fats were given to asymptomatic middle-aged men with selected risk factors have shown a 10 to 15% reduction in serum cholesterol levels. In most trials, this reduction has been associated with a decrease in the incidence of major cardiac events such as MI and sudden death [3].

Controversy also exists as to the specific amounts of dietary fats needed to lower the risk of atherosclerosis. The NIH panel [12] stated the following:

> After carefully considering the extensive scientific evidence linking blood cholesterol, atherosclerosis, CHD, and diet, this panel concludes that excessive intakes of saturated fatty acids, total fat, and dietary cholesterol, together with excessive body weight, all contribute importantly to biologically unnecessary and undesirable elevations of blood cholesterol. The panel concluded that Americans should change their eating patterns to reduce the average intake of saturated fatty acids and total and dietary cholesterol, and to eliminate excess body weight.

The expert panel recommendation from the NCEP is less than 10% of total calories from saturated fat, an average of 30% of total calories or less from fat, dietary energy levels needed to reach or maintain desirable body weight, and less than 300 mg cholesterol per day.

Interestingly, six recent, randomized clinical trials have assessed the effects of interventions on coronary atherosclerosis and found that patients in control groups who consumed a diet consisting of 30% fat and 200 to 300 mg cholesterol per day showed progression of coronary atherosclerosis in all studies. Those patients who consumed a diet of 10% fat that was devoid of cholesterol demonstrated regression of atherosclerosis [15]. The NCEP recommendations may represent a "transition" diet, one that may be easier to follow for the majority of our culture. However, in high-risk individuals, particularly those who have had a recent MI, or who have documented severe CAD, a very low fat/no-cholesterol diet appears to be the most prudent.

It is highly likely that occupational physicians will be called on to advise on both the practicality of *screening* workers for elevated cholesterol and the appropriate *clinical* management of certain levels. Routine issues related to screening will surface, including the reliability and validity of the screening device, including the analytic technique; availability and efficacy of treatment measures; and appropriate follow-up study.

New analytic methods have been developed for determining level of cholesterol, including those that can formulate results on a "fingerstick" blood sample. Considerable variability exists, however, in the results obtained from various techniques [16]. One study showed that a serum cholesterol of 240 mg/100 ml (LRC method) would yield a value of 275 mg/100 ml on the standard SMAC Technicon analyzer and 290 mg/100 ml on the Dupont analyzer [17]. The discrepancies apparently result from the use of different reagents and alternate standards for equipment calibration. One study showed that the fingerstick method tended to *underestimate* the actual cholesterol level (i.e., the value obtained by a reference laboratory), and thus tended to produce false-negative results [18].

Additionally, even if the same technique is used, measurements of total or low-density lipoprotein (LDL) cholesterol on the same person may vary greatly at different times. Analytic and biologic variability account for the discrepancy in results. It is essential to know by how much and in what direction laboratories differ from the standardized values of the Centers for Disease Control [19, 20].

Despite potential inaccuracies in measurement of serum cholesterol levels, the NCEP recommends the classification shown in Table 14-3, based on total and LDL cholesterol levels [12].

Table 14-3. Guidelines for patient referral based on cholesterol levels

Classification	Cholesterol level	LDL cholesterol level
High	>240 mg/100 ml	>160 mg/100 ml
Borderline high	200–239 mg/100 ml	130–159 mg/100 ml
Desirable	<200 mg/100 ml	<130 mg/100 ml

The NCEP panel developed the following guidelines for referral based on blood cholesterol level.

Classification	Recommended action
High (>240 mg/100 ml)	Refer to physician for follow-up*
Borderline high (200–239 mg/100 ml)	Refer to physician for follow-up* if history of coronary heart disease or if two or more other CHD risk factors (excluding high-density lipoprotein cholesterol) detected on interview; if no reported history of CHD or less than two other risk factors, refer to physician within one year for repeat cholesterol measurement
Desirable (>200 mg/100 ml)	Recommend a repeat cholesterol follow-up in 5 years

*Individuals should be seen by their physicians within 2 months.
Source: From NCEP *Report on Population Strategies for Blood Cholesterol Reduction*. Washington, DC: US Department of Health and Human Services, 1990. Pp. 8, 30.

Although the "severity of atherosclerosis rises linearly with increasing levels of plasma cholesterol, risk for coronary heart disease does not begin to increase markedly until the critical zone is reached" [21]. These guidelines, thus, were proposed with the understanding that the relationship between serum cholesterol and CHD is curvilinear (Fig. 14-1); this implies that a "threshold" appears to exist between the extent of atherosclerosis and appearance of clinical manifestations of CHD, presumably because a critical narrowing (60%) of coronary vessel must first be present.

Serum cholesterol is but one lipid parameter that is of value in predicting risk of CHD. Although the major components of lipoproteins include low-density lipoprotein cholesterol (LDL-C), very low density lipoprotein cholesterol (VLDL-C), chylomicrons, and high-density lipoprotein cholesterol (HDL-C), it is the last that appears to have the greatest value in cardiac risk assessment [22]. The total cholesterol/HDL ratio has been described as the most sensitive parameter for predicting risk of CHD.

High-density lipoprotein, by mobilizing free cholesterol for metabolism by the liver, exerts a beneficial effect by slowing atherosclerosis. Investigations of populations with aortocoronary bypass grafts, angiographic evidence of CHD, or history of MI have consistently shown an inverse relationship between severity of atherosclerosis and HDL-C concentration [23].

Another factor of interest are the apolipoproteins a and b, in which elevated levels are strongly associated with CHD. Reduction of this level through diet and medication can lead to regression of CAD independent of HDL levels [24, 25].

Because of newer analytic techniques, the potential for screening large groups of people to determine level of cholesterol has expanded dramatically. A program conducted in New York City screened over 12,000 participants [26]. It was interesting that of the group screened, only 10% smoked cigarettes (implying a relatively high level of health awareness), but only half had ever had a serum cholesterol measurement taken.

Physical Fitness

Physical fitness has also been promoted as beneficial in controlling CHD [27–29]. Even minimal increases in physical activity can improve cardiovascular fitness

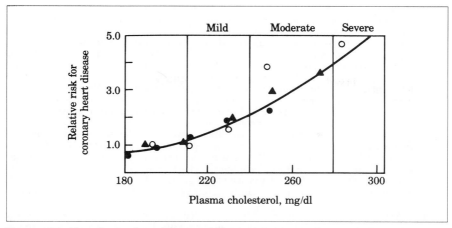

Figure 14-1. The relationship of plasma cholesterol level to relative risk for coronary heart disease as determined in three prospective population studies. Closed circles indicate Multiple Risk Factor Intervention Trial; open circles, Framingham Study; and triangles, Pooling Project. (From S. M. Grundy. Cholesterol and coronary heart disease: A new era. *J.A.M.A.* 256:2849, 1986. Copyright 1986, American Medical Association.)

among sedentary people. Although the precise amount of physical activity required to promote cardiovascular fitness is a matter of debate, sessions of 20- to 30-minute duration three times per week are routinely recommended (with the assumption that one exercises to about 75% of one's age-predicted maximal heart rate [220−AGE] for the exercise period). The current best estimate is that approximately 7 to 8% of adults participate three or more times a week for 20 minutes or more in an activity that requires 60% or more of VO_2 max [30]. Thus, an ideal opportunity exists in the occupational setting to promote the beneficial effects of various types of physical activity. (See Chap. 32 for a discussion on implementing an occupational fitness program.)

The clinical role for physicians overseeing a fitness program includes medical assessment of participants and ancillary and laboratory tests for monitoring the program. Guidelines need to be established concerning the type of exercise testing, if any, that will be conducted at the onset. Routine recommendations that require all participants to undergo an exercise electrocardiogram (ECG) should be discouraged. More restricted guidelines that focus on the presence of cardiac risk factors, past medical history, and symptoms reflective of CHD are more suitable [31]. On the other hand, submaximal exercise testing on a bicycle-like ergometer has been used to estimate maximal oxygen uptake (the most sensitive indicator of cardiovascular fitness). Maximal effort, however, must be expended in exercise to estimate maximal oxygen uptake. Many American adults who are not accustomed to bicycling experience leg fatigue (due to poor conditioning) before reaching their maximal cardiovascular potential. Thus, where feasible, treadmill exercise testing will yield more reliable results. Periodic testing can help monitor the progress of one's performance in an exercise or fitness program.

Ancillary testing of value in fitness programs includes measurement of serum lipids, such as total cholesterol and HDL-C, to aid in the estimation of cardiac risk factor. It may be helpful to measure concentration of apolipoprotein A-1, which has been hailed as offering "superior discriminatory ability over HDL-C" [32].

Assessing Work Capabilities Following a Major Cardiac Event

Over 1.5 million Americans suffer an MI each year, and upwards of 190,000 people undergo coronary artery bypass graft (CABG) surgery. Issues related to the ability of these people to return to work present challenges to the clinician. Coronary artery bypass graft surgery has resulted in the following benefits [33]: relief of angina in

80 to 90% of people with attendant improvement in functional capacity, reduction or elimination of significant ST depression on ECG, and improvement in left ventricular function.

One's ability to resume occupational activities following a major cardiac event depends on medical, social, and psychological factors [34]. In general, over 80% of people who suffer an MI or undergo CABG surgery return to their original positions. The major adverse medical "prognosticators" for failure to return to work include left ventricular dysfunction and persistence of ischemia [35]. Nonmedical factors, however, appear to present the greatest impediment for people to resume occupational activities [36] (Table 14-4). In fact, many people do not resume work, despite significant improvements in functional capacity [34].

Investigations regarding ability to return to work have led to inconsistent results. In a review of 893 men who underwent a CABG, the major factor involved in return to work was the *type* of job [37]. Age plays an important role, and in a German study 73% of patients in the 30- to 49-year-old age group returned to work, compared with only 56% in the 50- to 54-year-old age group and 7% in the 60- to 64-year-old age group [38]. Data from the United States found percentages of 68, 64, and 38, respectively [38].

Another study of 350 people, however, failed to show substantial improvement in level of employment following CABG surgery [39]. Those who worked prior to surgery tended to work thereafter. The authors suggested that in many cases there was little *financial incentive* for people to return to work.

Relief of anginal pain is another factor. If angina was completely or partially relieved postoperatively, 88% of patients less than 49 years of age returned to work versus 53% if angina was not relieved [40]. This difference remained consistent for older age groups.

One's level of self-assessed "disability" may affect ability to return to work. Even

Table 14-4. Factors involved in returning to work after a major cardiac event

Medical
    Severity and extent of CHD
    Effort angina/post-CABG chest wall or leg pain
    Physical capacity
Psychological
    Preevent and postevent anxiety/depression/coping styles/personality
Sociodemographic, economic, and cultural
    Age, gender, education level
    Disposable income, pension/retirement/disability benefits
    National customs
    Economic conditions
Individual's history and perception of prior work
    Type of work/physical environment
    Employment history
    Physical demands of job/perceived stress on job
    Job satisfaction
    Work limitations prior to event
    Availability of previous job/job change/retraining
Individual's perception of health and risk to life
    Attribution of MI/CHD to previous job
Individual's perception of self
    Self-confidence
Influence of and constraints on others
    Family
    Employer's reluctance to rehire
    Union practices or fears
    Government/legislation
    Physician advice
Individual's expectations and predictions

Source: Adapted from D. M. Davidson. Return to work after cardiac events: A review. *J. Cardiac Rehabil.* 3:60, 1983; and T. Kavanagh and V. Matosevic. Assessment of work capacity in patients with ischaemic heart disease: Methods and practices. *Eur. Heart J.* 9 (Suppl. L):68, 1988.

low physical capacity, for example, may not interfere with one's ability to handle routine household chores, such as shopping, maintenance, and certain leisure activities [41]. An Italian investigation demonstrated similar results: Nearly 25% of 118 patients who underwent valvular or CABG surgery showed no improvement in psychological attributes [42]. Most predictive of poor psychological outcome was evidence of hypochondriasis, anxiety, and depression. Psychological factors play a very important role in return to work after a cardiac event, and assessment and management of these factors must be a part of total patient care in order to optimize return to work [43].

Clinical Assessment of Work Capabilities

The physician overseeing an occupational medicine program is likely to be asked to evaluate a person's work capabilities following a major cardiac event. A thorough analysis includes a review of the disorder, including medical records and diagnostic studies; current status of the person, including presence of symptoms, physical findings, and appropriate laboratory testing, especially an exercise ECG; and a job analysis.

History/Physical Examination

A review of the nature of the MI or CABG surgery is necessary with attention to complications, such as congestive heart failure, persistence of ischemia, or dysrhythmias. A review of prior cardiac-related problems, medications, and current status, such as exertional chest pain, orthopnea, or ankle swelling, can help assess level of improvement. An inquiry into tolerance for routine activities is necessary to gauge the person's potential to assume occupational responsibilities safely.

The physical examination should be directed to signs of congestive heart failure, such as ankle swelling (pitting edema), hepatomegaly, jugular venous distention, or an S3 gallop at the myocardial apex. The character of the pulse should be assessed for regularity to determine the presence of altered rhythms or ectopy. A systolic murmur consistent with mitral insufficiency may indicate decompensation of cardiac function, if it was not present earlier.

Based on the evaluation and a review of records from the hospitalization, the need for additional ancillary testing can be determined. In some cases decisions regarding cardiac status can be made at this time, especially if an exercise ECG has recently been performed. In other cases, an ECG or chest film may be necessary if it appears that symptoms or physical findings have changed since the last evaluation. Situations vary as to whether the occupational physician or attending physician conducts these tests. Communication between the occupational physician, attending physician, and business enterprise is essential, with attention to local protocol.

Exercise Electrocardiogram

A symptom-limited exercise test is considered the most sensitive predictor of future reinfarction and death if the test is performed within 6 weeks after an acute MI [44]. Myocardial ischemia and left ventricular dysfunction, however, are the major determinants of both prognosis and functional capacity after an MI.

Clinical judgment about resumption of occupational activities can be refined through the use of an exercise ECG. For example, most people can generate up to 8 to 9 METs* of energy within 3 months of an uncomplicated acute MI; this level of energy is similar to that for most healthy men between the ages of 50 and 59 [45].

Although the work environment is often presumed to be more stressful than home, reinfarction and death do not appear to occur more frequently at work [35]. Actually, few jobs today require demanding physical effort, since automation has reduced the need thereof in many settings. Moreover, most people who have suffered a major cardiac event are older workers (>50 years), who have usually moved into more sedentary roles, even in labor-intensive industries. A review of the person's exercise ECG will yield information related to duration of the test, development of dysrhythmias, ischemia, hypo- or hypertension, fatigue, or shortness of breath. Energy expenditure in METs can then be compared to standard references to approximate the individual's physical capacity [46] (Table 14-5).

---

*An MET is the energy expenditure at rest, equivalent to approximately 3.5 ml O_2/kg body weight/min.

Table 14-5. Approximate metabolic cost of certain physical activities

	Occupational	Recreational
1.5–2.0 METs	Desk work Auto driving Typing Electric calculating machine operation	Standing Walking (strolling 1.6 km/hour) Flying, motorcycling Playing cards Sewing, knitting
2–3 METs	Auto repair Radio, TV repair Janitorial work Typing, manual Bartending	Level walking (3.2 km/hour) Level bicycling (8.0 km/hour) Riding lawn mower Billiards, bowling Skeet, shuffleboard Woodworking (light) Powerboat driving Golf (power cart) Canoeing (4 km/hour) Horseback riding (walk) Playing piano and many musical instruments
3–4 METs	Bricklaying, plastering Wheelbarrow (45.4-kg load) Machine assembly Trailer-truck in traffic Welding (moderate load) Cleaning windows	Walking (4.8 km/hour) Cycling (9.7 km/hour) Horseshoe pitching Volleyball (6-man noncompetitive) Golf (pulling bag cart) Archery Sailing (handling small boat) Fly fishing (standing with waders) Horseback (sitting trot) Badminton (social double) Pushing light power mower Energetic musician
4–5 METs	Painting, masonry Paperhanging Light carpentry	Walking (5.6 km/hour) Cycling (12.9 km/hour) Table tennis Golf (carrying clubs) Dancing (foxtrot) Badminton (singles) Tennis (doubles) Raking leaves Hoeing Many calisthenics
5–6 METs	Digging garden Shoveling light earth	Walking (6.4 km/hour) Cycling (16.1 km/hour) Canoeing (6.4 km/hour) Horseback (posting trot) Stream fishing (walking in light current in waters) Ice or roller skating (14.5 km/hour)
6–7 METs	Shoveling 10 loads/ minute (4.5 kg)	Walking (8.0 km/hour) Cycling (17.7 km/hour) Badminton (competitive) Tennis (singles) Splitting wood Snow shoveling Hand lawn mowing Folk (square) dancing Light downhill skiing Ski touring (4.0 km/hour) (loose snow) Water skiing

(continued)

Table 14-5 (continued)

	Occupational	Recreational
7–8 METs	Digging ditches Carrying 36.3 kg Sawing hardwood	Jogging (8.0 km/hour) Cycling (19.3 km/hour) Horseback (gallop) Vigorous downhill skiing Basketball Mountain climbing Ice hockey Canoeing (8.0 km/hour) Touch football Paddleball
8–9 METs	Shoveling 10 loads/ minute (6.4 kg)	Running (8.9 km/hour) Cycling (20.9 km/hour) Ski touring (6.4 km/hour) Squash racquets (social) Handball (social) Fencing Basketball (vigorous)
9–10 METs	Shoveling 10 loads/ minute (7.3 kg)	Running (9.6–16 km/hour) Ski touring (8 + km/hour) Handball (competitive) Squash (competitive)

Source: Adapted from S. M. Fox, J. P. Naughton, and W. L. Haskell. Physical activity and the prevention of coronary heart disease. *Ann. Clin. Res.* 3:404, 1971.

The following are caveats regarding the use of these tables [47]:

1. Figures represent *average* oxygen uptake values, which may vary depending on the *pace* at which the person performs the activity and previous training and work efficiency.
2. Figures were obtained during continuous *steady-state* work, whereas most occupational duties are *intermittent* in nature.
3. Figures were obtained based on oxygen uptake for *leg* exercise predominantly, which may *not* accurately reflect cardiac demands of positions with low somatic oxygen requirements but high myocardial demands due to psychological stress. Examples include positions such as air traffic controllers, taxi drivers, and some executive roles.

Job Analysis

At the minimum, the physician should request a job description, especially if physical activity is frequently required. Physical work can be classified into *static* and *dynamic,* which present different hemodynamic challenges. A heavy *static* load, for example, results in a *pressure* load on the heart, whereas heavy *dynamic* work produces a *volume* load [48]. Energy requirements of the job may also need to be assessed, as well as the presence of temperature or psychological stress. In some settings, simulated work testing such as a weight-carrying test or a repetitive weight-lifting test can be used in conjunction with a routine exercise ECG to enhance the assessment of work capabilities. Simulated testing offers more objective data and can aid in stimulating confidence in the patient for assuming occupational activities.

Cardiac Rehabilitation

Cardiac rehabilitation, especially prescribed physical activity, is accepted treatment for many patients with cardiovascular disease [49]. Benefits include improvement in physical capacity, psychosocial attributes, and lipoprotein patterns. The goals of cardiac rehabilitation have been well summarized and include the following [50]:

1. Delay or prevent cardiovascular complications
2. Improve physical conditioning to enable return to work and resumption of normal activities

3. Reduce risk factors
4. Enhance psychological adjustment

One investigation [50] of 31 patients following CABG surgery showed substantial improvements in physical work capacity and reduction in resting pulse. People exercised three times per week, with the sessions increasing from 20-minute sessions to 60 minutes over the first 6 weeks of the program. In a 5-year study (1980–1984) of 167 randomly selected cardiac rehabilitation programs, only 3 fatal cardiac arrests occurred among 51,303 patients [51]. This translated to one death/783,972 hours of patient exercise. Typically, patients in whom life-threatening arrhythmias or MI develop during exercise training demonstrate exercise-induced ischemia; have severe, nonaltered coronary disease; and choose to exceed their prescribed upper-limit heart rate during the exercise session [52]. The current cardiac rehabilitative process that allows prescribed and supervised exercise appears to be associated with an extremely low rate of cardiovascular complications. Other benefits include improvements in quality of life, which has been measured using the Sickness Impact Profile as an assessment tool [53].

While cardiac exercise is generally safe, there are circumstances in which monitored exercise is prudent. The American College of Cardiology has suggested that telemetry be employed when the following conditions exist: (1) severely depressed left ventricular function (ejection fraction < 30%); (2) resting complex ventricular arrhythmia (Lown type 4 or 5); (3) ventricular arrhythmias appearing or increasing with exercise; (4) systolic blood pressure decreasing with exercise; (5) previous cardiac arrest; (6) after MI complicated by congestive heart failure, cardiogenic shock, or serious ventricular arrhythmias; (7) severe CAD and marked exercise-induced ischemia (ST-segment depression $\geq$ 2 mm); or (8) inability to self-monitor heart rate due to physical or intellectual impairment [54].

Occupational Agents that Cause or Aggravate Heart Disease

People who have worked in dry-cleaning establishments, in explosives factories, and in the production of rayon have all suffered various types of cardiovascular disease as a result of their work. Carbon disulfide, nitrates, and carbon monoxide are firmly accepted as causative factors in heart disease. Heart disease, however, is so prevalent in Western society that occupational factors may be overlooked in clinical management. The point of this section is to review accepted occupational hazards to the cardiovascular system and to propose guidelines for the clinical evaluation and placement of workers exposed to these hazards.

The clinician is likely to be faced with two distinct scenarios regarding work situations hazardous to the cardiovascular system: the evaluation of symptoms or disease experienced by a person in a work setting and the proper placement of people with cardiovascular disease. The following examples are based on experiences in providing occupational medical services to small businesses.

1. A truck driver complains of headaches whenever he remains in his cabin for over an hour. He does not smoke, and the problem only seems to occur during the winter months.
2. An owner of an automobile repair shop experiences palpitations toward the end of the workday. He had been using cleaning solvents in an unventilated area of the shop.
3. A worker with CHD is referred for an evaluation concerning his ability to work as a degreaser at a jewelry firm. Although only 43 years old, he had experienced an MI and now suffers from atrial fibrillation.

In each of these situations, the work setting has a pronounced effect on the manifestation of heart disease. The cases represent examples of how carbon monoxide and solvents, in particular, can affect the heart. Although occupational cardiotoxins are few in number (compared, for example, to pulmonary toxins or neurotoxins), the effects of these agents are often life threatening.

Clinical Evaluation

In conducting an evaluation of chest pain, especially angina, an inquiry should be directed toward the activity associated with the onset of the discomfort, especially if it occurs at work. Symptoms that occur during or immediately after work may be due to carbon monoxide, methylene chloride, or perhaps overexertion. Extremes of temperature, whether heat or cold, may precipitate symptoms in some people.

When evaluating cardiovascular symptoms that may be due to work, it is helpful to consider associated signs and symptoms. For example, light-headedness and dizziness can occur with solvent exposure, especially methylene chloride, which is metabolized to carbon monoxide.

The physical examination and laboratory evaluation should be consistent with routine medical practice. Occupational cardiovascular disorders differ from the nonoccupational type only in etiology. Clinical manifestations and management are similar. Routine diagnostic studies are recommended, with special attention to the work setting. For example, a 24-hour ambulatory ECG monitor should be worn at work if symptoms of palpitations are suspected as being due to solvents.

To formulate these assessments, a thorough occupational history is essential. If an occupational agent is suspected of causing or aggravating a cardiovascular disorder, special attention can be directed to its specific toxicity. A review of the medical literature and industrial hygiene sampling may be necessary to form a refined opinion. A full discussion of all the agents suspected of cardiotoxicity is beyond the scope of this chapter, but common examples are described. More comprehensive reviews are available for further reading [55–57].

Cardiotoxic Agents

Carbon Monoxide

People exposed to automobile exhaust, furnaces, the incomplete combustion of carbonaceous material, and methylene chloride may experience adverse health effects of carbon monoxide. People with CHD appear especially sensitive to the effects of carboxyhemoglobin, the substance formed when carbon monoxide combines with hemoglobin.

Carbon monoxide can cause headaches, light-headedness, and dizziness as well as chest pain secondary to myocardial ischemia. The headache experienced by the truck driver described at the beginning of this section was due to carbon monoxide from a faulty exhaust system. A carboxyhemoglobin of 12% in a nonsmoker was convincing evidence of carbon monoxide toxicity, especially when symptoms resolved and carboxyhemoglobin declined when the exhaust system was repaired.

Further increases in carboxyhemoglobin (up to 25%) have been associated with ECG abnormalities, and greater vulnerability to cardiac rhythm disturbances—supraventricular and ventricular extrasystoles and atrial fibrillation. In fact, a rather striking dose-response relationship exists between level of carboxyhemoglobin and a variety of symptoms, with the more serious manifestations occurring at higher levels of exposure.

Individuals with CAD may exhibit symptoms at far lower levels, at carboxyhemoglobin levels as low as 3 to 5% [57]. Carbon monoxide can aggravate anginal symptoms in those with CHD. One study of Los Angeles freeway drivers demonstrated such an exacerbation of symptoms when ambient levels of carbon monoxide increased [58].

Clinical implications of carbon monoxide include proper job placement of people with angina and other symptoms of CHD. For example, can a person who has recently suffered an MI return to work as a tollbooth operator or clerk at an underground garage? Proper clinical assessment may require an exercise ECG and ambient measurements of carbon monoxide levels. In some cases, it may be of value to propose a trial period of observation. The approach suitable for each situation will depend on a number of factors, including availability of other positions and income replacement benefits. Unfortunately, no specific guidelines are available. Thus, thoughtful and practical considerations are necessary.

Solvents

Solvents refer to substances, usually liquid, that are used as cleaning agents. Examples include routine household products, such as paint thinner, and industrial materials used in degreasing operations, such as trichloroethylene or methylene chloride.

The major cardiovascular risk of solvents appears to be dysrhythmias, although methylene chloride has the unique property of being converted to carbon monoxide in vivo. Exposure to high concentrations of methylene chloride can also result in central nervous system narcosis, apart from the carbon monoxide effects, with the resulting respiratory depression predisposing to cardiac disturbances [59]. Both halogenated and nonhalogenated compounds have been associated with sudden death. Trichloroethylene, for example, has been implicated in sudden death apparently through the induction of ventricular dysrhythmias. Another type of solvent, fluorocarbons, was associated with palpitations in the course of workers preparing frozen sections from surgical specimens [60].

Clinical decisions may focus on whether symptoms of palpitations or irregular rhythms are due to work with solvents. A thorough evaluation focuses on nonoccupational as well as occupational factors and includes the use of a 24-hour ambulatory ECG monitor. Combined with industrial hygiene sampling, 24-hour Holter monitoring results can help determine whether the solvent is causing or contributing to the disorder.

Proper placement of the patient with a dysrhythmia can be problematic, especially if alternative positions are unavailable. The owner of the repair shop described earlier in the chapter had just purchased the business and did not want to give up his chosen type of work.

Carbon Disulfide
Carbon disulfide, a substance used in the viscose rayon industry, has been associated with increasing the rate of atherosclerosis [61]. A proposed mechanism for this adverse effect is through a decrease in fibrinolytic activity. The material is also used in chemical laboratories and in the manufacture of carbon tetrachloride.

Cross-cultural studies of Japanese, Finnish, Belgian, and American workers confirm the assertion that carbon disulfide can cause atherosclerosis, but apparently only in populations with a "Western diet." A Japanese study, for example, showed no unusual increase in CHD but a marked elevation in retinal hemorrhages (25%) compared to the Finnish group (4%). No difference was seen among unexposed Japanese and Finnish workers. Another study of male textile workers showed a significant and positive linear trend in LDL cholesterol and diastolic blood pressure [62]. These results may suggest another means by which carbon disulfide may influence ischemic heart disease.

Clinical evaluations of a person suspected of having carbon disulfide exposure might include urinary measurement of metabolites (positive iodine-azide reaction) in addition to routine diagnostic measures.

Nitro Compounds
Occupational exposure to nitroglycerin and other aliphatic nitrates has been associated with angina-like pain, MI, and cardiovascular death. Although exposure to these compounds also occurs in the pharmaceutical industry, studies have been directed primarily toward workers in the explosives industry [63].

Since nitroglycerin and ethylene glycol dinitrate can be absorbed through the skin, estimates of level of exposure associated with toxic effects are lacking. The anecdotal occurrence of sudden death in these workers has been dubbed "Monday morning death" because it often develops, as do other symptoms of coronary insufficiency, after being away from work for a brief period of time. This manifestation is presumed to be due to rebound coronary spasm as a result of withdrawal of nitrates. However, the increased mortality due to coronary disease in occupational cohorts principally occurred months and years after exposure ceased (which may suggest the presence of an additional pathogenic process). A recently published retrospective cohort mortality study from Scandinavia looked at over 5000 workers exposed to nitroglycerin, dinitrotoluene, and controls, and did *not* show a chronic effect of either on cardiovascular disease risk [64].

Clinical evaluation of workers exposed to nitrates might include determination of serum methemoglobin, in addition to standard diagnostic studies.

Miscellaneous Agents

The scope of this chapter limits a comprehensive review of suspected cardiotoxins, but other agents have been considered potentially harmful (Table 14-6). If an appropriate clinical evaluation is conducted, however, further review of toxicologic literature can shed light on the role that occupational factors may have on the expression of CHD or cardiac dysrhythmias.

Table 14-6. Agents associated with work-related cardiovascular disease

Antimony	Fluorocarbons*
Arsenic	Heat
Carbon disulfide*	Hydrocarbons (solvents)*
Carbon monoxide*	Methylene chloride*
Cobalt	Nitrates*
Cold	Heavy metals (lead, cadmium)

*Well-supported medical evidence.
Source: Adapted from L. J. Fine. Cardiovascular Heart Disease. In W. Rom (ed.), *Environmental and Occupational Medicine* (2nd ed.). Boston: Little, Brown, 1992. Pp. 593–600.

References

1. American Heart Association. *1993 Heart and Stroke Facts Statistics.* Dallas: American Heart Association, 1992.
2. Gunby, P. Cardiovascular diseases remain nation's leading cause of death. *J.A.M.A.* 267:335, 1992.
3. US Preventive Services Task Force. *Guide to Clinical Preventive Services: An Assessment of the Effectiveness of 169 Interventions. Report of the US Preventive Services Task Force.* Baltimore: Williams & Wilkins, 1989.
4. Erfurt, J., and Foote, A. Cost effectiveness of work-site blood pressure control programs. *J.O.M.* 26:892, 1984.
5. Fielding, J. E. Frequency of health risk assessment activities at US worksites. *Am. J. Prev. Med.* 5:75, 1989.
6. Fielding, J. E. Effectiveness of employee health improvement programs. *J.O.M.* 24:907, 1982.
7. *Healthy People: National Health Promotion and Disease Prevention Objectives.* DHHS Publication no. (PHS)91-50212, 1990. P. 406.
8. American Heart Association. *Heart at Work.* Dallas: American Heart Association, 1984.
9. Fielding, J. E., and Piserchia, P. V. Frequency of worksite health promotion activities. *Am. J. Public Health* 79:16, 1989.
10. Fisher, K. J., Glascow, R. E., and Terborg, J. R. Work site smoking cessation: A meta-analysis of long-term quit rates from controlled studies. *J.O.M.* 32:429, 1990.
11. Fiore, M. C., et al. Methods used to quit smoking in the United States: Do cessation programs help? *J.A.M.A.* 263:2760, 1990.
12. National Cholesterol Education Program, *Report on Population Strategies for Blood Cholesterol Reduction.* Washington, DC: US Department of Health and Human Services, 1990.
13. Lipid Research Clinics Program. The Lipid Research Clinics Coronary Primary Prevention Trial results: II. The relationship of reduction in incidence of coronary heart disease to cholesterol lowering. *J.A.M.A.* 251:365, 1984.
14. Olson, R. E. Mass intervention vs. screening and selective intervention for the prevention of coronary heart disease. *J.A.M.A.* 255:2204, 1986.
15. Ornish, D. Letter to the editor. *J.A.M.A.* 267:362, 1992.
16. Kaufman, H. W., et al. How reliably can compact chemistry analyzers measure lipids? *J.A.M.A.* 263:1245, 1990.
17. Blank, D. W., et al. The method of determination must be considered in interpreting blood cholesterol levels. *J.A.M.A.* 256:2767, 1986.
18. Naughton, M. J., Luepker, R. V., and Strickland, D. The accuracy of portable cholesterol analyzers in public screening programs. *J.A.M.A.* 263:1213, 1990.
19. Gwynne, J. T. Measuring and knowing: The trouble with cholesterol and decision making. *J.A.M.A.* 266:1696, 1991.
20. Irwig, L., et al. Estimating an individual's true cholesterol level and response to intervention. *J.A.M.A.* 266:1678, 1991.
21. Grundy, S. M. Cholesterol and coronary heart disease: A new era. *J.A.M.A.* 256:2849, 1986.
22. Castelli, W. P., et al. HDL cholesterol and other lipids in coronary heart disease: The cooperative lipoprotein phenotyping study. *Circulation* 55:767, 1977.

23. McCunney, R. J. Fitness, heart disease and high-density lipoproteins: A look at the relationships. *Phys. Sports Med.* 15:67, 1987.

24. Seed, M., et al. Relation of serum lipoprotein(a) concentration and apolipoprotein(a) phenotype to coronary heart diseases in patients with familial hypercholesterolemia. *N. Engl. J. Med.* 322:1494, 1990.

25. Brown, G., et al. Regression of coronary artery disease as a result of intensive lipid-lowering therapy in men with high levels of apolipoprotein B. *N. Engl. J. Med.* 323:1289, 1990.

26. Wynder, E. L., Field, F., and Haley, N. J. Population screening for cholesterol determination. *J.A.M.A.* 256: 2839, 1986.

27. McCunney, R. J. The role of fitness in preventing heart disease. *Cardiovasc. Rev. Rep.* 6:776,1985.

28. Manson, J. E. The primary prevention of myocardial infarction. *N. Engl. J. Med.* 326:1409, 1992.

29. Harris, S. S., et al. Physical activity counseling for healthy adults as a primary preventive intervention in the clinical setting. *J.A.M.A.* 261:3590, 1989.

30. Powell, K. E., et al. The status of the 1990 objectives for physical fitness and exercise. *Public Health Rep.* 101:15, 1986.

31. McCunney, R. J. Are exercise programs needed prior to a fitness program? *Occup. Health Saf.* 53:23,1984.

32. Maciejko, J. J., et al. Apolipoprotein A-1 as a marker of angiographically assessed coronary artery disease. *N. Engl. J. Med.* 309:385, 1983.

33. American Heart Association. *Heart Facts.* Dallas: American Heart Association, 1986.

34. Davidson, D. M. Return to work after cardiac events: A review. *J. Cardiac Rehabil.* 3:60, 1983.

35. DeBusk, R. F., Blomguist, C. G., and Kouchoukos, N. T. Identification and treatment of low risk patients after acute myocardial infarction and coronary artery bypass graft surgery. *N. Engl. J. Med.* 314:161, 1986.

36. Franklin, B. A. Getting patients back to work after myocardial infarction or coronary artery bypass graft surgery. *Phys. Sports Med.* 14:183, 1986.

37. Rimm, A. A., et al. Changes in occupation after aorta coronary vein bypass operation. *J.A.M.A.* 236:361, 1976.

38. Walter, P. J. Return to work after coronary artery bypass surgery. *Eur. Heart J.* 9 (Suppl. L):61, 1988.

39. Barnes, G. K., et al. Changes in working status of patients following coronary bypass surgery. *J.A.M.A.* 238:1259, 1977.

40. Hacker, R. W., et al. Employment Status of Patients After Coronary Artery Bypass Surgery. In P. J. Walter (ed.), *Return to Work After Coronary Artery Bypass Surgery. Psychosocial and Economic Aspects.* Berlin: Springer, 1985.

41. Neill, W. A., Branch, L. G., and de Jong, G. Cardiac disability: The impact of coronary heart disease on patients' daily activities. *Arch. Intern. Med.* 145:1642, 1985.

42. Magni, G., et al. Psychosocial outcome one year after heart surgery: A prospective study. *Arch. Intern. Med.* 147:473 1987.

43. Cay, E. L., and Walker, D. D. Psychological factors and return to work. *Eur. Heart J.* 9 (Suppl. L):74, 1988.

44. DeBusk, R. F., and Dennis, C. A. "Submaximal" predischarge exercise testing after acute myocardial infarction: Who needs it? *Am. J. Cardiol.* 55:499, 1985.

45. American Heart Association. *Exercise Testing and Training of Apparently Healthy Individuals: A Handbook for Physicians.* Dallas: American Heart Association, 1972.

46. Fox, S. M., Naughton, J. P., and Haskell, W. L. Physical activity and the prevention of coronary heart disease. *Ann. Clin. Res.* 3:404, 1971.

47. Hellerstein, H. K., and Franklin, B. A. *Exercise Testing and Prescription in Rehabilitation of the Coronary Patient* (2nd ed.). New York: Wiley, 1984. Pp. 197–284.

48. Sheldahl, I. M., Wilke, N. A., and Tristani, F. E. Exercise prescription for return to work. *J. Cardiopulm. Rehabil.* 5:567,1985.

49. Squires, R. W. Cardiovascular rehabilitation: Status, 1990. *Mayo Clin. Proc.* 65:731, 1990.

50. Greenland, P., and Broidy, M. E. Rehabilitation of the MI survivor: Management options to maximize post hospital outcome. *Postgrad. Med.* 75:79, 1984.

51. Van Camp, S. P., and Peterson, R. A. Cardiovascular complications of outpatient cardiac rehabilitation programs. *J.A.M.A.* 256:1160,1986.

52. Hossack, K. F., and Hartwig, R. Cardiac arrest associated with supervised cardiac rehabilitation. *J. Cardiac Rehabil.* 2:402, 1982.

53. Ott, C. R., Sivarajan, E. S., and Newton, K. M. A controlled randomized study of

early cardiac rehabilitation: The sickness Impact Profile as an assessment tool. *Heart Lung* 12:162,1983.

54. Position report on cardiac rehabilitation. Recommendations of the American College of Cardiology. *J. Am. Coll. Cardiol.* 7:451, 1986.

55. Rosenman, K. D. Cardiovascular disease and environmental exposure. *Br. J. Ind. Med.* 36:85, 1979.

56. Fin, L. J. Occupational Heart Disease. In W. Rom (ed.), *Environmental and Occupational Medicine.* Boston: Little, Brown, 1983. Pp. 359–365.

57. Petronio, L. Chemical and physical agents of work-related cardiovascular diseases. *Eur. Heart J.* 9 (Suppl. L):26, 1988.

58. Goldsmith, J. R., and Aronow, W. S. Carbon monoxide and coronary heart disease: A review. *Environ. Res.* 10:236, 1975.

59. Leikin, J. B., et al. Methylene chloride: Report of five exposures and two deaths. *Am. J. Emerg. Med.* 8:534, 1990.

60. Speizer, F. E., Wegman, D. H., and Ramirez, A. Palpitation rates associated with fluorocarbon exposure in a hospital setting. *N. Engl. J. Med.* 292:624, 1975.

61. Davidson, M., and Feinleib, M. Carbon disulfide poisoning: A review. *Am. Heart J.* 83:100, 1972.

62. Egeland, G. M. Effects of exposure to carbon disulphide on low density lipoprotein cholesterol concentration and diastolic blood pressure. *Br. J. Ind. Med.* 49:287, 1992.

63. Hogstedt, C., and Axelson, O. Nitroglycerine-nitroglycol exposure and the mortality in cardiocerebrovascular diseases among dynamite workers. *J.O.M.* 19:675, 1977.

64. Stayner, L. T., et al. Cardiovascular mortality among munitions workers exposed to nitroglycerine and dinitrotoluene. *Scand. J. Work Environ. Health* 18:34, 1992.

Further Information

DeBusk, R. F., et al. Identification and treatment of low risk patients after acute myocardial infarction and coronary artery bypass graft surgery. *N. Engl. J. Med.* 314:161,1986.
An excellent review of factors involved in determining the prognosis of people who have suffered MIs or who have undergone CABG surgery.

Eur. Heart J. 9 (Suppl. L), 1988.
An extremely informative issue devoted entirely to occupational cardiovascular disease. This issue includes a review article on chemical and physical agents of work-related cardiovascular disease.

Fielding, J. E. Smoking control at the workplace. *Annu. Rev. Public Health* 12:209, 1991.
An excellent review of worksite smoking control issues.

J.A.M.A. 264(23), 1990.
The entire issue is devoted to cholesterol, and includes original articles and two review articles on lipoproteins and atherosclerosis, and the role of cholesterol in coronary heart disease.

National Cholesterol Education Program Report of the Expert Panel on Population Strategies for Blood Cholesterol Reduction. US Department of Health and Human Services, November 1990.
A well-written and heavily referenced document (over 600 references) that represents the consensus view on cholesterol reduction.

Olson, R. E. Mass intervention vs. screening and selective intervention for the prevention of coronary heart disease. *J.A.M.A.* 255:2204,1986.
A review of the major studies (Lipid Research Clinics, MRFIT, Framingham) regarding the role of dietary factors and serum cholesterol in the development of CHD.

Rosenman, K. Cardiovascular disease and environmental exposure. *Br. J. Ind. Med.* 36:85, 1979.
A thorough review of the major studies that have investigated occupational cardiovascular hazards.

Neurotoxic Disorders

Robert G. Feldman and
Chang-Ming Chern

As with most occupational illnesses, the clinician is often the first to be consulted in the evaluation of a neurologic disorder that may be related to exposure to an environmental or occupational hazard. Although neurologic dysfunction secondary to toxic substances often results in typical histologic patterns, the clinical manifestations generally resemble those of primary neurologic disorders. Thus, the clinician needs to know (1) how a hazardous substance may contribute to a neurologic disorder and (2) how to evaluate whether exposure to a hazardous material has damaged the nervous system.

The clinician needs to be aware that literally thousands of new commercial substances are introduced into the economy each year. Barely 25% of currently used substances have been tested in some capacity regarding their toxicity. Thus, one needs to be aware of potential neurotoxic effects secondary to the production and use of certain materials.

Extensive educational efforts directed toward the toxic manifestations of a variety of substances have increased awareness among not only workers but also the general public. People know that insecticides and cleaning fluids can be harmful. They often present to their clinician concerned about whether damage to their health has occurred. This chapter addresses these issues, by describing acknowledged manifestations of neurotoxicity, citing the use and interpretation of diagnostic studies, and suggesting guidelines for the clinician about the need for specialty evaluation.

The clinician should evaluate whether certain symptoms may be manifestations of a neurotoxin before diagnosing a primary neurologic condition. Ataxia and tremor similar to that seen in degenerative diseases of the cerebellum (Friedreich's ataxia) can result from exposure to toluene, mercury, and acrylamide. Spinal cord lesions, such as those seen in neurosyphilis, vitamin B_{12} deficiency, and multiple sclerosis (in which the posterior columns are affected) can be caused by triorthocresylphosphate poisoning. Spasticity, impotence, and urinary retention, commonly associated with a diagnosis of multiple sclerosis, have been seen following leptophos poisoning or exposure to diethylaminopropionitrile.

Parkinson's disease, a disturbance of posture with rigidity and tremor, may actually be the result of the toxic effects on the substantia nigra and striatal structures from exposure to carbon monoxide, carbon disulfide, manganese, or n-methyl-4-phenyltetrahydropyridine (MPTP).

Accurate differential diagnosis requires analysis of the work history as well as a complete neurologic examination. Exposure information concerning neurotoxic substances is necessary when trying to identify possible causative agents. Toxicologic information from human and animal investigations can help the clinician recognize early manifestations of some neurotoxic disorders. With a good occupational and environmental history and a high degree of suspicion, a patient with neurologic symptoms may not only be recognized correctly as a victim of neurotoxicity but also serve as a sentinel case pointing to a hazard in the workplace for other individuals who may have similar exposures.

The *critical effect* is defined as an observable biologic disturbance that occurs as the first manifestation of a toxic effect of a given substance. The *critical organ* is the body part that is the first to manifest the effects of toxicity. Standards of acceptable exposure are determined by ascertaining the critical effect on the critical organ and associating it with determined levels of the neurotoxic substance in blood, urine, or the environment. Although a clinical diagnosis of neurotoxicity can be made based on symptoms and objective neurologic findings, confirmation of neurologic dysfunction should be obtained by physiologic, neuropsychological, and chemical means.

Documentation of the presence of a suspected toxin in the environment in which the subject may have been exposed is of utmost importance. The coexistence of underlying systemic disease, diabetes, and a history of previous exposures may influence the response of an organism to a neurotoxic substance. Indeed, the mere presence of a substance known to be capable of producing neurotoxic effects does *not* mean that each exposed individual will develop these reactions. Individual susceptibility and duration and intensity of exposure are the major factors involved in the development of neurotoxic effect.

Neurotoxicity is the adverse effect of a given substance on the functioning of the basic elements of the nervous system or its supportive structures. Clinical manifestations of neurotoxic effects depend on the region of the nervous system that is affected. Central nervous system effects occur when a toxin reaches neuronal systems, after passing the blood-brain barrier. Other substances cause toxic effects that are limited to the peripheral nervous system because the blood-brain barrier prevents access of certain chemical molecules to the neuron, its cell membrane, or subcellular organelles. Altered structures and function of cell membranes, myelin coverings, or intraneuronal cytoplasm result in failure of normal performance and interference with the initiation and transmission of nerve impulses. The clinical features of disturbed neurologic function, however, may resemble those common neurologic syndromes.

Peripheral Nervous System and Toxic Effects

Neurologic effects of toxic exposure may be direct or indirect, reversible or irreversible, depending on the specific substance, the nature and duration of exposure, and the selective vulnerability of the particular elements of the peripheral and central nervous systems. Neurologic dysfunctions such as motor weakness, sensory loss, or altered mental status result from damage to specialized neurons of the brain, spinal cord, and peripheral nerves. Clinical manifestations are *determined by the site of neurotoxicity*. The peripheral nervous system consists of nerve cell bodies located in the spinal cord. Peripheral axons extend distally and follow a predictable distribution to the extremities, which facilitates a diagnosis directed to a particular anatomic site.

Motor fibers originate in large neurons in the anterior gray matter of the cord and join other fibers to form the ventral root. Sensory fibers originate in the unipolar cells of the dorsal root ganglia. Information from the extremities is brought to the dorsal root ganglia by the afferent fibers of these sensory nerves. The sensory fibers and the ventral root fibers of the motor neurons travel together to skeletal muscles and skin as *bundles* of nerve fibers. The diameter of various nerve fibers is dependent on the quantity of myelin that covers them. The largest fibers convey impulses most rapidly; the smaller fibers, which contain less myelin, conduct more slowly. The smallest group of fibers, however, conduct impulses most slowly and are considered "unmyelinated" fibers. Nerve fibers are held together in bundles by connective tissue and are supplied by blood vessels with nutrients. The autonomic nervous system is distributed to smooth muscle, including that of blood vessels and glands throughout the body.

Disorders of Peripheral Nerves

Disorders of peripheral nerves are manifested clinically by a decrease in the ability to perceive sensation, spontaneous sensations (tingling), and painful sensations (dysesthesiae). Reflex activity, such that follows tapping a knee tendon or ankle tendon, occurs when the nerve fibers are able to conduct an impulse from the periphery to the spinal cord and back to the antagonist muscle group. Interruption in function of this pathway eliminates the reflex response and is a sign of peripheral nerve disorder.

When a widespread and bilateral peripheral nerve process results from toxic causes, the condition is referred to as *polyneuropathy*. The deficits in function may be motor, sensory, sensory-motor, or autonomic; they may be proximal, distal, or generalized in distribution. When the small thinly myelinated and unmyelinated fibers are affected, the condition is referred to as *small-fiber neuropathy*. In this condition, there is relative preservation of motor power and sensory functions of touch-pressure, vibration, and joint sensation, since these functions are carried by larger *myelinated* fibers. Sensations of pain and temperature are usually lost in small-fiber neuropathy.

In *large-fiber neuropathy,* there is weakness as well as loss of sensation of position, vibration, and touch-pressure. Toxic damage to myelin results in large-fiber neuropathy. When the toxic substance primarily affects the *axon,* conduction velocity may be less affected than is the *amplitude* of the response because the ability to conduct is preserved in the unaffected fibers. Damage to the myelin may be incomplete, and recovery may ensue when exposure is stopped. Destruction of the nerve cell or axon, however, results in *irreversible* deficits in function.

Electrodiagnostic Studies of Peripheral Nerve Function

Electrodiagnostic studies are used to evaluate peripheral nerve function. Measures of peripheral nerve conduction velocity depend on the ability of sufficient nerve fibers to conduct a stimulus applied to the nerve through the skin. Electrically, the fastest firing fibers (those with the most myelin) determine the measurable conduction velocity and response to a supramaximal stimulus. In moderately affected fibers, the conduction velocity is decreased; in severely affected fibers, a full block of conduction occurs. If conduction is completely blocked, no information is transmitted beyond the site of demyelination. Although remyelination of damaged peripheral nerve fibers can occur, recovery of nerve conduction is usually associated with decreased conduction velocities. Incomplete remyelination of some fibers may in turn account for abnormal clinical function such as weakness and abnormal sensation.

Modern electronic equipment has provided a way to study physiologic function of the peripheral nervous system. The conduction characteristics of a nerve fiber are determined by the nerve cell body and axons, its axoplasm, and its myelin covering. Transcutaneous electrical stimulation of a particular nerve can result in contraction of the muscle to which it conducts the induced impulses. The twitch of the responding muscle can be recorded by electrodes attached to the skin over the muscle or by inserting a recording needle electrode into the muscle belly. The muscle action response is conveyed by wires from the electrodes to an amplifier system and then, as an electrical potential, is displayed on a screen or printed out by a permanent recording device. By stimulating a nerve at two places (A and B) along its course, *the latency* (time between stimulus and response) can be determined between the points of applied stimuli and the muscle belly from which the twitch response is recorded. By subtracting the latency measured from point A (distal) from the latency measured from point B (proximal), the difference in latencies, expressed in milliseconds, is determined. The number (the difference in latencies) is divided into the distance between points A and B, expressed in millimeters, to calculate the motor nerve conduction velocity, expressed as meters per second.

Similar measurements of conduction velocity can be made for nerve fibers that conduct sensory information (sensory nerve conduction velocity). To measure *sensory conduction,* the distal portion of a nerve is stimulated transcutaneously, and then the evoked potential at a proximal site of the same nerve is recorded.

It is essential that standardized procedures be used in all studies of peripheral nerve conduction. Although many studies in the occupational medical and epidemiologic literature have not followed the strictest conventions, recent work reflects efforts to use standardized techniques so that interstudy comparisons can be made. The reader is referred to current textbooks of electromyography for appropriate methodology and use of control values.

Central Nervous System and Neurotoxic Effects

Central nervous system manifestations of neurotoxicity vary depending on different neurotoxicants and conditions of exposure such as concentration of the toxicants and duration and route of exposure. Acute exposure may cause drowsiness, somnolence, dizziness, or loss of consciousness, resulting from neurodepression. However, in acute organic solvent exposure, these are preceded by neurostimulation with euphoria, lack of inhibition, interrupted speech, and unsteady walking in a preliminary phase.

Vivid and pleasant hallucinations may occur in case of massive exposure. The neurostimulation phase lasts a few minutes to 1 or 2 hours. If exposure continues, it leads to the phase of clinical neurodepression. Exposure to high concentrations of organic solvent vapors in closed and poorly ventilated locations leads to simple asphyxia. The resulting anoxia can cause death in a few minutes [1]. Chronic low-dose exposures can lead to behavioral or cognitive dysfunction. Different neurotoxicants may have predilection for different parts of the central nervous system. Damage to Purkinje cells of the cerebellum results in ataxia; destruction of the neurons of the substantia nigra results in changes in *postural* activities. Spinal cord neurons and pathways, components of the central nervous system, are vulnerable to toxic insults that result in motor and sensory dysfunctions. *Indirect effects* on the central nervous system occur as a result of changes in the cerebral vasculature. Acute convulsions might even take place.

The term *myeloencephalopathy* refers to a disturbance of function of the entire brain and spinal cord. *Encephalopathy* is the term used to describe disturbances of function of the brain itself. The exact localization of damage, however, whether it is cerebral cortex, basal ganglia, limbic system, or white matter, is usually not specified. The *clinical manifestations* of the encephalopathies include disturbances of memory, behavior, problem solving, orientation, and attentiveness, and, at times, psychotic-like behavior. The terms *psychoorganic syndrome* and *neurasthenia* have been applied to toxic encephalopathies, which often result in fatigue, affect lability, depression, and memory disturbances. Subtle changes in mental function due to intoxication often go unrecognized unless sophisticated neuropsychological test batteries are employed [2–4].

Tests of Neurobehavioral Effects of Neurotoxicity

When a patient is suspected of experiencing central nervous system toxicity to agents such as solvents or heavy metals, neuropsychiatric testing can aid in the diagnosis. Many of these symptoms may be nonspecific and difficult to differentiate from those of functional or more benign disorders. By referring the patient to a professional appropriately trained in the administration of these tests, valuable information about memory, fine motor skills, and reasoning ability can be obtained. This can be very helpful in some clinical conditions. For instance, neuropsychological tests have been successfully applied in the differential diagnosis of senile dementia and chronic solvent encephalopathy in older workers [5]

The application of formal neuropsychological testing in assessing effects of subtle neurotoxicity offers a number of advantages. Specific, standardized rules for administering and scoring these tests exist. Results can be analyzed in terms of published "normative" scores based on age, sex, and education. These tests have been validated and found reliable in both research and clinical settings, allowing clear interpretation of results by independent neuropsychologists. Batteries of tests can be designed for clinical diagnosis of encephalopathy in individual patients and for screening large groups of workers. Skill areas assessed by these tests include attention (including vigilance, as well as ability to hold and manipulate information), motor skills and reaction time, concept formation (reasoning), language, visuospatial abilities, and mood and personality.

The most commonly used criterion for inclusion of a test in a battery is its confirmed sensitivity to particular neurotoxins. Since the mean differences between data obtained from the studies of exposed and nonexposed groups in research populations may be quite small, they may not always be applicable to the study of individual patients. In clinical situations, it is generally more appropriate to select neuropsychological tests that will assess as many functions as possible [4]. The battery is designed to cover a wide area of functions and to deal with as many manifestations of neurotoxic encephalopathy as possible (Table 15-1).

Perhaps the most difficult situation arises with respect to estimating the severity of past exposure. Evaluation of deficits often occurs at a time when body burden of the suspected substance is no longer elevated or environmental levels can no longer be ascertained. Obtaining an occupational/environmental history to estimate the extent of exposure (duration and intensity) is of the utmost importance. Essential to this inquiry are questions about the patient's current and previous occupations, job tasks, places of residence and employment, and hobbies.

Table 15-1. Neuropsychological test battery

Test	Description	Function
1. Wechsler Adult Intelligence Scale, Wechsler Adult Intelligence Scale—Revised		
Information	Questions of an academic nature	Basic academic verbal skills
Digit span	Digits forward and backward	Attention
Vocabulary*	Word definitions	Verbal concept formation
Arithmetic	Oral calculations	Attention, calculation
Comprehension	Questions involving problem solving, judgment, social knowledge, proverb interpretation	Verbal concept formation
Similarities*	Deduction of similarities between nouns	Verbal concept formation
Picture completion	Identification of missing parts of pictures	Visuospatial (analysis)
Picture arrangement	Sequencing pictures to tell a story	Sequencing, visuospatial (reasoning)
Block design*	Replicating designs of red and white blocks	Visuospatial (organization)
Object assembly	Puzzle assembly	Visuospatial (organization)
Digit symbol* (with incidental learning task)	Coding	Motor speed (visual short-term memory)
2. Wechsler Memory Scale, Wechsler Memory Scale—Revised		
Information	Personal information and political names	
Orientation	Time and place	
Mental control	Count backwards 20–1, recite alphabet, count by 3s beginning with 1	Cognitive tracking, attention
Digit span*	Digits forward and backward	Attention
Visual spans	Pointing span on visual array	Attention (visual)
Logical memories with delayed recall	Recall of narrative material presented in two paragraphs	Verbal memory acquisition, retention
Visual reproductions with delayed recall*	Drawing visual designs from immediate recall	Visual memory acquisition, retention
Verbal paired associates	Learning of 10 paired associates	Verbal memory acquisition, retention
Visual paired associates	Recognition memory for colors paired with designs	Visual memory
Figural memory	Multiple-choice memory for visual designs	Visual memory
3. Continuous Performance Testing*	Subject sees rapidly presented letters, must press button when X appears	Attention, reaction time
4. Trails	Connecting numbered dots, then alternating between numbered and lettered dots	Attention, tracking, sequencing

(continued)

Table 15-1 (continued)

Test	Description	Function
5. Wisconsin Card Sorting Test	Categorical sorting of cards	Concept formation
6. FAS—Verbal Fluency	Production of words with F, A, and S in one minute each	Language (fluency)
7. Boston Naming Test	Naming objects depicted in line drawings	Language
8. Reading Comprehension Subtest, Boston Diagnostic Aphasia Examination	Screening test of reading comprehension	Language (reading)
9. Wide Range Achievement Test	Reading, spelling, arithmetic	Basic academic skills
10. Boston Visuospatial Quantitative Battery	Drawing objects spontaneously and to copy clocks, US map locations	Visuospatial
11. Santa Ana Form Board Test	Turn pegs 90 degrees with each hand separately and with both hands	Motor speed
12. Milner Facial Recognition Test	Matching and remembering similar unknown faces	Visual memory, visuospatial (analysis)
13. Benton Visual Retention Test*	Multiple choice recall of visual designs	Visual memory
14. Difficult Paired Learning	10 paired associates low in associative value	Verbal memory
15. Albert's Famous Faces Test	Recall of famous faces from past decades	Retrograde memory
16. Profile of Mood States*	Mood testing on six dimensions: anger, vigor, tension, depression, fatigue, confusion	Affect
17. Minnesota Multiphasic Personality Inventory, MMPI-R	Personality test	Personality, affect
18. Interview	Extensive clinical interview re medical and cognitive symptoms, psychiatric symptoms, personal background, and work and educational history	

*Test included in lead battery.
Source: From R. F. White, R. G. Feldman, and P. H. Travers. Neurobehavioral effects of toxicity due to metals, solvents, and insecticides. *Clin. Neuropharmacol.* 13:392, 1990.

Clinical Evaluation of Neurotoxic Symptoms

The diagnosis of a neurotoxic disorder should be considered if a person exposed to a hazardous material experiences symptoms reflective of the agent's toxicity. Review of neurologic systems may suggest disturbances of memory, mood, or peripheral symptoms of abnormal sensation or strength. An analytic approach to the diagnosis of occupationally related neurotoxic syndrome has been suggested by Juntunen [6] (Table 15-2). Clinical, neurophysiologic, and psychological data for each patient suspected of having neurotoxic disease will aid in the confirmation of the disorder [7].

Evidence of exposure should be obtained, including the toxin levels in the environment of exposure and the toxin or its metabolites, or both, in various biologic media, such as blood or urine. Exhaled breath, hair, and nails may also serve as biologic indicators of exposure in certain instances. Oftentimes the environmental data are not available or the levels in certain tissues are not increased simply because the patients have already been removed from exposures due to health problems or retirement. In these conditions, exposure surrogates, such as previous job title at the exposure site, can be used in conjunction with current industrial hygiene data to assess the previous exposure status.

One should inquire whether similar disturbances of functions in other exposed individuals have occurred and whether the neurologic findings noted are similar to those that have been reported in relation to the agent of concern. The source of toxin, its molecular form, route of entry, and dose of exposure all determine the acuteness and severity of symptoms. Before forming a final opinion regarding the presence of a neurotoxic disorder, however, the clinician should be aware that such illnesses are generally considered only when acknowledged causes of the symptom complex are eliminated. Since patients present with symptoms, rather than diagnostic labels, it is helpful to consider occupationally related disease and neurotoxic effects from a symptomatic approach.

Headache

Headache, a common neurologic complaint, arises from distention, traction, or irritation of intracranial pain-sensitive structures, such as medium- to large-sized blood vessels, dura, falx, meninges, and mucous membranes of the sinuses. Increased intracranial pressure, elevated blood pressure, or chemical irritation of the mem-

Table 15-2. Diagnostic criteria for identifying neurotoxic effects

1. Verified quantitative and qualitative *presence of suspected substance* in the environment
2. Verified quantitative and *qualitative exposure* of the subject(s) to the suspected substance
3. Presence of *clinical manifestations* of central and/or peripheral nervous system dysfunction:
   a. "Typical" subjective symptoms
   b. Pathologic findings in one or more of the following:
      1. Clinical examination
      2. Electroencephalogram
      3. Electromyography
      4. Nerve conduction studies
      5. Evoked potentials and reflex studies
      6. Neuropsychological tests
      7. Computed axial tomography and/or magnetic resonance imaging
      8. Tissue content of toxin (biopsy)
4. *Exclusion of other neuropathologic conditions* attributed to nontoxic causes to explain clinical manifestations (in item 3), including primary psychiatric and/or sociopathic disorders

Source: Modified from J. Juntunen. Alcoholism in occupational neurology: Diagnostic difficulties with special reference to the neurological syndromes caused by exposure to organic solvents. *Acta Neurol. Scand.* 66 (Suppl. 92):89, 1982.

branes can cause headache. In some instances, headache results from brain swelling (tin, lead), while in others, transient hypoxia or vasodilatation may account for the pain that is experienced. Despite the vagueness of this symptom, the differential diagnosis of headache must include the effects of exposures to noxious substances. For example, headache can occur following exposure to zinc, tellurium, tin, manganese, lead, cadmium, and aluminum [8]. Solvents and other aromatic hydrocarbons, propellants, insecticides, and herbicides can also cause headaches on acute exposure as a result of irritation of mucous membranes of the nasopharynx and vasodilatation of intracranial vasculature. Headaches can also be due to inhalation of metal dust or fumes.

Chronic Toxic Encephalopathy

Chronic low-dose exposure to a variety of neurotoxicants can be associated with behavioral disturbances, mood changes, and a variety of cognitive dysfunctions, which are all indications of encephalopathy. These symptoms may also be present as sequelae after acute exposure. In addition, they are not specific to toxic encephalopathy, and other conditions, such as degenerative or metabolic encephalopathy, must be carefully excluded.

Lead

Overt manifestations of lead-related encephalopathy include ataxia, confusion, convulsions, fatigue, and mood changes [9]. As cases of severe acute lead intoxication become less frequent, increasing attention has been focused on the "subclinical" manifestations of lead exposure. Exposure to inorganic lead has resulted in characteristic changes in behavior and cognitive functioning in patients with blood lead levels less than 70 μg/100 ml. As lead levels rise about 40 μg/100 ml, short-term verbal memory skills have been found to be consistently impaired [8]. The Occupational Safety and Health Administration (OSHA) lead standard requires that workers receive a medical evaluation at a blood level of 40 μg/100 ml. Studies of subclinical and asymptomatic lead poisonings have shown that workers with blood lead levels in the range of 40 to 60 μg/ml not only show neurologic abnormalities but also have symptoms when asked [10]. Although studies of adults with blood lead levels greater than 90 μg/100 ml have shown inconsistent results, available evidence suggests that lead exposure in this range can lead to impairment in affect, attention, psychomotor function, verbal concept formation, short-term memory, and visuospatial abilities [2, 9–13]. Mood disorders resulting in apathy, irritability, and diminished ability to control anger are apparently common. The details of neuropsychological testing in the diagnosis of various toxic conditions have recently been reviewed [4].

Arsenic

Acute or chronic exposure has been linked with specific neurobehavioral effects, especially affective and cognitive impairment. Frank psychosis with vivid auditory and visual hallucination has been reported [14]. In addition, a symptom complex of malaise, emotional lability, insomnia, and depression have been identified in patients with arsenic poisoning. Other reported cases showed less specific complaints such as weakness, dizziness, fatigue, and progressive anxiety along with nausea, vomiting, diarrhea, and hot flashes [15–17]. Recently, with the availability of neuropsychological tests, more cases of subtle cognitive disturbances, such as recent memory impairment or concentration deficits, are more frequently recognized [18].

Manganese

Of the neurotoxic effects of metals, manganese is especially known for its acute behavioral manifestations. Neurotoxicity of manganese was recognized after manganese miners developed irritability, nervousness, and emotional lability. Some experienced visual and auditory hallucinations, whereas others had compulsive, repetitive, and uncontrollable actions. In fact, this initial phase of agitation in workers exposed to manganese ore was described as "manganese madness" [19–21], which heralded the prodromal phase of chronic manganese poisoning. Following or concomitant with these symptoms, signs suggesting a disturbance in basal ganglia also appeared. This intermediate phase of poisoning is further discussed in the section on neurotoxic parkinsonism. The final established phase exhibits muscular rigidity, fine tremors, and cock walk. Spasmodic laughter and excessive sweating also are reported in some patients [22].

Mercury

Mercury poisoning can occur from either inorganic or organic mercury. Signs and symptoms vary by type of mercury or mercurial compound and by type of exposure (acute or chronic). Chronic exposure to organic mercury can produce tremor, paresthesias (tingling sensations), dysarthria (slurred speech), ataxia, decreased visual fields, and mental disturbances [23]. The most notorious epidemics were those that occurred in Minamata and Niigata, Japan, in the 1950s [24]. The classic triad of chronic inorganic mercury poisoning includes tremor, psychological instability, and stomatitis [23].

Organic Solvents

Because most organic solvents contain mixtures of ingredients, it is difficult to attribute specific behavioral changes to a specific substance. When the predominant ingredient in a mixed solvent preparation is toluene, however, the principal health effect appears to be a reduction in performance associated with fatigue and dizziness even at relatively low levels of exposure. In situations involving high levels of exposure to toluene, excitatory effects such as euphoria, exhilaration, and excitement have resulted. Since the inhaled vapors usually induce a temporary euphoria, the substance has been abused; in fact, addition can result and lead to serious damage to the nervous system [25].

A broad range of psychological effects due to solvents has been reported by Hanninen and colleagues [26, 27]. These changes were noted by neuropsychological testing; workers exposed to carbon disulfide showed disturbances in speech, psychomotor functioning, dexterity, and alertness. In turn, most investigations of the effects of carbon disulfide have focused on these functions. "Pseudoneurasthenic" difficulties, including changes in mood or personality; excessive irritability; increased physical complaints such as headache, dizziness, weakness, and fatigue; and memory loss, have also been related to carbon disulfide exposure [28]. These complaints usually *precede the onset of more obvious neurologic involvements* such as postural changes and peripheral neuropathy. Frequently, depressive symptoms are presented.

Typical manifestations of *trichloroethylene* include visual disturbances, mental confusion, fatigue, and impaired concentration, which can occur secondary to acute, chronic, or subacute exposure. Decrements in manual dexterity, complex reaction time, and memory have been reported in volunteers exposed to an average trichloroethylene vapor concentration of 110 parts per million (ppm). (The current Threshold Limit Value for trichloroethylene is 50 ppm [29]).

The residual effects of a previous exposure to trichloroethylene intoxication have been reported in a carburetor cleaner [30]. The patient was seen acutely at the time of the accident and followed for 18 years after the exposure. Persistent difficulties in attempts to solve multiple-step problems and make business decisions have been observed throughout this time. Moreover, there is evidence of moderate depression on the Minnesota Multiphasic Personality Inventory as well as attentional, visuospatial, and short-term memory deficits. Neuropsychological testing in other patients after exposure to trichloroethylene has revealed memory deficits that were especially pronounced when comparing immediate recall of new information to delayed recall on both visual and verbal tasks. Recall of visual designs (Visual Reproduction Subtests, Wechsler Memory Scale), narrative material presented in two paragraphs (Logical Memory Subtest, Wechsler Memory Scale), and difficult paired associates was consistently impaired. Less consistent memory deficits were observed in delayed recall under multiple-choice conditions of faces (Milner Facial Recognition Test) and a simpler paired associate learning test (Wechsler Memory Scale Subtest). Moderate to severe visuospatial deficits were frequently seen in these patients, as evidenced by the performance subtests of the Wechsler Adult Intelligence Scale. Visual construction tasks involving puzzles, block designs, and sequencing of stories (object assembly, picture arrangement, and block design subtests of the Wechsler Adult Intelligence Scale–Revised) were especially affected.

Trichloroethylene can also lead to acute encephalopathy in settings with airborne levels of less than 50 ppm (current Threshold Limit Value). A worker in a machine shop who continually dipped his hands into trichloroethylene used as a degreaser experienced paranoia, behavioral changes, and memory deficits, documented by neuropsychiatric testing [31]. Improved work habits led to resolution of the symptoms.

Conclusions about neurobehavioral effects of solvents are difficult to draw. Caution must be used in the generalization of results from epidemiologic studies, since exact exposure levels and knowledge of other concomitant exposures are not always known. As a result, it may be difficult to identify one single causative agent. Many solvents and mixtures are commonly used in the workplace. Exposures to mixed solvents are a particularly common occupational hazard. Extensive studies of Scandinavian workers exposed to mixed solvents, including paints, degreasing fluids, and dry-cleaning fluids, suggest the potential for the development of neurotoxic disorders that appear to be related to the level and degree of exposure. Finnish investigators have extensively assessed neuropsychological functioning in subjects with chronic exposure to solvents. Although findings vary somewhat among study samples [32–35], the results consistently suggest that chronic solvent exposure can be associated with cognitive changes on tests of reasoning, visual constructive abilities, short-term memory, motor coordination and speed, and attention. Exposure to paints, carbon disulfide, and mixed solvents has been found to affect a particularly large number of cognitive abilities [34]. Impairment in reaction times, motor abilities, and short-term memories (but not reasoning or spatial skills) was reported in Swedish painters [36]. Scandinavian investigators have consistently identified psychiatric disorders of mood and behavior secondary to work with solvents [37, 38]. These encephalopathic changes have been attributed to solvent-induced diffuse brain damage [33]. Damage to central white matter and/or supportive structures is suspected.

Organophosphate Insecticides

Organophosphate insecticides alter nervous system function by affecting the availability of acetylcholine. Acute agitation, impaired vigilance and memory, reduced concentration, slowed psychomotor speed and information processing, linguistic disturbances, anxiety, and depression can be due to organophosphate insecticides [39]. Numerous case reports suggest the possibility of *persistent psychiatric symptoms following acute intoxication*. Common complaints include impaired concentration, emotional outbursts, anxiety, headaches, irritability, and memory difficulties [40–42].

Neurotoxic Parkinsonism

Parkinsonism may develop following exposure to certain neurotoxicants, namely, carbon monoxide, carbon disulfide, manganese, and MPTP. Another agent, beta-N-methylamino-L-alanine (BMAA), has been suggested as the underlying cause for parkinsonism–amyotrophic lateral sclerosis (ALS)–dementia complex in Guam [43]. The parkinsonian features of these disorders, such as bradykinesia, cogwheel rigidity, shuffling gaits, tremor, and poor postural reflexes, closely resemble those of idiopathic Parkinson's disease. This has led to the suspicion that Parkinson's disease or parkinsonism may be caused by environmental agents [44–46]. However, they have different neuropathologic changes. The major neuropathologic loci responsible for their parkinsonian features are globus pallidus for carbon monoxide, striatum pallidum for manganese, pallidonigral degeneration for carbon disulfide, and substantia nigra for MPTP; that is, except for MPTP intoxication, the output structures of the basal ganglia (i.e., the striatum and globus pallidus), rather than the substantia nigra, are predominantly affected [44]. In addition, Lewy body, typical of idiopathic Parkinson's disease, cannot be found in these patients, unless a patient with Parkinson's disease has these superimposed exposures. Patients with MPTP-induced parkinsonism respond to the full array of antiparkinsonian agents in a manner quite analogous to that seen in Parkinson's disease, including the side effects of the antiparkinsonian medications, whereas patients with other exposures do not [44]. Positron emission tomography (PET) scan has been used successfully to differentiate parkinsonism caused by manganese exposure and the idiopathic Parkinson's disease [47].

Peripheral Neuropathy

Numbness, tingling, weakness, and reduced reflexes are indicators of peripheral neuropathy. LeQuesne [48] pointed out the importance of understanding the pathophysiology of a suspected toxic effect when reviewing clinical neuropathies. In neuropathy caused by n-*hexane* and *methyl* n-*butyl ketone,* for example, motor *nerve conduction velocity is usually reduced,* but in some cases, it may be perfectly normal. Neurotoxic damage from hexacarbon solvents usually causes *axonal degeneration,* but sufficient secondary changes in the myelin may explain an overall reduction in conduction velocity (if not frank decreases). In acrylamide neuropathy, motor nerve conduction velocity may also be either normal or show little change. Similarly, sensory nerve *action potentials* may be normal, but reduced in amplitude. Although acrylamide has a selective destructive action on large-diameter fibers, and, thus, conduction velocity is not affected either. In triorthocresylphosphate (TOCP) neuropathy in baboons, reduced amplitude of muscle action potential is noted without apparent effect on conduction velocity. The appropriate electrophysiologic technique should be selected in order that the specific evidence needed to confirm a diagnosis in an individual patient can be obtained. *Speed of conduction is affected in demyelinating neuropathies,* while amplitude of the nerve *action potential is the essential* in ascertaining *presence of axonal neuropathies.*

Lead
The characteristic "wrist drop" has been considered pathognomonic of the diagnosis of lead poisoning. Recent studies of probable adult lead neuropathy describe progressive generalized weakness, mild distal atrophy, reflex loss, and occasional fasciculation. Lower limb weakness is prominent in childhood cases [49]. Subclinical diagnoses, however, have been detected in lead workers exposed for 5 to 13 years when their electrophysiologic characteristics were studied. Catton and associates [50] found no differences in the maximal velocity of motor fibers but noted a smaller amplitude of the patellar reflex in lead workers compared to controls. *In lead intoxication, motor nerve conduction velocity is affected more than sensory nerve conduction velocity* because the toxic effect involves segmental demyelination and remyelination [51]. When axonal changes occur as a later response, the slower fibers will then be affected.

Triebig and colleagues [52] correlated nerve conduction velocity to blood lead measures at levels of about 70 mg/100 ml. In contrast, lead foundry workers with blood levels of 90 mg or less had normal motor conduction velocity in the ulnar and peroneal nerves [9]. Amplitude of the ulnar motor response and sural sensory evoked potential, however, was reduced. Modest slowing of sensory conduction was also recorded. These peripheral nerve system effects of lead exposure are similar to those of other studies, which suggests that compared to control groups, people with high levels of lead exposure have slower nerve conduction velocities. It is unclear whether such decreases, noted on electrophysiologic testing, have clinical manifestations or increase the risk for permanent neurologic damage.

Arsenic
Most patients with arsenic neuropathy have mixed sensorimotor polyneuropathy [53]. However, sensory nerves are often involved earlier and to a greater extent; thus, the use of sensory nerve conduction velocity determinations can be more helpful than the motor conduction velocities [54]. A study of arsenic smelter workers [55] demonstrated more peripheral neuropathy than among nonarsenic workers; in fact, clinical neuropathy demonstrated by electrophysiologic methods was correlated with tissue levels of the toxic agent. The results of that study pointed out that nerve conduction velocity values should not be relied on entirely to diagnose a peripheral neuropathy. Accurate assessment depends also on a more detailed analysis of all data, including clinical findings and tissue levels, as well as electrophysiologic measurements. For all nerves tested ($n = 109$), with the exception of the sural amplitude, the lowest values were always found in the arsenic groups. Another study of smelter workers (47 copper workers) exposed to airborne arsenic for 8 to 40 years showed only minor neurologic abnormalities [56]. Significant differences were detected between exposed persons and the reference subjects when the data from all nerves were included in a statistical evaluation. Similar studies were done in a population in which arsenic had been found in concentrations ranging from 1 to 4781 µg/liter in well water [57]. Of 147 persons examined, only 6 had symptoms of physical findings compatible with mild sensory peripheral neuropathy. Two of the 6 had diabetes. In this study, none of the conduction velocities were slowed. The authors suggested that conduction velocity findings were insensitive in screening for subclinical neuropathy in persons exposed to inorganic arsenic.

Solvents

Symmetric polyneuropathy in humans exposed to toxic amounts of n-hexane and methyl n-butyl ketone has been found in the selective accumulation of neurofilaments in the distal axons. Similar accumulations of neurofilaments occur from intoxication by iminodipropionitrile (IDPN), acrylamide, and carbon disulfide [58, 59]. These chemicals also have the ability to produce central-peripheral distal axonopathy, in which there is swelling of the axon at the area of the node of Ranvier, subsequent distention of paranodal myelin, and eventual myelin retraction, which causes widening of the nodal distance between the myelin segments [60]. Conduction of nerve impulses is delayed or cannot occur when this paranodal area is demyelinated [61]. Motor and sensory conduction velocity in central peripheral axonopathy is slowed because of the secondary changes in myelin. Amplitude of sensory evoked responses in an affected nerve will be reduced because of damage to axons [62]. The long fibers of the low extremities show earlier slowing than the upper extremities because of the larger number of internodal segments that are vulnerable to the toxic effect, as well as the greater distance from the nerve cell body to the distal portion of the nerve.

Cranial neuropathy has been observed following exposure to trichloroethylene (TCE); the effects are primarily on the trigeminal nerve, and exposure has been associated with motor and sensory losses in the face. Blink reflex has been successfully used to detect TCE-induced trigeminal neuropathy [63].

Seppalainen and Antti-Polka [64] studied the long-term effects of solvent exposure on peripheral nerves in workers exposed to solvent mixtures containing aliphatic hydrocarbons and variable amounts of aromatic hydrocarbons, mainly ethyl, toluene, and trimethyl benzenes. Most of the workers had also been exposed to paint thinners (toluene, methyl isobutyl ketone, isobutanol, ethylene glycol, petroleum benzene, isopropanol, acetone, xylene, and butyl acetate). The results, based on observed findings on electromyography, suggested axonal changes rather than segmental demyelination. Although the duration of exposure to the substances was not related to the prevalence of illness, results of some electrodiagnostic parameters appeared related to the type of chemical exposure. Patients exposed to a *mixture* of solvents plus trichloroethylene or perchloroethylene, for example, experienced neuropathic findings more frequently than did people exposed *only* to the *mixed* solvents *without* trichloroethylene or perchloroethylene.

Organophosphorus Esters

Delayed-onset central-peripheral distal axonopathy can occur 7 to 10 days after acute, even single, exposure to certain organophosphorus esters [24]. Triorthocresylphosphate is the most infamous organophosphate. Other compounds in this category known to produce delayed distal axonopathy include letophos, mipafox, and trichlorphon. Both the axons in the peripheral nerves and the long tracts of the spinal cord are involved. The axonal lesion in the peripheral nerve becomes refractory to degeneration after repeated dose, whereas the lesion in the spinal cord is progressive, resulting in a clinical picture that may resemble multiple sclerosis [65]. Neuropathy target esterase (NTE), a nervous system esterase distinct from cholinesterase, is strongly suggested to be the target responsible for the delayed neurotoxic effect [65].

2,4-Dichlorophenoxyacetic Acid

Similar findings have been reported in patients exposed to certain herbicides, such as 2,4-dichlorophenoxyacetic acid (2,4-D). This substance appears to have its major effect on skeletal muscle because of interference at the neuromuscular junction. Several cases of peripheral neuropathy had been reported following exposure to 2,4-D or its close structural analogues. Patients suffering from acute intoxication to this herbicide exhibit fibrillary changes and paralysis of the intercostal muscles [66]. The mechanism of toxicity on subacute dose of 2,4-D appears to be a decrease in acetylcholinesterase activity in the diaphragm and other muscles (at least in the rat) [67]. It has been suggested that decreased activity in acetylcholinesterase may be the initial step in the development of *myopathy* that occurs after acute intoxication with 2,4-D. It is quite difficult to be certain, however, that a given individual exposed to amounts of a known neurotoxin that are above the previously recognized standards of safety will experience toxic effects. Likewise, toxic effects may be observed in individuals even though measurable levels of the given substance may be considerably below recognized standards.

References

1. Montoya, M. A. Neurotoxicology in Mexico and its Relation to the General and Work Environment. In B. L. Johnson (ed.), *Advances in Neurobehavioral Toxicology: Applications in Environmental and Occupational Health.* Chelsea, MI: Lewis, 1990.
2. Feldman, R. G. Ricks, N. L., and Baker, E. L. Neuropsychological effects of industrial toxins: A review. *Am J. Ind. Med.* 1:211, 1980.
3. Valciukas, J. A., et al. Lead exposure and behavioral changes: Comparison of four occupation groups with different levels of lead absorption. *Am. J. Ind. Med.* 1:421, 1980.
4. Feldman, R. G., White, R. F., and Travers, P. H. Neurobehavioral Effects of Toxicity Due to Metals, Solvents, and Insecticides. In A. B. Tarcher (ed.), *An Introduction to Environmental Medicine.* New York: Plenum, 1987.
5. White, R. F. Differential Diagnosis of Alzheimer's Disease and Solvent Encephalopathy in Older Workers. In B. L. Johnson (ed.), *Advances in Neurobehavioral Toxicology: Applications in Environmental and Occupational Health.* Chelsea, MI: Lewis, 1990.
6. Juntunen, J. Alcoholism in occupational neurology: Diagnostic difficulties with special reference to the neurological syndromes caused by exposure to organic solvents. *Acta Neurol. Scand.* 66 (Suppl. 92):89, 1982.
7. Feldman, R. G., and Travers, P. H. Environmental and Occupational Neurology. In R. G. Feldman (ed.), *Neurology: The Physician's Guide.* New York: Thieme-Stratton, 1984. Pp. 191–212.
8. Feldman, R. G. Effects of Toxins and Physical Agents on the Nervous System. In W. G. Bradley et al. (eds.), *Neurology in Clinical Practice,* Vol. 2. Stoneham, MA: Butterworth-Heinemann, 1991. Pp. 1185–1209.
9. Baker, E. L., et al. Occupational lead neurotoxicity—a behavioral and electrophysiologic evaluation: I. Study design and year one results. *Br. J. Ind. Med.* 41:352, 1984.
10. APHA. Lead Poisoning. In J. L. Weeks, B. S. Levy, and G. R. Wagner (eds.), *Preventing Occupational Disease and Injury.* Washington, DC: APHA, 1991.
11. Grandjean, P., Arnvig, E., and Beckman, J. Psychological dysfunctions in lead-exposed workers: Relation to biological parameters of exposure. *Scand. J. Work Environ. Health* 4:295, 1978.
12. Hanninen, H. Behavioral effects of occupational exposure to mercury and lead. *Acta Neurol. Scand.* 66 (Suppl. 92): 167, 1982.
13. Valciukas, J. A., et al. Behavioral indicators of lead neurotoxicity: Results of a clinical survey. *Int. Arch. Occup. Environ. Health* 41:217, 1978.
14. Landrigan, P. Arsenic. In W. N. Rom (ed.). *Environmental and Occupational Medicine.* (2nd ed.). Boston: Little, Brown, 1992. Pp. 773–780.
15. Frank, G. Neurologische und psychiatrische folgesymptome bei akuter Arsen-Wasserstoff-Vergiftung. *J. Neurol.* 213:59, 1976.
16. McCrutchen, J. J., and Utterback, R. A. Chronic arsenic poisoning resembling muscular dystrophy. *South. Med. J.* 59:1139, 1966.
17. Bolla-Wilson, K., and Bleecker, M. L. Neuropsychological impairment following inorganic arsenic exposure. *J.O.M.* 29:500, 1987.
18. Morton, W., and Caron, G. Encephalopathy: An uncommon manifestation of workplace arsenic exposure. *Am. J. Ind. Med.* 15:1, 1989.
19. Whitlock, C. M., Amuso, S. J., and Bittenbender, J. B. Chronic neurological disease in two manganese steel workers. *Am. Ind. Hyg. Assoc. J.* 27:454, 1966.
20. Mena, L., et al. Chronic manganese poisoning: Clinical picture and manganese turnover. *Neurology* 17:128, 1967.
21. Cook, D. G., Fahn, S., and Brait, K. A. Chronic manganese intoxication. *Arch. Neurol.* 30:59, 1974.
22. Seth, P. K., and Chandra, S. V. Neurotoxic Effects of Manganese. In S. C. Bondy and K. N. Prasad (eds.), *Metal Neurotoxicity.* Boca Raton, FL: CRC, 1988.
23. APHA. Mercury Poisoning. In J. L. Weeks, B. S. Levy, and G. R. Wagner (eds.), *Preventing Occupational Disease and Injury.* Washington, DC: APHA, 1991.
24. Schaumburg, H. H., and Spencer, P. S. Selected Outbreaks of Neurotoxic Disease. In P. S. Spencer and H. H. Schaumburg (eds.), *Experimental and Clinical Neurotoxicology.* Baltimore/London: Williams & Wilkins, 1980.
25. Boor, J. W., and Hurtiig, H. I. Persistent cerebellar ataxia after exposure to toluene. *Ann. Neurol.* 2(5):440, 1977.

26. Hanninen, H. Behavioral Study of the Effects of Carbon Disulfide. In C. Xintaras, B. L. Johnson, and I. de Groot (eds.), *Behavioral Toxicology: Early Detection of Occupational Hazards.* NIOSH Publication no. 74-126. Washington, DC: US Government Printing Office, 1974. Pp. 73–80.
27. Hanninen, H., et al. Psychological tests as indicators of excessive exposure to carbon disulfide. *Scand. J. Psychol.* 19:163, 1978.
28. Lilis, R. Behavioral Effects of Occupational Carbon Disulfide Exposure. In C. Xintaras, B. L. Johnson, and I. de Groot (eds.), *Behavioral Toxicology: Early Detection of Occupational Hazards.* NIOSH Publications no. 74-126. Washington, DC: US Government Printing Office, 1974. Pp. 51–59.
29. Salvani, M., Binaschi, S., and Riva, M. Evaluation of the psychophysiological functions in humans exposed to trichloroethylene. *Br. J. Ind. Med.* 28:293, 1971.
30. Feldman, R. G., et al. Long-term follow-up after single exposure to trichloroethylene. *Am. J. Ind. Med.* 8:119, 1985.
31. McCunney, R. J. Diverse manifestations of trichloroethylene. *Br. J. Ind. Med.* 45:122, 1988.
32. Hanninen, H., et al. Behavioral effects of long-term exposure to a mixture of organic solvents. *Scand. J. Work Environ. Health* 4:240, 1976.
33. Lindstrom, K. Changes in psychological performances of solvent poisoned and solvent-exposed workers. *Am. J. Ind. Med.* 1:69, 1980.
34. Lindstrom, K. Behavioral changes after long-term exposure to organic solvents and their mixtures. *Scand. J. Work Environ. Health* 4 (Suppl.):48, 1981.
35. Seppalainen, A. M., Lindstrom, K., and Martelin, T. Neurophysiological and psychological picture of solvent poisoning. *Am. J. Ind. Med.* 1:31, 1980.
36. Elofsson, S., et al. Exposure to organic solvents. *Scand. J. Work Environ. Health* 6:239, 1980.
37. Axelson, O., Hane, M., and Hogstedt, C. A case-referent study on neuropsychiatric disorders among workers exposed to solvents. *Scand. J. Work Environ. Health* 2:14, 1976.
38. Struwe, G., Mindus, P., and Jonsson, B. Psychiatric ratings in occupational health research: A study of mental symptoms in lacquerers. *Am. J. Ind. Med.* 1:23, 1980.
39. Ecobichon, D. J., and Joy, R. M. (eds.). *Pesticides and Neurological Diseases.* Boca Raton, FL: CRC, 1982.
40. Dille, J. R., and Smith, P. W. Central nervous system effects of chronic exposure to organophosphate insecticide. *Aerospace Med.* 35:475, 1964.
41. Gershon, S., and Shaw, F. B. Psychiatric sequelae of chronic exposure to organophosphorous insecticides. *Lancet* 1:1371, 1961.
42. Xintaras, C., Johnson, B. L., and de Groot, I. (eds.), *Behavioral Toxicology: Early Detection of Occupational Hazards.* NIOSH Publication no. 74–126. Washington, DC: US Government Printing Office, 1974.
43. Spencer, P. S., et al. Guam amyotrophic lateral sclerosis–parkinsonism–dementia linked to a plant excitant neurotoxin. *Science* 237:517, 1987.
44. Bleecker, M. L. Parkinsonism: A clinical marker of exposure to neurotoxins. *Neurotoxicol. Teratol.* 10:475, 1988.
45. Lewin, R. Parkinson's disease: An environmental cause? *Science* 229: 257, 1985.
46. Tanner, C. M., and Langston, J. W. Do environmental toxins cause Parkinson's disease? A critical review. *Neurology* 40 (Suppl. 3): 17, 1990.
47. Wolters, E., et al. Positron emission tomography in manganese intoxication. *Ann. Neurol.* 26:647, 1989.
48. LeQuesne, P. M. Electrophysiological investigation of toxic neuropathies. In J. Juntunen (ed.), Occupational Neurology. *Acta Neurol. Scand.* 66 (Suppl. 92): 75, 1982.
49. Schaumburg, H. H., Berger, A. R., and Thomas, P. K. Toxic Neuropathy. In H. H. Schaumburg, A. R. Berger, and P. K. Thomas (eds.), *Disorders of Peripheral Nerves.* Philadelphia: Davis, 1992.
50. Catton, M. J., et al. Subclinical neuropathy in lead workers. *Br. J. Ind. Med.* 2:80, 1970.
51. Bouldin, T. W., et al. Differential vulnerability of mixed and cutaneous nerves in lead neuropathy. *J. Neuropathol. Exp. Neurol.* 49:384, 1985.
52. Triebig, G., Weltle, D., and Valentin, H. Investigations on neurotoxicity of chemical substances at the workplace. Determination of the motor and sensory nerve conduction velocity in persons occupationally exposed to lead. *Int. Arch. Occup. Environ. Health* 53:189, 1984.
53. Jenkins, R. Inorganic arsenic and the nervous system. *Brain* 89:479, 1966.

54. Murphy, M. J., Lyon, J. W. and Taylor, J. W. Subacute arsenic neuropathy: Clinical and electrophysiological observations. *J. Neurol. Neurosurg. Psych.* 44:896, 1981.
55. Feldman, R. G., et al. Peripheral neuropathy in arsenic smelter workers. *Neurology* 29:939, 1979.
56. Blom, S., Lagerkvist, B., and Linderholm, H. Arsenic exposure to smelter workers clinical and neurophysiological studies. *Scand. J. Work Environ. Health* 11:265, 1985.
57. Kriess, K., et al. Neurologic evaluation of a population exposed to arsenic in Alaskan well water. *Arch. Environ. Health* 38:116, 1983.
58. Cavanagh, J. B. Neurotoxicology of acrylamides, hexacarbons, IDPN and carbon disulfide: Summarizing remarks. *Neurotoxicology* 6(4):97, 1985.
59. Seppalainen, A. M. Neurophysiological aspects of the toxicity of organic solvents. *Scand. J. Work Environ. Health* 11 (Suppl. 1):61, 1985.
60. Spencer, P. S., and Schaumberg, H. H. Cerebral-peripheral distal axonopathy: The pathology of dying back polyneuropathies. *Prog. Neuropathol.* 3:253, 1976.
61. LeQuesne, P. M. Clinical and morphological findings in acrylamide toxicity. *Neurotoxicology* 6(4):17, 1985.
62. Seppalainen, A. M. The Use of EMG Techniques in Solvent Exposure. In R. Gilioli, M. G. Cassitto, and V. Foa (eds.), *Neurobehavioral Methods in Occupational Health.* Oxford, Engl.: Pergamon, 1983. Pp. 177–182.
63. Feldman, R. G., et al. Blink reflex measurement of effects of trichloroethylene exposure on the trigeminal nerve. *Muscle Nerve* 15:490, 1992.
64. Seppalainen, A. M., and Antti-Polka, M. Time course of electrophysiological findings for patients with solvent poisoning. *Scand. J. Work Environ. Health* 9:15, 1983.
65. Anthony, D. C., and Graham, D. G. Toxic responses of the Nervous System. In C. D. Klaxon, M. O. Admire, and J. Doll (eds.), *Cassarett and Doul's Toxicology.* New York: Macmillan, 1991. Pp. 407–429.
66. Boack, P. 2,4-D poisoning in man. *J.A.M.A.* 214:1114, 1970.
67. Bernard, P. A., et al. 2,4-Dichlorophenoxyacetic acid (2,4-D) reduces acetylcholinesterase activity in rat muscle. *Exp. Neurol.* 87:544, 1985.

Further Information

Clayton, G. D., and Clayton, F. E. (eds.). *Patty's Industrial Hygiene and Toxicology* (3rd rev. ed.). New York: Wiley, 1981. Vols. 2A, B, and C.
These volumes provide an extensive encyclopedia-type reference for chemical information: usage, occupational standards, animal and human toxicology data, and exposure effects.

Cone, J. E., et al. Medical surveillance for neurologic endpoints. *Occup. Med. State of the Art Rev.* 5:547, 1990.

Ecobichon, D. J., and Joy, R. M. (eds.), *Pesticides and Neurological Disease.* Boca Raton, FL: CRC, 1982.
A review of the functioning of the nervous system followed by a chapter discussion of four major types of pesticides—chlorinated hydrocarbons, organophosphate esters, carbamate ester, and mercurial fungicides.

Goetz, C. G. *Neurotoxins in Clinical Practice.* New York: Spectrum, 1985.
Basic information on neurotoxins as seen in a clinical setting, but lacking in depth of reference sources.

Marquis, J. K. Contemporary Issues in Pesticide Toxicology and Pharmacology. In *Concepts in Toxicology.* New York: Karger, 1986. Vol. 2.
A discussion of pesticide mechanisms of action and their effects on the environment at large. Contains a chapter on the neurotoxicity of the organophosphate pesticides.

O'Donoghue, J. L. (ed.). *Neurotoxicity of Industrial and Commercial Chemicals.* Boca Raton, FL: CRC, 1985. Vols. 1 and 2.
Two-volume discussion of the neurotoxic action of chemicals seen in industry, each chapter dealing with a specific structurally related set of compounds.

Schaumburg, H. H., Berger, A. R., and Thomas, P. K. Toxic Neuropathy. In H. H. Schaumburg, A. R. Berger, and P. K. Thomas (eds.). *Disorders of Peripheral Nerves.* Philadelphia: Davis, 1992.

Spencer, P. S., and Schaumberg, H. H. (eds.). *Experimental and Clinical Neurotoxicology.* Baltimore: Williams & Wilkins, 1980.
The most extensive review on the classification, pathophysiology, epidemiology, and experimental information of the "classic" neurotoxins, i.e., acrylamide, n-hexane, metals (lead, mercury, aluminum, cadmium), carbon monoxide, and carbon disulfide.

White, R. F., Feldman, R. G., and Travers, P. H. Neurobehavioral effects of toxicity due to metals, solvents, and insecticides: Review. *Clin. Neuropharmacol.* 139:392, 1990.

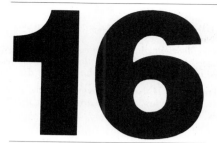

Noise-Induced Hearing Loss

Donald C. Gasaway

Overview

Cumulative overexposures to hazardous sounds and noises cause millions of people to lose hearing. Losses in hearing associated with overexposures are called *noise-induced* and such occurrences are mostly preventable. Therefore, solutions lie clearly within the province of occupational and preventive medicine. In the not too distant past, primary causes of this type of hearing loss were gunfire, blast, and military and occupational activities [1–3]. Today, sources of potentially damaging noises are kaleidoscopic, including many not associated with occupational or military environments. Even many recreational activities contribute to the problem, for example, target shooting, rock music, motorcycling, and others [4].

Noise-induced auditory damage is incremental. Small but irreversible damage occurs during the earliest stages without a person being cognizant that physical injury has taken place. Losses in auditory function ordinarily result from a lifetime of cumulative overexposures. Unfortunately, many young people develop some degree of noise-induced hearing loss *before* they encounter noise in an occupational setting. Although the human hearing system can accommodate a multitude of occurrences of loud sounds without sustaining permanent damage (given a reasonable period of auditory rest between intervals of exposure), the growing number and variety of potentially hazardous noises encountered during modern times and increasing numbers of people with noise-induced losses present a formidable challenge [5].

Since no treatment is available to mend noise-induced hearing loss, *preventive measures* are paramount. Preplacement physical examinations should include audiometric examinations to discover noise-induced hearing losses *prior to* assigning a person to work in a noisy job. This audiometric record may serve as a baseline (especially if the person receiving the audio was free from noise exposure before the test) against which later examinations can be compared. Also, the preplacement audiogram documents the status of hearing before a new employee encounters noise in the work environment, a potential legal consideration. When results of periodic audiometric examinations and noise exposure histories are reviewed, measures can be taken to prevent additional and more serious injury. Abnormal findings attributable to noise, once confirmed, should prompt careful *counseling* concerning the potential seriousness of repeated unprotected exposures.

Audiometry, measuring hearing thresholds for different discrete pure-tone signals ranging from 500 to 6000 or 8000 Hertz (Hz), furnishes valuable insight concerning the status of hearing. Although the normal frequency range of hearing is 20 to 20,000 Hz, most occupational audiometric examinations measure thresholds from 500 through either 6000 or 8000 Hz. The lowest intensity level at which a sound (pure-tone signals) can be detected at a given test frequency is known as audiometric threshold, which is recorded in decibels (dB), with 0 dB to 25 dB considered in the normal range. Most audiometers provide threshold measurements ranging from 0 to 100 or 110 dB. The higher the numeric decibel hearing level (dB hearing threshold level [dB, HTL]), the greater the deviation from "normal." Generally, "normal hearing" is represented within a range from 0 to 25 dB (HTL). The most critical frequency range for human audition is between 500 through 2000 or 3000 hZ—the range indispensable for hearing and understanding normal conversational speech [5–7].

Noise in Industry

The Occupational Safety and Health Administration (OSHA) [8] estimates that approximately 9,400,000 *production workers* in the United States either work or have worked in jobs in which the noise exposures are 80 dBA[1] (A-weighted noise levels) or higher. This estimate does not include people working in construction, agriculture, mining, transportation, oil well drilling and servicing, or federal and state government (also excludes military services of the Department of Defense and the Coast Guard of the Department of Transportation).

Insight into noise-exposed work groups can be obtained from study of state and federal OSHA citations for noncompliance with provisions of regulatory hearing conservation acts (known as Code of Federal Regulations, part 1910.95, or state equivalent). Job categories within "manufacturing" account for 90.0% of all employee work groups cited at facilities where failures or deficiencies, or both, have been observed [author's data: sampled January 1988 through March 31, 1990]. These findings are contained in Table 16-1. Category descriptions of US Standard Industrial Classification (SIC) Codes that represent those included within 20 to 39 (manufacturing) are identified, along with relative percentage distributions and rank order. Half (50.9%) of all citations include 4 subgroups: prefabricated metal products, primary metal products, lumber and wood products, and food and kindred products. With the addition of 4 subgroups (rubber and miscellaneous plastic products; transportation equipment; machinery, except electrical; and stone, clay, and glass products), only 8 of 20 subgroups within "manufacturing" account for 77.0% of all noncompliance citations observed within 20 categories.

Prevalence of Noise-Induced Hearing Loss

According to OSHA, using the average hearing levels at 1000 through 3000 Hz as a basis for classifying hearing impairment, 1,624,000 (17%) of production workers

Table 16-1. Summary of Standard Industrial Classification (SIC) Codes within *manufacturing* group (SIC Codes 20XX–39XX) receiving hearing conservation noncompliance citations during January 1988 through March 1990

SIC manufacturing subgroup	Two-digit SIC Code	Citations (relative %)	Rank order
Food and kindred products	20	9.2	4
Tobacco manufacturers	21	0.0	20
Textile mill products	22	2.1	14
Apparel/other textile products	23	0.6	17
Lumber and wood products	24	10.6	3
Furniture and fixtures	25	4.5	9
Paper and allied products	26	4.1	10
Printing and publishing	27	2.3	13
Chemicals and allied products	28	1.8	15
Petroleum and coal products	29	0.7	16
Rubber and miscellaneous plastic products	30	7.4	5
Leather and leather products	31	0.3	19
Stone, clay, and glass products	32	5.0	8
Primary metal industries	33	12.5	2
Prefabricated metal products	34	18.6	1
Machinery, except electrical	35	6.8	7
Electronic and electronic equipment	36	3.9	11
Transportation equipment	37	6.9	6
Instruments and related products	38	0.4	18
Miscellaneous manufacturing industries	39	2.4	12

[1]The dBA, or A-weighted level, a measurement of noise obtained using a sound measuring instrument, is commonly used to define degrees of auditory risk. The A-weighting is an electronic measurement that closely parallels the auditory characteristics of human hearing exhibited among normal subjects. The dBA is widely used in the US for expressing degrees of risk and other types of auditory correlations, such as noisiness and speech interference.

have at least mild degrees of hearing loss, 1,060,000 (11%) reveal material impairments in hearing, and 473,000 (5%) show moderate degrees of hearing impairment, comprising a total of 33% with some degree of hearing impairment [8]. Using similar data, the National Institute for Occupational Safety and Health (NIOSH) estimates that one fourth of workers 55 years of age or older exposed over their work life to noise levels of 90 dBA or higher have developed a material hearing impairment [9].

NIOSH, in a classic document used to form the foundation for OSHA auditory risk criteria, reported the number of workers in different industries in which noise exposures exceeded 90 dBA [3]. Using results of noise studies and worker population statistics, NIOSH estimated that 44% of employees in textile manufacturing routinely encountered noises above 90 dBA. Proportions of the other workforce studied who are similarly exposed are contained in Table 16-2. Industries included in the NIOSH study represent only a portion of the workforce, however, who routinely encounter potentially hazardous noise in the United States.

Roles and Challenges for Clinicians

Physicians who provide occupational health services face several challenges dealing with noise-induced hearing loss: (1) how to evaluate the need for an occupational hearing conservation program (OHCP); (2) how to evaluate audiometric results and identify changes attributable to noise; (3) how to structure elements of an OHCP to conserve hearing; (4) how to select appropriate hearing protection devices and monitor and ensure their long-term effectiveness; (5) how to recognize when referrals to otologists or audiologists, or both, are required; (6) how to structure feedback to employees that ensures their willingness to conserve their hearing, both on and off the job; and (7) how to evaluate initial and ongoing effectiveness of an OHCP and provide services and support to affected employees, managers, owners, and other safety/health providers.

Example of Progressive Noise-Induced Hearing Impairment

An example of a progressive noise-induced hearing loss will help set the stage for a better understanding of the nature of this basically preventable problem. Table 16-3 illustrates audiometric results for an employee who worked for 11 years in a noisy environment and used hearing protection sporadically. The reference (or baseline) audiogram was performed when this individual began work at 24 years of age. The baseline hearing levels reveal normal hearing in both ears across all test frequencies,

Table 16-2. Proportions of workforce in industries in which noise levels may exceed 90 dBA

Industry	Percent
Petroleum and coal products and processing	29
Lumber and wood products	26
Food processing, packaging, and canning	25
Furniture and fixtures manufacturing	18
Metal fabricating	17
Stone, clay, and glass products	17
Primary metal industries	15
Rubber and plastic products	14
Transportation equipment	12
Electrical equipment and supplies	11
Chemical and allied products	11
Apparel and other textile products	9
Ordnance and accessories	9
Instruments and related products	6
Nonelectrical machinery	4
Printing and publishing	4

Source: From *Criteria for a Recommended Standard—Occupational Exposure to Noise.* HSM 73-11001. Washington, DC: National Institute for Occupational Safety and Health, 1972.

Table 16-3. Example of audiometric thresholds obtained on worker who exhibited progressive noise-induced hearing loss

Hearing thresholds on:	Frequency (Hz)*											
	Left ear						Right ear					
	500	1000	2000	3000	4000	6000	500	1000	2000	3000	4000	6000
Reference	5	0	0	10	10	5	0	5	5	10	10	10
1st annual	0	0	0	10	10	10	5	5	5	10	15	10
2nd annual	5	5	0	10	15	10	0	5	5	15	20	15
3rd annual	0	5	5	15	15	15	5	5	5	15	25	10
4th annual	5	5	10	15	20	20	0	5	5	20	25	15
5th annual	0	5	15	25	30	25	10	10	10	15	25	20
6th annual	5	10	20	35	40	30	10	10	15	20	35	25
7th annual	0	10	30	45	50	40	15	15	20	30	40	35
8th annual	5	15	35	50	55	40	15	20	30	45	55	40
9th annual	10	25	40	60	70	50	15	35	45	55	65	50
10th annual	10	35	55	70	85	60	20	40	50	65	80	55
11th annual	15	40	65	80	95	80	10	45	60	75	90	70

*Frequency is a measure of the pitch of a sound and is expressed in Hertz (Hz). Higher frequencies (3000–6000 Hz) are usually first affected in noise-induced hearing impairments. Thresholds are recorded in decibels (dB), and the quantities shown under frequency indicate the softest intensity level at which the person could hear the different test tones. (Note: 0 dB is audiometric "zero," and deviations from optimum "normal" are recorded in dB hearing threshold levels greater than 0.)

that is, 500 through 6000 Hz (normal hearing is usually defined as decibel levels ≥ 25 dB at each test frequency). By the fourth annual examination, changes in thresholds from the baseline, especially within the range from 3000 through 6000 Hz, uncover a *trend*. The early so-called threshold shifts in hearing suggest damage due to noise. Subsequent examinations disclosed that the deterioration continued within the higher as well as the lower frequency ranges (below 3000 Hz). By the time the damage involved hearing acuity below 3000 Hz, the person's ability to hear and understand spoken communications has been compromised. Thus, this person acquired a significant amount of hearing impairment within a relatively short span of life and at a relatively young age—35 years. If the OSHA criterion for monitoring audiometric evaluations had been followed (i.e., *an average shift of 10 dB or more at 2000–4000 Hz for either ear from the reference* [8]), damaged hearing would have been identified during the fifth annual monitoring. At this point, actions should have been taken to prevent further impairment.

Hearing and Noise

Normal Hearing

Hearing is a marvelous sense. The normal ear can hear frequencies as low as approximately 20 Hz and as high as about 20,000 Hz, a range that allows us to hear the vast majority of sounds important to humans. The initial range of hearing most susceptible to noise damage is between 3000 and 8000 Hz, frequencies above the range at which primary conversational speech sounds are customarily heard. One with normal human hearing can discern even the softest utterances. The amplitude of sounds distinguished by a normal ear range from that of a leaf falling against grass to the blast of artillery. The capacity to hear the multitude of softer less intense sounds is progressively disrupted as noise-induced hearing loss continues [2, 6, 7, 10].

Nature of Damage to Hearing

Excessive noise exposures damage the intricate microscopic structures within the inner ear, particularly those comprising the organ of Corti. Hair cells, including pillar and supporting cells, blood vessels, the stria vascularis, and even the nerve fibers and cilia, are physically damaged, presumably as a result of both altered biochemical change and mechanical destruction [5]. During the early progressive stages of physical injury, the damage mostly involves structures located within the basal turn of the cochlea, but, with continued overexposure to noise, the damage affects structures within the medial and apical area [5].

Differences Between Noise-Induced Temporary and Permanent Changes in Hearing

Observations of noise-induced hearing losses are classified into two categories: *temporary* and *permanent*. *Noise-induced temporary threshold shifts* (NITTS) are changes in hearing associated with *transient* overexposures to noise that can be observed and documented by sequential audiometric examinations. NITTS may persist for minutes, hours, or even several days following an episode of overexposure. The greater the magnitude of noise exposures that produced the shifts, the longer the interval of time (auditory rest) required for hearing to return to normal. Given an adequate period of auditory rest, hearing usually returns to preexposure levels unless some degree of permanent damage has occurred.

Typically, the person experiencing a NITTS notices diminished hearing that is most pronounced immediately after a noise encounter. Generally, most audiometric examinations should not be attempted until at least 14 hours have elapsed since the last unprotected encounter with potentially hazardous exposures [8].

Day-to-day overexposures to auditory stresses may go unheeded because hearing appears to "return" to normal. Repeated episodes of NITTS may permanently damage hearing so that no amount of auditory rest can restore preexposure levels of audition. *Noise-induced permanent threshold shifts* (NIPTS) refers to an *irreversible* condition in which, despite a prolonged period of auditory rest, hearing does not return to normal [1, 5]. NITTS is a precursor of NIPTS. Therefore, evidence of temporary shifts following an encounter with noise can serve as a valuable clue to changes that may eventually become permanent.

Importance of Audiometric Changes Due to Noise

Typically, both NITTS and NIPTS changes, even though one is temporary and the other permanent, reveal disruptions in hearing that are most evident within the higher frequency ranges, that is, above 4000 Hz. Although these early stages of permanent damage can be prevented, progressive overexposures eventually result in losses *below* 3000 Hz. When this occurs, perceiving and understanding speech has been compromised [5, 10, 11].

The development of NIPTS is dependent on frequency spectrum, intensity, and duration of noise exposure, but typically, several months or even years pass before permanent damage to hearing becomes manifest within the speech–hearing range [5, 10]. When audiometric results are reviewed longitudinally, evidence of early damage can be detected (see Table 16-3). If properly counseled, the person may then become more motivated to prevent further deterioration in hearing, especially in the most vital area (i.e., below 3000 Hz) [12]. When impairment occurs below 3000 Hz, the ability to easily understand conversations progressively deteriorates and is often manifested by difficulty in distinguishing consonants; people so afflicted confuse such words as "fish" for "fist" and so forth.

Unilateral Versus Bilateral Loss

During the early stages, NIPTS typically affects hearing in one ear more than the other. Generally, hearing in the left ear tends to sustain more initial damage from noise than is observed in the right ear. Continued unprotected overexposures to steady and/or intermittent type noises, however, eventually affect both ears more evenly.

Using Audiometric Monitoring Effectively

Determining the effects of noise on hearing can be accomplished by serial audiometry. The following precautions help ensure that audiometric results are valid: (1)

The audiometer is maintained in perfect working order and routinely calibrated, (2) background noise in the testing environment is controlled (usually with a booth) so as not to interfere with measurements of threshold levels of hearing, and (3) examiners are properly trained in standard audiometric testing procedures (also a requirement of the OSHA Hearing Conservation Standard) [8, 10, 11–14].

Unfortunately, too frequently, noise-induced hearing impairments go undetected (see Table 16-3). This oversight may be due to fundamental differences between clinical and preventive medicine. The status of hearing is usually not of concern to the *clinician* until the capacity to hear and understand speech has been compromised. On the other hand, occupational medicine, as a discipline of *preventive medicine,* is concerned with recognizing the unique and vitally important role of early changes in hearing *before* substantial impairment develops.

The clinician is thus advised to recognize that relatively minor changes between audiometric test results viewed over time may reflect potentially serious consequences regarding ultimate cumulative loss of functional hearing. Hearing is considered "abnormal" if threshold levels at 500 through 3000 Hz equal or exceed about 25 dB [11, 15, 16]. Significant damage typically occurs before permanent injury progresses beyond this arbitrary "fence."

How to Identify Hazardous Noise Exposures

The physician who provides occupational health services is likely to be asked to evaluate the need for a hearing conservation program (HCP). The initial step in this process is to perform noise measurements, a procedure conducted by an industrial hygienist or related professional. Noise analysis instruments include: (1) simple sound level meters with which A- and C-weighted measurements can be obtained; (2) individual noise dosimeters, which electronically integrate cumulative noise exposures during a typical work period; and (3) octave-band analyzers, which measure overall noise within select (discrete spectrum) frequency ranges. The most common measurements performed in occupational settings consist of overall (usually A-weighted) levels obtained utilizing either a sound level meter or noise dosimeter [8, 13, 17].

Noise Measurements

Typically, initial measurements consist of *area surveys* conducted with a stationary sound level meter or noise dosimeter. Results obtained during these surveys are commonly used to identify the need for more detailed measurements since these results direct attention to potentially hazardous exposures for workers in the area sampled. Additional and more definitive measurements are usually required when ambient noises equal or exceed 85 dBA. According to OSHA, area monitorings are required to (1) identify employees to be enrolled in the OHCP, (2) identify employees required to use hearing protection, (3) identify areas where engineering or noise control measures, or both, need investigation, (4) identify the amount of attenuation that hearing protectors must be able to provide to render exposures as "safe," and (5) familiarize both employees and employers with the degree of noise hazard [8]. The Occupational Safety and Health (OSH) Act further stipulates that area surveys may be used to define individual exposures only when it is apparent that the workforce in question is located in essentially the same area throughout the shift and the character of the noise is relatively stable and does not fluctuate (i.e., does not change throughout the work shift and/or contain impulse or impact exposures).

If these requirements cannot be assured, OSHA requires that more detailed *individual* assessments be performed, which usually require the use of *personal noise dosimeters*. If a simple sound level meter is used for personal sampling, an evaluator must accompany the worker for a period of time throughout the sampling to ensure representative assessments. The evaluator in turn must record the different levels and duration parameters observed to formulate a typical cumulative exposure noise pattern. This procedure, however, is time consuming and subject to considerable variability [8, 17]. The simplest method for performing personal sampling is to employ a noise dosimeter that is "worn" by the worker throughout the sampling session. In both types of personal sampling, the microphone of the measuring device should be located as close to the ear as feasible [8, 17].

All instruments used to measure noise, including the condition of the battery, should be maintained in perfect working order and calibrated prior to and during the sampling [8]. Since the results will be used to identify and delineate degrees of auditory risk, the quality of the instrumentation, skills of the evaluator, duration of sampling, and interpretation of the data should be optimum.

Behavioral Clues to Hazardous Noise

A simple technique for identifying a potentially unprotected hazardous noise is based on observation. If a person needs to "shout" at a distance of about 1 meter (about 3 ft), the noise should be considered hazardous to unprotected ears, an indicator of when either on- or off-the-job auditory risks are encountered that equal or exceed about 85 dBA [10].

Elements of an Occupational Hearing Conservation Program

Although the OSH Act can be used as a guide, some details and procedures within the OSHA regulatory document are needlessly complicated, and thus, one is advised to consult other references for more practical and applied overall guidance [10, 13, 17–19]. An OHCP should contain specific and well-defined functional elements: (1) education, motivation, supervision, and discipline; (2) assessment of potentially hazardous noise exposures; (3) assessing at-the-ear allowable exposures for those wearing HPDs; (4) monitoring audiometry; (5) personal hearing protection and noise control measures; (6) documentation of OHCP monitorings; and (7) disposition and follow-up actions [10, 18, 19].

Education, Motivation, Supervision, and Discipline

Basic education related to hearing and the damaging effects of noise must be provided to workers in hazardous noise environments. Employees should understand the hearing process, how noise damages hearing, and why hearing protection is necessary. Employees should recognize how the elements of the hearing conservation program are designed to conserve their hearing and comprehend why compliance with such requirements is for their personal benefit. Workers need to know when and how to use hearing protection properly, whom to contact if they experience problems, and the purpose of the audiometric examinations [12, 19].

Motivation is a key element that can be developed from effective education. To prevent hearing loss, workers must recognize the critical importance of properly and consistently using hearing protection devices. The foundations underlying most effective HCPs instill strong *supervisor* and *employee* motivation [10, 13, 14, 18]. Too frequently, however, workers have to lose substantial amounts of hearing before they recognize the serious nature of noise exposure threats and become motivated to protect their hearing [12]. *Supervision* is a critically important part of a program. Supervisors should enforce the proper and consistent wearing of hearing protection. When supervisors are properly trained and motivated, the effectiveness of the program improves [10, 18, 19]. Failures observed within programs, especially improper or lack of use of HPDs, can often be traced to poor supervision [12, 20, 21]. *Discipline* is another critical element. Although disciplinary action may be viewed as a poor approach to achieving adherence to safety practices, appropriate measures for non-compliance should be structured into a hearing conservation effort [12, 20]. The most common area requiring disciplinary actions concerns either not wearing or refusal to use hearing protectors properly, and, even though "solutions" to such refusals may involve disciplinary actions, the reasons for refusal should be investigated and mutually acceptable resolutions or alternatives attempted [12, 21].

Assessment of Potentially Hazardous Exposures

Although general noise surveys can identify areas or workers where potentially hazardous unprotected exposures exist, they only serve to identify basic types of jobs, areas, or activities where workers may encounter dangerous noises. "Assessing" at-the-ear noise exposures among those wearing HPDs more accurately reflects degrees of risk than indicated by evaluation of only ambient noise levels. When a potentially hazardous exposure is identified, workers are required to wear HPDs.

Therefore, a critically vital task is calculating *at-the-ear exposures encountered when hearing protection is worn* [8, 10, 21, 22]. These assessments require consolidation of two basic parameters: *auditory risk criteria* and values of *attenuation* afforded by the type(s) of HPDs used. Inspection of OSHA auditory risk criteria reveals that the "action level" (the exposure parameter requiring enrollment in the OHCP) begins at 85 dBA[2] for a typical 8-hour workday (82 dBA for 12-hour per day work shifts), and the allowable durations (minutes or hours) are *reduced* by half for each 5-dBA increase above this boundary [8]; for example (using the "action line" as the boundary for limits of daily unprotected exposure), 85 dBA for 8 hours/day, 4 hours/day at 90 dBA, 2 hours/day at 95 dBA, and up to 115 dBA, which corresponds to 7.5 minutes/day.

Assessing At-the-Ear Allowable Exposures for Those Wearing HPDs

Estimating the amount of attenuation (noise reduction) afforded by a specific type of hearing protector is critically important. The manufacturer reports a noise reduction rating (NRR) for each device that is obtained under "laboratory" type conditions, but, unfortunately, many users fail to obtain this level of protection in actual work settings [21, 23]. In the "real world," amounts of protection actually achieved among users has been observed as only half of the NRR values reported by manufacturers [21]. One procedure for "adjusting" NRRs in an attempt to more accurately reflect real world conditions is to *reduce* or *derate* the published NRR by 50% (cut in half) when deciding if the user is adequately protected [23, 24]. Procedures for calculating at-the-ear exposures using published NRR data are discussed in greater detail elsewhere [3, 10, 24]. If assessments of at-the-ear exposures are in error, however, months and sometimes years may follow before losses among "protected" employees are discovered and corrective action taken [10, 20, 22]. Due to the potential for inadequately functioning HPDs, close scrutiny of audiometric monitoring results, combined with periodic on-site HPD use inspections, is critical. Even slight threshold shift changes must be viewed as indicative of inadequate personal hearing protection until further investigation proves otherwise. Affected employees may not be wearing HPDs during all types of hazardous encounters (including off-the-job) or their devices may be defective, deliver inadequate amounts of protection, and/or reflect improper usage.

Monitoring Audiometry

The kingpin of any OHCP is monitoring audiometry [6, 19, 25, 26]. Since noise-induced hearing losses result from cumulative overexposures, results of sequential audiometric findings must be carefully compared to detect subtle but consistent shift trends. Basic types of audiometric examinations should be structured according to the purpose for which they are performed (Table 16-4). Each category of audiometric examination has its own set of guidelines (conditions and restrictions) that should be complied with prior to, during, and after each specific type of audiometric examination [25].

Time away from productive work makes audiometric monitoring one of the most expensive elements of an OHCP [10]. Audiometry can be one of the most cost-effective components, however, when properly conducted and when appropriate follow-up actions subsequently prevent further hearing impairment [27].

Personal Hearing Protection and Noise Control Measures

Effective control of noise-induced hearing loss depends on reducing the potential for noise to affect the hearing process, by controlling noise at its source, by implementing engineering controls and other acoustic treatments, and/or by using HPDs. (See Nabelek [17] for a comprehensive discussion of noise control.)

Hearing protectors consist of three basic types: insert (devices that insert into the

---

[2]NIOSH criteria document suggests that damage to hearing may occur at 80 dBA if encountered for prolonged periods [3].

Table 16-4. Types of audiometric examinations according to purpose of test

*1. *Reference.* The baseline against which subsequent audiometric examinations will be compared and should be performed following an appropriate period of noise-free activity; usually following 14 hours out-of-noise.

2. *Initial follow-up for new worker* assigned to noisy work areas. May be performed within 90 days following initial placement in noise area(s); may or may not require noise-free activity preceding test.

*3. *Annual.* Examination performed as part of routine sequential monitorings of workers enrolled in the hearing conservation program; may or may not require noise-free activity preceding test.

4. Significant threshold shift (STS) *validation audiograms* are performed to confirm STS findings *before* medical referral. These tests require a mandatory period away from noise (usually 14 hours) immediately beforehand to avoid possible effect of temporary noise-induced threshold shifts.

5. *Close scrutiny audiometric examinations* allow audiologists and/or physicians to ensure that further changes in hearing are not occurring among people who *have* exhibited STS, and are intended to be accomplished at shorter intervals (such as 1-, 2-, 3-, or 6-month intervals).

6. *Utility audiometric examinations* are used to gain insight concerning effectiveness of hearing protection and validity of risk assessments. Results may also be used to motivate workers. Typically, pre- and postexposure audiograms are compared for evidence of temporary threshold shifts.

*Required by OSHA CFR 1910.95 Act [8].

Table 16-5. Classifications for basic types of personal protection devices

Insert (interaural or earplugs)
  Premolded—molded in fixed shapes and sizes
  Custom molded—individually molded using impression material that, when set or hardened, or remolded by manufacturer, provides a device that conforms to wearer's ear canals
  User molded—pliable material conforming to anatomic shape and contour of ear canals; may be expandable or nonexpandable material(s)
Semi-insert (semi-aural or ear caps)
  Interaural ear caps (fitted to bands or attached to other type suspension)
  Supra-aural ear caps (cover only outer opening to canals and attached to bands or other suspension system)
Circumaural muffs
  Muffs attached to band (band may be fixed or swivel; may be worn over head, behind neck, or under chin)
  Muffs attached to hard hats, bump caps, or helmets
  Muffs fitted with communication devices (attached to bands or installed within helmets)

ear canal proper), semi-insert (devices covering the entry into the ear canal and held in place by a band or other type of suspension device), and muffs (devices completely encapsulating to auricle or pinna). Table 16-5 lists subgroups within each of these three major categories. Many different models are represented within each subgroup. Health professionals should acquire a comprehensive understanding of functional features associated with each specific device contemplated for issue. No single type is "best" for all users, and many factors affect overall functional compatibility and effectiveness [10, 13, 22].

A device that cannot accommodate the anatomic features of the wearer can interfere with or compromise obtainment of optimum protection [20–22]. Too frequently, people who have acquired a hearing loss are later discovered to have been issued HPDs that were improperly fitted and/or they failed to receive indoctrination concerning proper use and care [12, 20, 21]. Prudent practice requires that *no type of hearing protector should be selected or issued without a thorough examination of the ears and surrounding anatomic structures to ensure optimum compatibility with the specific devices being considered for issue* [10, 20].

Generally, the widest range of HPDs is available from safety suppliers or distributors (see Yellow Pages in the telephone directory under "Safety Supply" or "Safety Equipment"). Samples should be available to those guiding HPD selection and issue, however, to ensure the best possible selection and appropriate indoctrination for each wearer, that is, a guided choice.

Salient features to be considered in the selection of HPDs are represented in Table 16-6 [10, 20, 22]. OSHA [8] and others [20, 21] recommend that employees be allowed to make selections from two or more types of *appropriate* devices. Such choices should be guided by the physician or related professional who is responsible for ensuring adequacy of hearing protection.

Documentation of OHCP Monitorings

Since clinically significant *noise-induced* hearing loss develops over a period of time, contents of various documents and records are vitally important at some later date if a reviewer must attempt to investigate cause-effect relationships that may have contributed to the observed shifts in hearing [28]. Such documents include clinical records, results of noise surveys, individual noise risk assessments, records of OHCP training and education sessions received by each employee, audiometric monitorings, records pertaining to calibration of noise measurement devices and audiometers, ambient noise levels in audiometric testing areas, records of disposition and follow-up actions, and documents reflecting work site inspections of employees wearing protection [8, 19, 27, 28].

Each person responsible for recording clinical and related OHCP information and data on a daily basis should document information carefully to facilitate and clarify comprehensive review at a later date of all types of OHCP negotiations. When completing medical, noise exposure histories, and related OHCP management documents, the person entering such information should assure that spaces are not left blank (every item should have an entry; blank spaces represent missing or incomplete entries of information) and that legibility is comprehendible and understandable [19, 27, 28]. Avoiding use of abbreviations, symbols, and jargon helps ensure more precise and accurate interpretations. For example, "AS" and "AD" may be easily recognized as left and right ears by otolaryngologists, but such entries may be confusing to others.

Disposition and Follow-up Actions

When any medical examination, such as an audiometric test, is performed, decisions regarding specifics of follow-up actions should be clearly stated [19, 25, 28]. If an

Table 16-6. Considerations involved in choices of personal hearing protection devices

Attenuation (amount of noise reduction provided by hearing protector)
Ease of use and wearability (can user successfully and easily use and wear device?)
Comfort (short term and long term)
Performance while executing listening-in-noise tasks
Care, cleaning, and hygienic considerations
Personal preference
Temperature and humidity (climatic) compatibility considerations
Carrying case, container, and/or stowage (when not being worn)
Visibility (ease of checking HPD use compliance by supervisors, etc.)
Compatibility with other head and body clothing and safety gear
Compatibility with requirements for detection if device becomes a foreign object in processed material (food, drugs, paper manufacturing, etc.)
Storage life (does not deteriorate or change)
Compatibility when dual (plugs and muffs) hearing protection is required
Cost
Availability of replacements (entire unit or parts and replacement elements)
Manufacturer and/or distributor support and services

annual audiometric examination reveals a significant threshold shift (STS), follow-up action is clearly indicated. All "positive" shifts, however, should be reevaluated following a reasonable period of auditory rest to rule out possible occurrence of noise-induced auditory fatigue as a cause of the observed abnormalities. Follow-up and disposition actions regarding abnormal examinations form a vital part of any OHCP monitoring effort. Flow charts can be helpful in this regard, especially for guiding technicians who perform audiometric testing on a routine basis [30].

Otologic/Audiologic Referral Criteria

Occasions will arise when the physician who reviews and/or manages OHCP moni-torings will need to make referrals to specialists. The following provides guidance to help physicians decide when referral actions may be indicated. Although physi-cians are obligated to comply with the OSHA critera for identifying STS, this does not preclude using another type of criterion as long as the one chosen is equal to, or more stringent than, those that OSHA dictate [8, 30].

The American Academy of Otolaryngology–Head and Neck Surgery (AAO-HNS) [11] provides guidance for *identifying a significant threshold shift* that speci-fies: ". . . a change for the worse of 10 dB or more in the average of pure-tone thresholds at 0.5, 1, and 2 kHz (500, 1000, 2000 Hz), or the average of pure-tone thresholds at 3, 4, and 6 kHz (3000, 4000, 6000 Hz), in either ear." Although this STS criterion differs from the one specified by OSHA, clinicians may wish to consider guidance provided by specialists within the field of otolaryngology, especially since the AAO-HNS criterion is more stringent than the one in the federal OSH Act.

AAO-HNS also provides *otologic referral guidance,* which states, ". . . a change in audiometric hearing levels in either ear (1) more than 15 dB for the average of 0.5, 1, and 2 kHz (500, 1000, 2000 Hz), or (2) more than 20 dB at 3 kHz (3000 Hz), or (3) more than 30 dB at 4 kHz (4000 Hz) or 6 kHz (6000 Hz), from the baseline levels" [11]. This criterion pertains to alterations in hearing that may be indicative of otologic problems requiring assistance from a qualified specialist, regardless of the cause or causes of the apparent loss.

Situations will arise when a physician may have to recommend against initial assignment or continuance of certain workers in jobs involving potentially hazardous noise exposures. Observations that may prompt such actions include: (1) a person who possesses good hearing in only one ear (severe unilateral loss); (2) a person who exhibits moderate to severe bilateral hearing impairment that appears to be pro-gressive in spite of efforts to control subsequent exposures; (3) a person who has chronic otologic problems (such as chronic otitis media or chronic otitis externa), especially if the condition(s) prevent(s) use of personal hearing protection; and (4) a person who continues to demonstrate progressive shifts in hearing that are attrib-uted to causes other than noise [5, 28]. Consideration should be given to principles of the Americans with Disabilities Act in any of these placement decisions.

Using Results of Audiometric Monitorings to Detect Noise-Induced Losses

Comparing periodic audiometric thresholds over several months or years can suggest early evidence of noise-induced hearing loss. Longitudinal monitoring used to iden-tify noise-induced loss can involve one or a combination of two types of audiometric comparisons: (1) the current (usually annual or initial follow-up) examination versus a reference or baseline, or (2) the current examination versus the preceding test (usually obtained a year earlier) [6, 25, 26, 31].

Comparing STS Between Current and Reference/Baseline Audiograms

The first type, current versus baseline, is commonly used to identify *STS* that may exist between the annual (or follow-up) audiometric examination and the baseline or reference. This procedure is required for basic OSHA compliance [8]. OSHA considers an STS "positive" when hearing levels on a current examination, compared against the baseline, equal or exceed an *average* of 10 dB at the audiometric test frequencies of 2000, 3000, and 4000 Hz of either ear [8].

The OSH Act refers to this criterion as a "standard" threshold shift (still abbreviated as STS), since the word "significant" may be misleading from a medicolegal or compensation point of view. Threshold shifts are computed by taking the decibel differences noted separately for each ear between the *reference* and the current audiogram at these three frequencies (2000, 3000, and 4000 Hz). If the total hearing level difference observed between the current and reference at these three frequencies for either ear equals 30 dB (which would average 10), a finding of STS has occurred. Tables 16-7 and 16-8 demonstrate how these computations may be performed.

In Table 16-7, the thresholds obtained on the current (annual) examination are compared against those recorded on the baseline. Amounts of threshold shift are entered by indicating a positive value (+) when the decibel hearing level of the current audio exceeds (poorer than) the value recorded on the baseline. A negative decibel value (−) indicates that the hearing level on the current examination is less (better) than noted on the reference. If no difference is noted, 0 (zero) is entered. Although STS comparisons only *apply to hearing levels at 2000, 3000, and 4000 Hz,* clinicians should note possible changes at other test frequencies (i.e., 500, 1000, 6000 Hz), which may prompt one of the otologic referral criteria recommended by the AAO-HNS [11, 16]. Table 16-7 illustrates STS found to be "negative," and Table 16-8 represents STS found to be "positive." Figure 16-1 is a sample form that can be used for computing STS and entering reference/baseline and current audiometric results.

The first method, current versus reference, represents the *most commonly used method* utilized for compliance with the OSH Act of 1983 [8]. This technique does not consider differences between *each* periodic audiometric examination; that is, only hearing levels recorded on the current audiogram are compared against the baseline.

Comparing Threshold Shifts Between Sequential Audiograms

The second approach (current versus preceding test results), although not an OSHA compliance, may be employed in conjunction with the first [19, 25, 26, 28, 31]. *Hearing level differences between sequential records* are studied in an attempt to discover early STS "trends." Evidence of such trends can alert OHCP providers that slight but consistent alterations or shifts in hearing may be occurring *before* cumulative hearing shift increments would total enough to "trigger" STS [10, 18]. Table 16-9 illustrates how this "trend scheme" can reveal shifts *before* the boundary of OSHA STS is reached or exceeded.

Although STS computations noted between the fourth annual and baseline shown in Table 16-9 did not reveal a "standard shift," results of the hearing levels during each annual examination disclosed a consistent *trend.* Though subtle, an astute observer will note that the hearing levels reflect a progressive but consistent direction of change. Evidence of such a trend would suggest further analysis of the affected employee's auditory risk factors and adequacy of HPDs. Combining these two strategies can enhance the quality of the OHCP and more easily identify shifts in hearing [10].

Accounting for Presbycusis (Aging)

Although aging influences the status of hearing, generally its effects do not become apparent until an individual is 45 to 50 years of age [2, 5, 32]. The term *presbycusis* refers to changes in audition directly associated with aging. Studies that report hearing levels according to age as the only parameter (presbycusis) typically exclude hearing data reflecting diseases or disorders that can affect hearing, including noise. *Sociocusis,* a more appropriate name, refers not only to hearing affected by the aging process but includes acquired diseases and hazards (including noises) associated with modern living [2, 5].

If clinicians wish to assess the extent to which "aging" has contributed to observed thresholds for an individual, a set of presbycusis hearing data (separately for men and women) may be used to "adjust" the current thresholds at different test frequencies (see Tables F-1 for men, F-2 for women, p. 9782 in the Appendix of [8]).

Table 16-7. Comparison of an annual and reference (baseline) where STS finding is negative

Hearing thresholds on:	Frequency (Hz)*											
	Left ear						Right ear					
	500	1000	2000	3000	4000	6000	500	1000	2000	3000	4000	6000
Current (annual)	10	0	0	10	10	20	5	5	5	10	15	15
Reference	5	0	0	15	15	10	0	5	5	15	20	10
Threshold shifts	+5	0	0	-5	-5	+10	+5	0	0	-5	-5	+5
Av. @ 2/3/4 kHz*				-3.3						-3.3		

*2/3/4 kHz = 2000, 3000, 4000 Hz.

Table 16-8. Comparison of an annual and reference (baseline) where STS finding is positive

Hearing thresholds on:	Frequency (Hz)*											
	Left ear						Right ear					
	500	1000	2000	3000	4000	6000	500	1000	2000	3000	4000	6000
Current (annual)	10	0	0	25	40	25	5	5	5	20	55	20
Reference	5	0	0	15	15	20	0	5	5	15	20	15
Threshold shifts	+5	0	0	+10	+25	+5	+5	0	0	+5	+35	+5
Av. @ 2/3/4 kHz*				+11.7						+13.3		

*2/3/4 kHz = 2000, 3000, 4000 Hz.

Name (L/F/MI):		Date (M/D/Y):
Examiner's name:	Audiometer:	Date last cal.
Hours/minutes since last noise exposure: _____		Type of noise exposure:
Hearing protection worn while in noise prior to this current audiometric exam? [__] No; [__] Yes		

	Left ear						Right ear					
Freq. (Hz) =	500	1000	2000	3000	4000	6000	500	1000	2000	3000	4000	6000
Current audio												
Reference audio												
Subtract ref. from current*												
Total HTLs @ 2/3/4 kHz	xxxx xxxx	xxxx xxxx				xxxx xxxx	xxxx xxxx	xxxx xxxx				xxxx xxxx

* If HTL of current is poorer (greater) than reference, enter + before sum and if better (less) than reference, enter − before sum; if no difference, enter 0.
Note: To compute STS, add HTLs at 2000, 3000, and 4000 Hz separately for each ear. If totals for these three frequencies equal or exceed 30 dB, then STS is "yes," if 29 dB or less, then STS is "no."

Findings: STS (Check) [__] No; [__] Yes	Follow-up action; If STS is "No" [__] return in 12 mos; "Yes" [__] retest

If re-testing required, schedule audio following minimum of 14 hours of noise-free activity. Enter following:
1) Date rescheduled: _____; 2) Time: _____

Comments:

Figure 16-1. Sample form for computing standard threshold shift (STS) using the 1983 OSHA criterion.

Unless concerns related to compensation or legal factors are involved, however, corrections for aging when performing routine STS comparisons are not usually recommended or performed [11].

Even casual inspection of equivalent age-related hearing data reveals poorer hearing among men than women. Aging tends to alter hearing more dramatically within the higher frequencies, but reveals relatively minor alterations within the primary speech-hearing range (i.e., at and below 2000 or 3000 Hz).

Correcting Noise-Induced Hearing Losses: Medical Alternatives

Unfortunately, little can be done to restore normal auditory function for those who have experienced noise-induced hearing losses. Many who have lost substantial hearing due to noise have discovered that a hearing aid fails to restore functionally "normal" hearing [6, 7]. These people also have considerable difficulty hearing in the presence of background noise and differentiating between competing messages [5].

Table 16-9. Results of sequential (longitudinal) audiometric monitoring revealing threshold shift trends before OSHA standard threshold shift achieved

Hearing thresholds on:	Frequency (Hz)*											
	Left ear						Right ear					
	500	1000	2000	3000	4000	6000	500	1000	2000	3000	4000	6000
Reference	5	0	0	10	10	5	0	5	5	10	10	10
1st annual	0	0	0	10	10	10	5	5	5	10	15	10
2nd annual	5	5	0	10	15	10	0	5	5	15	20	15
3rd annual	0	5	5	15	15	15	5	5	5	15	25	10
4th annual	5	5	10	15	20	20	0	5	5	20	25	15
Threshold shifts relative to 4th	0	+5	+10	+5	+10	+5	0	0	0	+10	+15	+5
Av. @ 2/3/4 kHz*				+8.3						+8.3		

*2/3/4 kHz = 2000, 3000, 4000 Hz.

The fields of medicine and electronics are severely limited in restoring normal hearing function for those whose hearing has been impaired by overexposures to noise. Most critical: Once a person has acquired a noticeable noise-induced hearing impairment, every encounter with loud sounds and noises must be avoided to ensure that further and more debilitating impairment does not occur.

Nonauditory Effects of Noise

Nonauditory effects of noise are neither well defined nor established; however, studies suggest that certain adverse health effects may be directly or indirectly associated with noise. Most people have experienced a startle response to sound, such as the screeching of brakes while crossing a busy intersection or the sudden sounding of a fire alarm in a building corridor. The response to such sounds may elicit mild to moderate physiologic responses, including fear reactions that may result in release of catecholamines associated with increased heart rate and elevated blood pressure. Although physiologic reactions can also be associated with noise, such as hearing a radio blaring in the next apartment or members of an audience speaking loudly during a performance, such reactions are difficult to measure and quantify objectively. It is obvious that different people respond differently. Similarly, noises in both work and nonwork settings, even recreational activities, may contribute to stressful reactions.

Noise can affect heart rate or rhythm, increase blood pressure, and cause temporary increases in blood cholesterol levels and certain hormones [33, 34]. Long-term effects may also be associated with cardiovascular and circulatory problems [33]. Disturbances in sleep secondary to noise can contribute to general fatigue, including lapses of attention or concentration during the next day. Mental health and ability to learn may be compromised if noise invades the learning area. Overall productivity and work efficiency can also be impaired [34].

The World Health Organization [33] summarized several nonauditory phenomena associated with noise: (1) interference with sleep and modifications of body functions during sleep; (2) stress-related responses, including adrenal gland secretions, such as epinephrine and norepinephrine; (3) circulatory system responses, such as vasoconstriction or vasodilation of blood vessels (during high levels of noise exposure) and increases in blood pressure; (4) startle responses and reflexes that may elicit catecholamine secretion; and (5) vestibular or equilibrium alterations.

The World Health Organization report also identified symptoms of nausea, headache, irritability, reduction in sexual drive, anxiety, nervousness, insomnia, irritability, abnormal somnolence, and loss of appetite [33]. These reactions, of course, may not be associated solely with noise, but nonetheless their presence should alert clinicians to consider noise when a patient exhibits symptoms or complaints that are otherwise not explainable.

Acute Acoustic Trauma

Unprotected exposure to very loud noises above about 140 dB, such as a ballistic blast or explosions, may damage the ear [1, 5, 35]. Typically, unprotected exposures in very high noise levels (above 140 dB) elicit physical discomfort and increase the potential for acoustic trauma. When a clinician evaluates a patient suffering from some type of acoustic trauma, the details of the event associated with the insult are generally unique and the source, time, and date of the occurrence can be determined [1, 5].

Clinical features of an acute acoustic trauma typically include a vivid recall of the exposure, a sudden change in the status of hearing immediately following the encounter, possibly dizziness, and/or evidence of physical injury to the tympanic membrane(s) [1, 5]. One distinguishing feature of acoustic trauma resulting from steady-state noise and impulse or impact (including blast or explosion) exposures is the difference in injury observed between ears. Generally, blasts or explosion type exposures tend to cause more damage to the ear closest to the source of the overpressures [1, 5], whereas a very loud steady-state type noise has more equal bilateral effects.

Physical injury to the tympanic membrane may also be accompanied by dislocation of the ossicular chain and may be accompanied by a permanent sensorineural hearing loss. In such instances, audiologic findings typically reveal both conductive and sensorineural effects. Fortunately, most acoustic trauma can be avoided with the use of HPDs. Therefore, noises from blasts, explosions, and rapid releases of air from pneumatic sources should be anticipated and hearing protection worn [10].

Following acute trauma, several days or months may be required before hearing stabilizes. Periodic audiometric examinations should be performed until a plateau is apparent and hearing has stabilized.

References

1. Ades, H. W., et al. *An Exploratory Study of the Biological Effects of Noise (BENOX Report).* Office of Naval Research Report of Project 144079. Chicago: University of Chicago, December 1, 1953.
2. Cohen, A., Anticaglia, J., and Jones, H. H. Sociocusis: Hearing loss from non-occupational noise exposure. *Sound Vibration* 4:12, 1970.
3. NIOSH. *Criteria for a Recommended Standard—Occupational Exposure to Noise.* HSM 73-11001. Washington, DC: National Institute of Occupational Safety and Health, 1972.
4. Davis, A. C., et al. *Damage to Hearing from Leisure Noise: A Review of the Literature.* MRC Institute of Hearing Research. Nottingham, England: University of Nottingham, 1985.
5. Alberti, P. W. Noise and the Ear. In J. Ballantyne and J. Groves (eds.), *Scott-Brown's Diseases of the Ear, Nose and Throat* (4th ed.). Boston: Butterworth, 1979, Vol. 2, Chap. 18, pp. 551–622.
6. Sprinkle, P. M., and Bodenheimier, W. G. The Otolaryngologists and the Occupational Safety and Health Act. In M. M. Paparella and D. A. Shumrick, *Otolaryngology* (2nd ed.). Philadelphia: Saunders, 1980. Vol. 2, sec. 2, pp. 1275–1286.
7. Silverman, S. R. Rehabilitative Audiology. In M. M. Paparella and D. A. Shumrick, *Otolaryngology* (2nd ed.). Philadelphia: Saunders, 1980. Vol. 2, sec. 2, pp. 1287–1300.
8. Occupational Noise Exposure; Hearing Conservation Amendment; final rule. *Fed. Register.* 48(46):9737, March 8, 1983.
9. Leading work-related diseases and injuries—United States. *J.A.M.A.* 255:2133, 1986.
10. Gasaway, D. C. *Hearing Conservation: A Practical Manual and Guide.* Englewood Cliffs, NJ: Prentice-Hall, 1985.
11. American Academy of Otolaryngology–Head and Neck Surgery Foundation, Inc. *Guide for Conservation of Hearing in Noise* (rev. ed.). Rochester, MN: Custom Printing, 1982 (with Addendum, 1983).

12. Gasaway, D. C. How to Successfully Educate, Indoctrinate, and Motivate Workers. In D. C. Gasaway, *Hearing Conservation: A Practical Manual and Guide.* Englewood Cliffs, NJ: Prentice-Hall, 1985. Chapter 6, pp. 85–102.
13. Berger, E., et al (eds.). *Noise and Hearing Conservation Manual* (4th ed.). Akron, OH: American Industrial Hygiene Association, 1986.
14. Feldman, A. S., and Grimes, C. I. (eds). *Hearing Conservation in Industry.* Baltimore: Williams & Wilkins, 1985.
15. *Guide to the Evaluation of Permanent Impairment* (2nd ed.). Chicago: American Medical Association, 1984.
16. Ogusthorpe, J. D. (ed.). *Guide for Conservation of Hearing in Noise* (4th rev.). Washington, DC: American Academy of Otolaryngology–Head and Neck Surgery Foundation, 1988.
17. Nabelek, I. V. Noise Measurement and Engineering Controls. In A. S. Feldman and C. I. Grimes (eds.), *Hearing Conservation in Industry.* Baltimore: Williams & Wilkins, 1985. Pp. 27–76.
18. Royster, J. D., and Royster, L. H. *Hearing Conservation Programs: Practical Guidelines for Success.* Chelsea, MI: Lewis, 1990.
19. Suter, A. H., and Franks, J. R. (eds.). *A Practical Guide to Effective Hearing Conservation Programs in the Workplace.* Report no. 90-120. Cincinnati: US Department of Health and Human Services, National Institute for Occupational Safety and Health, 1990.
20. Gasaway, D. C. Sabotage can wreck hearing conservation programs. *Natl. Saf. News* 129:56, 1984.
21. Royster, L. H., and Royster, J. D. Hearing Protection Devices. In A. S. Feldman and C. I. Grimes (eds.), *Hearing Conservation in Industry.* Baltimore: Williams & Wilkins, 1985. Chap. 6, pp. 103–155.
22. Gasaway, D. C. Thirteen steps to developing an effective hearing protection program. *Plant Engineering* 41:51, February 26, 1987.
23. Berger, E. H. Using the NRR to estimate the real world performance of hearing protectors. *Sound Vibration* 17:12, 1983.
24. Noise Survey Data (Chap. VI; Change 6, OSHA 3058). In *Industrial Hygiene Field Operations Manual.* Washington, DC: US Department of Labor (OSHA), March 30, 1984.
25. Gasaway, D. C. Purpose of audiometric tests important in defining procedures. *Occup. Health Saf.* 54:61, 1985.
26. Sataloff, R. T., and Sataloff, J. Improving hearing conservation in the industrial workplace setting. *Occup. Health Saf.* 56:35, 1987.
27. US General Accounting Office. *To Provide Proper Compensation for Hearing Impairments, the Labor Department Should Change its Criteria.* Report HRD-78-67. Washington, DC: US GAO, June 1978.
28. Gasaway, D. C. Documentation: The weak link in audiometric monitoring programs. *Occup. Health Saf.* 54:28, 1985.
29. Cooper, S. Making records work for you. *Spectrum* (National Hearing Conservation News Letter) 7:12, Winter 1990.
30. Gasaway, D. C. *Occupational Hearing Conservation: Practical Guidelines for Compliance with OSHA Standard. Labor Relations Guide.* Paramus, NJ: Prentice-Hall Information Services, March 13, 1987. Insert Chap. 40.058, pp. 40, 231–245.
31. Franks, J. R., Davis, R. R., and Kreig, E. F., Jr. Analysis of a hearing conservation program data base: Factors other than workplace noise. *Ear and Hearing* 10:273, 1989.
32. Dobie, R. A. The relative contributions of occupational noise and aging in individual cases of hearing loss. *Ear and Hearing* 13:19, 1992.
33. WHO. Noise: Environmental Health Criteria 12. Geneva, Switzerland: World Health Organization, 1980.
34. Jones, D. M., and Broadbent, D. E. Human Performance and Noise. In C. M. Harris (ed.), Handbook of Acoustical Measurements and Noise Control (3d ed.). New York: McGraw-Hill, 1991. Chap. 24, pp. 24.1–24.24.
35. Jansen, G. Physiological Effects of Noise. In C. M. Harris (ed.), Handbook of Acoustical Measurements and Noise Control (3d ed.). New York: McGraw-Hill, 1991. Chap. 25, pp. 25.1–25.19.

Further Information

Berger, E. H., et al. (eds.). *Noise and Hearing Conservation Manual* (4th ed.). Akron, OH: American Industrial Hygiene Association, 1986.
An updated and expanded version of one of the most frequently referred to guides for industrial hygienists and others who are seeking detailed and scientific summaries of noise measurement, analysis, and elements of occupational hearing conservation.

Royster, J. D., and Royster, L. H. *Hearing Conservation Programs: Practical Guidelines for Success.* Chelsea, MI: Lewis, 1990.
A guide that provides brief but pertinent considerations for establishing, conducting, and evaluating the effectiveness of an occupational hearing conservation program.

Suter, A. K., and Franks, J. R. (eds.). *A Practical Guide to Effective Hearing Conservation Programs in the Workplace.* Publication no. 90-120. Cincinnati: US Department of Health and Human Services (National Institute of Occupational Safety and Health), September 1990.
A guide that incorporates concepts and techniques considered important by a group of US hearing conservation authorities to ensure that an occupational hearing conservation program is effective. Contents are directed at employers, middle management, health and safety representatives, noise-exposed employees, and others involved in such programs.

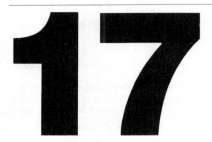

Occupational Skin Disorders

Steven K. Shama

Occupational dermatoses comprise those disorders of the skin *caused by or made worse by* components of the workplace environment. Physicians engaged in evaluating occupational dermatoses should be familiar with the importance of their appearance, causes, methods of evaluation, diagnosis, treatment, and prevention. This chapter reviews these topics; however, for a comprehensive discussion of occupational skin diseases the reader should seek other sources listed under Further Information. This chapter stresses contact dermatitis, which composes approximately 90% of all occupational skin afflictions. Table 17-1 reviews the various occupational skin diseases, which are discussed more completely elsewhere.

Significance of Occupational Dermatoses

Of all occupational illnesses, skin disorders are one of the most common and compose about 40% of all reported cases [1]. The cost to both workers and industry is great. Workers often lose pay for occasional days off because of skin disorders or may be transferred to job responsibilities that can result in a decrease in pay and loss of seniority. Some workers may be dismissed before an accurate assessment of the nature of their disease is made and may be unable to find similar work because of their history of skin problems. For industry, occupational skin disease may result in less productive workers, rehabilitation costs, workers' compensation litigation, and rehiring and retraining of new workers to fill open positions. Higher insurance costs may also result. The cost to industry for occupational skin disease is estimated to exceed $22 million per year; a figure of $200 million to $1 billion may be more accurate when underreporting is considered [2]. For example, in certain states, an occupational disorder is reported only if a skin disease is *caused* by work and not when a preexisting disease is *made worse* by work. In addition, in some states such as Massachusetts, problems due to work are reported only if they cause more than *5 successive days* of lost time; many skin disorders that are occupational in origin may not result in a lost workday but nevertheless can be troublesome to the worker. Underreporting may also be due to either the worker or physician, or both, failing to associate the skin disorder with workplace activities. Finally, workers may be afraid to report a skin condition for fear of losing their job.

Evaluation of Occupational Dermatoses

It is critical to evaluate a potential occupational skin disorder thoroughly to enable the worker to benefit from appropriate diagnosis and treatment. It is not unusual for both management and worker to want some quick answer to the worker's problem so that both can get on with the job and compensation claims. However, once the worker is labeled, whether properly or not, the label may be difficult to change and may make the worker ineligible for many other positions in the same or other industries. If the diagnosis is incorrect, the worker may be destined to have a chronic dermatitis that may never totally clear. The worker may wander from one industry to the next, one job to another, without a true understanding of why the skin eruption fails to clear. Therefore, the answer to many occupational skin diseases is not a simple job change but a *full* evaluation of the problem when it initially develops.

Evaluations of occupational skin disorders should be made by specialists whenever feasible; however, the primary care physician is often the first to be consulted.

Table 17-1. Causes of occupational dermatoses

Chemical
Irritant
  Absolute—immediate first-contact inflammatory reaction of skin—*strong bases and acid* (potassium hydroxide, ethylene oxide)
  Marginal—repeated contact (kerosene, various cutting fluids)
Allergens (epoxy resins, chemicals used in making of rubber, chromates, nickel)

Mechanical
Friction—calluses, abrasions, lichenification of skin (violinist's neck, knuckle pads in carpet layers), Koebner's phenomenon (development of lesions of psoriasis or lichen planus, in worker predisposed to having either of these skin disorders, in traumatized area of skin)
Pressure—blisters, nail dystrophy
Vibration—vibration-induced white fingers or Raynaud's disease (certain types of vibrating equipment)

Physical
Heat—burns, sweating (miliaria, intertriginous rashes)
Cold—frostbite, Raynaud's symptoms
Radiation—radiation dermatitis, skin cancers (x-ray exposure), photosensitivity eruptions—phytophotodermatitis (eruption from contact with plant containing furocoumarin in presence of light)

Biologic
Plants—poison ivy, oak, and sumac (forest fire fighters)
Insects—Lyme disease (from bite of tick in forester)
Animals—orf (viral eruption from infected sheep)
Microbiologic agents
  Viruses—herpetic whitlow (herpes simplex of finger in dentists)
  Bacterial—anthrax (contact with spores in contaminated goat hair)
  Fungal—*Mycobacterium marinum* (fish tank cleaners)
  Rickettsial—Rocky Mountain spotted fever (tick bite in dog handler)
  Protozoa—*Plasmodium* (Causing malaria from mosquito bite in laboratory worker)
  Helminthes—*Ancylostoma braziliense* (causing cutaneous larva migrans—skin eruption in workers who are exposed to organism from infected soil)

Source: Adapted from National Institute for Occupational Safety and Health. Occupational dermatoses: A program for physicians. 114 teaching slides on recognition, control and prevention of occupational skin disease.

Inherent difficulties in investigating occupational skin diseases include legal aspects of compensation cases such as report writing and dealing with lawyers and labor unions. In addition, since these investigations frequently need strong support from both management and labor, the potential for frustration on the part of the physician is great.

Skin disorders caused by work have a number of clinical patterns, including redness, scaling, vesicles, bullous lesions, and crusts (Table 17-2). Irritant and/or allergic contact dermatitis constitute 80 to 90% of all occupational skin diseases. Irritant contact dermatitis represents 80% of all of the contact dermatitis problems of industry. *Irritant reactions* are caused by substances that damage the skin at the *site of contact* by *nonimmunologic* mechanisms. Irritants, in general, are substances that cause injury to most individuals if given sufficient concentration and time of exposure. In contrast, *allergic contact reactions* require a *cell-mediated hypersensitivity* mechanism, and generally a smaller number of workers are affected. Patch testing can be, in many instances, proof that sensitization has taken place that has resulted in allergic contact dermatitis. On the other hand, there is no scientific test to establish the presence of an *irritant* reaction, which is established by clinical evaluation and knowledge of the toxicity of workplace substances. For the clinician, information regarding a substance's potential for causing a contact dermatitis of the

Table 17-2. Common clinical expressions of occupational skin diseases*

Skin disease	Clinical expression
Eczematous dermatitis	Irritant or allergic contact dermatitis—acute blistering reactions (hydrofluoric acid) to chronic rough scaling and thickened skin (chronic terpentine exposure)
Acneiform	Diffuse open and closed comedones and straw-colored cysts of face (chloracne—from certain halogenated aromatic compounds)
	Scattered open and closed comedones and cysts of face and chest (acne—heavy oil exposures)
Pigmentation changes	Hypopigmentation (especially hands—some phenolic compounds)
	Hyperpigmentation (any inflammatory process, especially in dark-skinned individuals)
Tumors	Malignant—squamous cell carcinoma (from x-ray exposure), basal cell carcinoma (from chronic sun exposure)
Miliaria	Diffuse papulovesicular eruption—usually trunk and intertriginous areas (from excessive heat exposure)
Urticarial	Local or generalized hives (from ammonium persulfate—hairdresser; acrylic monomer—plastics industry)
Granulomas	Nodules of skin
	Foreign body (silica)
	Allergic (beryllium)
	Infectious (sporotrichosis—*Sporotrichum schenckii*)
Ulcerations	Acute in onset (ethylene oxide)
	Insidious and chronic (chromic acid)

* See Plates 1–10.

skin can be obtained from the Material Safety Data Sheet. As discussed in Chap. 2, the Hazard Communication Standard stipulates that all workers in certain industries should be informed about the materials with which they work and their respective toxicity. In most cases, the first step in evaluating a potential occupational skin disease is to suggest that the worker bring in the data sheets for all substances the worker may use in the course of his or her job duties.

Allergic and irritant skin reactions generally cannot be differentiated by their clinical expressions. Both may have similar skin changes. Skin biopsies are also not generally useful. While it may be possible to separate an allergic from an irritant contact dermatitis during the first 24 to 48 hours after exposure by biopsy, most reactions are seen after this time when the classic pathologic differences overlap.

History and Physical Examination

Although the most common setting for the evaluation of an occupational skin disorder is the physician's office, a review of the workplace can be invaluable. It is the workplace where the physician can associate skin changes with certain hazardous substances with some certainty. A comprehensive history and physical examination, however, are always necessary to determine the cause of the skin eruption. In these often controversial settings, the physician is best considered an *objective* consultant. The *company does not lose* when the examining physician determines that an occupational skin disorder exists. Similarly, the *worker does not lose* when a skin disorder is attributed to nonoccupational causes. A proper diagnosis benefits both parties.

Questions To Ask (Table 17-3)

Where on Your Skin Is the Problem, and Where Did It Begin?

Many occupational skin eruptions begin on *exposed* skin. If seen in its earliest stages, a hand dermatitis may show a sharp cutoff at the wrist (where long-sleeved shirts protect the forearm). Similarly, facial eruptions may stop abruptly at the neck where the shirt collar begins (Fig. 17-1). However, as a dermatitis persists, it may involve *contiguous areas* of skin and *distant sites,* a process known as autoeczematization or an id reaction. If seen during this flare stage, the eruption can be misdiagnosed as a nonspecific eczema unless one is careful to ask *where the eruption began.* Knowing where the rash began can also rule out an occupational disorder. For example, if one is assuming an airborne contact as a cause and the first expression of the rash was in a covered area of the chest (and not the face or hands), the case for an airborne exposure is weakened.

Not all occupational skin disorders develop in exposed sites. If a worker is careful to wear gloves when handling corrosive or irritating liquids but has a habit of wiping soiled gloves on the trousers, the rash may initially develop on the thighs. A key question is to find out where the eruption began and to determine if known substances could have reached these sites.

When Did the Rash Begin?

Knowing the *date of onset* of the eruption helps in determining whether the eruption is related to some workplace activity such as a change in work practices or introduction of new materials. Skin eruptions may begin *insidiously,* thus requiring a number of weeks or months to become obvious. Try to find out when the *first signs* of skin irritation developed so that efforts can be made to relate them as closely as possible to some workplace activity or production change.

What Kind of Work Do You Do?

The worker needs to be *specific* so that the physician has a full understanding of job activities. All materials with potential for worker exposure, especially irritants or allergens, should be reviewed. Some workers may stress that they work with caustic liquids, but in fact one discovers that these substances are contained in totally enclosed systems and no skin contact is possible. Other workers may neglect to mention gross exposure to low-grade irritants, compounds they feel could not produce a skin rash. The physician should realize the importance of a thorough job history to avoid overlooking "trivial" exposures as a cause of the skin irritation. It is critical to establish whether the worker has the potential for a true contact with the materials in question and whether gloves or other personal protective equipment are used.

Table 17-3. Questions for a more effective history of occupational dermatoses

---

Where on your skin is the problem, and where did it begin?

When did the rash begin?

What kind of *work* do you do?

What happens to the skin condition on days off, on *vacations,* or when away from regular *job duties*?

What has been used to *treat* the condition?

Does the worker have any thoughts as to what might be the *cause* of the present skin problem?

Are *other workers* affected?

Have there been any *changes in work practices*?

Past history:
   Other skin disorders
   Previous contact allergies
   Previous jobs
   Hobbies
   Medications

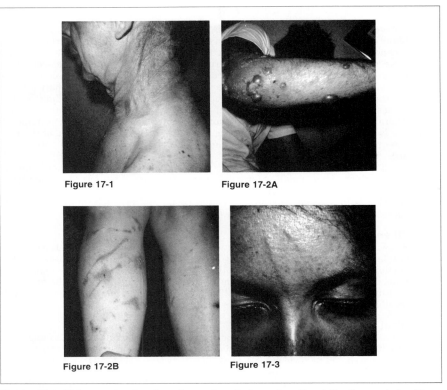

Figure 17-1   Figure 17-2A

Figure 17-2B   Figure 17-3

Figure 17-1. This eruption involves the neck and stops abruptly at the face and shoulders. The distribution suggests an airborne contactant, with the face protected by the full face mask the worker was using and the trunk protected by a shirt and collar.

Figure 17-2. The nature of this blistering rash on the forearm (A) is clearer when one notes the linear streaking on the leg (B)—a poison ivy contact dermatitis from a weekend hike in the woods.

Figure 17-3. This linear eruption in an office worker was caused by her habit of rubbing a pencil eraser on her face. An allergy to a rubber chemical was confirmed on patch testing.

What Happens to the Skin Condition on Days Off, on Vacations, or away from Job Duties?

In many cases of an occupational contact dermatitis, the eruption worsens as the work week progresses and stabilizes or lessens on weekends and vacations. However, after many months of recurrent eruptions, this pattern may change, and the skin irritation may not improve. The initial pattern of clearing following removal from certain job activities is helpful in establishing a potential link between the rash and an occupational substance.

What Has Been Used to Treat the Condition?

An eruption may not clear because of inadequate therapy or because the worker is using a preparation that is resulting in its own type of contact dermatitis. For example, Mycolog cream may have been effective for an innocent transient rash, but during its use the worker has become sensitized to the ethylenediamine, a preservative used in the cream. Continued use of the Mycolog prolongs the eruption, which is now due to an allergic contact dermatitis from ethylenediamine. (Mycolog II cream no longer contains ethylenediamine.) Therefore, all medication that has been used in an attempt to treat the eruption should be reviewed for possible secondary allergic contact dermatitis.

Does the Worker Have Any Thoughts as to What Might Be the Cause of the Present Skin Problem?

It is quite appropriate to ask the worker for whatever information he or she has with regard to the skin eruption. One should exercise judgment in sorting through the information that begins to accumulate, but never overlook the fact that it is often the worker who will suggest important possibilities that must be explored.

Are Other Workers Affected?

It is useful to know whether one is dealing with an *isolated* case (which may suggest an allergic contact dermatitis) or whether there are *numerous* cases (which suggest an irritant contact dermatitis). One should be cautioned, however, in evaluating alleged "cases," that interviews and examinations of these workers may uncover conditions not related to the present problem. In fact, these disorders may have antedated the current concern and be nonoccupational in origin [3].

Have There Been Any Changes in Work Practices?

A change in the rate of production may cause workers to work more quickly and overlook safe work practices. Sometimes, a *new material has been introduced* into the process, and shortly thereafter, a number of skin eruptions are noted.

One should also ask about protective gear that workers are using. Sometimes appropriate gloves are available, but replacement of the gloves is not done on a regular basis. Despite their wear, *gloves may be replaced only when workers feel they need to be replaced,* a practice that tends to allow for cracks to appear and thus contamination of the worker's skin.

One should also inquire about the kind of soap that is available in the workplace. Although a menagerie of work materials can cause a rash, recently introduced abrasive soaps may also be responsible for skin eruptions [4].

Past Medical History

Other skin disorders such as psoriasis should always be considered in the differential diagnosis. Always ask about past skin problems. A palmar eruption, for example, that one is labeling as an occupational contact dermatitis may, in fact, be an expression of psoriasis. Idiopathic lichen planus can also be confused with occupational skin eruptions.

Atopic individuals have a 13.5 times greater risk of developing an occupational skin problem, especially irritant reactions, than nonatopics. History of previous atopic dermatitis rather than previous respiratory allergies, is a better prognosticator of future work-related dermatitis [5].

Previous Contact Allergies

One should inquire about other contactants or substances that might have resulted in previous skin eruptions. Allergy to nickel has been associated with persistent and recurrent skin eruptions that are difficult to eliminate despite apparent cessation of contact [6].

Previous Jobs and Present Part-Time Jobs

A good occupational history of substances used in previous jobs can be helpful in evaluating the present eruption. For example, if a worker used an epoxy resin in the past (especially if there is a history of a rash during that time), one can focus on the role of the epoxy resin during the present job. A history of irritant dermatitis secondary to wet work in previous jobs can suggest that a similar problem is recurring.

One should also ask about part-time work a person may have. Although the physician may not uncover a cause for a skin eruption in company A where no obvious problems exist, finding out that the affected employee is a part-time hair stylist in company B (where numerous opportunities for irritant exposures exist) can uncover the problem.

Hobbies

More opportunities for the development of contact dermatitis may exist in many hobbies compared to industrial settings. Examples include epoxy resins and other glues used in model airplane building. Inquiring about what the person does in spare-time activities can yield valuable diagnostic clues.

Medications

Knowing what medications a worker is taking can occasionally be the answer to an unusual contact dermatitis. For example, a worker may have become sensitized to ethylenediamine from Mycolog cream that was used for a hand rash. Although the rash may have totally cleared (and been clear for a number of years), it may recur when this worker takes aminophylline for asthma. This subsequent hand rash may then be blamed on a workplace substance but in fact be due to aminophylline, a combination of theophylline and ethylenediamine. Ingestion of ethylenediamine in patients previously skin sensitized can result in dermatitis at the same site as the original sensitization. This phenomenon can also occur with other compounds, such as with the diphenhydramine (Benadryl) in Caladryl; ingestion of Benadryl then leads to the rash.

Physical Examination

A *complete skin examination* is necessary to determine the presence of other dermatologic conditions, such as psoriasis, lichen planus, or eczema, that may explain the present skin condition of alleged occupational origin. The physician should be advised, however, that the worker may not be aware of these conditions.

A thorough skin examination can determine the extent of the eruption, which will ultimately influence both the person's capability of returning to work and the aggressiveness of therapy. Mild local eruptions can be treated without interruption of job duties, but extensive rashes often require both time off and aggressive treatment. Determination of the distribution of the rash can aid in the diagnosis. Rashes involving the face and hands, for example, suggest contact dermatitis possibly due to an airborne contactant. Rashes that have the same shape as a piece of clothing (e.g., the waistband of underwear) suggest an allergy to the elastic and not an occupational exposure. Rashes with a linear or angular appearance suggest a contact dermatitis but not necessarily of occupational cause (Figs. 17-2 and 17-3).

Worksite Evaluation

The best place to evaluate an occupational skin disease is at the workplace. Planning a worksite visit, however, requires diplomacy to be successful. The physician must have a good working relationship with management and labor and avoid any hint of bias. The physician needs to emphasize that the goal is toward *health* and that a number of roles, including that of scientist, detective, industrial hygienist, and epidemiologist, are necessary. If one loses the trust of any member of the workforce, the investigation becomes more difficult and sometimes impossible.

Whenever possible, *the physician should tour the plant with representatives of all interested groups* but insist that someone familiar with both production and substances used be available to answer questions of a technical nature. It is important to get *an overview of the process of production,* including the various stages and potential for exposure to hazardous materials. Therefore, one needs to *tour the entire work facilities.* Then one can become more specific in the evaluation of the individual worker. Ideally, one should watch the worker perform the task, especially so-called normal operations. *It is also very helpful to see the "normal problems" that arise throughout the day.* There may be no physical contact with chemicals of concern during normal operations, but when a machine breaks down, which may be often, ample opportunity for gross exposure may exist. One should *note the protective gear* that a worker uses, as well as *personal hygiene,* such as eating and smoking habits. A sloppily attired worker who eats and smokes close to the work area may have more exposure to irritant chemicals during such activities than when operating machinery.

After a plant tour, the physician should have a thorough understanding of the potential for certain materials to cause skin irritations. A closing meeting with both management and labor is suggested so that the physician can summarize impressions, ask additional questions, and make appropriate recommendations. Specific conclusions, however, are not recommended at this time because additional information may need to be obtained and reviewed.

Based on an office evaluation and a worksite visit, one can formulate an opinion as to whether an occupational skin disease exists. This opinion is based on the history, appearance, and distribution of the rash; a review of workplace materials (including hobbies); and a physical examination. If an irritant or an allergic contact dermatitis is suspected, removal of the allergen or irritant is indicated. If the rash improves, the diagnostic accuracy of an occupational skin disorder is enhanced.

The Role of Patch Testing

If an *allergen* is believed to be the cause of an occupational skin disease, patch tests can be a valuable laboratory test to add scientific support to one's diagnosis. For this type of testing, the clinician is advised to refer the patient to a dermatologist who has experience in this area. The following discussion is designed to offer the physician an understanding of what one should expect from this procedure in terms of uncovering the cause of an unusual skin eruption. Patch tests reveal *only* allergic contact sensitization and cannot be used to determine the presence of an irritant contact dermatitis. Patch testing involves a standardized application of chemicals (in a nonirritating concentration) onto the skin of the patient. Either strips of cellulose disks (Al-test) or aluminum chambers (Finn Chambers) are applied to the skin, generally to the back for 48 hours, after which the test strips are removed and the areas examined. The test sites are reevaluated again after an additional 48 hours. True allergens have a fairly typical reaction at the site of application; however, both false-positive and false-negative reactions can occur, and thus a great deal of observer experience is necessary.

Patch testing has certain limitations. For example, one cannot simply take a number of unknown compounds from the worksite area and apply them to a worker's back. Such compounds may be primary irritants and can lead to false-positive reactions. Patch testing can also sensitize the worker to a number of different substances to which sensitization did not exist. The reader is referred to some excellent texts noted under Further Information for further discussion of the role of patch testing in diagnosing occupational skin diseases.

Exposure Prevention

After determining the presence of either allergic contact dermatitis or an irritant contact reaction and its respective cause, the physician should then advise that the worker avoid future exposure to the offending substance. A number of methods are available.

Engineering Controls

Material Selection
If a number of workers suffer from an allergy to an epoxy resin, it may be possible to use another substance that will not interfere with product quality.

Closed System
Rather than have a worker who is sensitized or irritated by certain chemicals directly handle such substances, a system can be designed that prevents any skin contact.

Ventilation
If an airborne contactant is the cause of the skin problem, the ventilation system may be altered to prevent or minimize skin contact.

Personal Protective Measures

In some cases, appropriate gloves can prevent skin irritations at work. Reasonable worker hygiene, such as not smoking, eating, or drinking at the work station, can be effective. Barrier creams, that is, *protective* creams or ointments, have been used in place of gloves in some settings. These creams, which may be used on the hands and other parts of the skin including the face, attempt to separate the skin from an irritating environment. At best, *barrier creams are a poor substitute for protective clothing* because the integrity of the so-called impenetrable barrier is difficult to maintain. The creams are much less effective than other types of skin protection. For example, they must be washed off during meals. On the other hand, such frequent washing also tends to keep the skin relatively free of irritating substances that might otherwise remain on the skin for many hours. Requiring workers to wash the barrier cream a number of times a day also increases their general cleanliness.

Administrative Controls

Certain managerial controls can be applied to decrease the possibility of an occupational skin disease. The *preplacement examination* is an excellent opportunity to sort out those workers who have a greater tendency of developing skin problems before they enter the workforce. Care should be exercised to make reasonable accommodations for workers who have a skin disorder disability recognized under the provisions of the Americans with Disabilities Act of 1990. An *atopic individual* who has had eczematous dermatitis, for example, may be at increased risk of skin irritation when working with certain materials. Similarly, a person with a *history of allergic reactions to certain substances* would be at risk of suffering an allergic response to related materials. In these types of situations, it would appear prudent to advise placement in another area. People with psoriasis, for example, especially of the hands, may suffer from more frequent and lengthy outbreaks if exposed to certain substances. It is advisable to review materials used in a facility to determine how serious the risk of skin irritation is and whether special measures are necessary.

When one is concerned about the potential for skin problems in a particular department that appears to be due to irritants, it may be possible to *rotate workers* on a regular basis out of the environment to prevent chronic skin irritation. Job rotations work, however, only when an irritant is involved. Allergy-based skin eruptions can only be prevented by absence of direct exposure. Finally, careful monitoring of the skin of workers exposed to skin irritants can uncover problems at a stage when intervention can prevent long-term consequences. Workers whose skin is adversely affected by certain materials can be treated early or removed from work for certain periods of time for a full evaluation and rest period.

Treatment

Topical Steroids

The nondermatologist often picks the lowest-potency topical steroid to treat a dramatic skin eruption, usually because the physician is not comfortable in prescribing higher-potency steroids. Unfortunately, this clinical approach may result in skin eruptions that would normally resolve in a few days taking weeks to clear. In fact, some eruptions may never clear because they were not treated aggressively initially. Occupational physicians are advised to become familiar with the broad range of *topical steroid creams* and to use high-potency steroids when appropriate (Table 17-4). Such potent steroids, however, should not be used to suppress a rash while a worker continues to work in the area in which the exposure to skin irritants may take place. If high-potency steroids are prescribed, the worker should be closely monitored; as soon as the eruption begins to clear, lower-potency steroids should be instituted.

In addition to topical steroids, the skin needs lubrication between applications of the steroid cream. Numerous lubricants are available; their effectiveness depends not so much on the type of lubricant but on the frequency of application. Some lubricants, for example, may be applied 10 to 15 times a day. On the other hand, topical steroids may become less effective if applied more than 3 times per day.

Antihistamines

Since many eczematous dermatitis eruptions itch, systemic antihistamines are often prescribed. However, such antihistamines are useful primarily for their antipruritic

Table 17-4. Topical steroids

Potency	Steroid (brand name)
Lowest	0.1% Dexamethasone (Decadron Phosphate, Decaderm)
	1.0% Hydrocortisone (Cort-Dome, Cortef, Penecort)
	2.5% Hydrocortisone (Penecort, Synacort, Hytone)
	0.25% Methylprednisolone acetate (Medrol)
	1.0% Methylprednisolone acetate (Medrol)
Low	0.01% Betamethasone valerate (Valisone)
	0.1% Clocortolone (Cloderm)
	0.05% Desonide (Desowen, Tridesilon)
	0.01% Fluocinolone acetonide (Synalar)
	0.025% Flurandrenolide (Cordran, Cordran SP)
	0.2% Hydrocortisone valerate (Westcort)
	0.025% Triamcinolone acetonide (Aristocort, Aristocort A, Kenalog)
Intermediate	0.1% Betamethasone valerate (Valisone)
	0.05% Desoximetasone (Topicort LP, Topicort Gel)
	0.025% Fluocinolone acetonide (Fluonid)
	0.05% Flurandrenolide (Cordran, Cordran SP)
	0.025% Halcinonide (Halog)
	0.12% Mometasone furoate (Elocon)
	0.1% Triamcinolone acetonide (Aristocort, Aristocort A, Kenalog)
High	0.1% Amcinonide (Cyclocort)
	0.05% Betamethasone dipropionate (Alphatrex, Diprosone)
	0.25% Desoximetasone (Topicort)
	0.05% Diflorasone diacetate (Florone, Maxiflor)
	0.2% Fluocinolone (Synalar HP)
	0.05% Fluocinonide (Lidex, Lidex-E)
	0.1% Halcinonide (Halog, Halog-E)
Highest (use should be supervised by a dermatologist)	0.05% Betamethasone dipropionate (Diprolene)
	0.05% Clobetasol propionate (Temovate)
	0.05% Diflorasone (Psorcon)
	0.05% Halobetasol propionate (Utravate)
	Treatment should be limited to 14 days and maximum of 50 g/week

Note: Only *lowest-potency steroids* should be used on face, neck, axilla, groin, perineum, and gluteal fold and any other intertriginous area. All topical steroids should be given for short periods of time and in limited quantities.
Source: Adapted from Topical corticosteroids. *Med. Lett.* 33:109, 1991.

effects, not for therapeutic effect on the rash. Therefore, to avoid sedation of the worker from the use of antihistamines, it is advisable to use potent topical steroids that have their own antipruritic effect.

Prednisone

In severe eruptions characterized by extensive involvement with weeping and inflammation, oral prednisone is a good choice. Generally if one prescribes 60 mg initially and then decreases the dosage by 5 mg each day over a 12-day period, almost all eczematous eruptions will clear, whether local or widespread. As with high-potency topical steroids, systemic prednisone therapy should not be given as a means of keeping a worker on the job when the environment is the cause of the persistent skin problems.

Hand Dermatitis

Hand dermatitis deserves special attention. Although the hand represents about 5% of the total body surface, when it is afflicted with dermatitis, one can become disabled from a variety of activities. When a weepy, blistery eruption leading to fissures occurs on the hand, for example, even if it occurs on only one or two fingers, the hand can be totally incapacitated. Therefore, any hand eruptions should be treated efficiently and aggressively.

In the general population, 1 to 2% of people have some type of hand dermatitis—for example, irritant and allergic contact dermatitis, atopic eczema, fungal infections, and others. When these people are followed over time, 34% of the hand eruptions are found to remain unchanged or to worsen [7]. The point to be recognized is that skin eruptions occur commonly in the general population, and they tend to become chronic, despite proper care and evaluation. Occupational hand dermatoses follow a similar pattern. Despite the best evaluations of occupational skin disease, some rashes may persist even after efforts to alter the job or work environment that was associated with the development of the skin eruption [8]. Therefore, one should not assume that a simple job change will necessarily eliminate the occupational skin disease. All efforts should be made to keep the worker on the same job if measures appear to be available to prevent recurrences of the skin reaction. Hand dermatitis may not improve because of improper diagnosis, failure to find the correct cause or to eliminate the cause completely, development of a secondary contact dermatitis not recognized, exposure to similar substances that cross-react with the primary allergen, or improper placing of the individual in a new irritating environment [9].

References

1. Wang, C. L. *The Problem of Skin Disease in Industry.* Office of Occupational Safety and Health Statistics. US Dept. of Labor, 1978.
2. Mathias, C. G. T. The cost of occupational skin disease. *Arch. Dermatol.* 121:332, 1985.
3. Rycroft, R. J. G. Occupational dermatoses in perspective. *Lancet* 2:24, 1980.
4. Mathias, C. G. T. Contact dermatitis from use or misuse of soaps, detergents and cleansers in the work place. *Occup. Med. State of the Art Rev.* 1:205, Apr–June 1986.
5. Shmunes, E., and Keil, J. E. The role of atopy in occupational dermatoses. *Contact Dermatitis* 2:174, 1984.
6. Christensen, O. B. Prognosis in nickel allergy and hand eczema. *Contact Dermatitis* 8:7, 1982.
7. Agrup, G. Hand eczema and other hand dermatoses in South Sweden. *Acta Derm. Venerol.* 49 (Suppl. 61):6, 1969.
8. Nethercott, J. R., and Gallant, C. Disability due to occupational contact dermatitis. *Occup. Med. State of the Art Rev.* 1:199, Apr–June 1986.
9. Committee on Occupational Dermatoses of the Council of Industrial Health. The problems of prolonged and recurrent industrial dermatitis. *J.A.M.A.* 168:516, 1958.

Further Information

Adams, R. M. *Occupational Skin Disease.* Philadelphia: Saunders, 1990.
This is an up-to-date major textbook on the subject. It is nicely written and includes chapters on most of the important topics, including patch testing, allergen concentration lists, and barrier creams. A must for those interested in occupational skin disease.

Arndt, K. A. *Manual of Dermatologic Therapeutics: With Essentials of Diagnosis* (4th ed.). Boston: Little, Brown, 1989.
A practical manual, discussing pathophysiology, diagnosis, and treatment of common skin disorders. Excellent discussions of products used in treatment, including numerous lubricants and topical steroid preparations.

Cronin, E. *Contact Dermatitis.* London: Churchill Livingstone, 1980.
Comprehensive text discussing many topics related to contact dermatitis in general and to occupational dermatoses specifically.

Epstein, E. Hand dermatitis: Practical management and current concepts. *J. Am. Dermatol.* 10:395, 1984.
A full and excellent discussion of hand dermatitis. Includes diagnostic possibilities and evaluation and extensive suggestions for therapy.

Fisher, A. A. *Contact Dermatitis* (3rd ed.). Philadelphia: Lea & Febiger, 1986. *A great general text on the subject with much relevance to occupational dermatitis; chapters on patch testing, allergen concentrations, and many other relevant topics.*

Leading work related diseases: Dermatologic conditions. *M.M.W.R.* 256:2312, 1986. *A summary of the major occupational skin disorders categorized by industry.*

The following articles relating to the practical aspects of occupational skin disease have been published in the *Occupational and Environmental Medicine Report.* Reprints are available from the publisher: OEM Press, 55 Tozer Road, Beverly, MA 01915.

Shama, S. K. *The dilemma of glove selection for industrial purposes. OEM Report* Vol. I, no. 3, 1987. P. 15.

Shama, S. K. *Connubial contact dermatitis. OEM Report* Vol. I, no. 5, 1987. P. 31.

Shama, S. K. *Occupational contact dermatitis in the electronics industry from soldering flux. OEM Report* Vol. II, no. 1, 1988. P. 2.

Shama, S. K. *Non-eczematous occupational dermatoses. OEM Report* Vol. II, no. 3, 1988. P. 22.

Shama, S. K. *Skin problems in video display terminal users. OEM Report* Vol. II, no. 5, 1988. P. 35.

Shama, S. K. *Glutaraldehyde: A cause of chronic hand dermatitis in health care workers. OEM Report* Vol. II, no. 10, 1988. P. 73.

Shama, S. K. *Skin and systemic reactions from carbonless copy paper. OEM Report* Vol. III, no. 1, 1989. P. 1.

Shama, S. K. *Chronic hand dermatitis in industry. OEM Report* Vol. III, no. 5, 1989. P. 38.

Shama, S. K. *Monitoring and updating patch test allergens used in the United States. OEM Report* Vol. III, no. 9, 1989. P. 69.

Shama, S. K. *When treatment becomes the cause: Corticosteroids as allergens in skin rashes. OEM Report* Vol. IV, no. 5, 1990. P. 35.

Shama, S. K. *Evaluating workers' disability claims for dermatitis. OEM Report* Vol. IV, no. 10, 1990. P. 73.

Shama, S. K. *Hand dermatitis from gloves. OEM Report* Vol. V, no. 5, 1991. P. 45.

Shama, S. K. *Reproducibility of patch test results. OEM Report* Vol. V, no. 11, 1991. P. 99.

Shama, S. K. *Education of the worker as a determinant of outcome in occupational contact dermatitis. OEM Report* 6:25,1992.

Shama, S. K. *The "paradoxical" rash of clothing dermatitis. OEM Report* 6:81,1992.

Appendix to Chapter 17: Some occupations and risk of dermatitis

Occupation	Irritants	Sensitizers	Contact urticaria
Agriculture (farmers, animal handlers, and keepers)	Artificial fertilizers, disinfectants and cleansers for milking utensils, petrol, diesel oil.	Rubber (boots, gloves, milking machines), cement, paints, local remedies for veterinary use, wood preservatives, plants, pesticides, antibiotics and preservatives in animal feed (quindoxin, ethoxyquine), penicillin for mastitis, cobalt in animal feed.	Animal hair.
Artists	Solvents, clay, plaster.	Turpentine, cobalt, nickel and chromate in pigments, azo dyes, colophony, epoxy-, acrylic-, formaldehyde-resins.	
Automobile mechanics	Solvents, oils, cutting oils, paints, hand cleansers.	Chromate (primers, anticorrosives, oils, welding fumes and cutting oils), nickel, cobalt, rubber, epoxy and acrylic resins, dipentene in thinners.	
Baking and pastrymaking	Flour, detergents.	Citrus fruits, flour improvers, thiamine, spices (cinnamon, cardamon), essential oils, food dyes.	
Bartenders	Detergents, citrus fruits.	Flavoring agents.	
Bathing attendants	Detergents.	Antimicrobial agents, formaldehyde, essential oils.	
Bookbinders	Glues, solvents, paper.	Glues, formaldehyde, plastic monomers.	
Building trade	Cement, chalk, hydrochloric and hydrofluoric acids, glasswool, wood preservatives, organic tin compounds.	Cement (chromate, cobalt), rubber and leather gloves, additives in shale oils, glues (phenol- or urea-formaldehyde resins), wood preservatives, teak, tar, epoxy resin, polyurethanes, rubber strip seals, joining material.	
Butchers	Detergents, meat, entrails.	Nickel	Animal tissues.
Canning industry	Brine, syrup, prawns and shrimps.	Asparagus, carrots, preservatives (hexamethylene tetramine in fish canning), rubber gloves.	Fruits, vegetables.
Carpenters, cabinetmakers, timbermen	French polish, solvents, glues, cleansers, wood preservatives (also phototoxic), glassfiber.	Exotic woods (teak, mahogany, rosewood, etc.) glues, polishes, turpentine, nickel, rubber (handles), colophony, epoxy-, acrylic- formaldehyde-, isocyanate-resins.	

(continued)

Occupation	Irritants	Sensitizers	Contact urticaria
Chemical and pharmaceutical industry	Numerous and specific for each working place.	Numerous and specific for each working place.	
Cleaning work	Detergents, solvents.	Rubber gloves, nickel, formaldehyde.	
Coal miners	Stone dust, coal dust, oil, grease, wood preservatives, cement, powdered limestone.	Rubber (boots), face masks, explosives, chromatic and cobalt in cement.	
Cooks, catering industry	Detergents, dressings, vinegar, fish, meat and vegetable juices.	Vegetables (onions, garlic, lemons, lettuce, artichokes), knife handles (exotic woods), spices, formaldehyde.	Meat, fish, fruits, vegetables.
Dentists and dental technicians	Soap, detergents, acrylic monomer, fluxes.	Local anesthetics (tetracaine, procaine), mercury, rubber, UV-hardening acrylates, acrylic monomer, disinfectants (formaldehyde, eugenol), nickel, epoxy resin (filling), methylmethacrylate, periodontal dressing (balsam of Peru, colophony, eugenol), the catalyst methyl-p-toluenesulfonate in plastics used for sealing teeth.	Saliva.
Dyers	Solvents, oxidizing and reducing agents, hypochlorite, hair removers.	Dyes, chromate, formaldehyde.	
Electricians	Soldering flux.	Soldering flux, insulating tape (rubber, resin, tar), rubber, nickel, bitumen, epoxy resins, glues (phenol-formaldehyde), polyurethanes.	
Enamel workers	Enamel powder.	Chromate, nickel, cobalt.	
Fishing	Wet work, friction, oils, petrol, redfeed from mackerel.	Tars, organic dyes in nets, rubber boots, rubber gloves.	Fish. "Aquatic irritant reactions" from toxins in sea organisms.
Floor layers	Solvents, detergents.	Chromate (cement), epoxy resin, glues (phenol- and urea-formaldehyde), exotic woods, acrylates, varnish (urea-formaldehyde), polyurethanes.	

(continued)

Occupation	Irritants	Sensitizers	Contact urticaria
Florists, gardeners, plant growers	Manure, bulbs, fertilizers, pesticides.	Plants (*Primula obconica*, chrysanthemum, tulips, narcissus, daffodils, alstromeria), formaldehyde, pesticides (e.g., thiuramsulfides), lichens (e.g., reindeer moss).	
Food industry, food handler	Detergents, vegetables.	Rubber gloves, spices, vegetables, preservatives.	Vegetables, fruit, meat, fish.
Foundry work	Oils, hand cleansers.	Phenol- and carbamide-formaldehyde-, furan-, epoxy-resins, chromate (cement, gloves, bricks).	
Glaziers	Rubber, epoxy resin, joining material, exotic wood.		
Hairdressers and barbers	Shampoos, soaps, permanent wave liquids, bleaching agents.	Hair and eyebrow dyes, rubber, nickel, perfumes.	Ammonium persulfate.
Histology technicians	Solvents, formaldehyde.	Formaldehyde, glutaraldehyde, organic dyes, acrylates.	
Hospital personnel	Disinfectants, quaternary ammonium compounds, hand creams, soaps, detergents.	Rubber gloves, formaldehyde, antibacterial agents, piperazine, phenothiazines, hand creams, nickel, glutaraldehyde, acrylic monomer, nitrogen mustard, local anesthetics.	
Household work	Detergents, wet work, solvents, polishes, vegetables.	Rubber (gloves), nickel, chromate, flowers and plants, turpentine (polishes), hand creams and lotions, handles of knives and irons, balsams, spices, citrus fruits.	Vegetables, fruit, meat, fish, spices.
Jewelers	Solvents, fluxes.	Nickel, epoxy resins, enamels (chromate, nickel, cobalt).	
Laundry workers	Detergents, bleaches, solvents.	Formaldehyde.	
Manicurists, beauticians	Wet work.	Formaldehyde, cosmetics, acrylic monomers (nails), nail polish (sulfonamide-formaldehyde plastic), perfume.	
Masons	Cement, chalk, bricks, acids.	Chromate and cobalt in cement, rubber and leather gloves, epoxy resin, exotic woods.	

(continued)

Plate 1 Eczema

An acute blistering irritant contact dermatitis to ethylene oxide is seen here. (NIOSH)

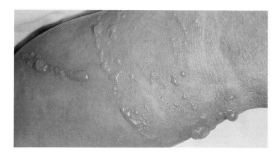

Plate 2 Eczema

These leathery-appearing hands are representative of chronic irritant dermatitis in a worker who uses kerosene to clean his hands. (NIOSH)

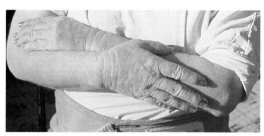

Plate 3 Acneiform

This car mechanic's forarms exhibit folliculitis from exposure to grease and lubricating oils. (NIOSH)

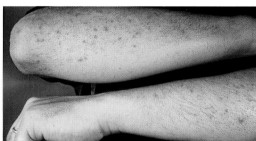
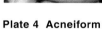

Plate 4 Acneiform

Exposure to certain halogenated aromatic chemicals by this worker led to this acne-like eruption, chloracne. It may be accompanied by stystemic toxicity. (*Cutis* 13:588, 1974)

Plate 5 Depigmentation

Depigmatation of hands of this hospital worker was the result of contact with phenolic germicidal detergent. (NIOSH)

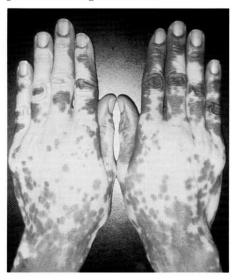
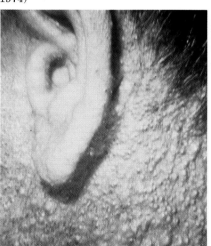

Plate 6 Tumors
Malignant tumors, such as this squamous cell carcinoma, can result from years of occupational exposure to both sunlight and coal tar (a carcinagen). (NIOSH)

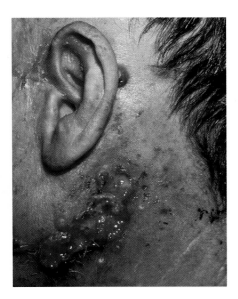

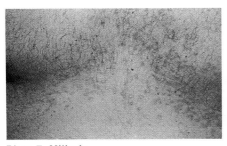

Plate 7 Miliaria
Excessive heat, leading to blockage of sweat ducts, can result in this bothersome eruption. (NIOSH)

Plate 8 Urticaria
Urticarial lesions develop on skin contact with a gypsy moth caterpillar. This worker in a forestry laboratory also had asthmatic attacks when in close proximity to this caterpillar (Courtesy of Dr. Shama).

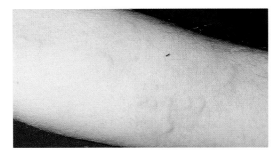

Plate 9 Granulomas
A chronic inflammatory allergic reaction to skin contact with beryllium can lead to granuloma formation. (NIOSH)

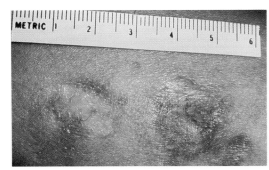

Plate 10 Ulcerations
Exposure to aerosolized chromic acid may result in painless ulceration of the nasal mucosa and septum. (NIOSH)

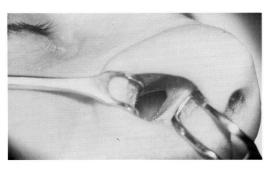

Occupation	Irritants	Sensitizers	Contact urticaria
Mechanics	Solvents, detergents, degreasers, lubricants, oils, cooling system fluids, battery acid, soldering flux.	Rubber, chromate, nickel, epoxy resin.	
Metal workers	Cutting and drilling oils, hand cleansers, solvents.	Nickel, chromate (antirust agents and dyes, welding fumes), cobalt, antibacterial agents and antioxidants in cutting oils. Chromate, cobalt, nickel may be found in cutting oil after it has been in use.	
Office workers	Photocopy paper, NCR paper.	Rubber (erasing rubber, mats, cords, finger stalls), nickel (clips, scissors, typewriters), copying papers, glue, feltpen dyes.	
Painters	Solvents, turpentine, thinner, paints, wallpaper adhesive.	Turpentine, thinner containing turpentine or dipentene (limonene), cobalt (dyes, driers), chromate (green, yellow), polyurethane-, epoxy-, acrylic-resins, glues (urea- and phenol-formaldehyde), varnish (colophony, urea-formaldehyde), preservatives in water-based paints and glues (e.g., chloracetamide, methylol-chloracetamide), putty (epoxy, acrylate, formaldehyde resins, polyurethane).	
Photography	Alkalis, reducing and oxidizing agents, solvents.	Metol (p-aminophenol), color developers (azo compounds), chromate, formaldehyde.	
Plastic industry	Solvents, styrene, oxidizing agents, acids.	Low molecular raw material, hardeners, additives, dyes.	
Platers	Solvents, paints.	Chromate in paints and on zinc galvanized sheets, glues.	
Plating industry, electroplating	Metal cleaners, alkalis, acids, detergents, heat, dust from metal blasting.	Chromate, nickel, cobalt, gold, mercury, rubber gloves.	
Plumbers	Oils, hand cleansers, soldering flux.	Rubber (gloves, packings, tubes), nickel, chromate (cement, antirust paint), glues, hydrazine.	

(continued)

Occupation	Irritants	Sensitizers	Contact urticaria
Printers	Solvents	Nickel, chromate, cobalt, colophony, paper finishes, glues, turpentine, azo dyes, formaldehyde, printing plates (acrylates and other chemicals), UV-hardening acrylates in printing ink, rubber gloves.	
Radio, television electronic repairmen	Soldering flux.	Soldering flux (hydrazine), epoxy resin, colophony (soldering), nickel, chromate.	
Restaurant personnel	Detergents, vegetables, citrus fruits, shrimps, herring.	Nickel, spices, vegetables, exotic wood (knife handle).	Vegetables, fruit, meat, fish.
Road workers	Sand/oil mixture, hand cleansers, asphalt (phototoxic).	Cement, gloves (leather, rubber), epoxy resin, tar, chromate in antirust paint.	
Rubber workers	Talcum, zinc stearate, solvents.	Rubber chemicals, organic dyes, tars, colophony, chromate, cobalt, phenol-formaldehyde resin.	
Shoemakers	Solvents.	Leather (formaldehyde, chromate, dyes), rubber, colophony, glues (e.g., p-tert. butylphenol-formaldehyde).	
Shop assistants	Detergents, vegetables, fruit, meat, fish.	Nickel.	Fruits, vegetables.
Tanners	Acids, alkalis, reducing and oxidizing agents.	Chromate, formaldehyde, vegetable tanning agents, glutaraldehyde, finishes, antimildew agents, dyes, resins.	
Textile workers	Solvents, bleaching agents, fibers.	Finishes (formaldehyde resins), dyes, mordants, nickel, diazo paper.	
Veterinarians	Hypochlorite, quaternary ammonium compounds, cresol, rectal and vaginal examination of cattle.	Rubber gloves, antibiotics (penicillin, streptomycin, neomycin, tylosine tartrate, virginiamycin), anti-mycotic agents. MBT in medicaments. (Tuberculin for injection in animals can elicit reactions on the hands.)	Animal hair and dander, cow placenta, animal tissues.
Welders	Oil.	Chromate (welding fumes, gloves), nickel, cobalt.	
Woodworkers		Woods, colophony, turpentine, balsams, tars, lacquers, Frullania, lichens, glues, wood preservatives.	

Source: Adapted from S. Fregert, *Manual of Contact Dermatitis* (2nd ed.). Chicago: Year Book, 1981.

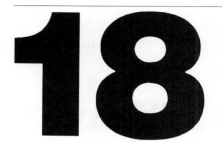

Psychiatric Aspects of Occupational Medicine

Peter J. Holland

The physician who practices occupational medicine will be faced with patients who exhibit a variety of psychiatric disorders. Often the patient will not recognize the psychiatric etiology of the disorder and will focus on any of a variety of other complaints. The purpose of this chapter is to acquaint the clinician with the appropriate evaluation of a person exhibiting psychiatric symptoms likely to be encountered in the occupational environment. A discussion of how certain psychiatric disorders can affect workplace functioning follows.

Mental Status Examination

Whether the physician is asked to evaluate a person exhibiting signs of emotional disturbance, alcohol abuse, or substance abuse, a uniform approach in evaluating the symptoms is necessary. The cornerstone of psychiatric diagnosis and evaluation is the *mental status examination,* an assessment of a patient's affect, appearance, speech pattern, thought processes, and cognition. Although the complexity and depth of the examination will depend on the nature of the problem and the expertise of the clinician, a routine approach is recommended.

Observation of the patient can tell the astute clinician a great deal about the patient's mental state. General appearance, alertness, and degree of cooperation are often a clue to a person's "mental status." As the patient reports his history, note the rate, clarity, tone, and rhythm of speech as well as whether the thoughts are coherent and logical. Ask *specifically* about *paranoid* ideation ("Do you ever feel people are plotting against you?"), *ideas of reference* ("Do you ever feel people on the television or radio are talking to you directly?"), *hallucinations* ("Do you ever hear things or see things that other people cannot hear or see?"), and so on. *Suicidal* and *homicidal* risk must always be assessed by direct questioning ("Does it ever seem so bad you think of hurting yourself?"). Often patients are relieved to be asked about thoughts of hurting themselves or others in a straightforward manner. If patients admit such thoughts, explore whether they have thought about *specific* ways to hurt themselves or others, whether they have thought out plans to do so, and whether they have taken any steps to implement their plan. Often depressed patients will have suicidal thoughts without suicide intent or will wish to be dead without having to take any action to cause their own death. If a patient appears to be a suicide or homicide risk, it is important to obtain psychiatric consultation before you allow him or her to leave your office.

A brief standardized and widely used screening tool for assessing cognitive dysfunction is the Mini-Mental State examination described by Folstein and Folstein [1]. Administration and scoring are straightforward (Fig. 18-1). Scores less than 25 correlate highly with the presence of cognitive deficits and may suggest the need for further evaluation.

Whenever serious psychopathology is suspected, consultation with a psychiatrist is essential. Any patient with a psychotic illness or a severe affective disorder is ideally followed at regular intervals by a psychiatrist.

Employee Assistance Programs

Employee assistance programs (EAPs) refer to the coordinating efforts of a variety of counseling and psychological services designed to assist employees who have

Patient's Name _____ Date _____

Age _____

Maximum
  Score   Score
                    ORIENTATION
     5   ( ) What is the (year) (season) (date) (day) (month)?
     5   ( ) Where are we? (state) (county) (town) (hospital) (floor)?

                    REGISTRATION
     3   ( ) Name 3 objects: 1 second to say each. Then ask the patient all 3
                    after you have said them.

                    Give 1 point for each correct answer. Then repeat them until he/
                    she learns all 3. Count trials and record.

                    ATTENTION AND CALCULATION
     5   ( ) Serial 7s. 1 point for each correct. Stop after 5 answers.
                    Alternatively spell "world" backwards.

                    RECALL
     3   ( ) Ask for 3 objects repeated above. Give 1 point for each correct.

                    LANGUAGE
     9   ( ) Name a pencil and watch. (2 points)

                    Repeat the following: "No ifs, ands, or buts." (1 point)

                    Follow a 3-stage command: "Take a paper in your right hand, fold
                    it in half, and put it on the floor." (3 points)

                    Read and obey the following: "Close your eyes." (1 point)

                    Write a sentence. (1 point)

                    Copy a design. (1 point)

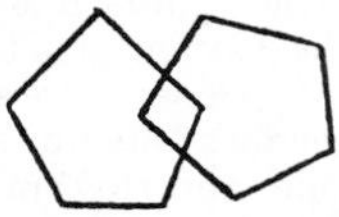

_____   Assess level of consciousness along a continuum.
Total Score
                    Alert   Drowsy   Stupor   Coma

Figure 18-1. Mini-Mental State examination. (From S. E. Folstein, and M. F. Folstein. "Mini-Mental State." *J. Psychiatr. Res.* 12:189, 1975.)

psychological or emotional problems that interfere with work. Employee assistance programs are growing in popularity in American industry. The Department of Transportation (DOT) drug-testing protocol has called for employees to be referred to an EAP counselor if the employee has a positive urine drug screen for drugs of abuse. Most often coordinated by psychiatric social workers, psychologists, or other trained professionals, they are intended to lower costs for employers while facilitating entrance into the mental health system. This model has been criticized for its reliance on nonmedical clinicians to perform the crucial tasks of diagnosis and triage. A comprehensive EAP should be able to offer primary counseling services with referral to appropriate health care professionals, including psychiatrists or facilities for treatment of alcoholism, drug abuse, financial problems, and family difficulties.

Physicians overseeing occupational health programs are urged to develop working relationships with the director of an EAP and an appropriate psychiatrist. Invariably, the physician will be requested to evaluate workers with various alcohol or substance abuse problems that may be affecting work performance. In other cases, it may be necessary to request a consultation regarding work capabilities in light of the presence of psychiatric disorders, such as posttraumatic stress disorders, depression, or mania.

Key aspects of EAPs include confidentiality, self-referral, and *aggregate* (not individual) reports. The most successful programs tend to make the services of an EAP readily available, usually during work duties.

Although they are widely utilized, the effectiveness of EAPs has not been objectively demonstrated. A recent review [2] of all previously published EAP evaluations found significant methodologic and conceptual flaws in these studies; positive outcomes are, therefore, *not* supported by the data available.

Stress

Stress refers to not a single event or reaction but a *process* that begins with a stressful event or series of events and ends with one's reaction to that event. The common factor seen in all stress is *change*. Stress is encountered whether the change is conceptualized as beneficial, as in promotion, or detrimental, as in being fired.

In moderate amounts, stress can be motivating and is known as "eustress." However, if the duration or intensity of the stress overloads a person's ability to manage the stress, it can lead to "distress," a spiral of emotional and physical ills. To illustrate these concepts, think of the metal spring of a watch. When stressed, the spring provides the force to keep the mechanism working. Without constant winding and stress, the watch will stop. If overwound, however, the metal becomes strained and may even break. This proper "spring tension" varies widely between individuals and also within one individual at different times.

Stressors, the factors involved in causing stress, can be divided into acute and chronic types. We have all experienced acute stress when we are traveling in a car and the vehicle in front of us makes a short and unexpected stop. The immediate release of epinephrine (the "adrenaline rush") causes the familiar "fight or flight" response that increases heart rate, blood pressure, and respiratory rate. Dissatisfying interpersonal relationships are usually responsible for chronic stress. The mechanism whereby chronic stressors exert their damage is primarily due to the increase of corticotropin-releasing factor and other mediators, which increase levels of circulating corticosteroid and increase blood pressure and heart rate, as well as possibly impairing immune response.

Occupational stress research has shown a clear relationship between stress and productivity (Fig. 18-2). All occupations have their own intrinsic characteristics including level of responsibility and degrees of authority, autonomy, and ambiguity. If one plots stress versus any of these characteristics, one finds that either extreme in characteristics can produce higher levels of stress. For example, a midlevel manager with responsibility for 20 employees (high level of responsibility) may be as stressed as an assemblyline worker (low level of responsibility). Although highly

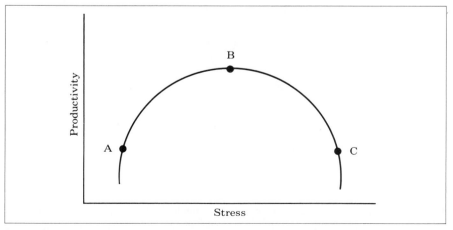

Figure 18-2. The relationship between productivity and stress. A. Stress is too low; therefore, productivity is low. B. Optimum stress and productivity. C. Stress is too high; therefore, productivity is low.

ambiguous occupations can be stressful, having no occupation at all is perhaps more stressful.

Although theories related to the cause of stress among people vary, one model described with some level of success is that of Alan McLean. Former eastern area Medical Director at IBM, he developed a model of three ever-changing circles to conceptualize an individual's relationship to stress (Fig. 18-3). Where there is overlap of the stress circles, unfavorable reactions occur. To use this conceptual tool, one must visualize the circles in a dynamic state; the circles are continually in motion, changing in size and in distance from one another. Only when conditions are "ripe" will a stressor produce symptoms.

Perhaps the most important consideration is the circle representing *individual vulnerability,* which includes personality, life stage, and recent life changes. Some personality types may be particularly sensitive to stressors. For example, a worker with an obsessive personality often has a rigid coping strategy for approaching new situations. If this strategy fails, the worker may lack the flexibility needed to find new solutions.

The influence of *life stage* on adaptation to "stressors" is demonstrated by a worker confronted with termination at age 45 compared to age 25. "Midlife crisis" also lowers one's ability to manage stress. The importance of recent life changes was first addressed by physician Adolph Meyer and more recently by Holmes and Rahe [3], who developed a "Schedule of Recent Life Events." They assigned "life change units" (LCUs) and ranked them according to commonly encountered life changes. Individuals who accumulate large amounts of LCUs appear to have increased risk of suffering stress-related illness (Table 18-1).

A second circle represents the *context* in which an individual faces a stressor. Context is made up of all the external factors in a person's life, including the world economy and one's family unit, friends, and work atmosphere, both people and the physical environment. The social/psychological support that one receives from co-workers and family does much to buffer the impact of the stressor.

A third circle represents the *stressor,* the factor involved in causing the adverse effect. Although every occupation has unique stressors, certain jobs are associated with high levels of so-called stressors, including shift work, work overload or work

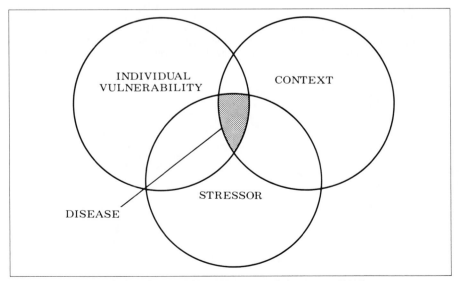

Figure 18-3. McLean's conceptual model of the individual's relationship to stress. Individual vulnerability includes internal factors such as personality, life stage, and recent life events. Context includes external factors such as physical environment, family, friends, and work atmosphere. Stressor is the factor causing an adverse result. The area of overlap of the three circles represents disease.

Table 18-1. The Holmes-Rahe Schedule of Recent Life Events

Rank	Event	Value (LCU)
1	Death of spouse	100
2	Divorce	73
3	Marital separation	65
4	Jail term	63
5	Death of a close family member	63
6	Personal injury or illness	53
7	Marriage	50
8	Fired from work	47
9	Marital reconciliation	45
10	Retirement	45
11	Change in family member's health	44
12	Pregnancy	40
13	Sex difficulties	39
14	Addition to family	39
15	Business readjustment	39
16	Change in financial status	38
17	Death of close friend	37
18	Change to different line of work	36
19	Change in number of marital arguments	35
20	Mortgage or loan over $10,000	31
21	Foreclosure of mortgage or loan	30
22	Change in work responsibilities	29
23	Son or daughter leaving home	29
24	Trouble with in-laws	29
25	Outstanding personal achievement	28
26	Spouse begins or stops work	26
27	Starting or finishing school	26
28	Change in living conditions	25
29	Revision of personal habits	24
30	Trouble with boss	23
31	Change in work hours, conditions	20
32	Change in residence	20
33	Change in schools	20
34	Change in recreational habits	19
35	Change in church activities	19
36	Change in social activities	18
37	Mortgage or loan under $10,000	17
38	Change in sleeping habits	16
39	Change in number of family gatherings	15
40	Change in eating habits	15
41	Vacation	13
42	Christmas season	12
43	Minor violation of the law	11

Key: LCU = life change units.
Source: From T. H. Holmes and R. H. Rahe. The social readjustment rating scale. *J. Psychosomatic Res.* 11:213, 1967. Copyright 1967, Pergamon Journals, Ltd.

underload, physical danger, noise and lighting, role ambiguity or conflict, high responsibility with low authority, and interpersonal conflicts.

It is not always possible or desirable to remove stressors that confront a patient. We can, however, help our patients modify their circles of individual vulnerability, context, and stressors so that overlap and thus symptoms are minimized. Substance abuse (alcohol, drugs, caffeine, nicotine) or chronic sleep deprivation will inhibit successful treatment; their presence must be addressed.

Engaging the Patient as Your Ally

The physician who delivers occupational health services is likely to be called on to evaluate people who may have symptoms due to stress. Necessary for any successful intervention is the establishment of the therapeutic alliance. The basic strategy is to create a nondefensive atmosphere where you can evoke a patient's willingness to work with you. The technique for achieving this outcome involves five simple but vital steps that cannot be overlooked [4]:

1. *Reduce defensiveness:* A good technique for reducing the patient's defensiveness is to externalize the patient's difficulty; rephrase the problem so that it is not coming from within the patient entirely. For example, you might ask, "What are the pressures on you at this time?"
2. *Inventory the patient's stress symptoms:* Your goal is to understand how stress is affecting the patient. Ask "What do these pressures do to you?" or, "How do you notice these pressures affecting you or your ability to handle life's problems?"
3. *Tap level of motivation:* It is imperative to determine whether the patient is truly interested in working on the problem before you undertake any stress management program. Ask the patient, "Are you willing to do something about it?"
4. *Review work environment:* Ask specifically about how work (i.e., job duties, physical environment, other workers) may be affecting the person. (This critical question, if overlooked, can result in failure to understand the broad dimensions of stress-related illnesses.)
5. *Willingness check:* Ask the patient, "Are you willing to work with me on solving this problem?"

Successfully completed, these steps result in an implicit contract between you and the patient to work together toward a common goal—the reduction of stress. Five commonly used stress management techniques (time management, relaxation training, physical exercise, increasing avocational interest, and spreading out life changes) will help you and your patient reach your goal.

Stress Management Techniques

Time Management
Structured time planning can help a patient who is overwhelmed by a task. Often, large tasks can be broken into manageable units. Have patients make up "to do" lists and set priorities among items on the list. Patients also need to decide what level of perfection is required for a particular task. Lists can be updated and priorities changed as needed.

Relaxation Training
Many people do not know how to relax because it is a skill that must be developed. For many, it is like learning to drive a stick-shift automobile. At first it is very awkward and unnatural, but with training and practice, it can become smooth and comfortable.

Relaxation training can take many forms. Commonly used techniques include biofeedback, transcendental meditation, self-hypnosis, and progressive muscle relaxation. Both patient and physician must be comfortable with the technique used. For example, a computer programmer may feel uncomfortable with the idea of hypnosis but intrigued with the hardware of biofeedback.

Exercise
Exercise is one of the simplest yet most effective antidotes to stress. Studies suggest that running has antidepressant qualities [5]. The better an activity is for cardiopulmonary training, the more powerful is its antistress effect. Walking, cycling, running, and swimming are all good cardiopulmonary training activities. For optimal effectiveness, an exercise program should be well integrated into a person's daily life. Although daily exercise is most desirable, 30-minute periods three times per week where one exercises to 75% of one's maximal heart rate appear to be beneficial (see Chap. 14).

Avocational Interests
Patients should be encouraged to expand their scope of gratifications. A person who depends on work as the sole source of self-esteem is heading for trouble. Placing a

few of one's eggs in the family, sports, and hobby baskets will help to avoid so-called burnout.

Spread Out Life Changes

This stress reduction strategy comes directly from the Holmes-Rahe Schedule of Life Change Events. Often we have no control over major life changes, but when a choice exists, major changes should be spread over several months. Good stress management skills are good health skills; strategies rely primarily on reducing one's circle of individual vulnerability.

Group Stress Management Programs

Group stress management programs can provide employees with an awareness of how stress affects their lives. For many employees, a 4- to 8-hour program enables them to begin to make changes to a healthier style of coping with stress. These programs are primarily educational in scope and are designed to acquaint people with stress, its adverse health effects, and means of control. Those employees with a large stressor load or rigid coping styles can benefit from an individualized stress management program.

Organizational change can challenge workers' ability to adapt to that change. This kind of stress can drastically affect employee morale and productivity. One technique of assaying this type of stress is through the administration of periodic "opinion surveys." Professional interpretation and analysis of such surveys can yield information pertinent to improving the situation and thus reduce stress.

Shift Work

"Shift work" implies either long-term night work or work involving rotation between day, evening, and night shifts. Over 27% of male workers and 16% of female workers have jobs that require them to rotate between day and night shifts [6]. Studies suggest that these workers, presumably due to a disruption in circadian rhythm, have increased morbidity and decreased work performance. Marked variability exists between people's vulnerability to the adverse effects of shift work, and vulnerability increases with advancing age. Workers who categorize themselves as "night people" and those who find it easy to sleep at unusual times are more likely to tolerate shift work. Although most studies can be criticized on some level, approximately 25% of workers are estimated to have significant difficulties in family, work, or social adaptation related to shift work [6] (Table 18-2).

Acute Time Shift Syndrome

Our circadian system can adapt to a phase delay of 2 hours or a phase advance of one-half hour without much disruption. Whenever a change in schedule occurs outside this limited "range of entrainment," an acute time shift syndrome may occur. During the process of readjustment to the new schedule, circadian rhythms in alertness, mood, and digestion are disrupted. Although short-lived, most common symptoms of acute time shift syndrome, that is, "jet lag," are insomnia, gastrointestinal distress, sleepiness, and fatigue. The intensity of the reaction is determined by the degree and direction of time shift. Since it is easier to adjust to a *delay in schedule* than an advance, workers adapt more readily to switching from day shift to night shift. Similarly, traveling westward across time zones (delay in time) has less potential for adverse effects than traveling eastward. Adequate hydration, avoidance of alcohol and cigarettes, and appropriate use of short-acting hypnotics to induce

Table 18-2. Guidelines on preventing the ill effects of shift work

Weekly rotating shifts—working 4 or 5 days on a particular shift before rotating to the next
Rotate shifts in the direction of delay of rhythms (working later)
Schedule mealtime ("lunchtime") halfway through a given shift
Maintain exposure to bright light during waking hours [7]
Sleep in a dark, quiet place [7]

sleep at the "new" bedtime may speed resolution of jet lag symptoms [8]. (Table 18-3 includes other measures designed to prevent jet lag.)

Chronic Shift Maladaptation Syndrome

Disturbance of the worker's "biologic clock" or circadian rhythms is responsible for a "shift maladaptation syndrome," which affects wakefulness, thermoregulation, and neuroendocrine regulation. The most common effects include gastrointestinal and cardiovascular disturbances and effects on level of alertness.

Disturbances on level of alertness are the *most commonly encountered consequence* of shift work. Night shift or rotating shift workers are more likely to suffer from insomnia and difficulty staying awake at work. The decreased total sleep time also results in a chronically sleep-deprived condition. This disrupted sleep pattern may be related to the higher incidence of both work and off-work accidents among shift workers.

Shift workers have a higher rate of gastrointestinal complaints and peptic ulcer disease than do day workers. Disturbed eating habits combined with disrupted diurnal control of intestinal enzymes are thought to contribute to these disturbances.

Several studies indicate that shift workers have higher than expected rates of cardiovascular disease and acute myocardial infarctions in particular [6].

Those who work nights or on evening rotation are less likely to be involved in political or social organizations. With fewer friends, they tend to have hobbies that are solitary in nature. Disruptions of family life among shift workers are often more problematic than the disruptions in community and social life. Marital disharmony may result from the shift worker's relative unavailability; a myriad of difficulties in parenting can also occur.

Malingering and Emotional Factors in Physical Symptoms (Somatoform Illness)

The emotional components of many medical illnesses are well recognized by astute physicians. The occupational physician must also be able to evaluate whether a *volitional* component plays a role in a worker's complaint. In most clinical settings, there is a tendency to consider a worker's illness as due to either a bona fide disease or a conscious attempt to deceive the physician. This view is overly simplistic, inaccurate, and not helpful when dealing with these workers. A more useful approach is to conceptualize a *continuum* of diagnostic entities. Generally, patients' symptoms do not fall into either extreme, but somewhere in the middle where there is an element of both conscious and unconscious motivation. It may be difficult to distinguish the degree of *voluntary control* a patient has over symptoms.

Occupational physicians should be familiar with the disorders noted in Fig. 18-4. At one end of the spectrum are disorders whereby psychological factors affect the expression of physical illness (e.g., asthma, irritable bowel syndrome). The midrange includes somatoform disorders, which refer to the presence of physical symptoms that suggest physical disorders but for which no organic basis can be established as the cause. Evidence often suggests that the symptoms are linked to psychological dysfunction. Examples of somatoform disorders include conversion reactions, psychogenic pain, and hypochondriasis. Somatization occurs when a patient expresses *psychological distress through a physical route;* the patient may not even be aware of the psychological distress or feel able to control the symptoms. Successful inter-

Table 18-3. How to prevent jet lag

Keep well hydrated
Avoid alcohol
Eat lightly on travel days
Avoid caffeine in the evening
Consider using short-acting benzodiazepines to help induce sleep at the "new" bedtime
Set your watch to the new time as soon as you get on the airplane

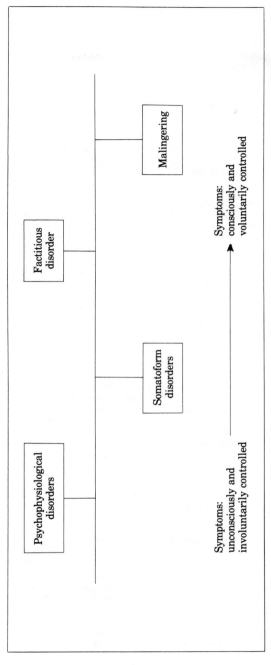

Figure 18-4. The continuum of psychological factors influencing physical symptoms.

ventions with patients suffering from somatoform disorders utilize the following techniques:

1. Establish a good *doctor-patient relationship*. Initially convey acceptance of the patient's problems, then gradually shift to exploration of psychological variables and "stress" in a patient's life that may contribute to the problems.
2. Avoid placing "cure" as the goal of your interventions. Focus rather on improved functioning or coping with symptoms.
3. Encourage exercise and physical therapy.
4. Treat any concomitant depression with antidepressant drugs at full therapeutic doses.
5. Accept the long-term chronic nature of these illnesses. It is more efficient to see patients for follow-up at regular intervals regardless of whether they are symptomatic. This approach is generally more beneficial than advising a return only if symptoms recur.

At the other end of the continuum (Fig. 18-3) are conditions in which symptoms are under the worker's voluntary control, such as malingering and factitious disorder.

In factitious disorders, the symptoms are "voluntary" in that they are deliberate and purposeful but not in the sense that they can be controlled; there is a compulsive quality to the simulation of illness. There is no apparent goal other than to assume the patient role. Often a severe personality disturbance exists.

In malingering, the "patient" is also in voluntary control of the symptoms, but the goal is based on environmental circumstances (rather than the patient's psychology). Under some circumstances, malingering may represent an adaptive behavior, such as feigning illness while a captive of an enemy during wartime. Malingering is not attributable to a mental disorder, although it is often associated with an antisocial personality.

The following are guidelines for identifying the patient who has a higher degree of voluntary conscious control of symptoms:

1. Carefully documented medical history.
2. Extensive legal involvement.
3. Angry and defensive during examinations.
4. Resists diagnostic procedures and prescribed treatment regimens.
5. Selectively excludes family or employer input to the evaluating doctor.
6. Inconsistencies in the reporting of physical symptoms.
7. When confronted with the nonorganic nature of the complaint, the malingerer will often develop a new problem.
8. Medical record appears to have been altered.
9. Patient reluctant to accept a favorable prognosis.

Posttraumatic Stress Disorder

Posttraumatic stress disorder (PTSD) is classified as an anxiety disorder by the American Psychiatric Association's *Diagnostic and Statistical Manual of Mental Disorders* (DSM-III-R) [9]. A subgroup of PTSD has been described as "atypical PTSD"; however, the condition closely resembles a somatoform disorder. Patients in whom atypical PTSD develops may have been exposed acutely or chronically to toxic substances that caused certain symptoms. They then experience recurrent symptoms or anxiety after subsequent exposure to innocuous substances or trivial amounts of toxic chemicals [10]. Treatment of atypical PTSD consists of supportive psychotherapy, including open discussion of the "traumatic" exposure. Occasionally, antidepressants are helpful, especially in the presence of insomnia or anxiety attacks.

Common Psychiatric Disturbances that Affect Occupational Functioning

Since psychiatric illnesses are ubiquitous, the occupational physician will encounter many workers impaired by these disorders. The following description of common psychiatric disorders is designed to acquaint the clinician with their effect in the occupational setting.

Affective Disorders

The chief characteristic of affective disorders is a disturbance of *mood.* Affecting approximately 10% of men and 20% of women during their lifetime [9], disturbances can be either elevated mood (mania) or depressed mood (depression). Some people have episodes of both abnormally elevated and abnormally lowered moods, such as manic-depressive disorder. Other patients suffer from one type of abnormality of mood, either mania or depression. Patients tend to have recurrent episodes throughout their lives, especially those suffering from manic-depressive illness. Although the prognosis for these disorders is generally good, the occupational disturbance during an acute phase can range from a mild decrease in performance to total disability. The vast majority of patients, however, obtain full recovery. Some patients may need continued medication, for example, lithium or antidepressants, to help decrease the chance of recurrences. Anticonvulsants are also used to stabilize mood. Patients with manic-depressive illness who have had a history of manic psychotic episodes should have regular visits to a psychiatrist to assure compliance with the medication regime. These patients frequently lose insight into their disease process and exercise poor judgment as they become ill.

Depression is commonly characterized by symptoms such as sadness, crying spells, sleep and eating disturbances, difficulty concentrating, suicidal ideation, indecisiveness, and somatic preoccupations. Occupational functioning decreases with increasing severity of depression. Mania is commonly characterized by an expansive mood, emotional lability, rapid loud speech, demanding behavior, grandiosity, paranoia, and poor judgment.

Psychotic Disorders

Psychosis implies a severe psychiatric disturbance in which the patient is out of touch with reality, which leads to an inability to function in daily life. The most common psychotic disorder is *schizophrenia,* with a lifetime prevalence in the United States of 1% [11]. Unlike affective disorders, complete recovery in schizophrenia is unusual. Most patients continue to have residual symptoms even between the acute psychotic episodes. Many symptoms can be controlled effectively with antipsychotic or neuroleptic medications. The prognosis is uncertain for schizophrenics whose ability to function deteriorates over time. Occupational limitations range from severe during acute psychotic episodes to mild during the residual phase early in the disease. Some schizophrenics may have no occupational impairments. Common symptoms of schizophrenia include delusions, which may be paranoid in nature, hallucinations, breakdown of logical thinking, social isolation, flattened affect, and bizarre behaviors.

Paranoia is one type of psychotic illness that has an insidious onset, usually beginning in midlife. Treatment is notoriously difficult, in part due to the patient's poor compliance with a treatment program. Occupational functioning may be severely affected, especially if the delusional system that characterizes this disorder involves the employer. Patients with paranoia do *not* have hallucinations, flattened affect, bizarre behavior, or social isolation as do schizophrenics; however, they suffer from well-organized delusions. For example, the patient may state, "The FBI is following me and tapping my phone calls" or "The company is trying to poison me."

Anxiety Disorders

Workers with anxiety disorders are plagued with extreme nervousness. An anxiety disorder can render a person totally disabled from daily activities, including work. In a *generalized anxiety disorder,* increased somatic manifestations, such as tachycardia, diarrhea, and sweating, are present. On the other hand, in *acute anxiety* states (panic attack), the patient decompensates from a period of normal functioning. Both forms of anxiety can lead to anticipatory anxiety, agoraphobia, and depression. Through the use of a combination of behavioral, cognitive, and pharmacological treatments, most patients can be "cured." No lasting occupational impairment should be expected.

Personality Disorders

According to the American Psychiatric Association [9], "Personality *traits* are enduring patterns of perceiving, relating to, and thinking about the environment and oneself, and are exhibited in a wide range of important social and personal contexts. It is only when *personality traits* are inflexible and maladaptive and cause either significant impairment in social or occupational functioning, or subjective distress that they constitute Personality Disorders. The manifestations of Personality Disorders are generally recognized by adolescence or earlier and continue throughout most of adult life, though they often become less obvious in middle or old age." Several discrete personality disorders are described: antisocial, histrionic, borderline, narcissistic, passive-aggressive, paranoid, schizoid, schizotypal, compulsive, avoidant, and dependent. Some patients have a mixture of two or more types. Workers with personality disorders frequently have marked occupational impairment. Interpersonal relationships are most severely affected. Because the maladaptive patterns are long-term traits that feel natural to the patient, treatment outcome is poor.

Mass Psychogenic Illness

Outbreaks of mass or epidemic psychogenic illness have been reported since the Middle Ages. These conditions have gained greater attention of late, primarily in the evaluation of indoor air complaints. Analysis of outbreaks reveals some common characteristics: inaccurate perception of a perceived hazardous exposure, absence of objective data to confirm etiologic causative factors, high female to male ratio, rapid spread followed by rapid remission of symptoms, hyperventilation, and syncopy. Victims are frequently under some kind of physical or emotional stress.

Victims of mass psychogenic illness do not necessarily have individual psychopathology, nor do they feign illness. On the contrary, the syndrome represents an understandable psychophysiologic response to a complex set of stimuli. Separating affected persons from one another may help speed resolution of the disorders.

Neuropsychiatric Disease Secondary to Toxic Exposure

Solvents, pesticides, and heavy metals are ubiquitous, and, thus, human exposure is inevitable. Workers, however, may be exposed to higher concentrations on the job. Although the exact amount required to produce symptoms is often unknown, marked variation in individual vulnerability appears to exist. Symptoms may be acute, resulting from brief, intense exposure, or chronic, secondary to many years of exposure at lower concentrations [12].

Acute intoxication syndromes depend on the particular agent; however, common symptoms include dizziness, light-headedness, and incoordination (see Chap. 15). In rare cases a florid psychosis may occur. Removal from exposure to the toxic substance usually clears the symptoms.

The *chronic* syndromes can be divided into three types: mild, moderate, and severe. The *mildest* syndrome type is an organic affective disorder, a reversible syndrome of depression identical to depression from other etiologies. Diagnosis is made by noting a temporal relationship between the *onset* of symptoms and the *exposure* to the toxic substance. (The diagnosis is considered by some to be one of "exclusion.") The organic affective disorder is often reversible if the offending substance is removed. The *moderate* severity type includes cognitive symptoms, such as short-term memory loss and psychomotor disturbances (slowness in response time, clumsy eye-hand coordination, or clumsy dexterity), in addition to the affective symptoms. The most *severe* type resembles dementia. As the severity of these conditions increases, withdrawal of the toxic substance is less likely to reverse the symptoms.

Measurement of cognitive function is particularly important when the possible effects of a toxic exposure are suspected. The Mini-Mental State examination is particularly helpful as a screening tool. When neuropsychiatric illness secondary to toxic exposure is suspected, *neuropsychological testing* by a psychologist trained in behavioral toxicology or neuropsychology may be helpful. Such testing can be used to assess a worker's level of psychological impairment. Serial testing can be used to measure change in functional level.

Multiple Chemical Sensitivities

Although "multiple chemical sensitivities" is also referred to as "20th century disease," it is not a new illness and perhaps has existed for centuries [13–15]. It is also sometimes referred to as "total allergy syndrome" or "environmental illness." In this syndrome, the patient attributes multiple ill-defined symptoms (for which no organic cause can be found) to exposure to chemicals to which the patient claims to be "allergic" or "hypersensitive." Although the recurrent somatic or psychological symptoms are attributed to chemical exposure, the symptoms are generally not consistent with the accepted toxicologic properties of the offending agent. The intensity and range of symptom complaints are often in excess of those expected based on the patient's exposure history.

The etiology and pathology of this syndrome have yet to be determined. Although symptoms of anxiety, stress, or depression are often present, it is not clear if the presence of psychiatric symptoms is one of the complex factors that contribute to production of the full syndrome or if psychiatric symptoms occur as sequelae to the syndrome itself [16]. This matter must be empathically appreciated while a complete evaluation of all complaints, both physical and psychological, is undertaken. Any attempt to attribute the patient's complaint to a "psychological" etiology will likely lead to hostility from the patient. However, if a good alliance with the physician exists, and the patient feels that each aspect of his or her complaints is taken seriously and investigated appropriately, the patient will more likely be receptive to psychiatric consultation as part of a comprehensive evaluation.

As with other patients who suffer from chronic illnesses for which there is no clear-cut treatment, establishment of a supportive doctor-patient relationship is essential. These patients clearly suffer real distress. The patient must feel both cared for and understood by the health care provider. Patients suffering from this syndrome are often very disillusioned with traditional medical care.

References

1. Folstein, S. E., and Folstein, M. F. "Mini-Mental State." *J. Psychiatr. Res.* 12:189, 1975.
2. Colantonio, A. Assessing the effects of Employee Assistance Programs: A review of Employee Assistance Program evaluations. *Yale J. Bio. Med.* 62:13, 1989.
3. Holmes, T. H., and Rahe, R. H. The social readjustment rating scale. *J. Psychosom. Res.* 11:213, 1967.
4. Personal communication, William Hollister, MD, University of North Carolina, Chapel Hill.
5. Mellion, M. Exercise therapy for anxiety and depression. *Postgrad. Med.* 77:3, 1985.
6. Moore-Ede, M. C., and Richardson, G. S. Medical implications of shift work. *Ann. Rev. Med.* 36:607, 1985.
7. Van Cauter, E., and Turek, F. Strategies for resetting the human circadian clock. *N. Engl. J. Med.* 322:18, 1990.
8. Nicholson, A. N., et al. Sleep after transmeridian flights. *Lancet* 2:1205, 1986.
9. *Diagnostic and Statistical Manual of Mental Disorders (DSM-III-R)*. Washington, DC: American Psychiatric Association, 1987. P. 217.
10. Schottenfeld, R. S., and Callen, M. R. Occupation-induced posttraumatic stress disorders. *Am. J. Psychiatry* 142:2, 1985.
11. Nicholi, A. M. (ed.). *The Harvard Guide to Modern Psychiatry*. Cambridge, MA: Belknap, 1978. P. 207.
12. Flodin, U., et al. Clinical studies of psycho-organic syndromes among workers with exposure to solvents. *Am. J. Ind. Med.* 5:287, 1984.
13. Kahn, E., and Letz, G. Clinical ecology: Environmental medicine or unsubstantiated theory. *Ann. Intern. Med.* 111:104, 1989.
14. California Medical Association Scientific Board Task Force on Clinical Ecology. Clinical ecology—A critical appraisal (information). *West J. Med.* 144:239, 1986.
15. American Academy of Allergy and Immunology. Clinical ecology. *J. Allergy Clin. Immunol.* 78:269, 1986.
16. Simon, G. E., Katon, W. J., and Sparks, P. J. Allergic to life: Psychological factors in environmental illness. *Am. J. Psychiatry* 147:7, 1990.

Further Information

Baker, E. Organic solvent neurotoxicity. *Ann. Rev. Public Health* 9:223, 1988.

Baker, E. L., and Fine, L. J. Solvent neurotoxicity: The current evidence. *J.O.M.* 28:126, 1986.

Benson, H. *The Relaxation Response.* New York: Morrow, 1975.

Collijan, M. J., and Pennebaker, J. W. (eds.). *Mass Psychogenic Illness.* Hillsdale, NJ: Erlbaum, 1982.

Diagnostic and Statistical Manual of Mental Disorders (DSM-III-R). Washington, DC: American Psychiatric Association, 1987.

Drugs that cause psychiatric symptoms. *Med. Lett.* 28:81, 1986.

Fiedler, N., Maccia, C., and Kipen, H. Evaluation of chemically sensitive patients. *J.O.M.* 34:5, 1992.

Florence, D., and Miller, T. Functional overlay in work-related injury. *Postgrad. Med.* 77:8, 1985.

Gamino, L., Elkins, G., and Hackney, K. Emergency management of mass psychogenic illness. *Psychosomatics* 30:4, 1989.

Harris, J. S. Stressors and stress in critical care. *Crit. Care Nurse* Feb. 1984.

Lande, R. Malingering *J.A.O.A.* 89:4, 1989.

McLean, A. *Work Stress.* Series on Occupational Stress. Reading, MA: Addison-Wesley, 1979.

Meja, S. Post-traumatic stress disorder: An overview of three etiological variables and psychopharmacological treatment. *Nurse Pract.* Aug. 15:41, 1990.

Moore, Ede, M. C., and Richardson, G. S. Medical implications of shift work. *Ann. Rev. Med.* 36:607, 1985.

Siebenaler, M. J. and McGovern, P. Shiftwork consequences and considerations. *A.A.O.H.N. J.* 39:12, 1991.

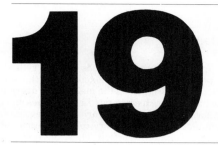

Allergy and Immunology

Donald Accetta and
Jack E. Farnham

Occupational Allergic Diseases

Occupational allergic diseases consist of allergic contact dermatitis, allergic respiratory diseases (allergic rhinitis, asthma, bronchitis, hypersensitivity pneumonitis, and broncho-pulmonary aspergillosis), and anaphylaxis. Of the more than 400,000 cases of occupational illnesses annually [1], about 20,000 are allergic contact dermatitis, which mostly result from contact with epoxy, *Rhus* oleoresin, chromates, nickel, and rubber products. These are fully described in Chap. 17, Occupational Skin Disorders, and are not evaluated further here.

Occupational allergic respiratory diseases comprise about 65,000 cases annually. In addition to the discussion in this chapter, the reader is referred to Chap. 11, Occupational Pulmonary Disease.

Occupational anaphylaxis is the same as the potentially life-threatening, acute anaphylactic reaction in general, with the exception that it is caused by occupationally related agents. The recorded incidence of occupational anaphylaxis is less than 200 cases a year.

Hypersensitivity Types

Proposed in 1975, the Gell and Coombs classification of hypersensitivity reactions [2] still remains the standard guide for types of immune responses. The four types of reactions are based on the presence or absence of humoral antibodies, the type of antibodies involved, whether or not complement is required to drive the reaction to completion, the target organ, and the cell types involved. Although the four types are described separately, they may occur in combination simultaneously.

Type I (allergic or anaphylactic) reactions require immunoglobulin E (IgE) antibody attached to mast cell receptors before antigen introduction. When the antigen cross-links with the specific antibody, the resulting reaction causes a release of histamine, serotonin, and other vasoactive amines from the mast cell. These chemical mediators induce the allergic reaction seen in allergic rhinitis, asthma, and anaphylaxis.

Type II reactions usually require IgG antibodies directed against antigen located on target cell surfaces (often red blood cells). Complement may be needed to drive the antigen antibody reaction, resulting in target cell destruction (immune hemolytic anemia, transfusion reaction, and some types of autoimmune disease).

Type III (immune complex) reactions occur when excessive antigen causes a precipitation of antigen-antibody (usually IgG or IgM) complex along the vascular endothelium, resulting in subsequent attraction of polymorphonuclear leukocytes that cause local damage. Examples of this type of reaction are hypersensitivity pneumonitis and some autoimmune diseases.

Type IV (delayed hypersensitivity) reactions require previously sensitized lymphocytes but no humoral antibodies or complement. Antigenic stimulation of lymphocytes causes release of lymphokines (interleukins and interferons). The lymphokines attract macrophages and leukocytes, which result in allergic contact dermatitis and granulomatous diseases such as tuberculosis.

The Allergic Reaction in Detail

After exposure to allergen, specific IgE is produced and binds to mast cells during the sensitizing phase, which may take 3 years. Upon reexposure to the same or similar antigen, the antigen binds to the IgE, triggering the mast cell to degranulate and release numerous preformed mediators (e.g., histamine). Leukotrienes and other inflammatory mediators are newly formed and released during the degranulation process and in the hours after degranulation. Inflammatory cells are recruited into the area and further accentuate the inflammatory reaction. Thus, the reaction may occur immediately, producing only an immediate hypersensitivity reaction, or may be delayed for several hours (late-phase allergic reaction). Frequently a dual (immediate and late) reaction occurs. It is the late or delayed reaction, occurring during the evening or nighttime hours, that can create confusion and difficulty in evaluating the person with a suspected occupational allergy. Further confusing the situation is the fact that the late-phase reaction, once initiated, can continue for hours, days, or even weeks with only minimal or even no further exposure to the inciting antigen.

The Allergic Workup

Assessing the atopic potential of a patient is important for a number of reasons. Some occupational diseases are more likely to occur in the allergic person (i.e., allergic people who are animal handlers) than in nonallergic workers. The latency period before symptoms develop is much shorter in the atopic person. Taking an allergy *history* is similar to taking any comprehensive history, although several areas are stressed. The timing of symptoms (including any seasonal variation) is important, although it may be misleading, for example, in a late-phase reaction (see previous section). A family history of atopic disease is significant because allergic diseases are genetically determined. Itching of mucous membranes, although rarely mentioned by the patient, is often a major complaint in the atopic patient.

In the *review of systems,* one should search for concomitant diseases that might mimic allergy. For example, chronic sinusitis is a very common disease in both atopic and nonatopic individuals. Many persons with this disease have only vague complaints of fatigue, nasal discharge or stuffiness, or a chronic cough. Sinusitis has been clearly shown to exacerbate preexisting asthma. Diagnosing sinusitis requires a high index of suspicion for the disease because its manifestations are often quite protean. Aggressive and often long-term treatment with broad-spectrum antibiotics and corticosteroid nasal sprays is necessary to promote resolution and prevent reoccurrences. Once the infection resolves, nasal and chest symptoms previously attributed to an "allergy" may disappear or subside.

In performing the *physical examination,* one should search for manifestations of atopic diseases, such as eczema, changes in the nasal membranes, and asthma. The person with chronic sinusitis may have severe nasal stuffiness, tenderness when the cheeks and forehead are palpated, halitosis, and frequently a thick, discolored nasal discharge. Eczematous changes in the skin, particularly in the popliteal, antecubital, postauricular, and palmar areas, indicate an atopic tendency. The presence of nasal polyps may indicate an underlying atopic condition (Sampter's triad—nasal polyposis, asthma, and aspirin hypersensitivity). Classic textbooks of medicine often associate specific coloration of the nasal mucosa with certain diseases. This is of little or no practical help in diagnosing allergic rhinitis, however. Wheezing may be absent on the physical examination of asthmatic individuals. Clubbing of the fingers is rarely present in asthma unless accompanied by other lung diseases.

Laboratory studies are often inconclusive. An elevated eosinophil count is frequently present in a patient with asthma or eczema. The IgE level is not a good screening test for atopy and a normal IgE level should not exclude the diagnosis of allergy. An extremely elevated eosinophil count or IgE level should prompt search for alternative diseases (such as broncho-pulmonary aspergillosis).

Skin testing remains the gold standard in determining the presence of specific IgE antibody. A wide variety of antigens are available and the procedure is quick, relatively inexpensive, and easy to perform. Interpreting the tests, however, requires a physician to correlate the test results with the history and physical examination; a positive skin test signifies only the presence of IgE and not an allergic disease.

The chief disadvantages of skin testing are the potential for anaphylaxis; the expertise necessary to perform, grade, and interpret the test; and the presence of severe skin disease in some people that prohibits skin testing.

An alternative to skin testing is the RAST test (radio-allergosorbent) or ELISA (enzyme-linked immunosorbent assay). In these tests, an allergen is bound to a solid-phase support system, the patient's serum is added, and, if antigen-specific IgE is present, it binds to the solid phase. Radioactively or enzyme-labeled anti-IgE is then added and radioactive counts or colorimetric changes are measured. The major advantages of these tests are the ease of testing and absence of anaphylaxis. The major disadvantages are lack of sensitivity (about 20% less sensitive than skin testing), the limited number of antigens available, and cost. Like skin testing, an elevated RAST or ELISA is a marker of exposure, not of disease.

Other laboratory tests employed in diagnosing asthma include spirometry (see Chap. 11, Occupational Pulmonary Disease) and peak flow measurements (see discussion under Occupational Asthma in this chapter).

Nasal *smear cytology* for eosinophils is often a help in diagnosing allergic rhinitis and allergic nasal conditions. This requires a technician experienced in interpreting thin mucus smears for cell types.

X-rays are usually of little benefit in the workup of allergic diseases, with the exception of sinus x-rays or computed tomographic (CT) scan of the sinuses. Chest x-rays are only of value in ruling out other types of diseases of the lungs that are masquerading as asthma.

Occupational Respiratory Diseases

Occupational allergic respiratory diseases include allergic rhinitis and allergic rhinosinusitis, occupational allergic asthma, hypersensitivity pneumonitis, and allergic bronchopulmonary aspergillosis.

Occupational rhinitis and rhinosinusitis may be irritative or allergic in nature. Irritation of the nasal mucosa occurs from physical (e.g., talc, coal dust) and chemical agents (e.g., aldehydes). Allergic reactions result from exposures to high or low molecular weight antigens. Most high molecular weight antigens are naturally occurring substances, such as dust mites, fungal spores, animal danders, and food substances. These antigens react with IgE antibodies present on the mast cells to result in a typical allergic reaction. The low molecular weight agents such as organic chemicals (isocyanates, acid anhydrides, aldehydes) and inorganic chemicals (chromium, platinum) cause allergy through IgE-IgG human serum albumin hapten complexes or poorly understood mechanisms. All antigens, whatever their molecular weight, cause sensitization (antibody formation after a latent period).

Symptoms are similar to those of spontaneous allergic rhinitis, that is, nasal congestion, sneeze, rhinorrhea, lacrimation, and itchy eyes. These usually appear in the workplace and clear shortly after leaving, unless an isolated late reaction occurs 6 to 8 hours after leaving the workplace. Examination usually reveals pale, boggy nasal turbinates with serous drainage. Rhinometry shows airway obstruction; nasal smear and nasal lavage show increased eosinophils and leukotriene levels. Permanent removal from the offending environment is required for a lasting relief, although antihistamines, decongestants, and nasal steroids may temporarily control the symptoms.

Occupational asthma has many causes and classifications. One theory recognizes three basic responsible mechanisms: pharmacologic, immunologic, and inflammatory. This chapter deals only with the immunologic factors; the reader is referred to Chap. 11, Occupational Pulmonary Disease, for discussion of other aspects of occupational asthma. Occupational asthma is defined as asthma caused by dusts, vapors, mists, and fumes in the workplace, even though symptoms may appear at a later time. Asthma resulting from high molecular weight antigens is expressed either as an immediate or an immediate and late (occurring 6–8 hours after exposure) reaction in over 95% of cases. Low molecular weight antigens are associated with an isolated late reaction in about 50% of cases, greatly confounding the search for the causative agent. When these late reactions occur at home in the evening several hours after the exposure, both patient and physician assume these are immediate reactions associated with an environmental antigen at home. The investigation is directed away from the workplace and much time is wasted and morbidity increased before the true cause is discovered.

High molecular weight antigens that cause immunologic occupational asthma come from three sources: plants, animals, and foods. *Plant* sources include fungal spores, grain dust, cereal dust, flour dust (wheat), green coffee bean, tea, green tobacco leaf, and vegetable gums, in addition to tree, grass, and weed pollens. *Animal* exposure occurs from dander, pelt, saliva, urinary proteins, scales, and feathers. Contact with animals occurs in occupations such as animal handlers, researchers, farmers, livestock workers, veterinarians, and others whose occupations require animal contact. These exposures may be complicated by pets at home. Inhalation sensitivity in the *food* industry can occur from exposure to eggs, mushrooms, shellfish, garlic, and many other foodstuffs. Occupational asthma to *enzymes* such as trypsin, chemotrypsin, and papain occurs in the pharmaceutical industry. The enzyme from *Bacillus subtilis* causes asthma in sensitized detergent industry workers. Most high molecular weight antigens can be detected by skin or RAST testing.

Risk factors in some, but not all, cases of high molecular weight asthma are atopy and bronchial hyperresponsiveness. Settipane [3] has shown that in atopic patients with allergic rhinitis, 50% have asymptomatic reductions in FEV_1 and 13% will develop overt asthma in 3 to 4 years.

The *low molecular weight antigens* are a varied group of agents that fall into three subdivisions: therapeutic drugs, organic chemicals, and inorganic chemicals. The first two groups generally cause asthma by means of the antigen–serum albumin (HSA) hapten interacting with antibody (usually IgG, occasionally IgE). Some of these can be evaluated by ELISA and RAST in vitro testing, a few by skin testing.

Therapeutic agents capable of causing allergic occupational asthma consist of antibiotics, other pharmaceuticals, and miscellaneous therapeutic agents. The beta-lactam antibiotics (penicillins, cephalosporins), the tetracyclines, and the sulfonamides, among others, are the most common causes of sensitivity. Other pharmaceuticals, such as methyldopa (Aldomet), psyllium, cimetidine, albuterol (Salbutamol), pentamidine, ipecac, and ethylene oxide, are capable of triggering allergic asthma. Miscellaneous agents such as piperazine and chloramine have also been implicated in immunologic asthma.

The major low molecular weight *organic chemicals* known or suspected of causing immune-mediated occupational asthma are listed in Table 19-1.

Abietic acid is the principal ingredient in colophony, which is produced from distillation of pine resin. Colophony is used as soldering flux (particularly in the electronics industry) and can be inhaled, causing suspected (but not proven) sensitization. It is possible that pine allergy may be a predisposing factor. Some workers are sensitized by inhaling pine dust, although there is no greater incidence of atopy in these workers.

Acid anhydrides are composed of several highly reactive low molecular weight compounds, notably phthalic anhydride (PA) and trimellitic anhydride (TMA). PA causes allergic rhinitis and asthma through anhydride—HSA hapten–specific IgE antibody (type I). TMA not only causes occupational asthma (type I), but also hypersensitivity pneumonitis (type III), late respiratory systemic syndrome (cough, dyspnea, fever, myalgia-arthralgia) through a TMA-HSA hapten–specific IgG or IgA (not IgE) (type I), and TMA pulmonary disease—anemia syndrome (cough, dyspnea, and hemoptysis) through TMA-HSA hapten–specific IgG.

Aldehydes (formaldehyde and glutaraldehyde) are airway irritants in most workers but can be sensitizers to a few through the IgE or IgG mechanism.

Isocyanates, along with acid anhydrides, are highly reactive compounds that cause sensitization in 5 to 10% of exposed workers. Allergen-specific IgE or IgG-HSA type reactions have been reported, but generally occupational asthma from isocyanates is believed to be multifactorial (pharmacologic, immunologic, and irritative).

Plicatic acid present in western red cedar wood dust can cause occupational asthma through a variety of pharmacologic, irritant, and specific and nonspecific immuno-

Table 19-1. Some organic agents that cause occupational asthma

Abietic acid (colophony)
Acid anhydrides
Aldehydes
Isocyanates
Plicatic acid (western red cedar)

logic mechanisms. It is not believed to be an IgE type allergen. Immediate, isolated, late, and dual asthmatic reactions can occur, which seem to implicate an immunologic basis. Much study is ongoing in an attempt to clarify this.

Inorganic chemicals, particularly the metals, can cause occupational asthma; however, the mechanisms are unclear at the present time. Similar to the situation with red cedar, an underlying immunologic mechanism is indicated.

Workup of Suspected Occupational Asthma

The evaluation of suspected immune-mediated occupational asthma must proceed in a logical step-wise fashion. As suggested by Becklake [4], the first step is to be certain that airflow limitation exists. This can be done by obtaining a history of dyspnea, wheeze, chest tightness, or cough; evidence of wheezing on physical examination (not always present); and evidence of an obstructive pattern on spirometry or a reduction in peak flow.

Second, hyperresponsiveness of the airways can be detected by a history of episodic nature of the symptoms and spirometry that shows reversibility after the use of bronchodilators. Third, the presence of atopy can be suggested by a history of allergic disease in the worker or family, positive skin or RAST tests, or elevation of total IgE.

Fourth, work-relatedness of the asthma can be suspected by a history of temporal relationship of symptoms to the worksite and either pre- and postshift expiratory flow comparisons or repeated worksite peak flow rates (PFRs) compared to non-workday PFRs. A common schedule is to measure PFRs every 2 hours during workdays for 2 weeks, followed by measurement every 2 hours during a week off work.

Fifth, to establish the presence of sensitivity to a specific workplace agent, several steps can be taken. Skin testing or measurement of specific IgE antibodies in vitro is possible with most of the high molecular weight antigens. Detection of IgE- or IgG-specific antibodies is possible through the ELISA technique in the case of some low molecular weight sensitizers (formaldehyde). In many cases of low molecular weight agents, however, the only definitive test is inhalation challenge with the specific antigen. Because of the variables of chemical concentration, worker sensitivity, and the strong possibility of an isolated late reaction occurring 6 to 8 hours after inhalation, specific inhalation challenge must only be done in a special chamber at a medical center with capabilities for emergency intervention and overnight observation of the patient.

Malo [5] suggests a questionnaire, skin or RAST testing, and pre- and postwork shift spirometry by the pulmonologist, allergist, or occupational medicine physician. Only if a 20% drop is seen in the FEV_1 at the end of the work shift does he recommend proceeding with repeated workplace PFRs, non-worksite PFRs, workplace inhalation test if feasible, or specific inhalation challenge in the medical center under a pulmonologist's supervision.

Peak Flowmeter Measurements

Peak flow measurement is a low-cost, effective way to help diagnose and monitor a worker's airway disease. Many peak flowmeters currently available provide sufficiently reproducible readings in a given patient to assist the physician in diagnosis and treatment of suspected bronchospastic lung disease. However, since the peak flow is effort dependent, a patient may not perform the test properly or may use it for secondary gain.

The physician should become familiar with one or two types of meters. Criteria used in selecting a particular meter include availability, cost (an adequate meter can be purchased for about $30), an easily readable scale, and durability.

Using a peak flowmeter is simple and easily mastered by almost all patients after minimal (5–10 minutes) training. Training must be conducted by an individual knowledgeable in the peak flow maneuver and the reading and charting of values. The patient should be observed while performing three peak flow measurements, but one should chart only the best (not the average) reading. Changes in medications and symptoms, as well as any changes in work schedule or duties, should also be noted on the chart. Ideally, the worker should take the first reading on arising and every 2 hours thereafter until bedtime. If the individual is taking a beta-adrenergic inhaler, all readings should be consistently taken before he or she uses the inhaler. Practically, however, it is probably sufficient to perform readings upon awakening and at preshift, midshift, end of shift, and bedtime. It is important to assess any important changes in readings (generally 20% change or greater) over the course of a day, as well as any significant differences between the different days of the work week, weekends, and vacations.

When the peak flow chart is reviewed, the physician should correlate the readings with the patient's symptoms and physical findings. A marked discrepancy between these factors suggests poor effort or technique in performing the maneuver. Fluctuations in the range of plus or minus 10% are usual, when comparing readings taken at the same time on different days. Too little variability suggests that the patient is not performing peak flow readings well.

Even with all the caveats noted above, peak flowmeters are a useful tool for the occupational medicine physician. In addition, the readings can provide useful feedback information for the patient in judging the degree of impairment and the need for medication.

Hypersensitivity Pneumonitis (Extrinsic Allergic Alveolitis)

Hypersensitivity pneumonitis occurs when inhaled antigens in the home or work environment cause an immunologic inflammatory reaction (type III, immune complex reaction) in the bronchioles, alveoli, and lung interstitium. The most frequent allergens are thermophilic actinomycetes, which are found in warm humid environments (such as soil, hay, or forced heating and cooling systems) in which the water has stagnated. Other causes of hypersensitivity pneumonitis include chemicals such as isocyanates and trimellitic anhydride. The prevalence of the disease is about 7 to 15% of exposed individuals.

Hypersensitivity pneumonitis (HP) can occur in an acute, subacute, or chronic form. The acute form appears as a flu-like illness 4 to 6 hours after heavy intermittent exposure. Symptoms abate after a few hours to a few days if exposure is avoided. Pulmonary function tests show a restrictive pattern. Hypoxemia and decreased diffusing capacity are found. The chest x-ray may be normal or show a granular or nodular pattern. The subacute and chronic forms occur with continued exposure. Progressive dyspnea, decreased exercise tolerance, productive cough, and weight loss develop gradually. Pulmonary function tests show a severe restrictive pattern. The chest x-ray findings are typical of diffuse interstitial fibrosis.

On physical examination, the lung auscultation reveals dry, crackling rales throughout the lungs that are more prominent at the bases. Wheezing generally does not occur, but if present, makes the differentiation between HP and occupational asthma quite difficult. Asthma may coexist with HP, especially in the atopic patient.

There is no single pathognomonic test for HP. Specific precipitating (IgG) antibodies to offending substances are helpful in making the diagnosis and are present in over 90% of individuals with the disease, but there are several points to remember. First, these antibodies are only a marker to exposure, not disease. Second, since the sensitivity of the test varies among commercial laboratories, negative tests in the context of strong clinical evidence suggesting the disease do not exclude the diagnosis. In addition, not all patients demonstrate antibodies to the same antigen and many patients have multiple precipitating antibodies. Finally, antibody levels begin to fall once exposure is terminated, although this fall in antibody levels does not correlate with disease remission or progression. Thus, the patient with severe, chronic HP may have no detectable precipitating antibodies. Since skin testing only detects IgE antibodies, it provides little or no help in confirming the diagnosis.

In treating the acute episodes, corticosteroids are often used to hasten recovery. There is no evidence that long-term corticosteroid usage protects against lung damage from chronic exposure. Avoidance of the offending antigen is the most important treatment. Masks, dust filters, and attention to the heating and air conditioning systems are all important. The patient may need to change occupations depending upon the degree of modification required to make the worker's environment safe and the specific antigen involved.

Acute Bronchopulmonary Aspergillosis

Acute bronchopulmonary aspergillosis (ABPA) is severe asthma associated with an elevated serum IgE and total eosinophil count. The condition results from colonization of the lower-respiratory tract with *Aspergillus fumigatus* spores (rarely other fungi). In addition to periodic episodes of severe bronchoconstriction, the patient demonstrates transient pulmonary infiltrates on x-ray and has thick, brown sputum plugs. Skin testing shows an immediate reaction to the fungal spores, with a late reaction appearing in about 4 hours in some patients. Serum precipitating IgG antibodies are also present. Damage to the bronchial walls occurs from the action of IgE and IgG *Aspergillus* antibody. This leads to central bronchiectasis and granulomas through type I, II, and IV reactions. Long-term use of corticosteroids is required for control.

Latex Hypersensitivity

Since the 1980s, numerous reports of immediate and delayed hypersensitivity reactions to latex and natural rubber have appeared in the literature. This increase coincided with the widespread use of latex in our culture. For the medical profession, for many workers, and for patients about to undergo any type of medical intervention, latex exposure is extremely difficult to avoid. True IgE-mediated allergic reactions are being reported with increasing frequency and have caused severe anaphylactic reactions and deaths. Allergic reactions may occur after direct contact with latex- or rubber-containing materials, or after exposure to aerosolized latex antigen.

Several groups are at *greatest risk:* (1) health care workers and workers in the rubber industry, (2) children with meningomyelocele or urogenital abnormalities who have undergone numerous manipulations with catheters and surgeries, and (3) any individuals who have a history of past latex reactions, a history of hand dermatitis from contact with latex, and a general atopic history, and those who have had unexplained anaphylactic reactions during surgery. In the past, it was assumed that these intraoperative reactions were due to allergic reactions to the anesthesia; now latex is suspected.

Types of allergic reactions include eczema, localized urticaria, allergic rhinitis or conjunctivitis, bronchospasm, and anaphylaxis. The route of exposure is often correlated with the type of allergic reaction. For example, latex exposure of the skin may cause a dermatitis, aerosolized particles from the latex gloves may produce rhinoconjunctivitis or bronchospasm, and latex exposure intraoperatively and during dental procedures can cause anaphylaxis as a result of the direct exposure of mucous membranes to the latex. Any worker with unexplained skin rash who has regular and frequent exposure to latex or rubber should be suspected of having latex hypersensitivity.

No standard screening evaluation to identify such patients currently exists. Recommendations taken in part from those made by the American Academy of Allergy and Immunology [6] include the following: (1) High-risk patients should be identified (see risk groups, above). (2) All patients should be asked about a possible history of latex sensitivity. (3) All high-risk patients should be offered testing for latex allergy. There is currently no standardized test for latex sensitivity. Skin testing using an extract made from a glove is quite sensitive, but should only be performed by physicians skilled in allergy testing. Anaphylactic reactions have occurred during testing. In vitro tests are available, but are not sensitive enough to identify all patients at risk. (4) Procedures on all patients with spina bifida and all history-positive patients regardless of risk group status should be performed in a latex-free environment. (5) Vinyl or synthetic latex-free rubber gloves, such as Neolon (neoprene; Becton-Dickinson, Franklin Lakes, NJ), Elastyren (a styrene polymer; Hermal Pharmaceuticals, Oakfield, NY), and Tactylon (a styrene polymer; Tactyl Technologies, Visa, CA) should be provided. (6) Persons who have serious reactions should wear a Medic-Alert tag and carry an epinephrine-containing emergency kit. The medical professional should teach the patient how to use it and provide scientific guidelines for when to use it. (7) Preoperative medication should be offered to any known latex-sensitive individual beginning 24 hours before surgery and continuing

24 hours after the operation. If a 24-hour wait is not possible, it is suggested that hydrocortisone be substituted for methylprednisolone. The following preoperative schedule is suggested [7]:

Diphenhydramine, 1 mg/kg q6h IV/PO
plus
Methylprednisolone, 1 mg/kg q6h IV/PO
plus
Cimetidine, 6 mg/kg q6h IV/PO
or
Terfenadine, 30–60 mg q12h PO
plus
Prednisone, 0.5 mg/kg q12h PO
plus
Ranitidine, 1–2 mg/kg/day PO divided q12h

Fungal Diseases

Of all the microbiologic agents, the fungi present particular problems, not only because of their ubiquity (greatest source of aeroallergens worldwide), but also because of their ability to cause hypersensitivity, infection, and toxicity. Fungal growth in the workplace is enhanced by dampness (standing water and high relative humidity), warm temperature, poor air circulation, and darkness. Source control requires attention to all these factors.

Hypersensitivity reactions result from the antigenic material released from fungal spore walls, mycelial walls, and submicronic airborne particles. All four types of *hypersensitivity* reactions can occur from fungal exposure: type I, immediate hypersensitivity (occupational rhinitis and asthma); type III, immune complex reactions (hypersensitivity pneumonitis) if spores are small and exposure is very intense; and a combination type I-II-IV reaction in ABPA.

Although fungal *infections* are usually limited to immune suppressed workers, overwhelming exposure to the spores of *Histo-plasma* and *Cryptococcus* may cause infections in otherwise healthy people.

Mycotoxins are a result of fungal metabolites that contaminate foods, particularly nuts, corn, rice, and other grains. These metabolites are toxic to animals and humans ingesting the contaminated foodstuffs. *Aspergillus flavus* produces aflatoxin, which is a powerful hepatocarcinogen. Trichothecenes are formed from *Fusarium*, *Trichoderma*, and *Cephalosporium* fungi and cause diarrhea, multiple hemorrhages, skin inflammation, and death if contaminated wheat is ingested. At present, no cases of mycotoxicity from inhalation have been reported.

Anaphylaxis

Anaphylaxis refers to a (potentially) life-threatening, acute IgE-mediated reaction that results in the release of large amounts of mediators. An anaphylactoid reaction produces physical findings and symptoms indistinguishable from those of an anaphylactic reaction, but without demonstrable IgE involvement (Table 19-2).

Symptoms may be limited to one organ system or involve multiple organs. Once the reaction begins, it may rapidly progress and become fatal. Nonfatal reactions resolve within 1 or 2 days.

Clinical manifestations of anaphylaxis present in three forms: mild sys-

Table 19-2. Common causes of anaphylactic and anaphylactoid reactions

Food	Blood products (human, animal)
Food additives	Local anesthetics
Antibiotics	Insect sting
Other drugs	Latex
Allergenic extracts	Exercise
Diagnostic agents	Temperature extremes (heat, cold)

temic reactions, moderate systemic reactions, and severe systemic reactions. Mild systemic reactions are characterized by peripheral tingling, a warm sensation throughout the body, fullness in the mouth and throat, nasal congestion, sneezing, facial swelling, and pruritus. Moderate systemic reactions usually involve respiratory distress (wheezing, dyspnea, hoarse voice, cough), anxiety, generalized hives, or angioedema. Severe systemic reactions are characterized by severe respiratory distress and inability to talk, cyanosis, swollen tongue, abdominal cramps, diarrhea, vomiting, hypotension, shock, and loss of consciousness.

Treatment consists of a rapid assessment since delay in therapy can result in a fatal outcome. Epinephrine (1 : 1000 0.3–0.5 ml subcutaneously) is the treatment of choice. Diphenhydramine (25–75 mg) intramuscularly may be given *in addition* to the epinephrine. (In patients with only skin rash, the physician may elect to use only the diphenhydramine.) If the reaction is the result of a medical injection or an insect sting (see below), a tourniquet should be applied above the injection site if possible. The patient should be observed for at least 30 minutes after symptoms subside and be told to contact his or her physician if symptoms reoccur over the next several hours. If symptoms progress or do not begin to subside quickly, one should consider transporting the patient by ambulance to an emergency facility. After the acute episode, the patient should be referred to an allergist for further evaluation.

Patients who are taking a beta-blocking drug may experience less effectiveness from epinephrine and a more severe or prolonged anaphylactic episode. Injection of glucagon has been advocated in such patients.

Allergy to insect stings is reported to be the cause of 40 to 60 deaths annually, although the actual number may be higher. A study of factory workers found that 5% had a history of significant reaction to an insect sting in the past. Outdoor workers such as agricultural workers or utility linemen may also experience reactions at a higher prevalence. The symptoms of insect sting anaphylaxis are no different than those outlined above. Although most cases of insect sting anaphylaxis occur soon after the sting, there have been several reports of late reactions, more than 24 hours following the sting.

Treatment of large local reactions to an insect sting consists of elevation of the limb, ice applied to the sting site, and oral antihistamines. One should consider a short course of prednisone for massive local reactions (reactions extending more than two joints beyond the sting site). Any patient who has had a generalized reaction should be assumed to be at risk for a serious anaphylactic reaction and, therefore, treated according to the protocol outlined above under anaphylaxis. In addition, any patient who has had a generalized reaction (*including* generalized hives) should be referred for an allergy evaluation. Insect venom immunotherapy is safe and extremely effective in preventing further systemic reactions. Also, any patient suspected of being venom allergic should be trained in the use of an emergency treatment kit containing epinephrine. ANA-Kit or ANA-Guard is available from Hollister-Steir (Spokane, WA), and Epi-Pen can be obtained from Center Laboratories (Port Washington, NY). Both companies have demonstration kits for health professionals.

Multiple Chemical Sensitivity

Multiple chemical sensitivity (MCS) is probably more correctly termed multiple chemical intolerance, because no evidence of hypersensitivity has yet been detected. At any rate, because of multiple definitions, much confusion has resulted. An all-encompassing *definition* by the Ontario Ministry of Health in 1989 is as follows:

> A chronic (i.e., continuous over three months) multisystem disorder, usually involving symptoms of the CNS and at least one other system. Affected persons are frequently intolerant to some foods and react adversely to some chemicals and environmental agents, singly or in combinations at levels generally tolerated by the majority of people. Affected individuals have varying degrees of morbidity, from mild discomfort to total disability. Upon physical exam, the patient is usually free from any abnormal or objective findings [8].

McClellan [9] lists five points that he considers necessary to make the diagnosis: (1) At least three organ systems are involved, with a plethora of symptoms; (2)

symptoms result from extremely low doses; (3) symptoms may start localized and then spread; (4) patients are more vocal about their symptoms; and (5) patients are more disabled than anticipated.

A variety of *symptoms,* including extreme sensitivity to odors, fatigue, headache, inability to concentrate, paresthesias, and other symptoms involving the respiratory, central nervous system (CNS), and gastrointestinal (GI) systems, are predominant. The symptom complex is usually identified by a well-defined event, either exposure to pesticides, petrochemicals, or generally innocuous substances. It is believed by proponents of this syndrome that total body load of "antigens" is exceeded, thus triggering the reaction. Once the illness occurs, however, almost any other natural or manmade substance at any dose may exacerbate the illness. Because of the self-imposed limitations on work and social activities, a feeling of isolation, depression, and frustration usually develops.

There are many *theories* regarding the underlying mechanisms, often in direct opposition. The three most common at the present time are immune dysregulation, limbic-olfactory hypersensitivity, and basic psychological disturbance. *The immune dysregulation theory* proposes that minuscule amounts of the offending chemical cause hyperreactivity of the immune system, leading to cellular damage [10]. *The limbic-olfactory theory* holds that low-level chemical stimulation of the olfactory nerve affects the limbic area of the brain, causing complex interactions between the immune, endocrine, and nervous systems (all of which are closely related in the limbic area) [11]. A third theory, based on psychometric testing, suggests that basic *psychological factors* (such as abuse in childhood, depression, or other psychological disorders) predispose individuals to development of some somatization of complaints after presumed exposure to chemicals [12]. At the present time, there is much controversy over the actual cause of this syndrome. No single theory is acceptable to all.

Because there are *no standard objective tests* that show a consistent abnormality in MCS, the diagnosis is based on history alone. Clinical ecologists, who are proponents of the syndrome, have failed to demonstrate well-controlled double-blind evidence that various tests and treatments (often using unproven and controversial techniques such as sublingual and neutralization tests) have any validity. Allergists-immunologists, on the other hand, are unable to detect any consistent abnormality in standard, universally accepted objective tests. Because of this, position statements by the American Academy of Allergy and Immunology [13] state the following: "An objective evaluation of the diagnostic and therapeutic principles used to support the concept of clinical ecology indicates that it is an unproven and experimental methodology. It is time consuming and places severe restrictions on the individual's life style. Individuals who are being treated in this manner should be fully informed of this experimental nature."

In another position paper regarding unproven techniques, the American Academy of Allergy Executive Committee [14] states that "Currently available procedures of proven effectiveness are sufficiently satisfactory for diagnosis and treatment of allergic and immunologic diseases, so that procedures of unproven effectiveness should not be used in routine fashion, but rather should be considered experimental . . ." In December 1992, the Council on Scientific Affairs, American Medical Association [15], concluded that "Based on reports in the Peer Reviewed Scientific Literature, the Council on Scientific Affairs finds that at this time, (1) there are no well-controlled studies establishing a clear mechanism or cause for multiple chemical sensitivity syndrome; and (2) there are no well-controlled studies providing confirmation of the efficacy of the diagnostic and therapeutic modalities relied on by those who practice clinical ecology."

Unfortunately, many patients are caught in the dilemma of becoming prisoners of their symptoms (imagined or real). This has led to an extremely restrictive limitation of work and social activities, loss of income from lack of gainful employment, and a frustrating search for adequate, compassionate medical care (either from traditional or alternative sources).

A *suggested approach* for the general occupational medicine physician at this time is as follows: (1) Listen to the patient's symptoms with an open mind; (2) carry out a complete examination; (3) do sufficient, standard, well-accepted tests to rule out allergic, endocrine, or neurologic diseases if suggested by the history; (4) refer to a specialist if necessary; and (5) treat with reassurance and appropriate medications, and, by all means, encourage physical activity and social interaction.

Immunotoxicology

Immunotoxicology is the study of toxic effects of xenobiotics on the cellular and humoral components of the immune system. The multiplicity of chemical and biologic agents in the home and workplace and their complex interactions within the immune system make this field confusing and difficult to assess.

The basic *functions of the immune system* are protection of the body from external agents and maintenance of internal homeostasis and surveillance. Several types of cells, organs, and humoral substances are utilized to accomplish these goals.

Components of the Immune System

Probably more than any other body system, the immune system consists of a great diversity of cells, organs, and humoral or secretory chemical messengers. The cellular components consist of lymphocytes, plasma cells, macrophages, mast cells, neutrophils, basophils, and eosinophils. The organs include the bone marrow, spleen, lymph nodes, and lymphoid tissue lining the GI tract. The humoral (acellular) elements consist of antibodies, leukotrienes, and complement.

The cellular elements arise from a common bone marrow–derived pluripotent stem cell that gives rise to the lymphoid and myeloid series. Some lymphoid stem cells are processed in the neonatal thymus and develop into *T lymphocytes;* others bypass the thymus and are processed in the "bursal equivalent tissues" (bone marrow, lymph nodes, appendix, and other GI tract–associated lymphoid tissue) to become *B lymphocytes.* A few lymphoid stem cells bypass both the thymus and bursal tissue to become *natural killer (NK) cells.* The T and B lymphocytes and plasma cells are involved with specific immunity and respond only to recognized antigens.

The myeloid stem cell develops into the macrophage, mast cell, or polymorphonuclear leukocyte (PMN), consisting of basophils, eosinophils, and neutrophils. The PMNs and NK cells are involved in nonspecific immunity and will interact with all foreign material.

An Overview of Function

On contact with the macrophage-processed antigen, T cells undergo transformation into helper (TH) or suppressor (TS) cells, which regulate antibody production from B lymphocytes. Still other T cells, when exposed to foreign antigens, become sensitized to liberate lymphokines (interleukins, interferons, and tumor necrosis factor), which set the stage for delayed-type hypersensitivity.

Contact with macrophage-processed antigens stimulates B lymphocytes to transform into antibody-producing plasma cells under the control of TH cells; the whole process is limited by the suppressing effect of TS cells. Plasma cells synthesize specific humoral antibodies of the immunoglobulin classes A, D, E, G, and M. ImmunoglobulinE is the allergy antibody. ImmunoglobulinM is formed initially after exposure to most foreign proteins; IgG is stimulated from exposure to viruses, bacteria, and toxins. Each clone of plasma cells will synthesize only one specific type of immunoglobulin. Circulating immunoglobulin antibodies attach to receptor sites on the surface of mast cells and remain there until specific antigens are attracted to them. As stated earlier, within the mast cells are packets of histamine and other vasoactive amines, which when liberated cause chemical inflammation in the surrounding tissue. At the time of specific antigen cross-linkage with two immunoglobulin molecules on the mast cell surface, the vasoactive material is released, causing the allergic reaction.

Interactions with antigens will result in specific reactions depending on the *immune status of the host.* As shown in Table 19-3, the hyperactive immune system will respond to external antigens (pollen, fungal spores, and animal dander) in the form of an allergic reaction. Antigens that resemble host proteins will cause autoimmune disease (e.g., lupus, scleroderma). In the hypoactive immune system, external antigens (bacteria, viruses) may cause infection or immunodeficiency syndromes, whereas internal antigens (tumor cells) can progress to malignancy.

The complement system consists of nine proteins, which interact in a cascade

Table 19-3. Host immune status

Immune status	External antigen	Internal antigen
Hyperactive	Allergy	Autoimmunity
Balanced	Normal	Normal
Hypoactive	Infection	Malignancy immune defect

fashion to facilitate the IgG and IgM antibody reactions with antigens of the Gell and Coombs class II and III type hypersensitivity.

Immunotoxicants

Many chemical, microbiologic, and physical agents can affect the immune system, some by nonspecific interactions and others by specific means. These complex interactions may result in stimulation or suppression manifested by different clinical syndromes representing all four Gell and Coombs categories.

Although the majority of immunotoxicants have a suppressive effect, some may stimulate the immune mechanism, resulting in allergy or autoimmunity, while others may cause uncontrolled cellular proliferation and altered host defense mechanisms.

Regarding *immunostimulation,* some metals (nickel, platinum, and beryllium) are capable of causing asthma (type I), pulmonary hypersensitivity syndromes (type III), and allergic contact dermatitis (type IV). Isocyanates can cause asthma (type I) and anhydrides can cause asthma (type I), pulmonary disease–anemia syndrome (type II), hypersensitivity pneumonitis (type III), and delayed-type hypersensitivity (type IV). Therapeutic drugs (especially beta-lactam antibiotics), food additives (sulfides and MSG), and pesticides (pyrethrum) are all capable of immunostimulation resulting in anaphylactic reactions (type I).

The low molecular weight compounds may bind with serum albumin to form haptens against which T and B cells misdirect antibodies, resulting in *autoimmune* destruction of autologous tissue. Dieldrin pesticide is associated with immune hemolytic anemia, hydrazine with lupus-like syndrome, monomeric vinyl chloride with scleroderma-like changes, and heavy metals (such as gold) with immune complex glomerulonephritis. Most of these autoimmune reactions are reversible upon removal of the offending chemicals.

The majority of immunotoxicants are *suppressive,* either dampening the whole immune apparatus or acting at specific points. For instance, benzine, although capable of general bone marrow suppression, specifically causes the reduced synthesis of IgG and IgE antibodies. Polychlorinated biphenyls (PCBs) depress both humoral (B cell) and delayed-type (T cell) immunity while the polycyclic aromatic hydrocarbon DMBA causes long-lasting immune suppression, mostly affecting the B cells. Urethane suppresses NK cell activity, allowing neoplastic cells to grow unchecked.

Many airborne pollutants, such as formaldehyde, ozone, asbestos, oxidant gases, and environmental tobacco smoke, depress nonspecific resistance to bacteria and viruses by suppressing macrophage, phagocytic, and enzymatic activity.

Microbiologics such as bacteria (thermophilic actinomycetes) and fungi (*Aspergillus*) can stimulate immune hypersensitivity lung reactions. Viruses (human immunodeficiency virus) can destroy T-cell clones, thus permitting opportunistic infections (*Pneumocystis carinii*) and unusual neoplasia (Kaposi's sarcoma).

Physical agents such as heat, cold, and vibration promote urticaria and angioedema through nonspecific immune aberrations.

Testing

The multitude of chemicals, complex interactions of the immune system, and confusing array of symptoms require a logical system of testing (in addition to a complete history and physical examination) to ensure that all major possibilities are investigated. The subcommittee on immunotoxicology of the National Research Council's Committee on Biological Markers has proposed a tiered testing approach [16].

Tier I (used in all people exposed to immunotoxicants) includes measurements of humoral antibody (such as pneumococcal or polio), total levels of the specific immunoglobulins (IgG, IgM, IgA, IgE) and isotope-specific antibody titration (ELISA), complete blood counts and differentials, lymphocyte enumeration and typing (T and B cells, T-cell subsets, and plasma cells), and measurements of delayed-type hypersensitivity (*Candida,* purified protein derivative, mumps, tetanus) and antibody titers (e.g., antinuclear antibody).

Tier II tests are only carried out in people with significant abnormalities in tier I. These tests include the induction of primary antibody response to injected protein or polysaccharide antigens, stimulation of lymphocyte proliferation with specific mitogens, additional T and B cell marker determinations, and measurement of cytokines (interleukins and interferons).

Tier III tests (limited to people with abnormalities in tier II) consist of tests for NK cell function (such as nonspecific killing of tumor cells in culture) and biopsy of lymphatic tissue, spleen, or bone marrow.

It should be pointed out that flow cytometry is not yet standardized and must be considered an experimental test at the time of this writing. All tests should correlate with the history and physical examination, and care should be taken to allow for individual ranges of variation. Indiscriminate use of biomarker assays may lead to misdiagnosis and erroneous associations.

Because of the complexity of techniques and multiple factors affecting the final laboratory results, it is important to have tier testing done and interpreted by certified immunologists at well-established, university-recognized immunotoxicologic laboratories.

References

1. Bureau of Labor Statistics, US Department of Labor, 1987.
2. Coombs, R. R. A., and Gell, P. G. H. (eds.). *Clinical Aspects of Immunology.* Philadelphia: Lippincott, 1975. P. 761.
3. Settipane, G. A. Rhinitis: Introduction in G. A. Settipane (ed.), *Rhinitis* (2nd ed.). Providence: Oceanside Press, 1991. P. 3.
4. Becklake, M. R. Features used to establish the clinical diagnosis of occupational asthma. *Chest* 98 (Suppl.):165S, 1990.
5. Malo, J. L. The case for confirming occupational asthma. *J. Allergy Clin. Immunol.* 91:967, 1993.
6. Slater, J. E. Allergic reactions to natural rubber. *Ann. Allergy* 68:203, 1992.
7. Kwitten, P. L., et al. Latex hypersensitivity reactions despite prophylaxis. *Allergy Proc.* 13:123, 1992.
8. Report of the Ad Hoc Committee on Environmental Hypersensitivity Disorders. Office of the Minister of Health, Toronto, Canada, 1989. Pp. 17–18.
9. McClellan, R. K. Biological intervention in the treatment of patients with multiple chemical sensitivity. *Occup. Med. State of the Art Rev.* 2:663, 1987.
10. Randolph, T. G., and Moss, R. W. *An Alternative Approach to Allergies.* New York: Lippincott and Cromwell, 1980.
11. Ashford, N. A., and Miller, C. S. *Chemical Exposures: Low Levels and High Stakes.* New York: Van Nostrand and Reinhold, 1991.
12. Schottenfeld, R. S. Workers with multiple chemical sensitivity: A psychiatric approach to diagnosis and treatment. *Occup. Med. State of the Art Rev.* 2:739, 1987.
13. American Academy of Allergy and Immunology position statement: Clinical ecology. *J. Allergy Clin. Immunol.* 78:269, 1986.
14. American Academy of Allergy and Immunology position statement: Unproven procedures for diagnosis and treatment of allergic and immunologic disease. *J. Allergy Clin. Immunol.* 78:275, 1986.
15. American Medical Association Council on Scientific Affairs. Multiple chemical sensitivity syndrome. *J.A.M.A.* 268:3465, 1992.
16. Goldstein, B., et al. *Biomarkers in Immunotoxicology.* Committee on Biological Markers, National Research Council. Washington, DC: National Academy Press, 1992.

Further Information

Bardana, E. L., Montanaro, A., and O'Halloran, M. T. *Occupational Asthma.* Philadelphia: Henley & Belfus, 1992.

An up-to-date text covering all types of occupational asthma, particularly strong on immune mediated types. Also has discussion of sick building syndrome and multiple chemical sensitivity.

Bernstein, I. L., et al. (eds.). *Asthma in the Workplace.* New York: Marcel Dekker, 1993.
A comprehensive text-reference that details the pathophysiology and step-by-step evaluation and treatment of occupational asthma with particular emphasis on immunology laboratory tests.

Dean, J. H., and Murray, M. J. Toxic Response of the Immune System. In Amdur, Doull, and Klassen (eds.), *Casarett and Doull's Toxicology* (4th ed.). New York: McGraw-Hill, 1991.
A detailed account of current knowledge of this specialized field. The text is a standard teaching and reference work for toxicology.

deShazo, R. D., and Smith, D. L. (eds.). Primer on allergic and immunologic diseases (3rd ed.). *J.A.M.A.* 260:2785, 1992.
A state-of-the-art update. Many articles, particularly those covering the "traditional" areas of allergy, are suitable for the generalist.

Lawlor, G. L., and Fischer, T. J. *Manual of Allergy and Immunology* (2nd ed.). Boston: Little, Brown, 1988.
An excellent "nuts and bolts" practical approach to diagnosis and treatment of common allergic and immunologic diseases.

20

Arm Pain in the Workplace

Nortin M. Hadler

The experience of discomfort in the upper extremity is commonplace. Some 30% of us will be forced to cope with this problem for at least one week each year [1–3]. Often these symptoms are exacerbated by usage of the affected limb or limb region so that performance in any setting is rendered less instinctive. Nonetheless, nearly all of us can find the personal resources to cope effectively until the symptoms subside spontaneously. There are occasions, however, when such coping becomes counterintuitive and guidance is sought. In the context of the workplace, the readily available resource is the medical department.

This chapter focuses on the plight of individuals with regional musculoskeletal illnesses of the upper extremity. These are individuals who would be well were it not for the particular musculoskeletal region that hurts. They can identify no forceful physical insult as a precipitant and have incurred no damage to the integument. Rather, their illness occurs in the course of activities that are customary and customarily comfortable. Regional musculoskeletal illnesses comprise the vast majority of disorders of the upper extremity; however, the clinician must be prepared to discern the patient whose upper-extremity symptoms follow no traumatic insult yet are not likely to reflect regional musculoskeletal illnesses (Table 20-1). In the presence of any of these clues, appropriate referral may be advisable, especially for some of the regional musculoskeletal illnesses. These conditions are exceptional, however, and are pointed out in discussions of those particular entities.

There are three common categories of regional musculoskeletal illness of the upper extremity: illness that relates to osteoarthritis, illness as a consequence of neuropathy, and soft-tissue illnesses. All three conditions can be recognized with confidence on the basis of history and physical examination, and there is a body of information for each upon which sound advice can be based.

Regional Musculoskeletal Illness that can be Ascribed to Osteoarthritis

Osteoarthritis refers to progressive changes in the biochemistry and anatomy of a joint that result in compromise in its structure and function. Although mild inflam-

Table 20-1. Upper-extremity symptoms and/or signs that suggest a systemic cause

Clinical clue	Diagnostic specter
Pain with ambulation	Angina
Pain with respiration	Pleural/diaphragmatic inflammation
Cramping with usage	Peripheral vascular disease
Writhing with pain	Aortic dissection
Erythema of tendon or joint *or* Swelling of tendon or joint *or* Bilaterality of symptoms *or* Cutaneous pathology *or* Raynaud's phenomenon	Systemic rheumatic diseases

matory symptoms and signs are frequent, a dearth of inflammatory changes is characteristic of the pathology. Involvement of the articulating structures, of the axial skeleton in osteoarthritis [2], is ubiquitous in the adult. Elsewhere, involvement is less predictable and seldom generalized so that patients with osteoarthritis of the hip need not be afflicted in the knee. Always, there is discordance between the pathoanatomy and symptoms. In fact, discordance with symptoms is a hallmark of osteoarthritis; many people with impressively damaged joints are totally asymptomatic and vice versa [4]. Furthermore, spontaneous regression of the symptoms—but not the anatomic damage—is the rule.

Osteoarthritis of the proximal joints of the upper extremity, the shoulder, and elbow is distinctly unusual and does not usually concern the occupational physician. Osteoarthritis of the hands, however, is common. The process afflicts all of us as we age but is most frequent and more advanced in the postmenopausal woman. Those people most severely afflicted are likely to remember similar conditions in their mother and grandmother. Osteoarthritis of the hands is readily recognized on examination. Degeneration of the joint spaces is associated with exuberant lateral growth of cartilage-covered osteophytes, but not all hand joints are involved. There is a predilection for the distal interphalangeal joints leading to decreased motion, malalignment, and osteophytes known as *Heberden's nodes.* The proximal interphalangeal joints are similarly involved but to a lesser degree, with excrescences termed *Bouchard's nodes.* No other joint in the hand or wrist is involved by osteoarthritis with one important and insufficiently recognized exception—the first carpometacarpal joint at the base of the thumb.

For most women, osteoarthritis of the hands is, to some degree, a cosmetic concern. Occasionally, an involved joint is inflamed, even slightly erythematous, but this affliction is usually intermittent and seldom is pharmacologic suppression of the inflammation warranted. The principal occupationally related compromise to which these women are at risk relates to power pinch. The forces of pinching are transduced to the base of the thumb, to the first carpometacarpal joint, which is often damaged, fixed in flexion to some degree, and tender. The symptoms can be reproduced readily. A contribution to the discomfort by the tendons that course across this joint can be excluded by stabilizing the carpometacarpal joint and demonstrating pain-free excursion of the overlying tendons when the interphalangeal joint is moved. Osteoarthritis of the first carpometacarpal joint is a far more common cause of discomfort at the base of the thumb than carpal tunnel syndrome or tendonitis in women beyond middle age. Management of this discomfort involves readjustment of tasks to obviate the need for power pinch. A classic intervention for individuals who do a lot of writing is to provide them with an implement that has a hefty diameter. Such a writing implement can be cradled in the length of the thumb and index finger so that pinching is no longer a prerequisite to writing.

The Neuropathic Syndromes

Cervical radiculopathies are common and present with pain that, whether localized or radiating, is *not usually exacerbated by limb motion,* although motion of the neck may exacerbate the symptoms. For that reason, maintenance of a neutral cervical posture is advisable. In the workplace, adjustment of the work station to avoid other than neutral postures may be necessary. The classic signs and symptoms of the radiculopathies are presented in Table 20-2. Variations are frequent and any uncertainty as to the diagnosis may justify referral to a specialist. There are few indications for aggressive intervention as nearly all radiculopathies are self-limited and leave little if any residua in their wake. Advice as to posture, antiinflammatory analgesic agents, warm showers, and reassurance is all that is indicated. Unusual severity; persistence beyond 6 weeks; any suggestion of *myelopathy,* such as a gait disorder, bowel or bladder dysfunction, or a Babinski's sign; or overt muscle weakness warrants additional diagnostic evaluation and perhaps a referral.

Entrapment neuropathies of the upper extremities are far less frequent than cervical radiculopathies. Most are rare indeed. The most common is carpal tunnel syndrome, with an incidence that approximates one case per thousand adults per year [5]. Entrapment neuropathies all share the features listed in Table 20-3, with varying sensitivity and specificity. The predictive value of the classic physical findings of carpal tunnel syndrome, if electrodiagnostic studies are used as the gold standard for diagnosis, is so marginal as to render them useless as screening tools [6]

Table 20-2. Signs and symptoms of cervical radiculopathies

Root	Pain, numbness	Sensory loss	Motor loss	Reflex loss
C3	Occipital region	Occiput	None	None
C4	Back of neck	Back of neck	None	None
C5	Neck to outer shoulder and arm	Over shoulder	Deltoid	Biceps supinator
C6	Outer arm to thumb and index fingers	Thumb and index fingers	Biceps (triceps) and wrist extensors	Triceps supinator Biceps
C7	Outer arm to middle finger	Index and middle fingers	Triceps	Triceps
C8	Inner arm to fourth and fifth fingers	Fourth and fifth fingers	Intrinsics Extrinsics	None

Table 20-3. Classic clinical features of an entrapment neuropathy

Dysesthesias are localized to the sensory distribution of the nerve.

Discomfort and paresthesia are more prominent at rest than with usage. Dysesthesias often interrupt sleep and may cause the patient to move the limb.

Sensory fibers are more susceptible to insult than motor fibers. Therefore, atrophy is a late sign and an indication for surgical intervention.

A Tinel's sign is frequently present; tapping the nerve at the site of entrapment elicits dysesthesias in the sensory distribution of the nerve.

Electrodiagnostic studies provide the gold standard for diagnosis.

in the workplace. Even electrodiagnostic studies leave much to be desired in that they are difficult to perform well, uncomfortable, and of limited sensitivity for radiculopathies and entrapment neuropathies other than carpal tunnel syndrome. Even in the setting of carpal tunnel syndrome, one needs to be wary of a minimal conduction delay as a basis for diagnosis given the considerable variability in the normal population. Conduction in the median nerve is normally delayed as a function of aging and obesity, particularly in women [7].

As a result, familiarity with sensory innervation of the upper extremity is essential to gain an appropriate index of suspicion when evaluating a patient with complaints of dysesthesias or pain not exacerbated by motion. Any evidence of muscle atrophy is cause for concern and warrants further diagnostic studies and perhaps consultation. In the absence of classic features of a neuropathic syndrome (Table 20-3), however, reassurance and observation are likely to be more beneficial than leaping to diagnostic inferences and empiric interventions. With persistence of symptoms, and any hint of atrophy, further guidance should be sought. Finally, surgical intervention for entrapment neuropathy without muscle atrophy should be discouraged. This remedy should be applied infrequently and only when the diagnosis is substantiated by unequivocal electrodiagnostic abnormality.

Soft-Tissue Regional Musculoskeletal Illnesses of the Upper Extremity

Soft-Tissue Illnesses

Soft-tissue illnesses represent the bulk of the regional musculoskeletal disorders of the upper extremity; however, labeling these illnesses as soft-tissue "syndromes" may not be appropriate. In fact, these labels—tendonitis, fasciitis, fibrositis, epicondylitis, tenovaginitis, tenosynovitis, and so forth—reflect noncritical thinking in the opinion of many authorities. They are obfuscating malaproprisms that should be avoided, especially in the context of patients with upper-extremity pain who lack objective signs of inflammation (see Table 20-1). Furthermore, no specific pathology can be demonstrated by any imaging or biochemical technique available. As a result, applying labels that sound ominous and imply inflammation or damage is inappropriate. These patients have localized discomfort, tenderness, and often exacerbation with motion of the painful region. Their prognosis is excellent even though the symptoms can take months to remit. Instead of using ominous-sounding terms such as "tendonitis" or "epicondylitis," one should advise patients that they have localized arm pain that will remit in time. Such a diagnosis takes advantage of the physician's ability to exclude more worrisome causes, and our ability to formulate a prognosis based on accumulated clinical experience. Furthermore, motions that might circumvent exacerbation can be suggested. In fact, tasks less likely to exacerbate symptoms can be proposed. Other interventions are trade-offs. In this author's opinion, acetaminophen is the only analgesic that makes sense (there is no role for nonsteroidal antiinflammatory agents in view of their potential for toxicity, let alone their expense). Prescribed physical modalities lack a convincing cost-benefit ratio, although they may provide temporary relief.

Regional Musculoskeletal Illnesses at the Shoulder

The shoulder region is the most frequent target for regional illness of the upper extremity. The approach to the patient is straightforward. If the patient can comfortably reach the occiput and the intrascapular region with the involved hand, the shoulder pain is referred; the differential diagnosis includes the entities displayed in Tables 20-1 and 20-2. If motion at the shoulder is impaired, one must next exclude a process involving the shoulder (glenohumeral) joint. The diagnostic maneuver is to have the patient stand with the arm dependent and the elbow flexed. Passive internal rotation isolates the glenohumeral joint that should be gliding and pain free. If this arc of motion is impaired or painful, inflammatory monoarthritis, reflex sympathetic dystrophy, avascular necrosis, and other disorders should be considered.

Very few patients with pain and impaired shoulder motion will manifest compromise in this arc of glenohumeral motion. Typically, external rotation in abduction is most difficult. Furthermore, there is clinical utility in discerning the sites of maximum tenderness about the shoulder because infiltration of such areas with nonabsorbable corticosteroid preparations has been palliative in controlled trials, although the intervention should be reserved for acute involvement and should seldom be repeated [8].

Regional Musculoskeletal Illnesses of the Elbow

The commonest elbow illness is discomfort with motion that lateralizes to the muscle mass around one or the other epicondyle (hence, the heuristic label of "epicondylitis"). Usually, there is tenderness to deep palpation. More specific signs involve the elicitation of discomfort when the lateral muscle masses are contracted against resistance. Flexion of the supinated wrist against resistance is the sign of "medial epicondylitis"; either supination of the forearm or extension of the pronated wrist against resistance is a sign of "lateral epicondylitis." Not only are the signs diagnostic but they also suggest advice that can be palliative, for example, patterns of usage to be avoided until the illness subsides. Intralesional steroid instillation has fleeting benefit at best [9].

Regional Musculoskeletal Illnesses of the Wrist

Discomfort about the wrist is an extremely common experience; well over 25% of people are aware of recent or recurrent episodes. Overt swelling or erythema is distinctly unusual and calls into question the diagnosis of regional illness. Rather there is tenderness localized to one or another compartment, usually of the dorsum of the wrist, and exacerbation in discomfort when that compartment is stressed. An appropriate diagnostic label for these symptoms is "benign localized discomfort" since the prognosis is so favorable.

"Benign localized discomfort" is managed conservatively with reassurance and consideration of the fashion in which dexterity can be maintained while avoiding stress of the involved region. The prognosis is excellent although, as is the case for most regional musculoskeletal illnesses, weeks or even months may pass before the region can be stressed without discomfort.

Regional Musculoskeletal Illnesses of the Hand

The hand is remarkable for the fashion in which it serves us without discomfort. (There are few regional illnesses, far fewer than proximally.) In some people a nodule develops, usually in a flexor tendon, and occasionally the nodule impedes glide through a fibrous tether that anchors that tendon in the hand. Motion of the finger served by the tendon can be impeded until the nodule suddenly pops through the tether, known as a "trigger finger." Triggering usually subsides spontaneously, although infiltration with corticosteroid preparations can be useful in the face of persistence [10].

Dupuytren's contractures are as common as trigger fingers and result in hyperplasia and hypertrophy of the palmar fascia with fibrotic nodule formation. Although painless, the process is progressive and disfiguring, and can interfere with finger extension. At that point, surgery offers a remedy.

When is a Regional Musculoskeletal Illness of the Upper Extremity an Injury?

The plight of individuals with regional musculoskeletal illnesses of the upper extremity is the focus of this chapter. Regional musculoskeletal illness challenges the comfort if not the effectiveness of the person's use of the involved region. Therefore, there is some risk of disability. Furthermore, particularly for the soft-tissue illnesses, usage may exacerbate discomfort.

During the mid-1980s, the regulatory and insurance establishment in the United States and much of the ergonomics and occupational medical community, came to accept two inferences regarding regional illness of the upper extremity. First, since the pain is exacerbated by usage, usage must be causal. Second, the regional pain is a manifestation of underlying damage so that the "illness," in fact, is a work-related injury that is a consequence of repetitive motion. "Cumulative trauma disorders" (CTDs) became compensable, and redress through litigation and regulation was necessary. As a consequence, people in the workforce with regional musculoskeletal symptoms often became claimants under workers' compensation insurance. Out of the turmoil that has followed has grown an appreciation that both inferences were wrong [11] and that their premature introduction has proved harmful.

The legislated approach for worker health and safety is designed to prevent trauma and to provide redress for tissue damage. If discomfort is used as a surrogate for damage, the legislated redress can backfire. The worker who hurts is drawn into the contest of causation. The pain becomes the evidence for a hazard, and the persistence of pain becomes prerequisite to carry forth the argument. Likewise, when pain is the cause of disability, persistence of pain is necessary to carry forth the argument. In either contest, the hurting worker is poorly served. To the contrary, they are at risk for getting sicker. They may become angry claimants willing to accept multiple unproven surgical interventions in defense of their claim. This same vortex has enveloped the industrial backache for decades [12], and now threatens to confound arm pain to the extreme of subjecting workers to multiple empiric surgical interventions [13]. This vortex is one of the major pitfalls of the format for disability determination that the West inherited from the Prussian statutes of 100 years ago [14]. Other countries have experimented with alternatives [15]. However, compassionate, major reform is long overdue to provide more efficient redress for work incapacity, whether a consequence of damage or of discomfort.

Regional musculoskeletal illness of the upper extremity or axial skeleton is an important target for improved worker comfort and workplace healthfulness. This predicament, like stress and unhappiness, colors all our lives at some time both in and out of the workplace. It is in the workplace, however, where salutary reform is feasible. We need to be able to complain when our own coping mechanisms are exhausted. Interpersonal relationships, fiscal and other rewards, information and misinformation, personal psychosocial confounders, and, yes, even ergonomics are relevant variables. Compassionate management should be the response to our plea—not contests, gauntlets, and ill-conceived medical and ergonomic interventions. The result will be the enlightenment of labor, management, and the individual worker.

References

1. Kelsey, J. L., et al. The impact of musculoskeletal disorders on the population of the United States. *J. Bone Jt. Surg.* 61A:959, 1979.
2. Hadler, N. M. Osteoarthritis as a public health problem. *Clin. Rheum. Dis.* 11:175, 1985.
3. Silverstein, B. A., Fine, L. J., and Armstrong, T. J. Occupational factors and carpal tunnel syndrome. *Am. J. Ind. Med.* 11:343, 1987.
4. Hadler, N. M. Knee pain is the malady—not osteoarthritis. *Ann. Intern. Med.* 116:598, 1992.
5. Stevens, J. C., et al. Carpal tunnel syndrome in Rochester, Minnesota, 1961 to 1980. *Neurology* 38:134, 1988.
6. Katz, J. N., et al. The carpal tunnel syndrome: Diagnostic utility of the history and physical examination findings. *Ann. Intern. Med.* 112:321, 1990.
7. Nathan, P. A., et al. Obesity as a risk factor for slowing of sensory conduction of the median nerve in industry. *J. Occup. Med.* 34:379, 1992.
8. Petri, M., et al. Randomized double-blind, placebo controlled study of the treatment of the painful shoulder. *Arthritis Rheum.* 30:1040, 1987.
9. Price, R., et al. Local injection treatment of tennis elbow—hydrocortisone, triamcinolone and lidocaine compared. *Br. J. Rheumatol.* 30:39, 1991.
10. Neustadt, D. H. Local corticosteroid injection therapy in soft tissue rheumatic conditions of the hand and wrist. *Arthritis Rheum.* 34:923, 1991.
11. Hadler, N. M. Cumulative trauma disorders. An iatrogenic concept. *J. Occup. Med.* 32:38, 1990.
12. Hadler, N. M. Back pain and the vortex of disability determination. *Semin. Spine Surg.* 4:35; 1992.
13. Hadler, N. M. Arm pain in the workplace. A small area analysis. *J. Occup. Med.* 34:113, 1992.
14. Hadler, N. M. Criteria for screening workers for the establishment of disability. *J. Occup. Med.* 28:940, 1986.
15. Hadler, N M. Disabling backache in France, Switzerland, and the Netherlands: Contrasting sociopolitical constraints on clinical judgment. *J. Occup. Med.* 31:823, 1989.

Further Information

Hadler, N. M. *Occupational Musculoskeletal Disorders.* New York: Raven, 1993.
A comprehensive and practical treatise on the scope of the impact of all the regional musculoskeletal disorders. The predicament suffered by each of us before we seek professional guidance, our fate should we choose medical care, the ramifications should we seek recourse under workers' compensation insurance, and the process of disability determination are all analyzed. In this monograph one can find a greatly expanded treatment of the topic of this chapter. Furthermore, the monograph treats other regional illnesses, including those of the axial skeleton and lower extremity, in a similarly comprehensive fashion.

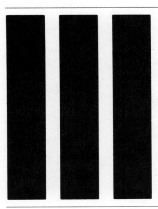

Evaluating a Health Hazard or Work Environment

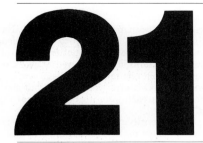

Suspecting Occupational Disease

Rose H. Goldman

Persons suffering from work-related illness enter clinicians' offices every day. Yet consideration of work-related etiologies rarely enters the practitioner's differential diagnosis. As a result, physicians may miss the chance to make diagnoses that might influence the course of a disease in some and might prevent disease in others (by stopping exposure). The following two cases illustrate the consequences of physician attention to (or lack of attention to) environmental exposures.

In the first instance, a man experienced retrosternal chest pain after applying a paint remover in his basement workshop [1]. On admission to the hospital, he showed the paint-remover container to his attending physician. The label cautioned that the product contained 80% methylene chloride and was to be used only with adequate ventilation. The physician made the diagnosis of anterior wall myocardial infarction but apparently did not look further into the health effects of methylene chloride. After discharge, the patient reused the solvent in a similar manner and suffered a fatal myocardial infarction. This tragic ending might have been averted if the history of solvent exposure had stimulated inquiry into the toxic properties of methylene chloride. If the practitioner had known that this substance is rapidly metabolized to carbon monoxide, which can stress the cardiovascular system [1–3], then he could have advised the patient not to use the solvent, particularly in an unventilated area.

In a contrasting situation, a young man reported fatigue, headache, and skin rash to his physician. He inquired if his problems could be related to his job, in which he machined metal parts and cleaned them with methylene chloride. The physician knew little about this solvent but was suspicious that it might be a contributing factor. He consulted with an occupational physician and learned that overexposure could cause dizziness, headache, excessive fatigue, and skin irritation. The physician then learned that the patient worked in a small, unventilated basement workshop over an open container of solvent. He dipped the part into the barrel, wetting his arms to the elbow, and then held the dripping part up to his eye for close inspection. The occupational physician discussed the dangers of these conditions with the patient and recommended methods for decreasing exposure. The employee persuaded the company to install a safer degreasing operation and also changed his own work practices. When those changes were made, his symptoms resolved.

These examples demonstrate how a physician's level of attention to potential environmental and occupational hazards can lead to strikingly different outcomes. These cases also raise certain questions about such disorders and how they can be detected.

It is difficult to estimate the extent of occupational illness in the United States because of the lack of accurate information. The Bureau of Labor Statistics (BLS) in the United States Department of Labor reports statistics based on surveys of private companies with greater than 11 employees, excluding the self-employed, farmers, and government employees. BLS showed that work-related illnesses and injuries in the United States increased by about 177,000 to nearly 6.8 million in 1990 [4]. The survey found nearly 332,000 new cases of occupational illness in 1990, with nearly 60% of these cases associated with repetitive motions such as vibrations and repeated pressure. Yet even these Department of Labor statistics are underestimates because of underreporting, lack of identification of cases, the tendency to report predominately acute rather than chronic cases, and failure to include all types of employers. In 1972, the President's Report on Occupational Safety and Health [5] estimated that 100,000 die annually in the United States because of occupational illness. To obtain more accurate estimates, a study was undertaken in 1986 of various data sources in New York State [6]. The best available data indicated that 5000 to

7000 deaths in New York State were attributable to occupational illnesses [6]. Based on these data, it was then estimated that approximately 50,000 to 70,000 deaths and 350,000 new cases of illness each year are caused by occupational exposures (excluding the approximately 10 million traumatic injuries suffered at work each year, or the 10,000 deaths per year that result from traumatic injuries at work) [7]. The number of cancers caused by work exposures is controversial [8, 9], but conservative estimates attribute 17,000 cancer deaths each year to occupational exposures [10].

Physicians have an important role to play in identifying potential workplace risks and possible work-related health problems in their patients [11, 12]. One obstacle to physicians' recognition of job-related health problems is insufficient education. A survey in 1983 showed that 50% of medical schools taught courses in occupational health, but the average curriculum time was only 4 hours [13]. The Institute of Medicine has issued a report on how to foster the role and education of the primary care physician in environmental and occupational medicine [14]. Important review articles [15–17], other useful paperback textbooks [18–21], and a recently published comprehensive textbook [22] are now available to help practitioners with their own educational efforts to learn more about recognizing and preventing occupational diseases and injuries.

Another impediment to the recognition of work-related illness is a *lack of uniqueness* in the clinical manifestations of many occupational illnesses. Wheezing caused by platinum salts, for example, is similar to wheezing due to animal dander or pollen. Oat-cell carcinoma caused by exposure to bischloromethyl ether behaves similarly to that due to cigarette smoking. Hepatitis secondary to hepatitis B virus contracted from contact with blood at work presents in the same way as community-acquired hepatitis.

A *long latency,* or the period from initial exposure to presentation of disease, also leads to underrecognition of some occupational diseases. Asbestosis, for example, can appear 15 to 20 years after one first works with the material. Occupational cancer such as mesothelioma can occur 40 years after exposure.

Despite these obstacles, physicians can enhance their recognition of occupational disease by taking a good *occupational history.* Patients can present with ordinary medical complaints, with neither the patient nor physician suspecting an underlying work-related etiology, or they can present with concerns about the relationship of certain symptoms to exposures or conditions at work. To detect cases of unsuspected occupational disease, an occupational history, even if brief, should be taken on *every* patient. This point is illustrated by a report of a young man who presented to an emergency room with abdominal pain and vomiting [23]. He underwent an appendectomy before it was learned that he removed *lead paint* from houses and that the actual cause of his symptoms was lead poisoning. Even a brief occupational history at the time of presentation could have provided clues to the correct diagnosis and might have avoided an unnecessary operation. His diagnosis of lead poisoning led to the screening of other workers, and modifications were then instituted to prevent lead intoxication in other workers.

Sometimes physicians observe an *unusual disease* in several patients. Searching for a connection among the cases may reveal that a work exposure is the common link. In fact, an occupational disease may be discovered that has not been previously described (see Chap. 33). Examples include the first description of *occupational cancer,* credited to Percival Potts, a surgeon who noted an increased frequency of scrotal cancer among chimney sweeps, which he attributed to the soot collected on their clothes and skin [24]; the observation of several cases of *angiosarcoma of the liver* in employees of a rubber company, which led to the discovery of the causative agent *vinyl chloride* monomer [25]; the detection of a bladder neurotoxin when a group of workers presented with urinary problems, which traced to the toxic effects of a newly introduced catalyst [26]; and a high prevalence of sarcoidosis in the Salem, Massachusetts, area ("Salem sarcoid"), linked to employees working in companies making light bulbs and eventually attributed to beryllium exposure (beryllium disease) [27]. In these cases, identification of the causative agents led to better control over exposures and reduction in associated diseases.

In another scenario, a patient might ask the physician whether certain symptoms could be related to certain materials. Sometimes a patient may complain of multiple symptoms (resembling a somatization disorder) that the patient attributes to workplace exposures.

Despite the type of presentation of an occupational illness, the practitioner needs an organized approach to arrive at an accurate diagnosis and to address possible connections to present or past exposures (Fig. 21-1) [28, 29]. The *occupational history* is the key preliminary step in determining the connection between an illness and the workplace.

Step I. Occupational History Survey

Symptoms related to hazardous exposures can appear as complaints involving *any body system* and mimicking ordinary medical diseases (Table 21-1) [19, 28]. To find

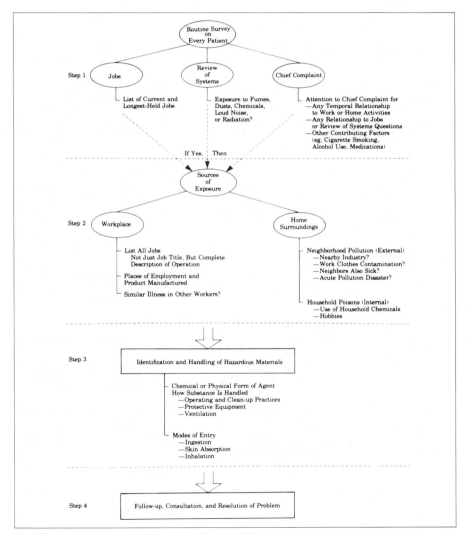

Figure 21-1. Systematic approach to history taking and diagnosis of occupational or environmental illness. (From R. H. Goldman and J. M. Peters. The occupational and environmental health history. *J.A.M.A.* 246:2831, 1981. Copyright 1981, American Medical Association.)

Table 21-1. Examples of environmental causes of medical problems

	Agent	Potential exposures
Immediate or short-term effects		
Dermatoses (allergic or irritant)	Metals (chromium, nickel), fibrous glass, epoxy resins, cutting oils, solvents, caustic alkali, soaps	Electroplating, metal cleaning, plastics, machining, leather tanning, housekeeping
Headache	Carbon monoxide, solvents	Firefighting, automobile exhaust, foundry, wood finishing, dry cleaning
Acute psychoses	Lead (especially organic) mercury, carbon disulfide	Handling gasoline, seed handling, fungicide, wood preserving, viscose rayon industry
Asthma or dry cough	Formaldehyde, toluene diisocyanate, animal dander	Textiles, plastics, polyurethane kits, lacquer use, animal handler
Pulmonary edema, pneumonitis	Nitrogen oxides, phosgene, halogen gases, cadmium	Welding, farming ("silo filler's disease") chemical operations, smelting
Cardiac arrhythmias	Solvents, fluorocarbons	Metal cleaning, solvents use, refrigerator maintenance
Angina	Carbon monoxide	Car repair, traffic exhaust, foundry, wood finishing
Abdominal pain	Lead	Battery making, enameling, smelting, painting, welding, ceramics, plumbing
Hepatitis (may become a long-term effect)	Halogenated hydrocarbons, e.g., carbon tetrachloride virus	Solvent use, lacquer use, hospital workers
Latent or long-term effects		
Chronic dyspnea		
Pulmonary fibrosis	Asbestos, silica, beryllium, coal, aluminum	Mining, insulation, pipefitting, sandblasting, quarrying, metal alloy work, aircraft or electrical parts
Chronic bronchitis emphysema	Cotton dust, cadmium coal dust, organic solvents, cigarettes	Textile industry, battery production, soldering, mining, solvent use
Lung cancer	Asbestos, arsenic, uranium, coke oven emissions	Insulation, pipefitting, smelting, coke ovens, shipyard workers, nickel refining, uranium mining
Bladder cancer	β-Naphthylamine, benzidine dyes	Dye industry, leather, rubber-working chemists
Peripheral neuropathy	Lead, arsenic, n-hexane, methyl butylketone, acrylamide	Battery production, plumbing, smelting, painting, shoemaking, solvent use, insecticides

(continued)

Table 21-1 continued

	Agent	Potential exposures
Behavioral changes	Lead, carbon disulfide, solvents, mercury, manganese	Battery makers, smelting, viscose rayon industry, degreasing, mfg/repair of scientific instruments, dental amalgam workers
Extrapyramidal syndrome	Carbon disulfide, manganese	Viscose rayon industry, steel production, battery production foundry
Aplastic anemia, leukemia	Benzene, ionizing radiation	Chemists, furniture refinishing, cleaning, degreasing, radiation workers

Source: From R. H. Goldman and J. M. Peters. The occupational and environmental health history. *J.A.M.A.* 246:2831, 1981. Copyright 1981, American Medical Association.

clues of such etiologies, a quick survey needs to be performed on all patients. *Three central points* can be incorporated into the routine medical history.

1. A short list of current and past longest held *jobs,* with a brief description if possible, including potential hazards or materials used.
2. A key question in the *review of systems* (ROS): Are you now (or have you ever been) exposed to fumes, chemicals, dust, loud noise, or radiation?
3. Attention to the chief complaint (or diagnosis) for (a) any *temporal relationship* to activities at work or at home, (b) any relationship to job titles and history of exposures, and (c) other contributing factors such as cigarette smoking, medications, or alcohol use.

These questions may trigger suspicion of occupationally related problems. Some diagnoses are more likely to be linked to current or past jobs, as indicated in the list of disorders called *"sentinel health events"* (SHE) that can be related to the workplace (see the chapter appendix). An SHE (occupational) is a disease, disability, or untimely death that is occupationally related and whose occurrence may provide the impetus for epidemiologic industrial hygiene surveys or serve as a warning signal that material substitution, engineering control, personal protection, or medical care may be required.

The recognition of a *temporal relationship* between the onset of symptoms and the performance of tasks at work (or at home) can provide important information. In general, symptoms that improve on the weekend or during vacation and reappear or worsen upon return to work suggest an occupational cause. As an example, an employee with a dry hacking cough that occurs at work or late in the day or evening and is worse during the work week than on weekends might be suffering delayed *bronchospasm* to a chemical at work such as toluene diisocyanate (TDI), a component of polyurethane [31]. It is important to note that allergic responses to certain agents may develop even after years of asymptomatic exposure.

Patterns of musculoskeletal symptoms are also worth noting. For example, if a worker develops hand pain shortly after starting on an assembly line for poultry processing, or after a period of prolonged data entry at a computer terminal, one would consider a diagnosis of tendonitis due to repetitive motion [32].

Exposure to occupational environmental substances can also *aggravate underlying medical conditions*. For example, carbon monoxide inhalation, even at the relatively modest levels of exposure encountered during commuter driving in heavy traffic, can precipitate *anginal* symptoms or decreased exercise tolerance in patients with coronary artery disease [2, 3, 33]. The expression of toxic symptoms is also influenced by the presence of other diseases, medications, and exposure to other hazardous substances. For example, the metabolism of certain poisons may be affected by liver disease, drugs, and chemicals (such as DDT) or any condition that alters the liver microsomal enzyme system.

The occupational history survey questions may raise the practitioner's suspicions that the patient's condition is related to an environmental or work exposure. The clinician then needs to gather more detailed information about work and home exposures.

Step II. Defining the Source of Exposure

Workplace

1. List *all* jobs.
2. Note places of employment and products manufactured.
3. Obtain a thorough description of the operations performed by the worker on the job.
4. Inquire about illnesses in other workers.

Although a brief list of job titles may be adequate as a part of the screening or initial medical examination, the practitioner evaluating potential occupational illness must take a more detailed history. In the case of latent diseases, an exposure occurring many years before the onset of symptoms may be responsible for the disorder. This point is illustrated by a 47-year-old worker with dyspnea whose roentgenogram showed bilateral pleural thickening and linear reticular parenchymal infiltrates consistent with asbestosis [34]. Sixteen years earlier he worked for 9 months in a factory making cigarette filters that contained asbestos.

A worker's description of job duties may reveal potential hazards not suggested by the job title. For more information about the type of hazardous exposures associated with certain jobs or work processes, the clinician can consult references that describe toxic substances associated with industrial processes [35–37].

The practitioner can also ask the patient for other sources such as the plant physician, manager, or union official who could be approached for more information and raise the possibility of requesting an evaluation by a governmental or private agency. It is also useful to ask the patient if similar illnesses have occurred in other persons at work or whether industrial hygiene evaluations have been conducted.

Home Surroundings

The routine survey questions may suggest that the symptoms relate to hazardous materials used in the home. Possible sources of toxic contamination in the home include

1. Neighborhood pollution produced by chronic low-level contamination, as from a nearby factory or chemical waste dump or, in rare cases, from the acute effects of a pollution disaster
2. Household contamination resulting from the use of household chemicals or from the performance of certain hobbies [38]

One source of external pollution is dust or chemicals carried into the home on work clothes. In this manner, children of employees at a lead storage battery plant showed excess blood lead levels [39], and mesothelioma developed in family members of asbestos workers [40]. Thus, it is useful to ask about the jobs of all occupants and if soiled clothes are brought home.

Industrial effluents emitted into the air or water can also lead to health problems. Community contamination is a growing public health concern in the United States, especially from toxic waste sites.

Examples of environmental contamination that aroused concern include polybrominated biphenyl in Michigan [41], toxic wastes at Love Canal, and methyl isocyanates in Bhopal [42]. Affected persons usually present to their local physician with their health complaints. To associate symptoms with environmental hazards, the clinician might inquire about whether similar symptoms have occurred in neighbors, the location of the home (near a factory, construction area, or dumpsite?), sources of water supply and possibility of contamination, or any noticeable changes in the neighborhood air quality. On rare occasions, sudden environmental disaster occurs, such as railroad or truck collisions that release toxic materials into the community. The practitioner then faces unique diagnostic and treatment dilemmas that may require appropriate consultation with specialists. Both immediate health problems and delayed effects often develop.

The home has internal hazards associated with the use of household chemicals and with the practice of some hobbies [38]. Increasing concern over "indoor air pollution" in the home has been directed to both the accumulation of toxic materials in the air and general poor air circulation as energy-saving insulation is installed without adequate ventilation [43] (see Chap. 44).

Due to inadequate labeling, home residents may be inadvertently exposed to hazardous chemicals in aerosol sprays, cleaning fluids, disinfectants, or insecticides (Table 21-2). Methylene chloride, for example, is a frequent component of many household products, such as paint "strippers." Rust removers may contain hydrofluoric acid, which can produce deep penetrating burns on skin contact. Without proper handling instructions, people may unsuspectingly develop a variety of symptoms and health problems from the use of these materials. Even mild exposure to certain materials causes allergic reactions in susceptible persons. Dangerous situations may arise when two substances are mixed to produce a more potent cleaning agent. Mixing ammonia and sodium hypochlorite (bleach) for example can lead to the generation of chloramine gas [44]. The effects include pulmonary problems secondary to toxic inhalation.

The growth and diversification of hobbies have introduced a multitude of hazardous substances into the household (Table 21-3). If the basement studio is poorly ventilated and unkempt, all family members may be exposed to toxic substances.

Even when evaluating a presumed occupational health problem, a good history concerning home exposures is essential. For example, in the investigation of elevated blood lead level in a foundry worker, one might learn that removing leaded paint at home was the major source of exposure to lead. This determination could be made by noting the absence of lead toxicity in other workers on that job and finding that there was a well-controlled work environment within Occupational Safety and Health Administration (OSHA) guidelines.

Whether exposure to a hazardous substance occurs in the home or at work, the next step is to identify and describe in detail the work process, including toxic agents and physical hazards.

Table 21-2. Examples of common dangerous household products

Product	Potentially hazardous agents
Disinfectants	Cresol; phenol; hexachlorophene
Cleaning agents and solvents	
Bleaches	Sodium hypochlorite (Clorox)
Window cleaner	Ammonia
Carpet cleaner	Ammonia, turpentine, naphthalene: 1.1.1-trichloroethane
Oven and drain cleaners	Potassium hydroxide, sodium hydroxide
Dry cleaning fluids, spot removers	1.1.1-Trichloroethane, perchloroethylene, petroleum distillates
Paint and varnish solvents	Turpentine, xylene, toluene, methanol, methylene, chloride, acetone
Pesticides	Malathion, dichlorvos, carbaryl, methoxychlor
Emissions from heating or cooling devices	
Gas stove pilot light	Nitrogen oxides
Indoor use of charcoal grill	Carbon monoxide
Leaks from refrigerator or air conditioner cooling systems	Freon
Microwave ovens	Microwave radiation
Sun lamps	Ultraviolet radiation

Source: From R. H. Goldman and J. M. Peters. The occupational and environmental health history. *J.A.M.A.* 246:2831, 1981. Copyright 1981, American Medical Association.

Table 21-3. Examples of hazards in hobbies

Activity	Potential hazard
Painting	Toxic pigments, e.g., arsenic (emerald green), cadmium, chromium, lead, mercury; acrylic emulsions; solvents
Ceramics	
Raw materials	Colors and glazes containing barium carbonate; lead, chromium, uranium, cadmium
Firing	Fumes of fluoride, chlorine, sulfur dioxide
Gas-fired kilns	Carbon monoxide
Sculpture and casting	
Grinding silica-containing stone	Silica (silicon dioxide)
Serpentine rock with asbestos	Asbestos
Woodworking	Wood dust
Metal casting	Metal fume, sand (silica) from molding, binders of phenol formaldehyde or urea formaldehyde
Welding	Metal fume, ultraviolet light exposure, welding fumes, carbon dioxide, carbon monoxide, nitrogen dioxide, ozone or phosgene (if solvents nearby)
Plastics	Monomers released during heating (polyvinyl chloride), methyl methacrylate, acrylic glues, polyurethane (toluene 2,4-diisocyanate), polystyrene (methyl chloride release), fiber glass, polyester, or epoxy resins
Woodworking	Solvents, especially methylene chloride
Photography	
Developer	Hydroquinone, metal
Stop bath	Weak acetic acid
Stop hardener	Potassium chrome alum (chromium)
Fixer	Sodium sulfite, acetic acid, sulfuric acid
Hardeners and stabilizers	Formaldehyde

Source: From R. H. Goldman and J. M. Peters. The occupational and environmental health history. *J.A.M.A.* 246:2831, 1981. Copyright 1981, American Medical Association.

Step III. Identification and Description of Hazard

The characterization of a hazardous exposure includes

1. Determining the *generic name,* if a chemical; describing the *physical form,* if a dust; or determining what form, if radiation.
2. Describing how a substance is handled: What are the operating or cleanup practices? What protective measures are used? Is a respirator worn and properly maintained? Is ventilation adequate?
3. Considering the mode of entry: Is it ingested by eating at the workplace or inhaled through cigarette smoking? Is protective clothing used to avoid skin absorption?

To characterize the health effects of a chemical substance, it is helpful to know its generic ingredients. To obtain this information, the practitioner can ask the worker or manufacturer for the *Material Safety Data Sheet* (MSDS), which usually lists the product's ingredients, physical properties, and some environmental protection information. The federal Chemical Hazard Communication Standard (29 CFR 1910.1200) and various state "right to know" laws [45] require that the employer provide employees with detailed information about hazardous chemicals used in the workplace. In general, the worker should be taught about the hazards of certain materials and properly trained in safe work practices. The standard stipulates that the employer must respond to an employee's request for an MSDS within 72 hours. *Clinical Toxicology of Commercial Products* [46] is one book that lists the ingredients of trade name products, toxicologic information, and recommendations for treatment of overexposures. Poison Control Centers are other sources of toxicologic information. Once a generic name or class of the substance is known, one can then consult other reference books that provide clinical descriptions of adverse health effects related to overexposure [37, 47, 48].

Step IV. Follow-up, Sources of Consultation, and Resolution of the Problem

One needs to determine if the symptoms and medical findings in the particular patient are consistent with the health effects and time course of toxicity associated with a particular hazardous exposure. Through the occupational history, information related to the job is obtained, but it may be necessary to get more accurate information by evaluating the worksite, taking environmental measurements, and conducting a literature search. The practitioner may also need more information about additional tests (e.g., biologic monitoring), methods of treatment, and details concerning future monitoring of the patient. In addition, the clinician may have concerns about the health of other similarly exposed workers or about other health hazards at the worksite.

To whom can the practitioner turn for additional consultation? The professional staff of the manufacturer often have substantial background in toxicology of many substances. Information is usually available from the MSDS. At the local level, state public health or labor departments often evaluate worksites and give information. OSHA also performs worksite inspections routinely on a priority basis or at the request of a current worker or management. In some cases, fines may be levied if OSHA standards are violated. Other consultative sources include academically affiliated occupational health clinics [49] and worker education groups such as Coalition for Occupational Safety and Health (COSH) groups. The National Institute for Occupational Safety and Health (NIOSH) in Cincinnati, Ohio, has a health hazard evaluation service in which large surveys of workers are performed to detect work-related health problems. NIOSH can also provide the practitioner with toxicologic and therapeutic information, published materials on various hazards, and recommendations for further medical care. Experts from any of these sources can investigate the problem further and suggest measures to prevent further exposure or illness in workers at the job site. Industrial hygienists from private consulting groups or from workers' compensation carriers can conduct worksite air monitoring.

The practitioner can also help an affected worker obtain workers' compensation when justified (see Chap. 2). The definition of "job related" may vary by state but usually implies that work responsibilities precipitated, hastened, aggravated, or contributed to the injury or illness. Workers' compensation provides benefits for work time lost, permanent disability, medical care expenses, and rehabilitation. The practitioner should become familiar with the state regulations related to workers' compensation through the medical society or department of health or labor.

In summary, the identification of work- or environmentally related disease is an important task for all practitioners. Thousands of chemical substances are commonly used in industry, and several hundred new substances are introduced to industrial processes each year. Unpredicted health hazards from new processes continue to emerge, and "well-known" toxins such as lead and certain solvents still escape surveillance and control. Equipped with an awareness and the approach outlined in this chapter, the practitioner can play an important role in the detection and prevention of occupational and environmental diseases.

References

1. Steward, R. D., and Hake, C. L. Paint-remover hazard. *J.A.M.A.* 235:398, 1976.
2. Allred, E. D., et al. Short term effects of carbon monoxide exposure on the exercise

performance of subjects with coronary artery disease. *N. Engl. J. Med.* 321:1426, 1989.

3. Sheps, D. S., et al. Production of arrhythmias by elevated carboxyhemoglobin in patients with coronary artery disease. *Ann. Intern. Med.* 113:343, 1990.

4. Bureau of Labor Statistics. *Results of Bureau of Labor Statistics Survey on U.S. Occupational Injuries, Illnesses in 1990.* Washington, DC: US Department of Labor, 1991.

5. President's Report on Occupational Safety and Health. Washington, DC: US Government Printing Office, 1972.

6. Markowitz, S. M., et al. Occupational disease in New York State: A comprehensive examination. *Am. J. Ind. Med.* 16:417, 1989.

7. Landrigan, P. J., and Markowitz, S. Current magnitude of occupational disease in the United States: Estimates from New York State. *Ann. NY Acad. Sci.* 572:27, 1989.

8. Doll, R., and Peto, R. The causes of cancer: Quantitative estimates of avoidable risks of cancer in the United States today. *J.N.C.I.* 66:1191, 1981.

9. Department of Health, Education and Welfare. *Estimates of the Fraction of Cancer in the United States Related to Occupational Factors.* Bethesda, MD: National Cancer Institute, National Institute of Environmental Health Sciences, National Institute for Occupational Safety and Health, 1978.

10. Millar, J. D. Summary of "Proposed National Strategies for the Prevention of Leading Work-Related Diseases and Injuries, Part 1." *Am. J. Ind. Med.* 13:223, 1988.

11. Health and Public Policy Committee, American College of Physicians. *The Role of the Internist in Occupational Medicine.* Philadelphia: American College of Physicians, 1984.

12. American College of Physicians. Occupational and environmental medicine: The internist's role. *Ann. Intern. Med.* 113:974, 1990.

13. Levy, B. S. The teaching of occupational health in United States medical schools: 5 year follow-up of an initial survey. *Am. J. Public Health* 75:79, 1985.

14. Institute of Medicine. *Role of the Primary Care Physician in Occupational and Environmental Medicine.* Washington, DC: National Academy Press, 1988.

15. Cullen, M. R., Cherniack, M. G., and Rosenstock, L. Occupational medicine, I. *N. Engl. J. Med.* 332:594, 1990.

16. Cullen, M. R., Cherniack, M. G., and Rosenstock, L. Occupational medicine, II. *N. Engl. J. Med.* 332:675, 1990.

17. Landrigan, P. J., and Baker, D. B. The recognition and control of occupational disease. *J.A.M.A.* 266:676, 1991.

18. Levy, B. S., and Wegman, D. H. *Occupational Health: Recognizing and Preventing Work-Related Disease.* Boston: Little, Brown, 1988.

19. Rosenstock, L., and Cullen, M. R. *Clinical Occupational Medicine.* Philadelphia: Saunders, 1986.

20. La Dou, J. (ed.). *Occupational Medicine.* Norwalk/San Mateo: Appleton & Lange, 1990.

21. Weeks, J. L., Levy B. S., and Wagner, G. R. (eds.). *Preventing Occupational Disease and Injury.* Washington, DC: American Public Health Association, 1991.

22. Rom, W. (ed.). *Environmental and Occupational Medicine.* Boston: Little, Brown, 1992.

23. Feldman, R. G. Urban lead mining: Lead intoxication among deleaders. *N. Engl. J. Med.* 298:1143, 1978.

24. Potts, P. Chirurgical observations relative to the cataract, polypus of the nose, the cancer of the scrotum, the different kinds of ruptures and the mortification of the toes and feet. *Natl. Cancer Inst. Monogr.* 10:7, 1963.

25. Makk, L., et al. Liver damage and angiosarcoma in vinylchloride workers: A systematic detection program. *J.A.M.A.* 230:64, 1974.

26. Kreiss, K., et al. Neurological dysfunction of the bladder in workers exposed to dimethylamino propionitrite. *J.A.M.A.* 243:741, 1980.

27. Hardy, H. L. Beryllium poisoning: Lessons in man-made disease. *N. Engl. J. Med.* 273:1188, 1965.

28. Goldman, R. H., and Peters, J. M. The occupational and environmental health history. *J.A.M.A.* 246:2831, 1981.

29. Occupational Environmental Health Committee of the American Lung Association of San Diego and Imperial Counties. Taking the occupational history. *Ann. Intern. Med* 99:641, 1983.

30. Mullan, R. J., and Murthy, L. I. Occupational sentinel health events: An up-dated list for physician recognition and public health surveillance. *Am. J. Ind. Med.* 19:775, 1991.
31. Peters, J. M., and Murphy, R. L. H. Pulmonary toxicity isocyanates. *Ann. Intern. Med.* 73:654, 1970.
32. Goldman, R. H. Cumulative trauma syndrome: An occupational hazard. *Emergency Med.* 23:45, 1991.
33. Aronow, W. S., et al. Effect of freeway travel in angina pectoris. *Ann. Intern. Med.* 77:669, 1972.
34. Goff, A. M., and Gaensler, E. A. Asbestosis following brief exposure in cigarette filter manufacture. *Respiration* 29:83, 1972.
35. Burgess, W. A. *Recognition of Health Hazards in Industry: A Review of Materials and Processes.* New York: Wiley, 1981.
36. Parmeggian, L. (tech. ed.). *International Labor Office Encyclopedia of Occupational Health and Safety* (3rd ed.). Geneva: International Labor Office, 1983.
37. Sullivan, J. B., and Krieger, G. R. (ed.). *Hazardous Materials Toxicology: Clinical Principles of Environmental Health.* Baltimore/Philadelphia: Williams & Wilkins, 1992.
38. Rossol, M. *The Artist's Complete Health and Safety Guide.* New York: Allworth Press, 1990.
39. Increased lead absorption in children of lead workers—Vermont. *Morbid. Mortal. Weekly Rep.* 26:61, 1977.
40. Anderson, H. A., et al. Household contact asbestos neoplastic risk. *Ann. NY Acad. Sci.* 271:311, 1976.
41. Carter, L. J. Michigan's PBB incident: Chemical mix-up leads to disaster. *Science* 192:250, 1976.
42. Andersson, N. et al. Exposure and response to methyl isocyanate: Results of a community based survey in Bhopal. *Br. J. Ind. Med.* 45:469, 1988.
43. Samet, J. M., Marbury, M. C., and Spengler, J. D. Health effects and sources of indoor air pollution, parts I, II. *Am. Rev. Respir. Dis.* 136:1486, 1987; 137:221, 1988.
44. Reisz, G. R., and Gammon, R. S. Toxic pneumonitis from mixing household cleaners. *Chest* 89:49, 1986.
45. Himmelstein, J. S., and Frumkin, H. The right to know about toxic exposures. *N. Engl. J. Med.* 312:687, 1985.
46. Gosselin, R. E., Smith, R. P., and Hodge, H. C. *Clinical Toxicology of Commercial Products* (5th ed.). Baltimore: Williams & Wilkins, 1984.
47. Hamilton, A., and Hardy, H. L. (reviewed by A. J. Finkel). *Industrial Toxicology* (4th ed.). Littleton, MA: Publishing Sciences Group, 1982.
48. Hathaway, G. J., et al. (eds.). *Proctor and Hughes' Chemical Hazards of the Workplace* (3rd ed.). New York: Van Nostrand Reinhold, 1991.
49. Rosenstock, L. Hospital based, academically affiliated occupational medicine clinics. *Am. J. Ind. Med.* 6:155, 1984.

Appendix to Chapter 21: Occupationally Related Unnecessary Disease, Disability, and Untimely Death[a]

ICD-9	Condition	A	B	C	Industry/process/ occupation	Agent
011	Pulmonary tuberculosis (O)	P	P,T	P,T	Physicians, medical personnel, medical lab workers	*Mycobacterium tuberculosis*
011, 502	Silicotuberculosis	P	P,T	P,T	Quarrymen, sandblasters, silica processors, mining, metal foundries, ceramic industry	Silica + *Mycobacterium tuberculosis*

(continued)

ICD-9	Condition	A	B	C	Industry/process/ occupation	Agent
020	Plague (O)	P	—	—	Shepherds, farmers, ranchers, hunters, field geologists	*Yersinia pestis*
021	Tularemia (O)	P	—	P,T	Hunters, fur handlers, sheep industry workers, cooks, vets, ranchers, vet pathologists, lab workers, soldiers	*Francisella tularensis, Pasteurella tularensis*
022	Anthrax (O)	P	—	P,T	Shepherds, farmers, butchers, handlers of imported hides or fibers, vets, vet pathologists, weavers, farmers	*Bacillus anthracis*
023	Brucellosis (O)	P	P	P	Farmers, shepherds, veterinarians, lab workers, slaughterhouse workers, field officers	*Brucella abortus, suis*
031.1[b]	Fish-fancier's finger (O)	P	P	P	Aquarium workers/ cleaners, breeders/ owners	*Mycobacterium marinum*
					Longshoremen	*Mycobacterium marinum*
054.6	Herpetic whitlow (O)	P	P	P	Surgical residents, student nurses, nurses, dental assistants, physicians, orthopedic scrub nurses, psychiatric nurses	Herpes simplex virus
037	Tetanus (O)	P	P	P	Farmers, ranchers	*Clostridium tetani*
042[c]	Human immunodeficiency virus (O)	P	P	P	Health care workers	Human immunodeficiency virus
056	Rubella (O)	P	P	P	Medical personnel, intensive care personnel	Rubella virus
070.0 .1	Hepatitis A (O)	P	P	P	Day care center staff, orphanage staff, mental retardation institution staff, medical personnel	Hepatitis A virus
070.2 .3	Hepatitis B (O)	P	P	P	Nurses and aides, anesthesiologists, orphanage and mental institution staff, medical lab personnel, general dentists, oral surgeons, physicians	Hepatitis B virus
070.4	Non-A, non-B hepatitis (O)	P	P	P	As above for hepatitis A and B	Unknown

(continued)

ICD-9	Condition	A	B	C	Industry/process/ occupation	Agent
071	Rabies (O)	P	—	P	Veterinarians, animal and game wardens, lab researchers, farmers, ranchers, trappers	Rabies virus
073	Ornithosis (O)	P	—	P,T	Psittacine bird breeders, pet shop staff, poultry producers, vets, zoo employees, duck processing and rearing	*Chlamydia psittaci*
082.0	Rocky Mountain spotted fever (O)	P	P	P,T	Laboratory technicians, tick breeders, virologists, microbiologists, physicians	*Rickettsia rickettsii*
100.8	Leptospirosis (O)	P	P	P,T	Farmers/laborers	*Leptospira*
115	Histoplasmosis (O)	P	P	P,T	Bridge maintenance workers	*Histoplasma capsulatum*
117.1	Sporotrichosis (O)	P	P	P	Nurserymen, foresters, florists, equipment operators	*Sporothrix schenckii*
147	Malignant neoplasm of nasopharynx (O)	P	P	P	Carpenters, cabinetmakers, sawmill workers, lumberjacks, electricians, fitters	Chlorophenols
155M[d,e]	Hemangiosarcoma of the liver	P	P	P	Vinyl chloride polymerization industry Vintners	Vinyl chloride monomer Arsenical pesticides
158, 163	Mesothelioma (MN of peritoneum and pleura)	P	—	P	Asbestos industries and utilizers	Asbestos
160.0	Malignant neoplasm of nasal cavities (O)	P	P,T	P,T	Woodworkers, cabinet and furniture makers	Hardwood dusts
					Boot and shoe industry	Unknown
					Radium chemists and processors, dial painters	Radium
					Chromium producers, processors, users	Chromates
					Nickel smelting and refining	Nickel
					Sawmill workers, carpenters	Chlorophenols
161	Malignant neoplasm of larynx (O)	P	P,T	P,T	Asbestos industry and utilizers	Asbestos

(continued)

ICD-9	Condition	A	B	C	Industry/process/ occupation	Agent
162	Malignant neoplasm of trachea, bronchus, and lung (O)	P	P	P	Asbestos industry and utilizers	Asbestos
					Topside coke oven workers	Coke oven emissions
					Uranium and fluorspar miners	Radon daughters
					Chromium producers, processors, users	Chromates
					Nickel smelters, processors, users	Nickel
					Smelters	Arsenic, arsenic trioxide
					Mustard gas formulators	Mustard gas
					Ion exchange resin makers, chemists	Bis(chloromethyl) ether, chloromethyl methyl ether
					Iron ore (underground) miners	Radon daughters
					Plant protection workers/agronomists	Pesticides, herbicides, fungicides, insecticides
					Welders	Unknown
					Copper smelter and roaster workers	Inorganic arsenic sulfur dioxide, copper, lead, sulfuric acid, arsenic trioxide
					Welders, gas cutters	Asbestos, hexavalent chromium
					Foundry—floor molders and casters	Polyaromatic hydrocarbons
					Dichromate production—floor molders/casters	Unknown
					Chromate production	Chromium dust
					Chromate pigment production workers	Lead chromate, zinc chromate
					Pigment production	Zinc chromate dust
					Steel industry—furnace/foundry workers	Unknown
					Rubber reclaim operations	Unknown
170	Malignant neoplasm of bone (O)	P	—	P	Radium chemists and processors, dial painters	Radium

(continued)

ICD-9	Condition	A	B	C	Industry/process/ occupation	Agent
187.7	Malignant neoplasm of scrotum	P	—	P,T	Automatic lathe operators, metal workers	Mineral/cutting oils
					Coke oven workers, petroleum refiners, tar distillers	Soots/tars/tar distillates
					Tool setters, fitters, cotton spinners, chimney sweeps, machine operators	Mineral oil, pitch, tar
188	Malignant neoplasm of bladder (O)	P	—	P	Rubber and dye workers	Benzidine, alpha- and beta-naphthylamine, magenta, auramine, 4-aminobiphenyl, 4-nitrophenyl
189	Malignant neoplasm of kidney, other, and unspecified urinary organs (O)	P	P	P	Coke oven workers	Coke oven emissions
204.0	Lymphoid leukemia, acute (O)	P	—	P	Rubber industry Radiologists	Unknown Ionizing radiation
205.0	Myeloid leukemia, acute (O)	P	—	P	Occupations with exposure to benzene Radiologists	Benzene Ionizing radiation
207.0	Erythroleukemia (O)	P	—	P	Occupations with exposure to benzene	Benzene
283.1	Hemolytic anemia, nonautoimmune (O)	P	—	P	Whitewashing and leather industry	Copper sulfate
					Electrolytic processes, arsenical ore smelting	Arsine
					Plastics industry	Trimellitic anhydride
					Dye, celluloid, resin industry	Naphthalene
284.8	Aplastic anemia (O)	P	—	P	Explosives manufacture	Trinitrotoluene
					Occupations with exposure to benzene	Benzene
					Radiologists, radium chemists and dial painters	Ionizing radiation

(continued)

ICD-9	Condition	A	B	C	Industry/process/occupation	Agent
288.0	Agranulocytosis or neutropenia (O)	P	—	P	Occupations with exposure to benzene	Benzene
					Explosives and pesticide industries	Phosphorus
					Pesticides, pigments, pharmaceuticals	Inorganic arsenic
289.7	Methemoglobinemia (O)	P	—	P,T	Explosives and dye industries	Aromatic amino and nitro compounds (e.g., aniline, trinitrotoluene, nitroglycerin)
					Rubber workers	Aniline, o-toluidine, nitrobenzene
323.7	Toxic encephalitis (O)	P	P	P	Battery, smelter, and foundry workers	Lead
					Electrolytic chlorine production, battery makers, fungicide formulators	Inorganic and organic mercury
332.1	Parkinson's disease (secondary) (O)	P	P	—	Manganese processing, battery makers, welders	Manganese
					Internal combustion engine industries	Carbon monoxide
334.3	Cerebellar ataxia (O)	P	P	—	Chemical industry using toluene	Toluene
					Electrolytic chlorine production, battery makers, fungicide formulators	Organic mercury
354M[f]	Carpal tunnel syndrome (O)	P	P	—	Meat packers, deboners	Cumulative trauma
354.0 .2 .3	Mononeuritis of upper limb and mononeuritis multiplex (O)	P	P	—	Dental technicians	Methyl methacrylate monomer
					Poultry processing—turkey	Cumulative trauma
					Meatpackers, deboners	Cumulative trauma
357.7	Inflammatory and toxic neuropathy (O)	P	P,T	P,T	Pesticide industry, pigments, pharmaceuticals formulators	Arsenic/arsenic compounds
					Furniture refinishers, degreasing operations	Hexane
					Plastic-coated fabric workers	Methyl n-butyl ketone

(continued)

ICD-9	Condition	A	B	C	Industry/process/occupation	Agent
					Explosives industry	Trinitrotoluene
					Rayon manufacturing	Carbon disulfide
					Plastics, hydraulics, coke industries	Tri-o-cresyl phosphate
					Battery, smelter, and foundry workers	Inorganic lead
					Dentists, chloralkali workers	Inorganic mercury
					Chloralkali plants, fungicide makers, battery makers	Organic mercury
					Plastics industry, paper manufacturing	Acrylamide
					Ethylene oxide sterilizer operator	Ethylene oxide
366.4	Cataract (O)	P	P,T	—	Microwave and radar technicians	Microwaves
					Explosives industries, trinitrotoluene workers	Trinitrotoluene
					Radiologists	Ionizing radiation
					Blacksmiths, glass blowers, bakers	Infrared radiation
					Moth repellant formulators, fumigators	Naphthalene
					Explosives, dye, herbicide and pesticide industries	Dinitrophenol, dinitro-o-cresol
					Ethylene oxide sterilizer operator, microbiology supervisors, inspectors	Ethylene oxide
388.1	Noise effects on inner ear (O)	P	P	—	Occupations with exposure to excessive noise	Excessive noise
443.0	Raynaud's phenomenon (secondary) (O)	P	—	—	Lumberjacks, chain sawyers, grinders, chippers, rock drillers, stone cutters, jackhammer operators, riveters	Whole body or segmental vibration
					Vinyl chloride polymerization industry	Vinyl chloride
493.0 507.8	Extrinsic astham (O)	P	P,T	P,T	Jewelry, alloy, and catalyst makers	Platinum
					Polyurethane, adhesive, paint workers	Isocyanates
					Alloy, catalyst, refinery workers	Chromium, cobalt
					Solderers	Aluminum soldering flux
					Plastic, dye, insecticide makers	Phthalic anhydride

(continued)

ICD-9	Condition	A	B	C	Industry/process/ occupation	Agent
					Foam workers, latex makers, biologists	Formaldehyde
					Printing industry	Gum arabic
					Nickel platers	Nickel sulfate
					Bakers	Flour
					Plastics industry, organic chemicals manufacture	Trimellitic anhydride
					Woodworkers, furniture makers	Red cedar (plicatic acid) and other wood dusts
					Detergent formulators	*Bacillus*-derived exoenzymes
					Crab processing workers	Unknown
					Hospital and geriatric department nurses	Psyllium dust
					Laxative manufacture and packing	Psyllium dust
					Prawn processing workers	Unknown
					Snow crab processing workers	Unknown
495.4	Maltworker's lung	P	P	—	Maltworkers	*Aspergillus clavatus*
495.5	Mushroom worker's lung	P	P	—	Mushroom farm/ spawning shed, farmers	Pasteurized compost
495.8	Grain handler's lung	P	P	—	Grain handlers	*Erwinia herbicola (Enterobacter agglomerans)*
	Sequoiosis	P	P	—	Red cedar mill workers, woodworkers, sawmill, joinery	Redwood sawdust. *Thuja plicata.*
495.9	Unspecified allergic alveolitis	P	P	—	Cinnamon processing workers	Cinnamon dust, cinnamaldehyde
					Distillery, vegetable compost plant workers	*Aspergillus fumigatus*
					Sawmill workers	Unknown
					Paper manufacture/ wood room	*Alternaria,* wood dust
					Snow crab processing workers	Unknown
500	Coalworker's pneumoconiosis	P	P	P	Coal miners	Coal dust
501	Asbestosis	P	P	P	Asbestos industries and utilizers	Asbestos

(continued)

ICD-9	Condition	A	B	C	Industry/process/ occupation	Agent
502M[g]	Silicosis	P	P	P	Quarrymen, sandblasters, silica processors, mining, metal, and ceramic industries	Silica
					Cryolite refining	Cryolite (Na_3AlF_6), quartz dust
	Talcosis	P	P	P	Talc processors, soapstone mining/milling, polishing, cosmetics industry	Talc
503M[h]	Chronic beryllium disease of the lung	P	P	P	Beryllium alloy workers, ceramic and cathode ray tube makers, nuclear reactor workers	Beryllium
504	Byssinosis	P	P	P	Cotton industry workers	Cotton, flax, hemp, and cotton-synthetic dusts
506.0 .1	Acute bronchitis, pneumonitis, and pulmonary edema due to fumes and vapors (O)	P,T	P,T	P,T	Refrigeration, fertilizer, oil refining industries	Ammonia
					Alkali and bleach industries	Chlorine
					Silo fillers, arc welders, nitric acid industry	Nitrogen oxides
					Paper and refrigeration industries, oil refining	Sulfur dioxide
					Cadmium smelters, processors	Cadmium
					Plastics industry	Trimellitic anhydride
					Boilermakers	Vanadium pentoxide
					Organic chemicals manufacture	Trimellitic anhydride
570, 573.3	Toxic hepatitis (O)	P	P	P	Solvent utilizers, dry cleaners, plastics industry	Carbon tetrachloride, chloroform, tetrachloroethane, trichloroethylene, tetrachloroethylene
					Explosives and dye industries	Phosphorus, trinitrotoluene
					Fire and waterproofing additive formulators	Chloronaphthalenes
					Plastics formulators	Methylenedianiline

(continued)

ICD-9	Condition	A	B	C	Industry/process/occupation	Agent
					Fumigators, gasoline and fire extinguisher formulators	Methyl bromide, ethylene dibromide
					Disinfectant, fumigant, synthetic resin formulators	Cresol
584, 585	Acute or chronic renal failure (O)	P	P,T	P,T	Battery makers, plumbers, solderers	Inorganic lead
					Electrolytic processes, arsenical ore smelting	Arsine
					Battery makers, jewelers, dentists	Inorganic mercury
					Fluorocarbon formulators, fire extinguisher makers	Carbon tetrachloride
					Antifreeze manufacture	Ethylene glycol.
					Chromate pigment production workers	Inorganic lead
606	Infertility, male (O)	P	P	—	Kepone formulators	Kepone
					DBCP producers, formulators, and applicators	Dibromochloropropane
692	Contact and allergic dermatitis (O)	P,T	P,T	—	Leather tanning, poultry dressing plants, fish packing, adhesives and sealants industry, boat building and repair	Irritants (e.g., cutting oils, phenol, solvents, acids, alkalis, detergents); allergens (e.g., nickel, chromates, formaldehyde, dyes, rubber products)
733-.9M[i]	Skeletal fluorosis (O)	P	P	—	Cryolite workers (grinding room)	Cryolite (Na_3AlF_6)
					Cryolite refining workers	Cryolite (Na_3AlF_6)

Key: A = unnecessary disease; B = unnecessary disability; C = unnecessary untimely death; P = prevention; T = treatment.
[a]External causes of injury and poisoning (occupational), including accidents, are classified in the *International Classification of Diseases,* 9th Revision, under the E codes.
[b]Original ICD rubric = Cutaneous Diseases Due to Other Mycobacteria.
[c]From the *International Classification Diseases,* 9th Revision, Clinical Modification (ICD-9-CM).
[d]M, modified ICD rubric.
[e]Original ICD rubric = Malignant Neoplasm of Liver and Intrahepatic Bile Ducts.
[f]Original ICD rubric = Mononeuritis of Upper Limb and Mononeuritis Multiplex.
[g]Original ICD rubric = Pneumoconiosis Due to Other Silica or Silicates.
[h]Original ICD rubric = Pneumoconiosis Due to Other Inorganic Dust.
[i]Original ICD rubric = Other Disorders of Bone and Cartilage.
Source: From R. J. Mullan and L. I. Murthy. Occupational sentinel health events: An updated list for physician recognition and public health surveillance. *Am. J. Ind. Med.* 19:775, 1991.

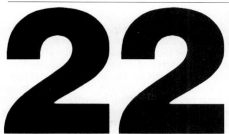

Industrial Hygiene

James M. McCunney

The physician who practices occupational medicine needs to have a working knowledge of many related disciplines, including epidemiology, toxicology, and industrial hygiene. The industrial hygienist, in particular, can offer valuable assistance to the physician who is asked to consider the health risks associated with certain work settings. The industrial hygienist, usually a graduate-level professional, can help in many areas, but most often in the following:

1. Determining the need for *medical surveillance* or special examinations of workers exposed to particular materials
2. Evaluating whether exposure to an occupational or environmental hazard may have contributed to the development of an *occupational illness*
3. Determining the presence of potential offending agents and the adequacy of ventilation systems in outbreaks of illness, such as *indoor air pollution* (see Chap. 44)
4. Complementing the efforts of a physician who has completed a preliminary *plant walk-through* (see Chap. 4)

This chapter is designed to acquaint the physician with an overview of industrial hygiene through a discussion of the types of hazards found in the workplace, their means of detection, and guidelines for interpretation of the results.

Industrial hygiene, a relatively new technical discipline when compared to medicine, is an area that will prove helpful to the physician in preventing and controlling occupational illness. Although new, it has accumulated a wealth of knowledge of the inner workings of the workplace. Conversely, important findings uncovered by astute physicians have steered the industrial hygienist in the right direction when searching for the offending agent. The relationship has proved valuable for both parties. A physician who suspects lead poisoning, for example, can ask an industrial hygienist to review the workplace for a source of lead. Joint efforts on behalf of the industrial hygienist and physician can reduce the time needed to reach an assessment. Ideally, the industrial hygienist's thorough knowledge of the workplace will be combined with the physician's knowledge of disease to solve workplace hazards and prevent occupational illnesses.

The profession of industrial hygiene has as its main goals the recognition, evaluation, and control of workplace health hazards. *Recognition* of a hazard requires knowledge of both the *processes* and the *hazards* of the materials used in the processes. A thorough grasp of these matters is essential as the foundation for a health hazard investigation. Reviewing the various hazardous materials used will reveal potential air contaminants. In addition, reviewing the process can also uncover air contaminants that may be released as an intermediate or as a decomposition product in the chemical reaction. The decomposition products, at times, may be more hazardous than the raw materials.

After the type of air contaminant that may be released is determined, a sampling strategy can be developed that will provide the information needed to *evaluate* the hazards. Selecting a sampling strategy will depend on the information that is sought. The data obtained from the monitoring of a person performing a process are then compared to exposure guidelines, for example, Occupational Safety and Health Administration (OSHA) permissible exposure limit (PEL), for the air contaminants of concern. This approach will determine whether the person is *overexposed* to any air contaminants and by how much.

If an overexposure exists or if there is a desire to reduce employee exposure, a *control* measure is then determined to bring the air contaminant concentration below the exposure guideline or to the desired level. Control can be implemented by controlling the contaminant at the source, the pathway, or the person.

If a less hazardous material is introduced into the process thereby eliminating the air contaminant exposure, the hazard is controlled *at the source*. A noise barrier or a local exhaust ventilation system that effectively removes the contaminant are examples of how control can be exercised *at the pathway* of the contaminant or hazard. Lastly, having people use personal protective equipment such as respiratory protection or work inside an enclosure will control the exposure *at the person*.

Any of these methods will control or limit the exposure because the contaminant does not reach the person or its concentration is reduced. Ideally, the most desirable approach would be to eliminate the hazard altogether, for example, by replacing the material with a nonhazardous material. Controlling the hazard at the person by using respiratory protection is the least desirable approach because it is dependent on the person's work habits. An enclosure, however, is desirable because it is independent of the worker's habits.

Types of Hazards

The hazards found in the workplace can be divided into five types: gases/vapors, dusts, fumes/mists, physical agents, and biologic agents. An understanding of these hazards can be helpful to the physician because routes of entry of the contaminant, applicable personal protective equipment, and appropriate sampling methods will be determined by the *type* of hazard. In some instances, many types of hazards will be present simultaneously. This situation not only makes evaluation more difficult for the industrial hygienist but it also presents the physician with a more complicated array of factors to consider in diagnosing an occupational health problem.

Gases and Vapors

Gases are substances that are normally in the *gaseous state* at room temperature; in contrast, *vapors* are the gaseous state of substances that are normally in the *liquid* state at room temperature. For example, carbon monoxide is a common gas found in the workplace that is produced as a result of incomplete combustion (i.e., propane-powered forklift trucks, gasoline-powered engines, kerosene heaters). Trichloroethylene, on the other hand, is normally a liquid but becomes vaporized when heated in a vapor degreaser. The main route of entry into the body for both gases and vapors is through *inhalation*. Some contaminants, however, will be absorbed through the skin. If the cutaneous route contributes to the exposure of the individual, the designation "skin" will appear next to the name of the substance in either the American Conference of Governmental Industrial Hygienist's (ACGIH) Threshold Limit Value (TLV) book or OSHA's permissible exposure limits.

Dusts

Many types of dust are found in the workplace, including nuisance-type dusts, toxic dusts, and pneumoconiosis-producing dusts. Dusts can be generated by a variety of means. For example, the handling or dumping of a crushed solid like limestone creates dust that, although considered a *nuisance* dust, will result in exposure to the lungs in most people. The use of lead oxide in the manufacture of automobile batteries creates a *toxic* lead dust exposure. Foundries that use green sand molds to make metal castings have the potential for crystalline silica dust exposures (pneumoconiosis-producing) in work areas involving molding, shake-out, and grinding.

The contaminant dust size depends on the material used and the respective process involved. Large dust particles that can be seen with the eye (50 μ or more in size) may coexist with respirable-sized dusts (< 10 μ in size). Most of the large dust particles, however, are trapped by the upper-respiratory tract, whereas the respirable dusts will reach the alveoli. Some fibers, such as fibrous glass and asbestos, can also be classified as dusts. Fibers are defined as particles having a length-to-width ratio (aspect ratio) of at least 3 to 1. The main route of entry for dusts is by inhalation.

Fumes and Mists

A *fume* is a *solid* that has been vaporized and subsequently condenses. In the process of welding steel, for example, iron oxide fume is produced. Zinc oxide fume is produced when welding galvanized metal. Excessive exposure to zinc and other metals can cause "metal fume fever," an acute illness with symptoms similar to those of influenza, which usually occur a few hours after initial exposure. Metallic taste in the mouth, dryness of nose and throat, weakness, fatigue, muscular and joint pain, fever, chills, and nausea usually last less than 24 hours. A temporary immunity usually follows; however, when workers return to the job after a weekend or a holiday, the symptoms may return.

A *mist* is a *liquid* that has been dispersed into the air as fine droplets. Cutting oils used in a machine shop become oil mists from the action of the metal-working machinery. Chromic acid mist can be generated during chrome-plating operations by the bursting of hydrogen gas bubbles. Fumes and mists enter the body by inhalation.

Physical Agents

Some physical agents encountered in the workplace are noise, heat, cold, ionizing and nonionizing radiation, lasers, and vibration. Since the physical agents involve a field of energy, the whole body can be at risk. Ionizing radiation is found in nuclear facilities and many other industrial processes in small doses, especially for instrumentation purposes. Microwaves, a form of nonionizing radiation, are found in areas near radar telecommunicating devices. Some physical agents mainly affect only a part of the body; for example, noise affects the ear and lasers the eye. Excessive vibration from pneumatic construction equipment can lead to "white finger" disease, now known as hand-arm vibration syndrome. Vibration, in addition to ergonomic factors, can lead to cumulative trauma disease (CTD) [1].

Biologic Agents

Relative newcomers to the industrial hygiene scene are the biologic agents, which include bacteria, viruses, and fungi. With the development of genetic engineering, resource recovery of municipal solid waste and indoor air pollutants, more attention is being paid to this area of occupational health. The use of biologic agents in research laboratories and hospitals has led to the development of indicator organisms, which can provide a measure of exposure to biological agents. Much more work has to be completed in this area to give physicians and industrial hygienists an understanding of the significance of exposure measurements, which at this time are of undefined significance.

Air sampling can be conducted for many organisms, but the interpretation of results can be problematic. For example, in outbreaks of hypersensitivity pneumonitis in an office setting, culturing of the filters from the air-handling system may yield a growth of *thermophilic actinomycetes*. It may also be demonstrated that afflicted individuals showed an antibody response (serum precipitation) to the same organism. Although it may appear logical to infer that the air-handling system caused the disease, this approach overlooks the fact that it is not uncommon to culture the same organism from environments without the disease and for people to show antibody responses though they do not have or never had the disease. The caveat emerges: Just because an organism is present does not mean it is causing a health problem. Sampling methods continue to be improved in an attempt to evaluate the extent of exposure to biologic agents in the workplace.

Monitoring

Monitoring employee exposure to air contaminants is the most visible aspect of the industrial hygienist's job. After the sampling strategy is determined, monitoring is performed to assess the extent of exposure to an air contaminant. Monitoring can be done by obtaining personal or area samples. In personal sampling, the sampling device or equipment, or both, is placed on the worker (Figs. 22-1 and 22-2) to ensure the most accurate exposure determination. For area sampling, the sampling appa-

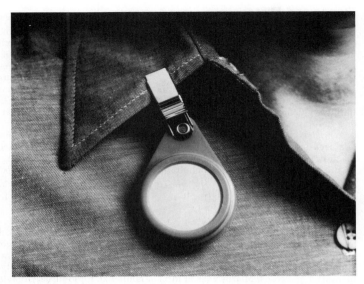

Figure 22-1. A passive dosimeter air monitoring badge. (Courtesy of Mine Safety Appliances Co.)

ratus is placed in the vicinity of the worker performing the job. Although more convenient, area monitoring often is less precise than personal monitoring. Methods for monitoring air contaminants are given below. For specific methods, the reader is referred to publications listed under Further Information.

Gases and Vapors

Organic gases and vapors can usually be collected with an adsorbing material, like activated charcoal or silica gel. The adsorbing material is contained in a small glass tube that is attached to a sampling pump, which draws a known volume of air. Passive dosimeters that do not require an air sampling pump are also used frequently. These devices consist of a collecting medium inside a badge. The air contaminant then diffuses from the air onto the collecting device. The concentration is determined based on the *time* the device was exposed to air and the *amount of contaminant* found on the collecting medium. Inorganic substances can be collected in an impinger or bubbler whereby the contaminant is drawn into a liquid collecting medium using an air pump.

All of these methods, however, require the assistance of a qualified laboratory to analyze the sampling medium for the presence of the contaminant. Some methods that do not require laboratory analysis include detector tubes or direct-reading instruments that can give an immediate measure of the concentration of the air contaminant (Figs. 22-3 and 22-4). Gases and vapors are usually reported in parts per million (ppm) units, a volume per volume measurement.

Dusts

Dusts, including asbestos, coal, wood, and silica, can be monitored using a variety of instruments. The method used will depend on the type of dust, the size of the dust, the PEL or TLV, and the cost of the method. The most common method is to collect the dust on a preweighed filter medium using an air sampling pump. The filter is then weighed after the sampling is completed and, along with the volume of air displaced during the sampling, the concentration of the contaminant can be

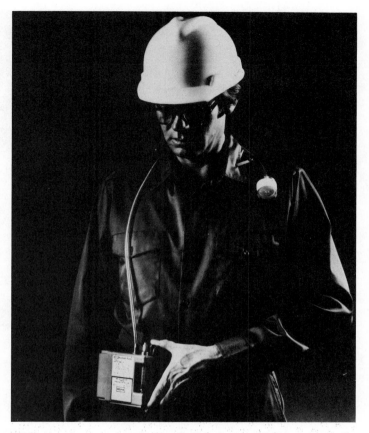

Figure 22-2. A worker wearing air sampling equipment: filter cassette connected to an air sampling pump. (Courtesy of Mine Safety Appliances Co.)

determined. This method, also known as a gravimetric analysis, is used with nuisance-type dusts and dusts that do not require identification.

The type of dust may determine the sampling method. Asbestos, for example, can be sampled with the filter method mentioned above. The filter medium is not weighed, however, as it is for nuisance dusts, but undergoes a microscopic analysis to determine the fiber count, rather than weight.

The size of the dust may also determine the sampling method. If a total dust measurement is desired, the gravimetric analysis mentioned above can be used. This will collect both large dust particles and small dust particles based on the filter pore size. Respirable dusts, those of 10 μ or less in size, are monitored differently. In addition to an air sampling pump, a cyclone is used to separate the respirable from the larger dusts. This method is used to monitor respirable dusts such as silica that affect the terminal parts of the lungs.

Cotton dust is sampled using a vertical elutriator, a sampling method specifically mentioned in the OSHA Cotton Dust Standard. In this case the PEL or TLV may determine the particular sampling method used.

Cost is also a consideration for air sampling. New electronic instruments such as fibrous aerosol monitors used for monitoring asbestos and other fibrous materials can be expensive to purchase. Electronic instruments are also available to monitor total and respirable dusts. More sophisticated sampling analyses can also be expensive. Reliability and accuracy of results also come into consideration when evaluating

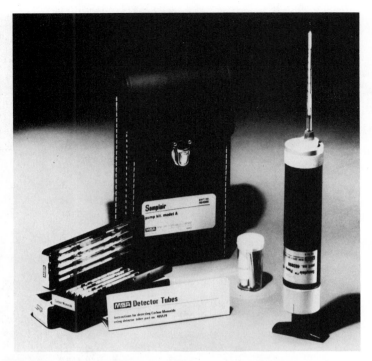

Figure 22-3. A colorimetric detector tube system that gives immediate results of air concentration. (Courtesy of Mine Safety Appliances Co.)

the different methods. The ultimate choice of a sampling and analytical method, therefore, will depend on consideration of all these various factors.

Fumes and Mists

Fumes and mists are collected on filters, like dusts, and analyzed in the laboratory. For example, a welder can be sampled for iron oxide fume through the use of a filter cassette, which is later analyzed by the chemist for the presence of iron.

Physical Agents

Physical agents such as noise and microwaves are usually monitored with an electronic instrument that responds to the energy field of the agent. Noise, for example, is monitored with a sound level meter or noise dosimeter. The sound level meter gives an immediate reading of the noise level, whereas the dosimeter accumulates the noise data over a period of time and reads out in an average decibel level or a percent dose. (The reference used for the dose calculation is the PEL, i.e., 90 dBA [decibel measured on the A scale] for 8 hours' duration = 100%) (see Chap. 16).

Biologic Agents

Microorganisms can be sampled using a variety of methods, but commonly with a particle sizing device. The various plates can then be incubated and counted to determine the airborne concentration. Sampling, however, is not usually recommended unless a source of a biologic agent is known to exist in the building or area.

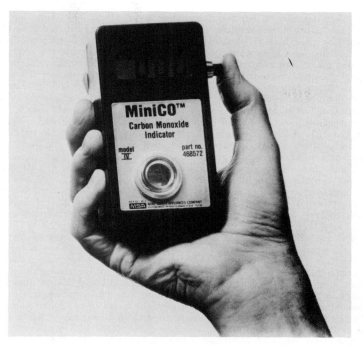

Figure 22-4. A direct-reading instrument for monitoring carbon monoxide. (Courtesy of Mine Safety Appliances Co.)

Table 22-1. Recognized exposure guidelines

ACGIH Threshold Limit Values (TLV)
ACGIH Biological Exposure Indices (BEI)
American Industrial Hygiene Association (AIHA) Workplace Environment
    Exposure Limit (WEEL)
National Institute for Occupational Safety and Health (NIOSH) Recommended
    Exposure Limits (REL)
OSHA Permissible Exposure Limits (PEL)

Exposure Guidelines

Several guidelines are available to the industrial hygienist to evaluate the significance of exposure levels to air contaminants (Table 22-1). All guidelines refer to *airborne* exposures except for the Biological Exposure Indices, which refer to safe *biologic* levels of the *substance* or *its metabolite* in body fluids or in expired air. Exposure guidelines can suggest to the occupational health professional how bad or good, in simplistic terms, a workplace exposure is. The TLVs developed by the ACGIH are updated annually and are meant to protect nearly all workers from adverse effects when they are repeatedly exposed to an agent. These values are the most comprehensive, have been in existence the longest, and are used by many regulatory authorities around the world. In the introduction to the TLVs, the TLV committee elaborates by stating that "because of wide variation in individual susceptibility, however, a small percentage of workers may experience discomfort from some substances at concentrations at or below the threshold limit; a smaller percentage may be affected by *aggravation* of a pre-existing condition or by development of an occupational illness" [2].

The TLV committee of the ACGIH points out that these levels are not to be used as a fine line between safe and dangerous concentrations. The committee also warns against the use of the guidelines as proof or disproof of an existing disease or physical condition. If a worker's exposure to an agent is below the guidelines, one cannot necessarily conclude that the exposure is safe for that person or that his or her symptoms are not related to the exposure. On the other hand, overexposure to an agent does not necessarily mean that the agent is responsible for the noted symptoms. Other factors, especially potential confounders such as cigarette smoking, should be considered.

Although officially the TLVs are *"guidelines* for good practices," they have assumed the power of law after OSHA adopted the 1968 TLVs as their PELs. The rationale for the TLV guidelines, which are based on industrial hygiene experience and experimental studies on animals and humans, can be found in the *Documentation of the Threshold Limit Values* published by the ACGIH [3].

The *Biological Exposure Indices* (BEI), also published by the ACGIH, are warning levels of biologic response to a chemical or its metabolite (Tables 22-2 and 22-3). These values may be of use to a physician in determining a *dose* to a worker because other routes of entry, besides inhalation, may be involved [3]. For example, blood lead analysis reflects the relative dose that the worker receives from all routes of exposure, including ingestion.

The use of biologic indices has been limited, however, because of the wide range in individual response to hazardous agents and the wide range in what is considered normal. In addition, sensitive analytic methods specific for certain materials are lacking. The BEIs are particularly useful, however, in evaluating situations where skin absorption may occur, as indicated by the notation "skin" next to a substance's entry in the TLV book. The BEIs are usually based on epidemiologic and/or pharmacokinetic analysis of the metabolism of the agent in controlled human studies. The BEIs should be used only when relating to an 8-hour exposure. (See discussion on Biologic Monitoring in Chap. 25.)

The OSHA PELs are published in the Code of Federal Regulations (29 CFR 1910) for general industry. These limits were adopted in 1971 along with the other OSHA safety and health regulations. Most of the exposure limits are found in subpart Z of the regulations, where over 400 PELs are listed. In addition, there are permissible exposure limits in specific standards, such as lead (CFR 1910.1025.) These standards cover other aspects of lead exposure, as well as the PEL.

In 1989, OSHA, through a generic rulemaking procedure, updated the 1971 permissible exposure limits and added some PELs for substances not previously regulated in the Air Contaminants Standard. This approach was a departure from their previous method of updating a PEL on an individual basis. At that time over 428 exposure limits were addressed.

On July 7, 1992, the United States Court of Appeals, Eleventh Circuit, issued a decision to vacate the Air Contaminants Standard. Since OSHA did not appeal this decision to the Supreme Court, the Eleventh Circuit Court's decision stands. It is uncertain, at the time of publication, what the ultimate effect of this development may be. At present, it has created a hodgepodge of permissible exposure limits in the country. For the states covered by the federal OSHA program, the PELs will revert to the original PELs adopted when OSHA began. In the states that are run by state OSHA programs, some will revert to the 1971 PELs and some will keep the updated PELs. OSHA, however, believes the 1989 PELs are more protective and encourages employers to continue compliance efforts to meet those levels particularly where engineering and work practice controls have already been implemented.

Most exposure limits are defined in 8-hour time-weighted averages. Other values refer to "ceiling" limits. A time-weighted average is usually based on an 8-hour work shift; however, some situations require appropriate adjustments for unusual work hours. The 8-hour time-weighted average is a method of calculating a *full-shift* average exposure by weighting short-term average concentrations by exposure time. For example, if an employee is exposed to carbon monoxide at 100 ppm for 4 hours and none for the remainder of the shift, the 8-hour time-weighted average would be 50 ppm. Ceiling values, which should never be exceeded, are usually assigned to strong irritants, cardiac sensitizers, and carcinogens. An STEL, short-term exposure limit, is another exposure limit used.

If a worker is exposed to more than one chemical that acts on the same organ system, the combined additive effect of the agents must be considered. To evaluate this situation the exposure concentrations are entered into a mixture formula, and if the result exceeds one, an overexposure situation exists. For example, if an em-

Table 22-2. Airborne chemicals for which biological exposure indices (BEI) have been adopted

Airborne chemical	Determinant
Aniline	Total p-aminophenol in urine Methemoglobin in blood
Benzene	Total phenol in urine Benzene in exhaled air
Cadmium	Cadmium in urine Cadmium in blood
Carbon disulfide	2-Thiothiazolidine-4-carboxylic acid in urine
Carbon monoxide	Carboxyhemoglobin in blood CO in end-exhaled air
Chlorobenzene	Total 4-chlorcatechol in urine Total p-chlorophenol in urine
Chromium (VI)	Total chromium in urine
N,N-Dimethylformamide	N-Methylformamide in urine
Ethyl benzene	Mandelic acid in urine Ethyl benzene in end-exhaled air
Fluorides	Fluorides in urine
Furfural	Total furoic acid in urine
n-Hexane	2,5-Hexanedione in urine n-Hexane in end-exhaled air
Lead	Lead in blood Lead in urine Zinc protoporphyrin in blood
Methanol	Methanol in urine Formic acid in urine
Methemoglobin inducers	Methemoglobin in blood
Methyl chloroform	Methyl chloroform in end-exhaled air Trichloroacetic acid in urine Total trichloroethanol in urine Total trichloroethanol in blood
Methyl ethyl ketone	MEK in urine
Nitrobenzene	Total p-nitrophenol in urine Methemoglobin in blood
Organophosphorus cholinesterase inhibitors	Cholinesterase activity in red cells
Parathion	Total p-nitrophenol in urine Cholinesterase activity in red cells
Pentachlorophenol (PCP)	Total PCP in urine Free PCP in plasma
Phenol	Total phenol in urine
Styrene	Mandelic acid in urine Phenylglyoxylic acid in urine Styrene in venous blood
Toluene	Hippuric acid in urine Toluene in venous blood Toluene in end-exhaled air
Trichloroethylene	Trichloroacetic acid in urine Trichloroacetic acid and trichloroethanol in urine Free trichloroethanol in blood Trichloroethylene in end-exhaled air
Xylenes	Methylhippuric acids in urine

Table 22-3. Airborne chemicals for which biological exposure indices are proposed

Airborne chemical	Determinant
Acetone	Acetone in urine
Arsenic and soluble compounds including arsine	Inorganic arsenic metabolites in urine
Cadmium	Cadmium in urine Cadmium in blood
Carbon monoxide	Carboxyhemoglobin in blood Carbon monoxide in end-exhaled air
2-Ethoxyethanol and 2-ethoxyethylacetate	2-Ethoxy acetic acid in urine
Mercury	Total inorganic mercury in urine Total inorganic mercury in blood
Methyl isobutyl ketone	MIBK in urine
Toluene	o-Cresol in urine
Trichloroethylene	Trichloroethylene in blood

ployee is exposed to 600 ppm acetone (PEL of 750 ppm) and 150 ppm methyl ethyl ketone (PEL of 200 ppm), the calculation is made as follows:

$$\frac{C_1}{L_1} + \frac{C_2}{L_2} + \frac{C_n}{L_n} = E_m$$

where:

E_m = the equivalent exposure for the mixture
C = the concentration of a particular contaminant
L = the exposure limit for that contaminant

$$\frac{600}{750} + \frac{150}{200} = 1.5$$

As evidenced by the example, neither acetone nor methyl ethyl ketone alone was above recommended guidelines (PELs), but their mixture suggests an overexposure.

The Workplace Environmental Exposure Limits (WEELs) and National Institute for Occupational Safety and Health (NIOSH) recommended limits are fewer in number but are also valuable guidelines to evaluate worker exposure. WEELs are published periodically in the *American Industrial Hygiene Association Journal.* NIOSH recommendations are found in the criteria documents and *Current Intelligence Bulletins.* Criteria Documents are summaries of the scientific literature on a specific chemical, which also include recommended exposure guidelines. These documents also contain information on *controlling* the hazard, appropriate *personal protective equipment,* and the rationale for selecting the recommended guideline.

Industrial Hygiene Services

If a patient's symptoms or illness is suspected as being caused by the workplace environment, industrial hygiene data should be reviewed, if available. By comparing the level of exposures in the workplace to the various guidelines, the physician can form a preliminary opinion regarding the contribution of the workplace environment to a particular illness. For example, OSHA states that if an employee's airborne exposure to lead is maintained at 50 mg/m^3, the blood lead concentration should be approximately 40 μg/100 g whole blood. If hygiene data indicate that the employee's exposure at work is not high enough to produce the elevated blood lead levels observed, personal habits, such as eating or smoking at the work station, or activities outside of work should be considered. The physician may learn that the individual was exposed to lead when stripping lead-based paint at home.

Industrial hygiene data may be available from various sources for a particular workplace. Federal or state OSHA offices or the workers' compensation insurance carrier may have conducted an investigation of the facility and have industrial hygiene data that may prove helpful to the physician. A call to the employer or to the OSHA office will help in locating the survey if one has been done.

An industrial hygiene consultant or company industrial hygienist may also have done a survey of the workplace. This information would have to be obtained from the employer. NIOSH, a research arm of the federal government, also conducts industrial hygiene surveys, which can be requested by interested parties including employees, unions, and physicians. Although fewer in number, these reports are comprehensive and can prove useful to a physician.

If industrial hygiene data do not exist for a particular operation or plant, the physician can ask the local OSHA office to conduct an inspection based on suspected occupational health problems. This request can be initiated by writing or calling the local office. OSHA will investigate the physician's concern and report conclusions of the findings to the physician. This option should be kept in mind, since the physician may be the only person suspecting the workplace hazard and the one who can then help correct the situation in the workplace for the patient and other workers.

Often a physician may evaluate a patient who works for a company that does not have an industrial hygienist on staff. In this case, an industrial hygiene *consultant* can perform the needed services, which may range from a complete industrial hygiene survey to selective air sampling for certain substances such as carbon monoxide. A listing of industrial hygiene consultants can be found each year in the January issue of the *American Industrial Hygiene Association Journal*. Certified industrial hygienists, those industrial hygienists with at least 4 years of experience and who have successfully completed a rigorous 2-day examination, will be listed with the designation "CIH" after their names.

References

1. McCunney R. J. Recognizing hand disorders due to vibrating tools. *J. Musculoskel. Med.* 9:91, 1992.
2. *Threshold Limit Values and Biological Exposure Indices for 1992–93*. Cincinnati: American Conference of Governmental Industrial Hygienists, 1992.
3. *Documentation of the Threshold Limit Values* (6th ed.). Cincinnati: American Conference of Governmental Industrial Hygienists, 1991.

Further Information

The American Industrial Hygiene Association can provide a host of educational material related to the recognition, evaluation, and control of workplace hazards. The Association can also help in locating industrial hygienists, who may serve as consultants. The AIHA office is located at 2700 Prosperity Ave., Suite 250, Fairfax, VA 22031; (703) 849-8888.

Baselt, R. C. *Biological Monitoring Methods for Industrial Chemicals* (2nd ed.). Davis, CA: Biomedical, 1988.
Contains information on blood concentrations, urine concentrations, metabolism and excretion, toxicity, biologic monitoring, and analytic procedures for many industrial chemicals.

Brief, R. S. *Basic Industrial Hygiene: A Training Manual*. Akron, OH: American Industrial Hygiene Association, 1975.
Exxon's industrial hygiene manual published by the AIHA gives a good short introduction to industrial hygiene.

Burgess, W. A. *Recognition of Health Hazards in Industry*. New York: Wiley, 1981.
An introduction to industrial processes and hazards.

Clayton, G. D., and Clayton, F. E. (eds.). *Patty's Industrial Hygiene and Toxicology* (4th ed.). New York: Wiley, 1991.
A comprehensive text in industrial hygiene.

Cook, W. A. *Occupational Exposure Limits—Worldwide*. Akron, OH: American Industrial Hygiene Association, 1987.
Exposure limits in other countries.

Documentation of the Threshold Limit Values (6th ed.). Cincinnati: American Conference of Government Industrial Hygienists, 1991.
Contains the rationale used in deciding on a specific TLV.

Hering, S. V. (ed.). *Air Sampling Instruments* (7th ed.). Cincinnati: American Conference of Governmental Industrial Hygienists, 1989.
Exhaustive guide to air sampling instrumentation.

Key, M. M., et al. (eds.). *Occupational Diseases: A Guide to Their Recognition* (rev. ed.). Washington, DC: US Government Printing Office, 1977.
A concise guide to occupational diseases, which contains permissible exposure limits and references.

OSHA General Industry Standards (29 CFR 1910). Washington, DC: US Government Printing Office, 1992.
Lists the OSHA regulations, both safety and health. Contains the permissible exposure limits, regulations for noise and radiation, and complete health regulations for substances such as asbestos and other carcinogens.

Plog, B. A. (ed.). *Fundamentals of Industrial Hygiene* (3rd ed.). Chicago: National Safety Council, 1988.

Threshold Limit Values and Biological Exposure Indices for 1992–93. Cincinnati: American Conference of Governmental Industrial Hygienists, 1992–1993.
Contains the TLVs that are published annually for limiting exposure. Handbook available from ACGIH, 6500 Glenway Ave., Bldg. D-7, Cincinnati, OH 45211-4438; (513) 661-7881.

US EPA and NIOSH. *Building Air Quality, 1991.* Publication no. 91-114.
A "self-help" guide to indoor building air quality. Helps identify causes, solutions, and control strategies.

23 Toxicology

David C. Logan

Toxicology is the study of the mechanisms of action and adverse effects of chemical agents in living organisms. The main objective of toxicology is to identify the nature of health damage that may be produced by a chemical substance and the range of doses over which damage is produced. This information can form a sound basis for predicting acceptable levels of exposure for humans who contact chemical substances during manufacture, use, and disposal.

Measuring the effects of a chemical exposure directly in humans either through epidemiologic or controlled clinical studies provides the best evidence of a chemical's toxicity in humans. However, in most instances, it is impossible to study toxic effects in humans directly, and indirect methods such as toxicologic testing in animals and cell systems are necessary. When properly conducted and evaluated, these toxicologic tests can accurately predict adverse health outcomes in humans. The underlying premise is that the final reaction of the chemical or its metabolite on the target cell within the animal or cell model is the same as that in humans.

The scope of toxicology is enormous, since virtually every known chemical, if present in sufficient amount, has the potential to produce injury or death. In our modern society, toxicologic tests are used to evaluate the potential health hazards that may result from exposure to environmental pollutants, food additives, pharmacologic agents, and occupational exposures among others.

The practicing physician will benefit from having an understanding of basic toxicologic principles. Whenever the physician suspects that an individual's illness, abnormal clinical findings, or symptoms are related to an environmental or occupational exposure, an understanding of absorption, metabolism, distribution, and excretion of the material in question will be of significant value in the diagnosis and management of the patient. In emergency situations, this knowledge can facilitate appropriate first aid and critical care management. Interpreting toxicologic data from Material Safety Data Sheets (MSDS), reference texts, and journals is important in evaluating whether an individual's findings might be related to a particular exposure and thereby can guide treatment. In addition, understanding the basic toxicologic tests that are in use today will enable the physician to evaluate more critically the use of this type of data in risk assessments and standard-setting activities at the Occupational Safety and Health Administration (OSHA) and other government agencies.

Exposure Considerations

The amount needed to produce an adverse effect varies considerably among materials. Some chemicals such as botulism toxin can produce death in microgram doses (much less than a drop) when ingested, whereas other chemicals may be relatively harmless following doses in excess of several grams. The critical factor is not the intrinsic toxicity of a substance but the associated degree of risk that the substance poses in a given circumstance. For example, a very toxic chemical when carefully handled may be less hazardous than a relatively nontoxic substance that is improperly used. Key elements in assessing the degree of human risk for any given chemical are the exposure, absorption, and metabolism of the substance.

Toxic effects of a chemical agent in humans or animal models are not produced unless the agent or its metabolites reach appropriate *receptors* in the body at a *concentration* and for a *length of time* sufficient to initiate the toxic manifestations. The most important factors influencing this critical event are the route of contact of the agent, the dose, and the duration and frequency of exposure.

Routes of Contact

The major routes by which toxic agents gain access to the body are the lungs (inhalation), the skin (absorption), the gastrointestinal tract (ingestion), and parenteral administration (blood). Toxic agents generally exhibit the greatest potency and produce the most rapid response when exposure is by the intravenous route, followed in approximate order by the inhalation, intraperitoneal, subcutaneous, intramuscular, intradermal, oral, and dermal routes. Industrial exposures to toxic agents occur most frequently by inhalation and dermal exposure. Inadvertent ingestion from contaminated hands can also occur. For example, intoxication from inorganic lead may be worsened if the worker is eating or smoking with inorganic lead dust on the hands.

Dose

The amount of exposure or dose is another important factor in determining a material's potential toxicity. Toxic manifestations usually occur with greater frequency and severity as the dose increases, a characteristic often described as a *dose-response relationship*. In a toxicologic study in which groups of animals are exposed to different dose levels of a chemical, evaluating whether there is dose-response relationship is an important element in determining the significance of the study results. Findings that are seen at low-dose levels but not at higher levels are usually not due to the chemical exposure. A dose-response relationship is not as relevant in situations where there is an immunologic reaction in the disease process. For example, in workers with extrinsic allergic alveolitis (hypersensitivity pneumonitis), the dose of antigenic material needed to initiate symptoms in the susceptible worker can be very low due to previous sensitization.

Duration and Frequency of Exposure

The time period over which the exposure occurs is also important in determining what toxicity is observed. In general, the adverse effect associated with a single dose is reduced when the total amount in the single dose is divided into two or more separately administered smaller doses. This reduced effect is the result of metabolism or excretion occurring between successive doses or partial or full repair of the injury prior to the next administration.

In addition to affecting the frequency and severity of toxic effects, the duration and timing of exposure often influence the *types of effects* that are observed. The toxic effects seen after an acute exposure (within a 24-hour time period) are usually immediate; however, delayed toxicity can also occur. Chronic exposure to the same material (exposure exceeding 24 hours) may also produce immediate effects in addition to long-term, delayed effects.

Because of these differences, toxicologic testing frequently incorporates several exposure regimens to identify the full range of effects that may be produced by the substance. These include single-dose exposures, short-term exposures administered over approximately a week, subchronic exposures of usually 3 months' duration, and long-term exposure regimens that involve a 2-year period or the lifetime of the animal.

Absorption, Distribution, Metabolism, and Excretion

Several factors influence whether a sufficient concentration of a toxic material reaches receptor sites within the body to initiate an adverse effect. These include the rate and amount of the material absorbed; the distribution of the toxicant within the body; the rate of metabolism or biochemical transformation, if any; and the rate of excretion of the toxicant or its metabolites.

Absorption Through the Lung

The process by which a material passes through body membranes and enters the bloodstream is referred to as absorption. Substances that are absorbed by the lungs are usually gases, such as hydrogen sulfide or carbon monoxide; mists of fine liquid droplets; and particulate dispersions, such as silica or asbestos dust. Most of the absorption occurs in the alveoli, which have a large total surface area, ranging from 50 to 100 square meters. Because of the very thin epithelial layer of the alveoli, gas in the alveoli equilibrates almost instantaneously with blood passing through the pulmonary capillary bed.

The amount of gas that enters the blood from the alveoli is dependent on the *solubility* of the gas in the blood. Highly soluble gases such as chloroform are rapidly taken up by the blood. A relatively large amount must be absorbed before the blood becomes saturated with the material and before a steady state or equilibrium is established, after which further net absorption from the lung does not occur. If the gas also has high lipid solubility, gas from the blood will rapidly enter body fat, and the time required to reach an equilibrium will be substantially longer. For highly soluble gases, the principal factors that govern absorption are the rate and depth of respiration and the concentration of the gas in inspired air.

For an insoluble gas such as ethylene, only a small amount can be dissolved in blood, and consequently an equilibrium is reached relatively quickly. Blood entering the lung rapidly takes up the amount that can be absorbed so that only a small percentage of the total gas in the lung is taken up by the blood during each respiration. In this case, increasing the respiratory rate or minute volume does not increase the transfer of gas to the blood. Increasing the rate of cardiac output, however, would markedly increase the rate of uptake of the gas.

For particulate matter and fogs or sprays of fine liquid droplets, the deposition within the pulmonary system depends to a great extent on the size of the particles. Particles of 5 μm or larger are usually deposited in the nasopharyngeal region and are carried by the mucous blanket of the ciliated nasal surface to the upper pharynx and eventually swallowed. Particles of 2 to 5 μm are deposited in the tracheobronchiolar regions of the lung, where they are rapidly and efficiently cleared by the upward movement of the mucous layer in the ciliated portions of the respiratory tract. Particles of 1 μm and below are able to reach the alveolar epithelium of the lung. In the alveoli, they may be absorbed into the blood or removed by two major routes, phagocytosis by phagocytes or macrophages or removal through the lymphatic system.

Removal of particulates from the alveoli is relatively inefficient and is dependent, in part, on the compound's solubility in alveolar fluid. Soluble compounds are removed at a faster rate than insoluble compounds. Some insoluble particles such as asbestos and silica may remain in the alveolus indefinitely when ingested by alveolar cells, which do not desquamate.

Absorption Through the Skin

The intact skin provides an excellent barrier to the absorption of toxic agents. However, some chemicals may be absorbed in sufficient quantities to produce systemic effects. For a chemical to be absorbed through the skin, it must pass either through the epidermal cells, the cells of the sweat glands or sebaceous glands, or the hair follicles. The epidermal cells are the most important route of absorption because they constitute the major surface area of the skin.

Materials that are absorbed through the epidermis first diffuse through the *stratum corneum,* which is the rate-limiting barrier for absorption. It appears that all toxicants move across the stratum corneum by passive diffusion with different molecular mechanisms for ionized and nonionized compounds. The stratum corneum differs significantly in thickness and degree of permeability from one region of the body to another. As a result, chemicals can cross the skin of the scrotum more easily than that of the abdomen, since the scrotal epidermis is extremely thin and relatively more permeable. Toxicants are absorbed with most difficulty through the sole of the foot due to the great thickness of the stratum corneum. Since the stratum corneum plays such a critical role in determining cutaneous permeability, abrasion injury or removal of this layer causes an abrupt increase in permeability.

After passing through the stratum corneum, chemicals can usually readily diffuse through the germinal layer of the epidermis, which contains a porous, nonselective, watery diffusion medium, and can then enter the bloodstream through capillaries.

Water plays an important role in absorption through the skin. Skin normally contains approximately 90 grams of water per gram of dry tissue. Upon additional contact with water, the stratum corneum can substantially increase its water content, resulting in a two- to threefold increase in permeability. Occlusion of the skin such as with work gloves can hydrate the stratum corneum and thereby greatly enhance the absorption of a material such as an organic solvent that inadvertently enters or penetrates the glove. Certain bipolar solvents such as dimethyl sulfoxide (DMSO) can also facilitate the penetration of toxicants through the skin.

Several animal species have been used to study the absorption of chemicals through the skin, and significant differences have been observed among them. For example, the permeability of the skin of the guinea pig, pig, and monkey is very similar to that of humans. The skin of the rat and rabbit is more permeable, and that of the cat is less permeable than human skin.

Absorption Through the Gastrointestinal Tract

Absorption through the gastrointestinal tract is an important route of entry for many environmental toxicants that enter the food chain, for suicide attempts, and for accidental poisoning, especially among children. Absorption of toxicants through the gastrointestinal tract can occur in certain occupational settings such as with accidental ingestions or when workers eat or smoke with contaminated hands, but ingestion is usually less common than dermal or inhalation routes of exposure. Absorption through the gastrointestinal tract is influenced by the solubility of the material, active transport mechanisms, gastrointestinal motility, and physical properties of the substance.

Most toxicants cross body membranes by simple diffusion. Since the body's membranes are high in lipid content, the rate of diffusion of most materials across these membranes depends in large part on their lipid solubility and their concentration gradient across the membrane. An important determinant of a chemical's lipid solubility is its ionization form in solution. As a general principle, nonionized molecules are more lipid soluble and therefore more likely to penetrate lipid membrane barriers. The acidity of gastric juice and the neutrality of intestinal contents influence the ionized or nonionized state of a material. Therefore, a material's lipid solubility and thus its potential for absorption can differ markedly in these two areas of the gastrointestinal tract.

The mammalian gastrointestinal tract has specialized transport systems for the absorption of nutrients and electrolytes. Some toxicants can also be absorbed by these same specialized transport systems.

Gastrointestinal motility will affect the absorption of materials. A decreased motility tends to increase the overall rate of absorption due to the longer retention time of the material in the proximal segment of the small intestine, which has a large total mucosal surface area and relatively high absorptive capacity.

The physical properties of the compound such as its particle size and its solubility are also important in determining the degree of absorption. If the toxicant is relatively water insoluble, the compound will have limited contact with the gastrointestinal mucosa and therefore will not be as well absorbed. Since the dissolution rate of a material is proportional to particle size, large particles are generally not as readily absorbed.

A number of other factors have been shown to alter absorption. For example, certain metals can alter the absorption of other metals. Cadmium decreases the absorption of zinc and copper, calcium decreases the absorption of cadmium, zinc decreases the absorption of copper, and magnesium decreases the absorption of fluoride. The nutritional status and age of the animal also appear to affect absorption.

Absorption Through Special Routes of Administration

In addition to gastrointestinal, lung, and dermal routes of exposure, toxicologists frequently administer chemical agents by various other routes, including intraperitoneal, subcutaneous, intramuscular, and intravenous. Each route has its own unique characteristics. The intravenous route introduces the toxicant directly into the bloodstream. The intraperitoneal route results in a rapid absorption of the material due to the rich blood supply and large surface area of the peritoneum. As this absorption is primarily through the portal circulation, the toxicant must pass through the liver before reaching other organs. Thus, substances that are metabolized or extracted by the liver and excreted into the bile do not have the same toxicity when administered intraperitoneally as by another route.

The route of administration determines the rate of absorption and therefore the concentration of the material at various organ tissues over time. The concentration level and time course of exposure to target receptor sites are important factors in determining the chemical's toxicity. The route of administration that is chosen for a toxicologic study is often based on the route of exposure expected in humans. Use of the same route can remove certain questions regarding applicability of a given toxicologic study in predicting human risk.

Distribution

Following absorption, distribution of a chemical toxicant occurs through the bloodstream. This distribution depends principally on the ability of the chemical to pass through the cell membranes of the various tissues of the body and the affinity of the various tissues in the body for the chemical. In general, lipid-soluble molecules with a molecular weight of 50 or less can readily permeate cell membranes. Water-soluble molecules can diffuse through aqueous channels on the cell membrane or enter the cell through active transport mechanisms.

Materials that readily pass through cell membranes often become distributed throughout the body. Other materials with less membrane permeability accumulate in various parts of the body as a result of binding, active transport, or high solubility in fat. The site of accumulation may determine where the material exerts its major toxicity. For example, inhaled asbestos and radioactive dusts accumulate in the lung, and this is the organ where toxicity is most often observed. When a material accumulates at sites that are toxicologically inactive, such as fat depots, the accumulation serves initially as a protective mechanism. As the material leaves its area of storage and is eliminated from the body, it may have a delayed action on target receptors. For example, individuals with large body burdens of inorganic lead can continue to have symptoms of lead toxicity after removal from exposure due to the slow release of lead from bone and other storage depots into the bloodstream.

After entering the bloodstream, the toxicant may distribute into one or more of the water compartments of the body, in addition to binding to various receptor sites or entering storage tissues in the body such as fat, liver, or bone. Within the compartments of the total body water, the chemical may remain in the plasma or enter the interstitial fluid or intracellular fluid of the body. In the plasma, the chemical might bind with one or more plasma proteins, the most important of which is albumin. This protein binding is an important consideration for evaluating a material's potential toxicity. Once bound, the high molecular weight of the protein prevents passage of the substance outside the vascular space, thereby preventing the material from entering a target organ to produce injury. However, the binding occurs in an equilibrium process with unbound chemical in the plasma. As the unbound chemical diffuses from the capillaries, bound chemical dissociates from the protein. This process continues until chemical in the extravascular fluid equilibrates with unbound chemical in the plasma. Severe toxic reactions may occur if the agent is displaced from the plasma protein by another chemical agent. For example, if a sulfonamide drug is given to a patient who is taking an oral hypoglycemic drug, the sulfonamide may displace the anti-diabetic drug from plasma proteins and induce hypoglycemic coma. The insecticide dieldrin is another example of a material that avidly binds to plasma proteins and that may compete with other chemicals or drugs for available binding sites.

The liver and kidney concentrate more toxicants than other organs, since they have a high capacity to bind chemicals. Active transport and binding to specific proteins of the kidney or liver are important factors in this process.

Most toxicants do not enter the brain in appreciable quantities because of three major factors. First, the capillary endothelial cells of the central nervous system (CNS) are tightly joined, leaving few or no pores between the cells. Second, the capillaries of the CNS are largely surrounded by astrocytes, which provide an additional barrier for penetration. Third, the protein concentration in the interstitial fluid of the CNS is much lower than elsewhere in the body, which further limits distribution. Materials that do enter the brain are usually lipid soluble, nonprotein bound, nonionized, and of relatively small molecular size. Since this relative CNS barrier is not completely developed at birth, newborns are more susceptible to the toxicity of some materials, such as lead.

The placenta is not as effective a barrier as the CNS. Many chemicals, viruses, proteins, and even blood cells can cross from the maternal circulation into the fetal circulation through the placenta. As with most transfers across body membranes, simple diffusion appears to be the mechanism by which most toxicants pass through the placenta.

Metabolism

Metabolism refers to the chemical transformation of compounds that can occur in an organism as a result of enzymatic reactions. The enzymes that metabolize foreign compounds are localized mainly in the liver; however, metabolism is also known to occur in the intestine, kidney, lung, brain, and skin. The types of enzymatic reactions that can occur within an organism include catabolic or breakdown reactions of oxidation, reduction, and hydrolysis, and synthetic conjugation reactions.

The most important group of oxidative enzymes involved in metabolism is the cytochrome P450-containing monooxygenases. Through various mechanisms, these monooxygenases introduce oxygen atoms into a number of different compounds. The enzyme system is widely distributed in various organ systems in many animal species. The same cytochrome P450 enzymes can also catalyze a number of reactions where azo and nitro compounds are reduced to the corresponding amines.

Conjugation reactions usually involve joining a parent material with another compound to form a third substance. The final product is usually more polar than the substrate, making it more water soluble and therefore more easily excretable. Probably the most important conjugation reactions in humans involve glucuronic acid found in the endoplasmic reticulum of many tissues, but most especially in the liver. Glucuronic acid can be conjugated to a number of compounds, including aliphatic and aromatic alcohols, mercaptans, certain acids, and primary and secondary aliphatic and aromatic amines.

A number of factors influence the rate of biotransformation. These include differences in age, nutritional status, sex, species and strain of animal, and the presence of underlying disease.

Another factor is the possible presence of enzyme-inducing or activating agents such as phenobarbital. Phenobarbital induces certain of the cytochrome P450 enzymes, which can greatly enhance the biotransformation of certain chemicals and drugs.

Excretion

Toxicants are primarily eliminated from the body through the kidney, but the liver and biliary systems, the lungs, sweat, tears, and even breast milk can all excrete chemicals from the body.

Chemical substances are excreted by the kidney through passive glomerular filtration, passive tubular diffusion, and active tubular secretion. Most toxic agents that are not protein bound are small enough to be filtered at the glomerulus. Once filtered, the chemical may remain in the filtrate or be passively resorbed through the tubular cells. Highly lipid-soluble nonionic molecules are much more likely to be passively resorbed through these lipid membranes than are polar or ionized molecules. Since the pH of the urine can dictate whether a given chemical is in a nonionic or ionic form, it is an important factor in determining how quickly a material will be excreted by the kidney. In addition to these processes, certain organic acids and organic bases can be excreted into the urine through active transport. Protein-bound chemicals that are not easily filtered are fully available for these active secretory processes. One of the characteristics of these active transport processes is that various compounds can compete with one another for secretion. This has important therapeutic implications, such as when probenecid is given to a patient to reduce the active secretion of penicillin.

The liver is another important organ where the excretion of toxic agents can occur. The blood from the gastrointestinal tract passes through the liver before reaching the systemic circulation. As a result, the liver can remove compounds absorbed from the gastrointestinal tract, limiting their distribution to other parts of the body. The material can be excreted by the liver cells into the bile and passed into the small intestine, where the substance may be excreted or resorbed. Many organic compounds are biotransformed into polar metabolites before being excreted into the bile. The compounds in turn become less lipid soluble and thus less likely to be resorbed in the gastrointestinal tract. As with renal tubular secretion, chemical agents that are bound to plasma proteins are fully available for biliary excretion, and many such protein-bound compounds are excreted into the bile. Some materials such as lead, arsenic, and manganese are rapidly concentrated and excreted into the bile. Other materials such as zinc, iron, gold, and chromium are poorly concentrated. Liver dysfunction can markedly reduce the liver's ability to excrete chemical substances. Conversely, as previously noted, pretreatment with some drugs such as phenobarbital increases the enzyme activity of a number of liver microsomal enzymes, which can thereby hasten metabolic breakdown of a particular toxicant. This increased rate of elimination appears to be due not only to an increased conjugation of certain chemicals and drugs, but also to an increase in bile flow and possibly blood flow through the liver.

The lungs are important in eliminating materials that exist predominantly in the gas phase at body temperature or that have a high vapor pressure. Elimination from the blood appears to be by simple diffusion into the alveolar space.

Excretion into the breast milk is an important route because toxic materials can be passed to a nursing child from the mother. Because of breast milk's high lipid content, lipid-soluble compounds such as DDT and polychlorinated and polybrominated biphenyls are easily transferred through passive diffusion into the lipid portion of milk. Elimination of chemical compounds through sweat, saliva, skin, hair, and nails can occur, but these routes are quantitatively of minor importance.

Measurement of exposure agents in these fluids and tissues can occasionally provide useful information regarding the degree of absorption of the material or the amount retained or bound to critical sites in the organisms. A discussion of biologic monitoring can be found in Chap. 25.

Toxicologic Testing Methodologies

Toxicology testing has become an important method to evaluate a chemical's potential toxicity. The Toxic Substances Control Act (TSCA) passed by Congress in 1976 has had an important influence on much of the toxicology testing that is currently conducted. The overall objectives of TSCA are to obtain information about chemicals, to assess their risks, and to regulate those materials that are found to have an unreasonable benefit-to-risk ratio. Under TSCA, the Environmental Protection Agency (EPA) may require data on mutagenic, carcinogenic, teratogenic, synergistic, or behavioral effects by epidemiologic, in vitro, or laboratory animal methods whenever an unreasonable risk to health or environment may exist and there are insufficient available data to determine the risk. In addition, under TSCA, a manufacturer must notify the EPA at least 90 days before the production of any new chemical substance. The manufacturer must submit test data and other information with this premanufacturing notice to show that the production poses an insignificant risk to health and the environment. Based on a review of the submitted data, the EPA may approve the production or new use or limit the manufacture or distribution of the substance until additional test data are available. TSCA has greatly increased the use of toxicology testing in these hazard evaluations.

Two fundamental assumptions underlie all animal toxicity testing. First, the effects produced by the compound in laboratory animals are often the same as the effects observed in humans. Second, the rate of adverse health effects increases as the dose or exposure increases. In toxicologic testing, relatively large doses of the material under study must be used, since the number of animals that can be studied is small. By using large doses, any toxicity that may relate to the material will occur frequently enough to be detected.

Despite phylogenetic differences, laboratory rodents have been found to be the most suitable test species for predicting human reactions to foreign chemicals. Larger mammals may occasionally be more appropriate as experimental species. If several unrelated species of vertebrates show a similar pattern of response to a test substance, humans are likely to react in the same way. *As a general principle, if the absorption, distribution, metabolism, and excretion of a material are similar in humans and a particular animal species, test results in that species are generally predictive of toxicity of the material in humans.* Because there are often important differences in these characteristics, toxicology studies must always be carefully interpreted. These differences and the fact that most chemicals in commerce today have not undergone extensive toxicology testing mean that the clinician should be alert to the possibility that a chemical may have toxicity not previously described.

The standard toxicology testing methods that are commonly used to assess chemical toxicity are described below.

Acute Toxicity Studies

Acute toxicity studies are performed by administering a test material to animals on one occasion and evaluating any resulting toxicity over the following hours, days, and even weeks. These studies can determine the median lethal dose for a chemical (LD50). An LD50 is defined as the dose that would predictably kill one half of the animal population experimentally exposed. For inhalation studies, the LC50, or lethal concentration required to produce death in 50% of the animals, is determined. In addition to determining a material's lethality, these tests are used to evaluate a number of other toxic effects, including behavior, response to stimuli, reflexes, and effects on bodily functions and vital signs. From these data, the experienced toxicologist can arrive at certain conclusions regarding the site and mechanisms of action of compounds undergoing the test.

The results of acute toxicity testing provide basic information about a material's relative potential to cause acute or immediate toxic effects. This relative potential is often expressed in terms of toxicity ratings or classes. An example of a classification system is given in Table 23-1. Discovery that a material has a "6" or "super toxic" rating using this classification system would help the clinician quickly appreciate the highly toxic nature of the material and its potential to severely injure or kill an individual at extremely low dose levels. Such classification systems are only qualitative, but they serve a practical and useful purpose in describing the acute toxicity of a material. Recommendations regarding the need for medical attention, the induction of vomiting, washing of exposed skin and laundry, or discarding of contaminated clothing and shoes are frequently based on such acute toxicity classification systems.

Dermal Irritation, Sensitization, and Phototoxicity

The ability of a chemical to irritate the skin is usually determined in the rabbit. The fur on the back of the rabbit is removed with clippers, and the chemical is applied to the skin under a covered patch for a period of usually 3 days. The degree of skin irritation is scored for erythema and eschar formation, edema formation, and corrosive action. These dermal observations are repeated at various intervals after the covered patch is removed.

Cutaneous sensitization is usually evaluated in guinea pigs. Through initial skin testing and testing with subsequent challenge doses, both irritant and challenge scores can be determined. A comparison of these scores is then used to determine the material's ability to sensitize.

Phototoxicity is assessed by irradiating the dosed skin with ultraviolet light and comparing the dermal effects with dosed skin not irradiated.

Eye Irritation

Most compounds that are generally available for human use are tested for irritant effects following topical application of the agents to the eyes of experimental animals.

Table 23-1. Numerical toxicity rating definitions

Toxicity rating or class	Probable oral lethal dose (human)	
	Dose	For 70-kg person (150 lb)
6 Super toxic	Less than 5 mg/kg	A taste (less than 7 drops)
5 Extremely toxic	5–50 mg/kg	Between 7 drops and 1 tsp
4 Very toxic	50–500 mg/kg	Between 1 tsp and 1 oz
3 Moderately toxic	0.5–5 g/kg	Between 1 oz and 1 pt (or 1 lb)
2 Slightly toxic	5–15 g/kg	Between 1 pt and 1 qt
1 Practically nontoxic	Above 15 g/kg	More than 1 qt (2.2 lb)

Source: From R. Gosselin et al. *Clinical Toxicology of Commercial Products* (5th ed.). Baltimore: Williams & Wilkins, 1984. P. I-2.

The test procedure involves applying material in liquid or solid form to the lower conjunctival sac of one eye in each of at least six rabbits. The eyes are then examined at 1, 2, and 3 days after exposure and scored according to the degree of irritation present. The irritation score for a particular material gives useful information regarding the material's potential to irritate human eyes on contact.

Subchronic Exposure

The objective of subchronic exposure studies is to evaluate and characterize the potential toxicity of a compound when administered to experimental animals on a daily basis over a period of 3 to 4 months. The subchronic study is usually performed in two animal species, using the same route of exposure that is expected in humans. Observations on the test animals include mortality, body weight changes, diet consumption, hematology, and clinical chemistry measurements. At the end of the experiment, the gross and microscopic condition of the animals and selected organs and tissues are evaluated and recorded. One of the objectives of the subchronic study is to attempt to demonstrate some form of toxic effect, at least in the high-dose group of experimental animals. Use of short-term acute toxicity studies prior to the subchronic test is helpful in planning an appropriate subchronic dose regimen. Subchronic studies also aim at determining the exposure level at which there is no adverse effect or adverse effects are not observable.

With appropriate modifications, the basic subchronic test can be used to evaluate mutagenesis, teratogenesis, and effects on reproductive capacity. Except for carcinogenesis and some forms of cytotoxicity, the subchronic test will usually reveal most forms of toxicity to adult animals. These findings form a reasonable basis to predict the material's potential toxicity to humans when exposed through the same route of exposure.

Lifetime Bioassay to Evaluate Carcinogenicity

Studies used to evaluate a material's potential to induce cancer are usually performed in rats and mice. Fifty animals are commonly used for each of three exposure groups along with a control group. Exposure is usually 30 months for rats and 24 months for mice. The test chemical can be administered in the diet, by gavage, or by inhalation. Gross and microscopic pathologic examinations are made on both the animals that survive the chronic exposure and those that die prematurely.

The bioassay is designed to assess whether the test chemical produces a carcinogenic effect, which is defined as

1. The development of *types of neoplasms* not seen in controls
2. An *increased incidence* of the types of neoplasms occurring in controls
3. The occurrence of neoplasms *earlier* than in controls
4. An *increased multiplicity* of neoplasms in individual animals

There appears to be a strong correlation between the results of well-conducted laboratory animal carcinogenicity experiments and epidemiologic studies of human carcinogenicity. With the possible exception of arsenic, all recognized human carcinogens are carcinogenic in appropriately conducted studies in laboratory animals. Even the one apparent exception, arsenic, has been reported to produce carcinomas of the respiratory tract in hamsters. Also, at least 19 carcinogens have been identified in which the target organ is the same in humans and experimental animals. Thus, in the absence of direct epidemiologic data, laboratory animal carcinogenicity studies currently provide the best experimental method for assessing a chemical's carcinogenic potential in humans.

Mouse-Skin Bioassay

The material to be tested is applied to the shaved dorsal skin of mice, two or three times per week, for 80 weeks or more. These studies usually employ groups of 50 male mice treated with a single dosage level of test material. Mice are observed for the development of dermal tumors at the application site.

In Vitro Assays

In vitro toxicology assays utilize cell cultures and bacterial systems outside the living animal. These assays provide a rapid and relatively inexpensive means of identifying mutagenicity and a material's ability to damage DNA. Mutagenesis is the ability of chemicals to cause changes in the genetic material in the nucleus of cells in ways that can be transmitted during cell division. Since mutations are thought to be an important mechanism for the initiation of cancer, mutagenic tests are often used to screen for potential carcinogens.

The most widely utilized bacterial test system for identifying mutagenicity is the *Salmonella typhimurium* microsome test developed by Dr. Bruce Ames and co-workers and commonly called the Ames assay. The marker utilized for the detection of gene mutations in these strains of *Salmonella* is the ability of the bacteria to synthesize histidine, an amino acid essential for bacterial division. The bacteria have mutations rendering them unable to synthesize histidine, and thus they must depend on histidine included in the culture medium to be able to multiply.

When these bacteria are exposed to a mutagenic chemical, some will back-mutate and regain their ability to synthesize histidine. These bacteria will therefore now be able to survive in a histidine-free medium. By counting the number of back-mutated colonies that develop after exposure to a particular chemical and comparing this number to spontaneous back-mutation rates, a chemical's mutagenic potential can be determined.

Use of Toxicologic Data

Understanding toxicologic principles and testing methods can assist the physician in evaluating patients who have symptoms or illness possibly caused by an occupational or environmental exposure.

In any such patient evaluation, a detailed and complete occupational history is of great importance. Knowing what exposures the patient may have encountered at work, the magnitude of these exposures, and over what time period they occurred will permit the physician to consider whether any of them may be a contributory factor in a particular illness. Nonoccupational exposures that could be related to the illness should also be carefully considered. These include a smoking and alcohol history, a history of exposure to materials through hobbies, and a history of possible exposures from living near a mine, plant, or smelter that could have contaminated the surrounding area.

Frequently, information concerning workplace exposures can be obtained through consultation with medical and industrial hygiene professionals at the individual's place of employment. The OSHA Hazard Communication Standard requires that information regarding the materials used or handled be made available to the employee. In addition, the OSHA Access to Employee Medical and Exposure Records regulation provides for employee access to exposure records that are applicable to the employee.

Evaluating whether the identified exposures may be of medical significance in a given circumstance is often a difficult process. Toxicologic information on the materials in question can contribute greatly to this assessment.

As an initial review, knowledge of how the material is absorbed, distributed in the body, metabolized, and excreted will assist in determining whether the exposure is of clinical significance. Such information will enable the clinician to determine if biologic monitoring might be appropriate in a given situation. For example, knowledge that the solvent trichloroethylene (TCE) is metabolized to a number of different products, including trichloroethanol and trichloroacetic acid, can enable the physician to consider whether measuring these metabolites in the urine of a patient might provide useful information. If exposure is questionable but important to establish, urinary measurement of trichloroethanol and trichloroacetic acid might be appropriate. However, knowledge that the biologic half-lives of trichloroethanol and trichloroacetic acid in urine are 10 to 15 hours and 70 to 100 hours, respectively, will help the clinician realize that conducting urinary measurements 1 week after exposure would not likely be of value.

Acute toxicity tests on the material can provide reliable information regarding its relative toxicity and the dose level that would predictably affect human health. Results of eye and skin irritation studies in animals are useful in assessing whether the material may irritate humans on exposure. Subchronic studies can identify potential systemic toxicity and the target organs that may be impacted after over-exposure. A well-conducted laboratory animal carcinogenicity experiment can be helpful in evaluating the material's carcinogenic potential in humans.

In reviewing toxicologic data, it is important to keep in mind the *animal model* that was used in the study, the *route of exposure,* the *dose levels* used, and the *time period* over which exposure took place. The relevance of animal test results to humans is increased when the route of exposure used in the animal study is the same as the route of exposure in humans. Otherwise, it is important to consider how this difference might alter the assessment of the study's significance to humans. An oral feeding study in animals may not have much significance if there is negligible potential for ingestion in humans. However, the results may be meaningful if the material can be absorbed through the lungs and reach the target organ where toxicity was demonstrated in the animal study.

The results of animal testing are more likely to be predictive of effects in humans when distribution, metabolism, and excretion in the animal model and humans are similar. These characteristics are frequently described as the *pharmacokinetics* of the material; because of their importance, toxicologic laboratories routinely incorporate pharmacokinetic studies as part of a chemical's total evaluation.

In reviewing a toxicologic study, it is important to evaluate the methods employed. For example, did the study use an *adequate number* of animals? Were *control animals* used to enable a comparison with exposure groups? Was the *proper animal model* selected? Was the laboratory qualified to conduct the test? In addition, it is important to consider whether the results of the study were properly presented and interpreted. Were the results *statistically significant*? Were potential *confounding variables* such as effects of other agents or laboratory procedures considered? Was there a *dose-response relationship* demonstrated in which the toxic effects increased in frequency or severity with the level of dose? Another important consideration is whether the results have been *replicated* in other studies. If several unrelated species of vertebrates show a similar pattern of response to a test substance, humans are likely to react in the same way.

The results of *epidemiologic studies* involving workers with exposure to the material under review can provide additional information to enable a proper assessment of the toxicologic data. Findings observed both in well-conducted animal tests and in well-conducted epidemiologic studies usually demonstrate a true toxicity of the material.

In evaluating a particular toxicologic test result, the limitations of animal studies should be kept in mind. Wide variations in the susceptibility of individual species and strains of animals may exist. Detecting certain manifestations in experimental animals such as neurobehavioral effects and memory deficits may not be possible. In addition, the sex, age, and nutritional status of the experimental animals can be important variables affecting the outcome of a study.

A comprehensive evaluation of a specific toxicologic test that considers the points enumerated above usually requires a great deal of experience and training. However, understanding the basic elements involved in toxicologic testing and the large number of considerations that are needed in interpreting test results will help the physician make preliminary judgments. In addition, because toxicologic data are being increasingly used as a basis for risk assessments and the promulgation of exposure standards at OSHA and other government agencies, knowledge of how toxicologic data are generated and interpreted will aid the physician in understanding these important activities.

Advice to the Clinician

The clinician will occasionally have inadequate information to evaluate the possible relationship of an occupational exposure to the symptoms or illness in a particular patient. For example, if a worker presents with elevated liver function studies and the history and initial workup has led the clinician to question whether a particular material at the employee's workplace may be responsible, the clinician often will need to obtain more information about the material before reaching a conclusion.

As discussed previously, a detailed occupational history will help assess the degree and nature of the individual's contact with the material. Knowledge of how the material is absorbed, distributed, metabolized, and excreted can help the physician reach an informed conclusion regarding the significance of an exposure in a given circumstance. If significant exposure seems likely, the clinician will usually want to obtain more information about the composition and toxicity of the material. If it is a trade-name product or a product that contains several constituents, obtaining the MSDS can provide important information. The appendix to this chapter outlines information that the OSHA Hazard Communication Final Rule (29 CFR 1910.1200) requires to be included on MSDS covered by the regulation.

In reviewing the MSDS for the material under consideration, the clinician will want to review the ingredients that are listed for the material. If some of the ingredients are not listed because of their proprietary nature, the clinician may find that more detailed information on the ingredients can be obtained by contacting the manufacturer listed on the MSDS.

Available toxicity data on the material will also be listed on the MSDS. Any acute toxicity data for the material can be reviewed, as well as available subchronic and chronic toxicity data. In addition, any epidemiologic data relevant to the material would be listed. Recommended handling practices and any personal protection recommendations can also be reviewed to see if the employee was using the material in a proper manner.

In this example, the clinician would want to know if any of the toxicologic tests described on the MSDS demonstrated any evidence of liver toxicity. If liver toxicity is described, the clinician would want to consider carefully all of the factors described under Use of Toxicologic Data in interpreting the study results.

Finally, if the MSDS is not available or does not provide sufficient information, the physician might consider reviewing the current literature on the material or its constituents. Reading the relevant sections of standard reference texts such as those listed under Further Information or performing a literature search using MEDLINE, TOXLINE, and/or NIOSH/TIC will frequently identify toxicologic data that can be of value in the clinical investigation. Knowledge of the toxicologic testing methods used in obtaining these data and the factors that need to be considered in interpreting toxicology study results will help the physician in the use and application of the data identified through these searches.

Further Information

Gosselin, R., et al. *Clinical Toxicology of Commercial Products.* Baltimore: Williams & Wilkins, 1984.
A comprehensive reference text that provides a list of trade-name products together with their ingredients, sample formulas of many types of products, toxicologic information including an appraisal of toxicity for individual ingredients, and recommendations for treatment and supportive care.

Klaassen, C., Amdur, M., and Doull, J. (eds.). *Casarett and Doull's Toxicology: The Basic Science of Poisons.* New York: Macmillan, 1986.
A standard textbook and reference that covers the basic principles of toxicology, the types of injury produced in specific organ systems by toxic substances, information on specific classes of toxic materials including environmental pollutants, and discussions of the applications of toxicology.

Lewis, R. (ed.). *Sax's Dangerous Properties of Industrial Materials.* New York: Van Nostrand Reinhold, 1992.
A comprehensive reference to more than 10,000 industrial and laboratory materials. A concise summary of relevant hazard information and a toxicity rating are provided for each substance.

Proctor, N., Hughes, J., and Fischman, M. (eds.). *Chemical Hazards of the Workplace.* Philadelphia: Lippincott, 1988.
A useful reference that presents basic information about the chemical, physical, and toxicologic characteristics of over 400 chemicals. Information is also provided on the diagnosis and treatment of medical conditions related to exposure to these materials.

TOMES.
An electronic database that supplies medical treatment information and hazardous materials handling advice, and offers access to several government databases and information from poison control centers.

Williams, P., and Burson, J. (eds.). *Industrial Toxicology: Safety and Health Applications in the Workplace.* New York: Van Nostrand Reinhold, 1985.
A practical reference that is structured for easy use by the health professional. In addition to presenting basic toxicologic principles and toxicity information on metals, pesticides, and solvents, case histories are used to demonstrate the application of toxicologic principles in the industrial setting.

Appendix to Chapter 23: Material Safety Data Sheets

The OSHA Hazard Communication Final Rule (29 CFR 1910.1200) requires the following information to be included on Material Safety Data Sheets for hazardous chemicals covered by the regulation:

1. The identity used on the label, and
   A. If the hazardous chemical is a single substance, its chemical and common name(s);
   B. If the hazardous chemical is a mixture that has been tested as a whole to determine its hazards, the chemical and common name(s) of the ingredients that contribute to these known hazards, and the common name(s) of the mixture itself; or
   C. If the hazardous chemical is a mixture that has not been tested as a whole:
      1) The chemical and common name(s) of all ingredients that have been determined to be health hazards, and that comprise 1% or greater of the composition, except that chemicals identified as carcinogens are to be listed if the concentrations are 0.1% or greater; and
      2) The chemical and common name(s) of all ingredients that have been determined to present a physical hazard when present in the mixture;
2. Physical and chemical characteristics of the hazardous chemical (such as vapor pressure, flash point);
3. The physical hazards of the hazardous chemical, including the potential for fire, explosion, and reactivity;
4. The health hazards of the hazardous chemical, including signs and symptoms of exposure, and any medical conditions that are generally recognized as being aggravated by exposure to the chemical;
5. The primary route(s) of entry;
6. The OSHA permissible exposure limit, ACGIH Threshold Limit Value, and any other exposure limit used or recommended by the chemical manufacturer, importer, or employer preparing the Material Safety Data Sheet, where available;
7. Whether the hazardous chemical is listed in the National Toxicology Program (NTP) Annual Report on Carcinogens (latest edition) or has been found to be a potential carcinogen in the International Agency for Research on Cancer (IARC) *Monographs* (latest editions), or by OSHA;
8. Any generally applicable precautions for safe handling and use that are known to the chemical manufacturer, importer, or employer preparing the Material Safety Data Sheet, including appropriate hygienic practices, protective measures during repair and maintenance of contaminated equipment, and procedures for cleanup of spills and leaks;
9. Any generally applicable control measures that are known to the chemical manufacturer, importer, or employer preparing the Material Safety Data Sheet, such as appropriate engineering controls, work practices, or personal protective equipment;
10. Emergency and first-aid procedures;
11. The date of preparation of the Material Safety Data Sheet or the last change to it; and,
12. The name, address, and telephone number of the chemical manufacturer, importer, employer, or other responsible party preparing or distributing the Material Safety Data Sheet, who can provide additional information on the hazardous chemical and appropriate emergency procedures, if necessary.

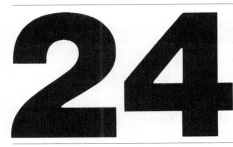

Epidemiology and Biostatistics

Joseph K. McLaughlin and
Ron Brookmeyer

Epidemiology is the study of distribution and determinants of disease in human populations [1]. Its approach is population based, as compared to a clinical or individual perspective. The object of this chapter is to introduce the epidemiologic approach as it applies to etiologic investigations in occupational medicine. The fundamental goal of these investigations is to obtain valid and reasonably precise estimates of exposure-disease associations in occupational groups. Case reports and other forms of anecdotal data may alert an investigator to potential health risks, but the epidemiologic approach provides a systematic method for identifying and quantifying such health risks.

Strengths and Limitations of Epidemiology

Epidemiology has made major contributions toward the understanding of the causes of diseases such as cancer, heart disease, and stroke, among others. A good deal of the success in these areas is because risk of disease is measured directly in human populations [2]. With the epidemiologic method, there is no need to rely on questionable extrapolations across species to estimate the impact of an exposure in humans. It is possible in epidemiology to examine the consequences of an occupational or environmental exposure in the manner in which it actually occurs in humans, not the artificial manner in which laboratory studies of animals are done [3]. The issues of dose, route of exposure, concomitant exposures, and host factors are also directly assessed [4]. It was epidemiology that demonstrated the serious health risks associated with tobacco, radiation, asbestos, and a number of other occupational exposures [5].

Although epidemiology may be the only direct way to evaluate harmful or potentially harmful exposures in humans, the method has several shortcomings [1, 2, 4, 5]. *Low-level risks* are difficult to detect using this method. Very small increases in risk of exposed compared with unexposed groups may be accounted for in epidemiologic studies by *bias* (systematic error), *confounding* (distortion of exposure-disease association by an extraneous variable), or by *chance*. Ten to fifty percent increases in risk are usually difficult to detect without very large, expensive epidemiologic studies. It should be added, however, that it is also difficult to demonstrate effects in experimental studies of laboratory animals at low exposure levels; hence, very high doses are usually given to animals in carcinogenicity studies. The long latency (time from exposure to disease) of most chronic diseases is another obstacle in epidemiologic research. Five- to fifty-year latency periods between initial exposure and disease occurrence make detection of exposure-disease associations quite difficult and render timely epidemiologic evaluation of new agents introduced into the environment or workplace virtually impossible. Furthermore, in occupational settings, there are often many concurrent exposures, and it can be quite difficult to disentangle them. Sometimes epidemiologists must use surrogate measures such as job title or place of employment instead of direct information on exposures, thus allowing the opportunity for misclassification. Another major difficulty with the epidemiologic approach is the inability to control for unknown confounding in the data. Analytic methods are available to control for known confounders, but unknown ones are free to distort risk estimates. Experimental studies have the distinct advantage of *randomization*, a procedure that distributes both known and unknown confounders equally between the test and control groups.

Observational Versus Experimental Studies

Since epidemiologists study disease in human populations, they are usually precluded from using experimental techniques to investigate the causes of disease. From an ethical point of view, researchers could not randomly assign humans to two groups, one to receive 300 rads of ionizing radiation and one to serve as a control group to assess the short- and long-term effects of radiation. As a result, they are left with studying how diseases actually occur in populations. Some situations can be considered to be "natural experiments," such as workers exposed to a particular agent during the course of their work or an ethnic or religious group with unusual dietary habits. In experimental studies, the problems of bias and confounding are controlled by the use of randomization, whereas in observational studies, these issues must be evaluated on a study-by-study basis. The major types of observational studies in epidemiology are the cohort, case-control, and cross-sectional designs.

Types of Observational Studies in Epidemiology

Cohort Study

The most common type of study in occupational epidemiology is the cohort study, in which information on a factor (or factors) is collected in a defined population that is followed over time for the occurrence of a disease (or diseases). The disease rate among those exposed to a particular factor is compared with the rate among the nonexposed in the cohort to assess if there is an association between the study factor and disease. This type of study is also known as a follow-up, longitudinal, or prospective study. The well-known cohort studies of cigarette smokers are examples of this type of study. The *prospective* or classic type of cohort study, however, takes a long time to complete and analyze, since the investigators usually have to wait many years before acquiring enough cases of disease (or deaths if disease outcome is measured by mortality).

To eliminate a possible 10- to 20-year follow-up period, a variant of the prospective cohort study has been developed, the retrospective cohort study. In a *retrospective* cohort study, the past records of individuals are used to characterize the exposure status of the study subjects, and the disease status (usually measured by mortality) is determined until the present (or until a particular date in the recent past). It is this variant that is most commonly found in the occupational literature, since the need to wait for a long follow-up period is eliminated, as it is already part of the design.

Often the most difficult issue to address in an observational study is choosing the comparison group. A comparison group should be from the same study base or source population as the study group. In cohort studies, this ideally means that the nonexposed group should be from the study cohort.

In practice, however, cohort comparisons are often derived from external sources such as from other employed populations that are similar to the study cohort or from the general population. The study base or *internal comparison* is closest to the ideal, since the workers in the cohort went through the same employment selection process and may be similar in a number of lifestyle factors, such as smoking, alcohol consumption, and diet. An *external* occupational comparison group may also meet some of these criteria of selection and comparability in lifestyle factors. Perhaps least satisfactory is the use of the general population (usually in the form of national disease rates) for comparison, since disease rates may vary by geographic area; if the exposed cohort is from an area with unusually high- or low-background rates and the national disease experience is used as a comparison, a misleading result may be reported. For this reason, it is more appropriate to use geographic units closer to the area of the study cohort, such as county, state, or perhaps regional rates (if available), before using national rates. When using general population rates, the potential for the "healthy worker effect" is high because both sick and well and employed and unemployed individuals make up the comparison group. Employed people, as a result of preplacement physical examinations and other selection factors, are generally healthier than the nonemployed population and have lower mortality for most of the major diseases [6]. Sometimes, if one of the comparison groups (e.g., general population) has a deficiency, it may be useful to have more than one comparison group. If the results are consistent using two comparison groups, the findings are thereby strengthened; however, if the results are not consistent the interpretation of the findings can be quite difficult [7].

Advantages and Disadvantages

The main methodologic advantage of the cohort design (both prospective and retrospective) is that information on exposure is recorded before the development of disease. The researcher knows that the exposure or hypothesized risk factor preceded the onset of the disease. This eliminates the *recall bias* (differential recall between ill and healthy individuals) to which case-control studies are potentially vulnerable [8]. A more complete picture of the health effects of a particular exposure that may cause more than one disease can be observed in a cohort study compared with a case-control study, which usually involves only one disease group. If the exposure is rare in the general population and causes only a small proportion of a particular disease, a cohort study is more suitable than a population-based case-control study, since the latter would have too few exposed cases for analysis [9].

For the *prospective cohort* design, the rates of disease can be calculated in both the exposed and unexposed groups for a direct measure of the absolute and relative risk. This cohort design, however, is very costly, and it can sometimes take decades before enough disease events occur to be analyzed meaningfully. It is, therefore, not an efficient way to study rare diseases. Also, because of the long time between the start and completion of such a study, loss to follow-up is a problem. In a mobile society such as the United States, a subject may move a number of times in a 10- to 20-year period. However, with this design predisease information can be collected, along with repeated measures of the study exposure over the course of the investigation. Increased information on the early stages of the natural history of the disease and advances in the precision of exposure measures over time make this design important in etiology research [9].

The *retrospective cohort* study design does not suffer from the disadvantage of a long time period before study results because all events have already taken place (i.e., the exposure and the disease). For a disease with long latency periods, such as cancer, this design is also more advantageous. Because they are relatively cheaper and faster than the prospective method, retrospective cohort studies are sometimes used to generate hypotheses, whereas the prospective cohort design is usually reserved for hypothesis testing. For these reasons the retrospective cohort design is commonly used in occupational studies. There are also disadvantages with the retrospective cohort design, however, such as difficulty in finding reasonably complete records to characterize the cohort, and there is usually little if any ability to control for confounding factors, such as cigarette smoking, alcohol consumption, and other lifestyle factors, which are normally collected at the start of a prospective cohort study. (This problem can be solved with a case-control within a cohort study design; see below.) Exposure information is usually of lower quality and less complete than in a prospective study. The study of rare diseases and loss to follow-up are also problems with the retrospective design. Since most of these studies are of occupational groups with unusually high exposures to a particular agent, an attributable risk estimate cannot be meaningfully interpreted, as the exposure level is unrepresentative of the general population [9].

Case-Control Study

In a case-control study, two groups are compared, one group consisting of people with a particular disease and the other consisting of those from the source population or study base without the disease [10]. From each person in the two groups, information regarding past exposures and habits is obtained (usually by interview). If the exposure of interest is reported by a larger proportion of cases than controls, an association between the exposure and disease can be said to exist.

In some occupational investigations, a case-control within a cohort study (sometimes called a nested case-control study) is initiated. This study is usually begun after the completion of a retrospective cohort study and is identical to the case-control study described above except that the source population is the occupational cohort under study. This methodologic maneuver is usually done when detailed personnel records are available for the cohort and an increased risk is suspected for a particular disease of interest. Employment records of individuals with the disease are analyzed by specific occupation titles along with any available exposure information and compared with the records of a sample of fellow workers without the disease. This comparison may help isolate or pinpoint a particular exposure or occupational process that may be responsible for the increased disease risk in the cohort and also provide the opportunity to assess confounding by lifestyle factors (e.g., smoking) by interview of the workers or their next of kin. A nested case-control study also reduces cost, as it is much less expensive to interview or examine only the records of the individuals with the disease of interest (and their controls) than to interview or examine the records of all the individuals in the cohort, which often can involve thousands of subjects.

The most difficult problem in case-control studies is the selection of an appropriate control or comparison group. The key principle, however, is to select the control subjects from the study base or source population from which the cases arose [10]. Thus, if one ascertains all the cases of a disease from a defined geographic area (a population-based study), the controls should similarly be population based, or if the cases were ascertained from a select number of hospitals, the control subjects should also be chosen from those hospitals. The case-control within a cohort approach can be seen as the paradigm for this principle, since the controls are chosen from within the cohort (the source of the cases). In the case-control approach, as in the cohort approach, a second control group can be used to address any shortcomings of the first, but an inconsistent result across control groups makes interpretation difficult [8].

Advantages and Disadvantages

Although there is often more criticism of case-control studies than cohort study designs, they do have distinct advantages [10]. They are more efficient and suitable for the study of *rare diseases* and diseases with long *latency periods* than the cohort designs. A much larger number of exposure variables can be evaluated with the case-control design, and such studies can be relatively inexpensive and quick compared to prospective cohort studies. Because exposure information is collected after the onset of disease, case-control studies may suffer from *recall bias* in which the patients, as the result of having a disease, may report exposures differently than do the control subjects. This usually is assumed to be in the direction of patients overreporting exposure experiences compared with controls, thus creating a spurious association between an exposure and the disease under study. Although this is a potential bias, there are few documented occurrences [8]. The use of hospital control subjects may help reduce the potential for recall bias, since they, too, have recently experienced a disease. Because of the ability to enroll large numbers of patients in relatively short periods of time, to adjust for confounding factors such as cigarette smoking, and to obtain lifetime job histories, case-control studies have proved useful in identifying occupational determinants of disease [6, 11].

Cross-Sectional Study

In a cross-sectional study design, people are selected regardless of exposure or disease status. Often this study design is called a survey or prevalence study. Usually cross-sectional studies use random or probability sampling procedures to select subjects. This allows for the examination of the prevalence of a disease in a representative sample of the population, and analysis by various combinations of age, sex, and the presence or absence of disease is obtained at the same time, usually by interview.

Advantages and Disadvantages

A cross-sectional study or prevalence survey has no methodologic advantage over the cohort or case-control design. Cross-sectional studies are useful for hypothesis generation and health services planning if done by random sampling. If the information is not gathered using a random sampling procedure, estimates of the prevalence of a disease or of an association between a factor and a disease are of little value, since they are not representative of a study base or source population and are subject to many biases. Since exposure and disease status are usually measured at the same time in a cross-sectional study, there is no way to ascertain the time sequence, that is, did the agent or exposure precede the disease or did individuals with particular medical conditions select certain jobs? This, however, is not inherent in cross-sectional studies, and the sequence of events can be ascertained as part of the investigation. Diseases of short duration (either because of cure or death) are not good candidates for this study design, as they on average are likely to be missed;

conversely, long-duration diseases are usually overrepresented in cross-sectional studies. In occupational settings, this type of study is likely to include information only on currently employed individuals, thereby missing retired employees and persons who may have quit due to ill health that may be related to the exposure under study [11].

Biostatistical Aspects of Epidemiologic Investigations

Sample Size and Power

A fundamental issue in planning a study is the number of subjects needed to assess the potential exposure-disease relationship. Ideally, there should be enough subjects to avoid inferring that the exposure is associated with the disease when in fact it is not (type I error) and to avoid stating that there is no association between the exposure and the disease when in fact there is (type II error). The *power of a study* is the probability of finding an association (risk) of a given magnitude between an exposure and a disease when in fact it exists. The larger the sample size, the greater the power to detect a specified difference in risk; conversely, the smaller the sample size, the lower the power to detect a difference in risk. Also, the smaller the magnitude of the association, the lower the power of a given study. Rare or very common exposures also require very large studies. Some study designs lend themselves to greater power when testing or evaluating a hypothesis. For example, if the disease is *rare*, greater power is generally available in a small- to moderate-sized case-control study than in a large cohort study. On the other hand, if the exposure is rare, it may be advantageous to follow a group exposed to the rare agent using a cohort design. Unfortunately, issues of sample size and power are usually constrained by practical concerns about time, money, and the availability of appropriate study subjects.

Assessing Chance Variation

The role of statistics in occupational epidemiology is to detect patterns (exposure-disease associations) in the data and to determine if these patterns (associations) could be accounted for by *chance*. The goal of the statistical analysis is to obtain a *valid comparison* of disease risk in an occupationally exposed group and in the comparable unexposed group. This comparison should be supplemented with an evaluation of the likelihood that the observed differences in disease rates are artifacts due to chance or represent a real exposure effect.

The scientific credibility of occupational studies requires that chance variation be accounted for. Chance variation refers to the natural variation in health outcomes observed among similarly exposed individuals. Two individuals who appear identical will not necessarily develop the same health problems. Two statistical tools for assessing the role of chance are the *P value* and the *confidence interval*. P value is the probability of obtaining by chance alone a difference in disease rates between the exposed and unexposed as large as or more extreme than what was observed, assuming the *null hypothesis*, that is, that the exposure has no effect on disease incidence rates and that differences in disease rates are due solely to natural variation. The smaller the P value the less consistent the data are with the null hypothesis that the exposure does not have an effect. For example, a P value of 0.005 means that the probability of obtaining by chance alone an exposure effect as large as or more extreme than what was observed is only 5 per 1000. Based on this result, one can conclude either that a rare "chance event" has occurred or, alternatively, reject the null hypothesis and conclude that the exposure has an effect of risk of disease.

Small P values (below 0.05) are sometimes referred to as "*statistically significant.*" This term is frequently overemphasized and by itself is not a very useful concept for interpreting data because it dichotomizes the results of a study into either significant or nonsignificant. Furthermore, the threshold P value below which the researcher calls the result "significant," often referred to as the alpha level (e.g., 0.05), is arbitrary. Rather than stating whether a result is significant, it is preferable to report the actual P value. However, a P value by itself also has serious limitations. It gives no indication of the magnitude of the effect of the exposure and does not distinguish between statistical and clinical or public health significance. Results from studies with very large sample size may be "statistically significant," but the effect of the exposure, although not zero, may be negligible and have no biologic or public health importance. Accordingly, it is important to present a quantitative estimate of the effect of exposure, along with a measure of the uncertainty of the estimate (the standard error). This is often presented in terms of a *confidence interval.*

The confidence interval gives the plausible values for the actual effect of exposure with a desired degree of confidence. For example, the 95% confidence interval for the (relative) risk associated with an occupational exposure is an interval in which the "true" *relative risk* will be included 95% of the time. The "true" relative risk is the risk that would be observed based on an infinite amount of data, that is, if sampling variability could be eliminated. A 95% confidence interval that includes 1.0 implies that a value of 1.0 for the relative risk is plausible and thus the null hypothesis of no exposure effect is consistent with the data at the alpha = 0.05 level of significance (if 1.0 is not included in the interval, the null hypothesis is rejected). Inspection of a confidence interval is a rapid method of evaluating statistical significance; however, *the actual P value cannot be immediately deduced from a confidence interval.* The P value and the confidence interval complement each other, and both are sometimes reported.

Multiple Hypothesis Testing

A problem that deserves special consideration is the issue of multiple hypothesis testing in epidemiology. Epidemiologic studies often involve the collection of large amounts of data on numerous potential risk factors. Interviews and questionnaires often include items of secondary importance for various reasons. For example, a researcher might simply want to be comprehensive and to consider as many factors as possible, or a researcher might want to obscure the real purpose of the questionnaire by asking about an assortment of other exposures or risk factors. In any event, once the data are collected, it is standard epidemiologic practice to analyze all the variables, to compute risk estimates, and to assess statistical significance.

If a large number of risk factors are tested for statistical significance, there is a high probability of declaring at least one risk factor significant, even if there is no real association between the disease and any of the risk factors. Several solutions have been proposed for dealing with the problem.

A classic solution is to require a smaller alpha level (P value) when testing each risk factor. For example, if one wants at most a 0.05 probability of finding any of N risk factors significant when actually none of the risk factors is associated with the disease, one may test each risk factor at the 0.05/N level of significance. The approach is often referred to as the *"Bonferroni approach"* [12, 13]. However, there are some intuitive difficulties with this approach. If N is large, one would require a very small P value before declaring any risk factors significant. Suppose, for example, that it was known that smoking was an important risk factor for a particular disease (based on previous research) and a sufficiently large number of secondary risk factors (e.g., 25) were also being evaluated. In this case a Bonferroni-type approach might lead us to declare the effect of smoking not statistically significant for any P value greater than 0.002 (0.05/25).

In an informal way, researchers use their prior beliefs of an exposure-disease association in the interpretation of new data. How this is done is unclear, but almost certainly no formal methodology is followed. The problem of integrating one's prior knowledge with the results of a new study is not a trivial one. It is fundamental to epidemiology, since no single epidemiologic study is conclusive or stands alone; rather, a series of studies are required before anything definitive can be inferred. Sometimes the amount of evidence required before accepting or rejecting a hypothesis is related to how strongly one believed the hypotheses before the study.

Analytic Techniques

We will focus on several statistical techniques commonly used in occupational epidemiology: the 2×2 table, the standardized mortality ratio, and the proportionate mortality ratio. Our purpose is to introduce some basic statistical indices of occupational risk and to describe the approaches for evaluating their chance variation. We attempt to unify the procedures by emphasizing that the essence of all the techniques is a comparison of the observed number of disease cases to the expected number of disease cases.

The 2 × 2 Table

The simplest statistical technique, the 2 × 2 table, is useful when occupationally exposed and unexposed individuals are followed for equal amounts of time for disease incidence. The data can be summarized in a 2 × 2 table:

	Disease (events)	Healthy	
Exposed	d_1	$n_1 - d_1$	n_1
Unexposed	d_2	$n_2 - d_2$	n_2
	d		N

In this table, d_1 is the number developing disease among the n_1 exposed individuals, and d_2 is the number developing disease among the n_2 unexposed individuals. The total number observed with disease is $d = d_1 + d_2$ from among the $N = n_1 + n_2$ individuals. The proportions developing the disease among the exposed and unexposed are d_1/n_1 and d_2/n_2, respectively. A useful measure of the risk of disease associated with exposure is the ratio of the two proportions, called the *relative risk*. For example, if 58 of 150 exposed individuals show abnormal pulmonary function while 27 of 200 unexposed individuals show abnormal pulmonary function, the relative risk associated with exposure is 2.9. This is interpreted to mean that an exposed individual is at nearly three times the risk of abnormal lung function of an unexposed individual.

To determine if this excess in risk can be explained away by chance variation, the well-known chi-square (χ^2) statistic is computed. The rationale for the statistic is essentially based on a comparison of the observed number of cases of disease in the exposed group (d_1) to the expected number, E. To calculate the expected number, the probability of disease is multiplied by the number exposed; that is, the expected number of cases of disease among the unexposed is $n_1 (d/N)$, where $d = d_1 + d_2$ is the total number of cases and $N = n_1 + n_2$ is the total sample size. *The larger the discrepancy between the observed and the expected, the stronger the evidence is that the observed exposure effect is real and not a chance occurrence.* The χ^2 statistic is the square of the discrepancy $(d_1 - E)^2$, divided by a quantity called the variance of d_1. The variance of d_1 is a measure of the uncertainty in the number of cases of disease that one might normally see among a sample of n_1 individuals. Division by the variance "standardizes" the statistic and accounts for the size of the samples; a discrepancy obtained from a large study represents more evidence in favor of an exposure effect than a discrepancy of the same magnitude from a small study. P values are obtained by referring the value of the statistic to a χ^2 table (with 1 degree of freedom). The degrees of freedom are essentially a measure of the size of our 2 × 2 table. If we had more than two rows or more than two columns, we would have more degrees of freedom. *The larger the value of the χ^2 statistic, the smaller the P value, and the less likely it is that the observed excess of disease is a result of chance.* For example, a χ^2 statistic greater than 2.71 only occurs 10% of the time by chance alone, and a χ^2 statistic greater than 3.84 only happens 5% of the time by chance. These probabilities have been derived mathematically but they could also be demonstrated empirically by performing a computer simulation. In the pulmonary function example, the value of the χ^2 statistic is 29.4, and the associated P value is less than 0.001.

There are several caveats with this statistical procedure. The most important caveat concerns confounding. The exposed and unexposed groups are assumed equivalent in every respect except for the exposure; however, there may be imbalance on an important variable that is related to disease (for example, smoking history or age). If there is an important potential confounding variable, the analysis should be stratified by that variable; that is, a separate analysis should be performed for those with and without the variable. For example, an observed excess of lung cancer deaths in an occupational group may be due solely to an excess in smoking among those workers and unrelated to any occupational exposure. In this case, a separate 2 × 2 table should be formed for smokers and one for nonsmokers. The Mantel-Haenszel statistical procedure [14] is a useful tool for combining the evidence from several 2 × 2 tables, also called strata. The importance of performing stratified analysis to control confounding cannot be overemphasized, as confounding can distort the results of a study. If the analysis has not been appropriately stratified, the unadjusted risk estimate or the single P value from the simple χ^2 analysis can be seriously misleading.

Cohort Methods

The statistical methods discussed above for the 2×2 table assume that all individuals were followed for the same amount of time. In occupational studies, however, the duration of follow-up is often variable, and this must be accounted for in the analysis. For example, if the exposed group was followed for a longer time, more cases of disease should be expected in this group, even if the exposure had no effect on disease. The most commonly used epidemiologic method that accounts for variable follow-up is the calculation of the *disease incidence rate*. It is calculated by dividing the observed number of cases of disease by the total person-years of follow-up:

	Number of Events	Total Observed Person-Years	Disease Incidence Rate
Exposed	d_1	T_1	$I_1 = d_1/T_1$
Unexposed	d_2	T_2	$I_2 = d_2/T_2$
	d	T	

The statistical procedure for assessing whether the difference in observed incidence rates could be due to chance is based on a comparison of the observed number of events in the exposed group and the expected number [13]. Again, the expected number refers to the background incidence of disease that could be expected if the exposure was harmless and thus neither increased nor decreased the risk of disease. The expected number of cases is the total person-years of the exposed group, T_1, multiplied by the incidence rate assuming no effect of exposure, $d/(T_1 + T_2)$. Thus, the expected number, E, is $dT_1/(T_1 + T_2)$. The larger the discrepancy between the observed and the expected number of events $(d_1 - dT_1/T)$, the less consistent the data are with the null hypothesis of no exposure effect. P values are obtained by computing the square of the discrepancy $(d_1 - E)^2$, divided by the variance of d_1, and comparing this value, often called a χ^2 statistic, to the critical value in a χ^2 table. (The formula to compute the variance is omitted but can be found in Breslow and Day [9].) For example, suppose 350 person-years are observed in an occupationally exposed group, producing 30 events, while 776 person-years are observed in an unexposed group, producing 40 events. A convenient summary statistic is the ratio of disease incidence rates ($[30/350]/[40/776] = 1.7$). This is interpreted to mean that the incidence in the exposed group is approximately 70% higher than in the unexposed. To assess whether the observed excess over the expected disease incidence could be due solely to chance, we calculate the χ^2 statistic described above. The numerator of the χ^2 statistic is $(30 - 70[350/1126])^2 = 67.9$. When divided by the variance, the χ^2 statistic becomes 4.52, with a P value slightly over 0.03, suggesting that there is less than a 4% chance that the excess in disease could be explained by chance.

There are a number of caveats and assumptions associated with this methodology. The most important is that it equates 10 individuals each followed for 1 year to 1 individual followed for 10 years; in both situations, 10 person-years of observations are contributed. This approach is justified only if it can be assumed that the disease incidence rate is constant over time, often referred to as the *exponential assumption*. However, in occupational settings, the disease may vary with time from the first exposure. Excess risk from a carcinogen may only be observed after a minimum latency period has elapsed. In these situations, it is important to examine how disease risk evolves over time. A simple approach for examining the effect of latency is to form time intervals; for example, categories of 0 to 5, 5 to 10, 10 to 15, and 15 to 20 years after exposure are often used. Separate incidence rates can be computed within each interval for the exposed and unexposed groups. Special care is needed to assign the events and person-years to each time interval correctly. For example, if disease develops 7 years after exposure, 5 person-years are assigned to the 0 to 5-year interval, and 2 person-years as well as the event are assigned to the 5 to 10-year interval.

As in the analysis of the 2×2 table, it is crucial to account for potential confounding factors. In particular, adjustment for age is essential. The analyses should be stratified by the confounder and summary measures such as the ratio of incidence rates in the exposed and unexposed groups reported.

The Standardized Mortality Ratio

The statistical methods discussed above made use of an internal control group; that is, data are collected on an occupational group in which some are exposed to a potentially hazardous substance and some are not. Unfortunately, such a study base or internal control group is not always available, and in these situations, we must rely on external comparisons. The observed number of cases in an exposed cohort are compared to the expected number using a set of known, standard disease rates. The estimate of the relative risk is called the standardized mortality ratio (SMR) [6, 9, 11] and is the ratio of the observed number of events (0) to the number expected if the exposure had no effect (E):

$$SMR = \frac{O}{E}$$

The expected number of events are computed by applying standard rates to the study cohort. The study cohort is usually stratified by age, sex, year of birth, and race. To obtain the expected number, the observed number of person-years in each age-year-race-sex stratum are totaled and then multiplied by the standard disease rate for that stratum. The expected number from each stratum are then summed to obtain the total expected number of events.

For example, suppose a retrospective cohort study is conducted to examine the cancer risks in an occupational group exposed to high airborne concentrations of a potential carcinogen. The expected number of cancer deaths is computed from the sum of the product of the number of observed person-years in each 5-year age and calendar-year period and the race-sex specific mortality in the community for the same calendar period. If 47 observed deaths from malignant neoplasms occurred, and 39.4 were expected, the SMR would be 1.2. This can be interpreted to mean that the occupationally exposed group is at 1.2 times the risk of cancer death compared with the reference population. To assess if this increase is explainable by chance, a statistic based on the difference between the observed and expected is computed:

$$\frac{(O - E)^2}{E}$$

P values are then obtained by comparison with the χ^2 table. In this example, the χ^2 statistic is 1.46, corresponding to a P value of 0.22. Therefore, the observed excess in cancer deaths can be explained by chance variation.

The Proportionate Mortality Ratio

Occasionally, the only information available for assessing occupational risks consists of the death certificates from individuals employed in an industry. A death certificate review can be a fast, economical method for alerting the epidemiologist to potential health risks. However, as we discuss below, the approach is not nearly as sound as the cohort or case-control methodology. The proportionate mortality ratio (PMR) [6, 9, 11] is useful for comparing the distributions of various causes of death, based on the death certificate review. To calculate the PMR, the relative frequency of death from a particular cause, such as leukemia, in an exposed population is compared to the relative frequency in a reference population. The rationale of this index is that an excess proportion of leukemia deaths among the total number of deaths may indicate an excess risk for leukemia. The PMR, however, is not a cause-specific death *rate* because there is no information on total years of exposure (denominator data). Results are based on the total number of deaths and not on the number of individuals at risk. An apparent excess of one cause of death may simply be a reflection of a deficit in risk from another cause of death, perhaps due to the healthy worker effect, an effect termed "borrowing" [15]. For example, an occupationally healthy group may make the percent of deaths due to leukemia appear excessive. As such, this occupational group may appear to be at higher risk of leukemia based on a proportionate mortality analysis, when in fact risk of death from leukemia may be no different than for an unexposed population. The apparent excess in risk of death from leukemia is an artifact and due to a lower risk of death from heart disease. If total mortality is the same in the exposed and reference populations, SMR and PMR analyses produce comparable results. However, if there is a difference in total mortality, the "borrowing effect" distorts risk estimates derived from a PMR study. In some situations, the artificial effects induced by borrowing can be eliminated by deleting some causes of death, such as heart disease, from PMR analysis. The proportionate cancer mortality ratio, for example, in a PMR analysis restricted only to cancer deaths.

Interpretation of Epidemiologic Data

When interpreting the results of an epidemiologic study, a reader must ask if the reported exposure-disease association is a result of bias, confounding, chance, or a causal association.

Bias

Bias or systematic error is usually a result of flaws in the study design or data collection and is of two basic types: selection and information [16]. *Selection biases* involve systematic differences in the study exposure between those selected and not selected for inclusion in the study. Examples may include enrolling only surviving cancer patients and ignoring the exposure experience of the deceased cases in a case-control study or having a high loss to follow-up among the exposed but not the unexposed in a cohort study.

Information biases involve differences in measuring the exposure of interest between the compared groups. Recall and interviewer biases would be examples of this kind of error. Selection and information biases often cannot be corrected in the analysis, since they are typically a result of the study design or its execution.

Confounding

Confounding refers to the effect of an extraneous variable that may partially or completely account for an apparent association between a study exposure and disease [16]. A confounding variable must be related to both the exposure and the disease. For example, in a case-control study of a blue-collar occupation and bladder cancer or a case-control study of alcohol consumption and heart disease, cigarette smoking would be an obvious confounding variable, since it is related to blue-collar employment and bladder cancer and also to alcohol consumption and heart disease. Confounding can usually be evaluated in the analysis phase of the study by stratification of the study subjects in the suspected confounding variable. In this manner, the effect of the study exposure in those with and without the confounding variable can be estimated. Confounding can also work in the other direction (negative confounding) to mask an association between an exposure and disease.

Chance

The role of chance is evaluated in epidemiologic studies by the use of significance testing and confidence limits. If a risk estimate is statistically significant at a specified level (e.g., 0.05) or if the lower bound of the confidence limit excludes 1.0, we can assume that chance is an unlikely explanation of our results. It does not completely exclude chance as an explanation; rather, it simply means that chance could explain the risk estimate we observe only 1 of 20 times.

Causality

If bias, confounding, and chance are excluded as likely explanations of the results, the issue of causality must be evaluated: Is the exposure factor causally related to the disease? Much has been written about the meaning and philosophic implications of causality, but we will focus mostly on practical ways to assess the likelihood of a causal association. A set of criteria or principles has been developed that is used by epidemiologists when confronted with a possible causal relationship between an exposure and disease. These principles were forged during the heated debate of the late 1950s and early 1960s over the association of cigarette smoking and lung cancer [17, 18].

Key Principles in Interpreting Epidemiologic Studies

1. *Strength of the association.* In general, the higher the risk estimate, the less likely the finding is a result of confounding or bias. An SMR of 450 is considerably more persuasive than an SMR of 125, since the latter (which is only a 25% increase in risk) may be more easily accounted for by bias, uncontrolled confounding, or chance.
2. *Dose-response effect.* If the risk of the disease rises with increasing exposure, a causal interpretation of the association is more plausible. This is sometimes referred to as the biologic gradient principle. The failure to demonstrate a dose-response effect does not necessarily rule out a causal interpretation, since there may exist the possibility of a threshold effect or a saturation effect [16].
3. *Time sequence.* The exposure or risk factor must precede the disease. There appears to be no exception to this principle. In studying chronic diseases with long latency periods, however, the temporal sequence is sometimes difficult to establish. To a great extent this difficulty arises from the particular study design employed; cohort designs, for example, ensure the proper temporal sequence.
4. *Consistency.* Results from other epidemiologic studies of the exposure-disease association should be similar. If similar results are found in different populations using various study designs, the plausibility of a causal interpretation is increased. Any alternative explanation of bias or confounding would have to apply to each of the different studies, a highly implausible explanation.
5. *Biologic coherence.* Does the exposure-disease association make biologic sense given what is known of the natural history of the disease? Do animal experiments support the association? Do other types of collateral evidence support the association, such as secular trends of the exposure factor and the disease? Unfortunately, for many diseases little is known about their etiologies, so the informational background by which to judge biologic coherence is often limited. Thus, failure of this broad principle does not necessarily weaken the plausibility of a causal interpretation.

The first three principles can be applied to an individual study and used to assess the findings. The last two principles refer to results outside a particular study and relate more to external issues of coherence and consistency. All of the criteria or principles should be viewed as guidelines. Except, perhaps, for time sequence, none is required for a causal interpretation.

References

1. MacMahon, B., and Pugh, T. F. *Epidemiology: Principles and Methods.* Boston: Little, Brown, 1970.
2. Hoover, R. N. Detection of environmental cancer hazards: Epidemiologic methods. *J. Med. Soc. N.J.* 75:746, 1978.
3. Ames, B. N., and Gold, L. S. Too many rodent carcinogens: Mitogenesis increases mutagenesis. *Science* 249:970, 1990.
4. Fraumeni, J. F., Jr., and Hoover, R. N. Current views of epidemiologic methods. *Fed. Register* Part II, March 14, 1985. Pp. 58–64.
5. Doll, R., and Peto, R. *The Causes of Cancer.* New York: Oxford University Press, 1981.
6. Monson, R. R. *Occupational Epidemiology* (2nd ed.). Boca Raton, FL: CRC, 1990.
7. Wacholder, S., et al. Selection of controls in case-control studies. II. Types of controls. *Am. J. Epidemiol.* 135:1029, 1992.
8. Wacholder, S., et al. Selection of controls in case-control studies. III. Design option. *Am. J. Epidemiol.* 135:1042, 1992.
9. Breslow, N. E., and Day, N. E. *Statistical Methods in Cancer Research.* Vol. II. *The Design and Analysis of Cohort Studies.* Lyon, France: International Agency for Research on Cancer, 1987.
10. Wacholder, S., et al. Selection of controls in case-control studies. I. Principles. *Am. J. Epidemiol.* 135:1019, 1992.
11. Chekoway, H., Pearce, N., and Crawford-Brown, D. J. *Research Methods in Occupational Epidemiology.* New York: Oxford University Press, 1989.
12. Cupples, L. A., et al. Multiple testing of hypotheses in comparing two groups. *Ann. Intern. Med.* 100:122, 1984.

13. Mantel, N. Assessing laboratory evidence for neoplastic activity. *Biometrics* 36:381, 1980.
14. Mantel, N., and Haenszel, W. Statistical aspects of the analysis of data from retrospective studies of disease. *J. Natl. Cancer Inst.* 22:719, 1959.
15. Walters, S. D. Cause-deleted proportional mortality analysis and the healthy worker effect. *Stat. Med.* 5:61, 1986.
16. Kleinbaum, D. G., Kupper, L. L., and Morgenstern, H. *Epidemiologic Research: Principles and Quantitative Methods.* Belmont, CA: Lifetime Learning, 1982.
17. Hill, A. B. The environment and disease: Association or causation? *Proc. Roy. Soc. Med.* 58:295, 1965.
18. US Department of Health, Education and Welfare. *Smoking and Health: Report of the Advisory Committee to the Surgeon General.* Public Health Service Publication no. 1103. Washington, DC: US Government Printing Office, 1964.

Further Information

Alderson, M. *Occupational Cancer.* London: Butterworth, 1986.

Anderson, S., et al. *Statistical Methods for Comparative Studies: Techniques for Bias Reduction.* New York: Wiley, 1980.

Armitage, P. *Statistical Methods in Medical Research.* New York: Wiley, 1971.

Breslow, N. E., and Day, N. E. *Statistical Methods in Cancer Research.* Vol. 1: *The Analysis of Case-Control Studies.* Lyon, France: International Agency for Research on Cancer, 1980; Vol. II: *Design and Analysis of Cohort Studies.* Lyon, France: International Agency for Research on Cancer, 1987.

Chekoway, H., Pearce, N., and Crawford-Brown, D. J. *Research Methods in Occupational Epidemiology.* New York: Oxford University Press, 1989.

Cochran, W. G. *Planning and Analysis of Observational Studies.* New York: Wiley, 1981.

Fleiss, J. L. *Statistical Methods for Rates and Proportion* (2nd ed.). New York: Wiley, 1981.

Kahn, H. A., and Sempos, C. T. *Statistical Methods in Epidemiology.* New York: Oxford University Press, 1989.

Kleinbaum, D. G., Kupper, L. L., and Morgenstern, H. *Epidemiologic Research: Principles and Quantitative Methods.* Belmont, CA: Lifetime Learning, 1982.

MacMahon, B., and Pugh, T. F. *Epidemiology: Principles and Methods.* Boston: Little, Brown, 1970.

Miettinen, O. S. *Theoretical Epidemiology: Principles of Occurrence Research in Medicine.* New York: Wiley, 1985.

Monson, R. R. *Occupational Epidemiology* (2nd ed.). Boca Raton, FL: CRC, 1990.

Rosener, B. *Fundamentals of Biostatistics.* Boston: Duxbury, 1982.

Rothman, K. J. *Modern Epidemiology.* Boston: Little, Brown, 1986.

Schlesselman, J. J. *Case-Control Studies: Design, Conduct, Analysis.* New York: Oxford University Press, 1982.

Siemiatycki, J. *Risk Factors for Cancer in the Workplace.* Boca Raton, FL: CRC, 1991.

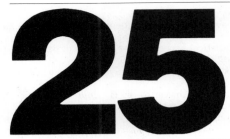

Medical Surveillance

Philip Harber,
Robert J. McCunney,
and Ira H. Monosson

Medical surveillance, the systematic collection, analysis and dissemination of disease data on groups of workers, is designed to detect early signs of work-related illness. A well-run program can aid in the early recognition of a relationship between exposure to a hazard and disease, in the assurance of the safety of new substances, and as an indicator of the effectiveness of existing control measures.

The primary purpose of medical surveillance is *to prevent disease,* rather than to diagnose and treat existing disease. Therefore, methods of interpreting results must be focused on this purpose. Surveillance testing is often, but not always, designed to be of benefit to the *individual* worker tested. However, in some situations, the testing is performed for the benefit of a *group* (occasionally not even including the specific workers tested). Medical surveillance is optimally linked with environmental surveillance, rather than being used in isolation. The utility is determined by the adequacy of interpretation of the results and the actions based upon them to prevent disease. Establishment of a careful plan for interpretation is as important as actual data collection. There are several phases of a successful program; these are listed in Table 25-1 and discussed in detail in this chapter. The chapter concludes with illustrations of surveillance programs.

Needs Assessment

The first stage of medical surveillance is *needs assessment.* Physicians who provide clinical services to business and industry are often confronted with questions such as, "Do certain workers need special tests?" This question is central to many areas of occupational and environmental medicine and can refer to the appropriate evaluation of hazardous waste workers, asbestos removal workers, and those at a lead foundry, among others. In many instances, medical surveillance is unlikely to be of benefit, whereas in others it can be of significant value.

In most cases, considerable judgment is required before a program can be designed and implemented. In Table 25-2, an approach to evaluating the need for medical surveillance is outlined. Every setting calls for the physician to have an understanding of the work process, job duties, and potential exposures to hazardous substances. A visit to the facility with an individual familiar with work duties is necessary.

The Worksite

During the plant visit, questions can be raised regarding previous problems and current concerns. Why is attention now being paid to medical surveillance? Has a

Table 25-1. Phases of medical surveillance programs

Needs assessment
Selecting programmatic goals and target population
Choosing testing modalities
Interpretation of data to benefit the individual
Intervention based on results
Identification of overexposures and disease patterns
Interpretation of data for the benefit of groups of workers
Communication of results
Program evaluation

Table 25-2. Needs assessment

I. Review process and potential for exposure
II. Review toxicity of materials
    A. Basic toxicology
    B. Available texts and databases
    C. Available guidelines
        1. Occupational Safety and Health Administration (OSHA) guidelines
        2. National Institute for Occupational Safety and Health (NIOSH) criteria documents
        3. American Conference of Governmental Industrial Hygienists (ACGIH)
    D. Medical literature
        1. Human studies
            a. Epidemiologic investigation
            b. Clinical case series and reports
        2. Animal studies
III. Does potential toxicity of material or job process require medical surveillance?
IV. Do ergonomic or other job stressors require medical surveillance?
V. Program design and feasibility
    A. Type of testing
    B. Frequency of administration
    C. Guides for further diagnostic evaluation and worksite review

new report appeared? Has a new Occupational Safety and Health Administration (OSHA) standard been introduced? Is there a change in the process? Has a new material been introduced? Is there a legitimate health risk? An understanding of these matters at the worksite can assist the physician in making a decision as to whether a program is needed, and, if so, what it is intended to accomplish.

After reviewing the worksite, the astute physician inquires as to whether an industrial hygiene audit has been conducted. Industrial hygienists, either from OSHA, the workers' compensation carrier, the plant, a consulting firm, or a corporate office will perform periodic evaluations of working conditions that often include air sampling and evaluation of other routes of potential exposure such as ingestion and skin contact. It may be necessary to request a reevaluation, however, if substantial changes have occurred in the work process.

Toxicity of Materials

Next, the toxicity of the materials used is reviewed. Guidelines are available from the American Conference of Governmental Industrial Hygienists (ACGIH) and from criteria documents prepared by the National Institute for Occupational Safety and Health (NIOSH). For some substances, an OSHA standard dictates the type of medical surveillance program required for certain work situations.

Review generally requires consultative help from a physician certified in occupational medicine. Results of human studies, especially large-scaled epidemiologic investigations, and clinical case series can also be of assistance in formulating an opinion as to the need for medical surveillance. A decision regarding the need for and type of medical surveillance program can now be made. Since few situations will conform to recommended guidelines, consideration should also be given to the potential for emergencies, results of animal studies, and public relations issues.

Selecting Programmatic Goals and Target Population

The next stage is deciding about *programmatic goals*. Table 25-3 lists general reasons for instituting medical surveillance programs. The target population must be carefully defined to be consistent with the goals chosen. For example, if the goal is to detect current exposures, then current workers represent the optimal target group. However, if the goal is to detect cancers, which generally have a long latency period (time from exposure to onset of disease), then focusing only on those currently

Table 25-3. Purposes of medical surveillance programs

For benefit of individual workers
1. Screening for disease
2. Risk factor for identification
3. Assessment of environmental exposures of the individual worker
4. Identifying overexposures
5. Fitness for duty
6. Preplacement testing
7. Worker selection
8. Job accommodation
9. Detection of nonoccupational disease
10. Health promotion
11. Baseline for future reference
12. Substance abuse detection

For benefit of groups of workers
1. Detection of new hazards
2. Identification of sites of exposure to known hazards
3. Assuring safety of current practices
4. Assessing absence patterns
5. Projecting health care resource needs
6. Planning of preventive programs

employed is usually inappropriate; that is, those who have retired are often at higher risk because of their longer latency. OSHA regulations typically do not address screening former rather than current employees.

Screening for Occupational Disease

When the purpose of medical surveillance is to identify work-related disease at an early stage, it is considered to be a type of screening. Screening is the search for a previously unrecognized disease or abnormal physiologic or pathologic condition at a stage at which intervention can slow, halt, or reverse the progression of the disorder. An effective screening program should identify disease at a stage at which intervention really matters.

Screening has been very effective in improving treatment and survivability of certain nonoccupational ailments such as hypertension and cervical and breast cancers. In fact, certain occupational disorders such as noise-induced hearing loss, bladder cancer, and some of the pneumoconioses lend themselves well to the principles of screening. On the other hand, screening efforts for certain malignancies such as lung cancer have consistently proved to be futile and at best only advance the point of diagnosis without improving outcome. In the latter setting, this advancement of the point of diagnosis is known from an epidemiologic perspective as "lead time artifact."

Screening is considered a *secondary* preventive measure in the control of occupational illness, since the primary control measure is to reduce the hazardous exposure. Screening is based on a number of principles, including the following:

1. The screening test must be selective and geared to the population at risk.
2. The disease should be identified in its latent stage, not when symptoms appear.
3. Adequate follow-up study is necessary.
4. The screening test is both valid and reliable.
5. Benefits outweigh the costs and, where feasible, tests are noninvasive.
6. Treatment should be both available and effective at a stage when the disease is detectable.

Screening for Nonoccupational Disease

Often, *screening* is conducted in the worksite *for nonoccupational disorders* (general medical screening). Occupational physicians have long played a role in evaluating the presence of unrecognized illness in an asymptomatic person. Periodic medical evaluations gained favor over 50 years ago as an effort toward reducing illness by early recognition of disease. As sophisticated diagnostic equipment became available, it was incorporated into the periodic medical evaluation. Now many preventive medicine and screening programs have become part of health promotion activities.

Unfortunately, consensus is lacking on the type and content of a periodic medical evaluation that physicians should offer the asymptomatic person. Guidelines, however, have been proposed [1]. The effectiveness of various ancillary procedures has also been critically reviewed. Not surprisingly, few of the ancillary procedures commonly used in medical practice today meet the full criteria of screening (see Chap. 40, Health Care Management, for a discussion of periodic medical examinations).

Screening programs are also plagued with difficulties involved in evaluating people with abnormal tests. False-positive results are inherent in most laboratory reference limits, simply because of the manner by which those limits are established. In general, 1 of every 20 "well people" has an abnormal test result—without evidence of illness.

Surveillance to Detect Exposure Rather than Disease

Medical surveillance is not limited to screening (in which the participant will *on the average* benefit). *In some settings, however, medical surveillance is designed to detect exposure* rather than disease. For example, biologic monitoring (discussed later) measures concentrations of chemical agents or their metabolites in biologic specimens. This type of testing may be useful for determining if exposure is occurring even at levels that do not imply the presence of disease. These techniques are discussed below.

Baseline for Future Reference

Another purpose of medical surveillance is to serve as a baseline for future evaluation. A previous electrocardiogram is often useful when interpreting a current one. Similar considerations apply to many other tests. Change over time is often more important than the actual value itself. For example, a worker whose forced expiratory volume in 1 second (FEV_1) declines from 119% of predicted to 81% of predicted over 1 year warrants review even though both results are "within normal limits."

Raw data, rather than interpretive conclusions (normal/not normal), should be kept on file for future reference. Documentation of the technique employed is essential to assure that future testing is performed by comparable methods.

Special considerations apply in tests subject to a "learning effect." Spirometry results, in particular, are subject to this problem because people perform better on the second test since they have "learned" how to improve their performance.

Risk Factor Identification

Medical surveillance programs are also used to detect precursors of disease or factors associated with disease. Unlike true screening, persons with "positive" results do not have specific, well-defined diseases, but a greater than average risk of developing disease without appropriate intervention. Here the interpretation is often more difficult than for screening, and the importance of carefully counseling the employee about the significance of the findings is paramount.

Choosing Testing Modalities

After establishing the need for medical surveillance and selecting general goals, the best "tools" must be selected. This section briefly reviews the major techniques. Physicians should avoid the temptation to recommend "tests" in a reflex-like fashion. Exposure to potentially hazardous substances does not necessarily indicate the need for special tests. Decisions should be based not only on the relative toxicity of the substance but also on the extent of control measures, sampling results, work practices, and usefulness of the tests themselves. Lay personnel who have responsibilities toward health and safety in the worksite may have unrealistic expectations about the value of medical monitoring and thus should be apprised of its limitations, in particular that medical surveillance is not a substitute for primary control measures.

In fact, "unnecessary" tests may lead to difficulties in assessing "false-positive" results and may also cause alarm among the well population and needlessly increase health care costs.

Questionnaires

Questionnaires are simple, inexpensive tools that for many disorders serve as a reasonably sensitive way to obtain an overview of a potential problem, which can provide the basis for further investigation. Most often, questionnaires are used in conjunction with other techniques. To be most effective, they should be directed to symptoms that may be associated with exposure to the substance under study.

Physical Examination

A physical examination is the time-honored method for detecting signs of illness. Although its effectiveness in screening settings is limited, some signs of illness might be uncovered. In asbestosis, for example, end inspiratory dry rales in the midaxillary line are a classic finding. A physical examination also offers people the personally perceived benefit of "being examined." Although this value can be overlooked, people generally appreciate the opportunity of discussing their health concerns with a qualified provider in an appropriate setting. In fact, effective physician counseling in these settings can help to motivate people to control health risks. A physical examination is relatively inexpensive and can also be performed by paramedical personnel. Its effectiveness increases if directed primarily toward the target organ. In many diseases, however, physical signs are a late finding.

Chest Radiography

Chest films gained favor as a screening device in the early detection of tuberculosis. They continue to find application in screening for nonmalignant lung disorders such as silicosis, asbestosis, and berylliosis. Annual chest films, especially in young workers, may be unnecessary in routine monitoring programs. For most occupational hazards, adequate information can be obtained if chest films are administered less frequently and programs include an annual review of symptoms and pulmonary function [2]. The method is discussed in more detail later in this chapter.

Pulmonary Function Testing

Pulmonary function testing is an integral component of most screening programs designed to detect nonmalignant occupational lung disorders. This procedure should be conducted in accordance with standard guidelines [3, 4]. Pulmonary function testing can be a sensitive screening device for some occupational lung disorders, but results can be affected by cigarette smoking and nonoccupational medical conditions, especially asthma and chronic obstructive lung disease. The test is most effective when results of the same individual are compared over time rather than with reference limits. An accurate, well-calibrated spirometer is essential. This is discussed further in Example 3 at the end of this chapter.

Assessment of Exposure: Biologic Monitoring

In biologic monitoring, tests are used to measure the extent of environmental exposures [5–8]. A biologic specimen (e.g., blood, urine, exhaled air) is analyzed for the quantity of an environmental chemical or one of its metabolites to provide an estimate of the worker's chemical exposure. Mere detection of a chemical, however, does not imply the presence of a disease or of toxicity. Other forms of biologic monitoring include measuring direct effects on red cell enzymes, protein-losing nephropathies (i.e., β_2=microglobulin in cadmium toxicity), or cholinesterase levels.

Biologic monitoring can be helpful when evaluating a hazardous exposure that a person may have experienced. For example, if people who live in a basement apartment are concerned about the presence of solvents thought to contain xylene, measurement of urinary levels of methyl-hippuric acid (a metabolic product of xylene) can indicate that exposure to xylene has occurred. Unfortunately, it is uncommon for a specific blood or urinary level of a hazardous material to be associated with particular adverse health effects. Certain substances such as inorganic lead, however, are notable exceptions.

Biologic monitoring data are used to assess exposure to a hazard rather than to make a "clinical" diagnosis. Therefore, interpretation mandates careful attention to timing of the specimen acquisition. Was it obtained in a worst-case situation, reflecting the highest possible exposure of the individual? Alternatively, was the specimen obtained during average work, which may not reflect peak exposures? Finally, was the specimen obtained when the person was not working or exposed, thus not reflecting actual exposure for materials that are cleared rapidly?

The biologic half-life of the agent determines whether it will be detectable following exposure. Measurement of substances with long half-lives (such as the blood lead level) reflects longer-term exposure, but rapidly disappearing agents (e.g., carbon monoxide) reflect the period immediately preceding acquisition of the sample. Timing of sample acquisition is most critical for substances that have a short half-life. Thus, obtaining a blood lead specimen after a 24-hour absence from work might be appropriate, whereas obtaining a carbon monoxide analysis of exhaled air after such a time lapse would be invalid.

Biologic monitoring, an attempt at evaluating the internal concentration of a toxic agent, accounts for factors that affect total exposure, including breathing capacity, work effort, and underlying medical conditions. Such factors may not be adequately reflected in routine air measurements conducted in an industrial hygiene audit.

Biologic monitoring offers other *advantages:*

1. It is an attempt to measure the parameter most directly related to potential health effects. Results can aid in formulating a more refined estimate of risk of illness secondary to exposure.
2. Nonoccupational exposures and individual variability are assessed.
3. Multiple exposures and other routes of exposure, such as dermal and ingestion, can be evaluated.

Biologic monitoring, however, has *limitations:*

1. Effectiveness is dependent on adequate toxicologic data. (For most substances used in commerce today, adequate toxicologic data do not exist.)
2. Test results can be affected by other factors such as alcohol and pregnancy. (At the same blood lead levels, women have higher levels of zinc protoporphyrin than men [9].) Dietary deficiencies can lead to enhanced toxicity of a variety of hazardous substances (see Table 25-2). Cigarette smoking can also interfere with monitoring results. Workers who smoke cigarettes, for example, may have levels of cadmium higher than their nonsmoking counterparts [10].
3. For some substances, relatively short biologic half-lives affect the monitoring. In monitoring for dimethylformamide, a solvent used in the production of adhesives, 24-hour urinary samples within the time of last exposure can indicate the level of exposure a worker has experienced. Beyond 48 hours from the time of last exposure, the major metabolite, N-methylformamide (NMF) is not detectable [11].
4. Monitoring is ineffective for surface-acting agents such as sulfur dioxide and ammonia.

Cancer Risk Screening

In the occupational setting, a number of techniques have been attempted to screen for cancer. Assuming that the development of environmentally related cancer proceeds in an orderly sequence [12], screening efforts theoretically may be focused at several points.

One technique is *assessment of exposure* to carcinogens. Persons with greater exposure have greater risk. Monitoring techniques include the assessment of mutagens in body fluids. Detection of urinary mutagens is the only assay that has shown some reliability in following groups of workers. The measurement of adducts created by binding of carcinogens or their metabolites to body chemicals (such as DNA or hemoglobin) can provide a measure of exposure. (See Chap. 29, Molecular Biology, for a more detailed discussion.)

Oncogene activation determination, although not currently useful, holds considerable promise. Activation of certain genes such as ras is believed to occur early in the malignant transformation process. Activation of such "oncogenes" may be determined by the detection of the protein products which are coded by the genes. For example, certain carcinogens (e.g., polycyclic aromatic hydrocarbons) activate the ras genes; these genes produce a protein known as p21. Testing for p21 in serum may be useful for early lung cancer detection [13].

Cytogenetic monitoring is the study of numerical and structural chromosomal aberrations, which may occur naturally or secondary to exposure to environmental agents. As an attempt to assess damage to the gross structure of chromosomes, cytogenetic monitoring has been used to determine increases in chromosomal abnormalities among groups exposed to carcinogens. To date, however, these results have proved to be of little value in the evaluation of individual risk of developing malignancy secondary to a toxic exposure (see Chap. 13, Occupational Cancers).

Cell surface antigens may change in the development of malignancy. Hence, immunologic studies of exfoliated cells such as those in sputum may permit earlier detection of lung cancers than traditional cytologic methods.

Cytologic morphology of malignant cells theoretically might be of benefit for tumors in locations that allow facile collection of shed cells (e.g., sputum, urine, or cervical cytology). Unfortunately, although routine cytopathology can detect cancers before development of symptoms, treatment options for some cancer sites may not always lead to improved survival.

Clinical testing methods have also been utilized. These aim at detecting malignancies at a stage that is more advanced than the stage addressed by the aforementioned methods. Radiographic screening for lung cancers in high-risk groups is controversial [14]. Other clinical techniques have included colonoscopy or cystoscopy for gastrointestinal and uroepithelial malignancies.

Data Type Should Guide Interpretation

The meaning of surveillance data depends on its source and type. Some surveillance data must automatically generate an investigation to find preventable factors (e.g., report of a fatality or of a highly work-specific disease). Other surveillance-based diagnoses are important only when they occur in excess or in time-space clusters (e.g., common cancers). Elevated rates of common diseases (e.g., hepatitis) or common symptoms (e.g., cough, back pain) warrant follow-up study.

It is important to interpret data in the context of the following:

1. Specific occupational diagnoses (e.g., confirmed TDI asthma)
2. Diagnoses often associated with work (e.g., nonviral hepatitis)
3. Nonspecific clinical diagnoses (e.g., bronchitis)
4. Indicators of symptoms rather than disease (e.g., hand-wrist pain, cough)
5. Exposure indicators (e.g., blood lead level)
6. Possible physiologic effect (e.g., spirometry)
7. Nonspecific genotoxic or genetic findings (e.g., cytogenetics)
8. Markers of personal sensitivity (e.g., atopic history in animal handlers)
9. Indications of possible *early disease* (e.g., β_2-microglobulin or *N*-acetylglucosaminidase in the urine of cadmium workers)

Interpretation of Data to Benefit the Individual

To benefit the individual worker, several questions should be asked. For screening, one asks, "Is a disease present?" For risk factor identification, the relevant question is, "Is a significant precursor of a disease present, and is there an appropriate intervention to prevent the disease from developing?" For work practices and environmental exposure assessment, the question should be, "Is this particular worker more highly exposed to an environmental agent (chemical or physical) than coworkers?"

A clear plan should be established for interpreting the *results* and presenting the findings to management and workers that avoids creation of either false anxiety or assurance. In general, ideal screening programs have high sensitivity (test is positive in a high percentage of persons with disease). The price paid for this high sensitivity is often low specificity (i.e., some workers with positive screening tests truly are free of disease). The predictive value of a test is of considerable interest because this represents the percentage of persons with a positive test who actually have the disease. For example, bilateral pleural thickening has an approximately 80% predictive value of being associated with previous exposure to asbestos. In reviewing these findings on a routine chest film, the physician can counsel the patient accordingly, especially if other causes such as pleurisy, obesity, and rib fractures have been considered [15].

The opposite problem must also be avoided—false assurance. The worker (and health care provider as well) must understand that a "negative" test result may not prove the absence of disease. The predictive value of a negative test (e.g., "If the test result is normal, what is the probability that the individual is truly free of disease?") is the relevant question in interpreting normal results. This figure depends on the sensitivity of the test and the prevalence of the disease.

Nonspecific Testing (such as Liver Function Testing)

A perplexing situation often arises when minor abnormalities may be "normal variants" or may be due to nonoccupational factors. Because many industrial materials, particularly at high dose, can cause liver function abnormalities, liver function testing frequently is included in surveillance testing [16, 17]. Unfortunately, many otherwise normal persons have slightly elevated concentrations of liver enzymes without disease. Furthermore, many nonoccupational factors such as obesity, alcohol use, and infections can cause minor liver enzyme elevations. Thus, interpreting liver function data from a surveillance program requires careful thought and planning. If relatively minor abnormalities are detected, one must consider an occupational cause rather than ascribing the abnormalities to "drinking." A careful examination with attention to occupational as well as nonoccupational factors is necessary. The physician should carefully and discreetly ask about hazardous exposures, even materials that the worker may be reticent to discuss (e.g., "Is work performed using unauthorized materials or in unauthorized manners?"). If there is any question about occupational hazards being contributing factors, a worksite visit, discussion with production supervisors, and industrial hygiene consultation may be needed. Minor functional abnormalities may allow intervention to prevent significant occupational disease, and an active approach is therefore needed in the occupational setting.

Intervention Based on Results

The intensity of intervention for risk factors must be chosen based on the gravity of the disease and the ability of the intervention to be effective. If an abnormality is found, a decision must be made about whether it was caused or aggravated by work conditions. Although the epidemiologic (group perspective) approach can help assess whether work conditions are contributing to disease in the population of workers, evaluating the individual case may be more problematic. For example, is a liver function abnormality a consequence of solvent exposure, nonoccupational disease (e.g., chronic active hepatitis), or lifestyle (e.g., alcohol use)? Implications for workers' compensation and employer liability should be addressed. In addition, reporting of certain diagnoses may be mandatory. The role of the director of the surveillance program in such determination of causality needs to be clearly defined in advance. Often, this physician may be more knowledgeable than the patient's personal physician or the specialist in understanding occupational toxicology and should therefore provide appropriate assistance in such decisions. The physician's ethical responsibility to the worker in this situation must be the foremost consideration, and a physician (no matter in whose employ) must never withhold any information for fear of adverse effects on the employer.

Several approaches to assuring follow-up may be employed. Workers found to have abnormalities may be referred to their personal physicians. A clear policy consistent with local, state, and federal laws should be stated regarding which costs will be borne by the employer and which are the responsibility of the individual worker or the worker's health insurer. In addition, the surveillance program director should establish a plan for referral of people who do not have a personal physician. Optimally, the physician to whom the patient is referred should prepare a report to the referring physician (surveillance program director) regarding the test results, nature of the diagnosis, treatment, and related information.

Identification of Overexposures and Disease Patterns

Physicians should encourage discussion during medical surveillance examinations because an employee may feel more comfortable reporting concerns about work to a health professional than to a line supervisor. Furthermore, because of the physician's role as "health advocate," workers often feel more comfortable in addressing concerns in a clinical setting [18, 19].

Medical surveillance may also detect patterns of illness. Sentinel health events–occupational (SHE-O) are medical diagnoses that are frequently associated with occupational causation [20]. When they occur, they should be investigated. Workers' compensation claims, although not necessarily accurate, may provide clues to show that a pattern of illness is developing; this has been successfully applied to skin disease surveillance [21]. Sentinel physicians, community-based clinicians who report disease of possible occupational origin, have been used for community-wide surveillance in the SENSOR program [22, 23], but this method is less applicable for the company-based than for public health agency–based programs.

Interpretation of Data for the Benefit of Groups of Workers

Analysis of aggregate data may reveal information that is useful for preventing occupational disease. Close interaction between the epidemiologist and the clinician can facilitate optimal use of such information. Formal statistical analysis of data, however, requires time, staff, and skills often not available in the clinical setting. Improvements in microcomputer equipment, however, are making data interpretation more efficient. Occupational health systems can provide information related to white blood cell counts at certain areas of a plant, for example.

There are several ways by which analysis of medical surveillance data can provide beneficial information to groups of workers, rather than just the person tested.

1. *Index case investigation.* In some instances, detection of a single case can alert the clinician to a preventable risk for a group of workers. For example, one case of TDI asthma (if confirmed) may indicate that exposures need control.
2. *Case clusters.* The occurrence of several cases in close spatial-temporal relationship warrants investigation, even if the illness is not specific for occupational causation. Case clusters can occur by chance, and proper investigation, not panic, should be employed.
3. *Temporal or geographic trends.* Even if individual results are "normal," aggregate data analysis may show a significant pattern. For example, an increase in average blood lead level over 1 to 2 years in a battery manufacturing plant may mean that work practices or process controls need reassessment. Similarly, if urinary mercury levels in one area of a thermometer plant are higher than in other areas, investigation is needed.
4. *Association with exposure status.* The clinical and laboratory results should be linked to exposure data. Where process descriptions or industrial hygiene sampling data are available, these should be linked with the medical data. This process requires joint planning of data collection and interpretation.

Health surveillance data can be used to detect new hazards through the review of rates of disease and abnormalities in groups of workers. If the rate of abnormality in an exposed group is higher than that of an unexposed group, an industrial hazard should be suspected. The reference (unexposed) group must be comparable to the exposed group, except for the exposure under consideration. For example, lung cancer rates or frequency of spirometric abnormality should not be compared between a plant employing many heavy smokers to one that has essentially a nonsmoking population.

Relatively small changes in a variable may be more important in an aggregate analysis than when evaluating one person [24]. For example, a 100-ml difference from predicted FEV_1 would hardly prompt a diagnosis of lung disease in an individual. On the other hand, if a population of exposed workers averages 100 ml less compared to an unexposed population, an occupational hazard could be present.

Aggregate analysis can identify new sites of known hazards. For example, although hazards of asbestos are well known, detection of pleural plaques on surveillance chest radiographs can lead to identifying processes not otherwise known **to** involve asbestos exposure or to contamination of raw materials (e.g., vermiculite ore) with asbestiform fibers. Similarly, although ergonomic factors associated with low back pain are well known, a geographic or temporal clustering of back injuries should prompt the clinician to suspect a particular area of the plant as having poor equipment design or work practices. Aggregate analysis of surveillance data can document the safety of materials and processes; in the absence of such data analysis, doubts may persist.

The ability to perform aggregate analysis depends on integration of various types of data. Personnel characteristics (e.g., job history) and industrial hygiene data (e.g., levels of exposures) in addition to the clinical information can be entered into computer programs for data analysis. However, confidentiality needs to be guarded in accordance with ethical and legal standards. When providing contractual service for a small employer without a corporate health department, the physician should urge aggregate as well as individual analysis of medical monitoring results.

Medical surveillance analysis ideally includes observation of absence patterns that may represent an occupational hazard. Some ergonomic hazards have been detected in this manner [25], and chemical exposure hazards may be pinpointed as well.

Communication of Results

Information about surveillance data may be directed to several different targets: the worker, the management, worker representatives (e.g., unions), and government.

The worker must be given surveillance testing results in a timely manner and in an understandable fashion [26]. Workers should be given a summary of their information, and access to the complete data must be assured. If values out of the "reference range" are noted, their significance should be explained in a clear and understandable manner. Interpretation (not just test values themselves) should be provided by a clinician (e.g., plant physician) whom they trust and who is accessible for additional discussion if needed. As a practical matter, it is often difficult to succinctly interpret data in an easily understandable manner. A blood lead level (BLL) of 35 is technically below the level at which OSHA mandates particular action, but it is indicative of exposure that should be limited. The communication to the worker should therefore avoid implying the diagnosis of "toxicity," but should also avoid giving the impression that everything is fine if it is below the OSHA standard of 40. Similarly, small-airway abnormality (isolated abnormality of the $FEF_{25-75\%}$) is unlikely to produce symptoms, but should not be ignored because it may be a harbinger of early abnormality (e.g., "Your breathing test showed normal FEV_1 and forced vital capacity [FVC], but one test, the $FEF_{25-75\%}$ was not in the normal range. This is not a major problem now, but it may be an indicator of an early problem. You should see Dr. X if you would like to discuss this.") It is important to avoid overemphasizing the importance of a borderline deviation in a test for which significance is uncertain [27].

Implications of certain test results must be reported to management. For example, detection of a medical condition that makes work unsafe for the individual, the public, or co-workers cannot be ignored. However, management is not generally entitled to the specific medical information, only the clinician's opinion about its implications. Therefore, physicians who perform testing must be prepared for this awkward situation.

Worker representatives (e.g., unions) also have limited access to medical data. Particularly if confidential data are involved, extreme caution is needed. Ethical considerations as well as the OSHA regulations should be considered.

When aggregate data analysis, in addition to interpretation of individual test results, is done, interpretations must clearly indicate the difference between group analysis and abnormalities in individuals. A smaller deviation from normality may be of greater concern in a group than in an individual. The results should not be construed to indicate the presence of "disease" in the traditional sense. Often, it is useful to indicate both the magnitude of the effect found and the estimated likelihood (considering all factors) that it is due to occupational exposure.

In reporting the interpretations, the clinician must be sensitive to the concerns of workers. Many may fear loss of jobs if any abnormality is found, whereas in other situations the workplace psychosocial environment might encourage inappropriate compensation claims that are not specifically occupational in origin.

Under certain circumstances, results must be reported to governmental agencies.

For example, if a specific occupational disease is diagnosed based on surveillance, it is mandatory to record it on the OSHA 200 log (see Chap. 2). Similarly, patterns of abnormalities, even if not absolutely proven, often must be reported to the Environmental Protection Agency and other agencies.

Many workers have personal physicians, some of whom may have very limited knowledge of the testing performed. Therefore, interpretation often must be done for the patient's physician as well as for the worker him/herself.

Program Evaluation

A final essential aspect of any medical surveillance program is assessment of the overall program efficacy. Thus, in addition to considering individual test results and aggregate analysis, the effectiveness of the program should be assessed. First, quality control must be considered. Are the results accurate and precise? For chemical tests, samples may be split and submitted to different laboratories. Known reference standards may be submitted in a blind fashion to the laboratory. For physiologic tests, such as spirometry, quality control can be assessed by reviewing hard copies of tracings or directly assessing the laboratory's quality assurance procedures. Often, the medical surveillance program clinician should personally conduct (or arrange for a consultant to conduct) a quality assurance audit of facilities used. In addition, the appropriateness of the target populations should be assessed. Of workers at risk, what percentage actually underwent medical surveillance? Conversely, how much testing, and so forth, was "wasted" on workers without specific risk factors warranting the testing? The effectiveness of the surveillance program can be gauged by determining if it was successful in leading to interventions that could decrease disease or injury rates. Often, surveillance programs include significant screening components, in which subsequently more detailed evaluations determine if disease is truly present. The sensitivity and specificity of the surveillance/screening testing can therefore be evaluated. This process requires that the "true" situation be ascertained. Finally, the cost of the program must be considered in interpreting its value.

Examples of Medical Surveillance

Example 1: A Well-Known Hazard with an Established OSHA Standard

The medical director of a multispecialty clinic is asked to evaluate the type of medical monitoring necessary to protect workers involved in removing asbestos from a local grade school.

Because of the hazards of asbestos, a regulatory process took place whereby a standard, enforceable by OSHA, was developed. OSHA standards have the force of law and apply to all occupational situations in which workers may be exposed to the respective material. Although asbestosis, the chronic irreversible pulmonary fibrosis secondary to exposure to asbestos, has been declining since the institution of better control measures, concern still exists about its potential to cause malignancies.

The OSHA Asbestos Standard has a special section directed toward medical surveillance. Workers exposed to asbestos more than 30 days a year at certain concentrations should be evaluated within 30 days of employment, at yearly intervals thereafter, and when terminating employment. Evaluations include an occupational history, a physical examination with attention to the pulmonary system, a chest film (posteroanterior), and pulmonary function studies. Dispute exists regarding the value of annual chest films in screening for asbestos and may be extended to 5-year intervals in some cases, such as the OSHA Asbestos Standard.

In helping to protect the asbestos removal workers, the physician overseeing the program should refer to requirements of the OSHA Asbestos Standard. The examining physician is also responsible for ensuring that workers are medically capable of safely using necessary respirator equipment. NIOSH and the American National Standard Institute have published guidelines for the use of respirators that include a discussion of training requirements. During the examination, the physician should counsel workers who smoke cigarettes about the importance of quitting because of the strong synergistic relationship between cigarette smoking and asbestos-induced malignancies.

Example 2: A Relatively New Commercial Substance with Limited Toxicologic Data

The family physician who has been conducting preplacement evaluations on workers at a research and development laboratory is asked to comment on special medical precautions necessary for workers involved in the production of gallium arsenide crystals.

Gallium arsenide has been heralded as an ultimate replacement for silicon chips in the semiconductor industry because of improved conductive qualities. Unfortunately, few toxicologic data are available on gallium arsenide, and, thus, the choice of the appropriate monitoring tool is problematic. In fact, OSHA has no standard, NIOSH no criteria document, and the ACGIH no recommended Threshold Limit Value (TLV). In this case, the physician inquires whether any corporate guidelines exist and whether consultive help is available.

After a review of the work process and appropriate air sampling, it was decided to consider gallium arsenide in the most serious light, that is, as an inorganic arsenic compound, for which an OSHA standard exists. In selecting urine as the monitoring specimen, attention was given to dietary influences that can elevate urinary excretion of arsenic.

Although medical monitoring is most often recommended in work situations in which exposures are above the "action level," monitoring was recommended even though the production process was "closed" and levels of arsenic and arsine, a gas that can be liberated in production, were undetectable. Since the process was a new development, monitoring was instituted as an added measure of safety.

Examples of Surveillance Targets

The scope of this book limits the extent of the discussion that can be given on the major hazardous substances used in commerce today. It can be instructive, however, to review four major types of hazardous situations encountered by workers: dust exposure, metal exposure, solvent work, and repetitive motion.

Example 3: Exposure to Dusts

Dusts may be considered either a nuisance or a toxic substance to the human body. Nuisance dusts are those substances that do not exert toxic effects, whereas toxic dusts, such as asbestos and silica, can be harmful. To demonstrate the principles of interpreting results of a program to assess adverse health effects secondary to dusts, nonmalignant respiratory disease will be used as an example.

Respiratory disease surveillance usually contains a combination of three components: the occupational and medical history, spirometry, and chest radiography. Physical examination of the chest, although usually included, does not play the same primary role that it does in clinical care.

Medical History

Certain symptoms, such as shortness of breath, cough, sputum production, and wheezing, may indicate lung disease; however, the manner in which the patient is asked about symptoms may affect the response. To record data in a uniform fashion, a specific means of coding responses is necessary; several standardized questionnaires have been developed that may be self-administered or administered by a trained interviewer. The protocol for administration should be followed according to routine guidelines. The American Thoracic Society/National Heart, Lung and Blood Institute questionnaire is commonly used in the United States to inquire about respiratory symptoms.

Bronchitis refers to a symptom of cough and sputum production. "Chronic bronchitis" is considered to be present if sputum (phlegm) production occurs at least 4 days a week for 3 consecutive months in 2 consecutive years and there is no other known cause for sputum production.

An occupational history is a critical ingredient in a surveillance program designed to detect effects of dust on lung function. (See Chap. 21 for a detailed description of the methods used to obtain a reliable occupational history.)

Because of the major impact that cigarette smoking exerts on lung function, it is essential to obtain information related to the amount (packs per day) and duration (years) of the smoking habit. Otherwise, interpretation of surveillance results will be problematic and open to the bias of confounding.

Pulmonary Function Testing

Properly performed and interpreted, spirometry is simple, economical, and reliable. Results depend in part on the manner in which the technician encourages the patient to perform the test. Calibration errors can also produce inaccurate spirometry. The person supervising the testing must be trained in principles of spirometry. Although such training is required only by selected OSHA standards (e.g., cotton dust), persons administering spirometry tests ideally should complete a course approved by NIOSH. The spirometer should be checked daily for accuracy, including the newer automated spirometers, which may lead to complacency because of ease of operation.

Since a variety of parameters may be derived from spirometry, the physician must decide in advance which factors are of significance. In general, the FEV_1, the FVC, and the FEV_1/FVC ratio are most important. An appropriate reference group should be chosen to compare each subject's value with the "predicted." Normal ranges are calculated through the use of gender-specific regression equations that employ age and height as the major variables. Adjustment of predicted values for race may be advisable, since blacks average 10 to 15% lower predicted values at the same age and height. If the automated spirometer prints predicted values as well as observed values, the interpreter must know the source of prediction equations and whether race adjustment has been accomplished (see Chap. 11).

Longitudinal testing is potentially valuable. After age 25, FEV_1 and FVC decline with age; acceleration of the annual decline (whether due to nonoccupational cause such as smoking or occupational cause) indicates significant risk of developing respiratory disability in the future. However, precise measurement of annual decline is difficult because the magnitude of the change is comparable to the variability of measurement. Estimates of rate of decline in individuals must be based on at least three measurements over a several-year period. Thus, although declines of FEV_1 of greater than 35 ml per year may further warrant medical evaluation, imprecision of estimating the annual decline rate requires caution in interpretation.

When spirometry data will be used for longitudinal comparisons, special attention to detail is necessary. Small changes over time, particularly in a large group of workers, might be significant. Unfortunately, small differences in technique (e.g., effort urged by the technician, differences in equipment, control groups, or time of day of the test) may similarly affect results. Attention to adjustment of the spirometer for barometric pressure and ambient temperature is needed.

To ensure repeatability, the original tracing rather than numeric summary should be kept on file. When workers are tested at several sites (e.g., different plants), another group of individuals should be tested at all sites to ensure comparability. For multisite surveillance programs, physicians who interpret tests are advised to do so according to a common algorithm.

Chest Radiographs

Effective chest radiography depends on quality control regarding technical factors such as contrast and penetration. The usual radiologist interpretation should be supplemented by a standardized coding system to ensure comparability between physicians performing the interpretation, to permit aggregate data analysis, and to allow comparison with past and future results. The International Labor Organization (ILO) has developed a standardized system for coding chest radiographs (the ILO/UC system) [28]. Under this system, posteroanterior (PA) films are interpreted in a standardized fashion. The shape and number (profusion) of opacities consistent with pneumoconiosis are described with a series of letters and numbers by comparing the patient's radiograph with a set of reference films supplied by the ILO. The presence of pleural disease and other abnormalities is coded in the standardized manner. Epidemiologic studies and comparisons over time are facilitated, since the number of opacities is described by a 12-point scale rather than a long verbal description. Where important decisions are based on interpretation of radiographic surveillance, each radiograph may be interpreted by several readers according to the ILO system; those readers who tend to overread or underread thus may be identified.

Radiologists, chest physicians, occupational medicine specialists, and others may be certified as B readers by NIOSH if they successfully complete a course and pass a standardized and exacting test. Lists of B readers in each geographic area can be obtained from NIOSH.

The occupational implications of abnormal chest radiographs must be considered carefully. According to the ILO system, a positive report indicates findings "consistent with" pneumoconiosis but does not indicate that such disease actually is present. The radiographic findings must be integrated with exposure information and other clinical findings to achieve an accurate diagnosis. Even though interpretation by B readers using the ILO system is useful, inconsistency may occur [29–31]. The ILO system was designed for epidemiologic purposes and not for establishing clinical diagnoses in individuals.

Radiography is a relatively sensitive method for detecting early pneumoconiotic changes. Workers who have abnormal radiographs and yet have no physiologic impairment raise difficult questions about job placement. For example, should a coal miner with early radiographic abnormality be precluded from any coal mine work (i.e., considered "disabled" for such work) even if pulmonary function is completely normal? The current consensus is that removal would be advisable to prevent the abnormality from possibly developing into progressive massive fibrosis (PMF) with attendant morbidity. Early pulmonary fibrotic changes viewed radiographically in asbestos-exposed workers raise similar questions; optimally, the worker without physiologic impairment can continue working if the work environment or work practices can be successfully modified to prevent any further asbestos exposure.

Example 4: Exposure to Metals

Occupational exposure to metals is common and can lead to adverse effects. Surveillance programs targeting workers exposed to the heavy metals (lead, mercury, and arsenic) have been effective at decreasing the morbidity associated with such exposures.

Lead

Inhalation or ingestion can result in inorganic lead accumulation. Metal smelting operations (e.g., during primary metal refining or during secondary smelting to recover lead from existing materials such as storage batteries) can produce significant exposures. Lead incorporated into paints can be ingested (especially by children) or may be inhaled if the surface is subjected to heat, sanding, or grinding. Nervous system effects are the main consequences of lead exposure. In children, lead encephalopathy (including apathy, coma, and seizure) may be seen, while adults tend to have peripheral nervous system effects (e.g., wrist drop and abnormalities of nerve conduction). More subtle effects on central nervous system functioning, particularly in children, are receiving considerable attention. Lead inhibits hemoglobin synthesis and therefore can produce anemia. Lead also produces renal disease; acute lead nephropathy is characterized by proximal tubular damage, while more chronic exposure can produce progressive renal fibrosis and renal failure. Hypertension may be related. Gastrointestinal symptoms (e.g., abdominal pain and constipation) also occur. Lead rarely can produce joint pain and also precipitate gout. Lead has adverse reproductive effects as well. Persons with lead exposure who have any of these health problems require both careful medical evaluation and assessment of the work environment to evaluate exposure.

Workers with significant potential exposure to lead must be placed in a medical surveillance program. The OSHA standard is very explicit about criteria for inclusion. Decisions regarding the need for medical surveillance depend on a number of factors, including the toxicity of the agent, working conditions, and level and degree of exposure. In general, situations that result in exposures over the "action level" prompt the need for surveillance. The action level usually refers to one half of the TLV established by ACGIH and generally followed by OSHA as the permissible exposure limit (PEL). In the OSHA Lead Standard, however, the action level represents approximately 60% of the upper exposure limit (8 hours, time-weighted average). Blood lead level determination is useful as a reflection of exposure. Zinc protoporphyrin (ZPP) levels are much more nonspecific (affected by many causes of interference with heme synthesis). Zinc protoporphyrin testing may be of some utility in reflecting long-term exposure and is performed because the requirement has not been deleted from the OSHA Lead Standard. Blood lead measurements should be performed by competent laboratories certified by the Centers for Disease Control and Prevention. In general, these measurements should be made every 6 months.

Detection of blood lead levels above 40 µg/100 ml in itself does not prove that clinical toxic effects are present but does indicate that significant overexposure has occurred. Although diagnosis of clinical toxicity is an individual matter, OSHA mandates certain implications of BLL surveillance: It requires that workers with BLL greater than 60 µg on one test or whose 6-month average BLL is greater than 50 µg/100 ml be removed from exposure until the lead concentration returns to legally acceptable levels (40 µg/100 ml); during such periods of removal, the mandated Medical Removal Protection requires that employers continue workers' pay at the usual rate.

As discussed earlier, interpretation of biologic monitoring data should be based on knowledge of the kinetics of disposition. Blood lead concentrations are indicative of recent and acute exposures, while urine measurements provide an integrated measure of more chronic exposure. However, elevated BLL may persist after cessation of exposure because of a high body burden of lead due to prior chronic overexposure. Zinc protoporphyrin and hematocrit levels may be affected by lead exposure, but the results may be difficult to interpret in the presence of chronic disorders (e.g., iron deficiency anemia and increased serum bilirubin).

Mercury
Mercury exposure occurs in many industrial processes. Chloralkali cells used for producing chlorine can lead to exposure, as can use of mercury in instrument production, dental offices, laboratories, and the paper pulp industry. After inhalation, ingestion, or uptake from the skin, mercury is widely distributed in the body and accumulates in the brain. Chronic exposure to inorganic mercury can produce tremors, a psychoaffective disorder known as erethism (a personality change with withdrawal, anxiety, irritability), gingivitis, and renal disorders. In contrast to inorganic mercury exposure, organic mercury leads to cerebellar findings, which are more prominent than the psychological effects.

As with many other parameters of biologic monitoring, there is only a loose association between clinical toxicity and measurement of blood and urine mercury. Nevertheless, blood and urinary levels of mercury do reflect exposure, and therefore, mercury-exposed workers should have such urine testing periodically. Hair levels, if specimens are obtained properly and analyzed carefully, may have utility in a small number of cases as a reflection of long-term or distant exposures.

Arsenic
Arsenic exposure is often a consequence of smelting of other metals, since arsenic is a common contaminant of ores of lead, copper, and zinc. It also is used in the chemical and pesticide industries. Chronic exposure produces dermatologic effects, including hyperkeratosis, eczematous dermatitis, increased pigmentation, and an increased risk of lung cancer. Hepatic toxicity and sensory neuropathy may occur from industrial arsenic exposures.

For surveillance purposes, urinary arsenic provides the best indicator of exposure. Arsenic has a short blood half-life, and therefore, blood levels rarely are useful except as an indicator of very recent exposure. Surveillance programs also may include periodic liver function testing and examination of the skin in arsenic-exposed workers. One must remember that since ingestion of ocean fish or shellfish can lead to brief but rather high urinary arsenic concentrations, a careful dietary history is important in any worker found to have an increased urinary arsenic level. In the evaluation of an increased concentration of urinary arsenic, it is advisable to recommend abstinence from seafood for a short period of time. Sputum cytology, despite being part of recommended surveillance for the OSHA Arsenic Standard, is not routinely considered an effective screening device.

Example 5: Exposure to Solvents

Solvent exposures are common in industrial and other settings. Optimal surveillance program design and interpretation should be tailored to the nature of the particular solvents involved. Details of the effects of individual solvents are available from several sources included under Further Information. Development and interpretation of surveillance programs must be based on knowledge of the specific solvent(s) involved. Several general categories of surveillance techniques to detect the effects of chronic exposures, however, may be considered (Table 25-4).

Dermatologic effects are common due to defatting of exposed skin. Hence, clinicians must pay particular attention to the hands and other solvent-exposed body parts during periodic examinations, carefully looking for dryness, flaking, cracking, or even weeping and erythema.

Table 25-4. Possible uses of biologic monitoring to assess solvent exposure

Toxic agent	Specimen	Substance monitored
Methylene chloride	Exhaled air	Carbon monoxide
	Blood	Carboxyhemoglobin
Benzene	Urine	Phenol
	Exhaled air	Benzene
Toluene	Urine	Hippuric acid
Trichloroethylene	Urine	Trichloroacetic acid
Tetrachloroethylene	Expired air	Tetrachloroethylene
Xylene	Urine	Methyl-hippuric acid

Hepatic toxicity occurs from several solvents (particularly the low molecular weight, aliphatic chlorinated hydrocarbons such as chloroform). Preplacement and periodic testing of liver function may be advisable for workers who are exposed to potentially hepatotoxic solvents.

Benzene, an aromatic hydrocarbon solvent, causes marrow hypoplasia and aplasia as well as leukemia. Benzene is a common contaminant of other aromatic hydrocarbon solvents. Therefore, benzene-exposed workers (including those with exposure to benzene as a contaminant) may need periodic blood counts (including red blood cells, hematocrit, platelet count, and white cell count). The leukocyte differential count may be of assistance in detecting early hematologic toxicity; increases in the proportion of basophils or of immature forms (e.g., bands) may warrant further medical attention. The reticulocyte count also is a good screening test for early depression of hematopoiesis and may well be the most sensitive of all the routine tests available.

At least three organic solvents, n-hexane, methyl n-butyl ketone, and carbon disulfide, are well-documented causes of peripheral neuropathy. For others, including methylethyl ketone and trichloroethylene, current clinical surveillance techniques cannot determine whether early peripheral neuropathy occurs. However, periodic clinical examination with referral of workers with possible abnormalities for more complex testing (e.g., nerve conduction testing) may be helpful, and the possibility of peripheral neuropathy should be kept in mind when evaluating any solvent-exposed worker.

Behavioral effects of long-term chronic solvent exposure have been reported in several epidemiologic studies. These effects include cognitive defects (e.g., decreased memory) and personality affective effects (e.g., apathy and depression). The research data are still controversial, however [32]. Interpretation of the results of surveillance programs for such cognitive and affective effects is extremely difficult because of the nascent state of knowledge about such solvent effects, which are quite nonspecific (e.g., alcohol causes many of the same effects). Therefore, clinicians examining such exposed workers must understand the possibility of these effects, but it appears premature to establish programs for routine testing of such functions except for research purposes. Standardized batteries of tests are being developed and validated to permit objective and efficient testing in the future.

Biologic monitoring may prove useful in assessing solvent exposure. For example, 50% of methylene chloride absorbed is metabolized to carbon monoxide; measurement of exhaled air and the carboxyhemoglobin therefore may permit detection of methylene chloride overexposure [33]. Urinary phenol concentration is related to exposure to benzene and several other organic solvents and may be useful as a biologic monitor. There is considerable current interest in developing biologic exposure indices (BEI) as reflections of workplace exposures to solvents.

In summary, many types of solvents are in use. Surveillance systems should be based on the solvents in use in a particular plant and on available testing and interpretation resources. Surveillance programs for solvent-exposed workers are likely to undergo significant changes over the next several years.

Example 6: Ergonomic Surveillance

Cumulative trauma disorders (CTDs) are increasingly recognized. Medical surveillance programs are essential for their detection and prevention. As an adjunct to worksite biomechanical analyses, worker-based clinical assessment can yield considerable useful information. Symptom surveys, either done specifically for this purpose or in the course of more routine examinations, may show a pattern of musculoskeletal symptoms in one area of a plant associated with one operation. Often the symptoms are not in themselves of sufficient specificity to make a traditional clinical diagnosis (e.g., "carpal tunnel syndrome"), but they can alert the clinician that further investigation of an area is necessary. Furthermore, clinicians must remember that symptom reporting of musculoskeletal symptoms can be affected by factors other than the workplace ergonomic hazard. Questions used should be very carefully worded, and if a questionnaire is used in written form, it should be pilot tested. Surprisingly high positive response rates are often obtained even in "control" groups.

Review of absence records, productivity data, and reports of clinical diagnoses may also be useful for ergonomic medical surveillance. On a research basis, several surveillance programs have been instituted in areas at high risk of cumulative injury, even including clinical examination. Unfortunately, reliance upon clinical signs is inappropriate. Even "classic" findings such as in Phalen's test actually have limited sensitivity and specificity.

Informal surveillance for ergonomic hazards can be effective. Workers often have better insight into the stresses of their job than do "experts," and the clinician should pointedly ask workers (when seeing patients) about whether there are any physical factors at the job that are "stressful." When the worker is asked in a nonthreatening manner with an appropriate plan for future investigation, problems that are easily preventable can be detected.

When ergonomic surveillance is performed, it is important to note that the "case definition" differs significantly from the usual clinical case definition. The "epidemiologic" (or surveillance) definition is not meant to be specifically interpreted as the presence of a clinical diagnosis; similarly, one should not wait until the establishment of firm clinical diagnoses to be concerned.

References

1. US Preventive Services Task Force. *Guide to Clinical Preventive Services: An Assessment of the Effectiveness of 169 Interventions. Report of the US Preventive Services Task Force.* Baltimore: William & Wilkins, 1989.
2. Kreiss, K. Approaches to assessing pulmonary dysfunction and susceptibility in workers. *J. Occup. Med.* 28:664, 1986.
3. Official Statement of the American Thoracic Society. Standardization of spirometry—1987 update. *Am. Rev. Respir. Dis.* 136:1285, 1987.
4. Committee on Occupational Lung Disorders of the American College of Occupational and Environmental Medicine (ACOEM). Spirometry in the occupational setting: Notes for guidance. *J. Occup. Med.* 34:559, 1992.
5. Monster, A. C. Biological monitoring of chlorinated hydrocarbon solvents. *J. Occup. Med.* 28:583, 1986.
6. Lowry, L. K. Biological exposure index as a complement to the TLV. *J. Occup. Med.* 28:578, 1986.
7. Lauwerys, R. R. *Industrial Chemical Exposure: Guidelines for Biological Monitoring.* Davis, CA: Biomedical, 1983.
8. Baselt, R. C. *Biological Monitoring Methods for Industrial Chemicals.* Davis, CA: Biomedical, 1980.
9. Wibowo, A. A. E., et al. Blood lead and serum iron level in non-occupationally exposed males and females. *Int. Arch. Occup. Environ. Health* 39:113, 1977.
10. Zeilhuis, R. L., et al. Smoking habits and levels of lead and cadmium in urban women. *Int. Arch. Occup. Environ. Health* 39:53, 1977.
11. Krivanek, N., McLaughlin, M., and Fayerweather, W. Monomethyl-formamide levels in human urine after repetitive exposure to dimethylformamide vapor. *J. Occup. Med.* 20:179, 1978.
12. National Research Council. Biological workers in environmental health research. *Environ. Health Perspect.* 74:1, 1987.
13. Brandt-Rauf, P. W. Advances in cancer biomarkers as applied to chemical exposures: The ras oncogene and p21 protein and pulmonary carcinogenesis. *J. Occup. Med.* 33:951, 1991.
14. Marfin, A. A., and Schenker, M. Screening for lung cancer: Effective tests awaiting effective treatment. *Occup. Med. State of the Art Rev.* 6:111, 1991.

15. Albelda, S. M., et al. Pleural thickening: Its significance and relationship to asbestos dust exposure. *Am. Rev. Respir. Dis.* 126:621, 1982.
16. Helzberg, J. H., and Spiro, H. M. "LFTs" test more than the liver. *J.A.M.A.* 256:21, 1986.
17. Hodgson, M. J., Goodman-Klein, B. M., and van Thiel, D. H. Evaluating the liver in hazardous waste workers. *Occup. Med. State of the Art Rev.* 5:67, 1990.
18. Welch, L. The role of occupational health clinics in surveillance of occupational disease. *Am. J. Public Health* 79:58, 1989.
19. Fontus, H. M., Levy, B. S., and Davis, L. K. Physician-based surveillance of occupational disease. Part II: Experience with a broader range of diagnoses and physicians. *J. Occup. Med.* 31:929, 1989.
20. Mullan, R. J., and Murthy, L. I. Occupational sentinel health events: An up-dated list for physician recognition and public health surveillance. *Am. J. Ind. Med.* 19:775, 1991.
21. Mathias, C. G. T., et al. Surveillance of occupational skin diseases: A method utilizing workers' compensation claims. *Am. J. Ind. Med.* 17:363, 1990.
22. Matte, T. D., et al. Surveillance of occupational asthma under the SENSOR model. *Chest* 98:173S, 1990.
23. Matte, T. D., Baker, E. L., and Honchar, P. A. The selection and definition of targeted work-related conditions for surveillance under SENSOR. *Am. J. Public Health* 79(S):21, 1989.
24. Harber, P. Interpretation of lung function tests. *Curr. Pulmonol.* 12:261, 1991.
25. Park, R. M., et al. Use of medical insurance claims for surveillance of occupational disease: An analysis of cumulative trauma in the auto industry. *J. Occup. Med.* 34:731, 1992.
26. Schulte, P. A., and Singal, M. Interpretation and communication of the results of medical field investigations. *J. Occup. Med.* 31:589, 1989.
27. American Thoracic Society. Lung function testing: Selection of reference values and interpretive strategies. *Am. Rev. Respir. Dis.* 144:1202, 1991.
28. International Labor Office. *Guidelines for the Use of the ILO International Classification of Pneumoconiosis.* Geneva: International Labor Office, 1980.
29. Wagner, G. R., et al. The NIOSH B reader certification program: An update report. *J. Occup. Med.* 34:879, 1992.
30. Ducatman, A. M., Yang, W. N., and Forman, S. A. "B-readers" and asbestos medical surveillance. *J. Occup. Med.* 30:644, 1988.
31. Balmes, J. R. To B-read or not to B-read (editorial). *J. Occup. Med.* 34:885, 1992.
32. Baker, E. L. Organic solvent neurotoxicity. *Annu. Rev. Public Health* 9:223, 1988.
33. Astrand, I., Ovrum, P., and Carlsson, A. Exposure to methylene chloride: I. Its concentration in alveolar air and blood during rest and exercise and its metabolism. *Scand. J. Work Environ. Health* 1:78, 1975.

Further Information

Baker, E. L. (ed.). Surveillance in occupational health and safety. *Am. J. Public Health* 79 (Suppl.), 1989.
Note: A major portion of the August 1986 and October 1986 issues of the Journal of Occupational Medicine *is devoted to the technical, ethical, and clinical aspects of medical surveillance. As of this writing, these issues of Volume 28 present the most comprehensive and current view of medical surveillance.*

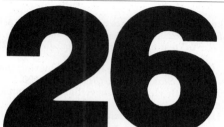

Risk Assessment

John Whysner and
Kenneth H. Chase

The workplace and the environment have always contained risks. Traditionally, accidents have been, and continue to be, the most important risks that must be assessed. However, the vast number of chemicals now used in the workplace and found in the environment have increased the complexity of assessing risk. In the past, certain jobs have been considered more hazardous than others based on risks that are clearly visible; however, the risks associated with exposures to chemicals are often hidden. The possibility of exposure may be hard to detect, and the effects of some chemicals may not develop until years or decades after exposure.

The practicing physician will be increasingly called on to provide guidance to individuals exposed to a variety of occupational and environmental hazards [1]. But how can the physician estimate the degree of risk that confronts a patient, and how can this risk be made understandable in a layperson's terms?

In this chapter, a general approach to this problem is given and illustrated by a case. This case provides a hypothetical situation in which sufficient information is available to make a reasonable risk calculation. Usually, such information is unavailable, or the time required for risk assessment calculations is prohibitive. However, by understanding the elements of the risk calculation, *those parameters that increase or decrease risk can be appreciated.* Such calculations are similar to those used by government agencies to determine regulatory limits for chemicals in the workplace or environment. For additional information on this subject, see References 2–5. (Regulatory bodies, such as the United States Environmental Protection Agency [EPA] have numerous risk assessment documents available.)

Clinical Approach to Evaluating Risk

The example given here is a hypothetical one involving a worker who has discovered that he has been exposed to compound X, by the dermal route, at his workplace. He has no clinical symptoms or abnormal laboratory findings, but he wants to know whether he can get cancer as a result of exposure. The approach to this patient should include the following three steps.

1. Risk assessment of *current and past exposure* based on actual dose, if available
2. *Modification of risk factors* in the workplace through counseling, personal protective equipment, and engineering controls
3. Reassessment of risks to provide the worker with input for determining acceptability of the risk

A review of the available information on compound X shows that it is a suspected carcinogen on the basis of animal toxicity studies and that a lifetime average daily dose (LADD) of 0.01 μg/kg/day corresponds to an upper-limit excess risk of cancer in humans of 1/100,000. (Such information is typically available from a regulatory agency such as the EPA.)

A call to the company where the employee is working reveals that the measured average surface concentration of compound X in his work area was 70 μg/100 cm². This was determined by taking various wipe samples with appropriate solvents. His job put him in the contaminated area for only one quarter of his working days. It is assumed that the work practices were constant over his work lifetime, which was 30 years.

The man was not a smoker, and other opportunities for oral exposure appear to have been minimal. Repeated measurements of air concentration (in this case) were negligible. For dermal absorption, a simplifying upper-limit assumption can be made that one half of the surface area of the hands and arms was in equilibrium with the contaminated surface area. Studies have shown that dermal absorption of compound X is about 10%. As can be seen from Fig. 26-1, the LADD, calculated based on the foregoing assumptions, exceeds 0.01 µg/kg/day by a factor of 10. Since 0.01 µg/kg/day corresponds to a risk of 1/100,000 additional cancer risk for a lifetime, the worker would have a 1/10,000 hypothetical additional risk of cancer over his lifetime. If the worker continues at the same job with the same exposure, each additional year will add an additional hypothetical cancer risk of approximately 1/300,000. (The 1/10,000 risk is accumulated over 30 years; one thirtieth of 1/10,000 is 1/300,000 per year.)

It is recognized that a physician will usually have neither the information nor the time to perform such a calculation. Also, there are numerous uncertainties in the assumptions involved in risk assessment. Consequently, this risk assessment represents, at best, a rough estimate, which may greatly overestimate risk. The correlation of 0.01 µg/kg/day with an excess cancer risk is an upper limit of risk, and some would argue that the human risk is 100 or 1000 times less or may even be zero at these low levels. This uncertainty is caused by the fact that high-dose animal cancer studies are used with linear-at-low-dose extrapolation methods. This extrapolation method may not be appropriate for certain types of carcinogens, as is discussed in Dose-Response Relationships.

```
Dermal Daily Dose Calculation:


    70 µg    X     1500 cm²    X     0.25 day
   100 cm²                             day


      X    0.1 µg absorbed/day     =      26 µg
              µg exposed                   day


Lifetime Average Daily Dose (LADD) calculation:


26 µg/day    X    240 working days/year    X    30 years
                  25,550 days/lifetime    X    70 kg

=        0.1 µg/kg-day



Where:

    70 µg    =    measured environmental surface level
   100 cm²


1500 cm²    =    one-half of the surface area of the arms


0.25 day/day    =    fraction of day exposed


   0.1 µg absorbed/day    =    absorption efficiency of 10%
        µg exposed
```

Figure 26-1. Calculation of cancer risk for a worker exposed to compound X.

Risk Communication and Hazard Reduction

Putting all of these uncertainties aside, how can an excess cancer risk of 1/300,000 per year be explained to the patient? By referring to Table 26-1,* the physician can explain that the risk of cancer from this exposure is about the same as the risk of dying in an earthquake if one lives in California or of dying in a flood. By further comparison, the risk is about 1/1000 that of smoking one pack of cigarettes per day.

Is this an acceptable risk? This is a complex issue. Government regulatory agencies have used 1/10,000 to 1/1,000,000 excess lifetime cancer risk as benchmarks for policy decisions. Such guidelines are for involuntary risks, however. For voluntary risks, as may be the case for those associated with certain occupational exposures, acceptability must be evaluated by the patient.

The next step is to consider ways to *reduce the current hazard*. Table 26-2 presents a number of factors that contribute to a risk. The patient should be counseled on the importance of personal hygiene and the use of protective equipment to reduce exposure. Steps such as approaching management, unions, or the shop foreman should also be considered to attempt reduction of exposure. For example, if the area of skin exposed can be reduced to one fifth by the use of protective clothing, and if surface contamination can be reduced to one fourth, the resulting incremental risk will be one twentieth of the 1/300,000 per year risk previously determined, or

Table 26-1. Risks

Situation	Deaths/person/yr (odds)
Motorcycling	1 in 50
Smoking (20 cigarettes/day)	1 in 200
Influenza	1 in 5000
Auto driving (UK)	1 in 5900
Leukemia	1 in 12,500
Drinking (1 bottle wine/day)	1 in 13,300
Struck by auto	1 in 20,000
Taking contraceptive pills	1 in 50,000
Floods	1 in 455,000
Earthquake (California)	1 in 588,000
Lightning (UK)	1 in 10,000,000
Release from nuclear reactor at site boundary	1 in 10,000,000

Source: From B. D. Dinman. Occupational health and the reality of risk: An external dilemma of tragic choices. *J.O.M.* 22:153, 1980. ©AOMA, 1980.

Table 26-2. Exposure factors that proportionally increase the calculated risk of cancer, assuming a linear-at-low-dose relationship.

For all routes
  Years of exposure
  Hours of exposure per day
  Concentration of toxic substance[a]
For dermal exposure
  Surface area of skin exposed[a]
  Length of time substance remains on skin[b]
For oral exposure
  Mouthing episodes from contaminated hands, cigarettes, food, etc.[b]

[a]Reduced by personal protective equipment and work practices.
[b]Reduced by hygiene.

*Some problems arise with the conversion of lifetime to yearly risks for hazards, such as carcinogens, that are cumulative. For the purpose of this discussion, this difficulty has been ignored, since both are approximations.

1/6,000,000 per year. As can be seen in Table 26-1, this is less than the risk of being struck by lightning and less than one thirteenth the risk of dying in a flood. Finally, the physician should attempt to discover whether the patient is exposed to other hazards in the workplace. Typically, multiple chemicals are present in the workplace, some of which may be of greater hazard than the chemical of concern to the worker.

Risk Assessment Methods and Terminology

Risk assessment is a statistical procedure employed by various regulatory agencies in an attempt to define an acceptable level of *risk* for exposure to a hazardous substance. Risk assessment uses available scientific evidence from human (epidemiology) and animal studies to develop models to predict toxicity of the various substances at *low* levels of exposure. Limitations inherent in this process include the reliability of the data, the accuracy of extrapolating results from animals to humans, and the legitimacy of assuming a linear relationship between low doses of a substance and the adverse health effect. This last problem manifests itself primarily in the evaluation of carcinogenic substances using information generated by US governmental agencies, which do not recognize the presence of a "threshold" dose below which exposure to a substance is not a health risk.

Dose-Response Relationships

The classic sigmoidal dose-response curve for most toxic effects appears in Fig. 26-2 (curve A) and exhibits a threshold at low doses below which the effect does not occur. For example, a very small dose of a chlorinated hydrocarbon will not produce chloracne; a minimal amount of exposure is required to alter the metabolism of the skin to produce these changes. The hatched area in the diagram is called a "no observed effect level" (NOEL). For regulatory purposes, limits on exposure are usually set at a fraction of the NOEL, usually 1/10 to 1/1000. This adjusted dosage

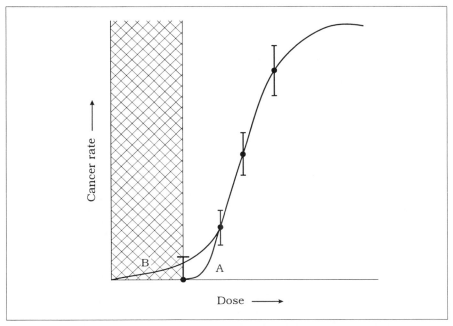

Figure 26-2. Alternative dose-response curves for carcinogenicity. In curve A, the data points are fitted to the curve with threshold. In curve B, the data points are fitted to the curve without threshold (linear model). The hatched area indicates no observed effect level (NOEL).

is called a "reference dose" (RFD) or an acceptable daily intake (ADI). The RFD is set well below the NOEL because the NOEL is usually based on animal studies rather than human epidemiology studies, and uncertainties exist in extrapolation from animals to sensitive humans. This approach is used by US Government agencies for noncarcinogenic effects and by other governments for many carcinogenic effects as well [2].

In contrast, for most carcinogenic effects, no threshold dose is assumed to exist by US governmental agencies, as shown in Fig. 26-2 (curve B). Only at zero dose is there assumed to be no effect [6]. For example, chemicals that cause tumors in rodents through increasing cell division, such as the food additives saccharin and butylated hydroxyanisole, appear to have a threshold dose [7, 8]. Also, chemicals that interact with hormone regulation only at high doses can result in organotropic effect, producing tumors [9]. This approach is controversial, since not all cancer-causing agents appear to fit this model. The "linear-at-low-dose" model predicts that the line can be extrapolated to smaller and smaller dose with declining risk of cancer. Various regulatory agencies have usually determined the range of 1/10,000 to 1/10,000,000 as an acceptable lifetime risk due to a chemical. The dosage associated with this risk is called a "virtually safe dose" (VSD).

The *"no-threshold" theory* of carcinogenesis is based on the premise that only one molecule of a carcinogen needs to interact with DNA to initiate cancer development. This theory, however, has been subject to considerable scientific challenge by authors who claim that large numbers of chemical molecules are required for a measurable response [10]. Presumably, the metabolic system can successfully detoxify small amounts of carcinogens. Additionally, chemical carcinogens act through different mechanisms. Many chemicals that act by a non-DNA-reactive mechanism exert their effects by enhancing the development of tumors rather than by creating neoplastic cells [11]. (See Chap. 13 for detailed discussion on occupational carcinogens.)

Calculation of Exposure

The assessment of risk requires an estimate of the patient's exposure. For this estimate, a measurement of the concentration of the chemical in the worker's environment is preferred. Depending on the exposure scenario, such a measurement may be the concentration of a substance in air, on a surface, or in a solid matrix such as soil.

To perform relevant measurements and estimate an exposure, it is first necessary to assess the routes and conditions by which a worker may be exposed. Such exposure scenarios are usually specific to an absorption route, which may be oral, dermal, or inhalation. Inhalation estimates are the easiest to perform; by knowing the airborne level, one can calculate the exposure, as shown in Fig. 26-3. The air concentration is usually measured in milligrams or micrograms per cubic meter (mg/m^3 or $\mu g/m^3$). For the respiratory route, it is often assumed that there is total absorption of the inspired toxic vapors, although this is not the case for most substances. For an adult, air is inhaled at a rate of 1 m^3 per hour at rest and 2 m^3 per hour for moderately vigorous activity. An exposure estimate (dose) can be calculated by simply taking the product of the measured concentration and the air volume inhaled over a specified time interval.

Dermal and oral absorption are more complicated to model. Dermal exposure is probably the most difficult to estimate, as evidenced by the sample calculation for the hypothetical worker in Fig. 26-1. The skin surface levels are assumed equal to the levels on environmental surfaces. The efficiency of absorption is usually less than unity, and can be 10% or less for exposures to particulate or soil-bound chemicals.

For oral exposure, the amount of ingestion must be estimated. For occupational exposures, there may be acute accidental ingestions that can be quantified. For chronic ingestions, the scenarios are more complex and generally occur by hand-to-mouth activities or "mouthing episodes" of smoking, eating, nail biting, or other personal habits. Soil ingestion directly from soil or from airborne soil particles has been estimated to average 25 mg per day for adults [12]. The calculation of daily oral exposure is performed as shown in Fig. 26-3.

For dermal absorption, a method has been developed that provides an upper limit of exposure. This method was used in the example given at the beginning of the chapter. In this method, the assumption is made that part of the skin is in contact with the concentration equal to the surface concentration of the toxic substance in

```
Inhalation:

Daily exposure  =  air level  X   1-2m³   X   hours
                                  hour         day


Oral (Soil):

Daily exposure  =  soil level  X  25 mg soil/day  X  % absorption


Dermal (Surfaces):

Daily exposure  =  surface level  X  1500 cm²  X

                      fraction of day exposed  X  % absorption

(The simplifying assumption of concentration equivalence between
of one-half the area of the arms and environment surface levels
will generally lead to an overestimation of exposure.)


All Routes:

Lifetime Average Daily Dose  =

     Daily exposure X days exposure/year  X  years exposure
           25,550 days/lifetime  X  70 kg
```

Figure 26-3. Formulas for calculating daily exposure by route. See text for explanation of terms.

the environment for a period of time. This assumption may be further refined by wipe samples utilizing an appropriate solvent. Then the equation for dermal exposure can be expressed as shown in Fig. 26-3. In this case, the absorption efficiency for a 24-hour contact must be known. Usually animal studies or in vitro studies of human skin are performed to determine this factor. The surface area exposed may include the hands only, the hands and forearms, or other exposed areas of the body.

The use of personal protective equipment will modify any of the above calculations. In fact, such calculations can be utilized to estimate the benefits of such protection. The presumed efficiency of air filtration devices or barrier clothing, which reduce exposures, can be included in these calculations.

Principles of Risk Assessment

Risk assessment is a *quantitative* approach to the risk of exposure from toxic chemicals. Usually it is not possible to perform all of these calculations on an individual patient. Such calculations are time consuming and are usually performed on groups or on an occasional patient involved in a litigation. However, an understanding of the risk factors can be useful in reducing hazards and in explaining risk to the patient. *Three principles of risk assessment* worth noting are the following:

1. For carcinogens, lowering the exposure can usually decrease the upper-limit risk of cancer to a level comparable to insignificant risks (see Table 26-1).
2. For most toxic effects and arguably for some carcinogens, keeping exposure below a certain level reduces the effect to zero.
3. Cancer risk is based on lifetime dose, which is determined by multiple factors (see Table 26-2). Reduction in these factors will reduce the risk of cancer proportionately.

For clinical purposes, it is important to realize that risk estimates are based on a number of statistical assumptions that may not be directly pertinent to the individual patient.

References

1. Bunn, W. B. Right-to-know laws and evaluation of toxicologic data. *Ann. Intern. Med.* 103:947, 1985.
2. Whysner, J. A., and Williams, G. M. International cancer risk assessment: The impact of biologic mechanisms. *Reg. Toxicol. Pharmacol.* 15:41, 1992.
3. National Research Council. *Risk Assessment in the Federal Government: Managing the Process.* Washington, DC: National Academy Press, 1983.
4. Office of Science and Technology Policy. Chemical carcinogens: Notice of review of the science and its associated principles. *Fed. Register* 49(100):21594, 1984.
5. Dinman, B. D. Occupational health and the reality of risk: An eternal dilemma of tragic choices. *J.O.M.* 22:153, 1980.
6. Anderson, E. L., and Carcinogenic Assessment Group. EPA quantitative approaches in use to assess cancer risk. *Risk Analysis* 3:277, 1983.
7. Cohen, S. M. and Ellwein, L. B. Cell proliferation in carcinogenesis. *Science* 249:1007, 1990.
8. Whysner, J. A. Mechanism-based cancer risk assessment of butylated hydroxyanisole. *Toxicology and Industrial Health* 9:283, 1993.
9. Hill, R. N., et al. Thyroid follicular cell carcinogenesis. *Fundamental and Applied Toxicology* 12:629, 1988.
10. Stokinger, H. E. Concepts of thresholds in standard setting. *Arch. Environ. Health* 25:153, 1972.
11. Williams, G. M., and Weisburger, J. H. Chemical Carcinogenesis. In M. O. Amdur, J. Doull, and C. D. Klaassen (eds.), *Toxicology. The Basic Science of Poisons* (4th ed.). New York: Pergamon, 1991. Pp. 127–200.
12. LaGoy, P. K. Estimated soil ingestion rates for use in risk assessment. *Risk Analysis* 7:355, 1987.

Further Information

Klaassen, C. D., and Eaton, D. L. Principles of Toxicology. In M. O. Amdur, J. Doull, and C. D. Klaassen (eds.), *Toxicology. The Basic Science of Poisons* (4th ed.). New York: Pergamon, 1991. Pp. 12–49.

National Research Council. *Improving Risk Communication.* Washington, DC: National Academy Press, 1989.

Slovic, P. Perception of risk. *Science* 280:5, April 17, 1987.

US Environmental Protection Agency. *Risk Assessment Guidance for Superfund,* Vol. 1. *Human Health Evaluation Manual,* Part A. EPA/540/1-89/002, 1989.

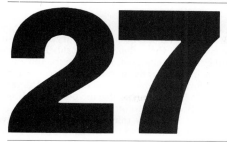

Searching the Occupational Medical Literature

Joseph Harzbecker, Jr.,
and William E. Browning, Jr.

The occupational health professional in today's world requires access to current information. In fact, it has become an essential aspect of occupational medical practice to be aware of potentially new associations between exposures to various agents and the development of a variety of illnesses. Active vigilance of risks associated with new technology and new materials places a responsibility on the occupational health physician to pursue certain clinical situations in more depth. Searching the literature is an exciting intellectual activity with interesting possibilities and important consequences.

In honor of the 200th anniversary of the United States Constitution (1987), the US Office of Technology Assessment published *Science Technology and the Constitution,* wherein it was stated "the pace of scientific and technological progress is relentless, offering us powers not dreamed of in 1787." The free flow of scientific information has been essential to all aspects of scientific progress. The toxicologist and practitioner of occupational medicine have benefited accordingly. Many of the sources listed in this section have been created by the US Government, a major disseminator of scientific information.

The intent of this chapter is to acquaint the occupational health professional with the means for reviewing the medical literature and to describe the process whereby a professional, through the use of either medical library services or a personal computer, can access publicly available information pertinent to occupational health practice.

The retrieval of toxicologic information is crucial to the formulation of an opinion that may have wide-ranging ramifications, but readers should recognize that access to information is only one component involved in the judgment process. Each situation has to be evaluated on its own merits in the light of principles in diagnosing occupational disease, as put forth in various other chapters of this book (see Chap. 21, Suspecting Occupational Disease, and Chap. 33, The Case Report: Discovery of Occupational Disease).

We cover the role and purpose of medical information resources, including books, reference texts, libraries, research librarians, national medical libraries, and electronic databases and their uses, and the classification of biomedical information.

The development of search strategies is treated by two approaches: (1) the use of a categorized system of medical subject headings (MeSH), in which descriptors are assigned by reviewers, and (2) direct searching of the words of the title, abstract, descriptors, and text (free-text searching), which depends on the ingenuity of the user to ascertain the terms used by the authors.

Finally, we illustrate the process of reviewing the literature in a clinical setting by considering two case histories. These examples are intended to serve as practical guides to enable the reader to become familiar with the sources and process available to obtain reliable information.

Medical Information Resources

A large variety of medical information resources are available to assist in searching both primary and secondary sources in the medical literature, including books and reference texts, medical libraries together with research librarians, the National Library of Medicine (NLM), electronic databases, and a system for the classification of biomedical information by the NLM.

The best example of a primary source is an article published in a scientific journal (the history of which dates back to the mid-seventeenth century). Today, nearly 100,000 journal publications are available throughout the world. Many types of information are published, including original observations, research, and editorials, among others. *Primary* sources also include trade journals and technical reports. Product, business, and advertising information may also be included. The technical report may describe research projects. Primary sources also include proceedings from conferences or symposia, doctoral dissertations, patents, and standards.

Secondary sources include abstracts, which may take two forms: descriptive, indicating what has been done, and analytical, in which interpretations regarding data are presented. Review articles, another secondary source, attempt to summarize existing knowledge into a concise, compact form. The well-done review article will identify existing knowledge gaps within a subject and provide an extensive bibliography on the subject. It is an excellent starting point for becoming familiar with a topic.

Medical Books and Reference Texts

In searching clinical questions, a review of basic medical textbooks can provide an overview of the problem. Occupational medicine texts may provide further clues to diseases of particular occupational groups. Thus, reference books should be considered part of the review process, even before one attempts to search the electronic databases. In the context of this chapter, however, it is assumed that the reader has addressed these sources and is primarily interested in the peer-reviewed literature and government documents on the topic.

Medical Libraries

Medical libraries, an essential resource in searching the occupational health and toxicology literature, may be found in various types of medical centers and some corporations. All libraries continue to evolve. The medical library mirrors the developments in particular health disciplines. Many exciting changes have taken place that have broadened the occupational health literature. The current structure of medical libraries in the United States provides accurate, timely, and comprehensive access to the world's health sciences literature. Difficult research questions are solved through the careful use of selected sources.

The first encounter in a medical library will likely be with the public service staff, including reference librarians, as well as the circulation desk staff. This public service staff will provide the necessary information required for that particular library, or provide referral service to other institutions. They will probably direct you to the library catalogue.

To many people, the mention of the term *library catalogue* conjures up images of dusty wooden drawers packed with 3×5-in. index cards. The vast majority of libraries, however, now possess on-line computer catalogues that enable them to update their holdings quickly and accurately. The on-line public access catalog (OPAC) is an evolving system. The typical catalogue allows the user access to thousands, if not millions of monograph titles. One may access through author, title, subject, or key word. Some systems allow the combination of author with title, subject with author, and so on. An entire university's book collection is searchable by this method. Many systems are available through on-line connection via a personal computer with a modem. As the OPAC evolves, more functions are added to its capabilities, including connections to other libraries in North America, Europe, and Australia. The OPAC is probably the best place to begin a search for monograph titles because of its flexibility and power.

The local medical library will have sources including specialized works, such as reference books and government publications. Reference books comprise a wide range of items, including dictionaries, encyclopedias, atlases, bibliographies, manuals, and handbooks. Encyclopedias, guides, and manuals provide factual information. Handbooks give specific information on chemicals, substances, and environmental pollutants. The addresses of government agencies, patient care groups, and associations may be found in many of these sources. Government publications, such as those prepared by the National Institute for Occupational Safety and Health (NIOSH), the Agency for Toxic Substances and Disease Registry (ATSDR), or the Environmental Protection Agency (EPA), have also contributed to the toxicology and occupational health literature. The medical library will also have many of the abstracts and indexes described in Appendix E. These sources can provide citations to articles on specific topics related to any particular search.

The National Library of Medicine

The National Library of Medicine (NLM), in Bethesda, Maryland, exists "to assist the advancement of medical and related sciences, and to aid in the dissemination and exchange of scientific and other information important to the progress of medicine and to public health" (Public Law 84-941). The NLM provides many services to the medical and library community through products such as Index Medicus, the Medical Literature Analysis and Retrieval System (MEDLARS), and the MeSH vocabulary, which is described in the next section.

Under the leadership of the NLM, these products are distributed to medical libraries and health professionals through the Regional Medical Library system. The Regional Library has certain duties in relation to NLM programs and the small- or medium-sized medical libraries located within each given region.

Three pieces of government legislation provided for the mandate and authorization of funding for the NLM's programs and services. Legislation included the Medical Library Assistance Act of 1956 (provided the basis of the mandate), the National Library of Medicine Act (the actual mandate), and the Medical Library Assistance Act of 1965 (authorized funding). These Acts form the basis of NLM operations and have provided an impetus for the evolving dissemination of biomedical, scientific literature throughout the past 35 years. The NLM and medical librarians have strived to provide health care professionals with accurate systems and quality programs to enable uncomplicated access to the medical literature.

The MeSH list is an evolving vocabulary system developed by the NLM to govern the classification and retrieval of biomedical information. It is the "central nervous system" for the NLM biomedical information database, MEDLARS. The MeSH list has three components: the Annotated Alphabetical List, the Tree Structure, and the Permuted Headings. In the Annotated Alphabetic List, subjects are arranged in alphabetical order with scope notes and alphanumeric codes for the tree structures. The Tree Structure is a subject-arranged listing of the over 14,000 terms from the annotated list. Subjects are grouped into 15 broad categories that are hierarchically arranged (hence the "tree structure"). Each entry in the list is given an alphanumeric code, which uniquely identifies a particular subject. The Permuted Headings serve as a thesaurus for the MeSH headings. In this highly readable, permuted display of all terms in the annotated MeSH, subjects are listed alphabetically by each significant word in the MeSH headings.

The MeSH is revised annually, and is used to index scientific articles listed in the Index Medicus, International Nursing Index, and Index to Dental Literature. All monograph titles, journal titles, and audiovisuals are classified with MeSH. The database file, MEDLINE, uses this indexing system. Although the MEDLINE system does not require users to read MeSH, it is helpful to become familiar with the system used to categorize medical information to fully appreciate how articles are indexed. The use of MeSH for searching the scientific literature is discussed in one later section of this chapter and is illustrated for specific applications in another section.

Electronic Databases

The most efficient, accurate, and comprehensive method to access scientific articles is through a search of electronic databases. Searching the literature in this way is an exciting area of library/information science because it is an intellectual activity with interesting possibilities. The term *literature* usually refers to scientific articles or research reports; however, book chapters and other forms of information are also included in databases. Some databases provide bibliographic identities, key words, and sometimes abstracts of articles. Others include the full text of articles, while still others may provide numeric nonbibliographic or simply statistical information.

It is crucial to determine which databases to include in a search. Many databases exist throughout the world. These constantly change, and it is often difficult to keep up with these changes. Appendix E section 7 provides a list of reference books that catalogue the availability of databases. The MEDLINE, TOXLINE, and TOXNET systems are basic to occupational medicine, yet some of the additional databases included in Appendix E may be useful.

The MEDLINE database (see Appendix E, 7.2) is one of the most heavily used databases in the health care field. MEDLINE is a "household" name among biomedical researchers and health care practitioners and is usually a good starting point for searching the literature on clinical questions. MEDLINE has always been a relatively low-cost database to search. The indexing system (MeSH) is flexible and specific and has enabled MEDLINE to become popular and successful. For the specifics on MEDLINE and some of its companion files, please refer to Appendix E.

TOXLINE is a companion file of MEDLINE, and should be included in searches in occupational medicine. The TOXLINE file contains citations from several small databases and the citations from MEDLINE that have the subheadings "adverse effects," "poisoning," and "toxicity." For the specific breakdown of the database, please refer to Appendix E section 7.5.

The TOXNET system (see Appendix E 7.6) is a factual database that includes data such as lethal dose, color, odor, and a wealth of information for thousands of compounds. This evolving reference source for substances includes an "integrated approach" to the development and review of records.

Biosis Previews (see Appendix E 7.7.2) is an extensive, comprehensive database covering the life sciences. This database is widely available and is very useful as a supplement to MEDLINE. Searches on occupational health subjects yield results that primarily duplicate those from MEDLINE, but the few additional reports found improve significantly the exhaustiveness of the search.

The National Technical Information Service (NTIS) database (see Appendix E 7.7.12) covers government-sponsored research, development, and engineering, including reports by the Hazard Evaluation and Technical Assistance Branch of NIOSH of investigations of suspected occupational disease or injury. These are very useful in searches for suspected associations between disease and agent.

It may be useful to supplement the information obtained from the above databases with statistics on the incidence, prevalence, morbidity, and mortality of diseases. Some of the specialized databases described in Appendix E can provide access to the epidemiologic literature, which has been of increasing importance to occupational health practitioners.

Health law sources may serve as valuable references for occupational health information, especially regarding regulations, statutes, and laws that apply to people at work. Federal, state, and local governments exercise a great degree of influence over the practice of health care and occupational medicine in particular. Drug testing, Medicare, and occupational safety are only a few subjects addressed by a plethora of statutes, regulations, codes, and public laws. Appendix E section 2 describes databases containing health law information.

Other databases mentioned in Appendix E serve specific purposes. These databases are intended primarily for English-speaking audiences; however, many others exist worldwide, and Germany and Scandinavia produce their own public health and medical databases. To learn more about the availability of these databases, one should consult some of the sources listed in Appendix E section 7.9.

You will probably conclude that you need a computer search of the literature. Searching may be done with a knowledgeable librarian or through a personal computer. There are several mechanisms for doing this. It is possible to access the biomedical databases on your own computer system. Access may vary depending on physical location, institution, and other considerations.

With the advent of personal computing in the late 1970s and early 1980s, more Americans have come to use computers in both the workplace and the home. In 1981, 0.75 million computers existed in US homes. By 1988, this figure rose to 22.38 million units. In the workplace the figure stood at 1.24 million units in 1981 and increased to 20.33 million in 1988 [1]. This trend was reflected in the health sciences; greater numbers of physicians, nurses, and allied health practitioners became involved in database searches.

For more than a decade, access to particular databases, chiefly MEDLINE, has been available to individuals, without an intermediary. It is easy to search from the office, laboratory, or home. A personal computer and modem (telephone modulator-demodulator) are necessary to have access to these databases. SMARTCOM and PROCOMM are two examples of the sort of software that would need to be installed in your personal computer, with a modem. It is beyond the scope of this chapter to list other specific products. Access is available through almost all personal computing setups.

Increasingly, more hospital floors and departments, in addition to library facilities, possess on-site terminals for accessing at least the MEDLINE database. The options for this activity are varied and may be confusing to the amateur. It is recommended that you talk with experienced medical librarians, who will provide neutral information. This group is always available for further consultation. Many medical school libraries and some hospitals, as well as the Regional Medical Libraries, offer introductory classes and "getting-started" programs.

The scope of database searching has expanded since on-line searching began in the 1960s. Accessibility has been improved and expanded. One may now access a database such as MEDLINE through direct connection to the National Library of Medicine's MEDLARS system, or through Compact Disc, Read-Only Memory (CD-ROM) work stations, or through an Internet or Bitnet connection. A clear trend has been the increased access by health professionals over the past 15 years. Members of this user group now even write articles on the advantages of such activity. (For a sample reference, see [2].)

To connect to MEDLINE and many other databases (see Appendix E), you will have to establish an account with a vendor, or gain access through a campus or hospital network (a local area network [LAN]) or the Internet (essentially an international "electronic highway"). Some vendors, for example, the NLM (the Grateful Med System) and PAPERCHASE, allow access to various databases other than MEDLINE. This technology changes rapidly; what you read here may not be the final word.

Databases such as MEDLINE and TOXLINE files are available in a variety of modes alternative to the traditional computer modem hookup discussed above, for example, CD-ROM or the Internet, or through a professional database searcher.

Some of the services offered through vendors such as DIALOG or BRS/Colleague contain full text from specific journals or books, for example, the Comprehensive Core Medical Library (CCML). Full-text databases have the convenience of providing on-line the full text of documents, but searches in them will not find documents for which the full text is not available. Searching in full-text databases requires slightly modified methods, which are discussed in the next section.

It is beyond the scope and purpose of this chapter to compare vendors and their services in providing access to common databases such as MEDLINE and TOXLINE. Many of these databases are listed in Appendix E, which also provides guides to databases, including information on availability.

Search Strategies

At the outset of the literature research process, it is crucial to think about what you truly wish to accomplish, a process that will save cost and valuable time. How comprehensive must you be? Will you be satisfied to find just a sampling of information? How important is it that you find everything that has been reported on the subject? What will be the consequences, if after you have delivered the results of your search, somebody discovers an additional report with results contrary to those you found? What are your constraints on cost and time to be spent on the search? These questions, and others that you may develop, are important in structuring the search.

To logically search for information, a sound strategy is essential. After developing a basic strategy, to be most effective requires an understanding of the source of the data or the manner in which the data have been stored. The strategy should define the types of sources to retrieve, either primary or secondary.

Finally, what would the title of the perfect article be?

You may find no relevant documents in your initial search. Whether you should accept such a result depends on the purpose of your search. If your client is considering testifying under oath that there have been no known cases of association between a certain agent and a certain disease, the cross-examining counsel and his or her information specialists will do all they can to find a document reporting such an association. You have to search more thoroughly than they do. You are testing the validity of a negative proposition. You will have to use all your ingenuity to discover other terms to use in your search, and you will have to explore all the databases that might have anything on the subject. This extra searching will add significantly to the cost of your project, but the consequences of an incomplete and erroneous result may be worse.

You may find important documents in foreign languages. Do not be deterred; very often abstracts in English are available. Often, translations have already been made and are available from commercial suppliers. It is also possible to commission translations of technical documents. Vendors of these services are listed in Appendix E section 12. The cost of previously prepared translations is not great and they are available without undue delay. Commissioned translations are much more expensive and involve significant delay; if your budget allows it and if the results are important enough, however, you should not allow your search to be incomplete just because of language problems.

If cost is an important factor, you can economize by breaking your search into brief sessions in which you do not have to stop to think about the next steps of your search. Plan several search statements, go on-line, and give the commands without pausing to read the results beyond verifying that the commands were accepted. Download the results onto your disc as you search, and go off-line quickly before the charges have accumulated very much. Then at your leisure on your word processor you can peruse the results to prepare the next set of search commands. You can also use your word processor to extract quotations from the reports for use in your report of the results of the search. Significant savings can be realized by searching off-peak during nights and weekends.

You may be tempted to sit down immediately at the computer and start searching. It is prudent to make full use of information that others have already assembled on the subject. Do not "reinvent the wheel." Reference books should be considered part of the review process, even before you attempt to search the electronic databases. A review of basic medical textbooks can provide an overview of the problem. Occupational medicine texts may provide further clues to diseases of particular occupational groups. Do you know of an author who is preeminent in the field of study? This preliminary survey can help define the problem and can identify concepts and vocabulary terms that will facilitate the search.

When the electronic search is actually begun, you should first try to retrieve reviews and monographs on the subject; then go off-line and read them for further guidance in composing the search. Review articles attempt to summarize existing knowledge into a concise, compact form, and provide extensive bibliographies on the subject. Monographs are books or chapters in books. They are excellent starting points for becoming sufficiently familiar with a topic to complete a purposeful search.

After gathering initial information, you need to answer several questions to set the bounds of the search. For example, are only articles in English going to be included in the final review? Perhaps articles with English translations of abstracts would be sufficient to decide for each foreign-language article whether translating is justified. Should animal investigations be considered or are you only interested in human studies? Which sexes or age or ethnic groups are you interested in? How many years do you wish to search?

Next, select databases, using the information discussed in the previous section. Your choices should maximize the number of relevant sources that fit the case. A wide variety of sources should be considered and prioritized during the search process. Unless there is an obvious reason otherwise, *MEDLINE is an effective initial choice.*

With this preparation, you are ready to begin developing search statements. The syntax for search commands varies between databases and between vendors. Vendors supply manuals and quick reference guides for the databases they provide. It is beyond the scope of this chapter to provide a complete manual for writing search commands.

The need to search the literature can take two major forms in contemporary occupational medical practice: (1) A patient is noted to have a disease, and concern is raised as to whether exposure to an occupational or environmental hazard may have caused or contributed to the ailment, and (2) a person may have been exposed to a potentially hazardous agent and concern is raised about potential health implications, either currently or in the future. Other aspects of occupational medical practice also may require a facility to obtain information, but these two components of occupational experience, disease and a potentially hazardous agent, are the customary purview of a specialized occupational medical practice.

Thus, you will usually be seeking information involving a combination of subjects. For example, if you want information on the association between a disease and an agent, you would first request a search on the disease and then ask for a second search on the agent. Each of these commands would yield hundreds or thousands of "hits," that is, documents that satisfy the criteria of the search command. Your computer screen will display only the number of hits, the information you need to pursue your search. Thus, you might find thousands of documents dealing with the agent in which you are interested. A third search command to combine the results of the first two could take the form: "1 and 2," meaning that you want the documents that are included in both the results of search 1 and search 2. If search 3 results in a small enough number of hits that you would be interested in looking at them, or at least at their titles or their abstracts, you are ready to request a display of the documents. A set of 5 or 10 documents is a very useful result at this stage.

If you have zero hits, then either no information has been published on your subject, a circumstance over which you have no control, or you have been unduly restrictive in composing your search. Instead of searching on specific diseases and agents, search on a slightly broader category of each. When you examine this larger set of hits, you will develop ideas about making your search more specific again.

If you have too many hits to look at, it may prove useful to look at a few of them and to note what kind of irrelevant documents are being retrieved. Then you can make your search commands more specific, or perhaps introduce a third factor in your search to narrow it as to date, age of subjects, details about the nature of exposure, and so forth. It is quite feasible to extract useful information from a set of several hundred documents. You can request the computer to display only the titles and roll a hundred of them across the screen of your computer in only a few minutes, selecting those few for which you would like to read the abstract.

When you have completed this aspect of the search process and have identified a set of documents you wish to see, you can give the command to display various parts of the documents, such as bibliographic information (title, author, and source) and possibly the abstract. For many purposes the abstract is a sufficient end product of a search. You can obtain full copies of the documents in various ways. In some databases, full texts are available on-line. Some vendors offer to send hard copies of published documents. Cost of searching and availability of space on your disc may be important considerations, and, depending on proximity, it may be better to visit your nearest medical library and to examine the report in their stacks.

When you have completed your search, examine in detail the retrieved documents to note their relevance and to identify other search terms that would have been more effective. Feedback in searching is important, for improving the present search and for developing better techniques for future searching.

Searches in MEDLINE use the MeSH system in combination with free-text searching; searches in other databases use free-text searching.

Searching Using MeSH

The MEDLINE database and its print counterparts, the Index to Dental Literature, Index Medicus, and International Nursing Index, are constructed on a system of medical subject headings. When a journal article is indexed by indexers at the NLM, appropriate MeSH terms are applied. These terms are used to index the paper. There is basically no single correct way to index an article and retrieve it. Each paper is usually assigned about 10 MeSH terms; the indexer cannot assign more than 25. Thus, if a paper has information on more subjects than the indexer assigns, that information will escape your search. As a searcher, you should use as many subject headings as possible to broaden your search and, therefore, not miss anything. It is effective to supplement your search with free-text searching that utilizes natural language as opposed to subject headings.

As was mentioned previously, the MeSH exists in three components: the Annotated Alphabetical list, the Tree Structures, and the Permuted Headings. The Annotated List contains all medical subject headings in alphabetical order, which are revised annually to conform to changes in biomedical terminology. The Tree Structure is simply a system of arranging the medical subject headings from the Annotated List by subject category. This alphanumeric (Table 27-1) structure displays subjects in order from broad to specific. In Table 27-1, you will notice that the category is Digestive Diseases; more specific than that is Liver Diseases, followed by Hepatitis,

Table 27-1. An example of the Medical Subject Headings Tree Structure*

C6: Diseases–Digestive

Digestive system diseases

Liver diseases	C6.552			
Hepatitis				
Hepatitis, toxic				
Hepatitis, toxic	C6.552.380.615	C21.613.512		
Hepatitis, viral, human	C6.552.380.705	C2.440		
Delta infection	C6.552.380.705.270	C2.440.270		
Hepatitis A	C6.552.380.705.422	C2.440.420	C2.782.687.	
Hepatitis B	C6.552.380.705.437	C2.256.435	C2.440.435	
Hepatitis C	C6.552.380.705.440	C2.440.440		
Hepatitis, chronic active	C6.552.380.705.460	C2.440.460		
Hepatitis E	C6.552.380.705.470	C2.440.470		
Hepatolenticular degeneration	C6.552.413	C10.228.140. C18.452.648.	C10.228.140.	
Hepatomegaly	C6.552.446			
Hepatorenal syndrome	C6.552.465	C12.777.419.		
Hypertension, portal	C6.552.494	C14.907.489.		
Cruveilhier-Baumgarten syndrome	C6.552.494.250			
Esophageal and gastric varices	C6.552.494.414	C6.306.240	C14.907.489.	
Liver abscess	C6.552.597	C1.539.26.		
Liver abscess, amebic	C6.552.597.517	C3.518.600 C6.552.664.	C3.752.700.	
Liver cirrhosis	C6.552.630			
Liver cirrhosis, alcoholic	C6.552.630.380	C6.552.645.	C21.613.53.	
Liver cirrhosis, biliary	C6.552.630.400	C6.130.450. C23.888.498.	C6.552.150.	
Liver cirrhosis, experimental	C6.552.630.467			
Liver diseases, alcoholic	C6.552.645	C21.613.53.		
Fatty liver, alcoholic	C6.552.645.390	C6.552.241.	C21.613.53.	
Hepatitis, alcoholic	C6.552.645.490	C6.552.380.	C21.613.53.	
Liver cirrhosis, alcoholic	C6.552.645.590	C6.552.630.	C21.613.53.	
Liver diseases, parasitic	C6.552.664	C3.518		
Echinococcosis, hepatic	C6.552.664.272	C3.335.190.	C3.518.314	
Fascioliasis	C6.552.664.424	C3.335.865.	C3.518.424	
Liver abscess, amebic	C6.552.664.642	C3.518.600 C6.552.597.	C3.752.700.	
Liver neoplasms	C6.552.697	C4.588.274.		
Peliosis hepatis	C6.552.802			
Tuberculosis, hepatic	C6.552.933	C1.252.410.		
Zellweger's syndrome	C6.552.970	C10.228.140. C16.131.77.	C12.777.419.	
Pancreatic diseases	C6.689			
Cystic fibrosis	C6.689.202	C8.381.187	C16.614.213	
Pancreatic cyst	C6.689.500	C4.182.640		
Pancreatic pseudocyst	C6.689.500.692	C4.182.640.		
Pancreatic fistula	C6.689.583	C6.185.800	C23.439.185.	
Pancreatic insufficiency	C6.689.612			
Pancreatic neoplasms	C6.689.667			

*A portion of one of the 15 broad subject categories of the Tree Structure is shown. Opposite each heading is the alphanumeric code for that heading. This portion, on liver diseases, is used in the search in one of the cases discussed in the text.

Hepatitis-Toxic, and so on. You are able to group related terms together with the broader and more general terms higher in the tree.

You could make a search for a very specific disease by giving the command "C6.522.630.400" (see Table 27-1), which designates the disease: liver cirrhosis, biliary. You would obtain the same result by the command "liver cirrhosis, biliary". You could retrieve all kinds of articles and citations on liver cirrhosis by requesting each of the diseases, separated by the Boolean connector, "or"; the advantage of the Tree Structure, however, is that the single command "C6.552.630," will accomplish the same thing. The command will take different forms in various databases from various vendors. "C6.552.630+" or "C6.552.630$" means any code designation that starts with the characters "C6.552.630," no matter what follows. Similarly, all liver diseases could be retrieved by requesting "C6.552." This process of retrieving all the more specific terms under a tree word by entering the single heading is called "exploding." MeSH headings can be exploded by commands such as "exp liver-cirrhosis" or "exp C6.552.630" for various systems.

The Medical Subject Heading also employs subheadings (or qualifiers) to specifically pinpoint an aspect of a subject. The power of subheadings is that you may use one or many to refine a search. With the term *Hepatitis-Toxic* you could apply mortality, chemically induced, and immunology subheadings in addition to many others.

Additional tools to focus your search may include the use of major and minor descriptors, check tags (age of subjects, sex, animal type), and details on the nature of exposure and type of report. It is recommended that you consult the system manual of the MEDLINE system of your choice.

Free-Text Searching

Free-text searching has access to every word in each document in the database. This type of search has the advantage of retrieving words that an author used. However, a disadvantage is that you may not choose the terms the author used. This can be compensated for by examining documents already retrieved to identify words that authors in the field actually use.

This style of searching is effective in combination with subject heading searching, or when a subject is so new or rare that the only way to retrieve it is through free text, or in databases in which the MeSH system is not available. Both MeSH and free-text searching have strengths and weaknesses. The factors that contribute to this are varied. In searching any database it is prudent to try various commands, strategies, and techniques. No two searches or searchers are identical.

Searches may be executed using words anywhere in the documents. Information such as author, title, source of publication, data, and type of document are contained in *fields*. The search for "cirrhosis" would retrieve all documents containing that word anywhere in the document. It would even retrieve a document stating that a patient had *not* been examined for cirrhosis. Searches may be more restrictive by specifying the field in which the word must occur. For example, "cirrhosis.ti." would restrict the search to documents in which cirrhosis appears somewhere in the title. The search "cirrhosis.ti. and solvent$1.ti." would retrieve those articles in which the word "cirrhosis" appeared in the title and in which the words "solvent" or "solvents" appeared anywhere in the article. The combination of "cirrhosis.ti. and (carbon tetrachloride or methylethyl ketone)" would be restricted *only* to those two solvents.

Case Histories

We will illustrate the application of searching the literature by considering two cases of suspected occupational disease. The first case is a cluster of two women in whom cataracts appear to have developed after exposure to a workplace incident. In the second, a patient who was diagnosed with cirrhosis, but who had no history of alcoholism, is concerned about whether a recent high-dose exposure to certain solvents may have caused his problem.

Our clinical questions on cataracts and cirrhosis were searched in the MEDLINE database back to 1988 on a proprietary CD-ROM system developed from CD-PLUS, Inc. They were also searched back to 1966 in MEDLINE on the Bibliographic Retrieval Services (BRS) system. The search strategies, with document retrieval

Table 27-2. Search for cataracts in workers with occupational exposure to solvents

Search no.	Command*	No. of hits	Comments
1	exp cataract	1,861	
2	exp occupational-diseases	11,191	
3	exp occupational-exposure	1,998	There are 2 similar phrases on exposure in the MeSH headings.
4	2 or 3	12,597	Documents on either of the occupational phrases
5	1 and 4	23	Documents dealing with cataracts and occupational exposure or cataracts and occupational diseases

*"exp" means that the search is to be "exploded" to include the MeSH heading specified and all the more specific headings below it.

Table 27-3. Search for Crohn's disease and liver disease in workers with occupational exposure to solvents

Search no.	Command[a]	No. of hits	Comments
1	exp crohn-disease	2,276	
2	exp liver-cirrhosis	5,357	
3	exp liver-hepatitis	10,000	
4	exp occupational-diseases	11,191	
5	exp occupational-exposure	1,998	
6	exp butanones	228	The MeSH heading that includes methylethyl ketone
7	exp solvents	1,897	
8	exp carbon-tetrachloride	547	
9	exp carbon-tetrachloride-poisoning	308	Another MeSH heading
10	2 or 3	12,000	Documents on either cirrhosis or hepatitis
11	4 or 5	12,597	Either of the occupational phrases
12	6 or 7 or 8 or 9	2,935	Any of the 4 chemicals
13	1 and 10	37	Documents dealing with both Crohn's disease and hepatitis or cirrhosis
14	10 and 12	425	The 2 liver diseases and the chemicals
15	1 and 12	0	No hits on Crohn's disease and the 4 chemicals
16	11 and 14	10	The 2 liver diseases and either solvent

[a]"exp" means that the search is to be "exploded" to include the MeSH heading specified and all the more specific headings below it.

postings, have been reproduced in Tables 27-2 and 27-3 to illustrate how many citations were retrieved for each term.

Cataracts

You are asked to evaluate development of cataracts in two middle-aged women who work at the same plant in the same department. Concern has been raised at the facility as to whether the eye disorders may be related to exposure to various solvents that have been used in the adjacent work area. Neither woman has any underlying medical risk factors associated with cataracts, and neither has had any previous exposure to traditional occupational risks of developing cataracts. As an occupational physician, you are asked to investigate whether a relationship between the exposure and eye disorder is plausible.

We begin searching MEDLINE in CD-PLUS with the command "exp cataract" (search 1 in Table 27-2), yielding 1861 documents in which the MeSH indexers have assigned that heading. Searches 2 and 3 for occupational diseases and occupational exposure yield 11,191 and 1998 hits, respectively. Search 4 uses an "or" operator to combine all the documents that have either occupational phrase, yielding 12,597 hits. This is less than the sum of results 2 and 3 because some of the documents can contain both phrases. Search 5, "1 and 4," selects those documents, each of which deals with both cataracts and one or both of the occupational phrases, yielding 23 citations. Several of the citations involve the effects of light, especially laser light, and are apparently not relevant to the case at hand. One citation describes occupational morbidity of ore miners, evidently involving cataracts.

A similar search, not shown, of MEDLINE in the BRS system over a longer time period, 1966 to May 1993, yielded 180 hits. Restricting these further to documents dealing with solvents reduced the number to 21. Several among these were of interest. One study of 92 car painters exposed to organic solvents showed a significant increase in the occurrence of cataracts [3]. Another study found that the solvent acetone produces cataracts in guinea pigs [4]. An earlier study had shown that cataracts do not develop in rabbits on exposure to acetone [5].

Thus, we have found three reports that may be relevant to the cataract case. It would be well to ascertain what solvents were involved and to compare them with the ones treated in these three studies.

Liver Disease

Hepatitis develops in a patient who has worked in a chemical laboratory and was exposed to solvents for a few years. The hepatitis proves to be negative for an infectious cause such as hepatitis A or B or for transfusion-related hepatitis such as hepatitis C. The worker has abstained from alcohol since his early college days. He also suffers from Crohn's disease that is associated with a number of extraintestinal effects, including cirrhosis of the liver. This patient has worked for 5 years with methylethyl ketone and carbon tetrachloride.

In addressing hepatitis of potential occupational origin in the context of the patient with Crohn's disease and cirrhosis of the liver, a firm understanding of the basic pathophysiology of these disorders, their respective causes, and the relationships between them is essential to guide us in developing a search strategy. Reference to the *Merck Manual* (see Appendix E) establishes that Crohn's disease is a chronic inflammation of unknown etiology that affects any part of the gastrointestinal system and may affect other systems. Hepatitis is an inflammatory process of the liver. Some inflammatory conditions of the liver of unknown etiology are associated with Crohn's disease. Cirrhosis is a diffuse disorganization of hepatic structure by regenerative nodules surrounded by fibrotic tissue. Thus, we need to find any reports of association between Crohn's disease and either hepatitis or cirrhosis, and also association with exposure to methylethyl ketone or carbon tetrachloride, or more generally to similar solvents.

The liver disease search, which was more involved than the cataract search, is illustrated in Table 27-3 using the MEDLINE database. More terms were used and the retrievals were included in five sets (sets 12 through 16). First, we will search on the diseases, then on the exposure conditions, and then combine the results. We find the heading "Crohn's Disease" in the MeSH Tree Structure in a part of subcategory C6, Digestive System Diseases, different from that illustrated in Table 27-1.

Command number 1, "exp crohn-disease," yields the result that there are approximately 2000 documents with that MeSH heading in the database. Similarly, searches 2 and 3 on cirrhosis and hepatitis yield about 5000 and 10,000 hits, respectively. Searches 4 and 5 on occupational diseases and occupational exposure yield about 11,000 and 2000 hits, respectively. The term "methylethyl ketone" does not appear as an MeSH heading, but the Permuted Medical Subject Headings, Supplementary Chemical Records, reveal that it is one of several butanones under which it would be indexed by reviewers. Carbon tetrachloride appears in two headings, one on carbon tetrachloride poisoning. Searches 6, 7, 8, and 9 on the four chemicals yield about 200, 2000, 500, and 300 hits respectively. We have now introduced all the terms we will need for our search.

Search 10, using the "or" operator, combines all the documents dealing with either of the two liver diseases; the resulting 12,000 hits are less than the sum of hits 2 and 3 because many of the documents refer to both diseases. Search 11 combines documents dealing with either of the two occupational terms, with approximately 13,000 terms. Search 12 combines all documents dealing with any of the four chemicals, with about 3000 hits. We have now assembled all the documents into four sets: number 1 representing Crohn's disease, number 10 representing the two liver diseases, number 11 representing the two occupational conditions, and number 12 representing the four chemicals.

At this point, by use of the "and" operator, we select documents in which two or more terms are present in each document. Search 13 selects those documents, each of which mentions Crohn's disease and either or both of the two liver diseases, yielding about 35 hits. Search 14 selects documents dealing with the liver diseases and one or more of the four chemicals, yielding about 400 hits. Search 15 looks for documents dealing with Crohn's disease and any of the four chemicals, yielding no hits. Search 16 adds a further restriction to search 14 by requiring one of the occupational terms to be included, yielding 10 hits. We have now selected in results 13, 14, 15, and 16 a small number of documents dealing with these subjects in various useful combinations.

Result 13 has about 35 documents dealing with both Crohn's disease and either of the two liver diseases. This would be very useful if we were interested in pursuing this combination of diseases without restriction as to work environment; that is off the track of our objective, however. Result 15 indicates that the literature found so far has little to tell us about an association of Crohn's disease with our specific chemicals. However, a further search, not shown in the table, in the BRS version of MEDLINE covering a longer time period (1966 to May 1993) yielded two hits for Crohn's disease together with occupational exposure but without restriction as to liver diseases. One of them is an epidemiologic study seeking risk factors for Crohn's disease [6]. This report identified occupational risk factors for Crohn's disease, including exposure to unspecified solvents, and should be of interest to our occupational medicine professional dealing with this case. The document was not indexed by the MeSH indexers for solvents, although the word appeared in the abstract. This points up the advantage of supplementing an MeSH search with a free-text search.

Results 14 and 16 contain potentially useful information on the liver diseases in combination with our chemicals, but result 16 should have the richer concentration of relevant information. Examining the 10 titles in result 16 revealed two documents that would appear to be relevant [7, 8]. Thus, we have found three journal articles suggesting the association of Crohn's disease and the two liver diseases with occupational exposure to solvents.

References

1. Domestic Personal Computers and Use: 1981 to 1988. In *Statistical Abstract of the United States: 1992* (112th ed.). Washington, DC: US Bureau of the Census, 1992.
2. Kelly, J. A., and Hillson, S. D. Searching for answers. Using computers to find the literature you need for patient care. *Minn. Med.* 75:39, 1992.
3. Raitta, C., Husman, K., and Tossavainen, A. Lens changes in car painters exposed to a mixture of organic solvents. *Albrecht von Graefes Arch. fuer Ophthalmol.* 200:149, 1976.
4. Taylor, A., et al. Relationships between acetone, cataracts and ascorbate in hairless guinea pigs. *Ophthalmic Res.* 25:30, 1993.

5. Rengstorff, R., Petrali, J., and Sim, V. Attempt to induce cataracts by cutaneous application of acetone. *Am. J. Optom. Physiol. Opt.* 53:41, 1976.
6. Lashner, B. A. Risk factors for small bowel cancer in Crohn's disease. *Dig. Dis. Sci.* 37:1179, 1992.
7. Bode, J. C., and Kuhn, C., Liver damage from organic solvents. *Deutsche Med. Wochenschr.* 117:1127, 1992.
8. Chen, J. D., et al. Exposure to mixtures of solvents among paint workers and biochemical alterations of liver function. *Br. J. Ind. Med.* 48:696, 1991.

Further Information

See Appendix E of this text for a detailed listing of books, references, and monographs available for searching a topic in occupational and environmental medicine.

See Chapter 36, Computers in Occupational Medical Practice for a discussion on the proper use of a computer system in accessing medical information.

28 Ergonomics

J. Steven Moore

Ergonomics is a broad field that covers issues such as biomechanics, work physiology, anthropometry, and man-machine interfaces. In terms of occupational medicine, ergonomics is most recognized as a discipline related to musculoskeletal disorders. Low back pain among workers has been recognized and studied for decades. In the 1980s, upper-extremity disorders, especially carpal tunnel syndrome, became a major concern for employers, employees, insurance providers, and health care providers. Unfortunately, scientific knowledge about these disorders and their causes is often limited, published in an unmanageable variety of journals, and follows the development (and sometimes the fixation) of beliefs. One purpose of this chapter is to provide readers with contemporary knowledge about the low back and upper extremity as they relate to work. The reader is cautioned, however, that knowledge is still growing. As a result, it may be necessary to reexamine one's theories and beliefs so that the current models used to analyze or rationalize the occurrence of musculoskeletal disorders among workers are consistent with valid observations.

As an adjective or adverb, the word *ergonomics* implies something favorable, for example, an ergonomically designed work station is good. It is a lack of ergonomic considerations that increases risk of discomfort or injury. As a result, there is no such thing as an *ergonomic disorder* because an ergonomically designed job would not have caused such a disorder.

A deficiency in ergonomic design or work organization may lead to the presence of risk factors, such as low back pain risk factors. Overexposure to these risk factors may contribute to a worker developing low back pain. These low back pain risk factors are not ergonomic factors. In ergonomics, risk factors are external sources of *stress* to the worker, and are often called *stressors*. The effect of such stresses on the body is called *strain*. For example, the strength requirements of a job reflect a stressor, while an overexertion injury would represent a manifestation of the strain.

In this chapter, we discuss ergonomics from the perspective of a physician. You may need to apply ergonomic knowledge and skills in the course of managing workers with musculoskeletal disorders, performing plant walk-throughs or serving as a member of an ergonomics team. In particular, we emphasize upper-extremity disorders and low back pain. The areas of ergonomics that correspond to this clinical context are called *occupational biomechanics* and *work physiology*. Like industrial hygiene, these are disciplines that emphasize assessment of exposure (stress), not disease (strain). The ergonomist can characterize the biomechanical and physiologic stresses of a job by using a variety of tools to estimate "exposure." Under ideal conditions, this estimate of exposure (akin to dose in toxicology) could be applied to a dose-response curve that would predict the risk of developing a corresponding disorder. Assessment of the effects of the job, such as the occurrence of a musculoskeletal condition, review of the Occupational Safety and Health Administration (OSHA) 200 Logs, or a symptom survey, reflects the response portion of the dose-response curve.

In practicing occupational medicine, several instances warrant consideration of exposure data as they relate to ergonomics, including determining work-relatedness and managing return to work. Musculoskeletal disorders are common and are not always related to employment. As a result, the physical demands of the job affect the determination of whether the condition was caused or aggravated by work—in essence, an exposure assessment. The exposure assessment defines whether a hazardous condition is present or absent, not the case itself. In assessing a person's ability to return to work, the physician should attempt to compare the physical capabilities of the patient with the physical demands of the job. Again, an exposure assessment is required.

In this chapter, we discuss principles and tools available for estimating exposure to the upper extremities and back. The purpose of this chapter is to acquaint practitioners with the fundamentals of occupational biomechanics so that they will be able to (1) understand the ergonomically related risk factors for certain types of musculoskeletal disorders and (2) develop a fundamental approach for the recognition and estimation of these risk factors, such as when conducting a walk-through survey or viewing a videotape.

Upper Extremity Disorders

To date, the evaluation of ergonomically related exposures to the upper extremity has focused on determining the presence of one or more generic risk factors [1–4]. Since there have been no guidelines for quantifying the intensity or degree of these risk factors, ergonomics evolved along the lines of subjective estimates of the importance of these stressors. Upper extremity exposure assessment lacks standardization. As a result, there are significant debates regarding whether ergonomic exposures are causally associated with upper extremity disorders, especially carpal tunnel syndrome [5–9]. Until further research is published and exposure analysis tools are validated, the assessment of upper extremity disorders will likely remain controversial. However, it is important for the occupational physician to develop a sense of context into which these disorders have been observed. In this section, we review the epidemiologic context of upper extremity disorders and physiologic and biomechanical models for estimating stresses to the upper extremity.

The Epidemiologic Context

As summarized in Table 28-1, several studies have been published that describe the spectrum of disorders associated with jobs or tasks that are believed to be hazardous to the upper extremities [10, 11]. These disorders are largely grouped into two categories: disorders of the muscle-tendon unit (tenosynovitis, peritendinitis, epicondylitis, etc.) and disorders of the nervous system (carpal tunnel syndrome, cervical spondylosis, etc.). Taken as a whole, these studies consistently demonstrate that disorders of the muscle-tendon unit are much more common than carpal tunnel syndrome and that carpal tunnel syndrome that is believed to be causally associated with work activities is almost always associated with other muscle-tendon unit

Table 28-1. Number and type of disorders reported in previous studies of upper-extremity morbidity

Study	Total disorders (no.)	Muscle-tendon* disorders (%)	CTS (%)
Hymovich and Lindholm (1966)	62	100	0
Ferguson (1971)	62	95	5
Kuorinka and Koskinen (1979)	17	100	0
Luopajarvi et al. (1979)	89	95	5
Armstrong and Langholf (1982)	78	87	13
Armstrong et al. (1982)	32	93	7
Viikari-Juntura (1983)	6	80	20
Silverstein (1985)	43	52	48
Amadio and Russoti (1990)	20	67	33
Moore and Garg (1993)	104	83	21

Key: CTS = carpal tunnel syndrome.
*Disorders of the muscle-tendon unit include some specific conditions, such as stenosing tenosynovitis, epicondylitis, peritendinitis, etc., and may include nonspecific conditions, such as hand-wrist pain.
Source: Adapted from J. S. Moore and A. Garg. The Spectrum of Upper Extremity Disorders Associated with Hazardous Work Tasks. In S. Kumar (ed.), *Advances in Industrial Ergonomics and Safety IV*. London, Taylor & Francis, 1992. Pp. 723–730.

disorders in the same individual or among other workers performing the same task [10, 11].

A Physiologic Model—Localized Muscle Fatigue

The physiologic model for assessment of upper-extremity exposures emphasizes minimizing localized muscle fatigue. Simonson [12] defined fatigue as the transient loss of work capacity resulting from preceding work. Localized muscle fatigue is a reversible physiologic state. Its exact cause is unknown, but may involve accumulation of waste products, depletion of energy reserves, or hypoxemia secondary to impaired blood flow into the contracted muscle [12]. Symptoms of localized muscle fatigue may include a sensation of exhaustion, discomfort, or fatigue; increased perceived exertion; decreased strength; and loss of neuromuscular control [13]. In addition, there are electromyographic manifestations of localized muscle fatigue that generally follow, rather than precede, the above symptoms [13].

Localized muscle fatigue is most commonly observed in the context of concentric or static work. A concentric activation of a muscle-tendon unit implies that the muscle shortens during the contractile phase. When curling a weight with the arm, the lifting phase (flexing the elbow) represents concentric activation of the biceps and brachialis muscles. In contrast, an eccentric exertion is one in which the muscle lengthens despite contraction. The eccentric component of the curling task is represented by lowering the weight (extending the elbow). Static work represents isometric contraction, that is, the muscle neither shortens nor lengthens. This would be represented by holding the weight at some fixed elbow angle. The onset of localized muscle fatigue takes longer to develop with dynamic than with static work [14].

Rohmert [15] studied localized muscle fatigue from the perspective of static isometric exertions. He demonstrated that the onset and degree of localized muscle fatigue is dependent upon the intensity of the exertion, expressed as percent maximal force, and the duration of the exertion. The definition of percent maximal force is represented by equation (1). It is important to note that the required force and worker's maximal force are task specific; that is, if the task requires gripping with the wrist flexed 45 degrees, the worker's maximal grip strength would have to be estimated or measured with the wrist flexed 45 degrees.

$$\% \ Maximal \ force \ = \ required \ force \ \div \ worker's \ maximal \ force \qquad (1)$$

The concept of percent maximal force is important. In general, strain increases and work capacity decreases with increasing percent maximal strength. In addition, strain increases and work capacity decreases with increasing duration of exertion. Let's consider a hypothetical task—carrying a heavy suitcase through the airport. Suppose it is determined that this task requires 50 lb grip force to hold the suitcase. For a traveller with 100 lb maximal grip force, the strength demand would be 50% maximal force. At this level of exertion, localized muscle fatigue would start to develop in about 1 minute. If the duration of the exertion is less than 1 minute, the traveler would not experience any effects of fatigue; however, if the exertion lasts longer, the traveler might perceive that it is a little more difficult to maintain the same grip force and may ultimately begin to lose grip strength, so that the suitcase might slip out of his/her hand.

In contrast, consider another person with only 50 lb maximal force (perhaps due to genetic endowment, gender, or impairment), who would be working at 100% capacity. At this level of exertion, the maximum duration of exertion is only 6 seconds. As a result, this person would experience a greater degree of strain in a shorter period of time and have a significantly reduced work capacity compared to the other traveler. This person would lift the suitcase, walk a few steps, then either drop or set the suitcase down and rest (to recover from the localized muscle fatigue). Once recovered, the person could again attempt to grasp, lift, and carry the suitcase, but would only last a few seconds. In this circumstance, this person should rent a luggage cart—an example of an *engineering control*.

Overall, the concept of percent maximal force is useful because it takes into account factors that affect either the numerator (required strength) or the denominator (worker's maximal strength). Some factors may increase the numerator, thus increasing the percent maximal force, for example, cold temperature, poorly fitting gloves, or use of a vibrating handheld tool. Other factors may reduce the denominator, also increasing the percent maximal force, for example, individual variability, gender, age, impairment, or awkward posture.

Mathematically, percent maximal force and duration of exertion are exponentially related [15] (Fig. 28-1). At very high percent maximal forces, the maximum duration of exertion is measured in seconds. At levels of percent maximal strength below 15%, it is possible to maintain this exertion for up to 10 minutes without developing localized muscle fatigue [15].

Aside from studying the onset of fatigue, Rohmert [15] also investigated recovery from fatigue. He developed a series of mathematical equations that allowed one to calculate the rest period required to recover from localized fatigue. For example, consider a gripping task that requires 50% maximal force to be maintained for 1 minute. According to Rohmert's equations, this would require a 10-minute rest interval to return to full capacity for work. Since the duration of exertion is 1 minute and the rest period is 10 minutes, the minimum cycle time for this task would be 11 minutes. This corresponds to a frequency of approximately 5.5 exertions per hour.

Dr. Suzanne Rodgers [16, 17] has developed a job analysis methodology based on Rohmert's work in localized muscle fatigue. As shown on her Ergonomic Job Analysis Form (Fig. 28-2), three critical variables in her system correspond to the variables described above. First, it is necessary to estimate the *intensity of effort* required by the job (the percent maximal force). Dr. Rodgers has defined three levels of effort for the major muscle groups of the body: "1" = light, "2" = moderate, and "3" = heavy. Her second variable is called *continuous effort time*. This variable corresponds to the duration of holding time (duration of exertion) and also has three rankings: "1" = < 6 seconds, "2" = 6–20 seconds, and "3" = > 20 seconds. Finally, Dr. Rodgers includes a category called *efforts per minute:* "1" = < 1/min, "2" = 1–5/min, and "3" = > 5–15/min.

Consider the following example: A job involves crimping two leads on an electronic subassembly. The work is delivered via conveyor at a rate of four subassemblies per

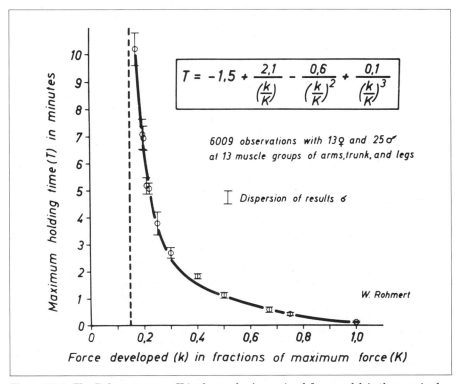

$$T = -1,5 + \frac{2,1}{\left(\frac{k}{K}\right)} - \frac{0,6}{\left(\frac{k}{K}\right)^2} + \frac{0,1}{\left(\frac{k}{K}\right)^3}$$

6009 observations with 13♀ and 25♂
at 13 muscle groups of arms, trunk, and legs

⊥ Dispersion of results ♂

W. Rohmert

Maximum holding time (T) in minutes

Force developed (k) in fractions of maximum force (K)

Figure 28-1. The Rohmert curve. K is the worker's maximal force and k is the required force for the task. The percent maximal force equals $100 \times k/K$. (From W. Rohmert. Physiologische Grundlagen der Erholungszeitbestimmung. *Zbl. Arb. Wiss* 19:1, 1965.)

Ergonomic Job Analysis

Body Part	Effort Level	Continuous Effort Time	Efforts/ Minute	Priority	Effort Categories
Neck/Shoulders	R ___ L ___	___ ___	___ ___	___ ___	1 = Light 2 = Moderate 3 = Heavy
Back	___	___	___	___	Continuous Effort Time Categories 1 = < 6 sec
Arms/Elbows	R ___ L ___	___ ___	___ ___	___ ___	2 = 6 to 20 sec 3 = > 20 sec
Wrists/Hands/ Fingers	R ___ L ___	___ ___	___ ___	___ ___	Efforts/Minute Categories
Legs/Knees	R ___ L ___	___ ___	___ ___	___ ___	1 = < 1/min 2 = 1 to 5/min 3 = > 5–15/min
Ankles/Feet/Toes	R ___ L ___	___ ___	___ ___	___ ___	

Priority for Change

Moderate =	123 132 213 222 231 232 312	Job Title: _____ Specific Task: _____ Job Number: _____ Department: _____ Location: _____
High =	223 313 321 322	Contact Person(s) _____ Phone: _____ Analyst: _____ Phone: _____
Very High =	323 331 332	Date of Analysis: _____

Figure 28-2. The Ergonomic Job Analysis Form used in Dr. Rodger's physiologic model. (From S. H. Rodgers. A functional job analysis technique. *Occup. Med. State of the Art Rev.* 7:679, 1992.)

minute. Worker feedback reveals that the intensity of effort is most appropriately rated as "2" (moderate). Using a videotape and stopwatch, you determine that duration of exertion (squeezing the handle of the crimping tool) is generally 2 seconds. As a result, the continuous effort time is rated as "1" since the duration of exertion is less than 6 seconds. The efforts per minute rating is "3" because there are eight exertions per minute (4 subassemblies with 2 leads per subassembly). As a result, this job is rated as "213." This corresponds to a "moderate" *priority for change* (other priority levels include "high" and "very high"). This system is also useful because it identifies the variables that would primarily improve the job. In this case, lowering the intensity of effort ranking to "1" or reducing the effort per minute ranking to "2" or "1" would eliminate it being assigned a priority for change rating.

While Dr. Rodgers' job analysis methodology appears functional in the field, there are no published validation studies to assess whether it is accurate, reproducible, and reliable. In addition, Dr. Rodgers' methodology is not designed to classify a job as hazardous or safe. Rather, the rating scheme is used to rank jobs in terms of priority for change. As a result, it may not be appropriate to use this tool to determine the work-relatedness of a particular condition or to predict risk of injury among exposed workers.

Another area of controversy regarding localized muscle fatigue is whether localized muscle fatigue has any relationship to disorders of the muscle-tendon units. In some instances, fatigue has been associated with tenosynovitis and peritendinitis; however, other mechanisms, such as blunt trauma followed by repetitive work, do not involve localized muscle fatigue. In the relationship with delayed-onset muscle soreness or nerve entrapment syndromes, such as carpal tunnel syndrome, the role of fatigue is unclear [18]. As a result, it is uncertain whether prevention of localized muscle fatigue would prevent most upper-extremity disorders identified by practitioners.

A Biomechanical Model

A muscle-tendon unit is comprised of an origin in bone, a proximal bone-tendon junction, tendon (usually called an aponeurosis near the origin), a proximal myotendinous junction, muscle tissue, a distal myotendinous junction, cord-like tendon tissue, a distal tendon-bone junction, and the bone of insertion. The responses of a muscle-tendon unit to stretching and compression have been reviewed and summarized [18]. If the two ends of the muscle-tendon unit are anchored, the forces along the longitudinal axis of the muscle-tendon unit can be increased by either increasing the contractile force of the muscle or stretching the two ends apart. Both of these circumstances produce *tensile load*. Numerous studies have examined the elastic characteristics of the muscle-tendon unit in the context of increasing tensile load to the point of failure as well as repeated applications of tensile load of various magnitudes. In terms of its elastic properties, connective tissue exhibits an *elastic limit*. If the tensile loads are below this limit, the tissue recovers to its original state without permanent deformation. However, if tensile loads exceed this limit, the structure is permanently stretched, or deformed, and does not return to its resting state. In terms of the tendinous tissue of a muscle-tendon unit, either the aponeurosis or the cord-like structure distally, physiologic levels of exertion are unlikely to exceed the elastic limit of the tendinous tissue; however, experimental data suggest that the myotendinous junction may be weaker than the tendinous tissue. In terms of a biomechanical model, it would be ideal if we could estimate the tensile load of individual muscle-tendon units. This process would require estimating the *magnitude of the applied tensile force* (a sum of the contractile force of the muscle plus the tensile force related to stretching of the muscle-tendon unit), the *duration of the applied force*, the *duration of the recovery period* to allow the tissues to return to their normal state, the *strain rate* or speed of increasing tensile force, and the *number of cycles* that the muscle-tendon unit is subjected to tensile load [18]. At this time, there is no feasible means of measuring the tensile load within the muscle-tendon unit in vivo.

The muscle-tendon unit is also exposed to a second type of force, called *compressive force*. This force acts perpendicular to the longitudinal axis of the muscle-tendon unit. Compressive forces can be categorized into extrinsic and intrinsic components [18]. Consider the compressive forces on the digital flexor tendons related to forcefully grasping a square-handled screwdriver. The edge of the square handle will be a source of *extrinsic compression* that is transmitted through the skin and subcutaneous tissue to the surface of the tendon and perhaps its tendon sheath. Blunt traumatic injuries are also examples of extrinsic compression, except that the time interval of the applied force is usually brief and much more localized.

As shown in Fig. 28-3, compressive forces may also arise from within. Consider the forces placed on the digital flexor tendons when the wrist is flexed or extended well beyond neutral posture. This can be modeled by a rope and pulley. Sources of compression arise where these flexor tendons rest against the flexor retinaculum or the carpal bones and associated structures. In estimating the magnitude of intrinsic compressive forces, it is necessary to know the *intensity of the tensile load* on the muscle-tendon unit, the *radius of curvature* of the surface around which the tendons angle, and the *length of arc of contact*. As a result, *intrinsic compressive forces* are related to the application of forces with deviated postures.

Aside from compressive forces, which can exist in static situations, a third type of interaction occurs when it is desired to move the tendon back and forth across an angled surface. In this situation, *frictional force* becomes important. Since most

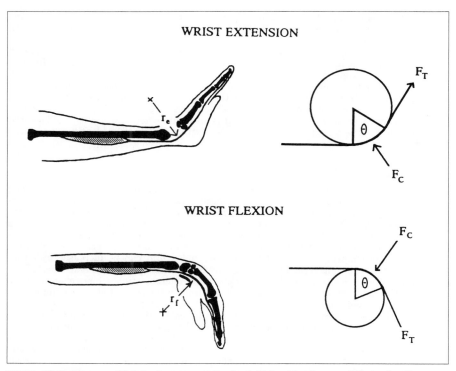

Figure 28-3. Sources of intrinsic compressive load (F_C) on tendons and their sheaths. F_T = tensile load. (From J. S. Moore. Function, structure, and responses of components of the muscle-tendon unit. *Occup. Med. State of the Art Rev.* 7:713, 1992.

tendons in the distal upper extremity are covered with sheaths as they cross joints, frictional forces are reduced by the low coefficient of friction of synovial fluid. If synovial fluid loses its viscous characteristics, the coefficient of friction could rise and lead to irritation of the tendon or its sheath across the deviated joint. The magnitude of the frictional force is related to the compressive force times the coefficient of friction.

Moore and Garg [19] are investigating a biomechanical model for estimating exposures to the distal upper extremity. The model is summarized in the following equation:

Strain index (SI) =
            F (force, duration of exertion, posture, efforts/min, speed, duration)   (2)

As in the model for localized muscle fatigue, force is estimated in terms of percent maximal force and is used to reflect the strain related to the tensile load in the muscle-tendon unit. Compressive forces are considered by adding an additional variable for posture. Additional variables include duration of exertion per work cycle, efforts per minute, and a variable that considers effects related to speed of work. As with the localized muscle fatigue model, this biomechanical model has not yet undergone thorough validation. This model will allow the user to identify the maximum sources of stressors to the upper extremity so that interventions can be appropriately targeted. In addition, preliminary results suggest that the model can be applied as a risk assessment tool. As a result, it is hoped that this model will enable physicians to incorporate exposure estimates into determinations of work-relatedness and provide a means of defining a job that does not need intervention, thereby allowing scarce resources to be applied appropriately to jobs that pose significant risk.

Generic Risk Factors

At this time, the most common method to analyze the ergonomic exposures of a job for the upper extremities involves the use of generic risk factors [1–4]. These risk factors are summarized in Table 28-2.

Force

The importance of force was demonstrated by incorporating variables of percent maximal strength into both the physiologic and biomechanical models. In addition, Silverstein and associates [20] demonstrated that risk of upper-extremity disorders was associated with increasingly forceful exertions. Moore and Garg [19] also observed that the forcefulness of jobs was the only exposure variable that was statistically significantly different between jobs associated with upper-extremity morbidity and jobs that were not associated with upper-extremity morbidity. Other measured variables, such as posture, cycle time, frequency, duration of exertion, percent exertion per cycle, duration of recovery, and percent recovery per cycle, were not statistically significantly different between these two groups. As a result, the *forcefulness* of a task may be the most significant risk factor.

Posture

Intrinsic compression forces are related to the magnitude of the tensile loads plus the effects of deviated postures. Awkward postures also affect maximal force. For example, assume a person has a grip force of 100 lb when measured with the wrist in neutral position. The maximal grip force decreases to approximately 60 lb if the wrist is flexed 45 degrees and decreases to approximately 75 lb if the wrist is extended 45 degrees; that is, maximal force decreases [21]. As a result, a significantly deviated wrist adversely affects the forcefulness of the task by increasing the percent maximal strength. This effect is demonstrated in Fig. 28-4. Current observations suggest that high or repeated compressive loads are the most probable explanations for disruptions of tendinous tissue (supraspinatus tendinitis) and disorders of the tendon sheath (DeQuervain's tenosynovitis and stenosing tenosynovitis of the digits) [18].

Posture also includes the *type of grasp* used to complete the task. Tensile loads of the flexor tendons to the fingers are much greater when using pinch grasp than power grasp [22]. As a result, posture, defined as type of grasp, also affects the magnitude of the forcefulness of the task.

In the distal upper extremity, posture alone may not be a significant risk factor in the development of disorders of the muscle-tendon unit. In the study of Silverstein and associates [20], neither wrist posture nor type of grasp was significantly associated with the prevalence of symptoms or disorders of the upper extremity. A similar finding was noted by Moore and Garg [19]. Given these observations, posture may primarily be important in its effects on the forcefulness of a job and, in particular, on its effects on increasing the tensile loads and compressive forces on varying components of the muscle-tendon unit.

Deviated wrist postures have also been associated with increased pressures in the carpal tunnel [23]. Control subjects, on average, had low carpal canal pressures in neutral posture (approximately 2.2 mmHg) and moderate increases in carpal canal pressure with extreme deviations of the wrist (approximately 30 mmHg). By contrast, patients with carpal tunnel syndrome (CTS), on average, have significantly elevated resting pressures (approximately 30 mmHg) as well as more marked excursions in pressure with similar degrees of wrist deviations (approximately 90

Table 28-2. Generic risk factors for upper-extremity disorders

Force
    Use of vibrating tools
    Cold temperature
    Poorly fitting or improper gloves
Repetitiveness
Posture
Localized mechanical compression

Source: Adapted from T. J. Armstrong. *An Ergonomics Guide to Carpal Tunnel Syndrome.* Cincinnati: American Industrial Hygiene Association, 1983.

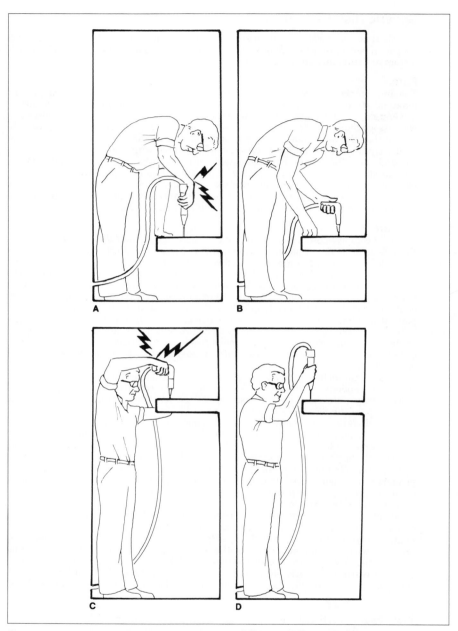

Figure 28-4. Effects of posture on the worker. In A and C, the deviated wrist is a source of intrinsic compression on the loaded flexor and extensor tendons that cross the wrist. In addition, the deviated posture reduces the worker's maximal grip force. It is noted that these stressors arise from the way the tool is used, not the tool per se. (From Health and Safety Department. *Strains and Sprains, A Worker's Guide to Job Design.* United Auto Workers, 1982.)

mmHg). Although this study demonstrates a difference between cases with carpal tunnel syndrome versus controls, it does *not* demonstrate a causal association between deviated wrist posture and the development of carpal tunnel syndrome.

Other work has shown that the *symptoms* of CTS are significantly associated with the magnitude of the pressure in the carpal canal and that these symptoms are likely a reversible manifestation of ischemia [24]. The data suggest that there is a *threshold of carpal canal pressure* below which one does not experience ischemia and, therefore, no symptoms (numbness and tingling) are present. Above this threshold, however, ischemia occurs and leads to symptoms. When the carpal canal pressure subsequently drops below the threshold, the ischemia and symptoms resolve. Considering the data of Gelberman and associates [23], people with CTS are more likely to cross this threshold than those without CTS. In addition, symptoms will probably develop whenever their wrists are held in a deviated posture for a sufficient period of time, whether at work or at home. As a result, activities associated with symptoms, such as sleep or driving, do not necessarily correlate with activities that may have caused the CTS. To infer causation or aggravation of CTS-based symptoms at work is naive. In terms of medical management, physicians often recommend wrist braces at night, which minimize symptoms; that is, the braces prevent assuming extreme wrist postures during sleep so that the carpal canal pressure is kept below the ischemia threshold. *Preventing the symptoms of CTS is quite different from preventing the development of carpal tunnel syndrome.* The indiscriminate use of wrist braces during work, especially when the work is associated with dextrous use of the wrist and hand as opposed to the extremes of wrist posture reported in the literature, may actually aggravate the problem.

Repetitiveness

A third generic risk factor for upper-extremity disorders is *repetitiveness*. Another way of thinking of this risk factor is in terms of the time characteristics of the job tasks. The durations of *exertion* and *rest* were both considered important in the physiologic model for localized muscle fatigue. Both of these variables have potential relevance in the biomechanical model. In the study by Silverstein and associates [20], "high repetitiveness" was defined as a cycle time greater than 30 seconds or performance of a fundamental cycle that lasted more than 50% of the cycle time. A job without either of these attributes was defined as "low repetitiveness." This definition of repetitiveness proved to be a significant predictor for risk of upper-extremity symptoms and disorders. However, defining exposures in terms of "high force" and "low force," in combination with these two levels of repetitiveness, was most appropriate. By contrast, Moore and Garg [19] noted that Silverstein and colleagues' definition of high versus low repetitiveness did not discriminate jobs that were not associated with upper-extremity morbidity. As a result, the *temporal characteristics* of a task are important, but must be considered in the context of the *forcefulness of the exertions* involved in the task.

Use of Vibrating Tools

Vibration has also been cited as a generic risk factor for upper-extremity disorders [1–3]. While the vibration characteristics of a handheld tool are causally associated with the development of hand-arm vibration syndrome, the role of vibration in the development of other upper-extremity disorders is less clear. A more accurate statement would be that upper-extremity disorders are associated with the *use of the hand to use vibrating tools*. Use of any tool, including a vibrating tool, implies that the tool must be held, grasped, activated, and applied to the piece or part. As a result, there are forces associated with the grasping, triggering, and applying of the tool to the part of interest. At times, a task may require a mechanically disadvantageous grasp or the use of an awkward posture, as shown in Fig. 28-4. As a result, the use of the tool would again be characterized in terms of forcefulness, posture, and the time characteristics of the hand use. Vibration per se may increase the forcefulness of a work task by two mechanisms: the tonic vibration reflex and impaired sensory feedback [1]. As a result, the fact that the tool vibrates only modifies the forcefulness of the task.

Other Modifying Factors

Cold temperatures and poorly fitting gloves can also modify the forcefulness of a task [1–3], since both impair sensory feedback regarding the forcefulness of the exertion. As a result, a person may grasp an object harder than is actually required, increasing forcefulness of the task. Neither of these factors is an independent risk factor for developing upper-extremity disorders. In fact, gloves may actually decrease the forcefulness of a task by improving the coefficient of friction.

Localized Mechanical Compression

Localized mechanical compression, the final generic risk factor, has been associated with compression of the thenar branch of the median nerve and, as a result, partial thenar atrophy, often without paresthesias [11]. The pathogenesis of this condition is believed to be related to the localized compression placed on this thenar branch as it exits the carpal tunnel by handheld tools that concentrate stresses in the area between the thenar and hypothenar eminences. Examples of localized mechanical compression of this nature involve using the palm of the hand as a hammer, such as when chiseling, where the end of the chisel fits within the space between the thenar eminences. Forcefully pressing on a screwdriver while inserting a difficult screw is another example.

Localized compressive forces are also important sources of extrinsic compression on the tendons and may cause trigger finger or trigger thumb [18]. Considering our previous analogy of the square-handled screwdriver, the edges would cause localized compression over the tendons or tendon sheaths and, as a secondary reaction, stenosing tenosynovitis of these flexor tendons. Whether placement of the volar surface of the wrist against a desk might also represent localized mechanical compression and, therefore, contribute to risk of CTS is unclear, but has not been shown to be a significant factor to date.

Summary

In this section, we have attempted to review current knowledge regarding ergonomic assessment of jobs for risk of upper-extremity disorders. Since knowledge in this area is evolving, the astute occupational physician should be aware of the epidemiologic setting within which upper-extremity disorders, especially CTS, occur. These settings may provide clues to understanding the association between the reported disorders and the work. In addition, two models of exposure assessment have been presented: a *physiologic model* derived from experimental observations from the laboratory and a *biomechanical model* based on laboratory and epidemiologic observations. Both models have merit, but neither has been sufficiently validated to predict whether a task poses a risk of injury to the upper extremity.

In general, contemporary exposure analysis for the upper extremity involves the subjective assessment of generic risk factors. The job evaluator should have some qualitative sense of to what degree these factors should be present before they become areas of concern. At this time, there is no feasible means to "calibrate" job evaluators so that their analyses would be accurate or consistent. As a result, there is often controversy because there may be insufficient understanding regarding how these generic risk factors actually affect risk of injury. It is common to see individuals unfamiliar with the work ascribe the hazard potential to the job's repetitiveness characteristics or posture. Neither of these factors alone, however, is a sufficient basis for such an attribution.

Ergonomic Considerations of Low Back Pain

We will discuss the ergonomics of low back pain in terms of its epidemiologic context and physiologic and biomechanical models. (See Chap. 12, Musculoskeletal Disorders, for a discussion of the diagnosis, treatment, and rehabilitation of back disorders.) The likelihood of identifying a specific cause for a patient's low back pain is approximately 5 to 10%; a definite structural diagnosis can be reached in no more than 50% of all cases [25, 26]. By contrast, it is usually possible to localize the signs and symptoms of an upper-extremity disorder to a particular muscle-tendon unit. In terms of job analysis, the available tools for upper-extremity exposure assessment are qualitative, subjective, and largely unvalidated. For the lower back, the available tools are more sophisticated, quantitative, and better validated.

Epidemiologic Context

There have been several recent comprehensive reviews of the epidemiology of low back pain [27, 28]. Approximately 10 to 17% of adults will have an episode of *back pain* each year. *Low back pain* is the second most common cause for physician visits and is the most common cause for decrease in work capacity among people aged 25 to 44 years. About 2% of all employees will have a *compensable back injury* each year. These injuries are associated with approximately 29 days lost per hundred workers per year. Low back injuries account for 21% of all injuries and illnesses in the workplace, but 33% of the workers' compensation payments and medical costs each year. *Overexertion* is considered the most common cause, with about 1 in 24 workers suffering an overexertion injury per year. Overexertion has been associated with 25% of all reported injuries. Sixty-seven percent of overexertion injury claims involve lifting, while 20% involve pulling or pushing. Sixty percent of people with low back pain report that overexertion was the cause. People with low back pain from overexertion, who have significant time loss from work, have a poor prognosis for return to their original job.

The exact anatomic cause for most forms of low back pain is unclear. One possible source could be a muscle strain. Recent studies suggest that muscle strains represent acute failure at the myotendinous junctions [29, 30]. These failures are believed to be associated with extremely high tensile loads in the muscle-tendon units. In general, these extreme tensile loads would be most likely associated with forceful eccentric actions of a muscle; for example, the muscles are contracted to near maximal tension and simultaneously stretched. No studies, however, have demonstrated that this myotendinous failure is relevant to low back pain.

Another major cause believed relevant to low back pain includes degenerative diseases of the spine [28]. Current models for low back pain emphasize the stimulation of nociceptors scattered throughout the various anatomic structures, such as the facet joint capsule and posterior longitudinal ligament. When stimulated, nociceptors produce the same perception of low back pain. Degenerative changes are typically classified according to two locations—disks and facets. It is *believed* that disk degeneration plays a central role in the etiology of most episodes of low back pain, especially if the physician has the opportunity to take care of the patient over a prolonged period of time. Disk degeneration per se is not necessarily symptomatic. As disk degeneration progresses, a permanent loss of disk height may elicit secondary changes in other structures, including the facet joints and ends of the vertebral bodies, which may stimulate nociceptors and cause the perception of low back pain.

Biomechanical Models for Estimating Low Back Pain Risk Factors

The biomechanical basis for low back pain has been reviewed by Garg [31]. The majority of studies used to understand the effects of stresses to the lower back have examined the *biomechanical* characteristics of the cadaver lumbar motion segment (Fig. 28-5). A lumbar motion segment is two vertebral bodies and the intervening disk, with or without intact posterior elements. These lumbar motion segments may be susceptible to compression, tension (or distraction), shear, and torsion. With increasing levels of disk compression forces, a level is reached that is associated with permanent deformation of the motion segment, primarily manifested as a cartilaginous end-plate fracture. In terms of healing, the cartilaginous surface is believed to be replaced by a fibrous scar. As a result, there is less efficient fluid transfer between the vertebral body and the disk, so that the disk loses its hydration characteristics and cells involved in the manufacture of critical chemical components of the disk lose their ability to maintain disk integrity. These effects may gradually lead to a permanent loss of disk height. It is unlikely that a single cartilaginous end-plate fracture is symptomatic or that a single episode would necessarily lead to end-stage disk degeneration. Repeated exposure to high disk compression forces is thought to lead to multiple cartilaginous end-plate fractures and, eventually, sclerosis of a significant portion of the end-plate. As a result, disk degeneration is better characterized as a *disease process* related to *repeated* episodes of high disk compression forces compared to the date of onset of low back pain. The maximum compressive strength of lumbar motion segments has been investigated [32]. Some studies include young males, while other may include females or elderly individuals. As a result, there is a wide degree of variability in the compressive strength of individual vertebral segments.

There have been a few experiments in which investigators were able to directly measure intradiscal pressure among "volunteers" while they assumed various postures or held various objects [31]. These types of studies formed the basis for bio-

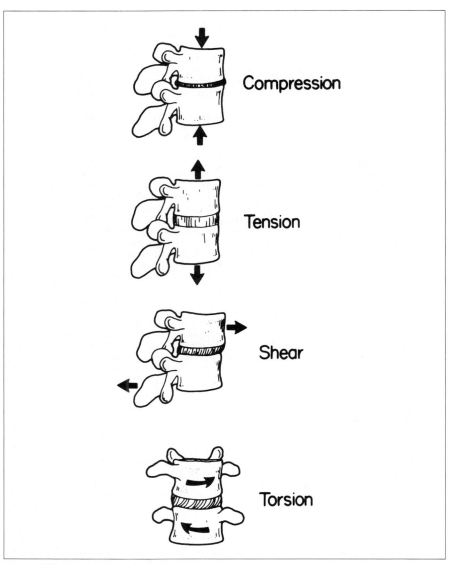

Figure 28-5. A lumbar motion segment. Compression, tension, shear, and torsion are the four primary forces that affect the lumbar spine. (From M. H. Pope et al. *Occupational Low-Back Pain: Assessment, Treatment and Prevention.* St. Louis: Mosby–Year Book, 1991.)

mechanical models that allow the estimation of disk compression forces in a manner that reproduces the observations from these experiments. Once validated, these models allow estimation of disk compression forces for other types of postures and lifting. Using two-dimensional estimates of disk compression forces, Chaffin and Park (1973) [33] demonstrated that the low back pain incidence rate was correlated with increasing predicted disk compression forces at the L5–S1 disk (Fig. 28-6). As a result, estimating risk of low back injury based on disk compression has undergone some validation. Based on considerations of the compression experiments on lumbar motion segments as well as the Chaffin and Park epidemiologic study, the National Institute for Occupational Safety and Health (NIOSH) adopted a disk compression

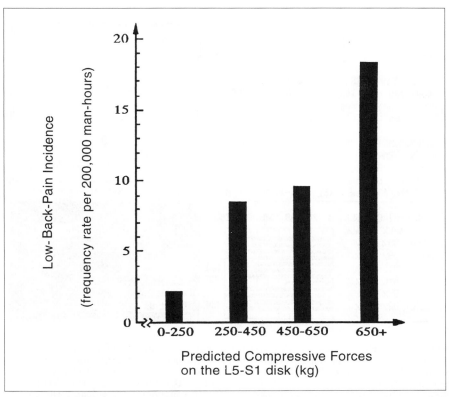

Figure 28-6. Relationship between incidence rate of low back pain and disk compression. (From D. B. Chaffin and K. S. Park. A longitudinal study of low-back pain as associated with occupational lifting factors. *Am. Ind. Hyg. Assoc. J.* 34:513, 1973.)

criterion called the Action Limit in their 1981 guide for manual lifting and the Recommended Weight Limit in the 1991 revised guide, according to which *compressive forces on the disk should not exceed 770 lb* (350 kg) [34, 35]. As noted above, disk compression forces are *estimated* using the two-dimensional and three-dimensional models. Multiple other models, however, have been developed. Figure 28-7 is a printout from a two-dimensional biomechanical model [36].

Psychophysical Criteria for Low Back Pain

Overexertion is a significant factor in many people with low back pain. One perspective of overexertion involves strength. In terms of strength, one is interested in comparing the strength required of the job to the worker's job-specific maximal strength. If the worker's capabilities exceed the demands of the job, the worker is considered capable of performing the task. On the other hand, if the demands of the job exceed the worker's capabilities, the worker may not be capable of performing the task, and, if it is attempted, might experience an overexertion injury. As with the disk compression estimates, epidemiologic evidence suggests that the strength demands, expressed as a ratio of job requirements to maximum strength, are also associated with increasing risk of injury [33] (Fig. 28-8). In particular, when the strength requirements exceed the worker's capabilities, the risk of musculoskeletal injury is three times greater than when the strength demands of the job are less than the worker's capabilities. Both the strength *requirements* and strength *capabilities* have been modeled in terms of *isometric* exertions; that is, both the job demands and the worker capabilities were assessed in terms of the static isometric

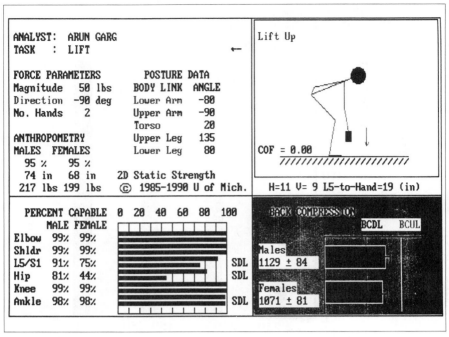

```
ANALYST:  ARUN GARG                              Lift Up
TASK   :  LIFT                          ←

FORCE PARAMETERS        POSTURE DATA
Magnitude    50 lbs     BODY LINK  ANGLE
Direction   -90 deg     Lower Arm   -80
No. Hands     2         Upper Arm   -90
                        Torso        20
ANTHROPOMETRY           Upper Leg   135
MALES  FEMALES          Lower Leg    80
  95 %    95 %                                COF = 0.00
  74 in   68 in         2D Static Strength
 217 lbs 199 lbs        © 1985-1990 U of Mich.   H=11 V= 9 L5-to-Hand=19 (in)

 PERCENT CAPABLE  0  20  40  60  80  100     BACK COMPRESSION
     MALE FEMALE                                         BCDL   BCUL
Elbow  99%  99%
Shldr  99%  99%                            Males
L5/S1  91%  75%                       SDL  1129 ± 84
Hip    81%  44%                       SDL
Knee   99%  99%                            Females
Ankle  98%  98%                       SDL  1071 ± 81
```

Figure 28-7. Printout from the University of Michigan 2-Dimensional Static Strength Model. *H* and *V* are the horizontal and vertical distances defined according to the NIOSH guide. *L5-to-hand* is the horizontal distance from the center of the L5–S1 disk to the center of the hands. SDL = strength design limit; BCDL = back compression design limit; BCUL =back compression upper limit. (From University of Michigan 2-Dimensional Static Strength Program. Center for Ergonomics, Ann Arbor, MI.)

exertion. Clearly, the majority of material-handling tasks performed in industry do not involve isometric exertions.

Other types of strength have also been investigated. In *isokinetic* strength, either the angular velocity of the torso is kept constant while the individual presses on a bar or the linear velocity of the object lifted is kept constant. While the technologies for measuring worker capabilities are well developed for these types of strength, the ability to analyze the job in terms of isokinetic variables is less clear. In addition, no published study has compared the isokinetic demands of the job to the isokinetic capabilities of the worker to estimate risk of injury.

A third type of strength is called *maximum acceptable weight*. In determining maximum acceptable weight, a person is instructed to lift a box of specified height at a specified frequency from specified origins to specified destinations during the course of approximately 45 to 60 minutes. During the trial, the subject adjusts the weight of the box by adding or removing load so as to derive a weight, called the maximum acceptable weight, that the person feels she/he could perform for an 8-hour day without undue fatigue. Snook and Cirello [37] at Liberty Mutual have developed the most comprehensive table of maximum acceptable weights. These tables, however, were developed as *design criteria* for jobs rather than ways to assess the work capacity of individuals. For example, in designing a lifting task that would accommodate 90% of women, the various parameters of the task, such as box size, lifting zone, distance of lift, and frequency, can be addressed in the table to determine the maximum acceptable weight. As a result, the weight of the object could be specified. Table 28-3 is an excerpt from the Liberty Mutual tables. These "mini-tables" provide maximum acceptable weights of lift for men and women for a box width of 13 in. (defined as the distance from the body) and a lifting height of 20 in. in the floor-to-knuckle height zone. When the frequency of lift and weight of the box

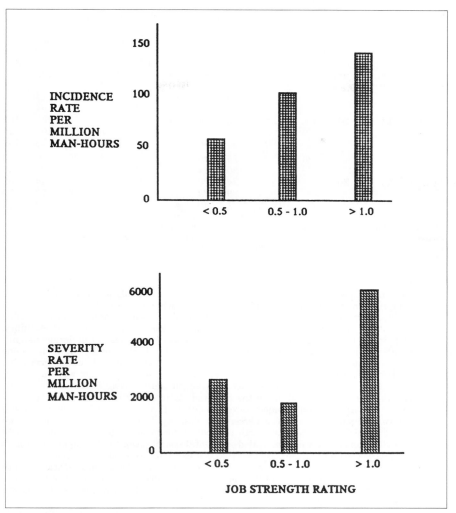

Figure 28-8. The incidence and severity rates for musculoskeletal injuries with increasing strength demands. The job strength rating is a ratio of the required strength divided by the worker's maximum strength. (From D. B. Chaffin and K. S. Park. A longitudinal study of low-back pain as associated with occupational lifting factors. *Am. Ind. Hyg. Assoc. J.* 34:513, 1973.)

are specified, the percent of capable men or women can be determined by looking up the weight in the table that corresponds to the specified frequency, and then reading left across the row to the percent capable. The fewer the percent capable, the more stressful the task. The tables can also be used for job design. In this case, the weight that would accommodate a specified percentage of capable men or women can be determined by selecting the desired percent capable, then reading across the row to the point where it intersects with the specified frequency of lift. The table value is the maximum acceptable weight of a box for the specified percent capable population and frequency.

There is one important caveat in using these tables. Some values are italicized (some high-frequency lifts). Even though these weights were considered acceptable, the energy expenditure (aerobic demands) exceeds recommended guidelines of 8 hours

Table 28-3. An excerpt from the maximum acceptable weight of lift tables

Gender	Box width (in.)	Distance of lift (in.)	Percent capable	Floor level to knuckle height*—One lift every:							
				5 sec	9 sec	14 sec	1 min	2 min	5 min	30 min	8 hr
Male	13	20	90	20	22	26	35	40	44	44	53
			75	26	33	40	51	57	62	64	75
			50	37	44	53	68	77	84	86	101
			25	46	55	66	86	97	106	108	125
			10	55	66	77	101	114	125	128	150
Female	13	20	90	15	20	20	24	26	26	29	40
			75	20	24	26	31	33	33	35	48
			50	24	29	31	35	40	40	44	59
			25	29	33	37	42	46	46	53	70
			10	31	40	42	48	53	53	59	79

*Italicized values exceed 8-hour physiologic criteria (energy expenditure).
Source: From S. H. Snook and V. M. Cirello. The design of manual handling tasks: Revised tables of maximum acceptable weights and forces. *Ergonomics* 34:1197, 1991.)

(see the following section). In addition, some heavier loads might exceed the disk compression criterion for safe lifting, especially when performed near the floor.

Whenever the strength requirements of a job exceed the maximum acceptable weights for the worker, the worker may be at increased risk for overexertion injury. This latter use of the maximum acceptable weight tables has not undergone significant validation, even though Snook and associates [38] estimated that up to one third of compensable low back pain incidents may have been related to performing exertions that exceeded the maximum acceptable weight for 75% of women.

We have now discussed two types of strength: *static strength* and *maximum acceptable weight*. Information on the required static strengths of the job is available in the two-dimensional biomechanical model. In fact, the output of the model will inform the job analyst of the percent capable population among men and women (see Fig. 28-7). The static strength is reported for various body parts, such as L5– S1 extension or elbow flexion, called segmental static strengths. This approach allows the analyst to identify the body part that is maximally stressed (in terms of strength). In 1981, NIOSH [34] defined the Action Limit as a level of segmental static strength such that 75% of women and 99% of men are capable of performing the task. The 1991 revision uses the same criterion, but now calls it the *Recommended Weight Limit* [35].

Physiologic Model for Estimating Risk for Low Back Pain

The physiologic model, often called the energy expenditure model, reflects the *aerobic demands* of a task [39]. Jobs with significant aerobic demands are believed to lead to whole body fatigue and, as a result, increase the risk for overexertion injury or loss of dexterity and slipping or falling [40]. An example of a job that would involve *high energy expenditure* would be carrying boxes repeatedly from a moving van to a second-story apartment. The weight of the boxes could be less than 10 lb and thus pose minimal stresses in terms of disk compression and strength; however, the carrying combined with walking and climbing would be a significant aerobic demand on the cardiovascular system. Another example of high energy expenditure would be repeated bending to the floor to pick up an object as trivial as a paper clip. When bending to the floor disk compression forces are likely to increase; if performed frequently, significant energy expenditure is used to raise and lower the upper body.

It is possible to exercise solely with the upper extremities. As a result, there is a different threshold for whole body fatigue when performing solely upper-extremity work [40]. NIOSH is recommending two criteria for energy expenditure for job design and analysis [35]. When activities are performed near the floor, thus requiring bending and lifting of the torso, the maximum energy expenditure should be less than 3.12 kcal per minute. When performing primarily arm work, the maximum energy expenditure should be less than 2.18 kcal per minute.

Energy expenditure can be estimated in several ways: One method is to look up a task reported in the literature, which is noted in standard tables. For example, it is easy to find estimates of energy expenditure associated with jogging, running, playing tennis, or other activities, which may not be relevant to the way the activity is done for each person. As a result, a more precise model was developed, called the *energy expenditure model,* which incorporates laboratory estimates for varying tasks that are then plugged into the model to generate the energy expenditure for the entire task [39]. Tasks may include lifting, walking, carrying, or lowering, among others. By entering the weight of the object and the distance and speed of the carrying or walking, as well as the origin and destination heights of lifting and lowering tasks, the energy expenditure of the job can be estimated more accurately. In addition, the major components of the task that contribute to the energy expenditure can also be identified so that intervention can be targeted as appropriate.

The NIOSH Guide for Manual Lifting

Before 1981, exposure assessment of manual handling tasks involved the estimation of (1) *disk forces and static strength demands* based on the two-dimensional model, (2) *strength demands* in comparison to maximum acceptable weights using the Liberty Mutual tables, and (3) *energy expenditure demands* of the job using either standardized tables or the energy expenditure model. Given the complexity of these job analysis techniques, a simplified method seemed more appropriate for widespread implementation. As a result, NIOSH convened a committee of experts to develop a guideline to meet these needs. The result was the 1981 NIOSH lifting guide [34]. The NIOSH guide was widely accepted and highly successful. It was quantitative, simple, easy to use, and effective, and greatly increased awareness of the ergonomic assessment and management of occupational low back pain. It also led to formal recognition that *prevention must include both engineering and administrative controls.* Unfortunately, the NIOSH guide did not meet all needs; it was limited to two-handed sagittal plane lifting and, as a result, could not contribute to the analysis of activities involving asymmetric lifting. The 1981 guide did not consider *compromised couplings* (e.g., box handles) or the *duration* of lifting, especially if lifting was performed intermittently. As a result, NIOSH convened another committee in the late 1980s to revise the 1981 guide [35].

The revised lifting guide continues to have limitations, including assumption of two-handed; smooth, continuous lifting motion; unrestricted lifting posture; adequate foot traction; moderate ambient environment; and an object length less than 25 in. It also assumes that a smooth, continuous lowering motion can be treated as lifting and that other manual handling activities are minimal. In the revised NIOSH lifting guide, the Action Limit (AL) and the Maximum Permissible Limit (MPL) terminology have been replaced by a single limit called the Recommended Weight Limit (RWL). The criteria for the RWL are (1) a compressive force less than 770 lb, (2) greater than 75% capability for women and 99% capability for men in terms of strength, (3) energy expenditure less than 3.12 kcal per minute near the floor or less than 2.18 kcal per minute above bench height, and (4) a nominal risk of low back pain based on epidemiologic data.

Both NIOSH lifting guides were based on the principle that *there is an acceptable weight limit for a standard lifting location.* The weight that corresponds to this standard lifting location is called the *load constant,* which, in the revised NIOSH lifting guide, is 51 lb. The load constant is then discounted (decreased) by multiplication with various multipliers that range between 0 and 1. There are six multipliers in the revised NIOSH guide. These include the *horizontal multiplier* (HM), the *vertical multiplier* (VM), the *distance multiplier* (DM), the *frequency multiplier* (FM), the *asymmetry multiplier* (AM), and the *coupling multiplier* (CM). The RWL is determined by the following equation:

$$RWL = (load\ constant) \times (HM) \times (VM) \times (DM) \times (FM) \times (AM) \times (CM) \qquad (3)$$

As shown in Fig. 28-9, the *horizontal distance* is defined as the distance from the midpoint between the ankles to the midpoint between the hands. In general, the horizontal multiplier is associated with the greatest degree of penalty as it deviates from the ideal location. The *vertical distance* is defined by the vertical location of

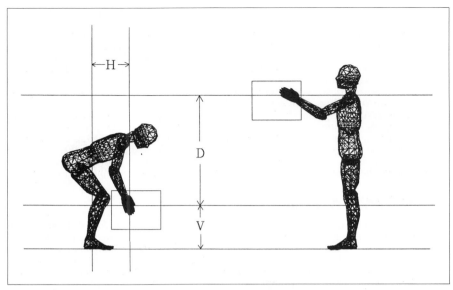

Figure 28-9. Definition of distances used in the NIOSH guide for manual lifting. In general, these distances are measured at the origin of the lift. *H* is the average distance between the malleoli and the center of the hands. The vertical distance, *V,* is the average distance from the floor to the center of the hands. The vertical travel distance, *D,* is the difference in vertical height between the origin and the destination.

the hands above the floor at the origin of the lift. If the hands are at separate heights, their vertical heights are averaged. The *vertical travel distance* is defined as the distance between the origin and destination at the lift. Asymmetry is defined by the *asymmetric angle,* which is the angle that the asymmetry line makes from the midsagittal plane, measured in degrees. The asymmetry line is defined as the line joining the midpoint between the angles with the midpoint of the hands as projected on the floor. As a result, the asymmetry angle does not necessarily measure torsional twisting, but is more of a reflection of the hands relative to the feet. *Couplings* are classified as good, fair, and poor according to a variety of criteria, including the length and height of the object; the types of handles available; whether objects are asymmetric, sagging, or unstable; and whether gloves are required. The *frequency multiplier* refers to the number of lifts per minute, measured over an interval of 5 minutes. In addition, another variable was defined as the *duration of lifting,* which is estimated by summing the duration of lifting episodes throughout the day. If the duration of lifting exceeds 2 hours, then the task is analyzed as if the lifting occurs all day. Other critical durations are less than or equal to 1 hour and less than or equal to 2 hours. For these brief episodes of lifting, an administrative control of resting time is allowed to enable a worker to recover primarily from the *physiologic demands* of the work.

Although the revised NIOSH lifting guide improves on the 1981 guide, there are many limitations in its applications. The single greatest source of difference arises from *inconsistent measurements of the horizontal distance.* The revised guide is a tool to estimate the demands of a job rather than an individual performing a particular job.

Postural Stresses

A fourth risk factor for low back pain, not previously addressed, is *static postural stresses,* which refer to prolonged awkward postures, such as bending over for several minutes to perform a task that is at or below knee height. These kinds of static work postures are associated with static muscular work, thus leading to localized muscle fatigue of the support structures of the spine. The effects of static postural stress can be estimated by using Rohmert's data [15].

Summary

A variety of methods are available to estimate the physical demands of jobs in terms of their effects (or potential effects) on the lumbar spine and associated structures. Disk compression forces may be estimated with a two-dimensional model [36]. Strength demands may be assessed in terms of static strength with a two-dimensional model and in terms of maximum acceptable weight using the Liberty Mutual tables [36, 37]. The energy expenditure model or standardized tables may be used to estimate the aerobic demands of tasks [39]. In addition, it is possible to integrate all three of these components to derive a more simple model that is reflected in the 1991 revised NIOSH lifting guide [35].

At this time, ergonomics is a combination of art and science. The assessment of jobs for risk of low back injury involves *quantitative* tools, thus representing the scientific aspect of the field. In contrast, the current method of subjective analysis of jobs in terms of generic risk factors reflects more of the art of the field. As a result, the experience of the practitioner in looking at jobs that may pose risk of injury is important. Practitioners should recognize the context within which manifestations of overexposure to ergonomic stresses occur.

Ergonomics is a much broader field than that related to the upper extremity and lower back. Ergonomics also includes the design of control panels as well as graphic user interfaces to optimize the interactions between a human and the work environment. Some aspects of ergonomics involve comfort, such as optimal office temperature and humidity, rather than risk of injury or disease. Another area evolving within ergonomics, especially in the workplace, deals with issues of participation and implementation. The topic of *participatory ergonomics* introduces organizational behavior variables as well as some of the principles, tools, and skills associated with some contemporary management philosophies, such as total quality management (TQM). The identification and/or assessment of a problem may be a legitimate role for an ergonomist, but the development and implementation of a solution usually requires team building and leadership skills.

On August 3, 1992, OSHA [41] published an Advanced Notice of Proposed Rulemaking (ANPR) regarding a potential standard for Ergonomics Safety and Health Management. It appears that OSHA is not pursuing a specification standard for particular risk factors. Rather, it is considering a rule that requires an employer to establish an ergonomics program with clear evidence of management commitment, employee participation, and certain required program components. The major program components include (1) worksite analysis and surveillance, (2) hazard prevention and control, (3) health management, and (4) training and education.

The ANPR seems to emphasize upper-extremity disorders. At this time, it is uncertain what shape the proposed rule might take or when it might be published. The Health Management and Training and Education sections may directly affect occupational medicine practitioners.

References

1. Armstrong, T. J. *An Ergonomics Guide to Carpal Tunnel Syndrome*. Cincinnati: American Industrial Hygiene Association, 1983.
2. Armstrong, T. J., and Lifshitz, Y. Evaluation and Design of Jobs for Control of Cumulative Trauma Disorders. In ACGIH, *Ergonomic Interventions to Prevent Musculoskeletal Injuries in Industry*. Chelsea: Lewis, 1987. Pp. 73–85.
3. Armstrong, T. J., et al. Repetitive trauma disorders: Job evaluation and design. *Hum. Factors* 28:325, 1986.
4. Silverstein, B. A., Fine, L. J., and Armstrong, T. J. Carpal tunnel syndrome: Causes and a preventive strategy. *Semin. Occup. Med.* 1:213, 1986.
5. Hadler, N. M. Is Carpal Tunnel Syndrome an Injury that Qualifies for Workers' Compensation Insurance? In N. M. Hadler (ed.), *Clinical Concepts in Regional Musculoskeletal Illness*. Orlando: Grune & Stratton, 1987. Pp. 355–360.
6. Hadler, N. M. Cumulative trauma disorders. An iatrogenic concept. *J. Occup. Med.* 32:38, 1990.

7. Nathan, P. A., Meadows, K. D., and Doyle, L. S. Occupation as a risk factor for impaired sensory conduction of the median nerve at the carpal tunnel. *J. Hand Surg.* 13B:167, 1988.

8. Nathan, P. A., et al. Location of impaired sensory conduction of the median nerve in carpal tunnel syndrome. *J. Hand Surg.* 15B:89, 1990.

9. Nathan, P. A., et al. Obesity as a risk factor for slowing of sensory conduction of the median nerve in industry: A cross-sectional and longitudinal study involving 429 workers. *J. Occup. Med.* 34:379, 1992.

10. Moore, J. S., and Garg, A. The Spectrum of Upper Extremity Disorders Associated with Hazardous Work Tasks. In S. Kumar (ed.), *Advances in Industrial Ergonomics and Safety IV.* London: Taylor & Francis, 1992. Pp. 723–730.

11. Moore, J. S. Carpal tunnel syndrome. In J. S. Moore and A. Garg (eds.), Ergonomics: Low-Back Pain, Carpal Tunnel Syndrome, and Upper Extremity Disorders in the Workplace. *Occup. Med. State of the Art Rev.* 7:741, 1992.

12. Simonson, E. Introduction. In E. Simonson (ed.), *Physiology of Work Capacity and Fatigue.* Springfield, IL: Thomas, 1971. P. xi.

13. Chaffin, D. B. Localized muscle fatigue—Definition and measurement. *J. Occup. Med.* 15:346, 1973.

14. Rohmert, W. Physiologische Grundlagen der Erholungszeitbestimmung. *Zbl. Arb. Wiss* 19:1, 1965.

15. Rohmert, W. Problems in determining rest allowances: Part 1. Use of modern methods to evaluate stress and strain in static muscular work. *Appl. Ergonomics* 4:91, 1973.

16. Rodgers, S. H. Job evaluation in worker fitness determination. *Occup. Med. State of the Art Rev.* 3:219, 1988.

17. Rodgers, S. H. A functional job analysis technique. In J. S. Moore and A. Garg (eds.), Ergonomics: Low-Back Pain, Carpal Tunnel Syndrome, and Upper Extremity Disorders in the Workplace. *Occup. Med. State of the Art Rev.* 7:679, 1992.

18. Moore, J. S. Function, structure, and responses of components of the muscle-tendon unit. In J. S. Moore and A. Garg (eds.), Ergonomics: Low-Back Pain, Carpal Tunnel Syndrome, and Upper Extremity Disorders in the Workplace. *Occup. Med. State of the Art Rev.* 7:713, 1992.

19. Moore, J. S., and Garg, A. A Job Analysis Method for Predicting Risk of Upper Extremity Disorders at Work: Preliminary Results. In R. Nielson and K. Jorgensen (eds.), *Advances in Industrial Ergonomics and Safety V.* London: Taylor & Francis. (In press.)

20. Silverstein, B. A., Fine, L. J., and Armstrong, T. J. Occupational factors and carpal tunnel syndrome. *Am. J. Ind. Med.* 11:343, 1987.

21. SUNYAB-IE. 1982/1983. Data from student laboratory projects for Industrial Engineering 436/536 (Physiological Basis for Human Factors) at the State University of New York at Buffalo, S. H. Rodgers, instructor. As cited by S. H. Rodgers (ed.), *Ergonomic Design for People at Work,* Vol. 2. New York: Van Nostrand Reinhold, 1986. P. 470.

22. Swansen, A. B., Matev, I. B., and DeGroot, G. The strength of the hand. *Bull. Prosthet. Res.* 1970. Pp. 145–153.

23. Gelberman, R. H., et al. The carpal tunnel syndrome: A study of carpal tunnel pressures. *J. Bone Joint Surg.* 63A:380, 1981.

24. Fullerton, P. M. The effect of ischaemia on nerve conduction in the carpal tunnel syndrome. *J. Neurol. Neurosurg. Psychiatry* 26:385, 1963.

25. Frymoyer, J. W., et al. Epidemiologic studies of low-back pain. *Spine* 5:419, 1980.

26. Pope, M. H., et al. Biomechanical testing as an aid to decision making in low-back pain patients. *Spine* 4:135, 1979.

27. Andersson, G. B. J. The Epidemiology of Spinal Disorders. In J. W. Frymoyer (ed.), *The Adult Spine: Principles and Practice.* New York: Raven, 1990. Pp. 107–146.

28. Garg, A., and Moore J. S. Epidemiology of low-back pain in industry. In J. S. Moore and A. Garg (eds.), Ergonomics: Low-Back Pain, Carpal Tunnel Syndrome, and Upper Extremity Disorders in the Workplace. *Occup. Med. State of the Art Rev.* 7:593, 1992.

29. McCully, K. K., and Faulkner J. A. Injury to skeletal muscle fibers of mice following lengthening contractions. *J. Appl. Physiol.* 59:119, 1985.

30. Nikolau, P. K., et al. Biomechanical and histological evaluation of muscle after controlled strain injury. *Am. J. Sports Med.* 15:9, 1987.

31. Garg, A. Occupational biomechanics and low-back pain. In J. S. Moore and A. Garg

(eds.), Ergonomics: Low-Back Pain, Carpal Tunnel Syndrome, and Upper Extremity Disorders in the Workplace. *Occup. Med. State of the Art Rev.* 7:609, 1992.

32. Jäger, M. Biomechanisches Modell des menschen zur Analyze und Beurteilung der Belastung der Wirbelsaule beider Handhabung von Lastten (PhD thesis). Dortmund, Germany: Universitat Dortmund, 1987.

33. Chaffin, D. B., and Park K. S. A longitudinal study of low-back pain as associated with occupational lifting factors. *Am. Ind. Hyg. Assoc. J.* 34:513, 1973.

34. National Institute for Occupational Safety and Health. *A Work Practices Guide for Manual Lifting.* US Department of Health and Human Services (NIOSH), 1981.

35. Putz-Anderson, V., and Waters, T. Revisions in NIOSH Guide for Manual Lifting. Paper presented at national conference entitled "A National Strategy for Occupational Musculoskeletal Injury Prevention—Implementation Issues and Research Needs." Ann Arbor, MI: University of Michigan, April 1991.

36. University of Michigan 2-Dimensional Static Strength Program. Center for Ergonomics, Ann Arbor, MI.

37. Snook, S. H., and Cirello V. M. The design of manual handling tasks: Revised tables of maximum acceptable weights and forces. *Ergonomics* 34:1197, 1991.

38. Snook, S. H., Campanelli, R. A., and Hart J. W. A study of three preventive approaches to low-back injury. *J. Occup. Med.* 20:478, 1978.

39. Garg, A., Chaffin, D. B., and Herrin, G. D. Prediction of metabolic rates for manual materials handling jobs. *Am. Ind. Hyg. Assoc. J.* 39:661, 1978.

40. Garg, A., Rodgers, S. F., and Yates, J. W. The Physiological Basis for Manual Lifting. In S. Kumar (ed.), *Advances in Industrial Ergonomics and Safety IV.* London: Taylor & Francis, 1992. Pp. 867–874.

41. US Department of Labor (Occupational Safety and Health Administration). Ergonomic safety and health management; proposed rule. *Fed. Register* 57:34192, August 3, 1992.

Further Information

Frymoyer, J. W. (ed.). *The Adult Spine: Principles and Practice.* New York: Raven, 1991.
This two-volume tome (> 2000 pages) is the most comprehensive summary of knowledge related to the adult spine. It includes sections addressing the cervical spine, the lumbar spine, and the sacrum and coccyx.

Kasdan, M. L. (ed.). *Occupational Hand and Upper Extremity Injuries and Diseases.* Philadelphia: Hanley & Belfus, 1991.
Dr. Kasdan's book offers a comprehensive overview of issues particularly pertinent to the treatment of a broad spectrum of upper-extremity disorders, including traumatic and nontraumatic injuries.

Moore, J. S., and Garg, A. (eds.). *Ergonomics: Low-Back Pain, Carpal Tunnel Syndrome, and Upper Extremity Disorders in the Workplace. Occup. Med. State of the Art Rev.* Vol. 7, no. 4, Oct.–Dec. 1992.
This is a compilation of review articles dealing with a variety of topics related to the lower back and upper extremity. Aside from topics discussed in this chapter, there are reviews of electrodiagnostic medicine, clinical management of low back pain, and the role of dynamic variables in ergonomics.

Pope, M. H., et al. *Occupational Low Back Pain: Assessment, Treatment, and Prevention.* St. Louis: Mosby–Year Book, 1991.
This book is a usable summary of contemporary concepts related to low back pain—especially issues related to pathogenesis, epidemiology, patient care, prevention, and legal aspects.

Rodgers, S. H. (ed.). *Ergonomic Design for People at Work,* Vols. 1 and 2. New York: Van Nostrand Reinhold, 1986.
To many, these two volumes are classics in the field of ergonomics. Dr. Rodgers and the Human Factors Section of Eastman Kodak provide an easy-to-read, yet scientifically rigorous, treatise on almost all of the major topics in ergonomics.

29

Molecular Genetics

Peter G. Shields

The genetic basis of disease and disease risk is the focus of many research laboratories. Such efforts have wide-ranging clinical importance and the results of genetic research have potential applications to the workplace. The lessons learned through molecular genetics will impact on medical decision-making, worker protection, risk assessment processes, and other parts of occupational medicine practice. Genetic biomarkers are being developed that reflect a spectrum of effects from internal exposure to disease and prognosis (Fig. 29-1). The ethical, legal, and social implications of genetic testing are complex and profound. Significant efforts are under way to ensure the proper uses of such testing, although many potential problems are only now being elucidated. These efforts cannot be separated from the research, development, and incorporation of genetic testing into the workplace. This chapter reviews some of the more commonly used molecular genetic methods of value in occupational practice and research, especially those of value in evaluating the potentially hazardous nature of certain materials and processes.

Occupational disease is caused by the interactions of exposure to exogenous agents, inheritable susceptibilities that determine the response to those agents, and endogenous processes that act independently of exposure. Each of these is important and dictates, for example, why one worker will develop an illness in response to a small exposure while another does not in spite of a large exposure. Genetic testing can be useful in several clinical areas (Table 29-1). It might predict which workers are at risk for specific diseases, identify who needs additional workplace protection, and suggest maximal allowable exposures, ethical issues notwithstanding. It also may be useful for finding an occupational etiology for a disease in a worker or provide prognostic information. However, the primary goal for biomarkers is to prevent disease and secondarily for early detection of disease.

Some currently available tests provide direct information about DNA sequence, structure, and expression of specific gene products. Other tests determine the phenotypic expression of a gene. For example, serum cholesterol testing reflects the phenotypic expression of several genes that determines the risk of heart disease. It is important to realize that phenotypes might not always accurately reflect genetic function because of exogenous influences; for example, lifestyle factors also affect serum cholesterol levels.

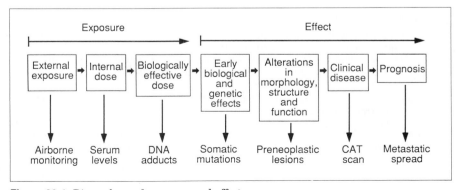

Figure 29-1. Biomarkers of exposure and effect.

Table 29-1. Examples of clinically applicable genetic tests in occupational medicine

Disease risk
Markers of inherited susceptibility
  Impaired metabolic activation or excretion of toxins
  Gene sequence or structure
Markers of acquired susceptibility
  Formation of DNA adducts
  Integration of viral DNA
  Mutations in critical genes
  Mutations in noncritical genes
  Altered gene expression
  Clastogenic abnormalities
  Antibodies to DNA adducts
  Urine mutagenesis

Preclinical disease
Markers of cellular alteration
  Altered morphology of cells
  Altered phenotypic expression of cells
  Clonal proliferation of cells
  Altered gene expression
  Antibodies to gene products

Clinical disease
Markers of cellular alteration
  Altered morphology of cells
  Altered phenotypic expression of cells
  Immunohistochemical staining
  Clonal proliferation of cells
  Altered gene expression
  Antibodies to gene products
Markers of prognosis
  Pathologic diagnosis
  Immunohistochemical staining
  Altered gene expression
  Cytogenetic abnormalities

The importance of molecular genetics is exemplified by the Human Genome Project [1]. This federally funded program, conceived in 1986 and formally established in 1990, is coordinated by the Department of Energy and the National Institutes of Health. Its goal is to map and sequence every human gene (approximately 100,000 genes consisting of three billion bases) within the next 15 years. To achieve this goal, a significant amount of research is focused on technology development, including improvement of molecular genetic techniques, information transfer, and training. The ultimate achievements of this project will greatly affect disease prevention, identification, and treatment. As the potential ethical, legal, and social implications of such research have been recognized, programs are being sponsored to foster an understanding and to develop policy options.

Background

Molecular genetics is the study of genes and gene structure. There are over 100,000 human genes located on 46 chromosomes. Genes are composed of deoxyribonucleic acid (DNA) sequences that provide a written language for genetic function. DNA is composed of two strands joined by nucleotide base pairing (guanine binds to cytosine and adenine to thymine). The genetic sequences are transcribed by enzymes that make complementary copies of messenger ribonucleic acid (mRNA). The mRNA is then translated into proteins that perform basic cellular functions. The genetic language that codes for the amino acid sequence in proteins is organized in triplets called codons. Each codon dictates which amino acid is to be incorporated into proteins and in what sequence. Not all of a gene or a chromosome codes for amino acids, however. Genes are composed of *exons,* which are transcribed, and *introns,* which are not.

Genes are the basic building blocks of heredity and control diverse body cellular functions and characteristics such as hair color, height, and facial features. This diversity is controlled through variations in DNA sequence. Any variation that occurs in more than 1% of the population is considered a *polymorphism.* Genetic polymorphisms might only result in one base change that fundamentally alters structure (i.e., sickle cell disease) or it may be reflected in all or part of the gene being altered or deleted. It is estimated that genetic polymorphisms occur in approximately every 500 bases.

Diseases in every organ and body system may be caused by genetic dysfunction due to point mutations (base substitutions and deletions), gene deletions, or gross chromosomal aberrations (loss of part of a chromosome or exchanging parts of a chromosome). Mutations in genes might result in altered transcription or protein production and activity, or both. Exogenous exposures such as viruses and chemicals also cause mutations. Here, dysfunction is acquired and not inherited. Finally, genetic dysfunction can be acquired through endogenous mutational mechanisms such as oxidative damage by chemicals released from neutrophils, errors during cell replication, and others. In fact, endogenous mutations are estimated to occur millions of times per day in any one person but are efficiently repaired by the body.

Molecular Genetic Assays

Several recently developed genetic tests are widely available (Table 29-2). Some of these are described below. These assays can detect mutations, determine susceptibilities through genetic polymorphism detection, use biochemical methods to detect carcinogens bound to DNA, and measure abnormal or altered gene products and others.

Restriction Enzyme Analysis

The use of restriction enzymes has aided genetic analysis in a multitude of ways. These enzymes identify short, specific DNA sequences, cutting the DNA at those sequences into uniquely sized fragments that can be separated electrophoretically. Restriction enzymes recognize palindromic sites where the sequence on each strand is identical to each other (when read in 5' to 3' direction). One use of restriction enzymes is for the detection of restriction fragment length polymorphisms (RFLP). Sometimes a polymorphic site coding for a particular trait might occur at a sequence recognized by restriction enzymes and in other cases it might be located between two sites so that the electrophoresis pattern changes.

The Polymerase Chain Reaction

Among the most important recent advances in molecular genetics is the ability to amplify small amounts of DNA for subsequent analyses. The polymerase chain reaction (PCR) is facile and inexpensive. It has been used in forensic medicine for DNA fingerprinting from a single hair follicle or blood stain [2], for mutation detection in single sperm cells to assess teratogenicity rates [3], and for amplification of DNA from paraffin-embedded tissue blocks [4], serum [5], or ancient DNA [6]. The method relies on a temperature-stable enzyme (*Taq* polymerase) that can replicate DNA when using primers that help begin the reaction at a previously chosen unique site and so are gene specific. While PCR is generally used for DNA amplification, it also can be used for RNA amplification using a different enzyme (reverse transcriptase) [7]. The major limitations for PCR lie in its sensitivity, which allows for contamination by unwanted DNA from other sources. It also is critical to choose primers carefully to ensure specificity and prevent amplifying the wrong gene.

There are many applications for PCR. It is being used directly without other techniques for diagnosing viral infections (e.g., human immunodeficiency virus in lymphocytes [8], hepatitis B virus in liver and serum [9], and papilloma virus in uterine cervix [10]). It can be used to amplify mutated and structurally altered

Table 29-2. Selected examples of molecular genetic assays

Assay	Description
Polymerase chain reaction	DNA is amplified from small amounts of DNA that can be coupled to other procedures or used by itself to detect the presence of a gene or mutation.
Southern blot analysis	DNA is subjected to restriction enzyme digestion and the resulting DNA fragments are separated by gel electrophoresis. The fragments are transferred to a membrane that is probed for a specific gene sequence. The presence and size of the fragment are then detected.
Northern blot analysis	RNA is resolved by gel electrophoresis and then transferred to a membrane that is probed for a specific gene sequence. The presence and size of the fragment are then detected. The amount of RNA can be quantitated to reflect gene transcription.
DNA sequencing	DNA is used as a template for the amplification of complementary strands of DNA, but 2,3′-dideoxynucleotides are also incorporated into the DNA, which causes the reaction to stop. The location of these labeled nucleotides reveals the genetic sequence when they are resolved electrophoretically.
32P postlabeling	This method is one of several used for the detection of DNA adducts. DNA is enzymatically digested to individual nucleotides. An enzyme is used to radiolabel each nucleotide, which is then resolved and quantitated by thin-layer chromatography.
Chromosomal assays	Each of the 46 chromosomes is isolated from cultured cells and identified. Deletions, additions, and translocations are detected by specific markers. Sister chromatid exchanges are used to detect abnormal DNA replication using nonspecific markers. Micronuclei are observed in cells where extra genetic material occurs outside the nucleus.

regions of a given gene (e.g., translocation of chromosomes by determining the breakpoint cluster region for the *bcr-abl* oncogene for the diagnosis of chronic myelogenous leukemia [11]). Other applications involve the identification of single base mutations or genetic polymorphisms by designing primers that anneal only if matched to the unique sequence (e.g., oligospecific PCR for the identification of polymorphisms in the *N*-acetyltransferase gene predictive of cancer risk in workers exposed to aromatic amines [12]). PCR also is combined with other techniques whereby PCR amplification products can be subjected to restriction enzyme digestion to identify genetic polymorphisms or mutations (e.g., RFLP analysis for cytochrome P450 genetic polymorphisms [13]) or used for hybridization with mutation-specific probes (e.g., oligonucleotide hybridization for the detection of ras mutations [14]). Another important application is the use of PCR to amplify sufficient quantities of DNA fragments for nucleotide sequencing. This method allows for the determination of specific sequences from unknown genes or for the detection of mutations [15].

Use of DNA Probes to Detect Genetic Sequences

The fortunate property of DNA, whereby each strand is complementary and annealed by nucleic acid base pairing (guanine to cytosine and adenine to thymine) can be taken advantage of to identify specific genetic sequences. Under experimental conditions, the two complementary DNA strands are separated and reannealed. Single-stranded probes of short DNA fragments are then used to identify a specific genetic sequence by exposing the DNA to the probe. If the probe is either radioactive or has a fluorescent marker, the DNA binding can be readily identified. This unique property allows for Southern blot analysis of DNA [16], which subjects DNA to restriction enzyme digestion, separation of the resulting fragments by electrophoresis, and then probing the fragments for the genetic sequence and measuring the lengths of the fragments. The method also is used for Northern blot analysis of mRNA [17], which is almost identical with Southern blot analysis except that RNA is used instead of DNA.

Southern blot analysis has many applications, such as RFLP detection [16], determining that a part of a gene has been deleted so as to suggest the location of a tumor suppressor gene (loss of heterozygosity) [18], detecting the presence of a malignant clone (T-cell gene receptor analysis where a predominant band is seen for the detection of malignant lymphomas), and identifying metabolic genotypes (capacity to metabolize medicines and environmental chemicals) [19]. A simpler approach for the detection of mutations (oligonucleotide hybridization) is to fix the DNA to a membrane, without electrophoretic separation, and use a probe that is specific for either the normal sequence (wild type) or a mutated sequence (e.g., detection of ras gene mutations [14]).

DNA Sequencing

The dideoxy-mediated chain termination method allows for the determination of a nucleic acid sequence of a gene [20]. For example, a PCR fragment is amplified and four dideoxy reactions are carried out for each of the four nucleotides. The amplified product, radiolabeled nucleotides, 2,3'-dideoxynucleotides, and a polymerase are mixed so that the 2,3'-dideoxynucleotide is randomly incorporated into the DNA. Based on the location of the dideoxynucleotide incorporation, the DNA sequence can be determined after electrophoretic separation. DNA sequencing remains the best method for identifying mutations and reveals unique sequences for gene identification.

DNA Adduct Detection

Chemicals or their reactive metabolites can specifically bind DNA, resulting in promutagenic lesions. The combination of the chemical and the nucleotide is an *adduct*. The measurement of DNA adducts allows the distinction between the measurement of chemicals in the environment and exposures inside the body at target organs, where the former is not always indicative of the latter. DNA adducts reflect the biologically effective dose of an exposure, resulting from the competition of exposure, absorption, activation, detoxification, and DNA repair. Thus, the measurement of DNA adducts reflects both exposure and inherited susceptibilities. Elevated levels of DNA adducts have been correlated with cigarette use [21], occupational exposures to polycyclic aromatic hydrocarbons [22], and air pollution [23].

Several methods are currently available for the measurement of DNA adducts, although all remain research tools. These include the 32P postlabeling assay, which uses hydrolytic enzymes to reduce DNA to individual nucleotides and then uses another enzyme to radiolabel the nucleotides [24]. Any adducts that are present are then resolved chromatographically and quantitated by measuring the radioactivity incorporated into the nucleotide. This assay can be used as a screening method to detect unknown adducts [24] or can be combined with purification techniques to identify specific compounds such as adducts formed from polycyclic aromatic hydrocarbons [25] and N-nitrosamines [26]. Several important immunologic assays are available for the detection of DNA adducts, such as enzyme-linked immunosorbent assays (ELISA) or radioimmunoassays [27–29].

Cytogenetic Assays

Several methods are available to analyze the gross structure of chromosomes in metaphase and prophase of mitosis. Aberrations can be observed by identifying each of the 23 chromosomal pairs for completeness and number [30]. Common uses of such analyses include the detection of trisomy 21, which is diagnostic for Down's syndrome, and detection of a translocation between chromosomes 9 and 21, which is diagnostic for the chronic myelogenous leukemia and the Philadelphia chromosome. The availability of specific chromosomal markers now makes this method more specific. Another gross chromosomal change detectable in human cells includes the sister chromatid exchange [31]. In this case, sister chromatids of one chromosome are switched, which can be counted using nonspecific markers and correlated with exposures to tobacco and certain chemicals (see below). A method of detecting DNA damage that does not require cell culture and examination of chromosomes during mitosis is the detection of micronuclei [32]. Small chromosomal fragments are sometimes found to exist outside the nucleus. This assay is rapid, relatively inexpensive, and quantitative, so that its potential is greater as a screening test in humans for mutagenic exposures. It can be used for white blood cells and epithelial cells (bladder, lung, oral mucosa).

Detection of Gene Products and Proteins

Methods are available for the detection of both mRNA and its protein products. For the former, Northern blot analysis [17] uses techniques similar to Southern blot analysis and also relies on complementary base pairing of DNA probes (see above). This technique might be used clinically for the detection of overexpression of a particular gene such as one that confers multidrug resistance in cancer cells. Another use of complementary binding of probes for RNA is called a slot blot or dot blot [17]. In this case, the RNA is not electrophoretically separated into different sized fragments but merely fixed to a membrane to quantitate the amount of mRNA.

A variety of methods are available for the detection of protein products and protein activity as they relate to genetic sequence, structure, and function. Induction and activity might be measured through functional phenotypic assays such as hydrocarbon hydroxylase activity in peripheral lymphocytes or lung cells [33]. This assay reflects the capacity of cells to metabolically activate polycyclic aromatic hydrocarbons and respond to compounds such as dioxins and polychlorinated biphenyls. The amount of a protein can be quantitated by immunoassays using specific antibodies directed against epitopes of the protein of interest. Abnormal presence or quantities of a protein can be observed using techniques such as ELISA's (detection of oncogene products in serum) [34] or immunohistochemical staining of cells (accumulation of p53 tumor suppressor gene protein or *erb-B2* protooncogene protein in lung and breast cancer [35, 36]).

Clinical Applications of Genetic Testing—Selected Examples

While most genetic assays are used in the research setting, several studies demonstrate how such research might be applied to the worker and his/her health. In general, the type of testing described is recently developed or applied to occupational cohorts. Research results should be carefully interpreted with regard to the study design and any methodologic limitations associated with the assay.

A potentially important clinical application of genetic testing will be the prediction of occupational lung disease in persons with decreased production of α_1-antitrypsin [37]. Absence of two functional copies of this gene leads to the development of premature emphysema, which is worsened by concurrent exposure to tobacco smoke. The absence of one of two copies might lead to a partial deficiency and an inability for natural lung defense mechanisms to work properly when challenged by pulmonary irritants, allergens, or inflammatory agents. This gene is polymorphic, with over 7% of the population carrying a defective gene. The presence of an inheritable abnormality is demonstrable by PCR and oligonucleotide hybridization. If studies indeed identify an increased genetic risk, then industrial hygiene and medical surveillance might change.

Several genetic polymorphisms for drug and carcinogen metabolism have suggested that some workers might be at increased risk for occupational cancers. For example, the *N-acetyltransferase enzyme* is responsible for activating and also detoxifying aromatic amines and heterocyclic amines, depending upon the organ and compound, and may place workers at increased risk of bladder cancer [38–40]. The activity of this gene can be directly measured by administering isoniazid, dapsone, or caffeine and measuring urinary metabolites [41, 42]. Another example is the genetic polymorphism for cytochrome P4502D6. This gene is responsible for *N*-oxidation of many medications (tricyclic antidepressants, antiarrhythmic agents, beta-blocking antihypertensive agents, and others). The activity can be assessed in individuals by administration of dextromethorphan (cough medicine) or debrisoquin. Rapid metabolizers (approximately 90% of Americans) are at increased risk of lung cancer compared to poor metabolizers. Cigarette smokers who are homozygous for the active gene have a relative risk of 7.9 for lung cancer, which increases to 18.4 with concurrent exposure to asbestos or polycyclic aromatic hydrocarbons [43].

Recent advances in PCR amplification and DNA sequencing have led to findings that chemicals cause specific point mutations in DNA that may be "fingerprints" of that exposure (mutational spectra). This type of testing might be useful in learning the etiology of cancer in an individual. The determination of mutations present in the *p53 tumor suppressor gene,* which is the most commonly mutated gene in cancer, has been used to suggest a particular chemical etiology. Persons who develop hepatocellular carcinoma in regions where aflatoxin, believed to be etiologically linked to this cancer, is a common dietary contaminant have a typical G to T transversion in codon 249 [15]. This type of transversion is also demonstrable in vitro and is not found in persons with the same tumor who reside in nonaflatoxin-contaminated areas [44]. For lung cancer, it has been observed that the p53 mutations detected in persons who smoke can display different patterns compared to those in smokers who also are uranium miners and exposed to radon [4].

Specific and nonspecific genetic markers of exposure might be useful for assessing industrial hygiene safeguards and indirectly assessing the inherited predispositions to DNA damage. Sister chromatid exchanges, micronuclei, and chromosomal aberrations are observed more frequently in persons exposed to radiation [45], benzene [46], cytostatic drugs [47], and vinyl chloride [48].

The detection of infectious agents in vivo and in environmental samples has been an important application for molecular genetics, in some cases entirely replacing culture techniques. Genital infections such as papilloma viruses, gonorrhea, and chlamydia can be screened using PCR and genetic probes. Hepatitis B virus can be detected in serum or liver DNA, in some cases even when serologies are negative.

Cancer screening may be enhanced in persons known to be at increased risk. Using specific probes, mutated ras oncogenes can be detected in the stool in persons with colon cancer [49]; this technique also is being applied in sputum, urine, and other body fluids. *Increased production of ras p21 proteins,* detectable in the blood of immunoassays, has been observed in persons developing lung cancer who have preexisting asbestosis or silicosis, in some cases predating the diagnosis of lung cancer [50].

Implications for Genetic Testing in the Workplace

Advances in technology will improve accuracy, cost, and speed of genetic testing. Further studies will elucidate mechanistic relationships of genetics to disease, while epidemiology will assist in the identification of relevant assays for human risk. Ultimately, the institution of any clinical test depends on its reliability, sensitivity, specificity, predictive value, and cost.

The ethical, legal, and social implications for the use of genetic assays has stimulated much debate, especially in the workplace. Employers and medical providers are mandated to avoid discriminatory practices, as addressed in part by the Americans with Disabilities Act [51]. Additional legislation related to inherited risks uncovered by genetic testing may be required. Other forms of discrimination, such as might occur in the insurance industry, remain to be adequately addressed [52]. The odds of never developing a disease in spite of having a specific genetic trait must be considered in the context of other commonly used actuarial predictors (e.g., cholesterol level, hypertension). Separately, the stigmatization of having a specific genotype needs to be addressed in a number of different forums. Providing results of genetic testing can avoid stigmatization, if accurate risks are presented clearly. Further, due to the large diversity in human genotypes (polymorphisms of individual nucleotides occur approximately every 500 bases), *no longer can one genotype be considered "normal;" rather, there are common and less common types.*

The potential harmful effects of genetic testing must be considered in light of the many potential benefits. Strategies for disease prevention can focus on persons most at risk, thereby enabling programs to be cost effective and enhancing chances for success. Chemoprevention trials might be directed toward persons with the best-defined risks. Industrial hygiene measures could be designed to protect all workers, or vary according to the characteristics of a particular workforce (different ethnic groups may have different risks so that allowable exposure limits might justifiably be very different across countries). Finally, medical surveillance projects might identify those workers who require more or less surveillance, depending on genotype and exposure. Significant efforts, such as those funded by the Human Genome Project [1] are now addressing many of the potential problems and benefits of genetic testing.

The risk assessment process relies on epidemiologic studies and mathematical modeling to predict risk in populations. However, for many hazardous exposures, adequate epidemiologic evidence is not available so that extrapolations from laboratory animal studies are required. The use of such studies has been problematic because of study design (e.g., use of maximally tolerated doses) and inherent differences between laboratory animals and humans. Even when epidemiologic studies are available, they are generally unable to distinguish persons with different sensitivities to a particular hazard. Further, as the carcinogenic process is significantly complex and multistaged, greater emphasis needs to be directed toward risk assessment methods that are biologically, physiologically, and genetically based. The use of genetic studies also might better identify which laboratory animal studies more closely approximate human responses. Molecular epidemiologic studies, such as the measurement of DNA adducts in exposed populations, might help to better approximate risk by including the degree of DNA damage in risk assessment models.

The use of genetic testing for evaluation of disease risk, diagnosis, and prognosis will be incorporated into many parts of our lives. It is important to note that the prevalence of genetic disease is not increasing, in contrast to those diseases caused by infectious agents, so that genetic testing should have no negative economic impact on society. In fact, there might be a reduction in the cost of health care and a positive influence on the workforce if preventable genetic diseases are appropriately addressed. The prevention of discriminatory practices, education and dissemination of information, and the best uses of such testing are still evolving.

References

1. US Department of Energy and Office of Health and Environmental Research. *Human Genome: 1991–92 Program Report*. Washington, DC: US Dept. of Energy, 1992. Pp. 1–248.
2. *PCR Technology. Principles and Applications for DNA Amplification*. New York: W. H. Freeman and Co., 1991. Pp. 1–246.
3. Zhang, L., et al. Whole genome amplification from a single cell: Implications for genetic analysis. *Proc. Natl. Acad. Sci. U.S.A.* 89:5847, 1992.
4. Vahakangas, K. H., et al. Mutations of p53 and ras genes in radon-associated lung cancer from uranium miners. *Lancet* 339:576, 1992.
5. Martin, M., Carrington, M., and Mann, D. A method for using serum or plasma as a source of DNA for HLA typing. *Hum. Immunol.* 33:108, 1992.
6. Paabo, S. Amplifying Ancient DNA. In M. A. Innis et al. (eds.), *PCR Protocols: A Guide to Methods and Applications*. San Diego: Academic, 1990. Pp. 159–166.
7. Kawasaki, E. S., et al. Diagnosis of chronic myeloid and acute lymphocytic leukemias by detection of leukemia-specific mRNA sequences amplified in vitro. *Proc. Natl. Acad. Sci. U.S.A.* 85:5698, 1988.
8. Hewlett, I. K., et al. Assessment by gene amplification and serological markers of transmission of HIV-1 from hemophiliacs to their sexual partners and secondarily to their children. *J. Acquir. Immune Defic. Syndr.* 3:714, 1990.
9. Kato, N., et al. Detection of hepatitis C virus ribonucleic acid in the serum by amplification with polymerase chain reaction. *J. Clin. Invest.* 86:1764, 1990.
10. Manos, M. M., et al. Cancer Cells: Molecular Diagnostics of Human Cancer. In M. Furth and M. Greaves (eds.), *Cancer Cells: Molecular Diagnostics of Human Cancer*. New York: Cold Spring Harbor Press, 1989. Pp. 209–214.
11. Kurzrock, R., et al. Molecular Diagnostics of Chronic Myelogenous Leukemia and Philadelphia-Positive Acute Leukemia. In M. Furth and M. Greaves (eds.), *Cancer Cells: Molecular Diagnostics of Human Cancer*. New York: Cold Spring Harbor Press, 1989. Pp. 9–13.
12. Blum, M., et al. Molecular mechanism of slow acetylation of drugs and carcinogens in humans. *Proc. Natl. Acad. Sci. U.S.A.* 88:5237, 1991.
13. Kawajiri, K., et al. Identification of genetically high risk individuals to lung cancer by DNA polymorphisms of the cytochrome P450IA1 gene. *FEBS* 263:131, 1990.

14. Rodenhuis, S., et al. Mutational activation of the K-ras oncogene. A possible pathogenetic factor in adenocarcinoma of the lung. *N. Engl. J. Med.* 317:929, 1987.
15. Hsu, I. C., et al. p53 gene mutational hotspot in human hepatocellular carcinomas from Qidong, China. *Nature* 350:427, 1991.
16. Southern, E. M. Detection of specific sequences among DNA fragments separated by gel electrophoresis. *J. Mol. Biol.* 98:503, 1975.
17. Maniatis, T., Fritsch, E. F., and Sambrook, J. *Molecular Cloning: A Laboratory Manual.* New York: Cold Spring Harbor Press, 1982.
18. Weston, A., et al. Differential DNA sequence deletions from chromosomes 3, 11, 13 and 17 in squamous cell carcinoma, large cell carcinoma and adenocarcinoma of the human lung. *Proc. Natl. Acad. Sci. U.S.A.* 86:5099, 1989.
19. Sugimura, H., et al. Human debrisoquine hydroxylase gene polymorphisms in cancer patients and controls. *Carcinogenesis* 11:1527, 1990.
20. Sanger, F., Nicklen, S., and Coulson, A. R. DNA sequencing with chain-terminating inhibitors. *Proc. Natl. Acad. Sci. U.S.A.* 74:5463, 1977.
21. Phillips, D. H., et al. Correlation of DNA adduct levels in human lung with cigarette smoking. *Nature* 336:790, 1988.
22. Savela, K., et al. Interlaboratory comparison of the ^{32}P-postlabelling assay for aromatic DNA adducts in white blood cells of iron foundry workers. *Mutat. Res.* 224:485, 1989.
23. Perera, F. P., et al. Molecular and genetic damage in humans from environmental pollution in Poland. *Nature* 360:256, 1992.
24. Randerath, E., et al. ^{32}P-postlabeling analysis of DNA adducts persisting for up to 42 weeks in the skin, epidermis and dermis of mice treated topically with 7,12-dimethylbenz[a]anthracene. *Carcinogenesis* 6:1117, 1985.
25. Shields, P. G., et al. Polycyclic aromatic hydrocarbon DNA adducts in human lung and cancer susceptibility genes. *Cancer Res.* 53:3486, 1993.
26. Shields, P. G., et al. Combined high performance liquid chromatography/^{32}P-postlabeling assay of N7-methyldeoxyguanosine. *Cancer Res.* 50:6580, 1990.
27. Van Schooten, F. J., et al. Polycyclic aromatic hydrocarbon-DNA adducts in lung tissue from lung cancer patients. *Carcinogenesis* 11:1677, 1990.
28. Perera, F., et al. Comparison of DNA adducts and sister chromatid exchange in lung cancer cases and controls. *Cancer Res.* 49:4446, 1989.
29. Perera, F. P., et al. Detection of polycyclic aromatic hydrocarbon-DNA adducts in white blood cells of foundry workers. *Cancer Res.* 48:2288, 1988.
30. Bender, M. A., et al. Current status of cytogenetic procedures to detect and quantify previous exposures to radiation. *Mutat. Res.* 196:103, 1988.
31. Latt, S. A. Microfluorometric detection of deoxyribonucleic acid replication in human metaphase chromosomes. *Proc. Natl. Acad. Sci. U.S.A.* 70:3395, 1973.
32. Heddle, J. A., et al. The induction of micronuclei as a measure of genotoxicity. A report of the U.S. Environmental Protection Agency Gene-Tox Program. *Mutat. Res.* 123:61, 1983.
33. Geneste, O., et al. Comparison of pulmonary DNA adduct levels, measured by ^{32}P-postlabelling and aryl hydrocarbon hydroxylase activity in lung parenchyma of smokers and ex-smokers. *Carcinogenesis* 12:1301, 1991.
34. Brandt-Rauf, P. W., and Niman, H. L. Serum screening for oncogene proteins in workers exposed to PCBs. *Br. J. Ind. Med.* 45:689, 1988.
35. Bennett, W. P., et al. Archival analysis of p53 genetic and protein alterations in Chinese esophageal cancer. *Oncogene* 6:1779, 1991.
36. Davidoff, A. M., et al. Relation between p53 overexpression and established prognostic factors in breast cancer. *Surgery* 110:259, 1991.
37. Lappë, M. Ethical issues in genetic screening for susceptibility to chronic lung disease. *J. Occup. Med.* 30:493, 1988.
38. Cartwright, R. A., et al. Role of N-acetyltransferase phenotypes in bladder carcinogenesis: A pharmacogenetic epidemiological approach to bladder cancer. *Lancet* 2:842, 1982.
39. Evans, D. A. N-acetyltransferase. *Pharmacol. Ther.* 42:157, 1989.
40. Ladero, J. M., et al. Hepatic acetylator phenotype in bladder cancer patients. *Ann. Clin. Res.* 17:96, 1985.
41. Weber, W. W., and Hein, D. W. N-acetylation pharmacogenetics. *Pharmacol. Rev.* 37:25, 1985.
42. Kadlubar, F. F., et al. Polymorphisms for aromatic amine metabolism in humans: Relevance for human carcinogenesis. *Environ. Health Perspect.* 98:69, 1992.

43. Caporaso, N., et al. Lung cancer risk, occupational exposure, and the debrisoquine metabolic phenotype. *Cancer Res.* 49:3675, 1989.
44. Ozturk, M. p53 mutation in hepatocellular carcinoma after aflatoxin exposure. *Lancet* 338:1356, 1991.
45. National Research Council. *The Effects on Populations of Exposure to Low Levels of Ionizing Radiation (BEIR III).* Washington, DC: National Academy Press, 1990.
46. Sarto, F., et al. A cytogenetic study on workers exposed to low concentrations of benzene. *Carcinogenesis* 5:827, 1984.
47. Sorsa, M., and Yager, J. W. Cytogenetic Surveillance of Occupational Exposures. In G. Obe and A. Basler (eds.), *Cytogenetics: Basic and Applied Aspects.* New York: Springer-Verlag, 1987. Pp. 345–360.
48. Au, W. W. Monitoring human populations for effects of radiation and chemical exposures using cytogenetic techniques. *Occup. Med.* 6:597, 1991.
49. Sidransky, D., et al. Identification of ras oncogene mutations in the stool of patients with curable colorectal tumors. *Science* 256:102, 1992.
50. Brandt-Rauf, P. W., et al. Serum oncoproteins and growth factors in asbestosis and silicosis patients. *Int. J. Cancer* 50:881, 1992.
51. Orentlicher, D. From the office of the General Counsel. Genetic screening by employers. *J.A.M.A.* 263:1005, 1008, 1990.
52. Harper, P. S. Insurance and genetic testing [see comments]. *Lancet* 341:224, 1993.

Further Information

Maniatis, T., Fritsch, E. F., and Sambrook, J. *Molecular Cloning: A Laboratory Manual.* New York: Cold Spring Harbor Press, 1982.

PCR Technology: Principles and Applications for DNA Amplification. New York: W. H. Freeman and Co., 1991. Pp. 1–246.

Shields, P. G. Inherited factors and environmental exposures in cancer risk. *J. Occup. Med.* 35:34, 1993.

Shields, P. G., and Harris, C. C. Environmental causes of cancer. *Med. Clin. North Am.* 74:263, 1990.

Shields, P. G., and Harris, C. C. Molecular epidemiology and the genetics of environmental cancer. *J.A.M.A.* 266:681, 1991.

Shields, P. G., and Harris, C. C. Principles of Carcinogenesis: Chemical. In V. T. DeVita, Jr., S. Hellman, and S. A. Rosenberg (eds.), *Cancer: Principles and Practices of Oncology.* Philadelphia: Lippincott, 1992.

Medical Center Occupational Health

John Howard

Medical centers today are complex workplace environments that pose an assortment of safety and health hazards for those who labor in them as health care workers (HCWs). Be they nurses, food service workers, physicians, laboratorians, therapists, housekeepers, or environmental services personnel, HCWs are potentially exposed to many different biologic, chemical, physical, and psychosocial hazards [1].

Many occupational hazards found in medical centers are similar to those hazards confronted by workers in industries commonly thought to be "dangerous," such as construction or manufacturing. It is not generally appreciated, however, that the occupational hazards faced daily by workers employed in the health care industry can be every bit as dangerous as those found in other industries.

Medical centers should be at the forefront of the effort to provide state-of-the-art occupational safety and health prevention services for their employees, but often they are not.

For the past decade, more medical centers have begun to provide occupational health services to businesses and industries in their geographic vicinity. Recognizing the value of providing occupational health services to outside organizations, hospitals have often begun to look more carefully at their own operations with respect to occupational safety and health risks. In fact, in light of workplace regulations and other contemporary workplace safety issues, such as acquired immunodeficiency syndrome (AIDS) and workers' compensation, many medical centers have evolved programs designed for "infection control" into more comprehensive occupational health services. These changes are mirrored in this book itself: In the first edition, *Handbook of Occupational Medicine,* hospitals were afforded but two pages.

The regulatory milieu of medical center occupational health can be relatively complicated. Not only does the Occupational Safety and Health Administration (OSHA) have jurisdiction over medical centers, as it does over any other type of workplace, but also the Food and Drug Administration (FDA), the Nuclear Regulatory Commission (NRC), the Joint Commission on Accreditation of Health Care Organizations (JCAHCO), and the National Institutes of Health (NIH) have all proposed regulations or guidelines that may affect medical center activities. Sometimes, the jurisdiction of these agencies overlaps. For example, the NRC oversees the use of radioactive materials in hospital radiology departments, but the FDA regulates naturally occurring radioisotopes such as radium and radon, which can also be used in radiology departments.

The JCAHCO requires hospitals to establish policies and procedures for monitoring and responding to workplace safety and health hazards. The NIH has published guidelines pertaining to a variety of medical center activities, including establishing occupational health programs for animal handlers and for researchers involved with recombinant deoxyribonucleic acid (DNA) research. Also, the federal Centers for Disease Control and Prevention (CDC), as well as state, county, and city health departments often monitor the hospital environment to ensure that proper precautions are being followed to prevent transmission of communicable diseases.

It is likely that a majority of occupational health physicians will become involved in some manner with medical center occupational health issues, either by providing consultative services to the institution itself, or by treating those people who work there. This chapter describes how an occupational health program can be implemented at a medical center; discusses the important types of occupational hazards facing medical center workers, including the effect that these hazards can have on worker health and safety; and highlights methods that are available to prevent these effects.

Medical Center Occupational Health Programs

Hazard Assessment

The traditional emphasis in medical centers is to provide medical care for patients, not to prevent injury and illness among their workers [2]. This emphasis has led to inattention to effective assessment of workplace hazards through inspection and monitoring, medical evaluations, and hazard control.

Every medical center should establish and maintain a comprehensive occupational safety and health program to monitor and protect the health of its employees [3]. An occupational safety and health program, in addition to ensuring a safe workplace for medical center employees, can also ensure compliance with the various requirements of the JCAHCO, federal or state OSHA programs, state and local health codes, and workers' compensation regulations [4].

Hazard assessment is the first step in maintaining an effective occupational injury and illness prevention program. Physical inspection of the medical center should be performed on a regularly scheduled basis by people capable of recognizing safety and health hazards.

In addition to inspecting patient care areas for hazards particular to patient care providers, nonpatient care areas, such as administration, the machine shop, the power plant, and kitchen facilities, should also be inspected carefully. Environmental or area monitoring, as well as personal or breathing zone monitoring for airborne contaminants, should be performed where appropriate as part of the medical center's ongoing hazard assessment program.

Hazard Control

In general, the hierarchy of hazard control strategies consists of (1) engineering controls; (2) work practice controls; and (3) personal protective equipment.

Engineering controls are the most effective since they "engineer" out the potential exposure. An example of this is a system to "scavenge" waste anesthetic gases at their source. Work practice controls alter the way work is performed in order to reduce exposure; for example, turning the anesthetic gas valve off immediately when the breathing system is disconnected from the patient. Personal protective equipment (PPE) is usually the "control of last resort," since exposure can still occur if the employee is not provided with, or declines to use, PPE; for example, a respirator to prevent inhalation of trace levels of waste anesthetic gas.

Medical Evaluations

A common misconception is that HCWs can maintain their own health without the assistance of an employee health service. An HCW may actually need more time off from work because of an occupational injury or illness than the average American worker [5].

Medical evaluations are an essential aspect of a medical center's overall occupational safety and health program. Most new medical center employees should have an initial job-specific medical evaluation before beginning work. After hire, medical surveillance needs to be performed for certain workers on a periodic basis to monitor job-related exposures to specific agents. Prompt diagnosis and treatment of occupational injuries and illnesses should also be provided to medical center workers, including return to work examinations. Documentation of these efforts can help ensure compliance with regulations and various guidelines. Health education, health promotion, stress reduction, and substance abuse counseling should supplement an effective program.

Biologic Hazards

Bloodborne Pathogens

Foremost among workplace biologic hazards are those associated with hepatitis B virus (HBV) and human immunodeficiency virus (HIV). Occupational transmission of these viruses, as well as other bloodborne pathogens such as hepatitis C and syphilis, among others, occurs primarily through parenteral inoculation of blood or other potentially infectious body fluids through a needlestick or other sharps injury. Transmission can also occur through direct deposition of blood or other infectious fluids into the eye, on mucous membranes, or on the skin.

Occupational HBV infection can lead directly to acute or fulminant hepatitis B infection as well as chronic hepatitis. Chronic hepatitis B infection can lead to cirrhosis of the liver and hepatoma. The adverse effects of HBV infection can be prevented by administration of the HBV vaccine.

Occupational HIV infection results in cell-mediated immunodeficiency, which is progressive and can lead to AIDS. Clinically, AIDS is characterized by the occurrence of one or more life-threatening opportunistic infections, such as *Pneumocystis carinii* pneumonia, or neoplasms, such as B-cell lymphoma or Kaposi's sarcoma. As yet, no effective vaccine exists to prevent HIV infection.

In 1991, OSHA published a new occupational health standard designed to prevent exposure to HBV, HIV, and other infectious agents transmitted by contact with blood and other body fluids [6]. The Bloodborne Pathogens Standard requires that employees with occupational exposure to blood, or other potentially infectious materials (OPIM), be protected through a variety of measures as specified in a written Exposure Control Plan.

Employers must adhere to (1) universal precautions as specified by the CDC [7]; (2) engineering controls and work practice controls, such as the use of self-sheathing needles and the proper disposal of needles and sharps; and (3) use of PPE, such as eye and face protection, gloves, and gowns.

Employers must make HBV vaccine available and provide it free of charge to all employees with potential occupational exposure to blood and body fluids. The employee can decline to be vaccinated, but must sign a declination statement specified in the Appendix of the Standard.

In some individuals who receive the three-dose HBV vaccination series, a measurable immune response does not develop. When these individuals are revaccinated, 15 to 25% produce an adequate antibody response after one additional dose, and 30 to 50% after three additional doses [8]. The remainder may have a genetic or acquired inability to respond to HBV vaccine.

The Standard also requires that if an employee sustains an exposure incident, that is, a specific eye, mouth, other mucous membrane, nonintact skin, or parenteral contact with blood or OPIM, the employer must provide postexposure medical and follow-up evaluation. Employers must also alert employees to the presence of blood in the workplace by the use of BIOHAZARD labels, and provide information through employee training.

Other Infectious Agents

Infectious agents other than HIV and HBV can be transmitted from patient to HCW in the medical center. These agents include enteric pathogens that cause acute diarrhea, hepatitis A, herpes simplex, *Staphylococcus aureus,* group A and B *Streptococcus,* tuberculosis, varicella-zoster virus, cytomegalovirus (CMV), *Neisseria meningitidis,* cryptosporidium, *Bordetella pertussis,* scabies, and an assortment of respiratory viruses such as influenza.

Development and implementation of an effective infection control program in the medical center is necessary to eliminate the risk of transmission of infectious agents from patient to HCW, as well as from HCW to patient [9] (Table 30-1). Important elements of hazard control of infectious agents include preplacement medical evaluations, monitoring for tuberculin skin test reactivity, adult immunization programs, access to health counseling, and training in infection control procedures, such as hand-washing practices, use of gloves and other protective clothing, and proper disposal of infectious wastes [10].

Three viral infections pose a teratogenic risk for pregnant medical center employees—rubella, cytomegalovirus, and varicella-zoster infections [11]. Infection control programs should include steps to prevent exposure of pregnant employees to these teratogenic viruses. In addition, male employees exposed to these infections who have contact with hospitalized pregnant patients should be included in the same exposure prevention program. A vaccination program against rubella and varicella should also be implemented to prevent infection in exposed workers.

Latex Allergy

The escalating use of latex gloves in the health care industry to minimize contact with bloodborne pathogens has resulted in an increasing number of complaints of latex allergy. Other items made from latex products, such as anesthetic tubing, ventilator bags, and intravenous lines, can also be encountered by HCWs.

Latex allergy in HCWs may be underreported because of a lack of awareness of the problem. Some reports suggest that between 5 and 10% of HCWs, who depend on latex gloves to perform their job duties, will develop sensitivity reactions [12]. Clinically, this sensitivity can be assessed by measurement of immunoglobulin E (IgE) antibodies and the radioallergosorbent test (RAST).

Allergic contact dermatitis involving the hands is the most common manifestation of latex allergy in HCWs. However, systemic reactions, such as asthma or anaphylaxis, can also occur. Health care workers with latex allergy should be provided with hypoallergenic, or nonlatex-type, gloves. They should also minimize their contact with medical equipment made from latex products (see Chap. 19).

Tuberculosis*

After 35 years of decline, tuberculosis (TB) has increased in frequency in the United States every year since 1985. In 1990, 25,701 new TB cases were reported, which represents 9883 more cases than expected based on trends of the early 1980s [13]. Of grave public health concern is the recent appearance of strains of *Mycobacterium tuberculosis,* which are resistant to multiple antibiotics. Multidrug-resistant TB (MDR TB) has emerged as a major public and occupational health problem in New York and Florida [14]. Cases of MDR TB are associated with a mortality of approximately 80% [15].

The increase in TB cases has been attributed to the HIV epidemic, inadequacies in the public health infrastructure for monitoring compliance with outpatient TB drug regimens, immigration from countries with a high TB prevalence, homelessness, and limited access to medical care [16]. Health care workers employed in urban medical centers that care for large numbers of TB patients are at risk of acquiring occupational TB infection. Every medical center should develop a TB exposure control plan based on traditional principles of TB control [17]. An important element in a TB control program is surveillance for new TB infections.

Employees who have not previously had a TB skin test, or whose test results were negative or unknown, should receive a skin test at time of hire and at least at 12-month intervals. People who have been immunized with bacillus Calmette-Guérin (BCG) in other countries may exhibit falsely positive tuberculin skin test reactions.

Employees who have regular prolonged contact with suspect or confirmed infectious TB cases should probably be skin-tested more often. Employees should be informed that HIV infection and other medical conditions may cause a TB skin test to be negative even when TB infection is present.

Prompt medical evaluation and atmospheric isolation of all patients suspected of having infectious (i.e., pulmonary or laryngeal) TB are important. Most commonly, atmospheric isolation can be accomplished by housing the patient in an isolation room that is maintained under negative atmospheric pressure.

Medical procedures such as sputum induction and bronchoscopy performed on a suspect or confirmed infectious TB case can aerosolize body fluids likely to be contaminated with TB bacteria. As a result, they should be done only with effective local exhaust ventilation, dilution ventilation, or high-efficiency particulate air (HEPA) filtration of the immediate area or room. Respiratory protection should be used when other means of exposure control are not effective.

Lastly, TB prevention training should be provided to all employees reasonably anticipated to be exposed to a suspect or confirmed infectious TB case. Such training should emphasize (1) the danger of TB exposure especially for those with HIV infection, (2) modes of TB transmission, and symptoms and consequences of TB infection, (3) methods of preventing TB exposure, and (4) the importance of TB surveillance and preventive therapy.

---

*Currently, OSHA is developing a standard regarding occupational exposure to TB. Readers are advised to obtain updated information as appropriate.

Table 30-1. Summary of important recommendations and work restrictions for personnel with infectious diseases

Disease/problem	Relieve from direct patient contact	Partial work restriction	Duration
Conjunctivitis, infectious	Yes		Until discharge ceases
Cytomegalovirus infections	No		
Diarrhea			
Acute stage (diarrhea with other symptoms)	Yes		Until symptoms resolve and infection with *Salmonella* is ruled out
Convalescent stage *Salmonella* (nontyphoidal)	No	Personnel should not take care of high-risk patients	Until stool is free of the infecting organism on 2 consecutive cultures not less than 24 hr apart
Other enteric pathogens	No		
Enteroviral infections	No	Personnel should not take care of infants and newborns	Until symptoms resolve
Group A streptococcal disease	Yes		Until 24 hr after adequate treatment is started
Heptatitis viral			
Hepatitis A	Yes		Until 7 days after onset of jaundice
Hepatitis B			
Acute	No	Personnel should wear gloves for procedures that involve trauma to tissues or contact with mucous membranes or nonintact skin	Until antigenemia resolves
Chronic antigenemia	No	Same as acute illness	Until antigenemia resolves
Hepatitis, non-A, non-B	No	Same as acute hepatitis B	Period of infectivity has not been determined
Herpes simplex			
Genital	No		
Hands (herpetic whitlow)	Yes	(Note: It is not known whether gloves prevent transmission)	Until lesions heal
Orofacial	No	Personnel should not take care of high-risk patients	Until lesions heal
Measles			
Active	Yes		Until 7 days after the rash appears
Postexposure (susceptible personnel)	Yes		From the 5th through the 21st day after exposure and/or 7 days after the rash appears
Mumps			
Active	Yes		Until 9 days after onset of parotitis

(continued)

Table 30-1 (continued)

Disease/problem	Relieve from direct patient contact	Partial work restriction	Duration
Postexposure	Yes*		From the 12th through the 26th day after exposure or until 9 days after onset of parotitis
Pertussis			
Active	Yes		From the beginning of the catarrhal stage through the 3rd week after onset of paroxysms or until 7 days after start of effective therapy
Postexposure (asymptomatic personnel)	No		
Postexposure (symptomatic personnel)	Yes		Same as active pertussis
Rubella			
Active	Yes		Until 5 days after the rash appears
Postexposure (susceptible personnel)	Yes		From the 7th through the 21st day after exposure and/or 5 days after rash appears
Scabies	Yes		Until treated
Staphylococcus aureus (skin lesions)	Yes		Until lesions have resolved
Upper-respiratory infections (high-risk patients)	Yes	Personnel with upper-respiratory infections should not take care of high-risk patients	Until acute symptoms resolve
Zoster (shingles)			
Active	No	Appropriate barrier desirable; personnel should not take care of high-risk patients	Until lesions dry and crust
Postexposure (susceptible personnel)	Yes		From the 10th through the 21st day after exposure or if varicella occurs until all lesions dry and crust
Varicella (chickenpox)			
Active	Yes		Until all lesions dry and crust
Postexposure	Yes		From the 10th through the 21st day after exposure or if varicella occurs until all lesions dry and crust

*Mumps vaccine may be offered to susceptible personnel. When given after exposure, mumps vaccine may not provide protection. However, if exposure did not result in infection, immunizing exposed personnel should protect against subsequent infection. Neither mumps immune globulin nor immune serum globulin (ISG) is of established value in postexposure prophylaxis. Transmission of mumps among personnel and patients has not been a major problem in hospitals in the United States, probably due to multiple factors, including high levels of natural and vaccine-induced immunity.

Laboratory Animal Allergy

Large medical centers frequently engage in medical research utilizing laboratory animals. Medical center personnel who work in close proximity to laboratory animals are at risk of developing laboratory animal allergy (LAA).

Laboratory animal allergy represents an immediate-type hypersensitivity reaction mediated through IgE antibody. It can occur when an employee is exposed through inhalation, or through direct skin contact, to allergens from an animal's fur or dander, saliva, urine, serum, or other body product. The clinical manifestations of LAA are similar to those of other type I hypersensitivity reactions and include rhinitis, conjunctivitis, and asthma [18]. As with other type I immune reactions, elevations in IgE antibodies may occur.

Predicting which employees will develop LAA is not well established, but a number of different factors have been the subject of study, including atopic history, the species of animal, and the type of allergen. Studies have shown that atopic individuals are at increased risk for LAA [19], but a significant number of nonatopic individuals also develop sensitivity to laboratory animals [20]. Cats have been implicated more often than other animals in LAA, but mice, rats, and rabbits are also associated with its development. Urine and saliva proteins may be more potent as LAA allergens than fur and dander.

Effective methods to prevent LAA in medical center workers who are exposed to animal allergens are not well established [21]. Maintenance of a clean environment to house the animals and development of work practices that reduce the amount of airborne particulates are important. The use of PPE does not seem to be effective, however. Requiring workers to wear respirators to prevent allergen access to the respiratory tract, and goggles and other clothing to prevent eye and skin contact, is often resisted.

Engineering controls would seem to be the most effective. Among these methods are (1) utilizing "nude," or hairless, animals for experimentation; (2) preventing escape of allergens from animal cages by the use of filter-topped cages; (3) use of laminar flow-cage racks; (4) independent room ventilation and local exhaust systems equipped with HEPA filters; (5) frequent room air changes with no recirculation; (6) use of dust-free bedding; and (7) use of biologic safety cabinets for animal handling or cage cleaning [22].

Depending on the research interests and capabilities of a medical center, extensive animal centers may be present that house not only mice and rodents but also primates, such as macaque monkeys, and even farm animals. In these specific settings, attention needs to be focused on the prevention of zoonoses, that is, animal diseases that are transmissible to humans [23].

Hazardous Waste Disposal

The modern medical center generates large amounts of infectious (human, animal, or biologic) and noninfectious (radioactive, chemical, flammable, and explosive) waste. All of this hazardous waste must be properly collected, packaged, transported, and disposed of to protect both the HCW and the environment. Every medical center should have a detailed hazardous waste management plan that complies with applicable state and local hazardous waste management requirements.

Hospital infectious waste management consists of the following basic elements: proper designation of the type of waste that should be managed as infectious, separation of infectious and noninfectious waste, and packaging, storage, treatment, and disposal of infectious wastes [24]. Workers engaged in these processes should be trained in infectious waste management, including an explanation of the hospital's waste management plan, proper waste-handling work practices, and the use of PPE. Training should include an explanation of the various methods used to treat infectious wastes and a demonstration of the proper operation of waste treatment equipment such as steam or radiation sterilization, incineration, and thermal inactivation.

A management plan for the hospital's noninfectious wastes should also be provided for in the medical center's overall hazardous waste management plan. Recommendations for the proper handling and disposal of the major categories of noninfectious wastes, for example, radioactive wastes, chemical wastes, and flammable and explosive wastes, are available from several different sources [25].

Chemical Hazards

Waste Anesthetic Gases

The halogenated anesthetics used in medical centers today do not pose the fire and explosion hazard that older anesthetics once did. Adverse health effects, however, can occur from exposure to trace levels of "waste" anesthetic gases in operating and recovery rooms, labor and delivery suites, and emergency areas and outpatient clinics.

The principal source of waste anesthetic gas in the medical center is leakage from anesthetic equipment. Gas may escape during hookup and check-out of the system, may seep over the lip of the patient's mask, or may collect in the operating room because of nonexistent or inoperable scavenging systems. Recovery room personnel can also be exposed to waste anesthetic gases if they breathe the exhaled air of recently anesthetized patients.

The acute effects of waste anesthetic gas inhalation are similar to those seen in anesthetized patients—drowsiness, fatigue, irritability, headache, nausea, and incoordination. Controversy exists over whether trace amounts of waste anesthetic gases can affect cognitive function and impair job performance [26, 27]. Some studies have suggested an increase in various cancers from chronic exposure to trace levels of anesthetic gas [28], but no firm causal relationship has been demonstrated. Similarly, adverse reproductive and teratogenic effects, such as an increased risk of spontaneous abortion [29] and congenital malformations [30], have been reported, but, as with cancer, no firm causal relationship has been demonstrated [31].

Prevention of exposure to trace anesthetic gas can be easily accomplished by the "scavenging" of fugitive gases. A scavenging system collects waste gases and disposes of them through either the use of a central vacuum system or a nonrecirculating exhaust system. In the presence of an effective scavenging system, respiratory protection is unnecessary. Other methods of exposure control include preventing equipment leaks, ensuring the use of proper delivery techniques, and maintaining an effective gas monitoring program. Worker training and medical surveillance are also important elements in an exposure control program for waste anesthetic gases [32].

Antineoplastic Agents

Antineoplastic agents can produce both acute and chronic health effects in HCWs who handle these agents. A direct irritant effect can result from skin, eye, or mucous membrane exposure. Systemic effects can also occur, including facial flushing, coughing, headache, lightheadedness, abdominal pain, nausea, and vomiting [33]. Many antineoplastic agents also have mutagenic, teratogenic, and carcinogenic properties [34].

To prevent the development of acute and chronic health effects, safe-handling work practices must be followed by all HCWs who come into contact with antineoplastic agents. The medical center should develop written procedures for the safe handling of antineoplastic agents and ensure that all workers who handle these agents are trained in these procedures [35].

Also, proper engineering controls should be used to minimize exposure. For instance, antineoplastic agents should be prepared under a laminar flow hood to minimize inhalational exposure. Appropriate PPE should be utilized to prevent skin contact. Also, goggles and face protection should be worn to prevent eye and mucous membrane exposure. Spill cleanup should be performed only when using appropriate gloves. A medical surveillance program for employees exposed to antineoplastic agents should also be implemented [35].

Sterilants

Ethylene oxide (EtO) is the most widely used chemical sterilizing agent in the medical center. It is a colorless gas with a distinctive sweet, ether-like odor and is used to sterilize medical instruments, especially those that are sensitive to heat or moisture.

The major route of exposure is inhalation and occurs during the operation of hospital sterilizing equipment. Workers in central supply and in surgical and dental suites can be briefly exposed to high EtO concentrations when items are removed from the sterilizer. These short-term exposures have been shown to produce chromosomal aberrations [36].

Ethylene oxide is an acute irritant to the eyes, respiratory tract, and skin. It is also a neurotoxin, producing central nervous system (CNS) depression and peripheral neuropathy in high doses [37]. Chronic effects include reproductive damage such as increased rates of spontaneous abortions [38] and the possibility of leukemia [39].

Another sterilant commonly found in the central supply room or the dialysis unit of any medical center is formaldehyde, which is often used for cold sterilization of medical equipment. Formaldehyde can also be encountered in the laboratory as a tissue preservative in the form of formalin, a 37 to 50% solution by weight of formaldehyde gas.

Formaldehyde is an irritant and acute exposure can result in conjunctival and respiratory tract irritation. Repeated exposure has been associated with sensitization. Some reports indicate that formaldehyde-induced asthma can occur [40], but others suggest otherwise [41]. Formaldehyde is a mutagen in many bioassay systems and has produced nasal cancer in laboratory animals [42]. The National Institute for Occupational Safety and Health (NIOSH) recommends that formaldehyde be handled as a suspect carcinogen in the workplace [43].

To prevent exposure to sterilants such as EtO and formaldehyde, control measures must be instituted. Environmental monitoring can identify areas of the medical center in which sterilant concentration exceeds the permissible exposure limit (PEL) set by OSHA. The PEL for EtO is 1 part per million (ppm) of air, as an 8-hour time-weighted average (TWA) [44]. In 1992, OSHA lowered the PEL for formaldehyde from 1.0 to 0.75 ppm [45].

Engineering controls should be implemented in areas in which sterilant exposure exceeds the PEL. All sterilizing operations can be centralized within the medical center, and all EtO sterilization chambers used in the medical center should be equipped with basic safety features. These features include an automatic door-locking mechanism, controlled release of EtO into the sterilization chamber, and an effective local exhaust system.

Procedures should be in place to alert workers to high levels of EtO through continuous area monitoring, coupled with an alarm system that is triggered when hazardous EtO levels are reached. Also, an emergency evacuation plan should be in place if controls fail or a large spill occurs.

Skin and eye contact with sterilants should be avoided and PPE, such as gloves, face shields and goggles, and protective clothing, should be provided to the worker. Medical surveillance of workers who may be exposed to sterilants is also necessary.

Disinfectants

Many different types of chemical disinfectants are in use in the medical center. Isopropyl alcohol, sodium hypochlorite, iodine, phenolics, and quaternary ammonium compounds are among those most commonly used. Most of these agents are eye, mucous membrane, skin, and respiratory tract irritants, and appropriate protective clothing, including gloves and face shields, should be used to limit employee exposure. Glutaraldehyde is used as a substitute for formaldehyde, but it can produce adverse health effects also [46].

Laboratory Safety

Among a medical center's specialized work environments, its laboratories may contain the greatest variety of chemical, biologic, and physical hazards. Every laboratory should develop a safety policy and procedures, with an emphasis on staff training, container labeling, and ready access for employees to Material Safety Data Sheets (MSDSs) on the agents used in the laboratory.

Management of chemical hazards in the laboratory should include safe storage of potentially explosive or flammable materials and attention to the dangers of mixing incompatible chemicals. Management of biohazards should include the use of biologic safety cabinets for experiments that can generate pathogenic aerosols and the use of measures to prevent laboratory workers from contracting zoonoses. Management of physical hazards includes development of procedures for safe handling of glassware and radionuclides.

The availability and use of PPE are essential to an effective laboratory safety program. Laboratory coats, eye and face protection, and respiratory protection should be used when appropriate. Emergency shower and eyewash facilities should be located in close proximity to areas in the laboratory in which corrosive or irritating chemicals are used.

Medical center laboratories may be subject to federal and state requirements pertaining to laboratory use of hazardous chemicals [47]. The OSHA "Laboratory Standard" applies to facilities engaged in the "laboratory use" of hazardous chemicals. Laboratory use means that a single person can easily manipulate the containers used for chemical reactions, multiple chemical procedures are used but are not a part of a production process, and protective laboratory practices are in use to minimize employee exposure. The Laboratory Standard requires employers to (1) perform exposure monitoring, (2) develop and carry out the provisions of a chemical hygiene plan, (3) provide information and training for employees about chemicals present in their work area, and (4) provide medical consultation and examinations under specified circumstances.

Physical Hazards

Exertion

Manual lifting tasks are responsible for a high frequency of acute and chronic back pain complaints among medical center workers, especially among nurses' aides, nurses, orderlies, custodians, and laundry and maintenance workers. Studies have consistently shown that nurses' aides rank in the top ten occupations at risk for back injury as measured by the number of workers' compensation claims filled per worker [48].

In general, lack of fitness, postural stress, and the performance of work exceeding a worker's strength are important factors in the development of back pain [49]. Specifically, patient handling is an important work-related factor in the development of back pain in HCWs [50]. Patients, as objects to be lifted, are heavy, often cannot be held close to the body while being lifted, frequently resist being lifted, and often have to be lifted from awkward angles in cramped spaces [51].

Strategies to prevent back injury in the medical center include job modification, use of mechanical lifting equipment, and adherence to recommended work practice guidelines for lifting [52]. The use of low-back-support belts is popular, but of unproven efficacy.

Heat

The laundry area, boiler room, and kitchen facilities are environments in which medical center workers may be exposed to heat stress. Heat stress occurs most often during the warm summer months or when the hospital's ventilation system fails. Excessive heat exposure can produce a number of different adverse health effects, such as dermatitis, syncope, heat cramps, heat exhaustion, and heat stroke.

Strategies to prevent heat stress include (1) scheduling of work during the coolest part of the day and allowing frequent rest breaks, (2) insulating sources of heat production from the worker or installing reflective shielding, (3) ventilating and cooling hot work areas, (4) providing an ample supply of cool water to exposed workers and encouraging frequent ingestion, (5) training workers to recognize symptoms and signs of heat stress, and (6) allowing new employees or employees returning from vacation to become acclimatized to the hot environment before attempting strenuous work [53].

Noise

The modern medical center can be a noisy environment. Even though the ambient sound pressure level in a hospital does not approach the average 80- to 95-decibel (dB) level on the A-weighted scale found in many manufacturing environments, the measured levels are surprisingly high—in the 50- to 70-dB(A) range [54]. Indeed, patients commonly complain about hospital noise levels, and some may suffer from noise-induced sleep disorders while hospitalized [55].

Medical center noise is diverse and includes the sounds from pocket pagers, patient-activity monitors, telemetric monitoring devices, ventilator alarms, electronic intravenous delivery systems, computer printers, clanging food service carts, and ringing telephones. All of these "noise-emitters" contribute to the overall hospital noise problem, but the most important contributors may be the increasing number of staff who work in the modern medical center.

Noise exposure can produce both acute and chronic hearing loss by damaging the sensitive hair cells in the cochlea of the inner ear. Noise exposure can also produce adverse physiologic and psychological effects, which are just as deleterious to the health of HCWs as hearing loss. For example, since noise is an arousal stimulus, excessive noise can increase blood pressure, pulse rate, and muscle tension [56]. Noisy environments interfere with cognition and decrease the annoyance threshold [57]. They also increase errors and lead to a deterioration in worker performance [58].

The EPA has recommended that noise levels in hospitals not exceed an average of 45 dB(A) in daytime and 35 dB(A) at night [59]. Efforts should be made to reduce the ambient noise level in hospitals by the use of engineering controls and changes in work practices, and through education. Ambient noise levels should be monitored by acoustical sampling, and, when required [60], a hearing conservation program should be implemented.

Radiation

Electromagnetic radiation can be divided into two categories depending on its energy content. Ionizing radiation (alpha and beta particles, gamma and x-rays, and neutrons) has enough energy to ionize atoms, causing serious irreversible tissue damage. Nonionizing radiation (radio and microwaves, infrared, visible and ultraviolet light) has only enough energy to vibrate molecules, causing minor reversible damage. Health care worker exposure to ionizing radiation occurs from scatter of x-ray beams from diagnostic or therapeutic x-ray equipment, or from the emission of gamma rays by patients who are being treated with radionuclides.

The acute and chronic effects from overexposure to ionizing radiation are well known [61]. Acute, high-dose exposure can produce acute radiation syndrome, which can lead to death within a few weeks. A very high dose can produce cerebral edema and death within 24 hours. Exposure to ionizing radiation causes genetic mutation and chromosomal damage, cancer, lung and kidney fibrosis, cataracts, aplastic anemia, and sterility, and accelerates the aging process.

A radiation protection program includes source shielding, limiting exposure time, increasing the distance between the radiation source and the worker, the avoidance of unnecessary exposure, and exposure monitoring by environmental surveillance and personal dosimetry. Several different federal regulatory agencies are involved with the prevention of radiation exposure, including OSHA, the FDA, and the NRC. Worker exposure is subject to an OSHA standard [62], the performance of radiation equipment is regulated by the Center for Radiologic Devices of the FDA, and the use of certain radionuclides is regulated by the NRC. Individual states also have laws pertaining to radiation protection.

More common than exposure to ionizing radiation is exposure to nonionizing radiation. Sources of nonionizing radiation in the medical center include (1) ultraviolet (UV) radiation sources, such as germicidal lamps, nursery incubators, and some air filters; (2) infrared radiation (IR) sources, such as heating or warming equipment; (3) radiofrequency (RF)/microwave sources, such as diathermy, and sterilizing and food preparation equipment; and (4) lasers. Exposure to nonionizing radiation can result in local heat production, which primarily affects the eyes and the skin.

Lasers

Although not often thought of as a type of nonionizing radiation, laser (*light amplification by simulated emission of radiation*) equipment emits electromagnetic radiation in either the UV, IR, or visible spectrum. Lasers are used in the operating room as well as in many different outpatient clinics, such as dermatology, gynecology, ophthalmology, gastroenterology, and podiatry clinics.

No matter where they are used, lasers pose an ocular and cutaneous hazard to medical center workers. They produce extremely high-intensity light radiation in a very narrow beam (usually of a single wavelength). When such light is inadvertently focused on the retina, it can cause cellular damage and functional loss of vision. When focused on the skin, laser effects range from erythema to blistering to incineration of the skin. In addition to direct skin and eye damage, airborne contaminants in the laser "plume" can produce respiratory symptoms [63].

Laser hazard control is aimed at preventing ocular and cutaneous exposure to the direct laser beam and its specular reflections. No OSHA standards exist that regulate employee exposure to lasers, but the performance of laser equipment is regulated by the FDA. Several private organizations such as the American National Standards Institute (ANSI) [64] and the American Conference of Governmental Industrial Hygienists (ACGIH) [65] have published recommendations for the safe use of lasers.

Laser safety is an important adjunct to every medical center's safety and health program. Medical center personnel who may come into contact with an operational laser should be trained in laser safety measures. Prevention of laser exposure depends primarily on engineering controls such as shielding of the laser beam from view and the use of PPE-like effective eye protection. Work practice controls are also important. Lasers should never be left unattended during operation and warning labels should be prominently displayed when the laser is operational. Lastly, personnel who work with lasers should receive preplacement, periodic, and termination eye examinations.

Indoor Air Quality

The medical center exhibits several unique features with respect to indoor air quality. Hospitals house patients who may be more susceptible to various indoor air pollutants than the occupants of nonhospital buildings. Patients who are immunocompromised either through illness or medication tend to be at greater risk for infection with certain opportunistic organisms, such as fungal species of the *Aspergillus* family. In fact, contaminated air-conditioning systems, including cooling towers, have been the source of infections among these patients. As a result, continued vigilance by safety and industrial hygiene personnel of hospital areas where immunocompromised patients are treated is essential to prevent these types of infections.

Unlike workers in nonmedical center buildings, medical center workers are exposed to bioeffluents generated by patient care activities. As a result, special attention should be paid to the effective performance of the medical center's heating, ventilation, and air-conditioning (HVAC) system.

Psychosocial Hazards

Stress

Stress disorders are common in HCWs, and workers in intensive care units, burn units, emergency rooms, and operating suites frequently exhibit a high prevalence of stress-related disorders [66]. Most studies of workplace stress focus on subjective worker perceptions and individual coping mechanisms rather than on objective aspects of the work environment that are "stress-producers" and candidates for environmental control [67]. Factors associated with the development of stress in medical center workers include (1) chronic understaffing, (2) role ambiguity, (3) interprofessional and interpersonal conflicts, (4) working in unfamiliar areas, (5) shift work, and (6) the physical condition of the workplace [68].

Efforts to prevent job-related stress in the medical center should be aimed at identifying and controlling job stressors. Also, institution of stress management programs, promotion of regular staff meetings, provision of adequate staffing, arranging prompt employee assistance when needed, and establishing more flexibility in work scheduling have all been shown to be effective in preventing workplace stress.

Chemical Dependency

Chemical dependency among HCWs is higher than that seen in the general population. Drug abuse rates among health care professionals, such as physicians [69] and nurses [70], exceed those found in the general population. Job stress and easy drug availability make chemical dependency one of the most frequent occupational illnesses to affect the medical center professional.

Recognition by an HCW of chemical dependency in a fellow HCW may be difficult because the affected HCW usually preferentially protects his or her job performance over other life activities. An HCW's job performance may not deteriorate until quite late in the course of chemical dependency. Behavioral changes that may indicate the presence of chemical dependency include social withdrawal, mood swings including unexpected anger, poorly excused absences, dishonesty, and deteriorating job performance [71].

Both inpatient and outpatient programs are available that are specifically designed for treatment of medical professionals once substance abuse is identified. Preventing chemical dependency among HCWs can be promoted by limiting workplace access to addictive drugs, reducing job stressors, and providing unrestricted access to employee assistance programs.

Conclusion

The modern medical center is a complex and potentially hazardous workplace environment. Many different types of biologic, chemical, physical, and psychosocial hazards exist in every medical center. Meeting the challenge of protecting medical center workers from exposure to these hazards is often complicated by the dedication that every medical center employee has to providing quality patient care. Striking the balance between patient and worker safety is the challenge for those with the responsibility to ensure worker safety in a modern medical center.

References

1. Patterson, W., et al. Occupational hazards to hospital personnel. *Ann. Intern. Med.* 102:658, 1985.
2. Emmett, E., and Baetz, J. H. Health in the health care industries? *Occup. Med. State of the Art Rev.* 2:ix, 1987.
3. Guidelines for employee health services in health care institutions. *J.O.M.* 28:518, 1986.
4. NIOSH. *Guidelines for Protecting the Safety and Health of Health Care Workers.* Department of Health and Human Services, National Institute for Occupational Safety and Health, Publication no. 88-119, 1988.
5. Lewy, R. Prevention strategies in hospital occupational medicine. *J.O.M.* 23:109, 1981.
6. OSHA. Bloodborne Pathogens. 29 CFR 1910.1030.
7. CDC. Update: Universal precautions for prevention of transmission of human immunodeficiency virus, hepatitis B virus, and other bloodborne pathogens in health-care settings. *M.M.W.R.* 37:377, 1988.
8. Hadler, S. C. et al. Long-term immunogenicity and efficacy of hepatitis B vaccine in homosexual men. *N. Engl. J. Med.* 315:209, 1986.
9. Williams, W. CDC guidelines for infection control in hospital personnel. *Infect. Control* 4:326, 1983.
10. Garner, J. S., and Simmons, B. P. CDC guideline for isolation precautions in hospitals. *Infect. Control* 4:245, 1983.
11. Nelson, K., and Sullivan-Bolyal, J. Z. Preventing teratogenic viral infection in hospital employees: The case of rubella, cytomegalovirus and varicella-zoster virus. *Occup. Med. State of the Art Rev.* 2:471, 1987.
12. Latex allergy growing among patients and health care workers. *Infect. Dis. News* 6:19, 1993.
13. Tuberculosis morbidity in the United States: final data, 1990. *M.M.W.R. CDC Surveill. Summ.* 40 (SS-3):23, 1991.
14. CDC. Nosocomial transmission of multidrug-resistant tuberculosis among HIV-infected persons—Florida and New York, 1988–1991. *M.M.W.R.* 40:585, 1991.
15. Goble, M., et al. Treatment of 171 patients with pulmonary tuberculosis resistant to isoniazid and rifampin. *N. Engl. J. Med.* 328:527, 1993.

16. Frieden, T. R. et al. The emergence of drug-resistant tuberculosis in New York City. *N. Engl. J. Med.* 328:521, 1993.
17. CDC. Guidelines for preventing the transmission of tuberculosis in health-care settings, with special focus on HIV-related issues. *M.M.W.R.* 39-17, 1990.
18. Beeson, M. F., et al. Prevalence and diagnosis of laboratory animal allergy. *Clin. Allergy* 13:433, 1983.
19. Gross, N. J. Allergy to laboratory animals, epidemiologic, clinical and physiologic aspects and a trial of chromolyn in its management. *J. Allergy Clin. Immunol.* 66:158, 1980.
20. Nordman, H. Atopy and work. *Scand. J. Work Environ. Health* 10:481, 1984.
21. Lincoln, T. A., Bolton, N. E., and Garrett, A. S. Occupational allergy to animal dander and sera. *J.O.M.* 16:465, 1974.
22. Bland, S. M., et al. Allergy to laboratory animals in health care personnel. *Occup. Med. State of the Art Rev.* 2:525, 1987.
23. Hubbert, W. T., et al. *Diseases Transmissible from Animals to Man.* Springfield, IL: Thomas, 1975.
24. EPA. *EPA Guide for Infectious Waste Management.* Washington, DC: US Environmental Protection Agency. Office of Solid Waste, NTIS no. PB 86-199130.
25. Stoner, D. L., et al. *Engineering a Safe Hospital Environment.* New York: Wiley, 1982.
26. Gamberale, F., and Svensson, G. The effect of anesthetic gases on the psychomotor and perceptual functions of anesthetic nurses. *Work Environ. Health* 11:108, 1974.
27. Bruce, D. L., and Bach, M. J. Psychological studies of human performance as affected by traces of enflurane and nitrous oxide. *Anesthesiology* 42:194, 1975.
28. Corbett, T. H., et al. Incidence of cancer among Michigan nurse anesthetists. *Anesthesiology* 38:260, 1973.
29. Cohen, E. N., et al. A survey of anesthetic health hazards among dentists. *J. Am. Dent. Assoc.* 90:1291, 1975.
30. Pharaoh, P. O. D., et al. Outcome of pregnancy among women in anesthetic practice. *Lancet* 1:34, 1977.
31. Tannenbaum, T., and Goldberg, R. Exposure to anesthetic gas and reproductive outcome: A review of the epidemiologic literature. *J.O.M.* 27:659, 1985.
32. Popic, P. M., and Kruel, J. F. Control of Trace Anesthetic Gas Contamination. In W. Charney and J. Schirmer (eds.), *Essentials of Modern Hospital Safety.* Chelsea, MI: Lewis, 1990. Pp. 37–49.
33. Rodgers, B. Health hazards to personnel handling antineoplastic agents. *Occup. Med. State of the Art Rev.* 2:513, 1987.
34. Chabner, B. Second neoplasm—a complication of cancer chemotherapy. *N. Engl. J. Med.* 297:213, 1977.
35. Yodiaken, R. E., and Bennett, D. OSHA work-practice guidelines for personnel dealing with cytotoxic (antineoplastic) drugs. *Am. J. Hosp. Pharm.* 43:1193, 1986.
36. Yager, J. W., et al. Exposures to ethylene oxide at work increase sister chromatid exchanges in human peripheral leukocytes. *Science* 219:1221, 1983.
37. Gross, J. A., et al. Ethylene oxide neurotoxicity: Report of four cases and review of the literature. *Neurology* 29:978, 1979.
38. Hemminiki, K. Spontaneous abortions in hospital staff engaged in sterilizing instruments with chemical agents. *Br. Med. J.* 285:1461, 1982.
39. Landrigan, P. J. Ethylene oxide: An overview of toxicologic and epidemiologic research. *Am. J. Ind. Med.* 6:103, 1984.
40. Hendrick, D. J., et al. Formaldehyde asthma: Challenge exposure levels and fate after five years. *J.O.M.* 24:893, 1982.
41. Sheppard, D., et al. Lack of bronchomotor response to up to 3 ppm formaldehyde in subjects with asthma. *Environ Res.* 35:133, 1984.
42. Kerns, W., et al. Carcinogenicity of formaldehyde in rats and mice after long-term inhalation exposure. *Cancer Res.* 43:4382, 1983.
43. NIOSH. *Current Intelligence Bulletin 35—Evidence on the Carcinogenicity of Formaldehyde.* Cincinnati, OH: US Department of Health and Human Services, Public Health Service, Centers for Disease Control, NIOSH. Publication no. 81-111.
44. OSHA. Ethylene Oxide. 29 CFR 1910.1047(c).
45. OSHA. Formaldehyde. 29 CFR 1910.1048(c).
46. Bardazzi, F. Glutaraldehyde dermatitis in nurses. *Contact Dermatitis* 14:319, 1986.
47. OSHA. Occupational Exposure to Hazardous Chemicals in Laboratories. 29 CFR 1910.1460.

48. Klein, B. P., et al. Assessment of workers' compensation claims for back strains/pains. *J.O.M.* 26:443, 1984.

49. Chaffin, D. B., and Park, K. S. A longitudinal study of low-back pain as associated with occupational weight lifting factors. *Am. Ind. Hyg. Assoc. J.* 33:513, 1973.

50. Stubbs, D. A., et al. Back pain in the nursing profession. I. Epidemiology and pilot methodology. *Ergonomics* 26:755, 1983.

51. Harber, P., et al. Occupational low-back pain in hospital nurses. *J.O.M.* 27:518, 1985.

52. NIOSH. *Work Practices Guide for Manual Lifting.* Cincinnati, OH: US Department of Health and Human Services, Public Health Service, Centers for Disease Control. Publication no. 81-122, 1981.

53. NIOSH. *Criteria for Recommended Standard: Occupational Exposure to Hot Environments.* National Institute for Occupational Safety and Health, 1986.

54. Grumet, G. W. Pandemonium in the modern hospital. *N. Engl. J. Med.* 328:433, 1993.

55. Soutar, R. L., and Wilson, J. A. Does hospital noise disturb patients? *Br. Med. J.* 292:305, 1986.

56. Kryter, K. D. *The Effects of Noise on Man* (2nd ed.). Orlando, FL: Academic, 1985.

57. Schultz, T. J. Synthesis of social surveys on noise annoyance. *J. Acous. Soc. Am.* 64:377, 1978.

58. Teichner, W. H., et al. Noise and human performance, a psycho-physiological approach. *Ergonomics* 6:83, 1963.

59. EPA. *Information on Levels of Environmental Noise Requisite to Protect Public Health and Welfare with an Adequate Margin of Safety.* Report no. 550-9-74-004. Washington, DC: US Government Printing Office, 1974.

60. OSHA. Occupational Exposure to Noise. 29 CFR 1910.95.

61. Ecker, M. D., and Bramesco, N. J. *Radiation: All You Need to Know About It.* New York: Vintage, 1981.

62. OSHA. Ionizing Radiation. 29 CFR 1910.96.

63. Charney, W., et al. Laser plume: Case study. In W. Charney and J. Schirmer (eds)., *Essentials of Modern Hospital Safety.* Chelsea, MI: Lewis, 1990. Pp. 261–271.

64. ANSI. *American National Standard for the Safe Use of Lasers in Health Care Facilities.* New York: American National Standards Institute, ANSI 2136.3., 1988.

65. ACGIH. *A Guide for Control of Laser Hazards.* Cincinnati, OH: ACGIH, 1976.

66. Smith, M. J., et al. Occupational incidence rates of mental health disorders. *J. Hum. Stress* 3:34, 1977.

67. Baker, D. B. The study of stress at work. *Ann. Rev. Public Health* 6:367, 1985.

68. Celetano, D. D., and Johnson, J. Stress in health care workers. *Occup. Med. State of the Art Rev.* 2:593, 1987.

69. Brewster, J. M. Prevalence of alcohol and other drug problems among physicians. *J.A.M.A.* 255:1913, 1986.

70. Bissell, L., and Haberman, P. W. Alcoholism in the professions. New York: Oxford University Press, 1984.

71. Talbot, G. D., and Wright, C. Chemical dependency in health care professionals. *Occup. Med. State of the Art Rev.* 2:581, 1987.

Further Information

Information on medical center occupational health activities can be obtained from a number of organizations:

American Hospital Association, 840 North Lake Shore Dr., Chicago, IL 60611
Joint Commission for Accreditation of Health Care Organizations, 875 North Michigan Ave., Chicago, IL 60611
American College of Occupational and Environmental Medicine, 56 West Seegers Rd., Arlington Heights, IL 60005

Guidelines for Protecting the Health and Safety of Health Care Workers, National Institute for Occupational Safety and Health.
This thorough document is a must on any medical center occupational health bookshelf.

Appendix to Chapter 30: Occupational Hazards by Location in the Hospital*

Location	Hazard	Location	Hazard
Central supply	Ethylene oxide		Carcinogens
	Infection		Teratogens
	Broken equipment (cuts)		Mutagens
	Soaps, detergents		Cryogenic hazards
	Steam		Wastes (chemical, radioactive, infectious)
	Flammable gases		
	Lifting		Radiation
	Noise	Laundry	Wet floors
	Asbestos insulation		Lifting
	Mercury		Noise
Dialysis units	Infection		Heat
	Formaldehyde		Burns
Dental service	Mercury		Infection
	Ethylene oxide		Needle punctures
	Anesthetic gases		Detergents, soaps
	Ionizing radiation		Bleaches
	Infection		Solvents
Food service	Wet floors		Wastes (chemical and radioactive)
	Sharp equipment		
	Noise	Maintenance and engineering	Electrical hazards
	Soaps, detergents		Tools, machinery
	Disinfectants		Noise
	Ammonia		Welding fumes
	Chlorine		Asbestos
	Solvents		Flammable liquids
	Drain cleaners		Solvents
	Oven cleaners		Mercury
	Caustic solutions		Pesticides
	Pesticides		Cleaners
	Microwave ovens		Ammonia
	Steam lines		Carbon monoxide
	Ovens		Ethylene oxide
	Heat		Freons
	Electrical hazards		Paints, adhesives
	Lifting		Water treatment chemicals
Housekeeping	Soaps, detergents		Sewage
	Cleaners		Heat stress
	Solvents		Cold stress (refrigeration units)
	Disinfectants		
	Glutaraldehyde		Falls
	Infection		Lifting
	Needle punctures		Climbing
	Wastes (chemical, radioactive, infectious)		Strains and sprains
	Electrical hazards	Nuclear medicine	Radionuclides
	Lifting		Infection
	Climbing		X-irradiation
	Slips, falls	Office areas and data processing	Video display terminals
Laboratory	Infectious diseases		Air quality
	Toxic chemicals		Ergonomic/body mechanics
	Benzene		Chemicals
	Ethylene oxide		Ozone
	Formaldehyde		
	Solvents		
	Flammable and explosive agents		

(continued)

Location	Hazard	Location	Hazard
Operating rooms	Anesthetics		Standing for long periods
	Antiseptics		Infectious diseases
	Methyl methacrylate		Needle punctures
	Compressed gases		Toxic substances
	Sterilizing gases		Chemotherapeutic agents
	Infection		Radiation
	Electrical		Radioactive patients
	Sharp instruments		Electrical hazards
	Lifting	Pharmacy	Pharmaceuticals
Pathology	Infectious diseases		Antineoplastic agents
	Formaldehyde		Mercury
	Glutaraldehyde		Slips, falls
	Flammable substances	Print shops	Inks
	Freons		Solvents
	Solvents		Noise
	Phenols		Fire
Patient care	Lifting	Radiology	Radiation
	Pushing, pulling		Infectious diseases
	Slips, falls		Lifting
			Pushing, pulling

*Although this list is not exhaustive, it demonstrates the variety of hazards that can exist in a hospital environment. Stress is reported by hospital workers in all job categories and is not listed separately by location.

Source: Adapted from NIOSH. Guidelines for Protecting the Safety and Health of Health Care Workers. Department of Health and Human Services, National Institute for Occupational Safety and Health, Publication no. 88–119, 1988.

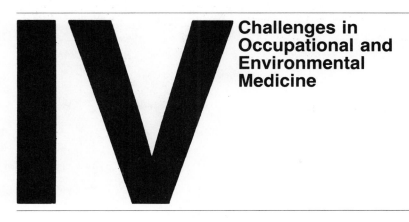

IV Challenges in Occupational and Environmental Medicine

31

Reproductive Hazards

William W. Greaves

The question, "Doctor, if I work with substance X, will it hurt my baby?" presents a physician with an often difficult task. The physician's response not only must incorporate the scientific literature on substance X and data on the work exposure but also must be sensitive to the fears and concerns of the patient. Even the manner used to inform the patient of the facts must be measured so misinterpretation or an irrational fear is not created. The answer to the patient's question should be designed to provide accurate information in proper perspective with the risks of everyday living and in a manner understandable to the patient.

Employee concerns about reproduction become important for three groups: pregnant women, women in the childbearing period, and men. The circumstances of their concerns may be varied. Maybe a relative, or even the patient, has had an inability to conceive, a fetal loss during pregnancy, or the birth of a malformed child. All are bitter disappointments and produce tremendous personal stress. Perhaps a chemical substance or video display terminals recently received media attention in the newspaper or on television, and now the patient is concerned because it is used in his or her workplace or work station. Determining the exact cause of the concern is important. All the factual information in the world will not alleviate the individual's concern if the root cause of that concern is not addressed. One cannot address emotional fears with only facts; the basis of the concern must be considered.

A 1991 Supreme Court decision [1] does not allow employers to keep pregnant or fertile women from working in jobs that may injure a fetus and cause an adverse reproductive outcome. Rather, employees decide as individuals whether they will perform potentially hazardous jobs after receiving information on potential risks. This presents a singular conundrum for the employer and the occupational physician in the event that the employee does not choose to act to avoid a specific exposure that scientific evidence links with an adverse reproductive outcome. Under section 5a(1), the "general duty clause" of the Occupational Safety and Health Act of 1970, an employer may be cited for failing to provide working conditions free from recognized hazards that are likely to cause serious harm. And, while with few exceptions employers cannot be held liable for recovery beyond workers' compensation, an injured child of an employee is apparently not bound by this limitation. At this time a prudent course of action for an employer is an approach based on the scientific literature, including both an employee educational and monitoring program for adverse reproductive outcomes and a policy to link employee removal from specific work activities to specific work performance.

This chapter helps the occupational physician respond to the woman or man concerned about reproductive hazards. The response should consider four areas:

1. The scientific literature on the substance(s) in question
2. The true and potential levels of exposure
3. The control measures used to assure safety
4. The specific concerns of the individual

These four areas are covered in later sections that describe the potential interferences with the normal reproductive process, the evaluation of a suspected problem, and guidelines useful for the practicing physician.

Case Example

Case 1: A 28-year-old married woman has been your patient for several years. You know her medical history well and recall that she has been employed in the data processing department of a large company for the past 6 years. Her husband has seen you for periodic maintenance visits only and has worked for a local foundry continuously since his military service in Vietnam. The young woman is visibly anxious and relates marital trouble as well as financial difficulties. She tells you that she and her husband have been trying to start a family for 3 years; she asks you if their work has made them sterile. What do you tell her?

Case 2: Over the past 5 years, you have been employed part-time by a company as their Medical Director. Initially, you were asked to provide preplacement and periodic examinations for the employees in addition to acute care both in-plant and at your office when necessary. Lately, the company has been asking you to address several policy decisions. You are now asked if the company should be concerned about potential hazards of substances used at a small chemical plant. Reproductive hazards are mentioned during the discussion. How do you respond?

These two case examples illustrate scenarios faced by physicians who practice occupational medicine: the concerned individual and the concerned company. Both address the issue of reproductive hazards in the workplace and both present a challenging task.

Reproductive Toxicology

An understanding of normal reproduction is a necessary foundation for the recognition of adverse effects to the reproductive processes of men and women. With this understanding of the normal or usual outcome, the actions of toxins or stressors can be more fully appreciated.

Male

Sexual differentiation begins about 7 weeks after conception and is completed by the fourth month in the male. Follicle-stimulating hormone (FSH) acts on the Sertoli cells in the testes to produce the release of a second hormone from the hypothalamic-pituitary axis, luteinizing hormone (LH). LH stimulates the testicular Leydig cells to produce testosterone. Although males and females have identical FSH and LH, it is the *hormonal* effects on sex-specific *target cells* that produce sexual differentiation.

In adult men, the high rate of cell division during the 70 to 80 days of spermatogenesis makes this process susceptible to adverse influences. Spermatogonia undergo mitosis into spermatocytes; spermatids are produced by further cell division through meiosis and mature into the characteristic head and tail shape of sperm. Normal sperm production is about 20 to 350 million per day, with human ejaculate containing from 50 to 150 million per milliliter. Less than 20 million sperm per milliliter is considered to be clinical infertility [2]. Fertility criteria have been defined as greater than 40% motile sperm, greater than 20 million sperm per milliliter of semen (normal sperm count is approximately 40–60 million/ml), and greater than 70% normal morphology [3].

Female

The entire complement of ova are present at birth, and their number gradually decreases with age. Only about 400 mature ova are released during ovulation in a lifetime. The release of specific factors from the hypothalamus and hormones from the pituitary produce the development of the ovarian follicle. The follicle expels the mature ovum at the peak of the estrogen and luteinizing hormone levels, approximately 14 days after the beginning of menses. Fertilization and early development occur during the ensuing few days and are followed by *implantation* onto the wall of the uterus.

The *embryonic stage* of development progresses from about the third through eighth weeks of pregnancy and includes *organogenesis*. Organ growth occurs during the ninth through fortieth weeks of fetal development. Adverse reproductive outcome can occur after harmful exposure during any of these stages, although the period of organogenesis is considered to be especially susceptible (Table 31-1).

Interference with the Reproductive Process

The potential interferences with the reproductive process are several. A healthy baby is the normal outcome if a healthy sperm fertilizes a healthy ovum that passes unimpeded through the fallopian tubes, implants in the uterus, develops normal organs, and grows to term. Interference with this basic process can occur with a change in libido or in the following steps, each with an example of an interfering exposure:

1. The *production of sperm*. Chromosomal or gene changes (nonlethal or lethal) can occur; fewer numbers may be produced (e.g., ionizing radiation).
2. The *production of ova*. Changes in hormonal patterns may interfere with ovulation (e.g., estrogen deficiency).
3. The fertilized ovum may not *pass through* the fallopian tube to the uterus (e.g., scar tissue from pelvic inflammatory disease). Effects on normal muscular, ciliary, and secretory activity may occur.
4. The fertilized ovum may not *implant* in the uterus. The endometrial lining may be altered, or the fertilized ovum may be damaged in the cleavage and blastocyst stages. This effect usually is lethal and produces an abortion recognized only as an abnormal menstrual period in humans but is the *equivalent to resorptions* in rats and mice and occasionally in rabbits (e.g., infectious diseases).
5. The embryo may be affected as its tissues *differentiate* or its organs develop. Congenital malformations, or structural aberrations, can occur during organogenesis, from day 21 to day 56 of gestation (e.g., rubella infection, thalidomide administration) [4].
6. The fetus may not grow normally, resulting in spontaneous abortions, stillbirths, or premature births. *A disease or toxic state in the mother* can affect the fetus (e.g., diabetes mellitus) and the risk of spontaneous abortion increases with maternal age and history of prior spontaneous abortions [5]. Postnatal growth and development may likewise be altered, the effect possibly not manifested until several years after birth (e.g., ethyl alcohol). In practice, of course, it is difficult to detect a pregnancy, even with good symptoms of morning sickness, until several weeks after conception. Because the woman is in fact pregnant but unaware of it, protection of the fetus at this stage can be a difficult task.

Teratogens

An agent or factor that causes physical birth defects or malformations in the developing embryo is termed a *teratogen*. The effects of a teratogen are dose related: A high dose is embryolethal, a moderate dose produces a defect, while a low dose may

Table 31-1. Stages of embryonic development and adverse outcome to toxic agents

Month	Stage	Adverse outcome
0	Conception and implantation	Embryonic death
1	Embryonic organogenesis	Birth defects
3	Fetal	Developmental deficits, metabolic dysfunction, cancer
9	Birth	
	Neonatal	Functional deficits

Source: Adapted from M. Radike. Reproductive Toxicology. In P. L. Williams and J. L. Burson (eds.), *Industrial Toxicology, Safety and Health Applications in the Workplace*. New York: Van Nostrand Reinhold, 1985. P. 353.

produce no effect. *Teratogens are substances that produce birth defects or congenital malformations without producing toxicity in the mother.* If a birth defect results from maternal toxicity, the defect may be caused by the *toxic effects* on the mother rather than a direct manifestation of the substance itself. The type of defect or malformation also depends on the day(s) during the period of organogenesis that exposure to the teratogen occurred.

General principles [6] *of teratology* are the following:

1. Susceptibility to teratogenesis depends on the *genotype of the conceptus* and the manner in which the genotype interacts with environmental factors.
2. Susceptibility to teratogenic agents varies with the developing *stage of the fetus* at the time of exposure.
3. Teratogenic agents act through specific mechanisms on developing cells and tissues, thus initiating *abnormal embryogenesis.*
4. The final manifestations of *abnormal development* are malformation, growth retardation, functional disorder, or death.
5. The access of adverse *environmental influences* to developing tissues depends on the nature of the influences (agents).
6. Manifestations of *abnormal development* increase from no effect to the totally lethal level as the dosage increases.

About 10 to 20% of normal conceptions (where the sperm has fertilized the ovum and pregnancy is recognized) fail to reach full growth and delivery. Similarly, 30 to 40% of spontaneous abortions have a chromosomal anomaly [7]. This relatively high level of "normal" spontaneous abortions needs to be recognized in evaluating rates of adverse reproductive outcome.

Congenital anomalies, or birth defects, have been reported in about 3% of all newborn children (Table 31-2); anomalies in another 3% of live births become manifest during postnatal or later development [8]. Two thirds of all congenital anomalies or malformations have no known cause, while drugs and chemicals are implicated in 3% (Table 31-3).

Table 31-2. Frequency of selected reproductive endpoints

Event	Frequency per 100	Unit
Azoospermia	1	Men
Birthweight* < 2500 g	7	Live births
Failure to conceive after one year of unprotected intercourse	10–15	Couples
Spontaneous abortion 8–28 weeks of gestation	10–20	Pregnancies or women
Chromosomal anomaly among spontaneously aborted conceptions 8–28 weeks	30–40	Spontaneous abortions
Chromosomal anomalies among amniocentesis specimens to unselected women over 35 yr	2	Amniocentesis specimens
Stillbirth	2–4	Stillbirths + live births
Birth defects	2–3	Live births
Chromosomal anomalies	0.2	Live births
Neural tube defects	0.01–1.00	Live births + stillbirths
Severe mental retardation	0.4	Children to age 15 yr

*More usefully analyzed as a continuous variable.
Source: Adapted from A. D. Bloom (ed.). *Guidelines for Studies of Human Populations Exposed to Mutagenic and Reproductive Hazards.* White Plains, NY: March of Dimes Birth Defects Foundation, 1981. P. 47.

Table 31-3. Causes of congenital anomalies

Cause	Percent
Maternal metabolic imbalance	1–2
Infections	2–3
Chromosomal aberrations	3–5
Drugs and environmental agents	
Radiation	1
Drugs and chemicals	3
Known genetic transmission (autosomal dominant, autosomal recessive, sex-linked recessive)	20
Combinations and interactions	Unknown
Unknown factors	69–73

Source: From American Medical Association Council on Scientific Affairs. Effect of toxic chemicals on the reproductive system. *J.A.M.A.* 253:3431, 1985. Copyright 1985, American Medical Association.

Human Data

The medical literature provides the primary source of information to the physician confronted with a reproductive outcome issue. Like any epidemiologic literature, that on reproductive outcomes must be assessed for its scientific merit as well as for what it has to say on the subject. Textbooks, such as those listed in the References and Further Information at the end of this chapter, detail aspects of study design and interpretation that should be considered in a critical review. Major points to consider include [9]

1. *Exposure levels.* Frequently, good industrial hygiene data are not available, and proper grouping of potentially exposed employee populations by time of exposure cannot be performed. Because reproductive effects are dose dependent, lack of exposure data may become a major limitation of an otherwise good study.
2. *Selection of controls.* Important variables that can also affect reproductive outcome include age, parity, nutritional and socioeconomic status, and smoking and alcohol habits.
3. *Background incidence of events.* Relatively common events of everyday living, such as infertility, menstrual disorders, and spontaneous abortions, require a large sample size and a large total number of cases to detect an increased incidence of the condition in the population under study. Rare events, such as a specific congenital malformation, require a smaller total number of cases to detect an effect, but rare events also require a larger population at risk to obtain that smaller number of cases.
4. *Reliability of ascertainment.* Once an abnormal outcome has occurred, determining the nature of the disorder becomes of paramount importance in the search for a cause. Early abortion, frequently recognized as a late heavy menses, or a change in libido are subject to self-assessment, which may confound the outcome evaluation.
5. *Multiple exposures.* When multiple exposures may be exerting effects, the points noted above may severely limit the inferences that can be made regarding a specific compound. In such a case, a valid assessment may still be made of the production process or work activity that involves the multiple exposures.
6. *Interpretation of findings.* Answering such questions as whether sufficient data are available to reach a final decision, whether a hazard exists, and what kind of action needs to be taken can be challenging tasks. Potentially confounding factors (Table 31-4), comparability of cases and controls, and the other points noted above must be evaluated.

Epidemiologic data provide the information necessary to take action on a potential reproductive hazard. For the practicing physician, these data come from two primary

Table 31-4. Potentially confounding factors for a number of adverse reproductive effects

Adverse reproductive effect	Potentially confounding factors
Impaired spermatogenesis	Surgical procedures such as vasectomy; diseases and illnesses such as varicocele, fever, mumps, and diabetes; certain therapeutic drugs
Reduced fertility	Contraceptive use
Spontaneous abortion	Maternal age, cigarette smoking, alcohol consumption, history of spontaneous abortions
Low birth weight	Race, cigarette smoking, parity, maternal nutrition
Birth defects: e.g.,	
Down's syndrome	Maternal age
Neural tube defects	Ethnic factors

Source: From I. C. T. Nisbet and N. J. Karch. *Chemical Hazards to Human Reproduction.* Park Ridge, NJ: Noyes Data Corp., 1983. P. 44.

Table 31-5. Reproductive endpoints for which population estimates are available

Endpoint	Population survey*
1. Infertility of male and female origin	NSFG, PYS
2. Conception delay	NSFG, PYS
3. Birth rate	NSFG, NNS, NFMS, PYS
4. Pregnancy complications	NSFG, NNS, NFMS, PYS
5. Gestation at delivery (prematurity, postmaturity)	NSFG, NNS, NFMS
6. Early fetal loss (<28 weeks gestation)	NSFG, NNS, NFMS, PYS
7. Late fetal loss (>28 weeks gestation)	NSFG, NNS, NFMS, PYS
8. Sex ratio	NSFG, NNS, PYS
9. Birth weight	NSFG, NNS
10. Apgar score	NNS
11. Congenital defect	NNS
12. Infant morbidity and mortality	NSFG, NNS
13. Childhood morbidity and mortality	NNS, NFMS, PYS

Key: NSFG = 1982 National Survey of Family Growth; NNS = 1980 National Natality Survey; NFMS = 1980 National Fetal Mortality Survey; PYS = Parnes Youth Survey.
*These surveys also contain data on the following related topics: onset of menses, fertility expectations, birth spacing, contraceptive use, sterilization, care-seeking for infertility, prenatal care, spontaneous and induced abortions, maternal smoking and alcohol consumption, chronic diseases and venereal infections in pregnancy.
Source: From US Congress, Office of Technology Assessment. *Reproductive Health Hazards in the Workplace.* OTA-BA-266. Washington, DC: US Government Printing Office, 1985. P. 165.

sources: the medical literature and monitoring programs on a plant- or company-wide basis.

A first step in assessing the role of the workplace in affecting reproductive experience is to apply simple and straightforward techniques to monitor reproductive experience. Monitoring can assure the safety of the workplace, focus industrial hygiene and safety efforts, and assist in employee health promotion. Monitoring allows reproductive outcome to be viewed dispassionately. If attention is focused on reproductive hazards at the time an unfortunate event has occurred, it is extremely difficult to obtain unbiased data.

A useful approach to *reproductive surveillance,* or monitoring, has two major steps:
 I. *Establish objectives*
  A. Assess outcome for normality during pregnancy, delivery, or postnatal development
  B. If not normal, determine type of abnormality (Table 31-5)
 II. *Explore etiology*
  A. Past and family history

B. Lifestyle and substance use
C. Nonoccupational influences
  1) Diseases
  2) Injuries
  3) Hobbies
D. On-the-job substance exposure

The *essential objective of monitoring* is to answer one principal question: Is there an unusually high incidence of an *abnormality*? This question is answered by assessing reproductive outcome and comparing the results to what would be expected. If the concern deals with the ability to reproduce, the ability to reproduce itself must be assessed. If the concern deals with an outcome such as birth defects, this outcome must be assessed. Then, if an abnormality is detected, the specific type of abnormality is determined and the reason it happened is explored.

Determining the precise abnormality may require extensive study of the individuals involved, including both parents and the fetus or newborn. The occupational physician will usually obtain the services of other medical specialists for the clinical evaluation of these individuals. The usual incidence of adverse reproductive outcomes by type of abnormality can be compared to that from various population monitoring surveys (Table 31-5). Whether an abnormal incidence is present among a specific group of workers and/or their spouses can then be determined.

Assessing etiologic factors that may result in abnormalities of the reproductive process requires consideration of several items. Both past medical history and family history are extremely important, as are lifestyle and substance use. The prior reproductive experience of both employees and spouses, as well as blood relatives, must be investigated. Smoking and alcohol use, and medications taken before or during a pregnancy, are as important to assess as substances an individual may encounter on the job.

Virtually all the data required to monitor reproduction adequately are *historical*. Other than the laboratory tests that may be needed to specify the type of abnormality that occurred on the occasion that a pregnancy outcome is abnormal and the data needed to indicate on-the-job substance exposure, everything else is obtainable by history or *questionnaire*.

Most questionnaires contain a great deal of information that is not needed and may omit the information required. A good history form should be clear, nonbiased, codable, and time specific from both a preemployment and postemployment standpoint. Basic questionnaires developed by the Chemical Industry Institute of Toxicology for men and women focus on the most recent marriage of the employee and can be expanded to include all partners (Fig. 31-1). The Institute has more elaborate questionnaires, but these require a trained interviewer for their administration.

Once baseline information has been obtained, periodic updates ensure data reliability and timeliness in the event a problem is detected. Data are ideally analyzed by job type or department, and if a pattern emerges, special studies can be conducted. Adverse reproductive outcomes occur at a relatively predictable rate, just as causes of death or illness occur at a relatively predictable rate in a population. If an unusual amount of an adverse outcome is encountered in a specific group of employees, vigorous investigation is required. If the rate of occurrence in a company or plant is consistent with usual experience, however, and no discernible differences occur among employees with different work experiences, assurance can be given that the work environment is not the source of an adverse health outcome. If a true hazard is uncovered, steps must be taken to abate it. A monitoring system can then serve to demonstrate the effectiveness of the abatement efforts.

Animal Data

In many cases, results on human populations will be unavailable; consequently, animal studies will need to be reviewed. Animal data can suggest estimates of possible human effects, although extrapolation to human experience is problematic. Ideally, human data from epidemiologic studies on reproductive experience should be reviewed to form a reliable assessment.

Items of importance to reproductive studies on test animals include

1. *Species.* Studies on humans, nonhuman primates, and nonprimates may show marked variations in the rate of biotransformation. For example, the amount

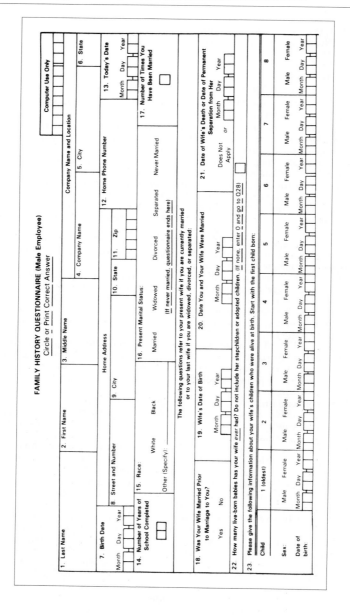

24. How many of your wife's children who were alive at birth had an abnormality or defect? *All* abnormalities or defects should be included even if you do not think they are relevant or if they were not discovered at birth. (If none, enter 0 and go to Q26) ☐

25. Please give the following information about your wife's children with an abnormality or defect:

Sex:	Male Female	Male Female	Male Female
Date of birth:	Month Day Year	Month Day Year	Month Day Year
Abnormality or defect (describe):			
How many months pregnant was your wife at his/her birth?	Months Pregnant: ☐	Months Pregnant: ☐	Months Pregnant: ☐

26. How many of your wife's children who were born alive are no longer living? (If none, enter 0 and go to Q28) ☐

27. Please give the following information about your wife's children who are no longer living:

Sex:	Male Female	Male Female	Male Female
Date of birth:	Month Day Year	Month Day Year	Month Day Year
Date of death:	Month Day Year	Month Day Year	Month Day Year
Cause of death (describe):			
How many months pregnant was your wife at his/her birth?	Months Pregnant: ☐	Months Pregnant: ☐	Months Pregnant: ☐

28. How many miscarriages or stillborn children has your wife *ever* had? (If none, enter 0 and go to Q30) ☐

Figure 31-1. Reproductive history questionnaire. (From R. J. Levine and P. B. Blunden, Family History Questionnaire, CIIT:FSA.1 3-83. Chemical Industry Institute of Toxicology, PO Box 12137, Research Triangle Park, NC 27709.)

of phenylacetic acid excreted in the urine after conjugation to glutamine is almost 100% in humans, 30 to 90% in nonhuman primates, and none in non-primates [10].

2. *Dose-response.* Measurable responses increase as the dosage frequency, duration, and intensity increase. Accurate dosage data are necessary to correlate dosage levels to the adverse outcome responses. For example, the concentration of a substance in parts per million (ppm) in a test animal's drinking water or feed may be known, but because the amount of water or feed the animal actually consumed may not be known, the total dose ingested is unknown. Higher doses in water or feed produce maternal toxicity and subsequent decreased maternal intake, which alters the dose delivered to the embryo or fetus. This altered dose cannot be accurately correlated to a response. A useful maximal dosage endpoint to determine whether the substance has an effect on the embryo or fetus is the dosage just below that which produces maternal toxicity.

3. *Route of administration.* The skin or dermal exposure LD_{50} (Lethal *D*ose for 50% of the test animals in the experiment) of many substances is about 10 times that for ingestion, and ingestion itself is about 10 times that for intravenous exposure. Occupational exposures occur frequently through the lung or inhalation route. Inhalation is a more efficient route of exposure than all others except intravenous.

4. *Period of the reproductive process* during which the animal is exposed to the substance. The first day of gestation may be referred to as day 0 or day 1, which introduces 1 day of error, a factor that becomes important during extrapolation of animal effects to humans. For example, a heart defect in animals is often assumed to produce a heart defect in humans when exposure occurs during the appropriate period of heart organogenesis.

5. *Summary of effects.* Adverse effects are generally described, along with a test of statistical significance. Often little consideration is given to biologic significance.

Outcome effects noted in animal studies include anatomic, biochemical, and functional changes. External appearance, gross pathologic weight, and gross volume of reproductive organs (e.g., ovary, testes, prostate) and the pituitary and adrenal glands are noted. Microscopy of these tissues is performed, and the numbers per milliliter and gross microscopic appearance of sperm can be determined. Biochemically, the synthesis and total content of nucleic acids and the activities of various enzymes contained within reproductive organs have been investigated. Circulating levels of hormones such as FSH and LH can be noted. Abnormalities of these parameters may suggest interference with the reproductive process, but their actual impact is uncertain in most cases.

Effects of reproductive outcome can be identified through single-generation and multigeneration studies. The Food and Drug Administration (FDA) protocol established in 1966 for *single-generation studies* is widely used to assess new drugs. Segment 1 studies (fertility studies) are characterized by *treatment occurring before mating;* theoretically, they can be used as a summary *outcome* assessment of all stages of reproduction. Segment 2 studies (teratology studies) have *treatment* occurring *during organogenesis.* Segment 3 studies test the effect on parturition and the postnatal period.

Multigeneration studies frequently follow the FDA protocol for food additives. Time consuming and expensive to complete, these studies begin by treating males and/or females, then by mating to produce two litters, F1a and F1b. The F1a litter is killed and examined, while some of the F1b litter are mated to form the second-generation litters, F2a and F2b. The F2a is examined; the F2b is mated to produce the third-generation litters, F3a and F3b, which are both examined for abnormalities. Both single-generation and multigeneration studies use rats or mice as the usual test animal at several exposure levels of the test compound. The lowest level produces neither adverse reproductive effects nor parental toxicity. The highest level produces maternal toxicity. In pregnant rats, the maximum tolerated dosage is defined as the exposure producing 10% maternal deaths. *The usual indicator for maternal toxicity* is a less than expected weight gain during pregnancy. The no-effect level of a compound (in a given species by a given route of exposure under laboratory conditions) is the highest dosage level, or exposure, producing neither maternal toxicity nor adverse reproductive outcome. *For the great majority of compounds, adverse reproductive outcomes tend to occur very close to the adult toxic dose.*

Clinical Aspects

Some physicians respond to the woman who asks, "Will compound X hurt my baby?" by writing "No chemical use allowed" on a slip that is returned to the place of employment. Unfortunately, this blanket response may needlessly heighten the patient's charged emotions and create volatile workplace situations and employee relations problems. This "reflex-type" response overlooks the myriad of chemicals present in the home environment, in addition to neglecting a critical review of available information. Guidelines and methods for setting policy [11, 12] and for determining if an individual may work in a job have been proposed (Fig. 31-2).

The algorithm of Fig. 31-2 provides a step-by-step process for assessing the work capability of the pregnant employee. This algorithm refers to four major categories of medical management outcome for the pregnant worker: (1) woman may continue working; (2) woman may continue working, job modification is desirable; (3) woman may continue working only with job modification; and (4) woman may not work.

These categories are dependent to an extent on exposure limits. The published Occupational Safety and Health Administration (OSHA) standards and American Conference of Governmental Industrial Hygienists (ACGIH) recommended Threshold Limit Values (TLVs) can be used as starting points for exposure limit guidelines. When reviewing toxicologic and epidemiologic studies, a search for no-effect levels, the highest dose level at which a toxic effect is not observed, is of value. When neither published standards nor apparently safe levels in animals are available, caution is suggested. If available, a no-effect level can be reduced by a safety factor of 10, 100, 1000, or more to set an acceptable exposure level in humans.

One set of guidelines [13] suggesting caution concerning potential exposure utilizes three terms: "avoid," "minimize," and "limit." By *avoid,* it is suggested that no

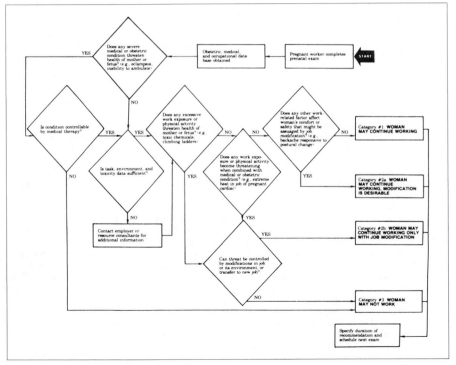

Figure 31-2. Algorithm for medical management of the pregnant worker. (From United States Department of Health and Human Services. *Guidelines on Pregnancy and Work.* NIOSH Publication no. 78-118, 1977. P. 14.)

exposure should occur. The term is used where there are no data on a no-effect level. By *minimize,* it is suggested that exposure should be kept at the lowest feasible level. The term is used in those instances where a no-effect level is apparently present in animals, but such a level in humans has not been reported. By *limit,* the exercise of caution in degree of exposure or frequency of exposure is suggested. The term is used for those substances for which human studies indicate a level of nonhazardous exposure. One should then keep exposure below the level at which hazardous effects have been noted. The guidelines refer, of course, only to the workplace, where exposure may be expected to occur throughout the workday and over a period of time, and do not refer to an occasional or infrequent exposure to minimal amounts of substances intended for consumer use.

Another decision faced by the physician regards the length of time into a pregnancy that an employee may continue to work without harming herself or her child. For the uncomplicated situation, the guidelines for continuation of various job tasks during pregnancy listed in Table 31-6 are very useful. These guidelines are generally recognized and have been produced by the American Medical Association's Council on Scientific Affairs [14].

A final issue requires elaboration. How does a physician determine work-relatedness of an adverse reproductive outcome? Occupational physicians are frequently called on to ascertain whether a disease or injury is related to the patient's work. The legal implications of the decision require a greater degree of certainty than do usual treatment situations; the cause must be established "to a reasonable degree

Table 31-6. Guidelines for continuation of various job tasks during pregnancy

Job task	Week of gestation
Secretarial and light clerical	40
Professional and managerial	40
Sitting with light tasks	
Prolonged (more than 4 hours)	40
Intermittent	40
Standing	
Prolonged (more than 4 hours)	24
Intermittent	
More than 30 minutes per hour	32
Less than 30 minutes per hour	40
Stooping and bending below knee level	
Repetitive (more than 10 times per hour)	20
Intermittent	
2 to 20 times per hour	28
Less than 2 times per hour	40
Climbing	
Vertical ladders and poles	
Repetitive (4 or more times per 8-hour shift)	20
Intermittent (less than 4 times per 8-hour shift)	28
Stairs	
Repetitive (4 or more times per 8-hour shift)	28
Intermittent (less than 4 times per 8-hour shift)	40
Lifting	
Repetitive	
Less than 25 lb	40
25 to 50 lb	24
More than 50 lb	20
Intermittent	
Less than 25 lb	40
25 to 50 lb	40
More than 50 lb	30

Source: From American Medical Association Council on Scientific Affairs. Effect of pregnancy on work performance. *J.A.M.A.* 251:1995, 1984. Copyright 1984, American Medical Association.

of medical certainty." Physicians can better respond to the demands of this situation if they understand how an examination for impairment, disability, or work-relatedness of a condition differs from an examination for treatment.

In an examination for treatment, the physician's primary responsibility is the patient's welfare; in contrast, in an examination for impairment, the physician also has increased responsibility to society. This different responsibility in the examination for impairment requires total objectivity and a legal requirement of truth that may at times conflict with the patient's interest. A great deal of miscommunication between the physician and patient can occur if these different roles are not understood. Determining the goal of the examination before seeing the patient assists the physician in structuring the evaluation.

Three steps may be used to determine the cause of a medical condition such as an adverse reproductive outcome and whether the cause is *work related* when sufficient evidence is available. *First,* a review of the historical, physical, and laboratory data must meet the necessary *criteria* to establish a diagnosis. Sometimes medical conditions unrelated to work can be aggravated by occupational factors. In such cases, a review of the natural history of the preexisting condition is conducted to determine whether it has been altered adversely by exposure. *Second,* a search of the medical literature can reveal whether there is any evidence that the substance or situation in question is *capable* of producing the established medical condition. The epidemiologic literature defines the *circumstances of exposure* under which the condition can result. A well-established diagnosis based on objective criteria will allow a meaningful literature search; going to the literature without an established diagnosis, with only disparate symptoms and signs, rarely provides useful information.

If the diagnosis and initial literature search suggest an occupational reason for the adverse reproductive outcome, *the third step* is to *evaluate the workplace.* The physician can either visit the workplace or obtain necessary data from the workplace. The medical, safety, industrial hygiene, or personnel department at the workplace may be able to give exposure information. If this information is not available, an industrial hygienist from a consulting firm, insurance carrier, or the state or local government can perform the necessary testing. With these data, the physician must then determine if exposure to the specific substance at the recorded level matches the circumstances of exposure sufficient to produce the patient's condition, as defined by the scientific literature.

Case Example Update

Case 1: A 28-year-old woman has asked you if her work or her husband's work has made them sterile. What do you tell her?

A first question to be addressed is whether she or her husband is in fact sterile. Establishing the diagnosis with an infertility clinical examination by an appropriate consultant produces two alternatives for the practitioner. (1) The patient and her husband may not be sterile: Address the patient's concerns and fears regarding workplace exposures by providing factual information in an understandable manner with the risks of everyday living. The latest information on the risks associated with video display terminals in an office, dioxin from Agent Orange in Vietnam, lead and other heavy metals in a foundry, and stress from marital and financial difficulties in one's personal life can be addressed. (2) The patient or her husband probably is sterile: Perform a complete investigation into the specific cause by determining the circumstances of exposure with data from the medical literature and the workplace.

Case 2: As a company physician you are asked about potential hazards of substances used at a chemical plant. How do you respond?

The company has a responsibility to protect its employees from hazardous workplace exposures. An overall corporate policy on health and safety can address this issue. The policy would cover legal requirements and medical standards. Medical standards can include a monitoring program to provide unbiased data to assure the safety of the workplace or to address a hazard at the earliest moment. For this case, do a complete *exposure inventory* within the specific departmental unit of concern, or the entire company, and compare this to a *scientific literature* review of the substances in the inventory to determine the level of evidence linking those substances with any *specific potential adverse reproductive outcome.* Then, *monitor* the reproductive outcomes of the employees, with particular attention to the specific outcomes or endpoints identified by linking the exposure inventory and the scientific literature.

References

1. *International Union v. Johnson Controls,* 111 US 1196 (1991).
2. Radike, M. Reproductive Toxicology. In P. L. Williams and J. L. Burson (eds.), *Industrial Toxicology, Safety and Health Applications in the Workplace.* New York: Van Nostrand Reinhold, 1985. P. 345.
3. McLeod, J., and Ving, W. Male fertility potential in terms of semen quality. A review of the past, a study of the present. *Fertil. Steril.* 31:103, 1979.
4. Manson, J. M., and Wise, L. D. Teratogens. In M. O. Amdur, J. Doull, and C. D. Klaassen (eds.), *Casarett and Doull's Toxicology: The Basic Science of Poisons* (4th ed.). New York: Pergamon, 1991. P. 235.
5. Kline, J. K. Maternal Occupation: Effects on Spontaneous Abortions and Malformations, In Z. A. Stein and M. C. Hatch (eds.), Reproductive Problems in the Workplace. *Occup. Med. State of the Art Rev.* Philadelphia: Hanley & Belfus, 1986. Pp. 381–403.
6. American Medical Association Council on Scientific Affairs. Effects of toxic chemicals on the reproductive system. *J.A.M.A.* 253:3431, 1985.
7. Bloom, A. D. (ed.). *Guidelines for Studies of Human Populations Exposed to Mutagenic and Reproductive Hazards.* White Plains, NY: March of Dimes Birth Defects Foundation, 1981. P. 47.
8. Kalter, H., and Warkany, J. Congenital malformations: Etiologic factors and their role in prevention. *N. Engl. J. Med.* 308:424, 1983.
9. Barlow, S. M., and Sullivan, F. M. *Reproductive Hazards of Industrial Chemicals, An Evaluation of Animal and Human Data.* London: Academic, 1982. Pp. 23–27.
10. O'Flaherty, E. J. Absorption, Distribution, and Elimination of Toxic Agents. In P. L. Williams and J. L. Burson (eds.), *Industrial Toxicology, Safety and Health Applications in the Workplace.* New York: Van Nostrand Reinhold, 1985. Pp. 47–48.
11. Bond, M. B. Role of corporate policy in the control of reproductive hazards of the workplace. *J.O.M.* 28:193, 1986.
12. Logan, D. C. Reproduction and the Workplace: An Industry Perspective. In Z. A. Stein and M. C. Hatch (eds.), Reproductive Problems in the Workplace. *Occup. Med. State of the Art Rev.* Philadelphia: Hanley & Belfus, 1986. Pp. 473–481.
13. Greaves, W. W. *Teratogenicity and Fetotoxicity Assessments.* Milwaukee: Ergotopology, 1983.
14. American Medical Association Council on Scientific Affairs. Effect of pregnancy on work performance. *J.A.M.A.* 251:1995, 1984.

Further Information

American Medical Association Council on Scientific Affairs. Effects of physical forces on the reproductive cycle. *J.A.M.A.* 251:247, 1984.
A referenced summary of known hazardous physical forces. Little support for adverse reproductive outcomes due to physical forces was reported. Hazards are known for atmospheric pressure (over 12,000 ft above sea level), hyperthermia (greater than 40°C), and ionizing radiation (depends on dose and duration).

CDC leading work-related diseases and injuries—United States: Disorders of reproduction. *M.M.W.R.* 34:537, 1985.
A hypothesis-generating summary of possible causes of adverse reproductive outcome estimates.

Christian, M. S., et al. *Assessment of Reproductive and Teratogenic Hazards.* Vol. III. *Advances in Modern Environmental Toxicology.* Princeton: Princeton Scientific Publishers, 1983.
A discussion of historical incidents, specific environmental exposures, and systems for rapid detection of potential hazards, and a description of toxicity and screening texts.

Freedman, A. *Industry Response to Health Risk*. Report no. 811. New York: Conference Board, 1981.
An extensive compilation of interviews and data from corporate executives and health staff on corporate response to public health needs. It is synthesized and written well, presenting practical points for the practice of occupational medicine.

Kline, J., Stein, Z., and Susser, M. *Conception to Birth. Epidemiology of Prenatal Development*. Vol. 14. *Monographs in Epidemiology and Biostatistics*. New York: Oxford University Press, 1989.
An extensively referenced and critical review of prenatal development. The text presents a synthesis and evaluation of current knowledge.

Levine, R. J., et al. A method for monitoring the fertility of workers: I. Method and pilot studies. *J.O.M.*, 22:781, 1980.
Surveillance for adverse reproductive outcome using an excellent questionnaire is reported. This directs more intensive investigation if an abnormality is detected.

Lewis, R. J., Sr. *Reproductively Active Chemicals. A Reference Guide*. New York: Van Nostrand Reinhold, 1991.
This reference work details experimental data on about 3000 chemicals and includes a Chemical Abstract Service number cross-index and a synonym cross-index.

Mattison, D. R. (ed.). *Reproductive Toxicology*. New York: Alan R. Liss, 1983.
A collection of papers addressing reproductive biology and toxicology, including male, female, prenatal, perinatal, and postnatal. The section on reproductive toxicology surveillance presents useful methods and data sources.

Office of Technology Assessment Task Force. *Reproductive Hazards in the Workplace*. Philadelphia: Lippincott, 1988.
Extensive introduction to the full range of issues and literature on the subject.

Paul, M. (ed.). *Occupational and Environmental Reproductive Hazards: A Guide for Clinicians*. Baltimore: Williams & Wilkins, 1993.
A comprehensive text covering a broad range of issues and questions arising from clinical practice.

Schardein, J. L. *Chemically Induced Birth Defects*. New York: Marcel Dekker, 1985.
A useful reference regarding acknowledged chemical hazards that may interfere with reproductive outcome.

Schnorr, T. M., Grajewski, B. A., and Hornung, R. W. Video display terminal and the risk of spontaneous abortion. *N. Engl. J. Med.* 324:727, 1991.
A study of 18- to 33-year-old telephone operators in eight Southeastern states found no significant differences in spontaneous abortion in women who did or did not work with video display terminals.

Stein, Z. A., and Hatch, M. C. *Reproductive Problems in the Workplace. Occup. Med. State of the Art Rev.*, July–Dec. 1986. Philadelphia: Hanloy & Belfus, 1986.
A review of the background and issues regarding occupational reproductive hazards.

Sweet, A. Y., and Brown, E. G. (eds.). *Fetal and Neonatal Effects of Maternal Disease*. St. Louis: Mosby–Year Book, 1991.
A detailed discussion of effects from a wide variety of infectious diseases and organ system disorders.

Appendix to Chapter 31: Agents Associated with Adverse Female Reproductive Capacity or Developmental Effects in Human and Animal Studies[a]

Agent	Human outcomes	Strength of association in humans	Animal outcomes	Strength of association in animals
Anesthetic gases[b]	Reduced fertility, spontaneous abortion	1,3	Birth defects	1,3
Arsenic	Spontaneous abortion, low birth weight	1	Birth defects, fetal loss	2
Benzo(a)pyrene	None	NA[c]	Birth defects	1
Cadmium	None	NA	Fetal loss, birth defects	2
Carbon disulfide	Menstrual disorders, spontaneous abortion	1	Birth defects	1
Carbon monoxide	Low birth weight, fetal death (high doses)	1	Birth defects, neonatal mortality	2
Chlordecone	None	NA	Fetal loss	2,3
Chloroform	None	NA	Fetal loss	1
Chloroprene	None	NA	Birth defects	2,3
Ethylene glycol ethers	Spontaneous abortion	1	Birth defects	2
Ethylene oxide	Spontaneous abortion	1	Fetal loss	1
Formamides	None	NA	Fetal loss, birth defects	2
Inorganic mercury[b]	Menstrual disorders, spontaneous abortion	1	Fetal loss, birth defects	1
Lead[b]	Spontaneous abortion, prematurity, neurologic dysfunction in child	2	Birth defects, fetal loss	2
Organic mercury	CNS malformation, cerebral palsy	2	Birth defects, fetal loss	2
Physical stress	Prematurity	2	None	NA
Polybrominated biphenyls (PBBs)	None	NA	Fetal loss	2
Polychlorinated biphenyls (PCBs)	Neonatal PCB syndrome (low birth weight, hyperpigmentation, eye abnormalities)	2	Low birth weight, fetal loss	2

(continued)

Agent	Human outcomes	Strength of association in humans	Animal outcomes	Strength of association in animals
Radiation, ionizing	Menstrual disorders, CNS defects, skeletal and eye anomalies, mental retardation, childhood cancer	2	Fetal loss, birth defects	2
Selenium	Spontaneous abortion	3	Low birth weight, birth defects	2
Tellurium	None	NA	Birth defects	2
2,4-Dichlorophenoxyacetic acid (2,4-D)	Skeletal defects	4	Birth defects	1
2,4,5-Trichlorophenoxyacetic acid (2,4,5-T)	Skeletal defects	4	Birth defects	1
Video display terminals	Spontaneous abortion	4	Birth defects	1
Vinyl chloride[b]	CNS defects	1	Birth defects	1,4
Xylene	Menstrual disorders, fetal loss	1	Fetal loss, birth defects	1

Key: 1 = limited positive data; 2 = strong positive data; 3 = limited negative data; 4 = strong negative data; CNS = central nervous system.
[a]Major studies of the reproductive health effects of exposure to dioxin are currently in progress.
[b]May have male-mediated effects.
[c]Not applicable because no adverse outcomes were observed.
Source: Adapted from *Reproductive and Developmental Hazards, Case Studies in Environmental Medicine*. Atlanta: Agency for Toxic Substances and Disease Registry, 1993.

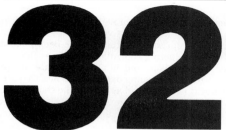

Health Promotion

Molly J. McCauley and
Robert J. McCunney

Health promotion is now recognized as an important part of the practice of occupational health, as shown by the number of worksites with health promotion activities. This integration of activities is evidenced in the findings of the 1992 national survey, conducted by the United States Office of Disease Prevention and Health Promotion, documenting that 81% of worksites with 50 or more employees offer at least one health promotion activity, as compared to 65% of worksites in 1985 [1]. Healthy People 2000, a compilation of health promotion and disease prevention objectives for the year 2000 published by the US Department of Health and Human Services, has set forth a challenge for continued growth by setting a goal to increase to at least 85% the number of worksites with 50 or more employees that offer health promotion activities [2].

This growth since 1985, and the challenge for future growth of worksite health promotion, is certainly not born exclusively of established national goals. It is driven by the desire of employers to manage health care costs, impact absence, and contribute to the health and well-being of their human resources. Yet, while such results of health promotion programming are desirable, definitive reports regarding cost effectiveness of programs are just beginning to appear.

The percentage of employers offering worksite health promotion is not the only thing that has evolved over recent years. The definition of health promotion has also. The historical view of health promotion maintained an individual focus and was characterized as wellness. Wellness programs have five dimensions: self-responsibility, nutritional awareness, physical fitness, stress management, and environmental sensitivity [3]. Today, however, the definition is much more inclusive and extends far beyond these five dimensions. Health promotion is the science and art of helping people change their lifestyle through a combination of efforts to enhance awareness, encourage behavior change, and create environments that support good health practices [4]. The goal of health promotion is individual movement toward a state of optimal health, which is a balance of physical, emotional, social, spiritual, and intellectual health [4].

Present-day programs that are comprehensive in nature best reflect the latter definition. Comprehensive programs give equal emphasis to establishing management support for health promotion activities, building a health-supporting work environment, fostering health activities as a viable business strategy, and helping employees identify health risks and behaviors in order to determine ways to change and improve.

The health professionals who deliver occupational health services will be asked to assess, design, develop, implement, and evaluate health promotion programs. In support of those work efforts, this chapter describes:

The rationale and justification for health promotion
Methods and strategies for getting started
The scope of comprehensive programs
Implementation options—what works and what doesn't
Evaluation approaches
Challenges and opportunities for worksite health promotion

Rationale and Justification for Worksite Health Promotion

In general, increased attention has been directed to the potential of workplace health promotion programs to control health care costs, impact utilization of medical care, decrease absenteeism, reduce health risks, and improve health- and work-related attitudes.

Specifically, since 1986, the findings from several studies have been published in the literature. Given the difficulty of conducting controlled studies at the worksite, evidence of cost savings, reduced absenteeism, and improved morale are promising [5]. Indeed, there has never been a recommendation that health promotion prevail as a stand-alone strategy, but it is recognized as part of the solution, thereby providing substantive rationale to invest in programming.

Health Care Costs

Controlling health care costs paid by employers is complex and part of an ever growing national dilemma [6–8]. Of the $838 billion the US spent on health care in 1992, 33% of the bill was paid by private health insurance [9], most of which is supported by employers. Assuming that health care costs continue to increase at a rate of 20 to 21% per year and that payroll continues to increase at a rate of 5 to 7% per year, by the year 2003 the salary line and health care cost line will cross, with health care costs becoming the number one cost of doing business [10]. The bottom line is that business profitability will be impacted, employee wages may decline, and jobs will be at risk.

There was early evidence that health promotion and positive health behaviors can reduce health care costs. Live for Life, Johnson & Johnson's program, documented a mean annual inpatient cost increase for active program participants of $42, as compared to a $76 increase for nonparticipants [11]. Control Data's cross-sectional study of insurance data showed that smokers experience 18% higher medical claims and that people with hypertension are 68% more likely to incur claims in excess of $5,000 per year [12]. However, a reconsideration of the Blue Cross and Blue Shield Indiana study concludes that program participation was *not* associated with reduced health care costs 5 years postprogram and that it is prudent to remain guarded about the health care cost savings of worksite health promotion programs [13].

With such ambiguity about the impact on health care costs, it remains essential that the rationale for initiating and retaining health promotion programs does not rest exclusively on health care cost outcomes.

Absenteeism

Employees who are absent from the job are not productive employees. Business not only pays the health care bill for an ill or injured employee, but it also incurs the cost of salary continuation when an employee is absent. The impact that health promotion has on absenteeism is therefore significant.

Johnson & Johnson examined absence in terms of sick hours and found that Live for Life participants report 20 fewer hours of sick time per year than nonparticipants [14]. Avoiding payment for two and one-half days of absence per employee per year across an entire employee population would dramatically reduce payment of salary dollars that are not associated with productivity.

Likewise, at DuPont, a study of 41 sites with a health promotion program as compared to 19 control sites without any health promotion documented a 14% decline in sickness-absence-disability days at the program sites and only a 5.8% decline at control sites [15].

Health Risks

One premise on which health promotion programs are justified is the ability to focus on the preventable aspects of morbidity and mortality in the US. The leading causes of death and disease today have been linked to major risk factors. It is estimated that many years of life are lost to premature death [16] and there are examples that the prevalence and levels of preventable risk factors in employed populations are high [17]. Efforts directed towards these risk factors are the essence of worksite health promotion.

The fact that actual health risks are reduced has been the easiest to document. AT&T's Total Life Concept (TLC) program reported significantly greater improvements among study group participants than control group participants for diastolic blood pressure, serum cholesterol, type A behavior, and body weight after just 1 year [18]. After 2 years, the significant improvements were maintained and resulted in a decrease in health age, as well as reduced population scores for total mortality, heart attack morbidity, and cancer morbidity [19].

If short-term risk reduction does translate to actual reduction of morbidity and mortality over time, companies will couple the short-term benefit of a healthier workforce with the long-term savings from reduced health care utilization and disability absence.

Attitudes Toward Health and the Company

Positive attitudes toward the employer, a necessary ingredient of high morale in the workforce, were a highly valued outcome by key corporate executives in the early 1980s. Companies, experiencing change and transition and equally concerned about the well-being of the employees, sought to document attitude change. Did employees feel better about the employer as a result of having the opportunity to participate in health promotion programs? Did employees have a better attitude toward health and did it make a difference? The answer is yes and no.

Johnson & Johnson found a significant attitudinal improvement in employees at participating Live for Life companies. Measures were favorable for organizational commitment, supervision, working conditions, job competence, pay and fringe benefits, and job security [20]. AT&T documented attitudinal changes as well. After 1 year of ongoing Total Life Concept programming, participants reported a belief that they could affect their own health and were committed to change health behaviors [18]. Additionally, participants perceived that AT&T cared about their welfare, were enthused about their work, and were satisfied with working conditions [18]. However, the positive job-related effects attained after 1 year were negated at 2 years, likely due to the organizational and operational changes that occurred during that time. This finding suggests that, while health promotion can positively influence attitudes toward the company, the presence of a program cannot eliminate the consequences of job/work-related transition, ambiguity, and uncertainty.

Strategic Planning Process

The options for program delivery are many; the appropriate choices depend on the characteristics of the employee population coupled with the goals of the business. A systematic planning process is the key to immediate and ongoing success and includes establishing vision, mission, and goals; assessing data; choosing interventions; and determining how results will be measured. The occupational health professional is in the unique position to champion this process.

Establishing the Vision, Mission, and Goals

At the outset of planning, a clear description of the expectations of the health promotion program is most essential. The stakeholders, key executives, and managers need to articulate the vision for the future in light of the initiation of health promotion. How will the program link to the business strategy; how will it contribute to the management of human resources? With that direction and support from top management, the mission and goals for the program can be formulated and endorsed.

Data Collection

Employee assessments, taking the form of surveys and focus groups, are a good place to begin. The goal is to understand the wants and needs of the population, as well as the ethnic, cultural, social, and organizational characteristics. Such assessment activities offer employees an opportunity to comment during the development stage, which may enhance interest and participation. Focus groups will identify a myriad of issues and highlight the barriers and helpers that the program may face. During focus groups, unofficial leaders may emerge who will be invaluable as employee committee members and in soliciting co-workers' participation.

Management interviews gather another perspective, that of the leadership and supervision in the company. It is critical that the needs of the business are understood and that the issues of managers are taken into consideration. The concern of "what's in this for me?" cannot be ignored; anything short of a win-win for both the employee and the manager sets the stage for failure. Interviews give valuable insights into the level of commitment within the organization and the degree to which financial support and personal involvement can be expected.

Health care cost data, illness/injury absence data, and demographic data should be used to determine the prominent disease categories that are driving costs, and for which groups of employees. A demographic overview can portray specific groups that may benefit from targeted interventions. For example, a young female population with a high rate of complications from pregnancy would benefit from a pregnancy program.

Finally, data from health risk appraisals (HRA) can be used to develop and aggregate a view of population risk, information that is essential to program planning. Computerized versions use a set of algorithms developed from investigations of large populations as the basis for interpretation. While some authors have suggested that employee populations have risks similar to those of the general population [21], company-specific data are more readily accepted by management, thereby building a case for the administration of the HRA, even if on a random selection basis. Baseline administration of an HRA and interval readministration can help gauge the effect of the program on employee risk factors.

Once all the data noted above have been collected, it is time to assimilate this information and begin molding a plan that will (1) include content acceptable to both the employees and management, (2) allow for implementation within the scope of the resources available, (3) incorporate strategies and methods that take into consideration employee preferences and the needs of the operation of the business, and (4) have specific measures indicative of both short-term and long-term results. Suggested program options and evaluation considerations are delineated in the next two sections of this chapter.

Scope of Programs for Health Promotion

Programs can range from health awareness campaigns, to educational seminars, to biologic screenings, to behavioral change modules. The important feature of all approaches is individual behavioral changes supported by the workplace environment. Whatever the topic of interest, the goal is the achievement and maintenance of positive health behaviors.

To choose a specific intervention, one needs to weigh factors pertaining to time availability of vendors and staff to deliver programs; time availability for employees to attend—on-work time, off-work time, and shared time; and costs—whether the employee pays a part, all, or no portion of the established cost.

This section discusses some of the more popular programs offered in the business setting: smoking cessation, exercise/aerobics, nutrition/cholesterol/weight management, blood pressure control, stress management, employee assistance programs, and preventive examinations. Although the nature of this chapter limits the depth of discussion on each particular program component, more detailed descriptions are available in the material listed under Further Information.

Screening Examinations

Appropriate screening examinations are essential, as they are the single program segment that focuses on the collection of actual physiologic measurements. These measures potentially can establish the teachable moment for the participant and the basis for evaluation for program managers. Past evaluations have pointed out the importance of age-, risk-, and history-specific screenings [22], with this same position shared by the US Clinical Preventive Services Task Force (see Chap. 40). Based on screening over 1000 employees for a health promotion program, Harris and associates [17] have proposed a screening protocol that incorporates these guidelines.

No screening is complete without an educational component and follow-up. One study of cholesterol screening follow-up conducted by Blue Cross and Blue Shield of Maryland found that the most successful predictor of referral completion after the screening itself was a cholesterol level equal to or greater than 240 mg/100 ml [23]. Another study of referral compliance after public cholesterol screening found that individuals with prior history were 10 to 15% more likely to initiate follow-up [24]. These studies are but a few examples of follow-up action taken by participants and, in the future, additional study conclusions may help health professionals target participants least likely to act on screening results.

Smoking Cessation

No single lifestyle behavior has a greater impact on health than cigarette smoking. It remains the single most important preventable cause of death in our society [25]. Additionally, the difficulty faced when individuals attempt to stop smoking is greater than that for many other health-related behaviors. According to the 1989 Surgeon General's report, smoking causes 87% of all lung cancer deaths and 21% of all coronary heart disease (CHD) deaths [25]. Overall, one in six deaths each year is attributed to smoking [26], and, with a projection of 40 million smokers for the year 2000 [27], that death rate is not likely to be markedly different. The costs for employees attributed to smoking are also staggering. Smokers can cost the employer anywhere from $336 [28] to $4700 [29] per year in indirect costs (those not related to health care claims and coverage).

Since 80% of all smokers currently say they would like to quit [25], smoking cessation is a reasonable program component. Unfortunately, at any given time only 10% of the 80% are ready to quit and interested in joining a program to do so. That is why smoking cessation programming necessitates a wide array of options as well as ongoing support for those who elect to quit on their own.

Many structured programs that address the addictive and behavioral components of smoking are readily available through the American Cancer Society, the American Lung Association, the American Heart Association, and Smoke-Anon. These organizations provide program material and often group facilitators. Hospitals and health maintenance organizations are also resources for smoking cessation.

Selecting the appropriate program for the population necessitates consideration of program duration, educational content, and support mechanisms. Programs range in length from 2 consecutive days to once weekly for 8 to 10 weeks. Program content should address the physiologic as well as the psychosocial and addictive characteristics of smoking. The support strategies may include a buddy system, behavioral contracting, use of incentives, and use of a nicotine supplement. Since no one method works for everyone, several different programs offered over time afford smokers the opportunity to find the program that works for them.

Formal programs are not necessarily the only approach to smoking cessation. Some people respond better to self-help, self-paced learning methods. The inclusion of family members is strongly recommended regardless of the program options offered. Many individuals will also seek advice about hypnosis, acupuncture, and biofeedback, which are indeed personal alternatives.

In the workplace, the greatest support and the most visible message are established when a smoke-free workplace policy is in effect. New evidence of the impact of environmental smoke on nonsmokers [30] is a compelling reason to institute a smoking policy.

Fitness/Aerobics

The goal of a fitness/aerobics component is to improve cardiovascular fitness, increase strength, and improve flexibility. The psychosocial benefits, as well as improved morale, attitude, and productivity, also cannot be overlooked. In order to implement a fitness program, it is not necessary to have a fully equipped, on-site facility. Motivating employees to begin an exercise program and referring them to community facilities that have qualified staff and safe equipment are viable alternatives for most organizations. However, the convenience of on-site facilities does tend to increase the percentage of actively exercising employees.

Regardless of where employees exercise, individual exercise routines should be tailored to the needs of the person and of sufficient intensity and duration to be beneficial to health [31]. Exercise screening (risk factor review, personal health history, heart rate, blood pressure, and cholesterol) is recommended before entry into any program, with additional testing (submaximal or maximal electrocardiography) as indicated by a protocol that quantifies risk factors. Exercise testing can be conducted using a bicycle ergometer and guides the development of a safe and beneficial exercise program.

Sharing membership costs, negotiating waiver of initial fees, and setting up a partial or full reimbursement procedure can enhance participation. Although coordinating a fitness program is time and labor intensive, the well-documented physical, social, and emotional benefits make that resource investment worthwhile. Higher levels of physical activity have been associated with reduced incidence of coronary artery disease (CAD) [32], and all-cause mortality is 3.4 times greater for the least fit men and 4.6 times greater for the least fit women [33].

Nutrition/Cholesterol/Weight Management

Obesity affects 20 to 40% of adults. It is associated with high risk of hypertension, diabetes mellitus, cardiovascular disease, and certain cancers [34]. Programs designed to promote weight reduction, control cholesterol, and assure proper nutrition need to incorporate principles of balanced nutrition, regular exercise, and cholesterol/fat intake to be of optimal value.

Reports from the National Heart, Lung and Blood Institute (NHLBI), dietary guidelines of the National Cancer Society, and results of several clinical investigations support the role of nutritional programs as an aid in reducing preventable illness. NHLBI initiated a National Cholesterol Education Program in 1985 to increase public awareness of cholesterol as a risk factor. In fact, results of the MRFIT study substantiated that levels of cholesterol above 180 mg/100 ml needlessly increase the risk of CHD among middle-aged American men [34]. The Framingham Study confirmed that relationship; specifically, when plasma cholesterol levels increase, so does the incidence of CHD [35].

Therefore, a nutritional program that places emphasis on balanced dietary intake (acceptable intake of carbohydrates, proteins, and fats) and assures fat intake equal to or less than 30% of daily caloric total is desirable. Changing eating behaviors is very difficult and no program will be successful without maintenance strategies and continued reinforcement.

No single approach is effective with weight management. Participants tend to lose weight if properly counseled and given necessary support and follow-up. Individual motivation, however, is a prime determinant in weight reduction efforts. The combination of caloric restriction and exercise seems to work best, as long as the psychosocial and cultural influences are not ignored [36].

Blood Pressure

Screening for hypertension is not new to Occupational Health. In fact, worksite treatment and education programs have been shown to be more effective in achieving compliance and reduction of health care costs than treatment by any other type of community-based program. Specifically, studies have found that screening, case identification, and referral linked to rigorous worksite follow-up achieve optimal blood pressure control. A structured educational component is an essential adjunct to any hypertension detection and treatment program. Hypertension control requires adequate diagnosis and appropriate follow-up. Screening for hypertension often lacks strong educational and follow-up elements in which case participants do not seek the necessary diagnostic tests and treatment required to achieve control. Provision of follow-up care that includes behavioral contracting and support groups enhances compliance in 70 to 80% of cases [37].

Using reliable criteria and protocols, organizations can easily provide routine treatment for employees with high blood pressure, while continuing to assure that a relationship with the primary care provider is maintained. A periodic visit to an occupational health professional provides the opportunity for accurate monitoring coupled with counseling about diet, exercise, weight control, and stress management that can complement the care and treatment of the employee's personal physician.

Stress Management

Stress management, integral to any comprehensive health promotion program, is a highly sought intervention by employee and manager alike. Stress has been implicated as a factor in many illnesses, including cardiovascular disease, asthma, skin disorders, and peptic ulcers, among others. Effective stress management techniques can improve employees' ability to cope with stress, improve their sense of well-being, and reduce the likelihood of stress-related symptoms. The reader is referred to Chap. 18 for a detailed description of stress and appropriate interventions.

Employee Assistance Programs

The prevalence of alcohol abuse among employee populations has been estimated to be between 5 and 10% [38]. In addition, 20% of the adult population suffers from various types of psychiatric disorders that would benefit from treatment [38]. Since family, marital, social, and legal problems can interfere with both personal and work life, employee assistance programs (EAPs) have emerged as a viable method of early detection for these problems. EAPs, a confidential resource for employees, have their origins in occupational alcoholism programs of years past. The EAP concept has since broadened to include behavioral problems and drug abuse. The passage of the Federal Rehabilitation Act and the Americans with Disabilities Act, which both address the issues of alcoholism, adds credence to employer-supported EAP. The direct cost to American industry to treat and rehabilitate alcohol and chemical dependency, mental illness, and other emotional problems has been estimated to be between $58 and $102 million annually [39]. The rationale behind EAP is to provide early assessment and intervention and as needed determine the most appropriate, cost-effective referral. For alcohol-related issues, treatment resources range from self-help groups (e.g., Alcoholics Anonymous and Al-Anon) to inpatient psychiatric and rehabilitation services. Intensive outpatient programs are increasingly popular, as they are extremely cost effective and have the added benefit of allowing the rehabilitation to take place within the context of the home and family. Referrals to EAP commonly originate through management, peers, family members, or the medical community. In most programs approximately half of the people are self-referred.

Establishing an EAP needs to begin with a clear policy statement regarding how emotional/behavioral problems will be addressed. Guidelines for participation need to be developed at the same time. Voluntary participation that ensures confidentiality is essential. Case management practices as well as the responsibilities of the employee need to be clearly articulated.

A counselor can be made available in several ways. Small companies can contract with a mental health practitioner or organization to provide service either on- or off-site. Often this service is on a per capita basis; however, a fee-for-service arrangement can also be made. Larger companies may find it more cost effective to hire their own staff, and, indeed, this may bring value added as an internal resource that understands the company. Unionized companies have found it advantageous to make the EAP a joint labor/management initiative. Not only can a collaborative effort support relations between the union and the company, but it may foster participation.

Other EAP components can be valuable adjuncts to the existing secondary prevention strategies. Lectures and seminars on aging, child rearing, change, violence, relationships, career conflicts, and communications are excellent primary prevention initiatives. Addressing self-esteem, assertiveness, commitment, and self-efficacy enhances people's ability to make effective behavioral changes that promote health.

Employee assistance programs, as an integral part of an organization's occupational health services, contribute to the productivity of the business, as well as to the well-being of both the employee and the company.

Implementation Options: What Works and What Doesn't

The single most important measure of success during the initial implementation phase of health promotion programs is participation; in other words, do the target audiences do more than merely express interest? The issue is, do they actively attend programs, take advantage of reading health communications, and join support groups and committees that initiate change in the social climate? Only through participation, whatever the level of involvement, is awareness raised, new knowledge acquired, health skills established, and group support added. Therefore, success at the level of participation is the key ingredient to achieving desired program outcomes over time.

Having considered the rationale for programming (the why) and selected appropriate content (the what), it is time to weigh the implementation options—it is time to answer the "who, when, where, and how" questions. By thoroughly working through this part of planning, the very best determinants of success will be established.

Who?

For many years the employee was the primary target for health promotion programs, and, with few exceptions, executives, management, and white and pink collar workers compromised the audience. Today, program planners must carefully consider strategies for production workers, employees in remote work locations, shift workers, office employees, and telecommuters. Employee demographics can help define any need for special programs to reach subgroups by age, gender, ethnicity, type of work, and so forth. Additionally, the employee's family and company retirees should be considered because they contribute significantly to the company's health care expenditures. Families can provide support for employee behavioral change, while a focus on retirees can influence their lifestyle and the high demand they place on the health care system.

When?

It is often difficult, based on the needs and nature of the business, to select times for lectures, classes, screenings, special events, and counseling sessions. Finding a balance between the needs of the business and convenience and access for the employees is a way to guide decision-making. Times for sessions and appointments may range from 6 AM when drivers pick up vehicles at a central garage to 10:30 PM when third-shift employees arrive at the plant. Scheduling during breaktime, lunchtime, before work, and after work assures maximal access. However, what may indeed be optimal is during-work-hours scheduling, primarily because of the strong message of organizational support and commitment that this sends. Finally, nontraditional time frames should be considered. Examples of nontraditional time frames include Saturday mornings at the ball park or Sunday afternoons at the company picnic.

Where?

Location, long recognized as the number one variable in real estate, is equally important in the context of program implementation. If programs target special populations, their churches, clubs, and community centers may afford the greatest appeal. If programs are for retirees, reaching them in the home via print and audiovisual material or at their senior citizen clubs may work best. No longer is the worksite classroom or clinic the location of choice. The plant floor, the entrance to the cafeteria, and the break room are locations that enhance opportunities for health-related learning, discussions, and monitoring. When considering location, adhere to the paramount rule: "Meet them where they are."

How?

The "how" questions pose a degree of complexity, especially when dealing with questions such as:

How will the program be staffed?
How will the program be paid for?
How will behavioral change strategies by incorporated?
How will the environmental support for positive health practices be addressed?

Selecting staff may be as easy as turning over programming to existing staff who have the essential skills, or it could be as difficult as hiring a new staff or selecting qualified vendors, or both. Do not assume capability based on credentials, but screen to specific criteria, assuring that experience and knowledge are substantive and that effective interpersonal, writing, and presenting skills exist.

Adequate resources, committed at the outset, are needed for planning and development and are generally supported by the company. However, ongoing resources for implementation are equally important and can be derived in various ways. Management can pay full costs. Inherent to that approach is the fact that they support employee health and stand to benefit from both the health care cost savings and the human resource aspects of the program. Employees can pay full costs. Again, they stand to benefit, but in this scenario it is personal gain as a result of increased well-being and morale. The compromise is shared costs, wherein all parties who stand to accrue results make a financial commitment.

With change in health behavior and maintenance of positive health behaviors as objects of interest, it is critical to recognize the complexity and multidimensional nature of behavioral change. It occurs over time as a result of incremental learning, and requires the application of a variety of strategies. To effect change, people need to be made aware of health risks and issues, learn new information to change the cognitive frame of reference, build new skills, and eventually incorporate positive health behaviors to replace those that are negative. Indeed, this is a process and not an event. Classroom learning, self-help libraries, self-paced activities, multimedia communications, theme events, and support groups all contribute to the process. Incentives, work team involvement and management recognition are but a few ways to support maintenance of positive health behaviors.

Evaluating the Effectiveness of Health Promotion

General Characteristics

This section provides consideration for evaluating worksite health promotion programs. The depth of evaluation and level of analysis will vary, depending on the setting and available resources. Nonetheless, the evaluation component should be developed at the beginning of the program when considering the interests of all "stakeholders." Determinations about data points and intervals are elements of the evaluation component. Without an evaluation design, the effects of a health promotion program will not be systematically measured, and the ability to justify continuing a program may be lost. In addition, the data from evaluation can be used as continuous feedback for quality improvement efforts.

In designing the evaluation, the goals and objectives should be clearly stated. Management may be interested in lowering costs and rates of absenteeism; occupational health professionals may be most concerned with reducing risk factors and impacting morbidity and mortality. The evaluation plan, therefore, should reflect a consensus, with stated goals that satisfy the interest of all concerned parties. Evaluations can be focused on measures of process, impact, and outcomes [40].

Process evaluations measure the participant's perception of the program. A logical indicator of program success is participation and, during the process, what was helpful and what was not, what should be changed, and what could be improved. It is important to acknowledge that there is little correlation between positive perceptions and change in health risk. For example, although participants in a high blood pressure program may find the information valuable, attend regularly, and rate the instructor highly, the individual's blood pressure may not be lower at the end of the program. Nevertheless, such a measure is useful and provides information that can easily give immediate feedback to management.

Impact evaluation measures the extent to which an intervention has had an immediate effect on biometric measures and risk factors. These measures are more objective than those obtained in process evaluation as they can indeed be observed or measured. Impact evaluation is more difficult and expensive to conduct, as it encompasses measures such as blood pressure, cholesterol, weight, and body fat. Self-reported behavior that influences risk as a measure of impact should be used with caution. Although the behaviors are a measure of impact, the more reliable way of assessing impact is through observation, which is obviously labor intensive and tedious.

Outcome evaluation determines the effect of interventions on the company or employee population as a whole. It measures subsequent consequences in terms of quality of life and economic benefits of physiologic and psychological changes [41]. Health status improvements as measured by changes in morbidity and mortality and social benefits as measured by improved quality of life are examples of outcomes. Reduced health care costs, reduced absenteeism, fewer on-job accidents, and improved employee morale (based on factor analysis) serve as indicators of health status improvement and the social benefits of health promotion.

A major caution of designing outcome evaluation is that beneficial effects may take years to produce favorable results.

During the implementation phase of the program, *confounding factors* that may affect the measures of interest need to be monitored and recorded. For example, revisions in the medical benefits plan, a labor strike, changes in the workforce, and fluctuating business demands all have an effect. Changes in the local community and national events can also influence employee health practices and then have an influence on both impact and outcome evaluation. The influence of the media and national educational campaigns needs to be recognized, especially if there is a measurable impact that is unexplained by the scope of the company's interventions. The use of a similarly matched control group that does not receive any health promotion interventions may help account for the effect of confounding variables; however, the profession recognizes the barriers and limitations of conducting controlled worksite studies.

Specific Program Evaluation Considerations

The impact of *smoking cessation interventions* is among the easiest to evaluate because the essential information to be obtained is whether participants stop smoking on completion of a program. It is important, however, not to determine program success based on end-of-program cessation, but on continued abstinence after 18 to 24 months. While individuals generally self-report accurately about their smoking habits, biochemical measures can be used to validate self-report. Carboxyhemoglobin, urinary cotinine, and salivary thiocyanate can indicate the presence and degree of smoking. Associated morbidity and mortality, comparing smokers and nonsmokers, can also be monitored as a measure of outcome.

For *fitness/aerobics programs*, the benefits of interest are improved cardiovascular endurance, strength, and flexibility. Cardiovascular fitness is measured by resting blood pressure and heart rate as well as estimation of maximal oxygen uptake. Measures of strength and flexibility are estimated by using simple grip and sit and reach tests. Percentage of body fat, body weight, total serum cholesterol, and high-density lipoprotein (HDL) can also be used as impact indicators. Long-term morbidity and mortality, particularly for cardiovascular disease, are outcomes of interest.

The impact measures for *nutrition, cholesterol, and weight management* are changes in dietary habits and biometric indicators. Analysis of pre- and postdietary intake records allow evaluators to determine if actual changes in eating have taken place relative to intake of fats, fiber, salt, carbohydrates, fresh versus processed foods, and total calories. More reliable and valid indicators of impact are changes in weight, percentage of body fat, total serum cholesterol, and HDL. Body fat is a more useful indicator than total weight, since this value considers added muscle mass that results from increased exercise undertaken as part of a comprehensive weight management program. Given the major impact of serum cholesterol as a risk factor for CHD and the influence of diet on its level, serum cholesterol is an important impact measure. In light of the recommendations in the second report of the Expert Panel on Detection, Evaluation and Treatment of High Blood Cholesterol in Adults (ATPII), a determination of HDL/cholesterol should be a part of testing for total serum cholesterol [42]. This new report also specifically recommends greater emphasis on physical activity and weight loss in combination with dietary therapy [42]. Attention should be given to the variability of serum cholesterol measurements and, when comparisons over time are being made, similar analytic devices should be used to assure comparability of results. Again, analogous to smoking cessation results, success is a program by-product when changes in eating behavior and reductions in weight and cholesterol/HDL are maintained over time.

Blood pressure control is a single-impact measure, obviously a reduced level of blood pressure. Maintenance of reduced levels over time, using standard protocols, is the measure of success. Improved self-efficacy and increased quality of life are important for the hypertensive individual living with a chronic disease. Long-term effectiveness of hypertension control can be based on the avoidance of complications such as stroke, heart attack, and renal disease and their attendant medical costs.

The impact of a *stress management program* is difficult to measure. Unlike cigarettes smoked, body weight, or blood pressure, stress does not lend itself to easy quantification. Thus, stress management programs are ideally evaluated by participant self-report. Differences in pre- and poststress assessment scores, collected using a validated instrument, at least provide indicators of participants' perception of their stressors; their ability to recognize physical, cognitive, and emotional responses; and their success in implementing coping strategies. Interpretations of impact need to be approached with caution.

Employee assistance programs can be evaluated by measuring the functional status of individuals before and after treatment relative to their diagnosis. Further assessment can be made by analyzing absenteeism, use of the health care system, and health care costs for individuals before and after treatment. Certain impact measures, depending on the diagnosis, can be selected, such as liver function tests, urine and blood tests for the presence of substances, and job turnover. Particularly in this arena, improved well-being, job performance, and quality of life are significant markers. The cost effectiveness of EAPs can be determined by assessment of the investment against selected outcome variables. Typical cost-benefit ratios for EAP are reported as $2.50 to $4.00 saved for every dollar invested (see Chap. 34).

Challenges and Opportunities

Worksite health promotion faces many challenges in today's business environment. The challenges that occupational health professionals must confront fall into two basic categories: those put forth by the professional community and those presented by the stakeholders.

The professional community is concerned about the products and services of health promotion, the audience for health promotion, and the results. We are challenged to answer the following questions: Are the populations that need prevention most being reached? Are the correct concepts and theories being applied to the practice of health promotion? Are new theories evolving as a result of learnings in the workplace? Are the changes in employees' health behaviors maintained over time? Are the products and services of health promotion cost effective and cost beneficial? Maybe we should wonder if these are indeed the right questions, but we cannot question the fact that we are challenged every day to answer them.

The stakeholders, defined as the management of American companies willing to invest in worksite health promotion, are asking different questions but, nonetheless, challenging ones. Can health care costs be contained through an investment in prevention? Can health promotion increase worker productivity? Will health promotion help to enhance employee morale, well-being, and stress levels? Can rates of absenteeism, on-job accidents, and long-term disabilities be reduced?

As the year 2000 approaches, with the advent of some type of health care reform, the questions cited above are ours to answer. Therein lies the opportunity. Answering the above questions will solidify the posture of worksite health promotion, personally benefit the employee populations served, and strengthen the companies that invest in their human resources through worksite health promotion.

In order to seize the opportunities that are ahead, there is the need to:

Collaborate and cooperate on research and initiatives across companies and across the public/private sector

Document the most effective strategies for reaching special populations

Determine which current theories (and combination of theories) enhance the success of interventions

Evolve new theories so that "state of the art" is documented and widely applied

Collect and analyze data that will answer the prevailing evaluation questions

Make health promotion a quality process by using data and feedback to continuously improve products and services

Use existing evidence to establish the net worth of health promotion, quantifying that evidence within business cases to acquire needed resources

Strive for a win-win-win situation in which all parties benefit. Occupational health professionals will have the opportunity to advance disease prevention and health promotion. Stakeholders will see evidence of the merits of health promotion as a human resource investment. Employees will be able to access resources that enable them to modify and maintain positive health practices.

References

1. US Department of Health and Human Services, Office of Disease Prevention and Health Promotion. *1992 National Survey of Worksite Health Promotion Summary Report*. Washington, DC: US Department of Health and Human Services, 1993.
2. US Department of Health and Human Services, Office of Disease Prevention and Health Promotion. *Healthy People 2000: National Health Promotion and Disease Prevention Objectives*. Washington, DC: US Government Printing Office, 1990.
3. Ardell, D. B. *High Level Wellness*. New York: Bantam Books/Rodale Press, 1977.
4. O'Donnell, M. B., and Ainsworth, T. (eds.). *Health Promotion in the Workplace*. New York: Wiley, 1986.
5. Pelletier, K. R. (ed.). Data base research and evaluation results—a review and analysis of the health and cost effective outcome studies of comprehensive disease prevention programs. *Am. J. Health Promotion* 5:311, 1991.
6. Herzlinger, R. E., and Schwartz, J. How companies tackle health care costs: Part 1. *Harvard Business Rev.* July/Aug. 1995. Pp. 69–81.
7. Herzlinger, R. E. How companies tackle health care costs: Part II. *Harvard Business Rev.* Sept./Oct. 1985. Pp. 108–120.
8. Herzlinger, R. E., and Caulkins, D. How companies tackle health care costs: Part III. *Harvard Business Rev.* Jan./Feb. 1986. Pp. 70–80.
9. Health Care Financing Administration, Division of National Cost Estimates. *Health Care Financing Review*. Washington, DC: US Government Printing Office, June 1993.
10. Hembree, W. Managing Health Care Costs (unpublished). Health Research Institute, 1992.
11. Bly, J. L., Jones, R. C., and Richardson, J. E. Impact of worksite health promotion on health care costs and utilization. *J.A.M.A.* 256:3235, 1986.
12. Control Data. *Health Risks and Behavior: The Impact on Medical Costs*. Minneapolis: Milliman and Robertson, 1987.
13. Sciacca, J., et al. The impact of participation in health promotion on medical costs: A reconsideration of the Blue Cross and Blue Shield of Indiana study. *Am. J. Health Promotion:* 7:374–383, 395, 1993.
14. Jones, R. C., Bly, J. S., and Richardson, J. E. A study of a worksite health promotion program and absenteeism. *J.O.M.* 32:95, 1990.
15. Bertera, R. L. The effects of workplace health promotion on absenteeism and employment costs in a large industrial population. *Am. J. Public Health* 80:1101, 1990.
16. Centers for Disease Control. Premature mortality in the United States: Public health issues in the use of the years of potential life lost. *M.M.W.R.* 35 (Suppl. 25):1S, 1986.
17. Harris, J. S., Collins, B., and Majure, I. L. The prevalence of health risks in an employed population. *J.O.M.* 28(3):217, 1986.
18. Spilman, M. A., et al. Effects of a corporate health promotion program. *J.O.M.* 28:285, 1986.
19. Bellingham, R., et al. Projected cost savings from AT&T Communications Total Life Concept (TLC) process. *Health Promotion Evaluation*. Stevens Point, WI: National Wellness Association, 1987. Chapter 3.
20. Holzbach, R. L., et al. Effect of a comprehensive health promotion program on employee attitude. *J.O.M.* 32:973, 1990.
21. Dickerson, O. B., and Mandelbilt, C. A new model for employer-provided health education programs. *J.O.M.* 25(6):471, 1983.
22. American Medical Association Council on Scientific Affairs. Medical evaluations of healthy persons. *J.A.M.A.* 249:1626, 1983.
23. Fitzgerald, S. T., Gibbons, S., and Agnew, J. Evaluation of referral completion after a workplace cholesterol screening. *Am. J. Prev. Med.* 7:335, 1991.
24. Maiman, L. A., et al. Improving referral compliance after public cholesterol screening. *Am. J. Public Health* 82:805, 1992.
25. Centers for Disease Control. Cigarette smoking attributable mortality and years of potential life lost—United States, 1990. *M.M.W.R.* 42:33, 1993.

26. Centers for Disease Control. Cigarette smoking attributable mortality and years of potential life lost—United States, 1988. *M.M.W.R.* 40:62, 1991.
27. Pierce, J. P., et al. Trends in cigarette smoking in the U.S.: Projection to the year 2000. *J.A.M.A.* 261:61, 1989.
28. Kristein, M. M. How much can business expect to profit from smoking cessation? *Prev. Med.* 12:358, 1983.
29. Weis, W. L. No ifs, ands or butts—why workplace smoking should be banned. *Management World.* 10/9:39, 1981.
30. US Department of Health and Human Services. *The Health Consequences of Involuntary Smoking: A Report of the Surgeon General.* Washington, DC: USGPO (87-8398), 1986.
31. McCunney, R. J. The role of fitness in preventing heart disease. *Cardiovasc. Rev. Rep.* 6:776, 1985.
32. Paffenberger, R. S., et al. Physical activity, all cause mortality and longevity of college alumni. *N. Engl. J. Med.* 314:605, 1989.
33. Blair, S. N., et al. Physical fitness and all cause mortality: A prospective study of healthy men and women. *J.A.M.A.* 262:2395, 1990.
34. Stamber, J., et al. for the MRFIT Research Group. Is the relationship between serum cholesterol and the risk of premature death from heart disease continuous and graded? *J.A.M.A.* 256:2823, 1986.
35. Gundy, S. M. Cholesterol and coronary heart disease. *J.A.M.A.* 256:2849, 1986.
36. Brownell, K. D. Obesity: Understanding and treating a serious, prevalent and refractory disorder. *J. Consult. Clin. Psychol.* 50:820, 1982.
37. Alderman, M. Hypertension at the workplace. *Corporate Commentary.* 2:1, 1986.
38. Grant, B., Noble, J., and Malin, H. The epidemiologic catchment area program. *Alcohol Health Research World* 10:68, 1985.
39. Spicer, J., and Owen, R. *Finding the Bottom Line: The Cost Impact of Employee Assistance and Chemical Dependency Programs.* Center City, MN: Hazeldon Foundation, 1985.
40. Green, L. W., et al. *Health Education Planning: A Diagnostic Approach.* Palo Alto, CA: Mayfield Publishing Co., 1980.
41. Green, L. W., and Lewis, F. M. *Measurement and Evaluation in Health Education and Health Promotion.* Palo Alto, CA: Mayfield Publishing Company, 1986.
42. National Heart, Lung and Blood Institute. New cholesterol guidelines released. *Heart Memo* Fall 1993. Pp. 1–2.

Further Information

American Journal of Health Promotion, 746 Purdy St, Birmingham, MI 48009.
A recent professional journal directed solely to health promotion research and practical alternatives.

Anderson, K. M., Castelli, W. P., and Levy, D. Cholesterol and mortality: 30 years of follow-up from the Framingham Study. *J.A.M.A.* 257:2176, 1987.
A review of the relationship of cholesterol to mortality in one of the most important perspective studies conducted on this issue.

Cataldo, M. F., and Coates, T. J. (eds.). *Health and Industry: A Behavioral Medicine Approach.* New York: Wiley, 1986.
A comprehensive text that looks at the relationship between workplace health issues, existing health promotion programs, and the application of behavioral principles in the occupational setting.

Fielding, J. E. *Corporate Health Management.* Menlo Park, CA: Addison-Wesley, 1984.
A comprehensive overview of medical issues that affect the workplace. An excellent quantification of the human and financial cost of ill health and a presentation of how to develop programs to deal with these costs.

Kizer, W. M. *The Health Workplace.* New York: Wiley, 1986.
A practical guide written for the business leader who understands the importance of health promotion but does not know where to begin.

O'Donnell, M. P., and Harris, J. S. (eds.). *Health Promotion in the Workplace* (2nd ed.). Albany, NY: Delmar, 1993.

Scofield, M. E. (ed.). Worksite Health Promotion. *Occup. Med. State of the Art Rev.* Philadelphia: Hanley & Belfus, Oct.–Dec. 1990.

Shumaker, S. A., Schrow, E. B., and Ockene, J. K. (eds.). *The Handbook of Health Behavior Change.* New York: Springer, 1990.

Sloan R., Gruman, J., and Allegrante, J. P. *Investing in Employee Health: A Guide to Effective Health Promotion in the Workplace.* San Francisco: Jossey-Bass, 1987.

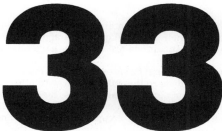

The Case Report: Discovery of Occupational Disease

William E. Wright

A patient relates that he thinks he has lung cancer, just like a number of other men with whom he works.

A doctor caring for a patient with cancer observes that the man was exposed to high levels of a chemical when a large volume of it spilled years ago. The patient's co-worker who helped clean up the spill is found to have an identical cancer.

A man has developed difficulty in urinating and asks his doctor whether he thinks that this condition is caused by his work.

Physicians are frequently faced with evaluating whether work has caused or aggravated illnesses [1]. The physician's inquiry, however, is usually hampered by insufficient information. The clinician may lack adequate information on exposure to industrial materials, may lack access to an entire working population for study, and usually lacks sufficient time for epidemiologic studies to test for suspected associations between work and illness. Yet, patients and society expect physicians to recognize occupational disease and, more recently, cumulative trauma, and be able to determine the cause. Unfortunately, few physicians are trained adequately to assess occupational components of disease. This challenge lies not only in assessing "traditional" or new occupational illnesses, but also in evaluating the occupational contribution, if any, to common musculoskeletal disorders and cumulative trauma, and stress-related symptoms. In either case, a firm understanding of the illness and job duties is essential. This chapter focuses on occupational illnesses, that is, medical disorders uniquely caused by a particular job environment or hazardous exposure. Readers interested in more detail on musculoskeletal disorders are referred to Chap. 7, The Disability/Impairment Evaluation. Stress is addressed in Chap. 18, Psychiatric Aspects of Occupational Medicine.

The small number of physicians trained in occupational medicine contrasts with the large potential for patients to develop occupational diseases. More than 5000 chemical substances are commonly used in the United States, and hundreds of new ones are introduced each year [1]. Our knowledge about the toxic properties of many of these substances is limited. Only a small proportion of the materials in use are covered by occupational health standards. The development of new commercial materials is proceeding at a pace beyond the capability to evaluate their toxicity adequately. The large number and wide variety of substances used and the continual changes in industrial technology create a situation in which new work-related illnesses will occur. The physician has both the challenge and responsibility of recognizing previously unrecognized health problems associated with exposure to workplace materials.

Identifying the cause of these illnesses is essential to their prevention through implementation of appropriate changes in the workplace. In addition to prevention, the benefits of recognizing the occupational components of illness include providing more effective treatment, assisting patients in obtaining appropriate workers' compensation benefits, and fulfilling the physician's legal obligation to report the occurrence of occupational disease. In the case of newly recognized or suspected associations of work and illness, publication of case reports can stimulate others to perform more formal evaluations to test and further define the association.

Physicians are often introduced to occupational medicine through questions from their patients. Sometimes the questions are directly related to work (e.g., "Doctor, do you think my hypertension is caused by my work?"). Sometimes clues related to work are provided by the patient's history (e.g., "I felt better when I was on vacation," or "My wheezing started after I took on the new job."). Sometimes a patient inadvertently suggests that work may be responsible (e.g., "Why me? Why should I have this cancer since I never smoked?"). Sometimes work as a cause of illness may be suggested by co-workers, employers, worker representatives, or legal counsel. Physicians should be prepared to answer their patients' questions and address their concerns by determining whether work conditions are likely to have affected the illness.

How can physicians identify new occupational diseases or unusual manifestations of traditional occupational afflictions and share this information with others? With a knowledge of epidemiology and common occupational diseases, the physician can employ a methodical approach to assessing possible interactions of work and illness. This chapter provides a framework for identifying occupational diseases and preparing case reports. The approach consists of a clinical diagnostic tool, the occupational history, and a series of questions, the answers to which will help organize data for decision-making. To attribute an illness accurately to a workplace substance or process, the questions should be answered thoroughly. Consultation may be needed with others who have specialty training in occupational medicine, clinical toxicology, or a related discipline. A review of pertinent medical literature is usually necessary and can help formulate an opinion that may serve as the basis of a case report.

Historically, for physicians to generate a case report of an occupational disease, the disease has been unusual, the number of cases has been large, or the association between the exposure and the disease has been strong. Identification of additional occupational ailments can be enhanced by routinely considering occupational exposures as possible causes in clinical evaluations, by considering the worker to be an important source of information, and by applying a logical and methodical approach to investigate work and health interactions. The occupational history is the cornerstone of the approach to recognition of occupational disease and generation of case reports.

The Occupational History

The *occupational history* is the clinical tool used to elicit and organize information about the workplace for any thorough diagnostic evaluation. Descriptions of the occupational history have been published in the medical literature and are highlighted in Chap. 21. A basic occupational history includes the following:

1. Description of *current and recent work,* including longest held job and years worked in each position.
2. Report of any *exposure* to chemicals, dusts, or fumes, including type, intensity, and duration; and information from manufacturers, employers, and Material Safety Data Sheets (MSDS). A request for exposure monitoring data, if available, is recommended.
3. *Relationship of symptoms to periods away from work* (e.g., weekends, holidays, vacations, or other absence) and to changes in work schedule.
4. Description of *any change in work activities,* production quotas, work processes, or other work routine preceding or coinciding with the development of symptoms.
5. Occurrence of *similar symptoms or illness in co-workers.*
6. *The patient's opinion* regarding the relationship of illness to work and reasons supporting the opinion.
7. History of *use of substances in avocational activities* and their relationship to symptoms or illness.
8. Contact with workplace or *worksite visit.*

The description of recent and longest held jobs, a screening question about exposures, and attention to the temporal relationship between the patient's chief complaint and work activities are suggested as part of a brief, routine survey provided to every patient [2, 3]. For illnesses likely to have a long latency between exposure to a hazardous substance and clinical presentation (e.g., cancer and chronic disorders), a complete chronologic occupational history is often needed to understand the relationships of work to illness. An example of a form that can be used to record an occupational history is shown in Fig. 33-1. After the occupational history is reviewed, *hypotheses* regarding the influence of work can be generated. The following steps can be used to assess more fully a possible association of work and illness and to prepare a *case report* for the medical literature.

1. Name _____   Date _____

2. Current position (job) _____
   Type of business _____
   Description of work activities _____
   _____

3. Are you exposed to or do you work with any chemicals, dusts, or
   fumes? Yes __ No __ Don't know __

4. Do any co-workers have medical complaints similar to yours?
   Yes __ No __ Don't know __

5. Do you think you have a medical problem related to or aggravated by
   your work? Yes __ No __ Don't know __

6. Have you ever worked with any of the following materials?

Asbestos	____	Plastics	____
Solvents	____	Radiation	____
Petroleum products	____	Lead	____
Vehicle or engine exhaust	____	Mercury	____
Degreasers	____	Other metals	____
Paints	____	Welding, brazing, soldering	____
Glues	____	Insulation	____
Grease and oil	____	Other dusts	____
Pesticides	____	Other gases	____
Silica	____	Noise	____

7. Have you ever done any of the following types of work?
   Plumbing or pipefitting   ____
   Shipyard work   ____
   Building construction   ____
   Mining   ____
   Forge or foundry work   ____
   Chemical plant work   ____

8. Have you worked in any other environments or with any other
   materials about which you are concerned? Yes ____ No ____
   If yes, describe: _____
   _____

9. Do you have any hobby activities that involve use of or exposure to
   dusts, chemicals, or fumes? Yes ____ No ____
   If yes, describe: _____
   _____

10. Starting with your first job, list your complete occupational history.
    Include summer jobs and part-time jobs.

   Dates (month/yr.)

From	To	Employer	Job	Exposures

Figure 33-1. Taking an occupational history requires using traditional techniques of
medical interviewing with prompts, follow-up questions, and interpretation by the physician. No form can provide a complete occupational history and yet be a convenient
length for use with all patients. The form shown here covers the essential elements of
the occupational history; questions numbered 1–6, 9, and 10 cover the outline of the
brief, routine survey that can easily be applied to all patients. The form can be shortened
or expanded to suit the user's needs.

Clinical Diagnostic Evaluation

The clinical diagnostic evaluation, which includes the occupational history, provides a starting point for decisions regarding the relation of work to illness. The following steps, expressed as questions to be addressed, can be used to evaluate a case or group of cases for which a diagnosis of occupational disease is entertained. An outline of this approach is shown in Table 33-1.

1. *What is the medical condition?* The *accuracy of the diagnosis* is essential. The physician must establish the presence of disease in accordance with standard diagnostic practices. If no actual disease is noted, a report of the presence of a constellation of symptoms or physiologic or laboratory abnormalities may be sufficient. When dealing with several cases, diagnostic criteria should be uniformly applied.

Where feasible, diagnoses should be reviewed and confirmed. Assuring the uniformity of diagnoses is important because criteria for diagnoses can change as understanding of the pathologic process evolves. For example, the association of asbestos exposure with malignant mesothelioma was first noted in a number of people, most of whom had been exposed to asbestos [4]. Malignant mesothelioma is now widely considered to be primarily of occupational origin, although as many as one third of patients lack specific exposure to asbestos. However, earlier in this century, pathologists debated whether primary tumors of the pleura occurred at all, and pathologists still differ on the criteria that should be used to diagnose the tumor with certainty [5].

Case reports of clusters of tumors of unusual type or at unusual anatomic sites have led to identification of occupational carcinogens. One example is the first report of an occupational cancer in 1775 by Pott [6], who noted that scrotal cancer occurred with an unusually high frequency among chimney sweeps. Contemporary examples include identification of the extremely rare tumor angiosarcoma of the liver in some workers at a plant where vinyl chloride was polymerized into polyvinyl chloride resins [7] and oat-cell carcinoma of the lung in a group of men who worked with bis-chloromethyl ether manufacturing ion exchange resins [8]. In addition to peculiar cancers, clusters of people with *unusual symptoms,* such as difficulty in urinating among foam workers exposed to a newly introduced catalyst, dimethylaminopropionitrile [9], and clusters of people with *unusual illness* (e.g., aspermia in workers exposed to the nematocide dibromochloropropane [10]) in groups sharing work experiences have led to case reports of new relationships between exposure and disease.

Some medical conditions may be more likely to be related to workplace factors than others. A way to increase the possibility of identifying occupational disease for case reports is to use the sentinel health event (SHE) approach described by Rutstein and associates [11, 12]. A SHE is a condition, already known to have occupational causes, that contributes to unnecessary disease, disability, or untimely death. Such conditions, when they occur in a practice setting, deserve special scrutiny of occupational factors. When used by practitioners, this approach has been shown to assist

Table 33-1. Summary of the evaluation of work-related disease

1. Determine the diagnosis accurately:
   a. Uniformity of diagnosis among cases.
   b. Standard diagnostic practices or clearly defined case definition.
2. Describe working conditions (occupational history).
3. Review toxicity of materials (literature review).
4. Evaluate information on dose and response:
   a. Consider dose-response relationships from epidemiologic studies.
   b. Consider factors that modify exposure.
   c. Consider exposure to analogous substances.
5. Consider plausible alternative explanations.
6. Review aggregate data related to the hypothesis that materials at work caused the illness:
   a. Features that substantiate the proposed relationship.
   b. Alternative explanations and their likelihood.
   c. Type of cause considered to be present (e.g., de novo, aggravation, predisposition).

with identification of occupational diseases. This area is covered in detail in another part of this book (see Chap. 21, Suspecting Occupational Disease).

2. *What are the working conditions, including level and degree of exposure to materials?* The occupational history should be taken in sufficient detail to identify the type, intensity, and duration of exposure to materials. If specific exposure information is not known, description of work activities and processes may be an adequate substitute. A good example of this is seen in a recent case report of pulmonary alveolar proteinosis in a cement truck operator [14]. The author lacked air monitoring to quantify exposure but used quantitative factors such as duration and frequency of exposure along with qualitative information such as verbal accounts of dust obscuring vision, the worker being covered with dust, and photographs of conditions to document significant exposure to dust.

Additional information obtained from an occupational health nurse, physician, industrial hygienist, plant engineer, or supervisor at the worksite can assist in characterizing the working conditions. Industrial hygiene monitoring data for similar jobs should be reviewed, if available. Manufacturers of substances may be able to provide information on chemical formulations and toxicity. A visit to the worksite and observation of work activities can be extremely valuable in determining the character and extent of exposure to certain materials.

A number of texts on industrial processes are useful for understanding work activities, potential for exposures, and chemical or physical agents that should be considered as potential causes of disease [15–19]. As a result of the Hazard Communication Standard, companies should have MSDS on file that describe materials used and their toxicity. Review of MSDS can yield clues for further investigation. One should recognize that a file of MSDS may not cover all substances that are used in industrial processes and that potential health effects of combined exposures, reactants, by-products, and contaminants may not be addressed. MSDS only cover known toxicity; additional effects not listed on the MSDS may occur, which may serve as the basis for a case report.

3. *Based on current knowledge, can the exposure, in any quantity, cause the disease?* Although obtaining the answer to this question may be time consuming, the process is straightforward and depends on a review of current information in the literature. In addition to the standard medical texts related to occupational medicine, the physician should become familiar with other available references that provide specific information regarding toxicity of materials [20–24].

A number of government agencies provide information on commercial substances and their effect on health. For example, the National Institute for Occupational Safety and Health (NIOSH) has regional offices that can provide current information. Criteria documents, medical advisories, and other bulletins are periodically published by NIOSH and are readily available to physicians upon request. The agency for Toxic Substances and Disease Registry (ATSDR) has developed a series entitled "Case Series in Environmental Medicine." This material, which describes an initial case, is followed by an overview of key considerations, such as toxicology and biologic monitoring. In addition, state governments and chemical manufacturers' associations can be sources of valuable information.

The *Index Medicus* and National Library of Medicine computerized literature searches (e.g., MEDLINE, TOXLINE) are becoming routine tools in this stage of the information-gathering process. A number of these databases are now available for access through personal computers at home, as well as at medical libraries and academic centers (see Chap. 27, Searching the Literature).

One should note that of many case reports related to occupational health issues that have attracted media attention recently [7–10], little or no relevant information was available on the toxicology of the suspected chemicals. In the case of dibromochloropropane [10], however, animal evidence of testicular toxicity could have been used as a basis for further evaluation or more cautious use. Some computerized literature services, such as TOXLINE, offer information on animal studies, significant results from which should not be ignored. On the other hand, in the case of dimethylaminopropionitrile [9], no industrial material was recognized to have the observed clinical effect in animals or humans (i.e., sacral autonomic neuropathy producing urinary bladder dysfunction).

4. *Based on current information, is the level of exposure sufficient to cause the disease?* When evaluating new substances or unrecognized effects of low exposure to familiar materials, this question usually cannot be answered with a desirable level of accuracy. In other situations, it is important to consider what is known about the

relationship between exposure and response. Characteristics of exposure, such as intensity, duration, and route, and personal characteristics, such as cigarette smoking, alcohol consumption, age, genetic susceptibility, intercurrent disease, and co-exposures, may interact to influence the ultimate effect on health.

Sometimes, simply relating timing of exposure and effects gives convincing evidence about sufficiency of exposure and work-relatedness. Several recent case reports lacking quantitative information on exposure emphasized that symptoms occurred at work or during work with a particular substance but did not occur on work-free days. This approach, which emphasizes a hallmark of occupational disease, was critical in linking epistaxis and dermatitis to use of glutaraldehyde for cold sterilization [25, 26], asthma to use of alkyl cyanoacrylate adhesives [27], allergic rhinitis to handling psyllium [28], and dermatitis to a non-bisphenol A epoxy used in preparation of tissue for electron microscopy [29].

The human body has the capacity to detoxify materials without recognizable ill effects. At some levels of exposure, homeostatic mechanisms allow transport, metabolism, and excretion of materials without discernible disruption of biochemical or physiologic function and without apparent clinical effects. For a clinical effect to become apparent due to exposure to a hazardous substance, the level of exposure must be sufficient to overwhelm homeostatic mechanisms and disrupt metabolic pathways so that damage occurs at the target tissue. In the case of alteration of genetic material as a target tissue for development of cancer, the damage must also be allowed sufficient time to be expressed. Unfortunately, adequate exposure information is not often available, and some plausible estimate is necessary. Toxicologic information related to the effect of dose on target organs is also usually unavailable. Results of animal studies may be available in some cases, but the validity of extrapolating results to humans is often subject to a variety of opinions.

Epidemiologic studies can be of considerable value in assessing the contribution of exposure to illness in individual patients if the studies demonstrate a dose-response relationship and if the working conditions of the patient under consideration resemble those described in the study. Investigations limited to only dichotomous exposure information (i.e., Exposed? Yes or No), job title, or employment in an industry without quantitation are more difficult to use. If the level of exposure under consideration seems insufficient to cause disease, it is also possible that the character of the exposure has not been accurately defined or personal characteristics of the patient have magnified the effect. In addition, some materials may affect the body through pathogenetic mechanisms, such as activation of the immune system, in which a graded response to increasing dose may not be apparent (e.g., as happens with industrial exposure to beryllium).

One should also be aware that simply because levels of exposure are *below* recommended standards, the exposure may *not* be safe. As new information becomes available, the American Conference of Governmental Industrial Hygienists (ACGIH) and regulatory bodies such as the Occupational Safety and Health Administration (OSHA) can be expected to revise the current recommendations and standards and historically usually has lowered Threshold Limit Values.

5. *Are there any factors that modify the exposures in some way?* Apparently harmless industrial processes can sometimes be modified by work practices or personal habits to lead to occupational disease. For example, the high temperature of burning cigarettes has been recognized to alter fluoropolymers into harmful fumes that produce flu-like polymer fume fever [30]. The occurrence of osteosarcoma of the jaw in painters of clock dials early in this century resulted in part from the work practice of using the tongue to point the tip of the paintbrushes laden with radium [31]. Personal techniques of job performance, hand washing, and preparation and consumption of food in a contaminated area should also be considered in assessing possible occupational exposures. One recent case report related an unusual exposure to carmustine from faulty equipment. The effects of the exposure may have been enhanced by prolonged contact with clothing that the drug had penetrated [32]. The pace of work and energy demands may also be important with some exposures, since mouth breathing, breath holding, and rapid, deep respirations may increase exposure to dusts and chemicals. Use of personal protective equipment may also modify exposure, but consultation with the worker and with an industrial hygienist may be necessary to assess whether the protective equipment being used is providing effective protection.

6. *Is the agent similar to any other recognized hazards?* A recent report of three cases of hematologic malignancy sharing exposure to 1,3-dichloropropene pointed out that

the chemical structure is similar to that of dibromochloropropane and vinyl chloride, two recognized carcinogens [33]. One clue to the presence of a potential toxic effect of a substance is whether its chemical structure is similar to that of other substances with recognized toxicity. An analysis of the Threshold Limit Values for chemical exposures set by the ACGIH emphasized that about one quarter of the chemicals for which exposure values were published were based on chemical analogy [1].

Although a review of the chemical structure is one way to assess a substance's potential for human toxicity, there are pitfalls in using this approach. The similarity of effects of organophosphate compounds on the nervous system, for example, appears to be due to the similarity in the *active site* of a number of otherwise dissimilar compounds. Another example is that among di-isocyanates that affect the respiratory system, the relevant similarity of structure also appears to be in the *active site* rather than in the entire molecule. Additional examples include toluene and xylene, which share the aromatic ring of benzene but apparently not its carcinogenicity. Undoubtedly, other chemical and physical features of chemicals, including polarity, molecular size, physical form, and metabolic pathways for activation or degradation, have important roles in determining potential for toxic effects. Metabolic conversion is recognized to be important in activating polycyclic aromatic hydrocarbons to carcinogenic epoxides that bind DNA and in degrading methylene chloride into carbon monoxide, which may be responsible for some of the acute toxic effects of this compound.

7. *Can other conditions or factors provide a plausible alternative explanation for the findings?* The history should be explored for the occurrence of other exposures during hobby or home activities that might be related to the condition under consideration [34]. A recent report relating a case of toxic epidermal necrolysis to work with plastic resins is a good example of an issue that is sometimes considered in attributing an illness to a workplace material [35]. The authors dealt with complexities of the workplace (mixed exposures, pyrolysis products) as well as the possibility that intercurrent infectious disease or medical treatment caused the observed illness. In assessing the relevance of work to the occurrence of similar conditions in a group of cases, the differential diagnosis should be explored sufficiently to assure that the conditions cannot be explained by coincident occurrence of different disease processes in each person (e.g., evaluating several people with neuropathy, alcohol consumption, diabetes mellitus, arteritis, trauma, or heavy metal poisoning, instead of a shared exposure, may account for the development of some of the cases). In addition, cigarette smoking, which is a common occupational and avocational exposure, can have an independent effect in causing disease that may be mixed with the effects of other substances (see Chap. 24, Epidemiology and Biostatistics).

8. *If current information does not support the hypothesis that the exposure caused the disease and no viable alternative exists, how should the data be interpreted?* Several features of a disease are often emphasized in case reports to substantiate a claim that the *exposure* of interest is related to the *disease* under consideration. Occasionally, available data can be used to estimate the likelihood of the number of observed cases in the exposed population. Presentation of figures of disease incidence was used in Figueroa and associates' report [8] of oat-cell carcinoma of the lung in chloromethyl methyl ether workers to emphasize the unusual nature of the case's occurrence. Other factors noted in case reports that are used to support claims of causality include (1) the exposure of interest precedes the occurrence of disease by a reasonable period of time; (2) the people proved or presumed to be the heaviest exposed are the ones to develop the disease, the first to develop the disease, or the ones to develop the most severe form of the disease; (3) signs and symptoms improve coincident with removal or reduction of exposure; (4) the exposure is relevant to the chronic disease under consideration because past high exposure was associated with severe acute illness; and (5) only chance provides a recognized viable alternative explanation. Most of these arguments are supported by information obtained from a thorough occupational history.

The diagnosis of an occupational illness is often one of exclusion; that is, the diagnosis is made after assuring that other well-known causes for the disorder are not present. However, the occurrence of disease in only one or several of a group of people who have shared exposure to a material should not detract from reporting a suspected association; not only are working conditions highly variable, but also people often react quite differently when exposed to the same material (see Chap. 24). As an analogy, even in infectious diseases, attack rates are usually far less than 100% [36].

Guidelines for Preparing the Case Report

Detailed descriptions of methods for preparation of medical research papers and reports have been published. If after a review of the case material using the steps suggested in this chapter, the physician believes that a new occupational illness or syndrome has been identified, the following guidelines, based on the format outlined by Huth [37], can be used to prepare the case report (Table 33-2).

Type of Case

First, decide on the type of case to be reported. Case reports in occupational medicine that contribute most to new and useful knowledge will usually be one of three types.

The Unique Case
Reporting of a unique illness resulting from an exposure may require extensive review of the literature to support the claim of uniqueness. In cases in which the pathophysiology of the condition is investigated using sophisticated medical technologies, the report may be best presented as a research paper rather than a case report [37].

New Association of an Illness with Exposure to a Material or Other Stressor (Mechanical or Psychological)
Many associations of illness with exposure to materials are likely to be coincidental. Support for the argument that a causal association exists may depend on either defining a plausible pathogenic mechanism or providing statistical evidence consistent with a low probability of a chance association (see Chap. 24). The coincidental occurrence of illness and exposure may still be an important factor in many cases. Symptoms that occur only with exposure or on workdays but not on work-free days, or allergic symptoms that occur after a period adequate for sensitization, lead to a strong presumption that some workplace factor is important in occurrence of illness.

Unexpected Course of an Illness
Unexpected improvement or deterioration of a patient's condition coincidental with exposure to a material may provide hints about the pathogenesis of the illness and about the metabolic fate and effects of the material. Support of the argument that a cause and effect relationship exists depends on excluding plausible alternative explanations, including chance, to the extent possible.

Unique or Unusual Circumstances of Exposure
Sometimes materials can produce occupational disease because of unusual circumstances of exposure. One of the case reports already cited focused on exposure to an antineoplastic drug that was probably enhanced by prolonged skin contact [32]. Pyrolysis of chemicals with cigarettes producing polymer fume fever represents

Table 33-2. Summary of case report preparation

I. Decide on *type of case* to be reported:
  A. Unique case.
  B. Previously unrecognized effect of a material.
  C. Unexpected course of an illness.
II. Decide on the *format* of the presentation:
  A. Use journal's guidelines to determine specific form.
  B. General outline for the single case:
    1. Introduction.
    2. Description of case.
    3. Discussion.
    4. Conclusion.
  C. Considerations for reports of multiple cases:
    1. More detailed section on methods.
    2. Tables or figures for presenting data.

another unusual circumstance [30]. A recent case report noted that when a material (phenoxyethanol), which could reasonably be expected to produce central nervous system depression, was used as an anesthetic for fish in a way that produced skin contact, serious chronic neurotoxicity ensued [38]. When unusual exposures occur they deserve consideration for case reports. These circumstances can provide opportunities for understanding mechanisms of injury and preventing occurrence of disease.

Clarification of Pathophysiology
Some case reports are produced because new or more sophisticated testing is available to define the disease or mechanisms of illness. Recent examples are found in two case reports of Schwartz and associates in which reactions to psyllium dust [28] and permanent wave solutions [39] were studied by using challenge tests and measuring nasal as well as lower-airway resistance.

Format of the Presentation

The journal to which the case report is submitted will determine the format to a large extent. The journal's guidelines will specify whether an abstract, summary, conclusion, or other special sections are required. In addition, the following format is usually sufficient and provides a concise framework for the case report.

Introduction
The introduction includes several paragraphs explaining how the case came to the author's attention, describing the illness and the material of interest or work setting in general terms to clarify the focus of the report, and stating why the case is of special interest.

Description of the Case
This section can be handled as a narrative account of the occurrence of illness, with flashbacks to prior events, illnesses, or work history that are relevant. The sequence of presentation of clinical and occupational information may vary depending on the author's preference for developing the narrative (e.g., chronologic versus presenting illness, course, and flashbacks) and on the nature of the case. The clinical evaluation and the details of the occupational history that provide a clear and coherent account of the workplace, job activities, and character and extent of exposure can be provided in this section. Any factors that may have modified the exposure to the material should be covered as well.

Other Considerations
Reports of multiple cases may require attention to additional detail or special sections. Case definition, uniformity of the cases, and methods used for case finding and for confirmation of the diagnoses and work histories may be addressed in the section describing the cases or in a separate section describing methods. Tables and figures may be used to illustrate the associations. For example, a case series of three workers exposed to trichloroethylene included a figure demonstrating symptoms corresponding to levels of urinary trichloroacetic acid [40]. The discussion section should address similarities among the cases and exclude, to the extent possible, plausible alternative diagnoses or explanations for the occurrence of the cases.

Discussion
This section provides the argument regarding the uniqueness of the case and the logical explanation of why the case is worth reporting. The literature reviewed and its support or conflict with the proposed association should be presented here. Information about the toxicology of the material of interest or about analogous materials should be presented. Critical analysis of the likelihood of associations being causal should be developed. An account of attempts to identify similar cases in the population at risk could also be included here. A conclusion can be placed at the end of this section or can be presented separately according to the journal format. The conclusion should cover the possibilities for further studies, the implications of the discovery for clinical medicine and public health, the opportunities for prevention, and the anticipated effects of preventive intervention for the population at risk.

Notes on Causation

A cause can be defined as an exposure to a substance that, if the exposure is modified, alters the rate of disease occurrence in populations. In occupational medicine, a case report may suggest either that a material presumed to be safe has adversely affected health or that an acknowledged hazard has resulted in a previously unrecognized effect. The reports are not definitive statements of cause. The case report, by the nature of the data on which it is based, involves a degree of uncertainty that can only be resolved by more extensive analytic studies.

Opinions among physicians vary regarding criteria considered valid to establish a *causal relationship.* For some, the term *cause* indicates a clear and generally accepted relationship between exposure and illness, for which no alternative explanation exists. This approach to formulating opinions regarding causes, however, may be considered restrictive and may lead to overlooking possible new associations. Even in medicolegal settings, cause is implied if exposure to an agent is considered to be more likely than not (i.e., 51% likely or more) to have caused the disease, based on available medical and epidemiologic data. Case reports, which are suggestions of causal relationships, are expected to have a lower level of certainty than might be required in other settings. This latitude in thinking is necessary to allow hypotheses to be tested so that new associations can be recognized. Clearly each situation should be evaluated based on careful consideration of the aggregate information, including all supportive and nonsupportive elements.

Hazardous substances can alter the rate of occurrence of disease in several ways. For example, a hazardous agent may be the *sole* cause of a *unique* disease. More commonly, an occupational illness does not have a unique clinical presentation or course that distinguishes it from a nonoccupational disease. What distinguishes an occupational disease is neither its histopathology nor its clinical, radiographic, or laboratory features, but its *etiology,* an occupational agent. Hazardous materials may cause disease de novo, alter a biologic function without apparent clinical effect, bring to light an existing subclinical condition, predispose individuals to develop a disease, or aggravate a preexisting disease. One should consider this range of adverse health effects that can result from exposure to materials. After presentation of the case report, universal acceptance of the proposed relationship between the illness and the agent will depend on confirmation by more refined epidemiologic studies.

One characteristic of case reports is that the number of cases reported may not include all cases that may have occurred. Furthermore, since the number of people at risk of developing the illness from the exposure may be unknown or poorly defined, the actual incidence rates or prevalence may not be obtainable. The case report, however, can provide useful information that can serve as the basis to investigate and prevent illness in other people exposed to the same agent.

References

1. Peters, J. M. Occupational Health: Working Yourself Sick. In R. L. Kane (ed.), *The Challenges of Community Medicine.* New York: Springer, 1974.
2. Guidotti, T. L. Taking the occupational history. *Ann. Intern. Med.* 99:641, 1983.
3. Goldman, R. H., and Peters, J. M. The occupational and environmental health history. *J.A.M.A.* 246:2831, 1981.
4. Wagner, J. C., Slegg, C. A., and Marchand, P. Diffuse pleural mesothelioma and asbestos exposure in the North Western Cape Province. *Br. J. Ind. Med.* 17:260, 1960.
5. Wright, W. E., et al. Malignant mesothelioma: Incidence, asbestos exposure, and reclassification of histopathology. *Br. J. Ind. Med.* 41:39, 1984.
6. Pott, P. Cancer Scroti. In *The Chirurgical Works of Percivall Pott.* London: Hawkes, Clark and Collins, 1775. Pp. 734–736.
7. Creech, J. L., Jr., and Johnson, M. N. Angiosarcoma of liver in the manufacture of polyvinyl chloride. *J.O.M.* 16:150, 1974.
8. Figueroa, W. G., Raszkowski, R., and Weiss, W. Lung cancer in chloromethyl methyl ether workers. *N. Engl. J. Med.* 288:1096, 1973.
9. Kreiss, K., et al. Neurological dysfunction of the bladder in workers exposed to dimethylaminopropionitrile. *J.A.M.A.* 243:741, 1980.

10. Whorton, M. D., et al. Infertility in male pesticide workers. *Lancet* 2:1259, 1977.
11. Rutstein, D. D., et al. Sentinel health events (occupational): A basis for physician recognition and public health surveillance. *Am. J. Public Health* 73:1054, 1983.
12. Mullen, R. J., and Murthy, L. I. Occupational sentinel health events: An up-dated list for physician recognition and public health surveillance. *Am. J. Ind. Med.* 19:775, 1991.
13. Fontus, H. M., Levy, B. S., and Davis, L. K. Physician-based surveillance of occupational disease. Part II: Experience with a broader range of diagnoses and physicians. *J.O.M.* 31:929, 1989.
14. McCunney, R. J., and Godefroi, R. Pulmonary alveolar proteinosis and cement dust: A case report. *J.O.M.* 31:233, 1989.
15. Burgess, W. A. *Recognition of Health Hazards in Industry—A Review of Materials and Processes.* New York: Wiley, 1981.
16. Considine, D. M. (ed.). *Chemical and Process Technology Encyclopedia.* New York: McGraw-Hill, 1974.
17. Cralley, L. V., and Cralley, L. J. (eds.). *Industrial Hygiene Aspects of Plant Operations.* Vol. 1, *Process Flows.* New York: Macmillan, 1982.
18. Cralley, L. J., and Cralley, L. V. (eds.). *Industrial Hygiene Aspects of Plant Operations.* Vol. 2, *Unit Operations and Product Fabrication.* New York: Macmillan, 1984.
19. *Encyclopedia of Occupational Health and Safety* (3rd ed.). Geneva: International Labour Organization, 1983. Vol. 1–2.
20. Key, M. M., et al. (eds.). *Occupational Diseases—A Guide to Their Recognition.* Public Health Service, NIOSH Publication no. 77-181. Washington, DC: US Department of Health, Education and Welfare, 1977.
21. Finkel, A. J. *Hamilton and Hardy's Industrial Toxicology* (4th ed.). Boston: Wright, PSG, 1983.
22. Mackison, F. W., et al. (eds.). *Occupational Health Guidelines for Chemical Hazards. NIOSH/OSHA,* Vol. 1–3. Department of Health and Human Services, NIOSH Publication no. 81-123, 1978.
23. Clayton, G. D., and Clayton, F. E. (eds.). *Patty's Industrial Hygiene and Toxicology* (3rd ed.). Vol. 2A-B-C, *Toxicology.* New York: Wiley, 1981.
24. Sax, N. I. *Dangerous Properties of Industrial Materials* (6th ed.). New York: Van Nostrand Reinhold, 1984.
25. Wiggins, P., McCurdy, S. A., and Zeidenberg, W. Epistaxis due to glutaraldehyde exposure. *J.O.M.* 31:854, 1989.
26. Fowler, J. F. Allergic contact dermatitis from glutaraldehyde exposure. *J.O.M.* 31:852, 1989.
27. Nakazawa, T. Occupational asthma due to alkyl cyanoacrylate. *J.O.M.* 32:709, 1990.
28. Schwartz, H. J., Arnold, J. L., and Strohl, K. P. Occupational allergic rhinitis reaction to psyllium. *J.O.M.* 31:624, 1989.
29. Dannaker, C. J. Allergic sensitization to a non-bisphenol A epoxy of the cycloaliphatic class. *J.O.M.* 30:641, 1988.
30. Wegman, D. H., and Peters, J. M. Polymer fume fever and cigarette smoking. *Ann. Intern. Med.* 81:55, 1974.
31. Rowland, R. E., Stehney, A. F., and Lucas, H. F., Jr. Dose-response relationships for female radium dial workers. *Radiat. Res.* 76:368, 1978.
32. McDiarmid, M., and Egan, T. Acute occupational exposure to antineoplastic agents. *J.O.M.* 30:984, 1988.
33. Markovitz, A., and Crosby, W. H. Chemical carcinogenesis: A solid fumigant, 1,3-dichloropropene, as possible cause of hematologic malignancies. *Arch. Intern. Med.* 144:1409, 1984.
34. McCunney, R. J., Russo, P. K., and Doyle, J. D. Occupational illness in the arts. *Am. Fam. Physician* 36:145, 1987.
35. House, R. A., et al. Work-related toxic epidermal necrolysis? *J.O.M.* 34:135, 1992.
36. Monson, R. R. *Occupational Epidemiology* (2nd ed.). Boca Raton, FL: CRC, 1990.
37. Huth, E. J. *How to Write and Publish Papers in the Medical Sciences.* Philadelphia: ISI, 1982.
38. Morton, W. E. Occupational phenoxyethanol neurotoxicity: A report of three cases. *J.O.M.* 32:42, 1990.
39. Schwartz, H. J., Arnold, J. L., and Strohl, K. P. Occupational allergic rhinitis in the hair care industry: Reactions to permanent wave solutions. *J.O.M.* 32:473, 1990.
40. McCunney, R. J. Diverse manifestations of trichloroethylene. *Br. J. Ind. Med.* 45:122, 1988.

Further Information

Huth, E. J. *How to Write and Publish Papers in the Medical Sciences.* Philadelphia: ISI, 1982.
Written by the editor of the Annals of Internal Medicine, *this book covers many of the dimensions of medical writing. This excellent reference includes guidance on many fundamentals, such as preparation of tables, figures, and references and conducting a search of the literature.*

Rutstein, D. D, et al. Sentinel health events (occupational): A basis for physician recognition and public health surveillance. *Am. J. Public Health* 73:1054, 1983.
This article introduces a list of diagnoses that can be used by practicing physicians for occupational health surveillance. Diseases on the list serve as warning signals that an occupational relationship may be likely and should be considered. Some details of the sentinel health events approach are also covered in Chap. 21, Suspecting Occupational Disease.

Specific Case Reports

The case reports referenced in this chapter can be used as models. Some of the more instructive reports are listed below by type of illness and exposure to help the reader identify reports of interest:

1. *Unusual illnesses attributed to specific chemicals*
   A. Oat-cell carcinoma—bis-chloromethyl ether [8]
   B. Angiocarcinoma—vinyl chloride [7]
   C. Difficult urination—dimethylaminopropionitrile [9]
   D. Aspermia—dibromochloropropane [10]
2. *Unusual illness attributed to mixed exposures*
   A. Pulmonary alveolar proteinosis—cement dust [14]
   B. Toxic epidermal necrolysis—plastic resins [35]
3. *Common illnesses attributed to specific chemicals*
   A. Asthma—alkyl cyanoacrylate [27]
   B. Dermatitis—glutaraldehyde, non-bisphenol A epoxy [29]
   C. Epistaxis—glutaraldehyde [25]
   D. Neuropathy, cognitive impairment—2-phenoxyethanol [38]
   E. Rhinitis—psyllium [28]
4. *Common illnesses attributed to mixed exposures*
   A. Rhinitis—permanent wave solutions [39]
5. *Unusual circumstances of exposure*
   A. Spill, prolonged skin contact of an antineoplastic drug [25]
   B. Exposure modified by pyrolysis in cigarettes [30]
   C. Unusual ingestion of materials [31]
   D. Prior chemical spill [33]

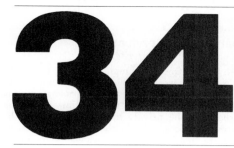

Economics of Occupational Medicine

Jeffrey S. Harris

Businesses and government organizations exist to produce specific goods and services. Typically, they have enunciated a mission and the way in which they want to produce those goods and services to satisfy their customers. The organizations' managers have goals framed in terms of output, market share, profit margin, customer service, and human resource management, among others. In well-run organizations, measurable objectives are set to meet these goals. The point of this chapter is to demonstrate how occupational health services can support the organizations they serve using business analysis and management.

The mission, goals, and objectives of the occupational health program (OHP) should be congruent with and support the mission, goals, and objectives of the organization. This consistency engenders organizational support for the programs, and clarifies why resources should be provided for different levels of occupational health. It is important to quantify the benefits provided to the organization, its employees, and their dependents to match resource needs with benefits provided, and to focus the operations of the OHP. In this context, the OHP can include medical liaison as well as treatment, consultation, and health management leadership. (See Chap. 40 for the definition of these levels.)

In the face of increasing medical care costs and significant questions about the value received for these massive outlays, occupational physicians are becoming more involved in benefits redesign and medical management (see Chap. 40). Occupational health professionals can act as liaisons with the private medical community to refer employees and dependents to high-quality, lower-cost providers (the two are inseparable) [1]. They may also act as internal consultants in evaluating medical care provided to employees and dependents, including operational management of vendors who provide services ranging from employee assistance, health promotion, and primary care to utilization management and managed care. Occupational health professionals, who have knowledge of epidemiology, practice parameters, technology assessment, and the research related to the effectiveness and appropriateness of various diagnostic and therapeutic modalities, are in a unique position to understand the organization's culture and the decision-making process, and to effectively provide an informed point of view, to the benefit of both management and employees [2].

Adverse health effects from the workplace should be prevented by medical surveillance and control of hazardous exposures (see Chap. 25). Strategic health management activities can also reduce morbidity, mortality, and disability caused by a number of diseases through informed co-management by the patient and health professionals (see Chap. 32, Health Promotion).

The economic benefits of any of these activities can be evaluated along a number of dimensions, including direct, indirect, and intangible costs. The information presented in this chapter should help occupational health professionals plan, manage, and monitor their programs of service. A number of the variables can be used to support continuous quality improvement efforts, which should increase the value of both the consultative and direct-service components of occupational health programs over a period of time.

Employers are often initially most interested in activities with an immediate economic benefit. Such activities include occupationally related medical treatment services, some aspects of health promotion, and the primary care of nonoccupational illnesses and injuries, which employers would otherwise pay for through their benefits plan. Management of the care purchased with medical benefits for optimal efficiency and effectiveness of care can also have a relatively quick payback, depending on the willingness of the provider organizations to work with health management specialists in company employ.

"Traditional" Occupational Medical Services

Employers are most familiar with the treatment and management of occupationally related illness and injury. In this section, we will review the economic benefits of those activities. We will also briefly discuss the other traditional role of occupational physicians and other health professionals—that of the "medical liaison." In this role, the occupational physician works with the private medical community through referral of employees to "preferred providers," ideally those who are high quality and cost effective. There is an interaction between the worksite professionals and community providers about issues such as limited duty, return to work policies, assistance that might be provided with rehabilitation after injury or illness, and perhaps reinforcement of instructions from a private treating physician. The key to these activities has been negotiating and assisting with job accommodation for those who have some degree of medical impairment, and assurance of quality care for those who have a variety of illnesses, injuries, and medically related impairments.

Preplacement, Disability, and Return to Work Examinations

The traditional cornerstone of clinical occupational health programs is the determination of the ability of an applicant or employee to perform the essential functions of a job as related to his or her health. This role has become more sharply focused with the passage of the Americans with Disabilities Act (ADA). Traditionally, preemployment examinations were an attempt to screen employees to prevent placing someone in a job that they were physically incapable of performing or in which they would become a threat to the health and safety of other employees. The ADA has changed the approach to these examinations to some extent, since they now must be performed *preplacement,* that is, after a conditional offer of employment, rather than preemployment. Employers are prohibited from asking a variety of medical questions which are not directly related to the functional requirements of the job. Complete medical histories, however, may be obtained by the examining physician on a voluntary basis.

In the past, a person might not have been considered fit for work if he or she

1. Was unable to perform the work for medical reasons, such as an impairment (for example, an inability to perform a specific required motion), or because of a history or potential for development of an adverse reaction to substances in the workplace
2. Posed a danger to the health or safety of the worker or co-workers
3. Had a reasonable and high probability of aggravation or recurrence of a preexisting condition
4. Was unable to attend work on a reasonable basis

The issue of regular attendance at work is in the purview of Human Resources, although serious illnesses that require frequent absence from work may constitute a significant problem for the employer, who, in some cases, can justify not placing such a person in the position sought. Nonplacement may also be justified when there is a question that the medical condition is correctly stated, or that the severity of the condition requires absence because of complete inability to perform essential or modified job functions.

The major change that occurred under the ADA is that a thorough attempt must be made to *reasonably accommodate* the applicant or employee if the person can perform the essential job functions with accommodation. For example, a careful analysis of the functions of the job must be performed before a statement can be made that a documented, measurable impairment prevents the applicant from performing the job without undue hazard to his or her health or safety or that of others. Further, economically viable attempts at reasonable accommodation, which might include splitting of job duties between this employee and others, reasonable assistance with minor aspects of the job, or the use of assistive devices or redesign of the job, must be made before disqualification. A number of the actions taken under the impetus of reasonable accommodation actually have made jobs safer for all employees. For example, changing the way in which weight is transferred or chemicals are handled should benefit anyone in that position by preventing cumulative trauma disorders (CTD) or reducing chemical exposures. In evaluating the economic effects of medical screening and placement programs, therefore, one would balance the cost of the program against decreases in real or projected cost of work-related illness or injuries. All direct and indirect costs, including the medical treatment, time lost from work, supervisory time, and so on, should be considered to obtain a proper analysis.

Failure to place employees after the above considerations have been taken into account may result in preventable costs for replacement and retraining, inefficiency, medical treatment, workers' compensation payments, fines under the ADA, actions under the Vocational Rehabilitation Act of 1974 or various state laws, as well as lost wages. In addition, grievance procedures may be filed and employers may be liable under tort law for pain and suffering as well as damages if willful negligence or recklessness can be demonstrated, thus invalidating the protection provided by workers' compensation statutes.

An example illustrating a number of such issues follows:

Joe Jones, a 46-year-old white man, has marginally compensated congestive heart failure. He applies for and obtains a higher-paying job forming packing molds using isocyanate resins. No preplacement examination is performed. Joe's congestive heart failure decompensates when he wears the respirator required for protection from isocyanate fumes. At first, he seems merely to be shirking work, but in fact he is severely hypoxic. He is disciplined for failing to do his job up to standards.

After his condition is detected by his private physician, Joe files a grievance for harassment. He applies for and receives workers' compensation and, on the advice of his union, sues the company for gross negligence as well as pain and suffering. His medical expenses are paid in part by the company's benefits plan. His replacement must be trained and brought up to speed. This situation (which has cost upward of $50,000 in similar real cases) would have been avoided had a preplacement examination, including certification for respirator use, been performed. Cases like this exist in many companies. These costs can be derived from company data or similar cases to calculate the total benefit of a medical placement program.

Although this example is anecdotal, it is cases such as this that provide the economic justification for preplacement evaluation programs. In the context of the ADA, consideration should also be given to savings from agency fines and litigation if accommodations were not provided for impairments.

Another example follows:

Suppose that an applicant with a previous history of back pain is denied employment for a position that involves lifting a 30- to 40-lb box, or "kit" to a table, after which the components in the box are assembled. There are a number of fairly obvious challenges to this assessment. First, if this task was relatively infrequent, other employees could be asked to help. A somewhat more expensive but probably more beneficial solution would be to install a device to raise the weight to the work surface, which can be done relatively inexpensively and therefore constitutes "reasonable accommodation." Another solution might be to break the components into smaller lots. In either of the latter situations, the frequency and severity of back strain in the entire population of employees performing this task would likely drop. Back strains are difficult to document and account for a large proportion of expensive and extended workers' compensation claims (see Chaps. 2 and 39).

The best demonstration of the effectiveness of a medical screening program would be to show decreases in illness and injury rates and their associated costs following the point at which the program was either installed or ungraded. The value of this type of program will depend on levels of hiring, placement needs, economic conditions (which can influence workers' compensation claims), and simple chance in smaller populations. The ultimate value of preplacement evaluations should be considered in light of a comprehensive program.

One example of clinical surveillance is early detection of CTDs, also known as repetitive strain injuries, which are typically preceded by symptoms of muscle or tendon overuse that may progress to permanent injury. The majority of cases filed under workers' compensation as carpal tunnel and other CTDs are precursor inflammation and pain syndromes, rather than disorders that meet the diagnostic criteria for carpal tunnel or other such disorders. Alert practitioners in regular contact with workers in repetitive motion jobs can screen for the discomfort that precedes disabling tendonitis, rotator cuff syndrome, and other CTDs, and recommend job redesign or other preventive interventions. Consistent monitoring, changes in job structure, and even on-site physical therapy are important modes to prevent progression of the disorders and to establish clear documentation of baseline physical condition. Surgical treatment of upper-extremity CTDs can cost upward of $12,000. One estimate showed direct costs for surgery and rehabilitation as $15,000 to $25,000 per case, and another estimated costs up to $100,000, including wage replacement, rehabilitation, retraining costs, and so on [3].

Many employees with these ailments find it difficult to return to the same job because of associated emotional trauma. Workers with intermittent back discomfort, for example, may fear a return to the position associated with the cause of their discomfort, even in the absence of serious illness. Stress claims for this type of problem, and more commonly for some mental trauma that occurred at the worksite, including violence and dysfunctional management practices, have become the most rapidly increasing cause of occupational *illness* claims, which are difficult to validate and are often filed late. In California, stress claims have increased rapidly and may occur in association with other employment-related activities.

A comprehensive or specific examination may need to be repeated periodically, especially in hazardous occupations and when an employee is considered for transfer to another job. The information then forms the database for a medical surveillance program (see Chap. 25, Medical Surveillance).

Medical Surveillance

A key duty of the occupational health professional is to monitor health-related data on members of the workforce exposed to chemical, radiation, and other physical hazards and to compare the values for exposed and unexposed groups periodically. If an increased prevalence of abnormal laboratory values or symptoms is detected in an exposed group, the exposure should be quantified and controlled through engineering measures, administrative efforts (i.e., rotating employees), or personal protective equipment, in that order. The economic value of this type of service depends on the cost of the disease avoided, which can be computed for a population of workers if the probability of illness is known for various levels of exposure. The probability at a given exposure is similar conceptually to the attack rate of an infectious disease (probability × number of exposed individuals = expected number of cases). The expected number is then multiplied by the average cost of treating such a case over the worker's lifetime to arrive at a total cost. Subtracting the cost of the surveillance program yields the net cost. (Although these measures may be beyond the capabilities of the average practitioner, such an economic analysis can be conducted by consulting firms or universities.)

For example, if 70% of a group of 4000 workers exposed to 50 fibers/cc asbestos for 10 years developed asbestosis, and 10% developed mesothelioma, the logic above could be followed to determine cost-effectiveness of the control program. There may be several levels of exposure that could be computed separately. The National Institute for Occupational Safety and Health (NIOSH) criteria documents that recommend Threshold Limit Values or Nuclear Regulatory Commission (NRC) exposure studies contain extrapolated or actual dose-response curves. Mortality costs may have been avoided also.

There are many examples of preventable occupationally related diseases that ultimately have caused great expense. Some authorities now believe that material-handling injuries without a specific inciting incident may be due to cumulative trauma as well. Alert practitioners can intervene in cases of back and other large-muscle pain with education, job change, conditioning exercises, and physical therapy before such cases become disabling or chronic.

Specific total costs avoided from this type of early detection and medical management programs can be determined from workers' compensation records. Direct costs include medical treatment and compensation payments to the employee. Indirect costs include reduced productivity of the impaired employee before definitive treatment, and replacement and retraining costs as well as probable retraining of the affected worker, since such injuries and illnesses may recur if the worker is placed back in the same job.

In many occupations, such as *health care* and *food service, transmission of infections* is a hazard to the business as well as to the individuals involved. Detection and control of infections is a vital service, especially at medical centers. The benefits include reduced medical costs and lost time; business interruption is also avoided.

Immunization

Immunization is an example of primary prevention resulting from a surveillance program. Workers in health care facilities, prisons, and waste disposal and sanitation are at high risk of hepatitis, influenza, and other blood-, body fluid-, or aerosol-borne diseases. The economic benefit of immunization of workers in these critical community services against influenza [4] and hepatitis B [5] has been demonstrated. Health care workers should also be primarily immunized against hepatitis B. Health care workers are at risk of acquiring and transmitting rubella. On-site or community occupational health services are more aware of the specific biologic hazards and able to ensure coverage and monitoring of the employed population [6].

Immunization of workers against tetanus will prevent many visits to medical facilities for prophylaxis of minor wounds. Diphtheria, influenza, and other routine immunizations will prevent considerable lost work time. Guidelines for adult immunizations are shown in Appendix 1.

Immunization and malaria prophylaxis for overseas travel is often more accurately and comprehensively done at the workplace because of the volume of cases and the need to avoid business interruption. Recommendations for immunization and prophylaxis for overseas travelers change frequently because disease distribution patterns often shift. The occupational physician should consult the Centers for Disease Control (CDC) or International Agency for Medical Assistance to Travelers for the latest recommendation by country. The CDC's *Health Information for International Travelers* [7] is a valuable guide, as is *Control of Communicable Diseases in Man* [8]. In general, travelers should have their primary immunizations for childhood diseases completed and updated. These illnesses are still quite common in developing countries. Generally, the manifestation of these illnesses is more severe in adults. In addition, travelers should be actively immunized against typhoid, cholera, yellow fever, influenza, hepatitis B, plague, and rabies, depending on their destination, occupation, and potential for contact with the respective pathogens. Prophylaxis against malaria and passive immunization against hepatitis A are also important to avoid unnecessary illness, business interruption, and emergency repatriation. Recommendations are listed in Appendix 2. (See Chap. 38, International Occupational Health, for a detailed discussion.)

Many employees can be reached at the worksite who would not otherwise have their immunizations up-to-date [9]. Cost savings per case of infectious disease prevented include avoidance of the cost of business interruption, repatriation expenses, and treatment, as well as replacement and retraining costs that would have resulted had workers not been immunized [10].

Treatment of Job-Related Injuries and Illnesses

Treatment of injuries and illnesses *on site* can be cost effective (see Chap. 39). Time lost to travel to a health facility and wait for treatment is avoided. The actual cost of treatment is usually less because the plant health center is not a for-profit operation. Finally, physicians and nurses who are familiar with the work environment usually have a better understanding of the toxicity of substances used, individual workers' backgrounds, attitudes and risks, and factors involved in injuries that may complicate the recovery process. The costs saved include differential prices between facilities, avoided time lost for workers and supervisors, reduced length of absence postincident, and the differential costs of more accurate treatment compared to cases managed elsewhere. In particular, it has been demonstrated that the quality and appropriateness of care delivered to many patients receiving workers' compensation is of significantly lower quality than that for general medical care [11]. On-site care may be of much greater quality.

Workers' compensation case rates may also be reduced because the employee is absent less than a half day (i.e., not a lost workday by Occupational Safety and Health Administration [OSHA] criteria), which can affect workers' compensation insurance premium rates, depending on the carrier's definitions and state workers' compensation regulations. Where on-site treatment is not feasible, community-based occupational health services can also save time by prompt treatment and effective management of work-related injuries.

There are a number of examples of very cost-effective on-site care, both for general medical care and for comprehensive care. These include the Gillette Company, which calculated a large savings based solely on decreases in absenteeism [12]. A comprehensive health management program at Northern Telecom, Inc., demonstrated significant decreases in cost for both work-related injuries and non–work-related illnesses [13].

Rehabilitation and Return to Work

Knowledge of the job is critical for appropriate placement of workers returning to work following an illness or injury. The occupational physician can prescribe modified duties in light of availability of proper assignment and medical limitations.

There are several advantages to early return to work. First, many employees, after a certain period of time, receive only partial wage replacement when absent for illness or injury of any sort. Second, with modified work of value, an employee who can work at 70% capacity costs only 30% in replacement, as opposed to 100% if absent. A return to work before full recovery can benefit the injured worker, who becomes a part of the work milieu again. Improvements in self-worth that result can aid in the recovery process. Unfortunately, the rate of return to work declines substantially after several months' absence and is very low after 6 months to a year. Many of these employees could work in some capacity if graduated accommodation were made (see Chap. 39) [14]. Savings in these cases derive from disability costs avoided (by comparison to similar unmanaged cases) and other intangible benefits. Successfully rehabilitated workers and their friends often have increased loyalty to the organization.

An example of the benefit of a "traditional" occupational health program should illustrate the cumulative effect of these measures. The key criterion used is the *absence rate,* or proportion of total available work hours lost to absence.

A major Canadian firm with three plants in Ontario and one in Quebec retained the services of an occupational health physician. The rate of absence for all illness and injury had been 9.5%, not uncommon for heavy industry. After 1 year of occupational medicine service in one plant, the absence rate was 8%, while it remained at 9.5% in the others. By year four, the rate had fallen to 6.5%. The health service was then extended to a second plant; its absence rate fell to 7.0% by year two. This meant that 1000 workers were required where 1025 were needed before. The health program cost $50,000 per 1000 employees; the savings were $650,000 for a net of $600,000, plus uncalculated savings for retraining, inefficient function of replacement workers, and business interruption.

Consulting Activities

Beyond the clinically based activities of placement, treatment, medical management, and rehabilitation, occupational medicine professionals often serve as internal consultants to an organization in areas of industrial hygiene, job modification, employee assistance, and other special problems. These activities can prevent health problems, both primarily and secondarily. The cost-effectiveness of consulting activities can be measured by savings resulting from the program recommendations. For example, if consultation results in prevention of exposure to a toxic substance, savings are the net of disease costs minus the cost of engineering controls. Or, if cases of alcoholism are treated early through an effective employee assistance program (EAP) that the physician recommended, part of the savings are due to the consultation activities.

Industrial Hygiene Consultation

Occupational health practitioners have the opportunity to prevent illnesses and injuries caused by chemical and physical hazards at the worksite in several ways. They can advise managers about the presence, nature, and magnitude of hazards. They can also evaluate the adequacy of barriers and procedures intended to protect employees from exposure, both by inspection and by epidemiologic surveillance of the workforce. The occupational physician should work closely with the industrial hygienist if one is available. The hygienist will usually measure air levels of toxins and evaluate barriers, while the physician can predict and monitor health effects based on analogous structures of chemicals, the literature, and surveillance examinations. The physician must be aware of industrial hygiene measures in his or her areas of responsibility and correlate them with observed health effects, if any. The object is to ensure that the workplace is safe (see Chap. 22, Industrial Hygiene).

Reductions in injury and disease rates attributable to improvements in industrial hygiene and safety can be calculated by measuring reductions in workers' compensation insurance costs and the value of enhanced productivity resulting from reduction of restricted and lost workdays. This latter figure can be derived by comparing restricted and lost workdays before and after the intervention on OSHA 200 Log or Workers' Compensation Board reports. The value of lost time should be multiplied by a factor of 3 to 10 to reflect the cost of business interruption, retraining, and associated costs. These savings should be offset against the cost of industrial hygiene controls (amortized over their expected useful life) and placement and biologic monitoring programs.

Workers' compensation insurance costs for fully insured companies will decrease only slowly because of a 10-year "tail" retained because the payouts in these cases often take that long to stop. Results can be seen much more rapidly in self-insured programs. In addition, if time-based management is used in these cases, and employees can be returned to work much more quickly, savings can be realized that much faster [15].

Intangible effects of control measures include corporate responsibility in not causing disease and injury, avoidance of liability for delayed or negligently caused health problems, and enhanced public image. These figures are difficult to pinpoint; however, they can be valued within broad limits.

Workers' compensation costs increased from $25 billion in 1980 to $60 billion in 1991. With greater awareness of issues such as chemically caused disease and repetitive strain injuries, as well as high inflation in medical care costs, this escalation is expected to continue. Prevention efforts, however, should modify this steeply rising curve.

Newer Occupational Services

Employee Assistance Programs

A small group of employees at most worksites use significantly more medical services than other employees and are absent a great deal because of somatization of psychological conflicts. Resolution of these somatization disorders by providing cognitive services has resulted in benefit-cost ratios of up to 10 : 1 [16].

One good example is a comprehensive program that is an extension of an EAP program. At First Chicago National Bank, the employee assistance program acts as a gatekeeper for a comprehensive mental health effort that includes concurrent psychiatric hospital utilization review, consulting psychiatrists, and some other features of case management. Mental health care costs have decreased as a proportion of total outlays, and the cost per covered employee was kept constant during a 5-year period while other benefits were inflating dramatically. The cost of inpatient mental health care dropped significantly during that time period [17].

Employee assistance programs provide savings by early intervention in mental health problems, which can prevent hospitalization and long-term illness. Nonproductive conflicts between employees and supervisors can be resolved early, as can performance problems due to stress or substance abuse (see Chap. 18) [18]. It should be noted that performance problems not related to an illness or injury are the province of the supervisor and not occupational health professionals, who should be careful to separate the two issues.

Work Hardening

Injury and reinjury in taxing jobs can be prevented by gradually increasing workload or time at the job. Protocols are available for acclimation schedules according to total workload over time. Medical personnel must work with supervisors to ensure that appropriate modified work is available. Reductions in injury rates and associated expenses can be costed in a manner similar to that described above. The value obtained from reconditioning workers appears to significantly outweigh the cost of professional time and lost production, although the evidence is primarily anecdotal.

On-Site Management of Nonoccupational Illness and Injuries

Many employers, especially those who are self-insured, have noted the advantages of providing comprehensive health care for both occupational and nonoccupational illnesses and injuries *at the worksite*. On-site treatment can be performed by physicians, and nurses, nurse practitioners, and physician assistants, under appropriate supervision. Advantages include earlier treatment with reduced morbidity, better health supervision, ready access to practitioners who understand the work environment, and lower unit cost. Access and quality can be improved in several ways. The employee, in turn, does not need to take half a day or more off from work to travel to a medical facility and wait in the waiting room; this scenario incurs lost wages and also interferes with production and work duties. Easier access to medical care frequently results in earlier treatment and reduction in severity of illness and resultant lost time. Physicians familiar with the work environment can be expected to recommend modified work duties that will be of benefit to the organization and the employee, and not aggravate or prolong the condition [19].

Allied health professionals such as nurse practitioners and physician assistants can provide many clinical and nonclinical services at significantly lower cost. The quality of care has repeatedly been demonstrated to be comparable to traditional services and often with evidence of better patient empathy on the part of the allied providers [20]. In the majority of cases treated by midlevel providers, the physician becomes a team leader rather than a direct provider of care.

According to the United States Chamber of Commerce, fewer than 40% of employed people have a primary care physician. Some patients may have trouble selecting an appropriate physician or gaining timely access to treatment. For these employees, on-site facilities improve access and may improve the quality of care. As an alternative to on-site treatment or for chronic or complex cases, the occupational physician can play a valuable role in facilitating referral to high-quality specialists and reduce anxiety and morbidity. Referred cases can also be tracked against a control group to assess the effects of the occupational health programs on total cost per case, including indirect costs.

Political difficulties can surface when an organization provides services on site or when an occupational health clinic for small business is established. Local physicians in particular may feel threatened with a loss of patient volume. Since fewer than half of employed people have a primary care physician, however, this fear is not justified. In fact, referral patterns from a well-run occupational health program greatly benefit the local medical community (see Chap. 1, Occupational Medical Services).

Occupational health programs designed to serve smaller companies in the immediate geographic area can have similar benefits to an organization. These programs focus on the work environment; thus, they are apt to be aware of special occupational medical concerns, in a manner similar to on-site programs.

Direct economic benefits of on-site treatment of both occupational and nonoccupational health problems include lost time saved and lower unit cost because of use of allied health professionals or contract arrangements with physicians at a community occupational health program. Indirect savings include decreased morbidity for specific cases, with imputed savings in absence and medical care costs. Whether on-site programs are appropriate or cost effective for any organization depends in large part on the number of employees, the type of business operation, and the resultant need for occupational medical services. At the Morgan Guarantee Trust, the on-site medical program provides primary care services and has been able to negotiate significant discounts for laboratory, x-ray, and consultative services from local medical providers, resulting in a significant savings to the company [21]. The Goodyear Tire and Rubber Company and Nestle's provide primary care to employees and dependents on site, apparently at significant savings [22]. Southern California Edison has integrated its on-site primary care clinics into its preferred provider organization. Apparently, by reducing overhead and medically unnecessary treatment, a savings also resulted [23]. At General Electric, on-site physical therapy decreased lost workdays by 32%, and overall cost by 37% for workers' compensation low back pain claims [24]. A similar saving was demonstrated at several plants at Northern Telecom, Inc.

Chronic Disease Management

Management of certain conditions such as hypercholesterolemia, diabetes, and hypertension may be more effective at the worksite, primarily because of ease of access to medical care, close follow-up, and coordination with managing physicians. Routine contact with allied health personnel and referral back to the primary care physician for medication have resulted in improved control of hypertension at lower cost [25]. Peer pressure also contributes to these success rates. Lost time for follow-up visits is also decreased when the services are provided on site. Further, work accommodations for disabilities in such patients can be made more efficiently.

Economic benefits of on-site chronic disease monitoring include reduced absence for treatment and increased compliance with treatment regimen, which reduces morbidity and mortality from the disorder. Over a period of several years, these benefits can be documented. In the shorter run, they can be determined from data available from federal and voluntary agencies applied to the demographics of the employee population.

Self-Care and Wise Use of Counseling/Education

Education of patients in self-care for minor illnesses and injuries has reduced health care costs. Benefit costs declined 17 to 35% in one study for those who participated in self-care education [26]. A variety of allied health care practitioners can effectively provide and coordinate this counseling and education. One interesting way of increasing awareness of the medical system, as well as saving a significant amount of money, is to have workers audit their hospital bills for accuracy. A reward can be given for errors discovered.

Educating employees in the best way to use the medical care system has resulted in increases in the quality of care and substantial decreases in inappropriate utilization. This training may take the form of print material or discussions with a health care professional [27].

Case Management

Close management of seriously ill, injured, or chronically ill employees or those undergoing treatment is also valuable to avoid unnecessary procedures, ensure appropriate therapy, and aid in proper discharge planning as well as early return to work. Savings of up to 10 : 1 have been reported over a 10-year period by one case management firm, which has followed over 130,000 cases on a computerized database, although such estimates bear careful analysis [28]. The 3M Corporation reported a $1.9 million savings after 2 years of careful case management. Examples from another source include savings in the range of $14,000 for coordination of medical care for an automobile injury victim with third-degree burns and a closed head injury, and $9,000 savings for arranging home treatment for a patient with a chronic skin condition. It should be noted that these savings are often based on projections from other cases or requests from physicians. Careful case control–type comparisons are needed to assure reasonably accurate estimates for care that was avoided. These figures will change as medical practices move to outpatient settings over time.

Health Promotion at the Worksite

Impact of Lifestyle on Health and Costs

Since the economic impact of lifestyle-related disease on health care costs has been more clearly recognized, health promotion programs have become increasingly common at the worksite. In fact, costs for lifestyle-related problems have been estimated at 10 to 15 times as much as work-related illness and injuries. Interactions between lifestyle and certain occupational exposures (e.g., smoking and asbestos) further compound the problem.

The leading causes of death as well as morbidity in the United States today are heart disease, cancer, stroke, injuries, chronic obstructive pulmonary disease, and influenza and pneumonia [29]. Heart disease accounts for 37.5% of all deaths, and cancer another 22.2%. Both of these disorders are lifestyle related. In terms of years of life lost before age 65, the leading lifestyle-related causes are unintentional injuries, cancer, heart disease, suicide and homicide, and human immunodeficiency virus (HIV) infection [30].

The effects of lifestyle on premature mortality are shown in Table 34-1 [31]. The prevalence of these risk factors in employed populations is shown in Table 34-2. The self-reported prevalence for some risks, such as uncontrolled hypertension, sedentary lifestyle, and nonuse of seat belts, has declined sharply in recent years. Others, such as cigarette smoking and obesity, have not changed significantly. The proportion of premature mortality due to risk factors in a typical employed group with a mean age of 35 years and a male-female ratio of 60 : 40 is shown in Table 34-3. These proportions are the result of multiplying the prevalence of a risk factor by the relative risk. Thus, a factor with a moderate risk but a high prevalence, such as a sedentary lifestyle (upward of 60% in many groups of older workers) would cause many more deaths than smoking (with a prevalence of less than 15%) in this age group (persons 60–69 years of age). Some diseases caused by smoking, such as cancer, cause the majority of attributable deaths in younger age groups, in which heart disease is not so prevalent. Excess mortality and morbidity in those with risk factors increase sharply after age 35 (Fig. 34-1).

Each case of heart disease that requires coronary bypass costs approximately $30,000 (depending on the part of the country in which it is performed) in direct costs, and as much as triple that in wage replacement and other indirect costs. In 1990, 284,000 bypass procedures were performed, almost all of them on employed adults. The treatment for lifestyle-related cancers such as lung cancer typically costs $30,000 per patient. There are one million new cases of cancer per year, of which over half are lifestyle related [32]. Life insurance costs should be added to these costs, significantly increasing the total outlay. There are additional indirect costs for retraining and replacement.

Medical care costs per nonfatal case for typical employee groups with lifestyle-related diseases are shown in Table 34-4 [32]. The data on the proportion of this morbidity that is preventable are not as well studied, but one review of medical records noted that the 13% of patients with one or more serious risk factors incurred the same medical care costs as the other 87% and had five times the number of major complications [33].

Effects of Health Promotion Efforts

There is evidence from both epidemiologic studies and clinical trials to show that morbidity and mortality are reduced if risk factors are decreased [33, 34]. Success rates for corporate programs are shown in Table 34-5. While the studies on the net cost effectiveness of health promotion programs have not been well designed, preliminary evidence appears to indicate that with a stable employee population, there is a significant positive benefit-to-cost ratio [34, 35]. A framework for the analysis of the cost effectiveness of health promotion programs has been provided in a recent publication [36].

Screening to Promote Health

While much of the risk screening done today is nonproductive, early detection of hypertension, hypercholesterolemia, and cervical and breast cancer has a significant benefit-cost ratio [32, 37]. In asymptomatic individuals, other tests, such as chest and back films, multichannel chemistries, and resting and stress electrocardiograms, are of minimal value and may result in unnecessary costs involved in ruling out false positives [38].

Cost for illnesses such as upper- and lower-respiratory infections, low birth rate, and some gastrointestinal diseases that could be affected by health promotion have been demonstrated [13]. Other studies demonstrating positive cost benefit include Johnson & Johnson's Live for Life Program [37] and Travelers' Taking Care Center [39]. It is frequently necessary to follow participants for up to 10 years to document long-term benefits [40]. Nonetheless, reductions in health risks can result in significant savings in benefits, retraining and replacement costs, business interruption, and improvements in performance and employee morale.

Table 34-1. Relative risk of death for a 35-year-old with designated risk factors

Risk factor	Heart disease		Cancer		Stroke		Injury		Chronic obstructive pulmonary disease		Influenza/pneumonia	
	M	F	M	F	M	F	M	F	M	F	M	F
Sedentary lifestyle	2.5	1.4	—	—	—	—	—	—	—	—	—	—
Cigarette smoking	2.0	2.0	10.0	10.0	1.2	1.5	7.0[a]	7.0[a]	4.0	4.0	3.2	1.2
Hypertension	2.0	2.2	—	[b]	2.0	2.2	[c]	[c]	—	—	—	—
Obesity	1.3	1.3	—	—	[d]	[d]	[c]	[c]	—	—	—	—
Diabetes	3.0	4.0	—	—	—	—	—	—	—	—	—	—
Elevated cholesterol	2.0	2.0	2.0	—	2.0	2.0	—	—	—	—	—	—
Positive stool occult blood	—	—	2.0	2.0	—	—	—	—	—	—	—	—
Failure to self-examine breasts	—	—	—	2.0	—	—	—	—	—	—	—	—
Failure to obtain Pap smears	—	—	—	7.0	—	—	—	—	—	—	—	—
Irregular use of seat belts	—	—	—	—	—	—	1.5	1.6	—	—	—	—
Heavy alcohol use	[d]	—	[e]	[e]	4.0	4.0	—	—	—	—	3.0	3.0

[a] Automobile injury.
[b] Elevated risk for some cancers, such as ovarian cancer.
[c] Elevated but unquantified risk in morbid obesity.
[d] Elevated risk; estimates vary.
[e] Elevated risk for cancers of pharynx, esophagus; synergistic with tobacco use.
Source: Adapted from J. Hall and J. D. Zwemmer. *Prospective Medicine.* Indianapolis: Methodist Hospital, 1979.

Table 34-2. Prevalence of health risks in employed populations

Risk factor	Men (%)	Women (%)
Acute heavy drinking	33.4	12.9
Chronic heavy drinking	13.8–23.4	04.0
Drinking and driving	09.2	03.3
Sedentary lifestyle*	12.1–41.0	11.9–30.8
Nonuse of seat belts	58.4–80.5	56.8–80.5
Uncontrolled hypertension	03.7–25.7	04.2–14.0
Smoking	17.0–37.0	15.0–52.0
Overweight	13.5–61.0	14.0–36.7
Lack of breast self-exam	—	37.3–43.2
Needs Pap smear	—	05.2–19.8

*Some estimates are as high as 50%. This also varies markedly by age, with older people exercising much less.
Source: Adapted from E. M. Gentry et al. The behavioral risk factor surveys: II. Design, methods, and estimates from combined state data. *Am. J. Prev. Med.* 1:9, 1985; J. S. Harris, B. Collins, and I. L. Majure. Prevalence of health risks in an employed population. *J. Occup. Med.* 28:217, 1986; and unpublished data.

Table 34-3. Premature deaths: Proportion of deaths due to various risk factors (in percents)*

	Age (yr)				
Risk factor	20–39	30–39	40–49	50–59	60–69
Men					
Smoking	7	15	20	14	7
Lack of exercise	19	46	59	57	73
High blood pressure	3	6	8	10	11
Cholesterol	0	3	4	4	5
Weight	0	1	1	0	2
Alcohol use	58	16	4	2	1
Nonuse of seat belts	13	13	4	2	0
No colon cancer check	0	0	0	11	1
Total	100	100	100	100	100
Women					
Smoking	8	25	36	30	18
Lack of exercise	2	13	11	27	40
High blood pressure	3	9	8	14	16
Cholesterol	4	5	6	6	7
Weight	5	4	4	19	18
Alcohol use	18	17	10	4	1
Nonuse of seat belts	60	27	9	0	0
No colon cancer check	—	—	16	0	0
Total	100	100	100	100	100

*Health risk appraisal computer simulation of mortality in a typical employed population. Risk factor prevalence varies by age.

Medical Benefits Quality and Cost Management

Benefit Design Consultation

Astute occupational medicine physicians can be of great value to a company's benefits organization by recommending appropriate medical services to be covered (including preventive services) and reimbursement schemes that discourage the use of medically unnecessary services. Conversely, the physicians can recommend and/or ar-

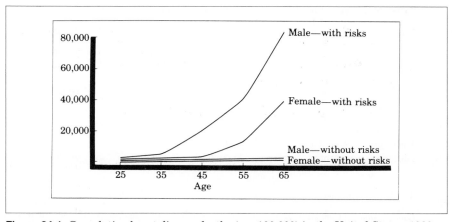

Figure 34-1. Cumulative heart disease deaths (per 100,000) in the United States, 1980 estimate. Risks include blood pressure, 160/100; weight, 50% over the ideal; cholesterol, 300 mg/100 ml; sedentary lifestyle; and one pack of cigarettes per day. (Data from J. Hall and J. D. Zwemmer. *Prospective Medicine*. Indianapolis: Methodist Hospital, 1979.)

Table 34-4. Hospitalization costs per episode of lifestyle-related disorders

Disease	Cost
Alcoholism	$12,000
Drug abuse	16,000
Mental disorders, other	12,000
Myocardial infarction	8,000
Ischemic heart disease	8,000
Malignancy	28,000
Digestive disease	6,000

Source: Based on Alexander and Alexander internal data. These costs are for 1992, and are mean values for inpatient and immediately pre- and posthospitalization outpatient diagnosis and treatment.

range for more appropriate services and audit fees considered inappropriate. They can also assist employees in auditing their hospital bills.

As described in Chap. 40, in the most comprehensive situation, occupational physicians can administer managed health care programs, which have been shown to provide significant decreases in costs or cost increase rates, and to improve the quality of care [41].

Utilization Management: The Gatekeeper Concept

Medical practice patterns vary significantly in different areas of the country, often with little discernible difference in treatment outcome. To curtail medically unnecessary services, some companies require employees to clear hospitalizations and diagnostic procedures or use defined practitioners; otherwise, benefits and coverage may be reduced. Other companies have authorized third-party services to review the need for hospitalization or surgery and to determine whether alternative measures, such as outpatient surgery, can be used.

Precertification and concurrent review of hospitalizations have led to steep drops in inpatient service use as criteria are tightened [38]. In one of the few controlled studies, private review of hospitalization decreased inpatient days by 11%, total hospital expenditures by 7%, and total expenditures by 6%. Admissions in this study dropped by about 13% [42]. Savings may have been offset to some extent by in-

Table 34-5. Typical health promotion results "for given participants"

Program	Result	Percent change
Fitness	Absences down	20–50
	Costs down	40–50
	Performance increased	
Smoking cessation	Smoking down	20–50
	Costs down	25
	Hospital days down	54
Medical self-care	Service use down	32
Blood pressure control	2 : 1 benefit-cost	
Employee assistances	Accidents down	50–80
	Lost time down	40–60
	Medical visits down	
Type A modification	Repeat myocardial infarctions down	50

Source: Adapted from W. N. Burton and D. J. Conti. Value of Managed Health Benefits. In J. S. Harris, H. D. Belk, and L. W. Wood. *Managing Employee Health Care Costs: Assuring Quality and Value.* Boston: OEM Press, 1992.

creased spending on outpatient cost and the cost of administration of the program. An Institute of Medicine study concluded that the evidence was not researched well enough to provide a definitive answer [43]. One study, published after the 10M report, of employers in the Houston area found that utilization review significantly reduced total monthly inpatient charges but increased total monthly outpatient charges, with a resulting net gain in cost [44]. It should be noted that the shift across from inpatient to outpatient settings can be controlled by using both inpatient and outpatient utilization management. It has also been noted that the program's impact is greatest at the onset, [45] because of a "sentinel" effect. If criteria and guidelines can be progressively tightened over a period of time, utilization will decrease. Case management of catastrophic and complex cases can have a significant effect on total costs, although many of the savings reports are anecdotal or deal with projected savings from "what might have been."

Second opinions regarding certain surgical procedures have resulted in nonconfirmation rates of 17 to 50%. Later reviews, however, show that the actual rate of avoided surgery was less than 1% in the Medicare program, prompting the Healthcare Financing Administration to focus on a few selected procedures (see Chap. 40). Level of care monitoring has resulted in savings of up to $500,000 per identified provider. These providers were outliers, identified by state peer review organizations, who changed their practice patterns after education. As the foregoing implies, a few providers often generate a tremendous amount of excess cost for little if any benefit to patients [38]. Savings in these areas can be calculated from company insurance payment rates compared to data for optimal case management for age, sex, and disease category.

Changes in Economic Incentives

Incentives in benefits plans that contribute to inappropriate utilization include full payment for services. Introduction of substantial deductibles and copayments can reduce costs by one third [46]. Full reimbursement for inpatient or emergency department treatment but partial or capped reimbursement for outpatient therapy or surgery also contributes to inappropriate care. Incentives for healthy lifestyles, such as reduced premiums or copayments for nonsmokers, have the potential to improve employee health.

Putting Providers at Risk

Capitated payment systems, whereby the provider of health care is at some risk for ordering testing and treatment of questionable benefit and in turn responsible for keeping patients healthy, have proved effective in managing health care costs [47]. The benefit of this change can be followed by comparing the capitation payment to the cost of the parallel conventional insurance plan. Another promising method of payment, which has price but not volume controls, is payment on the basis of diagnostic related groups (DRGs) [41]. Government programs have adopted both approaches in many areas. Since costs are now being shifted to private patients (i.e., employees), businesses may have to adopt cost management measures to prevent paying for patients receiving public funding [48, 49].

The author would like to acknowledge Jack Richman, M.D., for his contributions to the first edition of this chapter.

References

1. Donabedian, A. Quality and Cost: Choices and Responsibilities. In J. S. Harris, H. D. Belk, and L. W. Wood (eds.), *Managing Employee Health Care Costs: Assuring Quality and Value*. Boston: OEM Press, 1992. Pp. 13–18.
2. Buck, C. R., Jr. Assuring Value in Medical Care for Employees and Dependents: An Opportunity for Occupational Physicians. In J. S. Harris, H. D. Belk, and L. W. Wood (eds.), *Managing Employee Health Care Costs: Assuring Quality and Value*. Boston: OEM Press, 1992. Pp. 3–4.
3. National Safety Council, *Accident Facts*. Chicago: National Safety Council, 1992; National Safety Council, *Cumulative Trauma Disorders and Ergonomics: Causes, Treatment, and Preventive Measures*. Chicago: National Safety Council, 1984.
4. Recommendation of the Immunization Practice Advisory Committee. Prevention and control of influenza. *M.M.W.R.* 34:261, 1985.
5. Recommendations for protection against viral hepatitis. *M.M.W.R.* 34:23, 1985.
6. Harris, J. S. Blood Borne Diseases. In D. D. DiBenedetto, J. S. Harris, and R. J. McCunney, *The OEM Manual of Occupational Health and Safety*. Boston: OEM Health Information Press, 1993.
7. USDHHS, US Public Health Service, Centers for Disease Control. *Health Information for International Travelers, 1992*. HHS Publication no. (CDC)92-8280.
8. Benenson, A. S. (ed.), *Control of Communicable Diseases in Man* (15th ed.). Washington, DC: American Public Health Assoc., 1990.
9. Lewy, R. M. Occupational Health Program for Housestaff Physicians. *J.A.M.A.* 246:1432, 1981.
10. Koplan, J. P. Benefits, Risks, and Costs of Immunization Programmes. In CIBA Foundation, *The Value of Preventive Medicine*. London: Pitman, 1985.
11. Harris, J. S., et al. Business as Usual May Mean Going Out of Business. In *National Council on Compensation Insurance Digest*. 4:25, 1989.
12. Greer, W. T. Presentation to New England Medical Association, Boston, MA 1992.
13. Dalton, B. A., and Harris, J. S., A Comprehensive Approach to Corporate Health Management. In J. S. Harris, H. D. Belk, and L. W. Wood, (eds.), *Managing Employee Health Care Costs: Assuring Quality and Value*. Boston: OEM Press, 1992. Pp. 181–191.
14. Wickersham, J. F. Disability management: Key to cost savings at 3M. *Business and Health* 1:26, 1983.
15. Harris, J. S. Wise up to workers' compensation. *Financial Executive* November/December 1992.
16. Harris, J. S. Managing Health: What Employers Can Do About Health Care Costs. In J. Meyer and K. McLennon (eds.), *Care and Cost: Current Issues in Health Policy*. Boulder: Westview Press, 1989. Pp. 167–202.
17. Burton, W. N., and Conti, D. J. Value of Managed Mental Health Benefits. In J. S. Harris, H. D. Belk, and L. W. Wood (eds.), *Managing Employee Health Care Costs: Assuring Quality and Value*. Boston: OEM Press, 1992. Pp. 151–153.
18. Bureau of National Affairs. *Alcohol and Drugs in the Workplace: Costs, Controls, and Controversies*. Washington, DC: Bureau of National Affairs, 1986.
19. Walsh, D. C. Is there a doctor in the house? *Harvard Business Rev.* 62:84, 1984.
20. Scharon, G. M., and Bernacki, E. J. Corporate nurse practitioners. *Business and Health* 1:26, 1984.
21. Schneider, W. J. A Corporate Medical Department's Role in Medical Benefits. in J. S. Harris, H. D. Belk and L. W. Wood (eds.), *Managing Employee Health Care Costs: Assuring Quality and Value*. Boston: OEM Press, 1992. Pp. 171–174.
22. Bryant, M. Comeback for the company doc? *Business and Health* Feb, 1991. Pp. 44–58.
23. Geisel, J. Company-run clinics cutting health care costs: An interview with Jacques Sokolov. *Business Insurance* March 5, 1990.

24. Galvin, R. S. *Assuring Value in the Treatment of Low Back Pain,* 1994 in press.
25. Foote, A., and Erfurt, J. Hypertension control: Formula for success. *Business and Health* 1:13, 1984.
26. Vickery, D. M., et al. Effect of self-care education program on medical visits. *J.A.M.A.* 250:2952, 1983.
27. Gardner, H. H., and Schneiderman, C. A. Insuring Value by Supporting Consumer Decision-Making. In J. S. Harris, H. D. Belk, and L. W. Wood, (eds.), *Managing Employee Health Care Costs: Assuring Quality and Value.* Boston: OEM Press, 1992. Pp. 73–76; and Harris, J. S., Goldstein, J. R., and Tager, M. J., *Wise Moves.* Chicago: Great Performance, 1986.
28. Davis, D. H., One way to control disability expenses. *National Underwriter* November 19, 1982.
29. *Healthy People 2000: National Health Promotion and Disease Prevention Objectives.* Washington, DC: US Department of Health and Human Services, Public Health Service, 1990.
30. Fielding, J. E. Occupational Health Physicians and Prevention. In J. S. Harris, H. D. Belk, and L. W. Wood (eds.), *Managing Employee Health Care Costs: Assuring Quality and Value.* Boston: OEM Press, 1992. Pp. 154–166.
31. Hall, J., and Zwemmer, J. D. *Prospective Medicine.* Indianapolis: Methodist Hospital, 1979.
32. Harris, J. S., The Future of Health Promotion. In M. P. O'Donnell and J. S. Harris, *Health Promotion in the Workplace* (2nd ed.). Albany, NY: Delmar, 1994.
33. Zook, C. J., and Moore, F. D. High cost users of medical care. *N. Engl. J. Med.* 302:996, 1980.
34. O'Donnell, M. P. The Financial Benefits of Health Promotion. In M. P. O'Donnell and J. S. Harris, *Health Promotion in the Workplace* (2nd ed.). Albany, NY: Delmar, 1994.
35. Warner, K. E., et al. Economic implications of workplace health promotion programs: Review of the literature. *J. Occup. Med.* 30:106, 1988.
36. Harris, J. S. The Cost-Effectiveness of Health Promotion Programs. In J. S. Harris, H. D. Belk, and L. W. Wood (eds.), *Managing Employee Health Care Costs: Assuring Quality and Value.* Boston: OEM Press, 1992. Pp. 167–170.
37. Bly, J. L, Jones, R. C., and Richardson, J. E. Impact of worksite health promotion on healthcare cost and utilization: An evaluation of Johnson & Johnson's Live for Life Program. *J.A.M.A.* 256:3235, 1986.
38. Harris, J. S. *Cost Effective Health Care.* Nashville: Northern Telecom, Inc., 1988.
39. Lynch, W. D., et al. Impact of a facility-based fitness program on the number of absences from work due to illness. *J. Occup. Med.* 32:9, 1990.
40. The Multiple Risk Factor Intervention Trial Research Group. Mortality rates after 10.5 years for participants in Multiple Risk Factor Intervention Trial: Findings related to a priori hypotheses of the trial. *J.A.M.A.* 263:1795, 1990.
41. Gold, M. Health Maintenance Organizations: Structure, Performance and Current Issues for Employee Health Benefits Design. In J. S. Harris, H. D. Belk, and L. W. Wood, (eds.), *Managing Employee Health Care Costs: Assuring Quality and Value.* Boston: OEM Press, 1992. Pp. 117–125.
42. Feldstein, P. J., Wickizer, T. M., and Wheeler, J. R. C., Private cost containment: The effects of utilization review programs on health care use and expenditures. *N. Engl. J. Med.* 318:310, 1988.
43. Gray, B. H., and Field, M. J. *Controlling Cost in Changing Patient Care? The Role of Utilization Management.* Washington, DC: National Academy Press, 1989.
44. Custer, W. S. *Employer Healthcare Design, Plan Costs, and Healthcare Delivery.* Washington, DC: Employee Benefits Research Institute, 1989.
45. Khandker, R. K., Manning, W. G., and Ahmed, T. Utilization review savings at the micro level. *Med. Care* 30:1043, 1992.
46. Brook, R. H., et al. Does free care improve adult health? Results from a randomized clinical trial. *N. Engl. J. Med.* 309:1426, 1983.
47. Harris, J. S. Does Managed Care Manage Healthcare Costs Effectively?—It Depends. In J. S. Harris, H. D. Belk, and L. W. Wood, (eds.), *Managing Employee Health Care Costs: Assuring Quality and Value.* Boston: OEM Press, 1992. Pp. 131–135.
48. Davis, K., et al. Is cost containment working? *Health Affairs* 4:81, 1985.
49. Harris, J. S. *Strategic Health Management.* San Francisco: Jossey-Bass, 1994.

Appendix 1 to Chapter 34: Recommendations for adult immunizations

Vaccine	Target population	Dose	Frequency	Comments
Tetanus and diphtheria toxoids (Td)	All adults Pregnant women	0.5 ml IM	Every 10 years Every 5 years for severe wounds or burns	Contraindicated in person with previous severe hypersensitivity to Td. Persons with no history of immunizations should receive a 3-dose primary series.
Inactivated influenza virus vaccine	Those over 65, chronic medical conditions, smokers, persons in essential community services, the working population	0.5 ml SC or IM	Annually	Contraindicated with egg allergy. Useful to decrease morbidity and lost productivity.
Pneumococcal polysaccharide (23 type) vaccine	Persons over age 65; smokers, alcohol abusers, high-risk chronic disease patients, patients with splenic dysfunction	0.5 ml SC or IM	One time only	Can be given simultaneously with influenza vaccine at different site.
Hepatitis B vaccine	Preexposure: health care and laboratory workers, morticians, homosexuals, inmates and staff of correctional and mental institutions, persons with multiple sex contacts, IV drug users Postexposure: seronegative sexual and household contacts of hepatitis B patients and health care or sanitation workers with needlestick or other bloodborne exposure to blood of patients	10 µg 2 doses 1 month apart, then 3rd dose 5 months after second	Once	

(continued)

Vaccine	Target population	Dose	Frequency	Comments
Live rubella virus vaccine	Susceptible females of childbearing age; health care workers	0.5 ml SC	Once	Contraindicated in immunocompromised or pregnant women.
Live measles virus vaccine	Susceptible young adults or those given killed virus vaccine in the past; important in overseas travelers; health care workers	0.5 ml SC	Once	Contraindicated in pregnant women with egg or neomycin allergy.
Live mumps virus vaccine	All susceptible young adults; health care workers	0.5 ml SC	Once	Contraindicated in pregnant women with egg or neomycin allergy.
Human diploid cell rabies vaccine	Preexposure: veterinarians, animal handlers, field workers; travelers to high-incidence countries	1 ml IM	Initial 7 days 21–28 days	Likely carriers include skunks, foxes, raccoons, coyotes, bobcats, and bats. Rodents and Lepidopterae do not transmit rabies in the US. Unprovoked attack by domestic animals raises likelihood. Can be transmitted without bites through open wounds.
	Postexposure: individuals bitten by rabid or potentially rabid animal	1 ml with one dose HRIG 20 cc/kg	Initial 3 days 7 days 14 days 28 days	

Source: Adapted from N. M. Amin. Adult immunizations. *Am. Fam. Physician* 336:84, 1986; and P. Gardner and W. Schaffner. Immunization of adults. *New Engl. J. Med.* 328:1252, 1993.

Appendix 2 to Chapter 34: Recommended immunizations for travelers*

Vaccine	Dose/type	Comments
Tetanus and diphtheria	Booster; primary series if unimmunized	Both common in underdeveloped countries
Japanese B encephalitis	Primary series	Areas of risk, rural or prolonged exposures
Rabies	Preexposure series; booster every 2 years or with low antibody titer	For travel to areas with high incidence, particularly for children
Hepatitis B	Preexposure series	For travel to or residence in endemic areas, especially Arctic East Asia, and Sub-Saharan Africa
Measles, mumps, rubella	Trivalent live vaccine	If live vaccine not given previously; these diseases are endemic in the Third World and may be imported by unimmunized individuals
Poliovirus (OPV or IPV)	Give remaining doses for those not fully primarily immunized, orally or inactivated; booster for those fully immunized as children	For visitors to developing countries, particularly Africa or Asia. Inactivated virus, series SC preferred for primary in adults and travelers booster
Meningococcal polysaccharide	Tetravalent	Travel to areas with epidemic meningococcal disease
Killed typhoid	Two 0.5-ml doses IM 1 month apart. Booster every 3 years	Recommended for travelers to endemic areas such as rural Africa, Asia, Central and South America
Live, attenuated typhoid	4 oral doses; reimmunize every 5 years	Recommended for travelers to endemic areas such as rural Africa, Asia, Central and South America
Live, attenuated yellow fever	Two 0.5-ml doses SC	Available from a federally designated vaccination center; reported cases in Africa and South America
Plague	3 doses IM; intial dose of 0.1 ml, then 0.2 ml at 1 month and 5 months, booster at 6 months and then 1–2 years	Endemic in certain countries in Africa, Asia, and South America; consult CDC for specific recommendations
Smallpox		No longer recommended
Cholera		No longer recommended

*Consult the US Centers for Disease Control in Atlanta (404-329-3311); the International Health Care Services at Cornell University Medical Center, New York; or the International Association for Medical Assistance to Travelers, 736 Center St., Lewiston, NY, 14902, for the most current information by country.
Source: Adapted from N. M. Amin. Adult immunizations. *Am. Fam. Physician* 336:84, 1986; and P. Gardner and W. Schaffner. Immunization of adults. *New Engl. J. Med.* 328:1252, 1993.

35

Educational Opportunities

David J. Tollerud

In delivering quality medical care, physicians are aided by knowing what kind of work their patients do and how it may affect their health. Every week hundreds of thousands of workers visit their physicians for advice on work with reference to certain illnesses or injuries. Clinicians must decide when their patients have recovered sufficiently to return to work, whether their illness could have been caused or aggravated by work, and whether worksite modifications are necessary. To make these assessments, an understanding of the work environment is essential.

Occupational medicine in the United States remains a field in which most practitioners do not have formal training. In a study published in 1991 entitled *Addressing the Physician Shortage in Occupational and Environmental Medicine,* the Institute of Medicine estimated a current shortage of 3100 to 5500 physicians with special competence in occupational and environmental medicine [1]. This includes primary care physicians and other specialists who have undertaken some form of training or have acquired significant practical experience in occupational and environmental medicine. The estimated shortage of fully trained specialists in occupational and environmental medicine was 1600 to 3500. Based on these estimates, the Institute's Subcommittee on Physician Shortage recommended a series of measures to alleviate the shortage, most of which focus on increased education and training opportunities at all levels of medical education [1, 2]. In a separate report, the Institute of Medicine recommended that "all primary care physicians be able to identify possible occupationally or environmentally induced conditions and make appropriate referrals for follow-up" [3]. The fund of knowledge required to meet such a standard of care includes familiarity with principles of preventive medicine as well as occupational and environmental medicine, clinical skills in occupational history taking, a basic knowledge of common occupational and environmental diseases, and an understanding of the United States regulatory system and workers' compensation system.

Increasingly, US corporations are using external sources of medical care for their employees. Although large companies have well-staffed occupational medical programs at many of their plants and laboratories, the bulk of Americans work in small plants, in service organizations, or for themselves and do not have easy access to competent occupational medical advice. The result is that a growing number of primary care physicians and specialists are caring for employees with potentially work-related illnesses and injuries. For the clinician interested in providing occupational medical services, an understanding of the basic principles of the specialty is crucial.

An increased supply of physicians in the US, coupled with a change in funding of health care, has also motivated many physicians to seek alternative means to broaden their practices. The need for occupational medicine services has stimulated the development of occupational health "programs" at hospitals, emergency rooms, and group practices.

Recognizing this changing practice climate, the Accreditation Council for Graduate Medical Education (ACGME) now requires some element of occupational medicine training in accredited family medicine training programs [4]. Other boards and specialty areas such as internal medicine are likely to follow. National initiatives such as the Academic Award in Occupational/Environmental Medicine by the National Institute of Environmental Health Sciences (NIEHS) are aimed at developing occupational and environmental medicine faculty and curricula for medical schools to expose students to the field at an early stage in their medical education.

These approaches, however, only address the training of *new physicians.* A great need exists for educational opportunities for *established practitioners,* who provide the majority of occupational and environmental medicine services throughout the country. This chapter identifies educational options and sources of information for practicing physicians interested in expanding their knowledge and skills in the delivery of occupational and environmental medical services.

To understand the educational needs of practitioners, one must address the question: "What is *different* about occupational medicine?" The most fundamental distinction is that occupational and environmental medicine is a specialty that focuses on the *prevention* of illness and injury at work. The goal of the occupational and environmental medicine practitioner is to deliver consultative and clinical services designed to prevent illness and injury. Often a sentinel illness or injury will provide the lead for identifying a problem workplace. What sets the occupational and environmental medicine practitioner apart is the desire and expertise to go to the workplace and help formulate measures that will prevent recurrence of the condition among other workers. In instances in which illness is identified, the physician must have enough knowledge about the workplace and specific job activities of the person to render a judgment as to the relative contribution of the workplace.

To competently deliver occupational medical services, one must be more than just a good clinician. In most private practices, the clinician waits for the patient to come to the clinic with certain symptoms, makes a diagnosis, and prescribes a course of treatment. The occupational medicine physician deals primarily with a healthy workforce, and often focuses on medical surveillance of workers to identify potentially hazardous exposures at a stage when disease can be prevented (see Chap. 25). A large proportion of occupational medicine clinical practice also focuses on the treatment of acute injuries and their follow-up as well as treatment of extended soft-tissue pain. In this context, the physician needs to be aware of how work may have led to the illness or injury and the consequences or prevention. Other factors come to bear as well, including determination of a person's ability to work in light of an impairment.

The practitioner needs to think in terms of *populations of workers* and have an understanding of epidemiology and biostatistics to interpret *trends* in illness or presence of certain sentinel abnormalities in disease or laboratory surveillance measures [5]. The effective physician interacts comfortably with people from business, labor, and regulatory organizations in the day-to-day practice of the specialty.

Increasingly, occupational medicine practitioners are also called upon to develop policies regarding occupational and environmental health and safety issues. The ability to conceive and implement new programs requires a unique type of involvement on the part of the physician. To effectively carry out these complex tasks, clinical skills and a broad understanding of public health, business, and law are essential.

The purpose of this brief chapter is to list resources where information on occupational medicine training and education can be obtained. It is recognized that most physicians will not likely be able to take sufficient periods of time away from professional commitments to attend a residency training program. Thus, considerable attention has been directed toward shorter educational segments as well as professional societies, books, and periodicals.

Residency Training Programs

Occupational medicine training programs serve as the backbone for graduate medical education in occupational medicine. The current shortage of board-certified occupational physicians is due in large part to the small number of residency programs in existence before the late 1970s. At that time, the National Institute for Occupational Safety and Health (NIOSH) established 14 Educational Resource Centers across the country to address this shortage. Since then, many additional training programs have evolved.

Funding for occupational medicine residency training, although derived from a variety of sources, faces serious shortages if training centers are to fill the recognized void of specialists. NIOSH provides some degree of funding to most training programs through the Educational Resource Centers and Program Training Grants. However, such grants generally cover only a portion of training costs. Residency programs also rely on scholarships, corporate grants, income from consultative and clinical services, and a variety of innovative funding mechanisms. A significant source of scholarship support is the Occupational Physician's Scholarship Fund established with corporate support by the American College of Occupational and Environmental Medicine. The American College of Preventive Medicine has also created a task force to promote new mechanisms of funding, not only for occupational medicine but for other preventive disciplines as well. Unlike most graduate medical education, which receives significant support from hospitals in exchange for clinical services, occupational medicine residency programs are only rarely sponsored by hospitals [6]. Most are sponsored by schools of public health or medical schools, with limited resources for graduate training.

Oversight and accreditation for occupational medicine residencies are provided by the ACGME through its Residency Review Committee (RRC) for preventive medicine. The RRC develops special requirements for approved residency training programs and reviews their progress on an annual basis. A description of the special requirements for occupational medicine residency training can be found in the *Directory of Graduate Medical Education Programs* [4], which is updated annually.

In 1992, 37 residency training programs in occupational medicine were accredited by the ACGME in the United States, an increase from 25 in 1986 [4]. Occupational medicine residencies vary widely in size (ranging from 1 to over 10 residents). Nationwide, approximately 75 to 100 physicians graduate each year. The academic and clinical focus varies from program to program, but all provide trainees with the fundamental academic and practical knowledge to practice occupational medicine in a variety of settings.

Occupational medicine residency training includes three distinct components. The first year consists of an ACGME-accredited clinical internship. Many programs do not offer this clinical year, but require applicants to have completed at least one year of internship or residency before beginning the occupational medicine residency. The second year of the residency consists of a broad curriculum of study, generally leading to a Master of Public Health (MPH) degree or other master's degree. Required course work includes biostatistics, epidemiology, health services organization and administration, environmental and occupational health, and social and behavioral influences on health. An additional didactic component within the practicum phase must address environmental physiology, occupational disease, toxicology, industrial hygiene and safety, ergonomics, and topics in worker evaluation and clinical program administration. Many programs have added a focus in environmental medicine to address the increasing public concerns over the potential health impact of environmental chemicals and pollutants. The Agency for Toxic Substances Disease Registry (ATSDR), for example, publishes clinical case series in environmental medicine that some residency programs have incorporated into their curriculum (see Appendix B, Regulatory Agencies).

The third year of the typical residency program consists of a series of rotations provided at a variety of occupational medicine settings to gain practical experience. Termed the "practicum," this phase of training usually includes supervised training at industrial sites, occupational medicine clinics, labor organizations, and government agencies such as the Occupational Safety and Health Administration (OSHA), NIOSH, and ATSDR. Some residencies require additional training in certain specialties of importance to the practice of occupational medicine, such as dermatology, pulmonary medicine, and neurology.

Board certification in occupational medicine is administered through the American Board of Preventive Medicine (ABPM). Eligibility to sit for the annual certifying examination is determined by a thorough review of each applicant's credentials and experience [7]. Pathways to eligibility include completion of an accredited residency in occupational medicine followed by a period of relevant practice experience, or an increasingly restrictive alternative pathway for individuals who graduated from medical school before January 1, 1984. Effective January 1, 1993, applicants for the alternative pathway must successfully complete graduate-level courses in biostatistics, epidemiology, health services administration, and environmental health. Requirements for board certification are periodically revised. Potential applicants are urged to obtain current information from the ABPM.

Other Educational Opportunities

Educational Resource Centers

Educational Resource Centers (ERC) were established by NIOSH to provide multidisciplinary educational resources in occupational health. Each center was required to maintain at least three of the four educational components of occupational health as determined by NIOSH: occupational medicine, occupational nursing, safety, and industrial hygiene. These centers continue to provide an important educational resource for physicians and other health professionals seeking additional information and expertise in occupational medicine. In addition to their full-fledged training programs, ERCs provide continuing medical education (CME) opportunities, ranging from one-day conferences and short courses to extended educational programs of several weeks' duration. A catalogue of educational programs and courses can be obtained from each ERC.

Schools of Public Health

Schools of public health, of which 26 are accredited in the US, provide another important educational resource in areas such as epidemiology, biostatistics, toxicology, health services administration, environmental health, and behavioral sciences. Most schools offer curricula leading to the MPH degree, and many accept students on a part-time basis. In addition, many occupational medicine residency programs and ERCs are affiliated with schools of public health. Information on entrance requirements and admission procedures can be obtained by contacting the registrar at the school of interest.

Alternative Degree Programs

In addition to the part-time degree tracks offered by many universities, two innovative programs have been developed for people unable to enroll in a traditional residency program. The University of Michigan offers the "On Job/On Campus" Program, which affords practicing physicians in the region an opportunity to complete an accredited residency program on a part-time basis. The program includes a didactic component leading to an MPH degree in occupational health and a practicum component that may be taken independently. During the didactic component, students attend classes on one 4-day period (Thursday through Sunday) each month for 24 months. During the practicum component, students integrate practical experience on the job with residency training requirements during a 2-year work-study period. Students attend eight quarterly advanced workshops at the University of Michigan. They also complete a minimum of 4 months of field rotations in major industries that have a comprehensive program in occupational medicine and industrial hygiene. Field rotations are arranged and supervised by the University of Michigan faculty. Information can be obtained from the University of Michigan School of Public Health.

The Medical College of Wisconsin offers an MPH degree through its Academic Program in Occupational Medicine. After a one-day orientation session at the Medical College of Wisconsin in Milwaukee, students complete the program on a self-study basis, with curricular materials sent to the participants' homes. Interim examinations and review are accomplished by computer linkage (via modem) between the students' home computers and computers at the Medical College of Wisconsin. Course work is completed at the student's own pace, with computer quizzes taken (at home) after each segment. Final examinations are conducted at the Medical College of Wisconsin or at other cooperating institutions by special arrangement. Most students take several years to complete the degree program. Although the Medical College of Wisconsin also offers a formal occupational medicine residency, no practicum is offered in conjunction with this alternative degree program.

Professional Societies

The American College of Occupational and Environmental Medicine (ACOEM) sponsors seminars and courses related to the specialty. In addition to postgraduate seminars and courses offered at the national meetings in the spring and fall of each year, the college periodically sponsors 1- or 2-day courses of particular interest to practitioners. Recent examples include medical review officer (MRO) courses and seminars on the Americans with Disabilities Act (ADA). The ACOEM also offers the Basic Curriculum, a structured series of three 2-day segments designed to provide the nonoccupational medicine specialist with useful information and an introduction to occupational and environmental medicine. An outline of the basic curriculum presented at the Spring 1993 ACOEM meeting is presented in Table 35-1. Further information and registration forms for the basic curriculum can be obtained from the ACOEM Education Office, and membership information is available through the ACOEM Membership Office (55 W. Seegers Rd., Arlington Heights, IL 60005).

In addition to the national organization, regional groups have formed component societies of ACOEM. These components hold regular meetings and support continuing medical education (CME) activities at the local and regional level. Membership is coordinated through the ACOEM national office.

Many state and county medical societies also have active occupational medicine groups that sponsor informal meetings and CME programs. Information can be obtained by contacting the Medical Society branch or the American Medical Association.

A number of other professional and medical specialty organizations provide some educational programs related to occupational medicine. Many of these organizations include segments on occupational medicine in their national meeting programs with varying points of emphasis. Universities and medical schools also offer programs related to occupational and environmental medicine, including some extensive courses spanning 2 weeks or more. Interested practitioners are encouraged to contact the medical school or university in their area.

Federal and State Agencies

Educational programs are offered by federal, state, and local governmental agencies. The National Institute for Occupational Safety and Health has created a comprehensive curriculum for use by primary care residency training programs to teach the fundamentals of occupational and environmental medicine to nonspecialists.

Table 35-1. Basic Curriculum in Occupational Medicine*

Occupational Medicine I	Occupational Medicine II	Occupational Medicine III
Day 1		
Epidemiology and Biostatistics	Toxicology	Program Administration
Basic Principles and Methods	Basic Principles and Chronic Toxicity Studies; Population Monitoring	Environmental Health
Applications of Epidemiology in Industry (PMR, SMR, Cohort, Case Control); Establishing Causation	Standard Setting and Permissible Exposure Limits; Biologic Monitoring	Cost Containment and Surveillance
How to Critique Occupational Epidemiologic Studies; Computers in Data Management Systems	Industrial Toxicology	Occupational Diseases: Hearing, Pesticides, Low Back Pain, Radiation
Day 2		
Introduction to Occupational Medicine	Regulatory Issues	Industrial Hygiene and Ergonomics
Occupational Lung Disease	Employee Assistance Programs	Basic Principles; Walk-Through Surveys; Material Safety Data Sheets; Sampling and Analysis
	Occupational Diseases: Dermatology, Cancer, Metal Poisoning	Ionizing and Nonionizing Radiation
		Air Sampling and Personal Protection

*Presented at the spring 1993 ACOEM meeting.

This program, EPOCH-Envi, is currently being distributed through a series of "teach the teacher" seminars throughout the United States. It is anticipated that this material will also be used for CME offerings outside the formal residency programs. Additional information regarding the curriculum and a schedule of seminars can be obtained from the NIOSH Education Office. NIOSH and other programs in the Centers for Disease Control (CDC) also offer internships and fellowships, many of which are relevant to the practice of occupational and environment medicine.

NIOSH and other federal agencies, including OSHA, the Environmental Protection Agency (EPA), and (ATSDR) also provide educational materials and sponsor seminars that may be useful to the practitioner seeking additional information on selected aspects of occupational and environmental medicine (see Appendix B, Regulatory Agencies). Two particularly useful series are the NIOSH Current Intelligence Bulletins, which relate recent information on workplace hazards, and the Environmental Case Studies developed by ATSDR to illustrate a broad range of current environmental health issues. NIOSH also publishes a yearly update of current permissible exposure limits (PELs), available from the agency. A nongovernmental organization, the American Conference of Governmental Industrial Hygienists (ACGIH) publishes a pocket-sized booklet of Threshold Limit Values (TLVs) and Biological Exposure Indices (BEIs). The ACGIH also publishes documentation of the TLVs and BEIs, a useful reference for the theoretical basis for these standards and an extensive bibliography.

Journals and Computer Databases

Prominent journals with significant content in occupational and environmental medicine and related topics are listed in Table 35-2. The *Journal of Occupational Medicine,* founded in 1959, is the official publication of the American College of Occupational and Environmental Medicine. In addition, many specialty journals frequently contain articles relevant to the occupational medicine practitioner, particularly in the areas of pulmonary medicine, dermatology, allergy, and rehabilitation medicine. A useful review of selected occupational medicine literature can be found in the monthly publication *Occupational and Environmental Medicine Report.* The report contains reviews and comments on articles of general interest to occupational and environmental medicine practitioners (see Further Information).

Table 35-2. Journals with Significant Occupational Medicine Content

American Industrial Hygiene Association Journal
American Journal of Industrial Medicine
American Journal of Preventive Medicine
American Journal of Public Health
American Review of Respiratory Diseases
Applied Occupational and Environmental Hygiene
Archives of Environmental Contamination and Toxicology
Archives of Environmental Health
Chest
Clinical Toxicology
Environmental Health Perspectives
Health Physics
International Archives of Occupational and Environmental Health
Journal of the American Medical Association
Journal of Occupational Medicine
Journal of Risk Analysis
Journal of Toxicology
Journal of Toxicology and Environmental Health
Occupational and Environmental Medicine (formerly British Journal of Industrial Medicine)
Occupational Health and Safety
Occupational Medicine (published by the Society of Occupational Medicine)
Preventive Medicine
Scandinavian Journal of Work Environment and Health

Computerized databases such as the National Library of Medicine's MEDLARS on-line network provide a rapid, efficient mechanism for literature searches and data retrieval for specific topics. MEDLARS is an on-line network of approximately 20 bibliographic databases. (See Chap. 27 for a guide to retrieving medical literature.) This service is available directly from the National Library of Medicine or via subscription to commercial on-line services. Many medical libraries offer literature search services or assistance in preparing a search. The *Index Medicus* remains a practical alternative for manual searches. For medical literature, MEDLINE provides an excellent resource within the MEDLARS System. Other databases of potential interest for more specialized searches include CANCERLIT (cancer literature), CHEMLINE (chemical dictionary on-line) for information on specific chemical substances, and TOXLINE (toxicology information on-line) for information related to published human and animal toxicity studies.

Another source of information on occupational medicine and related topics are digital databases contained on compact disks, read-only memory (CD-ROM). Using laser technology similar to the popular music and video compact discs, CD-ROMs can hold enormous amounts of information that can be rapidly accessed by a computer fitted with a CD-ROM player. Discs are commercially available that contain listings of OSHA regulations, toxicology data, and selected complete textbooks. CD-ROM and related technology are improving rapidly and promise to have a major impact on information transfer and accessibility in the future.

Information on computer programs and databases can also be obtained from the ACOEM Computers in Occupational Medicine Section, which publishes a *Directory of Occupational Safety and Health Software*. For information or a copy of the catalogue, write to the ACOEM Office (55 W. Seegers Rd., Arlington Heights, IL 60005).

Books and Other Reference Materials

A "recommended library" for occupational physicians, developed by the publications committee of the ACOEM Council on Education, is included in Appendix F. A useful series of quarterly monographs entitled *Occupational Medicine: State of the Art Reviews*, provide current information on selected topics. Each issue consists of an in-depth review of a specific subject, with contributions by experts in the field (see Further Information).

Conclusion

The actual educational training needed for the practice of occupational medicine varies and depends on factors such as previous experiences, current responsibilities, and access to opportunities. Residency training is ideal, although other forms of education, including the ACOEM core curriculum, provide an introduction to the discipline. Keeping abreast of journals and attending local and national professional society meetings can be an invaluable means to stay current and meet colleagues who face similar challenges.

References

1. Institute of Medicine. *Addressing the Physician Shortage in Occupational and Environmental Medicine*. Washington, DC: National Academy Press, 1991.
2. Rosenstock, L., et al. Occupational and environmental medicine. Meeting the growing need for clinical services. *N. Engl. J. Med.* 325:924, 1991.
3. Institute of Medicine. *Role of the Primary Care Physician in Occupational and Environmental Medicine*. Washington, DC: National Academy Press, 1988.
4. American Medical Association. *Directory of Graduate Medical Education Programs*. Chicago: AMA, 1992.
5. Mullen, R. J., and Murthy, L. I., Occupational sentinel health effects: An updated list for physician recognition and public health surveillance. *Am. J. Ind. Med.* 19:775, 1991.
6. McCunney, R. J. A hospital-based occupational medicine residency program. *J. Occup. Med.* (In press.)

7. DeHart, R. L. Establishing eligibility for examination in the specialty of occupational medicine. *J.O.M.* 28:303, 1986.

Further Information

Occupational and Environmental Medicine Report. Published by OEM Health Information, 181 Elliot St., Beverly, MA, (508) 921-7300, (800) 533-8046.

Published since 1987, this monthly periodical critiques occupational medicine–related articles that appear in a wide range of professional journals. Each issue includes a "Special Report" focused on a practical aspect of occupational medicine.

Occupational Medicine: State of the Art Reviews. Published by Hanley & Belfus, 210 South 13th St., Philadelphia, PA 19107, 800-962-1892.

This quarterly publication addresses occupational and environmental medical topics in considerable depth. Each issue includes at least 6 to 10 scholarly and academic articles on one particular topic such as medical surveillance or occupational lung disease.

Computers in Occupational Medical Practice

Kent W. Peterson,
Barry A. Cooper, and
Todd D. Kissam

Computers offer an ever-expanding set of opportunities to improve the quality and cost effectiveness of occupational medical (OM) services. Yet the task of deciding when and how to use a computer can be daunting for confirmed computer hackers and computer-phobics alike.

There are two basic uses of computers in occupational medical practice. The *first* is office automation involving the use of software programs for word processing, spreadsheet, project planning, graphics, client contact, communication, personal assistance, computer utilities and similar functions. These programs, which can be linked together through local- and wide-area networks, serve as basic building blocks of an information system and can prove extremely useful to the OM practitioner. They are described in other publications and are not discussed here [1] (see Further Information).

Occupational medical applications are the *second* use, with a growing number of database management systems being tailored to the occupational health user. Some are focused on a single purpose (e.g., generating random numbers for drug testing or preparing the Occupational Safety and Health Administration [OSHA] report of first injury). Others handle multiple purposes and are usually described as an occupational health information system (OHIS). These systems are commonly designed for occupational health clinic use, either by employers or clinics serving many clients. A growing number of companies are moving toward development of an integrated health data management system (IHDMS) linking data from many different corporate functions (e.g., personnel, benefits, environmental health, and safety).

This chapter discusses (1) the benefits of computerization, presenting two case studies that show OM computer applications; (2) the establishment of an OHIS based on clear understanding of user processes and specifications; (3) currently available occupational health and safety software; (4) practical guidelines for evaluating, selecting, or developing a system; and (5) the future direction of hardware and software for occupational health information management technology.

This chapter has three target audiences:

1. *Individuals who currently have a computer system in use in an occupational medical setting.* This group will be able to compare their systems to the state of the art by reading the sections on OHISs and future directions.
2. *Individuals who are planning to purchase/develop a system.* This group will benefit by reading the entire chapter to understand how computers can help, what system components are available, and what the pros and cons are of different approaches to obtaining a system.
3. *Individuals without immediate plans to utilize a system.* This group will gain an understanding of future trends and when an OHIS would be appropriate for their situation.

Benefits of Computerization and Applications

Advantages of Automation

A growing number of corporate employers, hospitals, clinics, and consultants rely on computers for their practice management. The following list provides insight into some of the advantages they are experiencing.

Clerical costs at one clinic were reduced by 30% when it switched to a computerized clinic management system.

At many clinics, data entered once are now automatically incorporated into dozens of documents at multiple sites, without error.

Data from thousands of medical records are analyzed by providers to gain a greater understanding of individual practice profiles.

An OM clinic gained new business, due, in part, to its reputation for providing quick follow-up reports in a clear, standardized format.

A corporate medical director was able to target program interventions and demonstrate their cost effectiveness through an IHDMS.

Computers are quickly becoming essential management tools with valued applications in all aspects of OM. The use of a successful OHIS can significantly improve an organization's ability to achieve its goals through (1) improved efficiency and productivity, (2) enhanced quality and decision making (3) regulatory compliance and litigation assistance, and (4) the ability to inexpensively create additional supplemental and new services.

Efficiency, Accuracy, and Productivity

Tasks are accomplished faster and cheaper, with significant staffing economies possible. The consequent improvements in efficiency and accuracy result in greater productivity than that obtained using manual methods.

Computers provide users with instant access to vast amounts of data organized in a variety of standardized and customized formats. Using relational databases, information can be entered once and automatically duplicated in designated data fields on command. Standard forms and reports can be regularly generated to meet highly specific requirements. Efficiencies can also be achieved through direct electronic interface of test equipment and calculation programs, which help reduce errors while enhancing speed.

Warning: Many companies justify the implementation of an OHIS on the basis of projected cost savings from potential staffing cuts due to increased efficiency. A successful OHIS does increase efficiency, but affected staff are generally not eliminated. They are, instead, reassigned to other tasks that could not be accomplished previously.

Enhanced Quality and Decision Making

An OHIS can prove a valuable tool that provides higher levels of quality assurance and professional decision making than manual methods do. This is a tangible benefit that most companies undervalue when generating their OHIS requirements.

For example, the quality of decision making can improve by allowing more time and more immediate access to relevant information. Through the computer's powerful ability to organize and present data, managers and clinicians can analyze information from a variety of perspectives. The more quickly and easily data are transformed into information, the more effectively they can be used in analysis and in the development of more thoughtful decisions.

Regulatory Compliance and Litigation Assistance

With sophisticated computer-assisted analytical and reporting capabilities, regulatory compliance programs are more likely to remain on track, avoiding costly fines, penalties, and investigations. Litigation costs may also be reduced due to improved reporting and documentation, although some legal challenges continue regarding the admissibility of electronic medical records.

Provision of Supplemental Services

The use of an OHIS allows organizations to provide supplemental services with little additional cost. Virtually all OHIS components have a database kernel, which means that once a service is provided to an individual, the results of that service (the data) are stored in the computer within a database (an easy accessible file). Relational databases allow supplemental services to be provided to groups for almost no additional cost.

For example, for a hearing conservation program, after the computer has printed participant letters, the computer database can easily generate lists of participants who require medical follow-up, lists of participants who need education on hearing protection, and, if the needed data are available, a financial analysis of potential fiscal liability based on hearing test results and other analyses.

Occupational Clinic Management

To illustrate the favorable impact that computer technology can create for an OM practice, and some problems that the lack of such technology can create, we can compare the management of a typical work-related injury/illness in two clinics. One is a traditional clinic using manual systems; the other, a more automated clinic using state-of-the-art computer technology. In our examples, an employee, who had recently received a preplacement examination at the clinic, shows up without prior notice with an acute medical problem.

At the Traditional Industrial Medicine Clinic (TIMC), the patient is asked for much of the same information provided at his earlier visit. Retrieval of the medical record causes more delays because of a chronic filing backup. The admitting clerk completes several different records and forms, many calling for duplicative information, and makes a clerical error when copying a telephone number. Eventually, the patient is seen and a call is placed apprising the employer of the nature of the injury and the expected return-to-work date.

Client and insurance billing will be delayed as a consequence of the error. This will cause the employer significant inconvenience and exacerbate the TIMC's cash flow problems.

This example illustrates the following problems:

The patient is inconvenienced and treatment delayed. He wonders why the clinic is "so inefficient" when he is in so much pain.

His confidence in the clinic's quality of care is slightly diminished.

Due to the urgency of the case, a clinic physician begins treatment without the benefit of prior test results. When the medical record finally arrives, a revised treatment plan must be established, causing costly inefficiencies.

The clerk has become distressed because she is "continually behind in her paperwork." Her errors have become increasingly frequent and costly.

Chronic delays in the preparation of billing and insurance forms are causing serious problems for the clinic and its clients. Although these delays are caused by a variety of human factors (e.g., physician reluctance to complete forms), an OHIS could substantially improve overall efficiency.

A similar case is being treated at the State-Of-The-Art clinic (SOTA) across the street. This clinic's admitting clerk simply types the patient's name into the computer, confirms the identification number, locates the point in the database, and is able to automatically generate needed information and forms. These forms were streamlined during the intensive review that accompanied computerization. The patient is promptly evaluated and treated. Later in the visit, the treating physician enters a memo to the employer's workers' compensation manager regarding the nature of the injury and the expected return-to-work date. Once completed, this communication is instantaneously sent to the employer and its insurance company, who share an electronic data interchange network for the routine exchange of such information.

On completion of the visit, OSHA billing and insurance forms are automatically generated based on the *International Classification of Diseases,* 9th edition (ICD-9) and the *Current Procedural Terminology,* 4th edition (CPT-4) coding entered as part of the medical record. The clinic's accounts receivable file is updated, along with related financial statistics.

Although the SOTA's clinic management system develops occasional patient backlogs, these problems are far less severe because of their comprehensive OHIS. Thus, computerization has had the following impact:

The patient completes the paperwork more quickly, although he still wonders why he must complete forms when he is in discomfort.

Accuracy is enhanced because there are no copying errors; basic information is entered once and automatically shows up on subsequent applications.

Access to medical records is easier, because much of the task is automated.

Clients and insurers are better served through automated preparation of needed forms.

Financial management runs smoothly, with more timely billings and collections.

On the downside, the high level of automation has led the clinic to rely on written communications without personal staff follow-up.

This example suggests some of the more obvious benefits of using the computer in record keeping, forms, and financial management. It also alludes to the problems that can occur when there is an overreliance on automated processes, illustrated by the clinic's sending a follow-up employer memo without an accompanying personal telephone call.

Occupational Health Information Systems

Evolution of OHISs During 1970–1990

The development of OHISs has paralleled the evolution of general computer-based information systems.

First-Generation Mainframe Systems

The first generation of OHISs came on-line in the 1970s. Because these systems were mainframe based, only the largest companies could afford the millions of dollars for hardware and the even more millions for software development. Some of these companies tried to recoup their investment by selling the software to other companies. This tactic met with limited success because of lack of flexibility in meeting other companies' needs.

Most of these systems were large data storehouses. Tons of data (and money) were put in these systems, but limited provisions were made for getting the data out in usable form. This fatal flaw caused most systems to fail. Even extensive modification of these systems could not fully meet the users' needs, so these systems had to be scrapped. Mainframe systems that have survived use database software.

All mainframes (and their systems) have a closed architecture, which is proprietary to a single company and not accessible for outside vendors to use or enhance. The specifications are protected by patents. In an open-architecture system, the plans and specifications for the computer hardware are in the public domain, so any vendor can reproduce or improve the hardware. As a result of competitive pressure involved with open systems, they are cheaper and will continue to get even more so.

It was during this period that medical departments began to become prisoners of their data processing departments. When these departments implemented an OHIS, they applied the same methodology of back-charges used for other departments (e.g., accounting or engineering). This charge-back method turns data processing departments into internal profit centers, allowing them to build an empire by showing how much money they are making instead of answering to the criticism of how much money they are costing. The result was that most medical departments were charged for every page printed and for every medical record stored or accessed. One large chemical company's data processing department charged $1.65 each time a medical record was looked at. Instead of having a system that encouraged use and thereby increased the efficiency of the department, the system discouraged use by punishing the user.

Second-Generation Mini-Computer Systems

The second generation of OHISs came on-line in the late 1970s through the 1980s. In recognition of the limitations of proprietary, single-purpose mainframe systems, second-generation OHISs were based on mini-computers, which are cheaper than mainframes and easier to use, but not as powerful. Hospitals, mid-size companies, and the largest clinics and consultants could afford mini-computer hardware, but few could afford the investment in generating the software to create an OHIS.

Some mini-computer OHISs used early database technology, acquiring flexibility to meet different client needs. Unfortunately, the price of customization was prohibitive, and mini-computers did not allow a migration path that took advantage of new developments in database and PC technology.

Although mini-computers have a closed architecture, by using a UNIX operating system, they can allow the software to be independent of the hardware (see the section on future directions).

Third-Generation Micro-Computers

PCs, or micro-computers, first appeared in the 1970s, with the IBM PC (and compatibles and MacIntoshes) appearing in the 1980s. PCs were the first systems with inexpensive connections to modems, scanners, medical testing equipment, CD-ROM, etc. This has greatly enhanced the usability of these systems. The IBM-compatible PC represents an open architecture.

In the past decade, PCs and Macs have gained power at a rate never seen before in the computer industry. This increase of power and the ever-lower prices have resulted in the sale of over 100 million PCs and in increased software technology being available for PCs. The marketplace is so large that over 100,000 software packages are available.

OHISs have been implemented on both stand-alone and networked PCs. Most of these systems now use databases with fourth-generation languages. This results in more flexibility as well as in cheaper systems.

As the hardware has evolved from mainframe to mini to micro, the politics of OHISs has also evolved. Systems have migrated from being data processing–controlled to user-controlled. This shift has caused turf wars between the medical and other departments and the central data processing department within companies. This requires the OHIS user to become not only more technically competent but also more politically savvy.

Managed Care and the Growth of Information Management

Nowhere is the role of computers in OM more dramatic than in the managed care arena. As technology gets more sophisticated, elaborate expert systems can be applied to individual practice decisions. Expert systems are "rule-based" computer programs that can make sophisticated decisions while continually improving their performance based on the rules or principles programmed into them. If properly managed, these systems can contribute to sorely needed quality improvement and cost-containment initiatives. If poorly managed, they can prove counterproductive and limit the individual provider's ability to practice good medicine.

Understanding and responding to these fast-changing developments have become imperative for many providers as sophisticated systems are used to improve workers' compensation or short and long-term disability management. By applying utilization review and case management techniques previously used exclusively for major illnesses and injuries, computers are now being applied to more common OM cases, such as cumulative trauma disorders.

As the gatekeepers of a disability management system judged out of control (workers' compensation costs alone topped $70 billion in 1993), OM providers can be central players in a growing cost-containment movement that recognizes that wage-related benefit expenses are inexorably linked to medical decisions and costs. Large self-insured companies, major insurers and third-party administrators, a new generation of workers' compensation preferred provider organizations (PPOs), state workers' compensation systems, and a growing number of vendors and service companies are increasingly turning to computer-assisted solutions to stem the perceived cost crisis.

The new technology of OM managed care is beginning to take shape. It features utilization review and case management programs supported by medical guidelines, protocols, and databases. The medical community's charge is to use these sophisticated tools to help ensure the cost-effective delivery of care, carefully monitoring both resource use and quality.

The guidelines, protocols, and systems are usually based on ICD-9 and CPT-4 codes. Some are keyed to job demands and capabilities measures. Computerized case management systems can feature disability duration guidelines, medical protocols, and sophisticated scheduling and follow-up programs. They are increasingly available commercially through administrative services contracts, licensure, or as part of insurer and third-party–administered services. Ideally, as these tools evolve, they will also include coded elements of the history, physical, laboratory findings, and imaged x-rays, EKGs, and other documents.

The full impact of these developments on the practice of OM remains to be seen. Current systems do not provide sufficient information to establish the correct diagnosis and procedure. Further, forward-looking organizations recognize the variability of each case and the importance of individual patient reactions to psychosocial factors and treatment interventions. However, there have also been disturbing examples of the results of high technology being inappropriately applied in a field that defies simple solutions (e.g., overzealous case managers insisting that employees return to work by a designated date based on the use of absence duration guidelines).

The caveats are clear. The technology available through computer programs should be used to assist knowledgeable professionals to do their jobs more efficiently and accurately. Guidelines should be used as reference points—not to make complex, subjective decisions. A hierarchical decision-making process can help to ensure that the most appropriate professionals are involved in authorizing exceptions to expert system-generated recommendations. In a typical model, a registered nurse case manager with access to medical guidelines and treatment protocols is responsible for determining when additional input is needed (e.g., from a physician or vocational rehabilitation specialist).

Most clinical protocols are based on proprietary criteria, often not subject to public scrutiny or peer review. Yet, collectively, they may ultimately establish a new paradigm. As this technology evolves, the medical profession has a stake in ensuring that valid guidelines are developed and that they are applied with proper professional oversight.

Integrated Health Data Management Systems

Larger progressive corporations are turning to IHDMSs for help in making complex decisions. Implementation of an IHDMS can help to prevent unnecessary duplication of effort, foster coordination among units, and provide a clearer picture of the company's health expenditures and priorities. These systems may include disability and general health benefits; OM, wellness, and safety programs; and related databases (e.g., personnel) that cut across departmental lines for employees, dependents, and retirees.

It is important for the corporate medical department to take a central role as an IHDMS develops. Optimally, the medical director should assume a leadership role in the description of processes and user specifications (see below) to be supported by the system, ensuring that high-priority programs are included. Opportunities to better target and evaluate OM programs should be developed, with consideration given to systematically reengineering critical processes to ensure that they optimally contribute to the organization's mission and support departmental goals. Team-building processes inherent in establishing and maintaining an IHDMS should be employed in other aspects of corporate management. Minimally, the medical department should work with other departments and key vendors to help ensure that their computer systems evolve compatibly.

In the absence of an IHDMS, corporate health professionals should consider the need for establishing one. If a full system is not feasible, partial integration may be realistic. A workgroup should set out to review company and vendor databases with an eye to optimizing their utility.

OM clinic managers should be aware of opportunities to assist client corporations as they work toward health data system integration. For some clients, this will mean providing systems design assistance, while others may benefit from more active clinic participation in day-to-day data management and exchange. Clinics providing ongoing services to corporations have a vested interest in ensuring that the net effectiveness of their services is not masked by cost-shifting or tracking errors.

Establishing a Comprehensive OHIS/IHDMS

Developing an OHIS requires a clear understanding of the processes to be supported. Well-conceived user specifications will help ensure that the system will perform the necessary functions required. This is true for either off-the-shelf software programs or those developed in-house. If the system is to be custom-built, either by an in-house department or by consultants, system developers should develop preliminary system specifications documents based on the detailed user specification statement. This will help ensure that essential OM processes are optimally assisted by the software.

The following steps should be carefully considered (also see the section on practical guidelines for evaluating, selecting and/or developing software).

1. Identify the needs of each system user and follow through with precise requirements. The overall requirements for a system are generated from these needs.
    Example: A *need* is for the system to support a hearing conservation program by generating letters to employees who have had a temporary hearing threshold shift. A *requirement* is to generate up to 50 letters per day within 20 working days of the audio testing. Additional precise requirements would add the fol-

lowing qualifier: The system needs to generate up to 50 letters per day and be received by the employee (at home) within 20 working days of the audio testing for a cost (including data entry, processing, and quality control) not to exceed $2.00 per employee tested.

2. Employ a multidisciplinary approach in generating user specifications and system requirements. Requirements need to be generated by a task force with representatives of all affected departments in order to help ensure that systems will support commonly agreed upon processes and specifications.

3. Evaluate the implemented system against the goals/requirements. What if requirements are not met? What is the schedule for their implementation? The requirements need to be concise and complete enough so that the successes and the faults of the system are easily recognized.

4. Budget sufficient funds for on-going system modification. Unfortunately, most systems are never finished. Finishing the last 10% of a system can represent 50% of the entire systems cost, yet this last 10% frequently separates success from failure.

5. Build in flexibility to adjust to changes over time. (Here's where relational databases prove valuable.) If the system cannot adapt to a changing organization, then the system has failed. Restructuring, downsizing, acquisitions, new product development, and new business directions need to be part of the requirement discussions. "How will the system perform if . . . happens?" needs to be part of the finished requirements. This is another reason for a multidisciplinary approach.

6. Develop systems by using an open architecture to help ensure OHIS hardware and software flexibility. "Closed" systems can restrict flexibility and increase the ultimate cost of the system.

Components of an OHIS/IHDMS

Below, we discuss the many possible components of a comprehensive OHIS/IHDMS. Many of these components can be integrated within a single structured relational database or set of related relational databases sharing properly coded data elements to make retrieval and comparison possible.

General Office Automation

One of the most important components of an OHIS system—indeed, perhaps the most important component—is support of the office staff in the pursuit of everyday tasks. Document preparation (word processing), spreadsheets, contact and time managers, project timelines, and electronic mail are all important parts of general office automation support. Without integration of these functions, the OHIS may not be used. Most users already have these support programs on their desktop computers, and they do not want to (1) learn new systems, (2) have two computers on their desk, or (3) leave their desk in order to do their job.

Personnel Data

Almost every OHIS will require information about the company (e.g., sites) and employees (e.g., name, mailing address, date of birth, gender, social security number, and other demographic information). Because of employee turnover or relocation, this information must be able to be easily updated, indicating the last date information was changed. The most sophisticated systems now use data from company personnel databases, either through periodic "extracts" or from real-time linkages, where the actual data are stored in the personnel database.

Benefits Information

In an era of medical cost containment, linkage with benefits information can be valuable. Such information may include medically related absence and use of sick leave, health care utilization, workers' compensation, general health claims and costs, and detection of occult occupational diseases that are being treated by the general medical community.

Work History and Job Tracking

Current job titles, classifications, and prior job histories can become especially important in *medical surveillance studies* where test results or health outcomes are monitored for all workers in particular jobs, or those with selected exposures. Job histories can be particularly important when employees at the same locations are used as a control group to compare against workers exposed to hazardous substances.

Functional Job Requirements

Compliance with the Americans with Disabilities Act (ADA) requires OM professionals to have more information than a current job title. Understanding functional job requirements—including physical, psychological, social, and environmental demands—becomes critical in medical assessment. Such descriptions should distinguish between essential and marginal job functions. This area can be managed with a relatively simple computer application. Specialized software is available to help develop functional job requirements.

Job Capabilities and Work Restrictions

Traditionally, OM professionals have identified employee work restrictions (e.g., "unable to lift more than 50 lb," "blind," "sensitized to TDI [toluene diisocyanate]," or "may not operate hazardous equipment requiring use of upper extremities"). Job restrictions have often been systematized for use in medical or personnel information systems. The ADA challenges OM professionals to state an individual's capabilities rather than limitations (e.g., "able to lift up to 50 lb," "can be exposed to dust if uses a respirator," "can stand for 2 hours before requiring a 15-minute rest"). Contemporary systems will also list reasonable job accommodations.

Appointment Scheduling

In busy OM clinics, computerized appointment scheduling is a valuable asset, and can issue reminder and follow-up notices to employees and facilitate tracking those who miss scheduled appointments. Such a system can also schedule future appointment dates for people requiring periodic medical evaluations.

Regulatory Requirements

Through simple automated text-retrieval systems, computers can help track current company policies and state or federal medical requirements, including the periodicity of required examination procedures.

Medical Record Keeping and Retrieval

Computerized systems can summarize dates of past examinations and appointments, leaving actual medical information in hard copy or electronically imaged records. OM clinics are automating critically important information. A number of employers have actually adopted paperless medical records. Coding of health history (see below) and physical findings can significantly increase the value of these systems, but this development may be resisted by many clinicians who insist on using free text notes. The question of whether the electronic medical record is admissible as evidence in legal proceedings should be explored prior to converting from paper records. Procedures such as storing backup paper medical records signed by the health professional should be considered.

Health History

Most medical histories are completed on paper; however, key historical information is often entered into computers for archiving and comparison over time. Many employers have developed optically scannable health histories; some medical departments use interactive health histories. Interactive histories allow hundreds of questions to be included in a branching tree format, designed so that each employee only sees a fraction of the total available items. This approach requires use of key branch points (e.g., gender, use of tobacco, or key symptoms for each organ system). Automating health history information can help assure appropriate medical follow-up of positive symptoms, can even direct the physical examiner to do the most beneficial, cost-effective physical exam procedures, and can allow tailoring of periodic examinations to individual risk.

Medical Examination Results

Occupationally relevant test results are often automated (e.g., audiometry, spirometry, vision, respiratory fit, EKG, x-ray, specialized occupational tests, and the hands-on physical examination). Immunizations and medical treatment can be included as well. Automation allows comparison of results over time, and calculations, such as temporary threshold shifts for hearing, can be automatic. The computerization of medical examination results and related surveillance activities can be optimized by ensuring that they meet user specifications.

Health screening technology is moving toward direct computer interface of screening equipment, allowing greater efficiencies, immediate quality control, and even comparison with prior results at the time of testing.

Medical Problems and Treatments
As clinical care has moved toward the problem-oriented health record, master problem lists are increasingly sought. A problem-oriented occupational health record can include important medical diagnoses, required job-related examinations, medical surveillance, respirator clearance, risk factors, and other key information. Computers can be used to support this function through the use of coded problem lists.

Injury Monitoring and Management
Many computer systems record the federal and state OSHA reports of first injury or illness, generating forms to assure regulatory compliance. Tracking injuries by location and job can identify high-risk situations in need of follow-up and monitor patterns of injury and illness.

Case Management, Tracking, and Follow-Up
As disability costs skyrocket, computers are used to monitor absence and to compare absence against anticipated duration codes, flagging individuals whose absence has exceeded a threshold (i.e., outliers). Increasingly, these systems help to manage cases proactively in cooperation with clinical providers. Case managers seek computer support to help contact workers and supervisors, monitor clinical care, record anticipated return-to-work dates, schedule independent medical evaluations, and record free-text notes.

Health Promotion and Health Risk Appraisal
Automating risk factor information such as blood pressure, cholesterol, weight, fitness, and smoking status can assist health promotion programs. For example, individuals at high risk can be identified for targeted follow-up, health education mailings, and scheduled revisits. Computerized health risk appraisal ranges from inexpensive public domain software to highly sophisticated commercially available systems. Aggregate reports profile the health status of a population and can even project health benefit expenses related to modified risk factors. Specialized programs include diet and nutrition analysis, fitness evaluation, body composition, and stress profiles.

Drug and Alcohol Testing
Random drug testing requires use of random number generators to select individuals for testing on short notice. Specialized programs track individuals in a pool eligible for testing, urine collection procedures, laboratory test results, medical review of positive findings, and reporting of verified results to the employer. The extreme need for data security demands a high level of care in automating such information.

Employee Assistance Programs (EAP)
Separate medical records are often kept by EAP counselors. Automated EAP systems or EAP components of an OHIS with restricted access allow generation of activity reports, tracking and follow-up of individuals, and group reporting for evaluation purposes.

Medical Surveillance
A medical surveillance module tracks required examinations and assures that every employee has been tested. This can link to appointment scheduling systems and record pertinent test results.

Chemical Inventory
Manufacturers and users of chemicals must track chemicals used to comply with the OSHA Hazard Communication Standard (HazCom). More than 50,000 different chemicals are used in the United States. Tracking the ingredients of mixtures is challenging, especially when formulations are proprietary. This information is often linked to OHIS.

Exposure Monitoring
Because industrial hygiene measurements generate a high volume of data, they have become increasingly automated. Potentially hazardous substances, appropriate measurement techniques, required periodicity of sampling, and actual measured

exposures are included. Eight-hour time-weighted average exposures can be easily calculated. By linking industrial hygiene data with job and personnel information, individuals requiring medical surveillance can be identified. Flags can be set to identify any area exceeding allowable exposures, either by company action levels or by external standards. Workplace exposures can be tracked by location or groups of individuals.

Toxicology Information

Under the OSHA HazCom, employers must compile and make available to employees copies of Material Safety Data Sheets (MSDSs). Many companies have automated this information for substances that they manufacture, and a number of vendors have compiled large numbers of MSDSs. CD-ROM or telecommunications links to large databases allow rapid access to MSDSs and other toxicology information. These databases include CHEMINFO, Regulatory Information on Pesticides Products (RIPP), Transport of Dangerous Goods (TDG)/hazardous materials (49 Code of Federal Regulations), Chemical Evaluations Search and Retrieval System (CESARS), the National Institute for Occupational Safety and Health (NIOSH) Registry of Toxic Effects of Chemical Substances (RTECS), the Combined Health Information Database (CHID) of the National Institutes of Health, and the Superfund Amendments and Reauthorization Act (SARA) Title III.

Safety

Information frequently tracked by computer includes personnel protective equipment issued, employee training (e.g., hazard communication), audits and inspections, and fire and other safety information.

Administrative and Financial Information

OM clinics require information on clients, services rendered, invoicing, accounts payable and receivable, direct and indirect revenues, and other financial reports. Billing can be complicated when employers want a single consolidated invoice for multiple services provided by different elements of a hospital or clinic.

Analytic and Reporting Capabilities

While most OHISs still function largely as passive electronic storage cabinets, they must be able to report data in a variety of flexible formats. Increasingly, computer systems add features such as error checking, determining if values are beyond acceptable ranges and flagging situations that require follow-up. As total quality management becomes woven throughout OM, software systems are beginning to track variation in provider performance (e.g., variation in absence duration for selected conditions by provider). Systems are beginning to incorporate "decision support technology," which prompts the provider to make appropriate decisions. Examples include medical practice guidelines and protocols, such as those for diagnosing, treating, monitoring, and managing low back pain and soft-tissue injuries. Most OHIS products come with formatted standard reports. Customized reports generated by the user using ad hoc queries must be able to be easily generated.

Epidemiologic Analysis

The most demanding reporting capabilities are those of epidemiologic analysis. Epidemiologic studies require correlation of many data elements (e.g., numerator as well as denominator information on employee populations). Often test results or health outcomes are compared to workplace exposures or jobs. Standard and proportional mortality ratios require tracking of appropriate disease coding for all deaths. Cancer registries have often been maintained by selected industries that manufacture or use toxic substances. Software is available to help code medical diagnosis by ICD-9 or CPT-4.

Linkage to Other Systems and Databases

Increasingly, clinics and employers are moving toward the integration of health data within OHISs or IHDMSs. Users must consider whether data from inexpensive, single-purpose software programs can be imported into larger integrated systems. Similarly, occupational health clinic users may need to obtain selected data and share it with other corporate databases for purposes of industrial hygiene monitoring, chemical inventories, and safety and personnel data management.

Currently Available Software

Most occupational health and safety software products currently available fall into several general categories.

Multipurpose/Integrated Health Data Management Systems

Fewer than a dozen large-scale systems are available that track personnel, medical, industrial hygiene, safety, toxicology/MSDS, and, occasionally, benefits information. During the past decade, a number of expensive integrated systems have dropped out of the marketplace. These were mostly mainframe systems using second-generation database management software. The few surviving systems and most newer IHDMSs require mainframes or mini-computers. However, some systems now operate on a PC platform, with workstations linked by PC networks. Full-scale IHDMSs can cost many millions of dollars to develop, with licensing fees usually exceeding $100,000.

Clinic Management/Tracking/Medical Records/ Administration Systems

A second category of commercial software addresses the more focused needs of OM clinics. Almost two dozen commercial software programs are available, on PC platforms. Most include demographic and administrative information, appointment scheduling, injury/illness care and absence tracking, reporting capabilities, clinical results, accounting, and financial management. Some include alcohol and drug testing, hazard exposure and other environmental information, and ergonomics capabilities. Since most vendors have fewer than 100 installed clients, no software is dominant. Of interest is the continual entry of new software products into this competitive arena. Clinic management systems licensing fees are usually in the $5 to $25,000 range, with smaller annual maintenance/renewal fees.

Health Screening

A variety of much smaller software programs focus on health screening. Examples include human immunodeficiency virus testing, audiometric data storage and analysis, drug screening, pulmonary function, and respirator use. These programs usually cost a few thousand dollars.

Injury, Absence, and Disability Management/ADA Compliance

More than a dozen software products now focus on injury reporting and disability management, a rapidly burgeoning field. These range from simple programs that complete OSHA 200 Logs or provide absence duration guidelines to full-scale disability case management systems that support case managers.

Chemical and Environmental

Dozens of programs have been developed for safety, industrial hygiene, toxicology, emergency response, and environmental medicine needs. Many provide rapid access to large chemical databases by use of CD-ROM or telecommunications linkages. Others enable employers to comply with federal regulations, including OSHA, SARA II, and the Toxic Substances Control Act (TSCA). Some are PC based and others require mini- or mainframe computers.

Epidemiology/Statistical Analysis/Decision Support

More than 50 low-cost epidemiologic analysis software packages exist. Most of these build upon standard statistical analysis capabilities, but are tailored to the needs of epidemiologists.

Health Promotion/Fitness/Ergonomics

Almost a dozen software programs are available that perform health risk appraisal; most use algorithms promulgated by the Centers for Disease Control or the more recent Emory University Carter Center Update. A few have a more sophisticated risk computation science base and provide communication that motivates health behavior change. Other health promotion software performs dietary nutrition analysis, fitness evaluation, and ergonomics assessment, focused on the spine and upper extremities.

Bibliography/Education/Other

Software programs can track bibliographic information and medical references. They also provide health education information, drug information, computer-aided instruction, and continuing education with continuing medical education credit.

Practical Guidelines for Evaluating, Selecting, and/or Developing Software

The following recommendations are based on the authors' combined experience of over 50 years in the OM application of computers. This experience is spread over both consultations to, employment by, and management of corporations that were involved in implementing OHISs.

Evaluating and Selecting Software

1. *Define clearly your needs and intended use.* As is so often true in life, knowing yourself can make the critical difference in selecting one product over another. As the great American philosopher Moon Mullins once said, "If you don't know where you're going, any road will do." It is here that a clear understanding of user processes and specifications should begin.

   Areas to address include

   Program objectives, e.g., regulatory compliance, patient scheduling, tracking and billing, information storage and ready access, employee education, behavior change

   Users, e.g., degree of computer sophistication at all levels—end users, operators, systems managers

   Use, e.g., stand-alone task or part of integrated department or company-wide IHDMS

   Feedback: What specific information will be needed? What reports?

   Resources available—personnel, computers, software, other users

   Size of operation and volume of data processing

   Speed and turnaround time: How quickly are data entry and reports needed? Could data entry/processing be done off-site?

   Group data needs—management reports, measures of success

   Clear identification of needs can save a lot of time by helping to eliminate many products. Consider the analogy of house hunting: What would happen if a realtor had to show a buyer every property on the market? An internal or external consultant can help enormously.

2. *Explore the various available software packages and make the buy/build decision.* Evaluate your options in terms of how they meet your needs. Most vendors are product oriented (i.e., they will try to sell you what they have to offer, convincing you that they have just what you need). Look around thoroughly and be aware of the range of choices. None may suit your needs exactly and, hence, the potential need for customization. Even if one product meets your purposes today, your needs are likely to evolve, and the software must follow suit or be discarded. On the other hand, developing even the simplest program from scratch is fraught with hazard (e.g., time, money, and the frustration of re-creating the wheel). There is no magic bullet. If you elect to build your own software program, check the literature and contact organizations that have developed their own. Always become familiar with

commercially available alternatives and conduct a cost-benefit analysis before embarking on a major program development effort. Enlist the participation of other departments and establish an integrated program as appropriate. Beware of the many pitfalls of developing a system, described in the next section.

3. *Try out the software thoroughly and contact current users* once you are in the ball park. No amount of talking or reading of marketing materials will substitute for making arrangements with a vendor to have a few hours of actual hands-on work at the keyboard. Having a demonstration at an existing user site can be instructive. Run a number of sample employees, patients, examinations, or industrial hygiene measurements through the system; put it through the paces. Every vendor uses examples that put its best foot forward. What about the typical person in your intended audience? Try to discover the limitations of the system you are considering. Talk with several experienced users of the product.

4. *Look carefully at the organization and the key people* with whom you will be dealing. How long has the organization been in existence and what is its history? Is it stable? What is its financial condition? Will it be able to provide continued support after the next recession? How many clients does it have? How large is its programming staff? Are the annual renewal fees and number of current customers sufficient to support a programming staff? How long have the actual programmers worked with the vendor? What are the backgrounds and qualifications of the principals and of those with whom you will be dealing on a day-to-day basis? This is important because although many purchasers believe they are buying a product, in reality, they are buying a service and a relationship. Like most relationships, the true test comes after the purchase when the sky is dark, the winds are blowing, and hailstones are falling. Talk to other clients who will have similar uses as you. Does the organization come through and deliver as promised?

5. *Review the sample contract or agreement.* Are field tests, trial use of software, and a money-back guarantee offered if the system doesn't work or if you are not satisfied? Look at users' manuals and documentation; find out what kind of training, customer support, and software support is available. Is remote support provided, for example, linking your computer directly to the vendor's modem? Will you have access to the source code, possibly in an escrow account held by a third party, in case the company goes out of business?

6. *Is there enough flexibility to meet your needs?* Perhaps an off-the-shelf product is all you need. You may well want to customize things later on, however; this may be simple or complex, costing tens of thousand of dollars. For example, how easy is it to add variables (e.g., new questions to a questionnaire), to telecommunicate, or to export data for external storage or processing? What is the organization's track record in customizing its product for other clients? How close to budget and time did it come? What about data analysis, storage, transfer, software limitations, import/export capabilities, and compatibility?

7. *Look closely at group data as a valuable resource.* What group reports are available, and do they report what you need; for example, can they report employees by location, payroll code, job class, or other variables? Will they give you what you need to present to management, for example, on the health or illness of a defined population, or the potential cost savings or degree of improvement over time? What data summarization and query capabilities exist, and how complex is the query language? Many million-dollar systems have been developed or purchased without adequate consideration being given to analysis and reporting. How easy is report generation? Can you design your own reports without needing software customization?

8. *Regulatory compliance.* Does software meet current OSHA and other regulatory requirements? Does the vendor keep abreast of regulations?

Working with a Software Vendor

Once you have decided to purchase or develop a software system, the next challenge is how to work more effectively with a vendor or developer.

1. *Know your needs well; plan the program completely.* Again, the most important single thing you can do is to think through your needs as clearly as possible at the beginning. Plan the whole program as well as you can. It not only helps you to select the correct software package in the first place but aids enormously along the way. As health care professionals, we tend to be crisis oriented. Yet it often comes as a

surprise to hear we help create crisis around us. Careful planning—doing it right the first time—usually prevents turmoil and wasted effort, netting a large saving of time and money. For example, if you are asked to cost-justify a program or show its effectiveness in the workplace, you are more likely to succeed if the right data are collected from the beginning.

2. *Make your needs clear to internal developers and information system specialists.* Information system specialists can often help you think through program options and make good choices at the beginning (e.g., data needed for later program evaluation). However, manage their consultation. Beware of data processing departments motivated to extend or consolidate their empire.

3. *Clarify what you are buying.* What comes with the package and what will cost extra? What other services can the vendor provide? The price may never be lower than when you are negotiating the first dollar spent. What will cost extra? Get clarification in writing on such features as assistance in program design and evaluation, data analysis, graphics, and reporting.

4. *Cross-train two people to be liaisons with the vendor.* If you have multiple sites using software, it is useful to have all go through one coordinator. Developing in-house competence will become an asset. Have more than one person trained, however, so there is backup support in case of illness, absence, early retirement, or job transfer.

5. *Clarify customer support, periodic updates, and annual fees.* Be clear as to what services are covered under the basic licensing/purchase fee and what costs extra. Be willing to pay annual maintenance fees. Make certain that the vendor has a sufficient ongoing revenue stream to maintain the software and continuously improve it. You want to make sure that your vendor is in business in the future.

6. *Get to know the people; build a positive relationship.* Offer your questions, comments, and suggestions freely. The squeaky wheel gets the oil. More important, an interested customer can bring out the best in a software team.

Future Directions for Occupational Health Information Management Technology

In the information age, data become power, a form of currency. Unfortunately, OM is not at the forefront of this powerful new technology.

Quick access to the right information is the goal of all computer-based information systems. Currently, there are no standardized building blocks for assembling information age OHISs. The technologies described below represent the foundation stones of these building blocks. It may be 3 to 4 years before the foundation is complete and an OHIS/IHDMS begins to reach its full potential.

Legal Climate and Regulation

Food and Drug Administration Regulation of Medical Software

The Food and Drug Administration (FDA) has filed a position paper that would require all computer software and hardware that directly interact with a patient without a human as a gatekeeper to go through FDA approval. This measure predominantly affects medical instrumentation manufacturers. The position paper responds to severe injuries and several fatalities associated with automated radiation therapy device systems.

This policy will not affect an OHIS as long as a gatekeeper is involved. *Example:* Consider a system for hearing conservation that automatically interfaces the audiometer to the computer system that generates the follow-up letters. If the audio results are entered into the system without being flashed on the screen for technician acceptance or rejection (without a human seeing them first), the system would be subject to FDA approval.

Reasonable Accommodation Under the ADA

The ADA requires employers to provide accessible telephone and computer systems to employees, if needed, and to provide reasonable job accommodations. Potential enhancements for an OHIS might include image intensification of forms and video display terminals, and speech recognition for the visually impaired. The Job Accommodation Network, at 800-526-7234, is an excellent resource on available technology.

Computer Hardware

Growing Capacity and Shrinking Size

To appreciate the benefits of computer technology, consider that if the car had evolved like the computer chip, today's Rolls Royce would cost $100 and allow you to drive 10,000 years on one tank of gas.

Computer processors are doubling to tripling in performance every 3 years. In order to increase speed (electricity only travels 11.8 in. in a billionth of a second), everything must also get smaller.

Hard disk drives are also getting smaller and faster, and increasing in capacity (a 10:1 improvement in 10 years). Technologies under development ensure the continuing of this trend for at least the remainder of this decade.

One challenge is that the Internal Revenue Service still requires a minimum of 5 years on computer equipment depreciation. State-of-the-art PC-based systems require equipment replacement every 2 to 3 years.

Pricing Trends

In 1982, a basic office PC cost $7500 for the hardware and $750 for the software (software was 9.1% of total system cost). In 1993, a basic office system cost $1800 and the software $1200 (software was 40% of total system cost). *The good news:* The price of hardware decreased by 80%. *The bad news:* Not only did the cost of software increase by 60%, but the percentage that software represents as a part of the entire system increased from 10 to 40%.

Overall the combined price of software and hardware will continue to decrease. However, software will continue to take more and more of the pie.

Decentralizing from Mainframe to Mini to Micro

Virtually all Fortune 500 companies are involved with downsizing (the movement of systems from mainframe to mini-computer or micro-computer). There is a betting pool among computer journalists on when the last mainframe will be unplugged (the years 1996 to 2000 are the heavy favorites). Although this is hyperbole, the cost and performance advantages of PC-based systems make the movement from mainframes to PCs inevitable. The availability of multiple processor PCs and software that uses these machines will accelerate this trend. If a mini-computer–based system is to be used as an intermediate step, one should make sure that the mini-computer uses an open architecture.

Imaging

Computers do a cost-effective job of storing numbers and characters; however, the ability to store images (photographs, graphs, x-rays, etc.) is still expensive. A full-featured x-ray computerization system can cost $500,000. As economies of scale occur, the price of imaging systems will become a fraction of their current cost. This will result in new applications of imaging; within 5 years imaging will be a common feature of an OHIS.

The technology of scanning in pages of medical records and storing them as images is being successfully implemented by a number of corporate medical departments. These images are easily retrieved in digitized format that can take the place of hard-copy medical records. Notes can be attached that do not print out with the record. When signed, these paperless medical records are legally acceptable documents. Although imaged records can be indexed by type, they are not relational database files. Therefore, imaged information cannot be sorted or compared for analysis purposes.

Pen Computers

Pen computers are like clipboards with a computer underneath that can recognize your handwriting. They are useful for field data acquisition and for computerization (of the data entry) of forms (checking off boxes). Although current high prices of $3000 to $4000 prohibit widespread use, economies of scale will lower their price enough so that pen computers will replace scanners or keyed data entry in certain components of an OHIS. Physical examination and personal medical history are two examples.

Personal Data Assistants

Personal data assistants (PDAs) are just coming on the market. For OHISs they can be viewed as smaller versions of pen computers. Because they are targeted to the general public (vs. the workplace for pen computers) the price will be substantially lower. The lower price will have a trade-off with size and performance, but the PDAs may find a role in OHISs, where pen computers remain too expensive.

Software

Growing Storage and Memory Requirements

As the functions and features of an OHIS become more complicated and numerous and as users demand that systems be easier to use and work on different types of computer hardware, the software grows bigger and slower.

The bad news: Future software will continue this trend, doubling in size every few years. This means that faster systems with more memory (RAM) and larger disk systems will be required. *The good news:* The evolution of the hardware will more than make up for the above, still at prices lower than today's.

Fourth-Generation and Higher-Level Languages

It costs an estimated $100,000 per year to maintain "live-ware" (salary, benefits, office space, computer software/hardware for a programmer). In order to generate more complex OHISs, the productivity of the programming staff must increase. With each generation of language, there is a 5- to 10-fold increase in productivity. Fourth-generation level languages write much of the code based on simpler instructions. Many of the PC-based database languages are fourth generation. A fifth generation is being developed (it may become the holy grail of programming), but will not be available this decade.

Operating Systems

As users demand more easy-to-use features, the migration from character-based systems to graphical user interfaces will accelerate. This means that DOS and mainframe applications will migrate to Windows and OS/2 type systems.

DOS. Microsoft's DOS will continue to exist but will only be used in bare-boned systems (see Windows, below).

WINDOWS AND WINDOWS NT. Windows is evolving in several ways. First, it will add networking capabilities (from Windows for Workgroups). Second, it will become 32 bit (will run faster and bigger programs). Third, DOS will no longer be needed to run Windows. Windows will be the operating system used for most PCs through 1994, 1995, and perhaps 1996.

Windows NT will also evolve, first being used on network servers, or for complicated desktop applications. In 1994 through 1996, Windows NT may supplant Windows. Microsoft is still unclear on where Windows NT fits, but competitive pressure from IBM and Novell will decide where Windows NT is used and how much it will cost.

OS/2. IBM's more advanced and more powerful operating system for the PC was originally a joint project between IBM and Microsoft but is now a sole IBM effort. However, OS/2 will evolve because of Taligent, the IBM and Apple joint venture. OS/2 may become a niche product for users who are heavily using mainframes and other IBM-based systems.

UNIX. Originally this was a mini-computer operating system predominantly used in research. It is powerful (can handle multiple processors) and has good availability of software, but it is complicated to use.

UNIX is recommended for scientists and for large-scale database servers. Novell's recent purchase of UNIX indicates significant changes in how UNIX is marketed and how it is used in a client-server environment.

Networks

There are two types of PC-based networks.

SERVER BASED. This network is built around a centralized computer, which may be a PC. Data and software are obtained by the network nodes (desktop PCs) from this server. These networks tend to be complicated and usually require a dedicated staff person to maintain them. Examples of these server-based networks include Novell, LAN Manager, and Windows NT Server. This type of network provides higher levels of security and performance, and supports more connections (up to 1000 PCs connected together).

In the past decade, Novell has dominated this marketplace. However, Microsoft is challenging Novell's dominance with two products: LAN Manager and Windows NT Server. Novell will build on its purchase of UNIX to compete aggressively with

Microsoft's Windows NT Server. This will cause the marketplace to be volatile, probably through 1996. Competition will also result in better security and fault tolerance (the ability of a network or computer to continue to function even though partially broken) for the large-scale user. With the addition of client servers (see below), these two network environments can handle the vast majority of mainframe applications.

PEER-TO-PEER. A simple, easy-to-use network used by small companies or departments, peer-to-peer runs on top of DOS and is typically used by 2 to 20 computers but can support up to 200. Both security and the speed of information flow between computers are limited compared to server-based networks.

Until recently LanTastic had this part of the marketplace to itself. Novell with Novell lite and Microsoft with Windows for Workgroups have both attempted to penetrate this market. Their initial products have not been well received. For the next 2 years, LanTastic will still be the best choice. At the end of this time period, there will probably be only two vendors with products in the peer-to-peer area. It is still too early to tell who those vendors will be, however.

Client Servers

Computer networks often connect to large databases. These databases may be present on a different computer called a client server. Utilization of a client server approach is probably where most new OHISs will be developed. Information/data are requested from a server and then made available on the local PC in the user's choice of database software (e.g., Paradox, Dbase, Foxpro). The server may be another PC, a PC with multiple processors, a mini-computer, or even a mainframe. In most cases, the local PC will request the data needed in SQL, a standard relational database dialect. Client server system architecture allows greater performance and flexibility.

Object-Oriented Databases

The database system is often referred to as the key to an OHIS. Computer-based filing methods evolve over time. The indexed sequential access method (ISAM) data management method was commonly used in the 1960s. Although fast, ISAM required that all of the programs be changed whenever the format (variable added, modified, or deleted) changed. The first database (that allowed data formats to be changed without massive program changes) was hierarchical (IMS: IBM mainframe). This was followed by networking (IDMS: IBM mainframe) and then relational (e.g., SQL, Oracle, Focus, RBase). A new generation of databases seems to come along every 5 to 7 years. The object-oriented database is the currently available next generation, but it is not yet mainstream. This new generation of database will allow elemental modules of OHIS programs to be shared universally. Object-oriented databases are critical to the development of information age OHISs and will finally take companies out of the cycle of generating new systems from scratch every 5 to 7 years.

Artificial Intelligence/Expert Systems and Fuzzy Logic

Computers follow the general method of solving problems of "if this is true, then do that. . . ." Artificial intelligence (AI), expert systems, and fuzzy logic techniques allow a computer to follow a general-purpose approach in solving complicated problems and meet the need to learn by experience. Unfortunately, there are legal barriers to taking full advantage of these methods in an OHIS. Carnegie Mellon has had a computer program for over 10 years that can match or exceed the performance of an intern in medical diagnosis. The problem is that at least 2000 lawyers in the United States are waiting to sue a computer for malpractice in misdiagnosing a condition or disease.

Until this legal barrier is removed, AI will be confined to group data analysis under the supervision of a human professional, and not used in individual data analysis (see Managed Care and the Growth of Information Management).

Information Access

Telecommunications

High-speed nationwide data networks are part of the Clinton administration goals. We can expect the cost of remote data access to continue to decrease as these fiberoptic networks come on-line.

Dropping modem prices and faster transmission speed are dramatically increasing telecommunication's availability. Security has lagged behind this development but will be handled when Windows NT and planned upgrade versions of OS/2 become available.

Storage Devices (CD-ROM, WORM, Optical Disks)

Certain components of an OHIS, such as MSDSs and x-rays, require vast amounts of data. The following storage devices are durable and can handle large amounts of data.

CD-ROM drives cost $200 to $750, are capable of storing 650 megabytes (MB) like audio CDs, and are mostly read-only. Writing on a CD requires a $3500 system and can only be performed once. Data cannot be added later. CD-ROM drives are also relatively slow.

WORM (write once, read many) drives are more expensive ($2000) than CD-ROM but are faster and able to write on multiple occasions. The technology has been available for several years but has not gained wide acceptance. They are very good for archival data.

Optical disks, holding from 21 MB to over a gigabyte of memory, have the same advantages and disadvantages as WORM but can write more than once. Optical disks are the best future technology if the price comes down. CD-ROM, because of wide appeal, probably has the greatest realistic potential.

Connectivity

Medical Testing Equipment

As new models of medical testing equipment (e.g., audiometers, tonometers, spirometers) are introduced, they have added the necessary hardware and software to allow connection to an OHIS. Although most of these current interfaces are crude and require technical competence to be able to program, in 2 to 3 years these initial growing pains will fade.

Other Systems

Because much of the information needed by an OHIS is available on other computer systems within the company, OHISs tend to store duplicated data. Yet current systems can also be expensive to connect to other company systems so that data can be shared. Many of the previously mentioned technologies (e.g., client server, object-oriented database) will remove the difficulty and cost of these "data" connections.

Future state-of-the-art systems that utilize fax boards, modems, electronic mail, cellular telephones, and other technology will be heavily interconnected and may not require wire cabling to make these connections.

Centralized Data Processing Versus User Control

The turf wars over who controls and supports the OHIS within organizations will increase in intensity over the next 3 to 5 years. The resolution of conflict in most companies will be the narrowing of focus and breakup of the data processing empire that currently exists. The user will have increased options and responsibilities for systems, with the data processing department providing support on request.

Summary

The OHIS of the future will be PC based, utilizing a multiprocessor client server. Each of the nodes (connected desktop systems) will use a graphics user interface with a fourth-generation language and an object-oriented database as the underlying software. Much of the system software will be shared with other OHIS users, and system changes will be both inexpensive and quick to perform. Connections to other local company applications (other departments) and to keynote information sources will be transparent, eliminating data storage in more than one place. The system will store images of forms and x-rays using CD-ROM or optical technology. All equipment, whether testing or pen based, will be directly connected to the system. Employees and clients with disabilities will gain improved access to the system. The performance of the hardware will far exceed anything available today but will be cheaper than current systems. The software will be isolated from the hardware, allowing physical pieces of the system to be replaced, transparent to the user, as better technologies become available. All of the above will result in a system that is more productive and flexible.

Reference

1. Kissam, T. D. Selecting and Purchasing PC-Based Hardware and Generic PC Software. In K. W. Peterson and L. F. David (eds.), *Directory of Occupational Health and Safety Software* (version 6.0). Arlington Heights, IL: American College of Occupational and Environmental Medicine (ACOEM), 1993. Pp. 33–50.

Further Information

Perhaps the most in-depth source of OHIS software information is the *Directory of Occupational Health and Safety Software,* published by the Computers in Occupational Medicine Section of the ACOEM. The 6th edition lists detailed information for almost 100 software products. Most are commercial systems; a few are in the public domain. Available from ACOEM, the 450-page directory costs $75.00 ($50.00 to ACOEM/AAOHN members).

Briefer listings of occupational health and safety software are published in the annual software edition of the journal *Occupational Health and Safety* and *Software Packages in Occupational Health and Safety,* published by the Canadian Centre for Occupational Health and Safety.

Many useful books on generic hardware and software systems are available at bookstores and computer outlets, and by mail. These usually resemble readable user's manuals and focus on a particular software product. Quality publishers include Bantam Computer Books, Brady, McGraw-Hill, Microsoft Press, Norton, Osborne, SAMS, Sybex, and Que.

Computer magazines abound. Recommendations for the dabbler are *PC World* and *Computer Shopper.* More detail for the dilettante is contained in *Byte, InfoWorld, LAN, PC Magazine,* and *PC Week.* Software developers are encouraged to read *Computer Language* and *Dr. Dobb's Journal.*

The monograph *Putting the Pieces Together: A Guide to the Implementation of Integrated Health Data Management Systems* provides a comprehensive blueprint for IHDMSs, including three corporate case studies, checklists, and a bibliography. The guide was designed to help corporate decision-makers become more knowledgeable about the advantages of IHDMSs. Written by Sharon L. Yenney, it was published in 1992 by the Washington Business Group on Health, 202-408-9320.

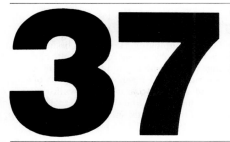

Training and Communications

Victor S. Roth and
David H. Garabrant

Many standards promulgated by the Occupational Safety and Health Administration (OSHA) explicitly require the employer to train employees in the safety and health aspects of their jobs.* Other OSHA standards make it the employer's responsibility to limit certain job assignments to employees who are "certified," "competent," or "qualified," in other words, those who have had special previous training, in or out of the workplace [1].

It is usually wise for the employer to keep a record of all safety and health training. Records can provide evidence of the employer's good faith and compliance with OSHA standards. Documentation can also supply an answer to one of the first questions an accident investigator will ask: "Was the injured employee trained to do the job?" [1]. Training in the proper performance of a job is time and money well spent, and the employer might regard it as an investment rather than an expense. An effective program of safety and health training for workers can result in fewer accidents and illnesses, better morale, and lower insurance premiums, among other benefits [1].

The purpose of this chapter is to compile the many settings for which training of employees is required in some aspect of occupational health and safety. Some general industry training requirements, including fire prevention, personal protection, and hearing conservation, are described, followed by highlighted examples related to the Hazard Communication Standard, Material Safety Data Sheets (MSDS), and the Laboratory Standard. Commentary regarding effective training and the role of the occupational health physician follows. It is recognized that the occupational health professional will have varying roles and responsibilities in providing training, either directly or in a supervisory manner. Many occupational health programs, whether hospital based or at an industry, include full-time trainers to address these regulations. The occupational physician's role can range from the development of a curriculum to giving presentations. The occupational health physician, in conducting a walk-through of a facility for occupational health risks, ought to be aware of the numerous training requirements that are often mandatory (see Chap. 3). Ideally, the well-trained worker will minimize risk of experiencing an injury or illness as a result of work responsibilities. Where prevention fails, training and education should help minimize adverse consequences.

Training Requirements in OSHA Standards

Training requirements of OSHA are found in the Code of Federal Regulations (CFR). This section, excerpted from those regulations, outlines general training requirements that apply to a wide range of industries. Though it is out of the scope of this book to detail training requirements for other more specific industries and chemical processes, mention is made of the equipment and chemicals that have required OSHA training guidelines, thus alerting those involved in such industries to reference such regulations in the more comprehensive Code of Federal Regulations.

---

*Training is an essential component of many OSHA standards. This chapter attempts to provide an overview of the basic requirements for training and to highlight major standards. Readers interested in the training components of the Bloodborne Pathogen Standard are referred to Chap. 30, Medical Center Occupational Health. Readers who are interested in more information regarding the Access to Medical Records Standard are referred to Chap. 2, Legal and Ethical Issues.

General Industry Training Requirements

At virtually any manufacturing facility employing 10 workers or more, some fundamental training requirements are mandatory. These requirements range from fire protection to respirator use, hearing, process safety management, and medical services, as well as related duties for contractors, the mechanical integrity of equipment, and appropriate prevention signs and tags. In conducting a walk-through of the facility, the occupational health professional may find it of value to develop a checklist to inquire as to whether training programs are currently performed for those areas.

Employee Emergency Plans and Fire Prevention Plans (CFR 1910.38)

The following elements, at a minimum, shall be included in the plan: (1) emergency escape procedures and emergency escape route assignments, (2) procedures to be followed by employees who remain to operate critical plant operations before they evacuate, (3) procedures to account for all employees after emergency evacuation has been completed, (4) rescue and medical duties for those employees who are to perform them, (5) the preferred means of reporting fires and other emergencies, (6) names or regular job titles of persons or departments who can be contacted for further information or explanation of duties under the plan. Although "medical duties" are mentioned above, availability of persons specifically trained in cardiopulmonary resuscitation is not noted as a requirement of this standard.

Before implementing the emergency action plan, the employer shall designate and train a sufficient number of persons to assist in the safe and orderly emergency evacuation of employees.

The employer shall review the plan with each employee covered by the plan at the following times: (1) initially when the plan is developed, (2) whenever the employee's responsibilities or designated actions under the plan change, and (3) whenever the plan is changed.

The written plan shall be kept at the workplace and made available for employee review. For those employers with 10 or fewer employees, the plan may be communicated orally to employees and the employer need not maintain a written plan.

The employer shall apprise employees of the fire hazards of the materials and processes to which they are exposed.

Personal Protective Equipment (CFR 1910.132–1910.140)

This standard includes requirements for eye and face protection, respiratory protection, occupational head protection, occupational foot protection, and electrical protective devices. Hearing protection is considered separately (CFR 1910.95) in OSHA regulations, as it is in this chapter. The major portion of this standard details respiratory protection.

All employees working in and around specific chemical or dust exposure for which personal protective equipment is mandated (such as respirators) must be instructed as to the hazards of their respective jobs, and in the personal protection and first-aid procedures applicable to the hazards of such exposure.

Respirators shall be used in accordance with OSHA regulations, and persons who may require them shall be trained in their use.

The correct respirator shall be specified for each job. The respirator type is usually specified in the work procedures by a qualified individual supervising the respiratory protective program. The individual issuing them shall be adequately instructed to ensure that the correct respirator is issued. Each respirator permanently assigned to an individual shall be durably marked to indicate to whom it was assigned. The mark shall not affect the respirator performance in any way. The date of issuance shall be recorded.

Written procedures shall be prepared covering safe use of respirators in dangerous atmospheres that might be encountered in normal operations or in emergencies. Personnel shall be familiar with these procedures and the available respirators.

Frequent random inspections shall be conducted by a qualified individual to assure that respirators are properly selected, used, cleaned, and maintained.

Supervisors and workers shall be instructed in respirator selection, use, and maintenance by competent persons. Training shall provide an opportunity to handle the respirator, have it fitted properly, test its face-piece to face-seal, wear it in normal air to become familiar with it, and wear it in a test atmosphere.

Every respirator wearer shall receive fitting instructions including demonstrations and practice in how the respirator should be worn, how to adjust it, and how to determine if it fits properly. Respirators shall not be worn when conditions such as beard growth, sideburns, skull cap, and absence of dentures prevent a good face-seal. Proper protection is assured if the worker checks respirator face-piece fit *each time* it is put on.

Employers are held accountable by OSHA to ensure that people who need to wear respirators in the course of their work are "medically certified." Although OSHA has considered implementing a standard on the use of personal protective equipment, there are presently no universal medical criteria to which this physician decision-making process must adhere. It is up to the judgment of the examining physician as to whether a person can be medically cleared for respirator use. Implementation of a questionnaire related to respiratory diseases or symptoms, and an updated pulmonary function test, are tools already in widespread use among occupational physicians in helping to make this decision. (See Chap. 11, Occupational Pulmonary Disease, for additional information on respirator clearance.) Many physicians exclude workers with forced expiratory volume in 1 second (FEV_1) or (FVC) of less than 70% of predicted from respirator use.

Hearing

The employer shall institute *a training program* for all employees who are exposed to noise at or above an 8-hour time-weighted average of 85 decibels, and shall ensure employee participation in such a program. The training program shall be repeated yearly for each employee included in the hearing conservation program (see Chap. 16, Noise-Induced Hearing Loss).

The training program should inform the employee about (1) the effects of noise on hearing; (2) the purpose of hearing protectors, as well as the advantages, disadvantages, and attentuation of various types and instructions on selection, fitting, use, and care; and (3) the purpose of audiometric testing and an explanation of the test procedure.

Process Safety Management of Highly Hazardous Chemicals

Concern over the safety of manufacturing, transporting, and using extremely hazardous chemicals is worldwide [13]. Some tragic statistics amplify this concern: more than 2000 dead at Bhopal; 24 dead, 132 injured at a Phillips Petroleum site; 17 dead at an Arco chemical plant. In the United States, there is an increased awareness and concern of process incidents involving hazardous materials. A great many people in the US think that a major chemical accident will occur domestically in the next 50 years. Fear also pervades the local level in communities where explosive or extremely toxic chemicals are made or handled. Large residential areas and institutional buildings have been built up around the chemical plants and storage tanks that have preceded the local population growth [2]. The Emergency Planning and Community Right-to-Know Act of 1986, known as Title III of the Superfund Amendments and Reauthorization Act (SARA), mandates that every facility using, storing, or manufacturing hazardous chemicals make public its inventory and report every release of a hazardous chemical to public officials and health personnel. Every facility must also cooperate with physicians who are treating victims of hazardous chemical exposure [3].

A recognition of the destruction that the above noted incidents have caused in recent years, and the fact that most of them are shown to be as preventable as they are tragic, has led OSHA to issue "Process Safety Management of Highly Hazardous Chemicals," one of the most far-reaching regulations it has ever set forth. Most of the provisions took effect on May 26, 1992 [1].

Initial training Each employee presently involved in operating process, and each employee before being involved in operating a newly assigned process, shall be trained in an overview of the process, and in the operating procedure. This training shall include specific safety and health hazards emergency operations including shutdown, and safe work practices applicable to the employee's job task. In lieu of initial training for those employees already involved in operating a process on May 26, 1992, an employer may certify in writing that the employee has the required knowledge, skills, and abilities to safely carry out the duties and responsibilities as specified in the operating procedure. At present, there is no requirement for posttraining certification of employee knowledge by the employer. Administration of a posttest for this purpose is quite variable. In most cases, the employer merely certifies that the employee attended the training session. This assumes retention by the employee of the information presented at these sessions.

Refresher training Refresher training shall be provided at least every 3 years, and more often if necessary, to each employee involved in operating a process to assure that the employee understands and adheres to the current operating procedure of the process. The employer, in consultation with the employees involved, shall determine the appropriate frequency of refresher training.

Training documentation. The employer shall ascertain that each employee involved in operating a process has received and understood the training required. The employer shall prepare a record that contains the identity of the employee, the date of training, and the means used to verify that the employee understood the training. There is no standard means to verify employee understanding of the training. In most cases, posttraining examinations are not administered. Employers usually maintain verification of employee attendance at the training sessions, and assume retention by the employee of the information presented at these sessions.

Medical Services and First Aid (CFR 1910.151 and 1926.50)

The occupational physician should utilize judgment on staffing and provision of supplies to the on-site dispensary. The staffing and supplies provided to the dispensary should take into account the type of operation in the workplace and the most common injuries that have previously occurred in the industry. Therefore, if burns are common because of the process carried out in the plant, medical supplies should be adequate to care for this type of injury.

The employer shall ensure the ready availability of medical personnel for advice and consultation on matters of plant health.

In the absence of an infirmary, clinic, or hospital in close proximity to the workplace, a person or persons shall be adequately trained to render first aid. First-aid supplies approved by the consulting physician shall be readily available.

Where the eyes or body of any person may be exposed to injurious corrosive materials, suitable facilities for quick drenching or flushing of the eyes and body shall be provided within the work area for immediate emergency use.

Contract Employer Responsibilities (CFR 1926.16)

Many recent legal decisions have been levied against employers for not properly overseeing the activities of the contractors that are hired. In short, an *employer* can be *held liable* for the negligence or other transgressions of the contractor.

The contract employer shall assure that each contract employee is trained in the work practices necessary to safely perform the job.

The contract employer shall assure that each contract employee is instructed in the known potential fire, explosion, or toxic release hazards related to his/her job and the process, and the applicable provisions of the emergency action plan.

The contract employer shall document that each contract employee has received and understood the training required. The contract employer shall prepare a record that contains the identity of the contract employee, the date of training, and the means used to verify that the employee understood the training.

Mechanical Integrity

The employer shall train each employee involved in maintaining the ongoing integrity of process equipment in an overview of that process and its hazards and in the procedures applicable to the employee's job tasks to assure that the employee can perform the job tasks in a safe manner.

Specifications for Accident Prevention Signs and Tags

All employees shall be instructed in the meaning of danger signs and that special precautions are necessary.

All employees shall be instructed that caution signs indicate a possible hazard against which proper precautions should be taken.

Safety instruction signs shall be used where there is a need for general instructions and suggestions relative to safety measures.

In addition to the above noted training guidelines that apply to numerous industries, there are more specific training recommendations listed in tabular form in the

Appendix to this chapter. These requirements are listed so that they can be easily located in the *Federal Register.*

In addition, there are specific training requirements for the maritime industry, construction industry, agricultural workers, and federal employees.

Hazard Communication Standard

In November 1983, OSHA promulgated the Hazard Communication Standard, a regulation covering a broad range of chemical hazards. This standard contains specific provisions regarding the evaluation of health hazards, labeling of containers, use of chemical information sheets called "Material Safety Data Sheets," and training of employees. Also known as *HazCom,* the standard originally applied only to chemical manufacturers, importers, and distributors, but was later expanded to cover many additional employers. Presently, all companies and employers that handle any hazardous substance in any form are required to comply with the standard [4].

The Hazard Communication Standard, commonly known as the "worker right to know" law, mandates that workers receive training and information on all potentially hazardous chemicals with which they work. It is a performance-based standard because it specifies what employers must do, but not *how* they must do it. The following list outlines the basic components of this standard [5]. (Chapter 2, Legal and Ethical Issues, and Chap. 23, Toxicology, discuss other aspects of the Hazard Communication Standard.)

1. Manufacturers must produce a MSDS for all hazardous chemicals that they produce and sell.
2. MSDSs must be shipped to all downstream users of the hazardous chemicals.
3. In all workplaces in which hazardous chemicals are present, the employer is responsible for the following:
   A. Labeling all hazardous chemicals in the workplace
   B. A written hazardous chemicals program that is accessible to employees who ask for it
   C. A system for managing MSDSs that gives workers access to them
   D. A training program for all employees who may experience an exposure to a potentially hazardous chemical
4. The training program must include information on the following:
   A. Location and identity of hazardous chemicals
   B. Physical hazards
   C. Health effects (acute and long term)
   D. Proper work practices and personal protection
   E. First aid
   F. Emergency response (including fire, leak, and spill)
   G. Workers' rights under the Hazard Communication Standard
   H. Labeling systems
   I. Material Safety Data Sheet systems

Many employers believe that compliance with the Hazard Communication Standard means obtaining and filing all of the MSDSs for their hazardous chemicals. In reality, this does the worker no good unless they have access to the information through training and access to MSDSs. The Hazard Communication Standard is really a proactive standard, and is explicit about employers' responsibility to train workers, not merely to respond to requests for information when workers ask for it [5].

Material Safety Data Sheets

Material Safety Data Sheets are a foundation of a successful safety and health program. They provide information that can be used during employee training and chemical exposure emergencies; they also give vital information to medical professionals caring for the affected employee. They inform employees of the health hazards of chemicals with which they are working and let them know what situations can produce explosion and decomposition hazards. Their purpose is to communicate critical facts about working safely with the material [6].

The primary function of the MSDS is to provide workers with enough information about a specific chemical substance to understand: (1) potential acute and chronic health effects; (2) recommended personal protective equipment; (3) proper work practices; (4) first-aid remedies; (5) spill, leak, and fire precautions and responses; and (6) any other information necessary to work safely with that potentially hazardous substance [5]. MSDSs vary with respect to thoroughness and the extent to which chemicals are tested and specified. Thus, a physician treating a patient with an exposure identified on the MSDS should realize that the information contained may be incomplete. Some chemicals may not be tested at all and others may be identified by the broad class of materials to which they belong. In some cases, it may be necessary to contact the manufacturer listed on the MSDS to get additional information.

The specific chemical identity of a hazardous substance may be withheld from the MSDS if it is determined that the information regarding this chemical is a trade secret (information used in one's business that gives that employer an opportunity to obtain an advantage over competitors who do not know how to use the chemical in this way). However, the MSDS must contain information concerning the *properties* and *effects* of the hazardous chemical and also *must indicate* that the specific chemical identity is being *withheld* as a trade secret. If a treating physician or nurse determines that a medical emergency exists that requires additional information about the specific chemical, the manufacturer, importer, or employer shall *immediately* disclose the specific chemical identity of a trade secret chemical to that physician or nurse. In nonemergency situations, health professionals must request information about trade secret chemicals in writing, detailing the need for such information. The health professional may be required to sign a confidentiality agreement, stating that information disclosed will not be used for any purpose other than for the health needs asserted.

Material Safety Data Sheets must be readily accessible to employees when they are in their work areas during their shifts. Some employers keep the MSDS in a binder in a central location. Others computerize the information and provide access through terminals. As long as employees can get information when they need it, any approach may be used [7].

As chemicals become more abundant in the workplace, and with new and more complex chemicals being developed, the MSDS is a valuable tool for the occupational physician in conducting occupational medical evaluations for surveillance purposes and evaluating exposure-related symptoms. It is therefore quite important that the physician advise potentially exposed workers and their employers that all pertinent MSDSs should accompany the employee when he or she is evaluated for chemical exposure.

Laboratory Standard

OSHA published the final rule of its laboratory standard, *Occupational Exposures to Hazardous Chemicals in Laboratories,* in the January 31, 1990, *Federal Register* (29 CFR 1910.1450).

The standard applies to all laboratories that use *hazardous chemicals* in accordance with the definition, "chemical for which there is statistical significant evidence based on at least one study conducted in accordance with established scientific principles that acute or chronic health effects may occur in exposed employees" [8]. This would include chemicals that are carcinogens, toxic or highly toxic agents, reproductive toxins, irritants, corrosives, sensitizers, hepatotoxins, nephrotoxins, neurotoxins, agents that affect the hematopoietic system, and agents that damage the lungs, skin, eyes, or mucous membranes. This is further detailed in the Hazard Communication Standard, and outlined in Table 37-1.

The following conditions pertain to the OSHA Laboratory Standard: (1) Chemical manipulations are carried out on a "laboratory scale," that is, work with substances in which the containers used for their handling are designed to be easily and safely manipulated by one person; (2) multiple chemical procedures or chemicals are used; (3) the procedures involved are not part of a production process, and do not in any way simulate a production process; and (4) "protective laboratory practices and equipment" are available and in common use to minimize the potential for employee exposure to hazardous chemicals. The Hazard Communication Standard (29 CFR 1910.1200) is to be consulted for guidance in defining the scope of health hazards

Table 37-1. Toxins and their effects

Toxin category	Definition	Signs/symptoms	Chemicals
Hepatoxin	Chemical that produces liver damage	Jaundice; liver enlargement	Carbon tetrachloride; nitrosamines
Nephrotoxin	Chemical that produces kidney damage	Edema; proteinuria	Halogenated hydrocarbons; uranium
Neurotoxin	Chemical that produces its primary toxic effects on the nervous system	Narcosis; behavioral changes; decreases in motor function	Mercury; carbon disulfide
Agents that act on the blood or hematopoietic system	Decrease hemoglobin function; deprive the body tissues of oxygen	Cyanosis; loss of consciousness	Carbon monoxide; cyanide
Agents that damage the lung	Chemicals that irritate or damage the pulmonary tissue	Cough; tightness in chest; shortness of breath	Silica; asbestos
Reproductive toxin	Chemical that affects the reproductive capabilities, including chromosomal damage (mutations) and effects on the fetus (teratogenesis)	Birth defects; sterility	Lead; dibromodichloropropane (DBCP)
Cutaneous hazard	Chemical that affects the dermal layer of the body	Defatting of the skin; rashes; irritation	Ketones; chlorinated compounds
Eye hazard	Chemical that affects the eye or visual capacity	Conjunctivitis; corneal damage	Organic solvents; acids

and in determining whether a chemical is considered hazardous for the purposes of the standard.

A major part of the Laboratory Standard is the *Chemical Hygiene Plan,* which must be made available to all employees and must be reviewed and updated annually by the employer. Necessary elements of this plan are:

Standard operating procedures relevant to safety and health that should be followed when using hazardous chemicals

Criteria to be used to determine and *implement controls* to reduce employee exposure to hazardous chemicals (engineering controls, personal protective equipment, hygiene practices), with special attention to chemicals known to be extremely hazardous

Requirement of *fume hoods* and other *protective equipment* to function properly and measures to be taken to ensure such proper operation

Circumstances under which a particular laboratory procedure shall require employer approval before implementation

Provisions for *medical consultations and examinations* (Unlike many OSHA standards, the Laboratory Standard does not require medical surveillance. On the other hand, if a laboratory worker develops symptoms or adverse health effects that may be related to workplace exposures, the employer must provide an appropriate medical evaluation.)

Specification of personnel responsible for implementation of the Chemical Hygiene Plan

Provisions for additional employee protection when working with particularly hazardous substances (e.g., select carcinogens, reproductive toxins, substances with a high degree of acute toxicity); such additional protection may include designated areas, containment devices such as fume hoods, procedures for removal of contaminated waste, and decontamination procedures

Provisions for *employee information and training:*

1. Employees should be apprised of the hazards of chemicals present in their work area
2. Information is to be provided on initial assignment to a work area in which hazardous chemicals are used and before assignments involving new hazardous exposures
3. Information given to employees is to include:
   A. Contents of the standard
   B. Location and availability of the Chemical Hygiene Plan
   C. Permissible Exposure Limits (PELs) for OSHA-regulated substances or recommended exposure limits where there is no standard
   D. Signs and symptoms of exposure
   E. Location and availability of references on the hazards including MSDS
4. Training should include:
   A. Methods and observations that may be used to detect the presence or release of a hazardous chemical
   B. The physical and health hazards of chemicals in the work area
   C. The measures employees can use to protect themselves from these hazards (work practices, personal protective equipment, emergency procedures)
   D. Details of the Chemical Hygiene Plan

Effective Training

During fiscal year 1991, OSHA cited general industry and construction employers for violations of the Hazard Communication Standard *more often than for any other regulation.* The majority of citations were for failure to have *a written hazard communication program.* Ineffective approaches to providing information and training were the most common shortcoming among employers who did have programs, according to OSHA [9].

Clearly, training must be effective to have any impact on worker health and safety. In a recent study [10] of training effectiveness, results suggested that not only *training content* but also implementation methods are critical to training success. A training delivery format based on relatively small groups (fewer than 25 employees), shorter training sessions involving the presentation of content material followed by question and answer periods, training scheduled before or at the beginning of work shifts, and a higher number of trainer contact hours were associated with more successful training outcomes.

An important element of the training session is the overview or introduction. Learning is easier if the broad picture is described first and the goal and objectives are defined [11]. The main body of the session should be presented in small chunks of information that can be assimilated easily. During this process, employees should be encouraged to participate in the learning process by means of practice exercises, small group problem-solving sessions, or review questions. It is motivational and practical if employees are encouraged to contribute examples from their own experiences. A critical component of training is a method for measuring its effectiveness.

Another study [12] suggested that it is important to tailor the training program as specifically as possible to the particular needs and issues that the trainee group encounters at the worksite. It was also implied that hands-on training and participatory exercises should be emphasized. It was believed that adult, working populations "learn better by doing." All trainees in this study stressed the importance of regular refresher training and training of all personnel at a given site. Other suggestions brought out in this study were that (1) employees should be consulted to assist in planning the course, (2) *all* employees at a given worksite should be trained, (3) more hands-on exercises should be included early to break up the lectures, (4) a posttraining test should be used, and (5) all of the topics in the questions should be covered in the sessions.

Frequently, different trainers conduct similar training sessions in the same or similar workplace settings. *Use of videotapes* as part of training sessions assures a certain basic level of material being presented to employees. With today's technologically advanced society, such videos should be high quality and sophisticated to maintain viewer interest. In addition, the videos should not be generic but *specific* for the industry and the jobs involved. Some training sessions have used actual videos of jobs performed at the worksite by the people attending the training session. The video is analyzed at the training course to effect changes in job performance and to increase safety.

Interactive laser videos have also been used for training. The participant responds to questions by touching different portions of the screen. This method, however, is relatively expensive and limited in use.

The Role of Occupational Physicians

Hazard communication requires teaching skills. Trainers must have training themselves to present information and answer questions. They also have to know where to refer employees for additional information [9].

Many experts believe that there may not be an "ideal trainer" and recommend a team approach, involving such varied resources as the production manager, shift supervisor, foreman, a hazardous waste expert, a safety and health director, and a shipping clerk [9].

A trained occupational health physician is well suited by education and interpersonal skills to head a training team. The physician's knowledge of different occupational exposures and their acute and long-term health effects is relevant to a major portion of employee concerns. The physician may find it helpful to call on the expertise of the plant foreman regarding the chemicals that are used and the types of jobs in which exposures occur, and on an industrial hygienist regarding the ways to measure and control exposures. The occupational physician's knowledge of the acute symptoms of exposure, different biologic measures available to determine body burdens, dose-response relationships, and long-term health risks in relation to specific jobs and corresponding exposures constitutes the essential core of the training information. Concern over acute and long-term health risks is the *major motivating factor* for employees in following specific recommendations brought out at training sessions.

References

1. *Training Requirements in OSHA Standards and Training Guidelines.* OSHA Publication no. 2254, revised. US Department of Labor, Occupational Safety and Health Administration, 1992.
2. Beddows, N. Chemical process safety needs effort from industry, government and public. *Occup. Health Saf.* June 1991. Pp. 66–67.
3. Leonard, R. B., et al. SARA, Title III: Implications for emergency physicians. *Ann. Emerg. Med.* 18:1212, 1989.
4. O'Neill, B. M., et al. Right-to-know laws: A guide to maintaining compliance. *Occup. Health Saf.* June 1988. Pp. 28–49.
5. Sattler, B. Rights and realities: A critical review of the accessibility of information on hazardous chemicals. *Occup. Med. State of the Art Rev.* 7:189, 1992.
6. Garbo, M. J., et al. OSHA Hazard Communication Standard, helping prevent chemical hazards. *A.A.O.H.N. J.* 36:366, 1988.
7. *Hazard Communication Guidelines for Compliance.* OSHA Publication no. 3111. US Department of Labor, Occupational Safety and Health Administration, 1988.
8. Kilby, J. A. New OSHA standard goes into effect regarding safety in laboratories. *Occup. Health Saf.* May 1990. Pp. 82.
9. LaBar, G. Hazard communication: A performing art. *Occup. Hazards* 7:35, 1992.
10. Robins, T. G. Implementation of the Federal Hazard Communication Standard: Does training work? *J. Occup. Med.* 32:1133, 1990.
11. Samways, M. C. OSHA voluntary guidelines provide blueprint for employee training; *Occup. Health Saf.* May 1987. Pp. 68–75.
12. The University of Michigan Evaluation Program of the Midwest Consortium of Hazardous Waste Worker Training. *Training Impact Evaluation Through In-Depth*

Site Follow-Up: Findings and Implications for Training and Training Evaluation, January 1992.

13. Auger, J. *Process Safety; Occupational Health and Safety,* May 1992. Pp. 60–66.

Further Information

US Department of Labor Occupational Safety and Health Administration (OSHA). *Training Requirements in OSHA Standards and Training Guidelines.* OSHA Publication no. 2254, revised. Washington, DC: OSHA, 1992.
The length and complexity of OSHA standards make it difficult to find all the references to training. OSHA's training-related requirements have been excerpted and collected in this booklet.

American Journal of Industrial Medicine, 22:619–784, 1992.
The entire issue of this journal is dedicated to innovative approaches to worker education in health and safety.

Appendix to Chapter 37:
Occupational Health Training Requirements

Subject	Standard number
Operations Training	1910.66
Ionizing Radiation	1910.96
Flammable and Combustible Liquids	1910.106
Explosives and Blasting Agents	1910.109
Storage and Handling of Liquefied Petroleum Gases	1910.110
Hazardous Waste Operations and Emergency Response	1910.120
New Technology Programs	1910.120
Temporary Labor Camps	1910.142
Control of Hazardous Energy (lock-out/tag-out)	1910.147
Fire Protection	1910.155
Fire Brigades	1910.156
Portable Fire Extinguishers	1910.157
Fire-Extinguishing Systems	1910.160
Fire Detection Systems	1910.164
Servicing of Multi-Piece and Single-Piece Rim Wheels	1910.177
Powered Industrial Trucks	1910.178
Moving Loads	1910.179
Crawler Locomotive and Truck Trains	1910.180
Mechanical Power Presses	1910.217
Forging Machines	1910.218
Oxygen-fuel Gas Welding and Cutting	1910.253
Arc Welding and Cutting	1910.254
Resistance Welding	1910.255
Pulp, Paper, and Paperboard Mills	1910.261
Laundry Machinery	1910.264
Sawmills	1910.265
Pulpwood Logging	1910.266
Telecommunications (including derrick trucks, cable fault locating, guarding manholes, joint power and telecommunications manholes, tree trimming, and electrical hazards)	1910.268
Grain-Handling Facilities	1910.272
Electrical Safety–Related Work Practices	1910.332
Qualification of a Dive Team	1910.410
Asbestos	1910.1001
4-Nitrobiphenyl	1910.1003
Alpha-Naphthylamine	1910.1004
Methylchloromethyl Ether	1910.1006
3,3'-Dichlorobenzidine	1910.1007

(continued)

Subject	Standard number
Bis-Chloromethyl Ether	1910.1008
Beta-Naphthylamine	1910.1009
Benzidine	1910.1010
4-Aminodiphenyl	1910.1011
Ethylenediamine	1910.1012
Beta-Propriolactone	1910.1013
2-Acetylaminofluorene	1910.1014
4-Dimethylaminoazobenzene	1910.1015
N-Nitrosodimethylamine	1910.1016
Vinyl Chloride	1910.1017
Inorganic Arsenic	1910.1018
Lead	1910.1025
Coke Oven Emissions	1910.1029
Bloodborne Pathogens	1910.1030
Cotton Dust	1910.1043
1,2-Dibromo-3-Chloropropane	1910.1044
Acrylonitrile (Vinyl Cyanide)	1910.1045
Ethylene Oxide	1910.1047
Occupational Exposure to Hazardous Chemicals in Laboratories	1910.1450

38

International Occupational Health

Craig Karpilow

The occupational medicine physician is likely to be called on to address a variety of international occupational health issues, including determining the availability of local medical care, addressing special needs for handicapped children, or simply obtaining a local physician. The physician may be asked to recommend immunizations or special precautions for a person who is traveling overseas on a work assignment. Another challenge might be apprising a person who is being transferred or taking employment in another country about unique health risks there.

Practical challenges related to preventing jet lag, preparing a medical kit, or recommending medical evaluation measures in the event of serious emergencies may face the occupational medicine physician who provides various aspects of international health care. The physician may need to evaluate the business traveler returning from an assignment as well as the one who experiences symptoms that may be related to endemic diseases in the host country.

An awareness of acquired immunodeficiency syndrome (AIDS), pollution, and physical safety is essential for the occupational medicine physician who deals with employees who go abroad. An additional responsibility for those who specialize in this emerging area of occupational medicine may involve setting up occupational health programs or participating in the development of local medical care for various facilities.

Employees required to travel and live in different nations have long tolerated medical annoyances that travel produces. They have been obliged to use existing medical systems of the country to which they travel with varying success. With international borders dissolving in the European community and economic and sociopolitical changes occurring at a rapid rate, corporations are becoming internationalized in their focus and attitudes. Medicine and its specialists, however, have not routinely crossed these international borders. Different methodologies, terminologies, and medical systems abound within the multitude of national borders.

The proliferation of international business has called upon occupational medicine physicians to become experts in international issues and to direct occupational programs at great distances. It has demanded that industrial hygienists bring technological expertise to developing nations and apply it in situations in which the basic infrastructure and finances are lacking for their techniques. It takes occupational health nurses, who are comfortable with and understand record-keeping and data-gathering techniques, and places them in a situation of dealing with more patients than they are accustomed to, significant language barriers, and a host of new health problems.

International occupational medicine necessitates an understanding of the global marketplace and its numerous cultural and socioeconomic variables. It involves developing appropriate programs to keep employees who live or work overseas healthy, and requires specialized planning. The patient population in international occupational medicine includes business travelers from multinational corporations and employees from educational institutions and private voluntary organizations, as well as health care workers who travel overseas and technical staff who repair facilities or remain in foreign locations to build industrial complexes.

This chapter addresses one aspect of the field: the business and technical travelers—their pretravel preparation, strategies for staying healthy while on the assignment overseas, and an outline of how to evaluate the returned employee. Readers interested in learning more about evaluating local conditions for medical facilities and program development in international occupational health are referred to the references at the end of this chapter [1].

Preparing Persons for Overseas Assignments

To appropriately advise the traveling employee, one must have a working knowledge of the specific operational issues of the country to which the employee is traveling. Legal, governmental, and other regulatory matters of the specific country must be addressed. A structured educational program for the expatriate or short-term business traveler before going overseas is appropriate. The occupational medicine physician can best serve employees internationally by providing appropriate protocols for common medical problems, baseline medical examinations, and country protocols for diseases that local physicians will treat. Working with the human resources department in developing guidelines for employee selection is another useful contribution that an occupational physician can make.

The Pretravel Consultation

In this setting, the physician evaluates the employee to ensure that the person's health will not be adversely affected by travel or living overseas [2]. Chronic diseases need to be identified and modifications made for those with various medical conditions, including pregnancy, diabetes, and autoimmune diseases. Current medications should be documented, and sufficient prescriptions, including extras for spoilage and/or loss, made available. Modifications of medication timing and dosage must be made for people with insulin-dependent diabetes mellitus (Table 38-1). The consultation includes a discussion of side effects of immunizations and the differences between recommended and required vaccines.

Depending on the country to which the person is traveling and the underlying medical history, medications may need to be prescribed for prevention of certain diseases (malaria, traveler's diarrhea, jet lag, high-altitude sickness). On-the-trip treatment of illnesses such as motion sickness, sinus infection, and bronchitis may also be necessary. Travel itself presents certain risks, such as thrombotic episodes and other medical emergencies [3, 4].

During this consultation, a physical examination and baseline blood work may be

Table 38-1. Insulin adjustment during jet travel across multiple time zones

		East Bound		
Daily insulin regimen	Day of departure	First morning at destination	10 hours after morning dose	Second day at destination
Single-dose schedule	Usual dose	2/3 usual dose	If blood sugar over 240, take remaining 1/3 of AM dose	Usual dose
Two-dose schedule	Usual morning and evening doses	2/3 usual dose	Usual evening dose, if blood sugar over 240, take remaining 1/3 of AM dose	Usual two doses

	West Bound		
Daily insulin regimen	Day of departure	18 hours after AM dose	First day at destination
Single-dose schedule	Usual dose	If blood sugar over 240, take 1/3 usual AM dose, followed by snack	Usual dose
Two-dose schedule	Usual morning and evening doses	If blood sugar over 240, take 1/3 usual AM dose, followed by snack	Usual two doses

Source: Courtesy of E. A. Benson, MD.

advisable if the person is traveling to a country with unique health risks or problematic medical systems. This information is designed to assist in medical evaluations overseas and provide a baseline from which to evaluate potential illness upon return.

Immunizations

Some countries *require* people to be vaccinated for various diseases, such as cholera, yellow fever, or plague, if they enter from a country considered contaminated by the illness. Although the World Health Organization has recommended that only yellow fever be required in this context, many countries still demand proof of cholera vaccination to enter their country. *Required* vaccines are designed to protect the host country's citizens from diseases brought in by foreigners.

Recommended vaccines ideally prevent travelers from contracting *endemic* diseases. Since the necessity for specific vaccines changes frequently, access to current information is essential. Various agencies provide recommendations, including the Centers for Disease Control (CDC) [5] and the World Health Organization [6]. The International Relations Division (DHSS) of the United Kingdom; Health and Welfare of Ontario, Canada; and the Commonwealth Department of Health in Australia are additional reliable sources (see Chapter Appendix 3).

Ideally, the traveling employee will be current on basic vaccinations and/or have sufficient time *before travel* to be immunized. *All* employees traveling overseas need to be updated on diphtheria/tetanus, polio, and measles vaccines (if born after 1956 and without documentation of measles). Influenza and hepatitis B vaccines (if dictated by the employee's job description) may also be advisable (Table 38-2).

Timing of the administration of the vaccine may be important. The cholera vaccine is a notable example and must be administered in two injections, one week to one month apart. Boosters are necessary every 6 months. Debate continues, however, between academicians and clinicians as to the usefulness of cholera vaccine. Theoretically, this vaccine is only 50 to 60% effective at preventing the disease if a person is exposed to contaminated food or water. A new cholera vaccine is being developed and should be available shortly. Until then, the standard cholera vaccine provides some protection. It will not only provide higher antigenicity than the *intramuscular* dosing but will also prevent many side effects (Table 38-3). Vaccine interactions, side effects, and allergic reactions also need to be considered in recommending the type of vaccination appropriate for designated countries (Table 38-4).

Medical Kits and Other Essentials

Some frequent business travelers have found value in including a medical kit along with their baggage. The components of such a kit will vary depending on a number of factors, including the country, local medical systems, the person's health, length of stay, and sociopolitical factors. Care must be taken to ensure that the person is properly informed of the use of the supplies and medications and knows to seek professional medical advice when appropriate.

Medical kits come in all sizes, from Band-Aid box sized novelty items to a 50-lb suitcase full of sophisticated materials. For the average business traveler, however, the latter is not practical. With some medical conditions, even the business traveler should carry a substantial medical kit. People working in a remote area, inaccessible to medical care, and performing risky operations should have a customized medical kit.

For the short-term business traveler who does not wish to spend valuable time looking for a pharmacy for medication, a useful medical kit is strategic. Even if the person can obtain medication, it might not be safe because many countries do not have strict labeling laws and quality assurance regulations regarding medications. Dating of medications is often not reviewed by small pharmacies. High temperatures in tropical climates may inactivate certain medications that sit in a hot non–air-conditioned pharmacy.

Kits are most effective if they are specific for the person's needs. A small amount of certain medications may be included in the medical kit for conditions that do not necessitate long-term treatment. Travelers should carry a letter signed by a physician on letterhead or prescription pad indicating the need for the medications and medical equipment contained in the medical kit. These papers should be kept with

Table 38-2. Dosing schedules for commonly used vaccines (1993)

Vaccine	Primary series	Booster interval
Diphtheria and Tetanus Toxoids and Pertussis vaccine adsorbed (DTP) (use in children < 7 years old)	4 doses[a] IM of vaccine, the first 3 doses given 4–8 weeks apart, dose 4 given 6–12 months after dose 3	Booster at 4–6 years of age
Haemophilus B conjugate[b]		
PRP-HbOC	3 doses[a] IM or SC at 2, 4, 6 months	Booster at 15 months
		Booster at 15 months
PRP-OMP	2 doses[a] IM or SC at 2, 4 months	None
PRP-D, PRP-HbOC, or PRP-OMP	1 dose[a] IM or SC at 15 months or older up to the 5th birthday	
Hepatitis B (Energix B) (accelerated schedule)	3 doses at 0, 30, and 60 days (1 ml IM in the deltoid area)	A fourth dose is recommended at 12 months if still at risk for hepatitis B exposure
Hepatitis B (Energix B) (standard schedule)	3 doses at 0, 1, and 6 months (1 ml IM in the deltoid area)	Need for booster not determined
Hepatitis B (Recombivax) (standard schedule)	3 doses at 0, 1, and 6 months (1 ml IM in the deltoid area)	Need for booster not determined
Influenza virus	1 dose[a] IM or SC annually	
Measles/mumps/rubella (MMR)[c]	1 dose[a] SC at 15 months or older	Booster measles vaccine at 12 years old; booster measles vaccine once in adult life before international travel for people born after 1957 but before 1980
Pneumococcus (23-valent)	1 dose[a] SC	None
Poliomyelitis, enhanced inactivated (E-IPV) (killed vaccine, safe for all ages)	Give doses[a] 1 and 2 SC or IM 4–8 weeks apart; give dose 3 at 6–12 months after dose 2; give dose 4 to children 4–6 years old	Give a dose once before travel in areas of risk
Poliomyelitis, oral (OPV) (attenuated live virus)[c]	Give doses[a] 1 and 2 orally 6–8 weeks apart; give dose 3 at 6 weeks after dose 2 (customarily at 8–12 months after dose 2); give dose 4 to children 4–6 years of age	Give a dose once to people less than 18 years old before travel in areas of risk
Tetanus and diphtheria Toxoids Adsorbed (Td) (for children > 7 years of age and for adults)	3 doses (0.5 ml SC or IM), doses 1 and 2 given 4–8 weeks apart, and dose 3 at 6–12 months later	Routine booster dose every 10 years

[a]See manufacturer's package insert for recommendations on dosage.
[b]Hib conjugate vaccines are not considered interchangeable for the primary immunization series.
[c]Caution: May be contraindicated in patients with any of the following conditions: pregnancy, leukemia, lymphoma, generalized malignancy, immunosuppression due to HIV infection or treatment with corticosteroids, alkylating drugs, antimetabolites, or radiation therapy.
Source: From Jong, E. C. Immunizations for International Travelers. In F. J. Bia (ed.), *Travel Medicine Advisor*. Atlanta: American Health Consultants, 1993.

Table 38-3. Dosing schedules for travel immunizations (1993)

Vaccine	Primary series	Booster interval
Cholera	2 doses 1 week or more apart (0.5 ml SC or IM) (pediatric dose 0.3 ml for 5–10 years of age, 0.2 ml for 6 months to 4 years)	6 months
Immune globulin (hepatitis A protection)	1 dose IM in the gluteus muscle (2-ml dose for 3 mo of protection; 5-ml divided dose for 5 mo); pediatric dose 0.02 ml/kg for 3-month, 0.06 ml/kg for 5-month trip	Boost at 3 to 5-month intervals depending on initial dose received
Japanese encephalitis (JE)	3 doses given on days 0, 7, and 30 (1 ml SC if > 3 years; 0.5 ml SC if < 3 years)	A booster dose may be given after 2 years
Meningococcus (A/C/Y/W-135)	1 dose[a] SC	None (variable immunogenic response in children < 4 years of age; revaccination for this group is recommended after 2–3 years for those who continue to be at high risk)
Plague	1st dose (1 ml IM); 2nd dose (0.2 ml IM) 4 weeks later; dose 3 (0.2 ml IM) 3–6 months after dose 2	Boost if the risk of exposure persists; give the first 2 booster doses (0.1–0.2 ml) 6 months apart, then give 1 booster dose at 1 to 2-year intervals as needed
Rabies, human diploid cell vaccine (HDCV)	3 doses (0.1 ml ID) on days 0, 7, and 21 or 28	Boost after 2 years or test serum for antibody level (must not use chloroquine prophylaxis until 3 weeks after completion of ID series)
Rabies (HDCV) or rabies vaccine absorbed (RVA)	3 doses (1 ml IM in the deltoid area) on days 0, 7, and 28	Boost after 2 years or test serum for antibody level
Tuberculosis (BCG vaccine)[b]	1 dose percutaneously with multiple-puncture disc; 1/2 strength for infants < 1 month old	Revaccination after 2–3 months in those who remain negative to 5 TU skin test
Typhoid, injectable	2 doses (0.5 ml SC or IC) 4 or more weeks apart; pediatric dose (< 10 years old), 0.25 ml	Boost after 3 years if there is continued risk of exposure
Typhoid, injectable (not acetone-killed and dried vaccine)		Boost with 0.1 ml ID every 3 years
Typhoid, oral	1 capsule PO every 2 days for 4 doses (> 6 years old)	5 years
Yellow fever[b]	1 dose (0.5 ml SC); pediatric dose 0.5 ml SC for > 6 months old	10 years

[a]See manufacturer's package insert for recommendations on dosage.
[b]*Caution:* May be contraindicated in patients with any of the following conditions: pregnancy, leukemia, lymphoma, generalized malignancy, immunosuppression due to HIV infection or treatment with corticosteroids, alkylating drugs, antimetabolites, or radiation therapy.
Source: From Jong, E. C. Immunizations for International Travelers. In F. J. Bia (ed.), *Travel Medicine Advisor.* Atlanta: American Health Consultants, 1993.

Table 38-4. Vaccine interactions

Vaccine	Interaction	Precaution
Immune globulin	Measles/mumps/rubella, (MMR) vaccine	Give these vaccines at least 2 weeks before immune globulin (IG), or 3–5 months after IG, depending on dose received.
Oral typhoid vaccine	Antibiotic therapy	Administer oral typhoid vaccine (OTV) at least 1 week after antibiotic therapy is completed. Do not take antibiotics for at least 3 weeks after OTV is completed.
Oral typhoid vaccine	Mefloquine malaria chemoprophylaxis	Schedule an interval of at least 8 hours between an oral typhoid dose and a mefloquine dose.
Oral typhoid vaccine	Oral polio vaccine	Oral polio vaccine (OPV) should not be taken at the same time as OTV, OPV can be given 7–10 days before or 10–14 days after OTV.
Rabies vaccine (HDCV) intradermal series	Chloroquine malaria chemoprophylaxis	Complete rabies vaccine (intradermal series) at least 3 weeks before starting chloroquine. Use the rabies vaccine IM series if the 3-week interval is not possible.
Virus vaccines, live (MMR, OPV, yellow fever)	Other live virus vaccines	Give live virus vaccines on the same day, or separate the doses by at least 1 month.
Virus vaccines, live (MMR, OPV, yellow fever)	Tuberculin skin test (PPD)	Do the skin test on the same day as receipt of a live virus vaccine, or 4–6 weeks after, because the virus vaccines can impair the response to the PPD skin test.
Yellow fever	Cholera vaccine	Give the two vaccines on the same day or at least 3 weeks apart.

Source: From Jong, E. C. Immunizations for International Travelers. In F. J. Bia (ed.), *Travel Medicine Advisor*. Atlanta: American Health Consultants, 1993.

the medical kit. ("This patient has been required to carry the following medication for medical reasons . . .") This measure will prevent the person from embarrassing and potentially long-term delays at international borders by curious customs agents. If routine medication is used, it is wise to state the patient's major health-related problems and the medication dosage on a prescription pad.

Other essentials include medication that the person normally takes and devices such as splints. An extra pair of glasses or contact lenses is recommended along with a lens prescription. Those going to excessively dirty or dusty areas should be encouraged to take eyeglasses in addition to contact lenses. (See Table 38-5, in which three different types of medical kits are proposed.)

A *Medic-Alert card* that includes basic medical information in wallet-size format is advisable if the patient has a serious medical condition. Some cards include vital health data, such as medications, blood pressure measurements, and copies of electrocardiogram tracings. A brief medical history and baseline blood results may benefit the employee on assignment overseas and aid the physician in the foreign country (see nos. 5 and 6, Chapter Appendix 1).

Malaria and Insect Protection

The degree of rural travel, intensity of exposure to mosquito bites, length of stay in an endemic area, and self-protection efforts will affect the possibility of contracting malaria. Antimalarial chemoprophylaxis should not lull the person into complacency

Table 38-5. Medical Kits

Kit A: Business travel to a temperate climate

Oral medications
1. Antihistamine/decongestant for colds or allergies
2. Bismuth-salicylate tablets II qid for prevention of traveler's diarrhea
3. Antibiotic and immodium for treatment of more serious traveler's diarrhea (e.g., ciprofloxacin, doxycycline)
4. Aspirin or acetaminophen for fever
5. Antacid/antiflatulence tablets for dietary indiscretions
6. Sleep medications, i.e., triazolam (Halcion) for noisy hotels or jet lag
7. Analgesic/nonsteroidal antiinflammatory agents: codeine, ibuprofen for minor injuries
8. Laxative (senna or bulk agent [Citrucel]) for constipation
9. Personal prescription medications[a]

Topical medications
1. Hemorrhoid suppositories
2. Saline eyedrops for dusty eyes
3. Povidone iodine individual pads or ointment for cuts and scratches
4. 1% Cortisone cream for minor rashes
5. Antifungal cream

Supplies
1. Alcohol swabs
2. Disposable syringes and needles[b]
3. Disposable thermometer
4. Cotton-tip swabs
5. Band-Aids, various sizes
6. Swiss army–type knife
7. Small scissors and forceps
8. Personal hygienic items
9. Latex gloves
10. Disposable masks
11. Water purifier

Kit B: Business travel to the tropics

All of the items included in kit A with the addition of:
1. High-numbered (25–35) SPF sunscreen
2. Sunglasses
3. Moleskin, pads, and other blister treatments
4. Antifungal cream, i.e., tolnaftate
5. Moisturizing lotion for sunburns
6. Insect repellent containing 35% DEET (ultrathon)
7. Permethrin spray for clothes and mosquito netting
8. Antimalarial tablets[c]
9. Oral rehydration (ORS) tablets or sachets
10. Anti-itch lotion (calamine)

Kit C: Business travel to high-altitude destinations

All of the items included in kit A with the addition of:
1. Sunglasses with good ultraviolet light filtration
2. Acetazolamide tablets (prevention of altitude sickness)
3. Dexamethasone tablets (acute mountain sickness)
4. Space blanket
5. High-numbered (50) SPF sunscreen

[a]Copies of prescriptions can also be helpful, especially for lengthy stays or for crossing international borders.
[b]As there is significant risk of bloodborne diseases, such as AIDS and hepatitis B, from contaminated syringes in certain countries, it is advisable to send disposables along with the traveler. A prescription indicating that the person needs to carry these items is sufficient to allay questions at customs checks.
[c]Depending on destination, the most commonly prescribed antimalarial medications are mefloquine, 250 mg, or chloroquine, 500 mg weekly, 1 week before, weekly during, and 4 weeks after return; and doxycycline, 100 mg, 3 days before, daily during, and 3 weeks after return.

about risks, since people can still contract this illness despite prophylaxis. Personal protective measures (repellants, clothing, nets) are essential adjuncts to the prevention of malaria.

Some malaria strains have become resistant to prophylactic drugs, in particular, chloroquine [7, 8]. Proguanil, mefloquine, and doxycycline are the most commonly used antimalarial prophylactic drugs for chloroquine-resistant malaria strains at this time. Sulfadoxine and pyrimethamine (Fansidar), and sulfisoxazole, are still used in other specific prophylactic regimes. Current recommendations for the area to which the person travels should be consulted. The potential side effects of the antimalarial drug need to be addressed. Mefloquine should not be used by airline pilots or others, in whom central nervous system side effects could be detrimental to performance or the safety of others. Drug interactions need to be considered (i.e., mefloquine should not be used with beta-blockers or calcium channel blockers, or with drugs that alter cardiac conduction). Treatment itself may result in adverse consequences, as noted by chloroquine's toxicity [9].

A coordinated approach to keeping mosquitos and other insects from attacking is essential in preventing not only malaria but also other insect-borne diseases (yellow fever, dengue fever, viral encephalitis, filariasis, leishmaniasis, trypanosomiasis, onchocercosis, etc.) [10]. Insect repellents with N-diethyl-meta-toluamide (DEET) may be used on the skin or clothing, or both. Repellents with more than 35% DEET can lead to neurologic symptoms because excessive amounts can be absorbed through the skin. Hexanediol is a viable alternative for those who may be sensitive to DEET. The commercially available moisturizer, "Skin-So-Soft," needs to be applied every 20 minutes to be an effective repellent. All persons traveling to endemic areas of malaria and other insect-borne diseases should wear long-sleeved shirts and long pants, especially after dusk. Clothes can be treated with DEET-containing repellents and the insecticide permethrin. Lightweight mesh jackets, hoods, and face-guards can be effective in highly infested areas. Mosquito bed netting is an important adjunct in malaria prevention. Numerous types of portable bed nets can be purchased in sports stores and from other suppliers to ensure appropriate protection while sleeping (see no. 14, Chapter Appendix 1). (See [11], [12], and [13] for a discussion on prevention and treatment of malaria.)

Water Precautions

For the traveler to the world's capitals, bottled water is usually available. You will rarely see local Parisians or Dubliners drinking tap water. Although usually safe, faulty "medieval" water pipes in certain sections of otherwise highly advanced cities allow for contamination. Travelers should be reminded to remove the plastic seal on any bottle sold as purified water. Carbonated water gives yet one more guarantee that the bottled water has not been tampered with. Heating water to 62°C for 10 minutes is sufficient to eliminate all strains of bacteria. Adding iodine or chlorine and allowing the water to sit for 30 minutes will disinfect the filtered water. Sediments should be filtered *before* adding the iodine or chlorine to ensure complete killing of the bacteria, parasites, worm larvae, and particularly viruses.

Water filtration systems that are effective on camping trips in North America may not be appropriate in developing nations since many do not filter bacteria and/ or viruses. The "PUR" brand of various-sized filters conveniently and efficiently combine 1.0-μ filters with a new technology—*tri-iodine resin matrix*—to eliminate bacteria, parasites, and viruses. The "Katadyn" filters come in individual and group filter formats. The latter is appropriate for the person staying in a foreign destination for some time. "Katadyn" filters to the 0.2 μ level. It is advisable to use iodine following this latter filtration process to eliminate the viruses [4, 10] (see Chapter Appendix 1).

Jet Lag

Short-term international travel involves rapid passage across great distances, often through several time zones. This rapid air travel can disrupt physiologic and psychological rhythms in the human body, which are referred to as *circadian rhythms* [14, 15]. *Circadian*, a term meaning "about a day," developed as the description of this process because it takes the human body 25 hours to cycle [16, 17].

The body and its biorhythms are tied much more closely to the solar day than to the 24-hour mechanical clock. The study of these cycles and their effects on the body is known as *chronobiology*. The signs and symptoms of jet lag are due to alterations of the circadian rhythm. This syndrome adversely affects millions of travelers by causing sleep disturbances, malaise, irritability, reduced mental and physical performance, apathy, depression, fatigue, loss of appetite, gastric distress, and altered bowel habits.

Exposure to light at particular intensities may be critical to both etiology and subsequent treatment of jet lag [18–22]. Light's intensity and *spectral quality* appear to initiate or block certain biochemical processes in the human and animal body. When a certain intensity of light is increased, melatonin production is suppressed [18, 23]. Melatonin is secreted by the pineal gland and regulates responses to changing daylight in many animal species. Other hormone and neurotransmitters may be implicated in the metabolic and neurochemical aspects of jet lag. Significant collaborative research indicates that exposure to light can reset the circadian clock [24].

When there is a difference between actual time and the body's internal "clock," *external dysynchrony* exists. The traveler who has a meeting at 10:00 AM local time may be functioning at 4:00 AM on the internal body clock. At 4:00 AM, however, the body is accustomed to a reduced physiologic and psychological state, which may not be appropriate for the person expected to be alert at a business meeting.

There are several ways of managing jet lag. For the fastidious person who has time to plan meals 3 days before travel, a diet that alternates a feast and fast of high carbohydrates and high proteins is available. Unfortunately, most travelers cannot adhere to this diet in a way that makes it effective. On a dietary basis, however, one may modify, to some extent, the symptoms of jet lag by eating a high-carbohydrate dinner the night before travel and, on the trip, eating salads, fruit plates, and other light dishes. Similarly, the employee should drink plenty of fluids before and during the air travel to reduce both jet lag and air travel fatigue. Alcohol before or during the trip should be avoided because it increases the effects of jet lag and suppresses the rapid eye movement (REM) phase of sleep, the most critical component of the sleep cycle.

Proverbial wisdom regarding light exposure and jet lag is to avoid exposure to morning light and maximize exposure to midday and late afternoon light. For example, if a person was leaving the East Coast of the United States on an evening flight to Europe, this approach would require avoiding daylight on the morning of departure and using dark sunglasses. Upon arrival in Europe, the person would avoid daylight until late morning and then spend as much time as possible in bright outdoor light or stare out the bright side of an office building. If, for example, that same person was flying west to the Hawaiian Islands on an afternoon flight, he or she would avoid daylight in the morning, take a window seat in order to adjust the light, and absorb as much afternoon sunlight as possible. A convenient computer program is now available, along with a tested headlamp, which provides the recommended amount of light to modify jet lag. (See no. 1, Chapter Appendix 1 for supplier.) For people who do not wish to use light as a modifier for jet lag symptoms, a formula of amino acids, vitamins, and hypnotics is available.

Triazolam (Halcion) has been used to reduce some of the effects of jet lag. It should not be taken, however, at altitude in conjunction with alcohol because of the risk of retrograde amnesia [25]. An antihistamine such as diphenhydramine at 50 to 100 mg will also produce an hypnotic effect. The patient should attempt in-flight exercises when traveling long distances to decrease fatigue and symptoms of jet lag.

Medical Evacuations and Medical Care Abroad

Several agencies provide lists of physicians knowledgeable in English who adhere to a financial agreement such that travelers are not charged outrageous sums for routine medical care. The International Association for Medical Assistance to Travelers (IAMAT), Inn Care, and Inter Continental Medical provide such services and lists of physicians overseas (see Chapter Appendix 1, nos. 7, 8, and 9, respectively).

If an IAMAT or Inn Care physician is not available, referral from fellow expatriates or business associates to their own personal physician is often an adequate method of obtaining medical care. Seeking advice for a physician from hotels or consulates/embassies is not recommended because political and economic incentives may override academic and clinical capabilities in the respective recommendations. Gaining access to medical care in some countries can be difficult because of language barriers, unfamiliar customs, government regulations, nonacceptance of foreign insurance carriers, and unfamiliarity with American medical practices.

In some countries, medical care is excellent and patterned after formats in which North American employers are familiar. In most countries, payment for services is expected at the time of service or before service. Consequently, people should be advised to take traveler's checks, cash, or credit cards to a hospital or physician's office and expect to pay, with possible reimbursement later on. It is also common practice in some countries to tip the receptionist or nurse so that waiting times decrease. In some countries, one pays the physician directly in the examination room.

Various travel insurance policies are available that cover two distinct areas: insurance for medical care overseas and insurance for evacuation from one area to a more appropriate medical facility. Occasionally, a combination of the two policies is available. It is a good idea for a traveler to carry one or both types of policies, since American insurance may not cover medical care overseas except for emergencies, and then often only after a protracted effort. Medicare, preferred provider organizations (PPOs), and most health maintenance organizations, in particular, do not offer coverage. It is often difficult to convince a medical insurance company in the United States that the care abroad was either appropriately priced or necessary, as translations may be problematic. (See Chapter Appendix 2 for insurance companies that provide this service.)

Several companies have expertise in the evacuation of ill and injured persons from areas where appropriate medical care is not available. Some organizations specialize in a particular region of the world, whereas others are worldwide in scope. Although a policy may be purchased from one corporation, the services of a local evacuation emergency service may be used as part of the arrangement. A wide variety of services are available from these companies, some of which have 24-hour availability and interpreter services. (See Chapter Appendix 2 for further description of these services.)

Screening the Traveler Upon Return

Except for the careful person who samples no local cuisine, meticulously boils or filters all liquids, and fastidiously washes hands before consuming food, it may be valuable to screen the returning traveler for "unwanted souvenirs" from his or her work assignment overseas [26]. For the traveler who has had contact with locals in a factory, health care facility, or private home, or had questionable dietary intake, and for those who may have reduced resistance to disease, *routine screening* is often recommended. Ancillary testing may vary from a complete blood count (CBC), erythrocyte sedimentation rate (ESR), and chemistry panel to urinalysis, tuberculin skin test, and stool for ova, parasites, and culture. These tests should be modified based on the countries visited and the person's symptoms. Serologic screening for hepatitis, schistosomiasis, filariasis, or dengue fever may be indicated [27, 28]. Certain tropically acquired diseases may remain latent for extended periods of time. As a result, earlier travel should be considered in the diagnosis of symptoms that appear months and occasionally years after the person's return.

A thorough skin examination should note rashes, edema, or unusual nodules. Examination of the eyes should concentrate on conjunctival migration of adult loiasis and other similar parasitic infections. Cutaneous mycoses, in particular tinea versicolor and tinea pedis, are the most common skin disorders acquired by travelers. Cutaneous myiasis may be brought home from Central and South America and tropical Africa. The botfly larva is the usual offending agent.

Traveler's Diarrhea

This ailment is pervasive among travelers. If the traveler is vigilant and meticulous in eating and drinking, as the CDC suggests, prophylactic antibiotics are not necessary. For the *short-term* visit to certain countries, such as North Americans traveling to Mexico, prophylactic antibiotics may be appropriate (i.e., doxycycline, 100 mg/day, or trimethoprim/sulfamethoxazole, 1 tablet/day) [29]. Prophylaxis and/or treatment of simple traveler's diarrhea can be achieved with bismuth-salicylate (Pepto-Bismol), 2 tablets qid). This treatment and prophylaxis is usually effective, but the patient should be cautioned that the tongue and stool may darken, and that no other aspirin-containing medications should be taken.

Oral rehydration with glucose and electrolyte solutions is the cornerstone of therapy for acute traveler's diarrhea since most cases are self-limited. Commercially available prepackaged mixes and tablets of oral rehydration salts (ORS) are available over-the-counter in most developing countries.

Recent studies have shown that various antibiotics alone or in combination with loperamide are highly effective in treating traveler's diarrhea [29]. Trimethoprim/ sulfamethoxazole (1 double-strength tablet) twice a day for 3 days taken along with two loperamide capsules at the onset of diarrhea, followed by one loperamide after every loose stool up to five per 24 hours, is usually effective.

Fluoroquinolone antibiotics are effective against *Shigella, Salmonella,* and *Clostridium jejuni* in addition to the most common *Escherichia coli*–induced traveler's diarrhea. Ciprofloxacin, 500-mg dose twice a day for 3 days, or a single 750-mg dose is also effective. One or two doses of loperamide, in addition to this antibiotic, may add some comfort. An alternative to ciprofloxacin is ofloxacin, 400 mg twice a day for 1 to 3 days.

Doxycycline, 100 mg twice a day for 1 to 3 days, will often cure traveler's diarrhea in people who are unable to take a quinoline or sulfa drug. In fact doxycycline, 100 mg per day, can act not only as a diarrheal preventive but also as a malarial prophylactic in certain *Plasmodium falciparum*–resistant areas, such as Thailand.

Metronidazole should only be used for microscopically diagnosed infections with *Giardia* or amebas (500 mg tid for 7–10 days). Outside the US, tinidazole is used for these two infections (2 g daily for 2–6 days).

Malaria

The person who returns with high fevers, chills, sweating, headache, and muscle aches may have contracted malaria. Not all cases, however, follow a classic pattern of fevers. Since there are many resistant strains of malaria, history of exposure to insect bites should raise the physician's level of suspicion. Blood smears, CBC, and liver function tests will often point to the diagnosis. If the level of suspicion is still high, and local laboratories have not diagnosed the organism, blood smears can be sent to a reference laboratory for potential identification. Depending on where the malaria was contracted, treatment with chloroquine, mefloquine, quinine, or doxycycline can be used.

Selected Issues

AIDS

AIDS has spread rapidly in Asia, West and East Africa, Latin America, and parts of Europe within the heterosexual population. Since sexual contact is the major route of human immunodeficiency virus (HIV) infection in the traveler, people should be advised about safe sex practices, especially with persons in whom the HIV infection status is unknown. Disposable syringes and needles should be available in the medical kit if injections or blood testing are necessary during travel in certain countries. A number of countries have rapidly changing policies regarding people with HIV infection entering their country. Some policies require proof of HIV testing for persons applying for visas that allow them to remain in a country for long periods of time. China, for example, at the time of this writing, requires AIDS testing for those remaining more than 3 months. It is customary to provide the traveler with a physician-signed (and in some cases notarized) copy of the laboratory slip indicating negative HIV testing. One may also place a note in the International Certificate of Vaccination (yellow book) in the "Other" section, indicating the date, address, and result of HIV testing. It is advisable that a business person be tested for HIV before assignment in a country where HIV is endemic, for personal knowledge and to reduce a corporation's liability.

If an employee is involved in an accident or requires surgical intervention and a transfusion, it should be recognized that the blood supply may not be *HIV free.* This problem is notable in Africa and other countries where HIV incidence is either not officially recognized or the financial means to test all blood supplies is absent. Consequently, it is often difficult to obtain accurate statistics. The National Red Cross organizations maintain some information worth pursuing before assignment. This topic emphasizes the importance of pretravel evaluation to decrease the necessity of uncertain medical interventions while overseas. Curtailment of certain risky sporting activities in remote areas is also advisable unless preparation has included appropriate medical kits and an insurance policy with provisions for evacuation from the country where blood supplies are questionable. Gathering blood from fellow expatriates for a scheduled surgery is becoming a common practice in some areas. Careful attention to the risks of HIV infection in some countries is advisable.

Pollution

Some large industrialized cities of the world have significant air pollution problems. Mexico City is one of the worst, although Bangkok, Seoul, Jakarta, Kiev, and Warsaw, among others, have pollution levels that can affect people with pulmonary disorders. One should evaluate and advise the person with a potential adverse reaction to highly polluted environments. In some major urban areas, people wear disposable cotton masks. For infection and pollution protection, this practice can assist by decreasing particulate contamination. In Mexico City, the air pollution is so bad that the city has actually installed oxygen booths in the city center.

Safety

More Americans die overseas from road traffic and pedestrian accidents than from infectious diseases. In most developing and newly industrialized nations, the number of people on the roads is overwhelming. Auto, bus, truck, rickshaw, bullock cart, and motorcycle drivers must weave their way among numerous pedestrians. One should remind the person to be vigilant of potential dangers when walking or crossing thoroughfare areas shared by various types of vehicles.

Physical Safety

Business travelers are at risk of being kidnapped, hijacked, taken hostage, or mugged. During travel to certain countries, it is inadvisable to dress like a high-profile business person or to carry expensive luggage or items that identify the person as an American. Travel to a high-risk country necessitates personal security training and a crisis management plan. Sensitive documents should be sent separately and the person should take a nonstop flight to the destination city. Various insurance companies will provide kidnap insurance (see Chapter Appendix 2).

International Organizations

As borders have become more fluid, the relationship between various international organizations has been enhanced. Occupational medicine physicians have opportunities to join colleagues in other countries to share ideas through meetings and organizations. (See Chapter Appendix 3 for specific organizations.)

Multinational Programs

Preparing the business traveler, administering vaccines, and preparing medical kits represent a small part of international occupational medicine. The specialist also sets up programs that challenge the internationally pervasive hazards inherent in the workplace, in a world in which old and new technologies persist simultaneously. These programs are developed within a framework of a multitude of cultures, medical systems, political intrigues, and regulations. In addressing multinational programs in Asia, Europe, Africa, Australia, the Middle East, and Central and South America, one must be aware of regional differences, social interactions, and endemic medical conditions.

When developing an occupational health program for a particular location, one must be knowledgeable of the risks related to socioeconomic conditions associated with caste systems, apartheid, and other artificially assigned work statuses. These conditions will affect how programs can be implemented. When sending an employee overseas, one must view all environmental and occupational health risks. The local conditions for a work situation or particular factory must be evaluated in light of the entire country or region's occupational health organization and available services.

References

1. Karpilow, C. *Occupational Medicine in the International Workplace.* New York: Van Nostrand Reinhold, 1991.
2. Green, B. M. Advice to Travelers. In Cecil (ed.), *Textbook of Medicine* (19th ed.). Philadelphia: Sanders, 1992. P. 1595.
3. Cottrell, J., et al. In flight medical emergencies: One year of experience with the enhanced medical kit. *J.A.M.A.* 262:12, 1989.
4. Cruikshank, J., Gorlin, R., and Jennett, B. Air travel and thrombotic episodes: The economy class syndrome. *Lancet* 27:497, 1988.
5. CDC. *Health Information for International Travel.* US Department of Health and Human Services, Public Health Department. Publication no. (CDC) 92-8280 annually updated for sale by the Superintendent of Documents, US Government Printing Office, Washington, DC, 20402.
6. WHO. *Vaccination Certificate Requirements and Health Advice for International Travel.* ISBN 92 4 158011 9. WHO, 1211 Geneva 27, Switzerland.
7. Moran, J. S., and Bernard, K. W. The spread of chloroquine resistant malaria in Africa. Implications for travelers. *J.A.M.A.* 262:245, 1989.
8. Lackritz, E. M. Imported *Plasmodium falciparum* malaria in American travelers to Africa. *J.A.M.A.* 265(3):383, 1991.
9. Riou, B., et al. Treatment of severe chloroquine poisoning. *N. Engl. J. Med.* 318:1, 1988.
10. Karpilow, C. Advice to travelers on malaria prevention. *Travel Med. Int. J.,* 9.1:35, 1991.
11. White, N. J. Treatment and prevention of malaria. *Eur. Clin. J. Pharmacol.* 34:1, 1988.
12. Recommendations for the prevention of malaria in travelers. Centers for Disease Control. *M.M.W.R.* 37:277, 1988.
13. Keystone, J. S. Prevention of malaria. *Drugs* 39:337, 1990.
14. Pool, R. Illuminating jet lag. *Science* 244:1256, 1989.
15. Minors, D. S., and Waterhouse, J. M. Circadian Rhythms in General Practice and Occupational Health. In J. Arend, D. S. Minors, and J. M. Waterhouse (eds.), *Biological Rhythms in Clinical Practice.* London: Butterworth, 1989. Pp. 207–224.
16. Moore-Ede, M. C. *The Twenty Four Hour Society.* Reading, MA: Addison-Wesley, 1993.
17. Moore-Ede, M. C., Sulzman, F. M., and Fuller C. A. *The Clocks That Time Us.* Cambridge, MA: Harvard University Press, 1982.
18. Lewy, A. J., et al. Light suppresses melatonin secretion in humans. *Science* 210:1267, 1980.
19. Czeisler, C. A., et al. Exposure to bright light and darkness to treat physiologic maladaptation to night work. *N. Engl. J. Med.* 322:1253, 1990.
20. Lewey, A. J., et al. Antidepressant and circadian phase shifting effects of light. *Science* 235:352, 1987.
21. Czeisler, C. A., et al. Bright light resets the human circadian pacemaker independent of the timing of the sleep wake cycle. *Science* 233:667, 1986.
22. Dawson, D., Lack, L., and Morris, M. Phase resetting of the human circadian pacemaker with use of a single pulse of bright light. *Chronobiol. Int.* 10:94, 1993.
23. Brainard, G. C., et al. Circadian rhythms of melatonin in primates' cerebral spinal fluid. *Natl. Register* 211:25A, 1985.
24. Van Cauter, E., and Turek, F. Strategies for resetting the human circadian clock. *N. Engl. J. Med.* 322:1306, 1990.
25. Morris, H. Travelers amnesia: Transient global amnesia secondary to triazolam. *J.A.M.A.* 258(7):945, 1987.
26. Gilles, H. M. Diseases of travelers returning from exotic areas. *J. Intern. Med.* 10(6), June 1989.

27. Gustatsson, L. L. *Handbook of Drugs for Tropical Parasitic Infections.* London: Taylor and Francis, 1987.
28. Warren, K. S. *Tropical and Geographical Medicine.* New York: McGraw-Hill, 1985.
29. Steffan, R., et al. Efficacy and side effects of six agents in the self-treatment of traveller's diarrhea. *Travel Med. Int. J.* 6:153, 1988.

Further Information

CDC. Hotline for International Travel (404-332-4559): Malaria (404-639-1610), Parasitic Drugs (404-639-3670), Rabies (404-639-3095), ETL (404-639-3311), PMs (404-639-2888).

Circadian Travel Technologies, 7315 Wisconsin Ave., Suite 1300W, Bethesda, MD 20814 (1-800-JETGUIDE; fax no. 301-907-8637).
Resource for jet lag headlamp or jet lag computer program.

Consumer Reports Travel Letter (1-800-525-0643).

Diabetic Traveler, PO Box 8223 Stamford, CT 06905.

Durgin, R. W. *The Physically Disabled Traveler's Guide Resources Directories.* 3103 Executive Parkway, Toledo, OH 43606.

The Journal of Emporiatrics Travel Medicine International. Croxted Mews, 288 Croxted Rd., London SE249DA, England. Hugh L. Etang, MD (ed.).

Moore, C. E. International Occupational Health Care. *J. Occup. Med.* 36:419, 1994. *A thorough article addressing health issues associated with expatriate assignments.*

Traveling Healthy. Karl Neumann, MD, 108-48 70th Rd., Forest Hills, NY 11375.

Travel Medicine Advisor, PO Box 740060, Atlanta, GA 30374.

US State Department travel advisories. Citizens Emergency Center, Washington, DC (202-647-5226).

World Press Review. PO Box 1997, Manon, OH 43305.

Appendix 1 to Chapter 38: Information and Supplies

1. Circadian Travel Technologies, 7315 Wisconsin Ave., Suite 1300W, Bethesda, MD 20814 (1-800-JET-GUIDE; fax no. 301-907-8637).
2. Computer Data Bases: Travel Health Information Service (1-800-443-5256); Immunization Alert (1-230-487-0002); Catis (1-416-340-3959).
3. Video: *How to Keep Your Employees Healthy When They Travel.* IPA, 509 Olive Way, Suite 803, Seattle, WA 98101.
4. "Polar Pure" and "PotableAqua" are iodine preparations that can be obtained in most sporting goods stores.
5. Medical Emergency/ID Cards: Medical Graphics Inc., PO Box 11687, St. Louis, MO 63105.
6. Medic-Alert Bracelet: 1-800-ID-ALERT.
7. International Association for Medical Assistance to Travelers (IMAT), 417 Center St., Lewiston, NY 14092 (716-754-4883) or (519-836-0102).
8. Inn Care, PO Box 1204, Clarksville, TN 37041 (1-800-489-6277).
9. Inter Continental Medical Ltd., 2720 Enterprise Pkwy. #106, Richmond, VA 23294 (804-527-1094).
10. Water Filters: *PUR* series of water filters (1-800-845-PURE) and *Katadyn* PF filter (602-990-3131).
11. Jet Lag Exercises: IPA, 509 Olive Way, Suite 803, Seattle, WA 98101.
12. Weather Reports: *USA Today* (1-900-555-5555) Weather, foreign country entry requirements, US dollar exchange rates, voltage requirements.
13. American Express (1-900-932-8437). Weather, 3-day forecast, passport and visa requirements, restaurant and hotel information.
14. Travel Supplies: Travel Medicine Inc. (1-800-TRAV-MED); Chinook Medical Gear Inc. (303-444-8689, Solumbra (1-800-882-7860).

Appendix 2 to Chapter 38: Evacuation Insurance Services

"World Access Australia," Second Floor, 178 Pacific Highway, St. Leonards NSW 2065, Australia, has gained a good reputation for these services in Asia. "International SOS Assistance," 1 Neshaminy Interplex, 310 Trevose, PA 19053, has particular expertise in Europe and North Africa. Several other services are available, including "Europe Assistance"; "Travelers Medical Service of London"; "Flying Doctors Society of Africa," Nairobi, Kenya (254-2-501-280); and "Swiss Air Rescue," Zurich, Switzerland (41-1-383-1111). Some of these policies can include multiple trips by a single employee.

The Overseas Security Advisory Council, a joint venture between the State Department and the private sector, PO Box 3590, Washington, DC 20007-0090 (202-663-0002) maintains an electronic bulletin board that provides information on overseas security conditions.

Insurance companies that provide *kidnap protection* include the Ackerman Group, Miami Beach, FL; Control Risks Ltd., Bethesda, MD; P. Argen Inc., New York; and Paul Chamberlain International, Beverly Hills, CA.

Insurance companies that provide *medical care insurance* overseas are TravMed (1-800-732-5309), Access America (1-800-284-8300), Travel Protection Plan (1-800-234-0375), Travelers Insurance (1-800-243-3174), Travel Assistance International (1-800-821-2828), and Health Care Abroad (1-800-237-6615).

Appendix 3 to Chapter 38: International Organizations

Administration de l'Hygiène et de la Médicin du Travail, 53 Rue Belliard, 1040 Brussels, Belgium.

The American College of Occupational and Environmental Medicine, 55 W. Seegers Rd., Arlington Heights, IL 60005, has an International Occupational Medicine Section and several committees dealing with international issues. The American College sponsors various educational programs dealing with international aspects of the field.

Australian Faculty of Occupational Medicine (Niki Ellis, MD FACOM, President), 44 Birtley Towers, 8 Birtley Pl., Elizabeth Bay, New South Wales 2011, Australia.

Australian and New Zealand Society of Occupational Medicine, 18 Fairfield Ave., Camberwell Vic. 3124, Australia.

Canadian Occupational Health Association, 1565 Carling Ave., Suite 400, Ottawa, Ontario K1Z 8R1, Canada.

Czechoslovakian Medical Societies sponsor a number of meetings in Eastern Europe. Czechoslovakian Medical Societies Sokolska 31120–26 Prague 2, Czechoslovakia.

The Department of Environmental Health, the Government of Egypt sponsors a number of conferences annually. The Department of Environmental Health, Fine Institute of Public Health, 165 El Horriya Ave., Alexandria, Egypt.

Finnish Association of Industrial Medicine, Makelankatu 2, SF 00500 Helsinki, Finland.

Global Environment Technology Network (GETNET) link specialists in environmental technology with each other and with the World Health Organization Information and Training resources. WHO Environmental Health Division (PEP), 1211 Geneva 27, Switzerland.

Greek Society of Medical Issues Studies, Spetson 93, Athens 113 63, Greece.

The Hungarian Society for Occupational Health, National Institute of Occupational Health, PO Box 22, Nagyvard Ter 2, Hungary.

The International Commission on Occupational Health incorporates many smaller international occupational medicine groups. Membership is open to all interested individuals. Address: Jerry Jeyaratnam, MD, Administrative Officer, ICOH, Department of Commerce, Occupational and Family Medicine, National University Hospital, Lower Kent Ridge Rd., S(0511), Republic of Singapore 0511 (65-772-4290; Fax no. 65-779-1489).

Japan Association of Industrial Health, Public Health Building, 11-29-8 Shinjuku Sinjuki-ku, Tokyo 160, Japan.

Korean Industrial Medical Centre, 1022-1 Bangbae-dong, Socho-ku, Seoul 137-063, Korea.

MEDICHEM,, an international organization of occupational health professionals concerned with health issues associated with the chemical industry. Information can be obtained from Dr. Andreas Flückiger, Corporate Health Services, F. Hoffman-LaRoche LDT, CH-4002 Basel, Switzerland. Medichem holds an annual Congress in a different country each year. Proceedings published by the World Health Organization.

The National Council for International Health, 1701 K St. NW, Suite 600, Washington, DC 20006.

The Overseas Security Advisory Council, a joint venture between the State Department and the private sector, PO Box 3590, Washington, DC 20007-0090 (202-663-0002) maintains an electronic bulletin board that provides information on overseas security conditions.

Philippine College of Occupational Medicine, PMA Building, North Ave., Quezon City, Philippines.

Sociedad de Medicina del Trabajo, C. de Correo 2, 1421 Buenos Aires, Argentina.

Sociedad Ecuatoriana de Salud Occupacional (SESO), Caasilla 7015, Guyaquil, Ecuador.

Sociedad Espanola de Medicina y Seguridad del Trabajo, Tapineria 10, Pralk, Barcelona 2, Spain.

Sociedad Portuguesa de Medicina do Trabalho, Av. Da Republica 34-1, P-1000 Lisboa, Portugal.

South African Society of Occupational Medicine, PO Box 6554, Johannesburg 2000, South Africa.

The Swedish Association of Occupational Health Physicians, Svenska Foretagslakarforeningen, PO Box 5610, Villagatan 5, S-114 86, Stockholm, Sweden.

39

Workers' Compensation

Jeffrey S. Harris

Workers' compensation management has become more visible in recent years because of an increase in the number of lost workdays per 100 employees and a rapid increase in the cost of both wage replacement and medical treatment. Wage replacement costs are increasing at almost twice the rate of the general wage index, and medical care costs are rising two to three times faster than the medical consumer price index. These costs have affected where companies locate, have driven a number of insurance companies to leave certain state markets, and have brought attention to the often fragmented management of real or allegedly occupationally related illness and injury, and the quality and quantity of medical care provided under workers' compensation statutes. Effective management of workers' compensation provides a challenge to the administrative and clinical skills of the occupational physician. The effort, however, can benefit both the injured worker with more effective medical care and the employer by increasing availability for work and decreasing unnecessary costs. This chapter discusses the history, provisions, and strategic management of workers' compensation from the perspective of the occupational physician.

Epidemiology of Occupational Death, Illness, and Injury

Mortality

Between 1912 and 1990, accidental work deaths per 100,000 population dropped 81% from 21 per 100,000 to 4 per 100,000 [1] (Fig. 39-1). The top five causes of deaths are motor vehicle accidents (35.5%), falls (12.7%), electric current accidents (3.6%), burns (3.5%), and noningestive poisoning (3.5%).

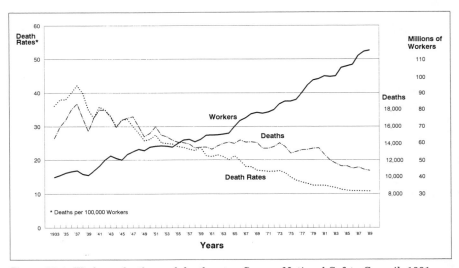

Figure 39-1. Workers, deaths, and death rates. Source: National Safety Council, 1991.

Although disagreement exists regarding the number of work-related fatalities in the United States, most authorities believe that the number of deaths is understated. The National Safety Council surveyed hospital discharge abstracts for the International Classification of Diseases (ICD) 9 E codes 800 to 949 in 1990, and estimated that there were 10,500 occupational deaths. The study covered all persons in the workforce [1].

The Bureau of Labor Statistics estimated that 36,000 were killed at work in 1989. This figure covers deaths due to injuries and illnesses that resulted from work acts and exposures in the work environment [2]. The National Institute for Occupational Safety and Health (NIOSH) estimated that there were 64,000 work-related fatalities in 1985, which covered traumatic injuries in persons 16 or older. This estimate was arrived at by counting death certificates obtained directly from the states [1].

Because of disagreements and limitations of these estimates, the Bureau of Labor Statistics has instituted a state and federal cooperative system that uses death certificates; state and federal workers' compensation reports; Occupational Safety and Health Administration (OSHA), Mine Safety and Health Administration (MSHA), and Federal Railway Administration (FRA) Act fatality reports; medical examiner's records; autopsy reports; and policy motor vehicle records to identify work-related deaths. This system is in operation in 27 states and became nationwide in 1992.

Morbidity

About 75 million workdays were lost to accidents in 1990 [1]. Of that figure, 35 million lost workdays were due to accidents that occurred in 1990 and 40 million were due to accidents from the previous year.

The most common causes of disabling injuries were overexertion, being struck by or against something, and falls, codes devised by the American National Standards Institute (ANSI) and commonly used for workers' compensation data, but typically not specific enough to allow epidemiologic analysis. As with fatalities, differences in estimates of frequency and severity of illnesses and injuries are found between the National Safety Council and the Bureau of Labor Statistics (see the Chapter Appendix).

Parts of Body Injured

Another ANSI coding scheme classifies injuries by the part of the body that was injured. Back "injuries," which are debatably injuries in the sense that there is infrequently a discrete acute event involved, and which may be due to nonwork events or cumulative trauma, have been the largest category of body parts injured for several years, accounting for 22% of cases and 31% of compensation costs [1] (Fig. 39-2). Back pain and cumulative trauma disorders are actually classified as diseases by OSHA. The next most common parts of the body to be injured are the legs, followed by fingers and arms.

Trends in Occupational Injury and Illness Incidence Rates

As noted in Fig. 39-3, the rate of occupationally related illness or injury dropped slightly from 1973 to 1989. The rate of nonfatal cases without lost workdays declined from 1973 to 1980 and then leveled off. The lost workday cases rate has increased only slightly, but the total lost workday rate has increased significantly over this time period. The latter rate is known as "severity" in workers' compensation circles, although it may not be correlated with the physical severity of an injury or illness. A number of theories have been put forward to account for this increase in lost workdays, but it is important to note that in almost all instances, absence from work is governed by a physician's note or certificate stating that the person is disabled. Many authorities believe that this increase in lost workdays is related to the accuracy of physician reports, and an employer laxness in verifying the medical necessity for absence. In addition, because of productivity goals, employers may not accept injured workers back unless they are completely able to do their original job. This results in significant adverse consequences, including apparently decreasing proportions of employees who return to work. In any event, it appears that much absence

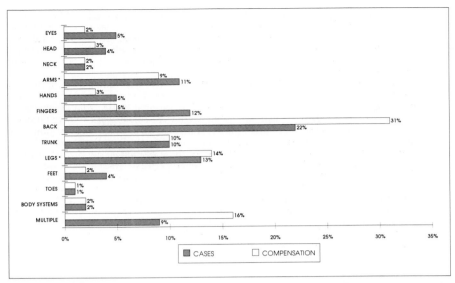

Figure 39-2. Part of the body injured in work accidents. *Includes multiple or not specifically classified injuries amounting to fewer than 2% of the total cases and compensation. Source: State Labor Departments, 1989–1990; cases—23 states; compensation—10 states.

from work is governed by medical opinion rather than objective assessment of impairment matched with the essential functions of the job.

In 1989, the OSHA recordable lost workday incident rate was 78.7 per 100 workers. During that same year, DuPont's lost workday rate was 0.05 and Johnson & Johnson, which had announced a goal of displacing DuPont as the corporate leader in safety, had a lost workday incidence of 0.14 lost workdays per 100 workers. In other words, the national lost workday incidence per 100 workers was approximately 1500 times worse than DuPont's, and 500 times worse than Johnson & Johnson's. Given the administrative barriers to effective medical management of workers' compensation claims, national health care cost escalation in general, as well as an increase in "breakthrough" lawsuits for gross negligence, one of the few effective approaches to managing workers' compensation is significant improvement in workplace safety.

The Evolution of Modern Workers' Compensation Laws

Workers have been injured or killed in the course of employment for centuries without compensation. The problem of loss of wage-earning capacity commanded more public attention during the industrial revolution. The *number* of industrial accidents and personal injury suits evolving from those accidents became larger as business enterprise and mechanical production increased. As modern production techniques were adopted, the amount of mechanical force and chemical energy used to produce products increased and the *rate* of injury increased as well [3].

As attitudes about the rights of workers and employers changed, common law in Europe and the United States evolved to enable workers to recover damages if a person was injured at work. By the turn of the century in the United States, workers could bring successful lawsuits against employers for injuries suffered on the job. Common law held that a "master" or employer was responsible for injury or death of employees "resulting from a negligent act by him" [3]. However, injured workers had to prove that their injuries were due to employer negligence, which resulted in a slow, costly, and uncertain legal process. As a result, workers often did not receive needed medical care or wage replacement in a timely manner.

In addition, there were a number of accepted common law defenses when an employer was sued by an employee. The employer could claim that the employee contributed to the injury, that he or she had assumed risk by taking the job, or that

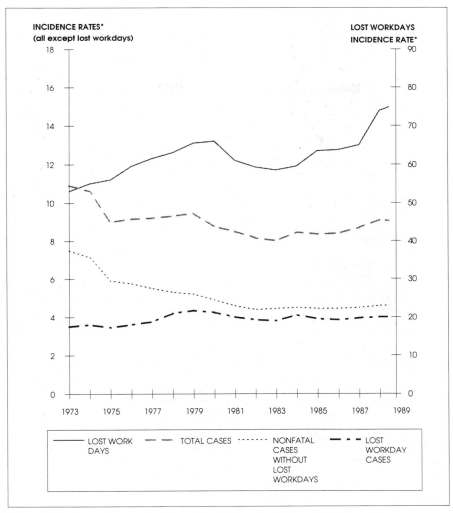

Figure 39-3. Rate of occupationally related illness and injury. *Number of days or cases per 100 full-time employees per year. Source: National Safety Council, 1991.

negligent acts of fellow workers were responsible for the injury. By the end of the nineteenth century it was generally accepted that these defenses and the employer's greater legal resources placed the employee at a significant disadvantage.

The situation changed between 1870 and 1910. First, there was an increased public awareness that placing the burden of industrial illness and injury on workers might be unfair. This attitude resulted in political pressure by reformers to make recovery of lost wages and lost earning capacity easier and faster. A countervailing trend between 1900 and 1920 involved the adoption of "employers' liability" laws in many states. These laws were intended to modify common law defenses and limit employers' liability.

Neither of these initiatives led to equitable and timely compensation for injured workers. As a result, a series of "no fault" workers' compensation laws were passed on a state-by-state basis. Workers' compensation laws represented a compromise or "lesser peril" for both employers and employees. These laws were supposed to ensure rapid payment to injured workers for lost wages and medical costs regardless of fault. In exchange, employers' liability for occupational injuries, illness, and death was limited if they participated in a compensation system. Under this system, employers generally were exempt from damage suits, unless gross negligence could be proved (see Chap. 2).

The first workers' compensation laws were passed by nine states in 1911. The first comprehensive Canadian laws were enacted in 1915. Today there are workers' compensation statutes in all 50 states, American Samoa, Puerto Rico, the US Virgin Islands, and all provinces in Canada. There are separate federal workers' compensation statutes, which include the District of Columbia Workers' Compensation Act, the Federal Employees Liability Act, and the Longshoremen's and Harborworkers' Compensation Act (the Jones Act). The latter provides workers' compensation for both public and private employees engaged in maritime work.

Occupational disease laws were not passed until 1917, starting in Massachusetts and California; all state laws did not cover occupational diseases until 1976. Part of the reason for the slow adoption of occupational disease compensation laws was a fear of liability because of the long latencies of disease and the lack of a definite onset of many occupational diseases. In addition, the sudden trauma of an occupational injury, which was generally used to define compensability, was missing, so that expansion of coverage required a change in thinking.

Coverage

All industrial and most service employment is covered by workers' compensation statutes; however, farm labor, domestic service and casual employees are usually exempted from the laws. As a result, only 85 to 87% of the American workforce is covered by these laws [3]. Many jurisdictions provide workers' compensation for all or certain classes of public employees. Minors, defined as those under the legal age of majority, are covered by workers' compensation; as an incentive to protect under-aged workers, some jurisdictions provide double coverage or penalties if minors are injured or killed at work.

Merchant marine and railroad workers are generally not covered by state workers' compensation acts, but may seek damages under the Federal Employee Liability Act (FELA). The Federal Black Lung Act (Title Four of the Federal Coal Mine Safety and Health Act of 1969 as amended in 1972, 1978, and 1981) provides benefits for total disability or death caused by black lung disease. This act is administered by the Division of Coal Mine Workers, the Department of Labor's workers' compensation programs, and the Social Security Administration.

The Federal Social Security Disability Program pays benefits to disabled workers under the age of 65 when disability is expected to last 12 months or longer or results in death. Benefits are financed by the Federal Social Security Tax. Combined Social Security, Disability, and Workers' Compensation benefits may not exceed 80% average current earnings before disability.

There is considerable dispute about the adequacy of workers' compensation coverage. In 1972, the National Commission on State Workers' Compensation Laws recommended 84 revisions in state systems to improve compensation, make the state laws more consistent, and remove certain inequities. However, most states have not completed these recommendations, 19 of which were considered essential. There have been recommendations for federal workers' compensation coverage to ensure equity and uniformity; however, these proposals have repeatedly been defeated. One of the more recent national health care reform proposals has included workers' compensation. Differences in benefits have created effective wage differentials between states based on workers' compensation premiums or payments, similar to cross-border differentials in labor costs.

Only a fraction of cases of work-related disease are thought to be covered by workers' compensation. The remainder of compensation for workers with these diseases comes from Social Security, welfare, pensions, veterans' benefits, and private insurance [4]. Provisions of occupational disease coverage require that death or disability result within 1 to 5 years after exposure. The latency period may be significantly longer than 5 years in many cases for illnesses such as asbestosis or pneumoconiosis. Further, several states pay benefits only if exposure lasts longer than a specified period. There are time limits on filing, which typically are 2 years after last exposure or onset of disability. These restrictions generally place the employee at a disadvantage since it is not always clear what the causal agent was, with the exception of certain unusual diseases such as mesothelioma [5].

Compensation laws are elective or compulsory. Under an elective law, the employer may accept or reject the compensation act. If the employer rejects it, he or she loses the common-law defenses of assumption of risk, negligence of fellow employees, and contributory negligence. While this approach used to mean that the laws were in effect compulsory, some of the highly restrictive regulations that prevented medical management of compensation cases in states such as Texas and New Jersey have meant that more employers are opting out of the compensation system. Currently, workers' compensation laws are elective only in New Jersey, South Carolina, and Texas. Opting out is under consideration in Louisiana.

Insurance Markets

Employers can purchase insurance from state funds or commercial insurers, or may self-insure. Self-insurance is permitted in all states and territories except Guam, Puerto Rico, the Virgin Islands, and Wyoming. In Texas, the insurance commission must approve self-insurance. The largest firms, which include about 1% of employers in the United States and employ 10 to 15% of the workforce, are self-insured. These employers are able to spread risk within their own workforce because of their size. Twenty-eight states and the Longshoremen's Act authorize group self-insurance for smaller employers, who pool their risks and liabilities.

Mid-sized firms (14% of employers, 70% of employees) generally purchase workers' compensation insurance on the commercial market. This insurance is risk rated according to the firm's own experience. The smallest firms (85% of employers, 15% of employees) are class rated, which is essentially a payroll tax based on industry-wide illness and injury history.

The administrative and legal frameworks of all workers' compensation programs are under state control. There are three fundamental provisions of all workers' compensation programs when claims are contested. First, the insurer or self-insured company is entitled to contest permanent disability claims and in most cases all claims. Second, all contested claims are adjudicated by state compensation boards or court systems. Third, the burden of proof is on the worker in any contested case.

Financial Condition of the Insurance Industry

In the last decade, the "loss ratios" or ratios of payout to premiums collected have averaged 110 to 120%. In other words, insurers were losing between 10 and 20% more than they were collecting. Many insurers therefore withdrew from the workers' compensation insurance market. In most states, a "residual market" enables uninsurable companies to obtain insurance. A surtax, known as a residual market load, is imposed on purchasers of commercial insurance. This surtax provides an incentive to self-insure, insure through an association, risk pool, or seek other methods of financing to avoid this tax.

Costs

There are various estimates of the actual cost of workers' compensation payouts. The National Council on Compensation Insurance [6] estimated that $60 billion was paid out in 1991 for wage replacement, administrative and legal costs, and medical costs. Wage replacement has been increasing at an average rate of 11% per year over the last decade. Medical expenses have been increasing at 14% per year. Both of these figures exceed both the average weekly wage and the medical consumer price index by at least a factor of two. Workers' compensation now averages 3% of payroll for most employers and 5% for manufacturers.

The National Safety Council has produced an analysis that has roughly the same total payout, although in its analysis approximately half of the payout is due to lost productivity and smaller fractions are due to losses such as fire damage.

The average medical cost per case for workers' compensation payments now exceeds $6000 [6]. If this trend continues, simple compounding will increase the cost over $20,000 per case by the year 2000 (Fig. 39-4). The proportion of total compensation payments for medical treatment has increased from less than 30% to almost 50% in some states.

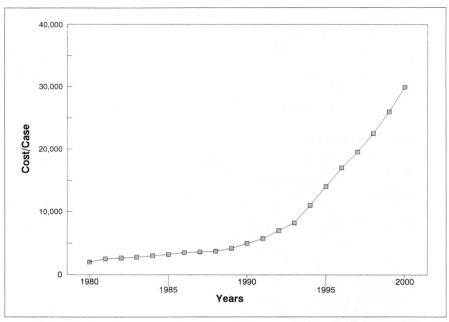

Figure 39-4. Projected workers' compensation costs. Source: Alexander & Alexander Projections using growth rates from NCCI, 1991.

It is widely believed that there is extensive cost shifting from Medicare, Medicaid, and other government programs, as well as from private insurance, because cost-containment programs have succeeded in those areas but have not been widely used in workers' compensation. This shifting is due in part to a confounding by administrative requirements and long time frames involved in workers' compensation. There is also a belief that all medical bills must be paid, although, in fact, few statutes or regulations make that statement. The correct statement is that medically necessary care must be reimbursed.

Benefits Provided

Benefits are provided for wage replacement, medical and legal expenses, and permanent impairment. Lump sum compensation is paid for certain scheduled physical damage or loss of function such as the loss of a body part, whereas medical and wage replacement payments are made whenever there is a wage loss related to work. A growing number of states are also requiring rehabilitation benefits. Impairment is defined as a loss of or damage to a body part or function due to illness or injury, whereas disability is defined as the inability to perform a specific task based on the functional requirements of the job, education, social factors, and other issues in addition to the medical impairment. In fact, one can be impaired but not disabled. Generally, physicians determine impairment and personnel administrators or supervisors determine disability.

Medical benefits are generally provided without dollar or time limits and are typically paid directly to providers. Many states have fee schedules for payments of medical costs. Most of these schedules apply to physician or chiropractic outpatient care only; inpatient care and facility fees are compensated at 100% of charges.

Many workers' compensation claims, called "medical only," require medical treatment but do not result in lost time or impairment. When there is lost time, income replacement payments are made on a weekly basis according to a formula expressed as a percentage of wages. Most states, have maximum and minimum limits; some states limit the total number of weeks payable. The highest weekly state payments are $630.65 in Illinois and $700.00 in Alaska. The maxima are increased periodically by either cost of living adjustments or legislative action.

"Disability" as used in workers' compensation is defined as "temporary and total" (i.e., the employee must be absent from work for a period of time), "permanent and total," "temporary and partial" (i.e., restricted work is possible), or "permanent partial." Lump sum awards are made for the permanent partial disability. Permanent partial is divided into nonscheduled and scheduled impairments. Most workers' compensation other than "medical only" involves temporary total disability or the need to be absent from work for more than one-half day (the OSHA definition). Temporary total disability definitions vary by state.

Most states limit compensation to two thirds of previous wages and cover all medical costs. Several states have more generous benefits. Self-insured employers must offer benefits at least equivalent to those required by state statutes. For a variety of reasons, some employers have elected to offer benefits equivalent to or coordinated with their short-term disability programs, which typically fully replace wages. Because these payments are tax exempt, they actually exceed the value of the average weekly wage. The Federal Employers' Liability Act (Jones Act), which applies to inland waterways and railroad workers; veterans' benefits for those injured while working in the military; and the Federal Black Lung Act, which pertains to occupational illness contracted while working in coal mines, have separate benefits.

The penalties for failure to provide workers' compensation insurance tend to be minimal. For example, in Delaware the fine is $10 per employee, per day. In general, most fines are in the range of $500 to $5000. In some states there are criminal penalties and jail terms and in Alaska, failure to insure is considered a class B or C felony. In New Mexico the employer may be enjoined from doing business in the state if compensation insurance is not provided [3].

Incentives and Disincentives

Workers' compensation insurance grew up as part of the property and casualty insurance sector. At the time the laws were enacted, there was little medicine could do for acute traumatic injuries, and health and life insurers were reluctant to write this coverage because of a perception that there might be "moral hazard," which means that the employee could seek unnecessary care for gain. The chief emphasis at the time the laws were passed was on loss.

Immediate versus Delayed Investment and Rating

One reason why workers' compensation costs have not led to an increased investment in loss control technology or prevention is that it is generally less expensive to buy insurance now than to install costly engineering controls. Due to the time value of money, paying insurance premiums over a 10-year period is less expensive in current dollars than paying a lump sum to install control technologies today. This is particularly true in the case of occupational diseases, which may take many years to appear.

Risk Spreading and Payment Lags

For those who are fully insured, compensation insurance premium calculations are a disincentive to improve loss control. Most premiums are calculated on a 3-year average of losses. There is also a significant retention of funds to cover the "payout" or "tail," which typically "runs off" in a long curve, peaking in the first or second year and tailing off over up to a 10-year period. The tail is apparently increasing. It is difficult, therefore, to see an immediate effect on cash outflow with a reduction in accident frequency.

By spreading risk through insurance, insurance pools, or large employee populations, financial incentives to avoid a catastrophe or other major losses have been diluted. Incentives to improve one's loss record in order to reduce costs have also been blunted. The situation has changed somewhat for self-insurers and experience-rated employers as workers' compensation costs have escalated rapidly. However, the attitude for diffusing or delaying costs remains and is subject to change [8].

Perverse Incentives Within Organizations

In many companies or nonprofit organizations, losses are not allocated back to the department in which they were incurred. This policy is an intracompany version of risk spreading that provides a disincentive to improvement and safety records.

Further, many managers have productivity incentives. They therefore prefer not to return employees to work on limited duty. This disincentive clearly prevents rapid return to work, which is associated with shorter recovery times and reduced payments. The availability of light work or modified duties is key to reducing accident severity rates. One study shows that absenteeism and disability with low back pain are significantly reduced when light duty is available [7].

Provider and Patient Incentives

With reductions in group health benefits, there has been a tendency to ascribe injuries to the worksite, since workers' compensation will pay 100% of the medical bills and provide wage replacement. As group health benefits continue to be reduced or are eliminated by smaller employers, this incentive to use the workers' compensation system is expected to increase.

There is also an economic incentive to undertake workers' compensation claims as benefits payments increase. The NCCI demonstrated that a 10% increase in indemnity benefits leads to a 4% increase in the frequency of claims [8].

Because workers' compensation pays 100% of charges, there has been an apparent increase in hospitalization rates as well as cost shifting. Managed care organizations seem to be very careful about assuring that compensable injuries are classified as such to ensure payment outside the prepayment system [9].

Dissatisfaction with one's job, monotonous and repetitive tasks, and the feeling of fatigue at the end of the workday are associated with greater absenteeism and disability leave [10, 11]. A study at the Boeing Corporation revealed that a major predictor of absence from work was poor performance evaluation and another was conflict with supervisors [12]. These studies also noted that workers who do not enjoy their jobs or communicate well with peers are more likely to file and maintain compensation claims.

Rehabilitation programs, which are mandated in many workers' compensation insurance programs, are based on a social service model that is in direct conflict with the compensation model. The goal of rehabilitation programs is to restore function, whereas one goal of workers' compensation, although probably an unintended one, is compensation for disability. In workers' compensation the law is construed as a right to benefits. Rehabilitation takes a clinical point of view, whereas workers' compensation may seem like a reward system to some. The incentives for rehabilitation are increased social rewards and self-esteem, whereas in workers' compensation the more disabled a person becomes the higher the award [13, 14]. Rehabilitation programs work best when they make as few changes in the client's pre-morbid life as possible, including transfer to the same job and the same occupation.

Legal Factors

Attorney involvement was the strongest predictor of disability in one extensive study [15]. In New York State an analysis of almost 3000 cases demonstrated that with attorney involvement much of the diagnostic testing conducted was frequently repetitious and unnecessary. The quality of medical records was poor [14]. In general, the probability of surgery was higher with attorney involvement, and when indications were less than clear, the outcome was poor [16, 17]. When comparing settlements for the same impairment, settlements were significantly greater with attorneys involved, but the claimants received less than half the settlements [18]. Because the amount of a settlement relates to the perception of disability, there is a financial incentive to portray the claimant as significantly disabled, which probably explains the increased use of tests and surgery. The proportion of litigated cases is increasing rapidly. It is now estimated that over 50% of the cases in California and Texas are represented by attorneys and in this supposedly "no fault" system.

The Occupational Physician's Role in the Management of Workers' Compensation

The occupational physician can contribute to the management of workers' compensation in areas ranging from clinical to administrative to organizational.

Formulation and Use of Standards and Criteria

There is a clear need for proactive medical management of workers' compensation cases because of the wide variations in the quality and quantity of medical care, and the absence of medical expertise under the present property and casualty insurance framework. Workers' compensation cases are typically managed by claims examiners or adjusters who are not medically trained; they are primarily concerned with complying with legal requirements of the workers' compensation system, including prompt payment, although they believe that they are managing medical care. Standards, criteria, and protocols have not been widely applied to those cases paid for by workers' compensation. The need for standards and criteria is made more urgent by the fact that many of the current major categories of occupational illness or injury are "nonspecific," subjective complaints such as back and wrist pain that can only be effectively managed with carefully constructed criteria and constant reference to physical signs. In many cases, imaging studies only confuse the issue unless they are applied judiciously; otherwise, the chances of a false-positive result and subsequent misdiagnosis and unnecessary surgery are extremely high [19, 20].

Time-based disability management of workers' compensation cases is also critical. For example, it has been demonstrated repeatedly that the average recovery time for uncomplicated low back pain is 2 days of bed rest and 8 days of partial disability before complete return to function [21]. However, comparison of a survey by the American College of Occupational and Environmental Medicine (unpublished data now used by Beech Street, Inc.) and several other consensus panels [22–24] revealed that while the average length of time absent from work for both back pain and wrist pain is in the range of 4 to 15 weeks, the expert consensus was 1 to 3 weeks.

In addition to management of existing cases by protocol and criteria, it is not infrequent for cases to be left open for long periods, up to years, without medical reevaluation or assessment of the employee's status. Many anecdotal studies have demonstrated that significant backlogs of cases have been left open without reexamination of liabilities amounting to millions of dollars for many mid-sized employers. A periodic medical review of these cases can be quite revealing. Additional medical evidence or reevaluation of the claimant may be in order. It is not infrequent for many disorders to resolve spontaneously, as this is the natural history of many nonspecific complaints, dermatitis, and other work-related complaints. Cases that do not meet criteria should be reevaluated immediately and attempts made to settle or close the cases as quickly as possible. Disability management can be based on either medical treatment or recovery guidelines or disability management guidelines, which are time based.

Assisting with creation of exclusive or preferred provider panels is an important area for physician involvement as well. Because of the highly variable patterns of diagnosis and treatment, which typically vary markedly from group health patterns of treatment [25], it is imperative that occupational physicians carefully screen and agree with specific providers in the evaluation and management of workers' compensation cases. It would be preferable if treating physicians and chiropractors would agree to protocols before treating a company's employees. Even in states with employee choice of physician, most employees do not have physicians and will use providers suggested by the employer, at least initially. It should be noted that the treating physicians should be very skilled at patient interaction so that they do not antagonize employees, who then choose other, probably less skilled and more variable, physicians or seek legal representation.

Another critical role for the occupational physician is to examine the record of the injury to determine if it is, in fact, causally related. This is not the "causality" used by claims examiners, but a question of whether an injury is mechanically or epidemiologically plausible based on exposure to the worksite during the time course of the injury. Some estimates are that over half of the occupationally related claims that are paid may not, in fact, be related to the worksite. Use of careful clinical judgment as well as standards and criteria should allow the occupational physician to state an informed opinion about the relationship of the inciting event to the alleged resultant injury.

Given the current complex, laborious, and expensive state of workers' compensation management, prevention and avoidance of the system are key. Attention to job design, job placement, education, and reduction of personal risk factors will result in significant reduction of injury rates. Preplacement evaluations directly related to the bona fide occupational qualifications of the job should be conducted, particularly in light of the Americans with Disabilities Act. One of the better ways of constructing functionally based accurate job descriptions that reflect the physical demands of the job is to use panels of workers who actually do that job [26]. It is not clear what the role of strength testing is at this point [27]. It is clear that physically fit individuals seem to have a lower rate of injury and recover more quickly [20].

Strategic Management

The occupational physician can provide leadership in strategic and tactical management of workers' compensation. This involves a series of strategic steps, which include assessing the present situation, visioning the desired future, gap analysis, strategic plan development, and tactical implementation.

Analysis of the present situation would involve bringing together disparate sources of data to obtain an accurate profile of the costs, sources, and treatment patterns for compensable injuries. One would also want to determine indirect costs such as supervisory time loss, retraining, and business interruption.

Other data that should be examined are the organizational location of workers' compensation management and flow of the process of injury management, including the management of the injured worker, information, and regulatory and administrative issues. An initial challenge to the management of compensable injuries and illnesses stems from the organizational fragmentation of the typical workers' compensation system within a company. It is frequently not clear who is in charge of the entire system. It may also be unclear who is in charge of the direct relationship with the injured worker. These processes therefore tend to move rather slowly, and workers can be "lost in the cracks." A third type of data that is critical to assess are the employee perceptions of treatment and compensation injuries, general attitude toward management, perceived management attitudes toward safety, perceived safety of the workplace, and other issues.

Once these data have been analyzed and presented to management, targets can be set and a vision of the organization of the program in the future can be established. Gap analysis is simply a comparison of the future vision with the current reality. It is entirely likely that a relatively major reorganization of the function would be appropriate if the typical degree of fragmentation and lack of medical management are discovered. However, it is also important to note that significant regulatory and administrative issues are involved with workers' compensation, so that all viewpoints must be taken into effect in designing a maximally effective system. Both preloss and postloss issues should be dealt with. System design would include the design of a more effective data management capability, which captures desired data elements and provides feedback to supervisors and providers.

Disability management should be assessed and improved. This system might include policies for disability management, institution of modified duty, and a feedback system to constantly assess how well disability is managed. Length of disability by diagnosis is a good initial statistic to track.

If the use of vendors is contemplated, proposals can be requested using a structured form based on the analysis of the current situation. Benchmarks can be established for performance, either from the current situation or from comparison with best-procedure companies. It is important to assure that data management is adequately taken care of. Once answers to very clear proposals are received, they can be assessed against predetermined evaluation criteria.

Using a strategic approach and process quality improvement techniques, management of workers' compensation can be significantly improved. The process flow map mentioned previously can provide the starting point for constant improvement using total quality management procedures. Employers and employees will benefit in many ways, including increased job satisfaction, better financial performance, and decreased mortality and morbidity.

References

1. National Safety Council. *Accident Facts.* Chicago: National Safety Council, 1992.
2. Bureau of Labor Statistics Supplementary Data System, 1988.
3. US Chamber of Commerce. *1991 Analysis of Workers' Compensation Laws.* Washington, DC: US Chamber of Commerce, 1992.
4. Ashford, N. A., and Andrews, R. A. Workers' Compensation. In W. Rom, *Environmental and Occupational Medicine.* Boston: Little, Brown, 1983.
5. Ashford, N. A. *Crisis in the Work Place: Occupational Disease and Injury.* Cambridge, MA: MIT Press, 1976. Chapter 8.
6. National Council on Compensation Insurance. *Issues Report,* 1992. New York: NCCI, 1992.
7. Wiesel, S. W., Feffer, H. L., and Rothman, R. H. Industrial low back pain: A prospective evaluation of a standardized diagnostic and treatment protocol. *Spine* 9:199, 1984.
8. Butler, R. J. Wage and Injury Rate Response to Shifting Levels of Workers' Compensation. In G. D. Worrall, *Safety in the Work Place: Incentives and Disincentives in Workers' Compensation.* Ithaca, NY: ILR Press, 1983. Pp. 61–86.
9. Ducatmann, A. M. Workers' compensation cost shifting: Unique concern of providers and purchasers of pre-paid health care. *J. Occup. Med.* 28:1174, 1988.
10. Vallfors, B. Acute, sub-acute and chronic low back pain: Clinical symptoms and absenteeism in the work environment. *Scand. J. Rehab. Med.* Supplement II:1, 1985.
11. Bigos, S. J., et al. Back injuries in industry: A retrospective study. III. Employee-related factors. *Spine* 11:252, 1986.
12. Bigos, S. J., et al. The prospective study of work perceptions and psycho-social factors affecting the report of back injury. *Spine* 16:1, 1991.
13. Berkowitz, M. Rehabilitation and Workers' Compensation: Incompatible or Inseparable? In P. Borba and D. Appel. *Benefits Costs and Cycles in Workers' Compensation.* Boston: Kluwer, Academic Publishers, 1990.
14. Haddad, G. H. Analysis of 2932 workers' compensation back injury cases: The impact on cost of the system. *Spine* 12:765, 1987.
15. Worrall, G. D., et al. *Age and Incentive Response: Low Back Pain Workers' Compensation Claims.* Presented at the Fourth Annual NCCI Seminar on Economic Issues in Workers' Compensation, 1985.
16. Fager, C. A. and Friedbert, S. R. Analysis of failure and poor results of lumbar spine surgery. *Spine* 5:87, 1980.
17. Long, D. M., et al. Clinical features of the failed back syndrome. *J. Neurosurg.* 69:61, 1988.
18. Derebery, B. J., and Tullis, R. H. Delayed recovery in the patient with a work compensable injury. *J. Occup. Med.* 24:829, 1981.
19. Borenstein, D. G., and Wiesel, S. W. *Low Back Pain: Medical Diagnosis and Comprehensive Management.* Philadelphia: Saunders, 1989. Chapter 6.
20. Brigham, C. R., and Harris, J. S. Low back pain part II: Administrative disability and workers' compensation issues. *Occup. Environ. Med. Rep.,* 4:92, 1990.
21. Deyo, R. A., Diehl, A. K., and Rosenthal, M. How many days of bed rest for acute low back pain? A randomized clinical trial. *N. Engl. J. Med.,* 315:1064, 1986.
22. Harris, J. S., et al. *Medical Disability Standards for Orthopaedic Disorders.* Brentwood, TN: Focus Health Care Management, 1989.
23. Doyle, R., et al. *Health Care Management Guidelines, Volume III. Ambulatory Care Guidelines.* Seattle: Milliman and Robertson, 1990.
24. Reed, P. R. *The Medical Disability Advisor.* New York: LRP Publishers, 1990.
25. Harris, J. S., et al. Business as usual may mean going out of business. *NCCI Dig.* 4:25, 1989.
26. Nylander, S. W., and Carmean, G. *Medical Standards Project Final Report* (3rd revised ed.). San Bernardino, CA: San Bernardino County, 1984.
27. Himmelstein, J. S., and Andersson, G. B. J. Low Back Pain: Risk Evaluation and Pre-Placement Screening. In J. S. Himmelstein and G. S. Pransky, Worker Fitness and Risk Evaluations. *Occup. Med. State of the Art Rev.* 3:255, 1988.

Appendix to Chapter 39: BLS Estimates of Occupational Injury and Illness Incidence Rates for Selected Industries, 1989

		Incidence rates			
Industry	SIC code	Total cases	Lost workday cases	Nonfatal cases without lost workdays	Lost work-days
Private sector		**8.6**	**4.0**	**4.6**	**78.7**
Agriculture, forestry, and fishing		**10.9**	**5.7**	**5.2**	**100.9**
Agricultural production	01–02	12.2	6.2	6.0	101.9
Agricultural services	07	9.7	5.3	4.5	99.8
Forestry	08	11.4	5.6	5.7	132.4
Mining		**8.5**	**4.8**	**3.7**	**137.2**
Metal mining	10	8.5	4.7	3.8	133.0
Coal mining	12	11.6	8.3	3.2	254.8
Oil and gas extraction	13	7.6	3.8	3.9	111.7
Crude petroleum and natural gas	131	3.3	1.6	1.8	41.6
Natural gas liquids	132	4.1	1.1	3.0	28.8
Oil and gas field services	138	12.1	6.0	6.0	184.7
Nonmetallic minerals, except fuels	14	7.9	4.4	3.5	90.2
Construction		**14.3**	**6.8**	**7.5**	**143.3**
General building contractors	15	13.9	6.5	7.4	137.3
Residential building construction	152	11.4	6.1	5.3	131.7
Nonresidential building construction	154	16.9	7.2	9.7	148.1
Heavy construction, except building	16	13.8	6.5	7.3	147.1
Highway and street construction	161	14.1	6.5	7.6	139.0
Heavy construction, except highway	162	13.7	6.5	7.1	150.6
Special trade contractors	17	14.6	6.9	7.7	144.9
Plumbing, heating, air conditioning	171	15.7	6.3	9.4	116.0
Painting and paper hanging	172	9.4	5.0	4.4	137.2
Electrical work	173	13.1	5.3	7.8	105.6
Masonry, stonework, and plastering	174	16.0	8.3	7.7	179.3
Carpentry and floor work	175	13.0	7.1	5.9	134.8
Roofing, siding, and sheet metal work	176	18.3	10.0	8.3	247.1
Manufacturing		**13.1**	**5.8**	**7.3**	**113.0**
Durable goods		*14.1*	*6.0*	*8.1*	*116.5*
Lumber and wood products	24	18.4	9.4	9.1	177.5
Logging	241	19.5	11.7	7.7	307.8
Sawmills and planing mills	242	18.6	9.6	9.0	187.3
Millwork, plywood, and structural members	243	17.7	8.8	8.9	151.2
Wood containers	244	16.2	9.0	7.2	180.9
Wood buildings and mobile homes	245	25.2	11.0	14.2	164.9
Furniture and fixtures	25	16.1	7.2	8.9	124.9
Household furniture	251	15.5	6.9	8.5	113.1
Office furniture	252	17.5	7.5	9.9	162.7
Public building and related furniture	253	19.6	8.5	11.0	163.5
Stone, clay, and glass products	32	15.5	7.4	8.1	149.8
Flat glass	321	21.9	7.3	14.5	116.6
Glass and glassware, pressed or blown	322	14.2	6.5	7.6	139.7
Products of purchased glass	323	16.9	6.7	10.1	120.8
Structural clay products	325	17.1	7.9	9.2	179.0

(continued)

Industry	SIC code	Total cases	Lost workday cases	Nonfatal cases without lost workdays	Lost work-days
				Incidence rates	
Pottery and related products	326	15.8	9.2	6.6	186.7
Concrete, gypsum, and plaster products	327	15.8	8.2	7.6	167.1
Miscellaneous nonmetallic mineral products	329	13.7	6.7	7.0	132.4
Primary metal industries	33	18.7	8.1	10.5	168.3
Blast furnace and basic steel products	331	16.7	6.8	9.8	166.8
Iron and steel foundries	332	25.4	10.8	14.7	183.6
Primary nonferrous metals	333	19.9	7.6	12.2	159.9
Nonferrous rolling and drawing	335	15.3	7.1	8.2	149.2
Nonferrous foundries (castings)	336	20.9	10.0	10.9	193.7
Fabricated metal products	34	18.5	7.9	10.7	147.6
Metal cans and shipping containers	341	16.2	6.5	9.7	128.1
Cutlery, hand tools, and hardware	342	14.8	6.2	8.5	131.7
Plumbing and heating, except electric	343	20.3	7.8	12.5	128.7
Fabricated structural metal products	344	21.3	9.6	11.7	167.9
Screw machine products, bolts, etc.	345	14.7	5.9	8.8	89.5
Metal forgings and stampings	346	23.1	8.7	14.4	186.8
Metal services	347	15.9	7.4	8.5	132.9
Ordnance and accessories	348	10.2	4.5	5.7	96.7
Miscellaneous fabricated metal products	349	16.7	7.5	9.2	138.3
Industrial machinery and equipment	35	12.1	4.8	7.3	86.8
Engines and turbines	351	13.9	5.2	8.6	112.3
Farm and garden machinery	352	18.7	6.8	11.8	102.7
Construction and related machinery	353	16.3	6.7	9.7	116.5
Metalworking machinery	354	12.7	4.6	8.1	78.4
Special industry machinery	355	13.9	5.3	8.6	89.5
General industrial machinery	356	13.7	5.4	8.3	98.0
Computer and office equipment	357	3.8	1.9	1.9	41.7
Refrigeration and service machinery	358	16.8	7.0	9.8	125.6
Industrial machinery, n.e.c.	359	12.9	5.1	7.9	94.8
Electronic and other electric equipment	36	9.1	3.9	5.1	77.5
Electric distribution equipment	361	12.0	4.8	7.2	92.0
Electrical industrial apparatus	362	11.1	4.6	6.4	98.4
Household appliances	363	18.0	7.1	10.9	127.3
Electric lighting and wiring equipment	364	10.8	4.8	6.0	100.8
Household audio and video equipment	365	10.0	4.6	5.4	96.3
Communications equipment	366	4.7	2.1	2.6	43.6
Electronic components and accessories	367	6.6	2.9	3.7	55.2
Transportation equipment	37	17.7	6.8	10.9	138.6
Motor vehicles and equipment	371	22.6	8.5	14.1	173.9
Aircraft and parts	372	10.1	3.7	6.4	70.2
Ship and boat building and repairing	373	38.0	15.6	22.4	343.9
Railroad equipment	374	20.9	9.7	11.2	181.0
Guided missiles, space vehicles, parts	376	4.8	2.2	2.6	39.7
Instruments and related products	38	5.6	2.5	3.1	55.4
Search and navigation equipment	381	3.6	1.6	2.1	35.6
Measuring and controlling devices	382	6.4	2.9	3.4	62.7
Medical instruments and supplies	384	7.4	3.4	4.0	74.3
Photographic equipment and supplies	386	5.2	2.2	3.1	49.3

(continued)

Industry	SIC code	Total cases	Lost workday cases	Nonfatal cases without lost workdays	Lost work-days
Miscellaneous manufacturing industries	39	11.1	5.1	6.0	97.6
Musical instruments	393	10.7	4.6	6.1	78.5
Toys and sporting goods	394	13.3	6.2	7.1	112.2
Pens, pencils, office, and art supplies	395	10.1	4.6	5.5	94.4
Costume jewelry and notions	396	7.2	3.4	3.8	82.7
Nondurable goods		*11.6*	*5.5*	*6.1*	*107.8*
Food and kindred products	20	18.5	9.3	9.2	174.7
Meat products	201	27.1	13.5	13.7	250.9
Dairy products	202	15.2	7.9	7.3	156.5
Preserved fruits and vegetables	203	17.5	8.3	9.2	148.8
Grain mill products	204	13.1	6.7	6.4	139.8
Bakery products	205	13.5	6.9	6.6	153.9
Sugar and confectionery products	206	14.2	6.9	7.3	118.8
Fats and oils	207	15.3	7.7	7.5	164.8
Beverages	208	17.7	9.1	8.6	165.1
Miscellaneous foods and kindred products	209	16.3	8.4	7.9	139.3
Tobacco products	21	8.7	3.4	5.3	64.2
Textile mill products	22	10.3	4.2	6.1	81.4
Broadwoven fabric mills, cotton	221	8.5	2.7	5.8	57.1
Broadwoven fabric mills, manmade	222	8.0	3.4	4.6	72.1
Broadwoven fabric mills, wool	223	9.7	5.2	4.5	118.8
Narrow fabric mills	224	11.5	5.4	6.0	96.7
Knitting mills	225	9.0	4.2	4.8	73.4
Textile finishing, except wool	226	11.6	5.1	6.5	89.2
Carpets and rugs	227	13.8	4.9	8.9	94.3
Yarn and thread mills	228	11.7	4.1	7.6	83.5
Apparel and other textile products	23	8.6	3.8	4.8	80.5
Men's and boys' suits and coats	231	8.9	4.3	4.6	98.8
Men's and boys' furnishings	232	11.3	5.5	5.8	126.9
Women's and misses' outerwear	233	4.9	1.8	3.0	45.1
Women's and children's undergarments	234	7.2	2.8	4.4	53.1
Hats, caps, and millinery	235	10.7	4.7	6.0	108.3
Girls' and children's outerwear	236	8.0	3.5	4.5	72.3
Miscellaneous apparel and accessories	238	6.9	3.3	3.6	60.9
Miscellaneous fabricated textile products	239	11.6	5.1	6.5	84.6
Paper and allied products	26	12.7	5.8	6.9	132.9
Paper mills	262	11.9	4.7	7.2	137.5
Paperboard mills	263	12.1	4.9	7.3	126.5
Paperboard containers and boxes	265	13.2	6.3	6.9	133.7
Printing and publishing	27	6.9	3.3	3.6	63.8
Newspapers	271	7.2	3.4	3.8	72.3
Periodicals	272	3.2	1.7	1.4	39.4
Books	273	6.5	3.1	3.4	55.5
Commercial printing	275	7.9	3.7	4.2	68.7
Manifold business forms	276	9.8	4.2	5.6	73.6
Blankbooks and bookbinding	278	9.6	5.0	4.7	88.9
Chemicals and allied products	28	7.0	3.2	3.7	63.4
Industrial inorganic chemicals	281	5.9	2.6	3.2	54.8
Plastics materials and synthetics	282	6.3	2.9	3.4	62.2

(continued)

				Incidence rates	
Industry	SIC code	Total cases	Lost workday cases	Nonfatal cases without lost workdays	Lost work-days
Drugs	283	5.8	2.9	2.9	55.0
Soap, cleaners, and toilet goods	284	8.5	4.0	4.5	72.4
Paints and allied products	285	10.4	5.0	5.4	85.3
Industrial organic chemicals	286	6.1	2.5	3.6	55.1
Agricultural chemicals	287	7.8	3.5	4.3	63.3
Miscellaneous chemical products	289	8.7	4.1	4.5	82.8
Petroleum and coal products	29	6.6	3.3	3.3	68.1
Petroleum refining	291	5.3	2.6	2.7	56.6
Asphalt paving and roofing materials	295	10.2	5.1	5.1	108.7
Rubber and miscellaneous plastics products	30	16.2	8.0	8.2	147.2
Tires and inner tubes	301	15.4	9.2	6.2	170.4
Rubber and plastic footwear	302	16.8	8.2	8.7	157.4
Hose and belting and gaskets and packing	305	13.8	6.4	7.4	110.1
Fabricated rubber products, n.e.c.	306	17.1	8.6	8.5	150.4
Miscellaneous plastics products, n.e.c.	308	16.4	7.9	8.5	146.8
Leather and leather products	31	13.6	6.5	7.1	130.4
Leather tanning and finishing	311	25.0	13.9	11.0	290.0
Footwear, except rubber	314	13.3	6.0	7.3	117.4
Transportation and public utilities		**9.2**	**5.3**	**3.9**	**121.5**
Railroad transportation	40	7.7	5.8	1.9	153.3
Local and interurban passenger transit	41	9.6	5.5	4.1	125.3
Local and suburban transportation	411	12.0	7.2	4.8	143.2
Taxicabs	412	4.9	3.0	1.9	77.9
School buses	415	9.0	4.3	4.7	88.9
Trucking and warehousing	42	13.5	7.9	5.6	205.0
Trucking and courier services, except air	421	13.4	7.9	5.5	210.0
Water transportation	44	12.1	7.3	4.8	263.1
Water transportation of freight, n.e.c.	444	10.0	6.4	3.6	167.1
Transportation by air	45	14.2	8.2	5.9	138.2
Air transportation, scheduled	451	14.5	8.5	6.0	142.3
Transportation services	47	4.3	2.4	1.9	47.9
Communications	48	3.1	1.7	1.4	33.2
Electric, gas, and sanitary services	49	8.0	4.0	3.9	73.0
Electric services	491	6.0	2.6	3.4	51.0
Gas production and distribution	492	7.2	3.5	3.7	53.8
Combination utility services	493	6.7	3.8	2.9	71.0
Water supply	494	10.6	5.9	4.7	81.3
Sanitary services	495	18.7	10.6	8.1	192.6
Wholesale and retail trade		**8.0**	**3.6**	**4.4**	**63.5**
Wholesale trade		*7.7*	*4.0*	*3.8*	*71.9*
Wholesale trade—durable goods	50	6.7	3.3	3.4	55.8
Lumber and construction materials	503	11.5	6.1	5.4	114.1
Electrical goods	506	4.3	2.2	2.1	37.1
Machinery, equipment, and supplies	508	7.7	3.6	4.1	55.3
Wholesale trade—nondurable goods	51	9.3	5.0	4.3	96.3
Groceries and related products	514	13.3	7.5	5.8	140.1
Petroleum and petroleum products	517	5.1	2.6	2.6	53.4

(continued)

			Incidence rates		
Industry	SIC code	Total cases	Lost workday cases	Nonfatal cases without lost workdays	Lost work-days
Retail trade		*8.1*	*3.4*	*4.6*	*60.0*
Building materials and garden supplies	52	9.8	4.8	5.0	78.1
General merchandise stores	53	10.7	5.0	5.7	82.6
Food stores	54	11.6	4.9	6.7	102.5
Automotive dealers and service stations	55	6.9	2.7	4.1	50.8
Apparel and accessory stores	56	3.0	1.3	1.7	21.7
Furniture and home furnishing stores	57	4.7	2.4	2.3	40.3
Eating and drinking places	58	8.5	3.2	5.3	49.4
Miscellaneous retail	59	4.2	1.9	2.3	37.5
Finance, insurance, and real estate		**2.0**	**0.9**	**1.1**	**17.6**
Depository institutions	60	1.4	0.6	0.9	12.2
Insurance carriers	63	1.7	0.7	1.0	14.0
Real estate	65	4.8	2.5	2.3	45.2
Services		**5.5**	**2.7**	**2.8**	**51.2**
Hotels and other lodging places	70	10.8	4.7	6.1	80.3
Personal services	72	3.6	1.9	1.7	42.9
Business services	73	4.7	2.4	2.3	48.3
Service to buildings	734	8.0	4.2	3.8	83.6
Auto repair, services, and parking	75	6.7	3.0	3.6	61.1
Miscellaneous repair services	76	8.6	4.4	4.2	73.8
Health services	80	7.3	3.8	3.5	76.7
Nursing and personal care facilities	805	15.5	8.8	6.6	181.8
Hospitals	806	8.5	4.2	4.2	78.7
Legal services	81	0.5	0.2	0.3	5.9
Educational services	82	3.5	1.5	2.0	26.8
Social services	83	5.7	2.8	2.9	46.5
Residential care	836	9.3	4.3	4.9	79.7
Museums, botanical, zoologic gardens	84	6.2	3.0	3.3	51.2
Engineering and management services	87	1.9	0.9	1.0	13.2

BLS = Bureau of Labor Statistics; SIC = Standard Industry Code; n.e.c. = not elsewhere classified.
Source: Adapted from Bureau of Labor Statistics Supplementary Data System, 1989.

40 Health Care Management

Robert Galvin

The staggering increases in health care costs in the United States have been well publicized. The latest figures show that total costs climbed 12% in 1991, to $838.5 billion. This represents more than 14% of the American economy, up from 9.4% of the gross national product (GNP) in 1980.

These rising health care costs represent a substantial threat to US business competitiveness. It is estimated that in 1992, health expenditures accounted for $1000 of the cost of a new automobile. One auto manufacturer claimed that, per automobile, more was spent for medical bills than for steel [1]. In response to a new regulation that changed the accounting methods used to declare retiree health benefits, General Motors Company made a fourth-quarter write-off of $22.2 billion in 1992, a sum that represents the largest annual loss ever reported by a US corporation.

Because occupational medicine is a field that concerns itself with health issues at the workplace, it would seem natural for occupational physicians to be deeply involved in the health cost problem. However, this has not been the case. Although there has been limited involvement with disability costs associated with work-related conditions, occupational doctors have had only a very minor role in the much greater cost problem associated with personal illness. This seems to be the result of a mutual reluctance, with occupational medicine largely perceiving health cost issues as outside its traditional scope of worksite health and safety, and business viewing physicians as having a "trained incapacity" to manage financial issues [2].

Nonetheless, there is reason to believe that this situation may change in the future. As employers become more involved with managing their investment in the highly technical field of health care, they will increasingly need medical experts to guide their decisions. And as health care management continues to develop from a pure cost-containment model to one characterized by a focus on outcomes, processes, and quality, occupational physicians may see this area as a natural expansion of their traditional role.

This chapter defines the specific issues for business in the health care cost problem, in particular quality and value; reviews the strategies that have been tried to date; and offers a model for involvement of the occupational physician in health care management. Business is concerned with two types of health costs: those associated with personal illness of employees and dependents and those linked to work-related injuries and illnesses of employees. Although there are indications that the health care management of these types of costs are being integrated, the financing mechanisms and underlying incentives of the two areas are distinctly different at this point. The health management issues are therefore treated separately in this chapter.

Personal Illness

Employer-Based Insurance

Most people with health insurance in the United States receive it through their employer. In 1990, 73% of all US citizens with health insurance had coverage through their jobs [3]. Despite the perception that many small employers do not offer medical benefits, 85% of those people who worked were covered by a health policy. The Health Care Financing Administration (HCFA) has estimated that business spent approximately $250 billion on health care in 1992 [4].

Health insurance in the United States has been linked to employment since the 1940s [5]. It is sometimes overlooked that medical insurance of any sort in the US is a phenomenon of only the past 60 years. The founding of Blue Cross in 1929 and

Blue Shield in 1939 was in part brought about by the Great Depression, as concerns over insolvency led hospitals and doctors to form third-party organizations to finance their operations. The linking of medical insurance to employment was a product of the statutory wage freezes of the World War II era, as both management and labor turned to health benefits as a popular alternative to increase compensation to employees. Health benefits have been tax exempt since their inception, creating a financial incentive for companies to keep offering them.

The responsibility for medical benefits did not become a problem for American business until the 1970s. As health care costs in general began to rise rapidly, so too did insurance premiums for employers. In 1976, health costs per employee rose 17%, and by the early 1980s, increases in per capita benefits were in the 20 to 24% per year range. The problem began to reach more serious proportions as medical inflation began to outstrip the general inflation rate. Despite the generally low rises of the consumer price index (CPI) in the late 1980s, health costs have risen 67% in real dollars since 1984 [4]. In 1990, health costs rose 17.1% and totaled $3217 per employee. According to the HCFA, actual employee health plan costs are predicted to be greater than the average annual wage within 10 years if the current rate of increase continues (Fig. 40-1). Figure 40-2 demonstrates the degree to which health benefits have risen more rapidly than other forms of employee compensation.

Cause of Rising Health Care Costs

The problem of rising health costs is not unique to the business community. Costs throughout the health care system have been increasing at comparable rates, creating a major problem for both government, which entered the health market with the establishment of Medicare and Medicaid in 1965 and pays a substantial amount for federal employees, and for individuals. The causes of the rise in health expenditures are many, and are listed in Table 40-1. The core of the problem is a rapidly expanding market that is essentially price insensitive. This has led both the supply and the demand sides of the system to grow with cancer-like speed. On the demand side, neither the individuals who use health services nor the physicians who order them face the costs of the resources they consume. While individuals pay on average about 20% of their health bill, providers do not bear any responsibility whatsoever for the cost. This creates a situation in which the consumer has a constant 80% discount: In this scenario, a $30,000 Cadillac can be purchased for $6000, with some invisible hand paying the additional $24,000. The $6000 fee is less than the cost of the least expensive automobile on the market, a clear incentive for the more expensive model to be consistently chosen.

The supply side of the system is not only price insensitive, but it is fueled by financial mechanisms that create incentives for utilization and price inflation. Hospitals have traditionally been paid on a cost-plus basis, meaning that the cost of an episode of care plus a certain profit margin was reimbursed by the payer. Since the

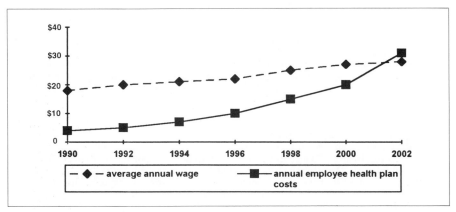

Figure 40-1. Average annual wages versus average annual health plan costs, based on an annual increase of 4% in wages and 25% in health plan costs. Source: Starr, P. *The Logic of Health Care Reform.* The Grand Rounds Press, 1992.

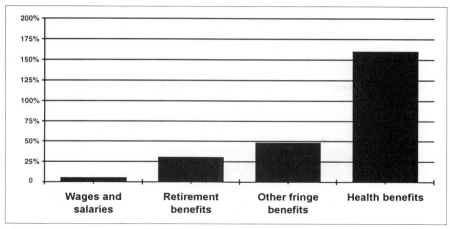

Figure 40-2. Rise in employer spending, 1970 to 1989 per full-time employee. Source: Starr, P. *The Logic of Health Care Reform*. The Grand Rounds Press, 1992.

Table 40-1. Causes of increasing health care costs

Price-insensitive economic market
Medical-industrial complex
Aging population
Oversupply of doctors and hospitals
High specialist/primary care ratio
Lack of knowledge about appropriate medical practice
Patient demand

hospitals determined their costs, this created incentives to do more services, and raise prices, while ignoring issues of efficiency. In addition, since capital expenditures were included as part of the cost of care, physical expansion was encouraged as well. Doctors have been paid with a similar inflationary mechanism known as fee-for-service. Essentially, any service performed by a physician has been reimbursed at a "usual, customary, and reasonable rate," which has been set at the 75th to 90th percentile of doctors' average charges in a region. Since doctors set their fees and were paid more if they did more, the incentive was clearly to charge more and to do more.

A phenomenon known as the medical-industrial complex has exacerbated these supply-side problems. As described by Relman [6], this refers to doctors increasingly owning medical supplies (e.g., laboratories or radiology units) that they control and from which they profit. Recent studies have shown that more tests are ordered by physicians who own facilities at which the tests are performed [7]. Recognizing this problem, the US Government has outlawed this practice for Medicare patients.

Two additional factors have contributed to increases in price and utilization: overcapacity in the health system and rapidly growing technology. The hospital industry for years has had an occupancy rate of approximately 70%, which has led to incentives both to have the empty beds filled and to raise prices to compensate for the unused equipment. Physician supply grew 40% between 1970 and 1987 (J. S. Harris; presented at ACOEM annual meeting, Spring 1991), largely as a result of a taskforce report that had predicted a physician shortage. However, the predicted shortage was for primary care physicians in rural areas, and the new doctors largely became specialists in large metropolitan areas. Studies have clearly shown that health care costs increase directly with both oversupply and specialization [8].

The paradoxical relationship between supply and demand in the health system, known as Roemer's law, is an important contributor to rising health care costs. It is characterized by a situation in which supply creates demand, the reverse of classic economic market theory. It is believed to result from the existence of an "imperfect" market, in which the usual constraints on supply and demand are not operative. In the health care system, this is due to many factors: an infinite desire for health, a highly technical field that makes it difficult for an individual to act as an informed consumer, and the aforementioned financing system, which disconnects the buyer from the payment [9].

A further factor in the rise of health costs has been the astounding growth in high-technology medical procedures. Services that are now commonplace, such as intensive care units, open-heart surgery, kidney dialysis, transplants, and endoscopies, are all phenomena of the past 25 years. This high-tech explosion has been fueled by the growth of National Institutes of Health (NIH) funding and academic medical centers in the post–World War II era. With little knowledge about what technologies were truly effective combined with the natural human predilection to choose health-promising procedures and a payment system that promoted use, the expenditure increases of the past 25 years were inevitable.

Cost Shifting

In addition to the factors listed in Table 40-1, business has faced the unique problem of cost shifting. As government increasingly controlled its health expenditures by statute (e.g., Medicare price freezes and hospital prospective payment), the providers of care shifted the burden of payment to the private employers. A consulting firm, Hewitt Associates, estimates that almost 30% of the increase in employer-based premiums of the past decade have been due to this cost shifting [4]. Figure 40-3 compares the relative growth of total health expenditures for the United States with those for business, clearly showing that employers have experienced a proportionally increased burden.

Small businesses have faced a second cost shift, as large employers often have been able to leverage their size to get discounts from providers and insurers. With the total size of the health care budget growing, and government and large business able to deflect their share of the growth, the burden has fallen increasingly on small and mid-sized business. When annual health cost increases for business as a whole are stratified by business size, it is seen that the smaller companies face increases two to three times those of the larger firms.

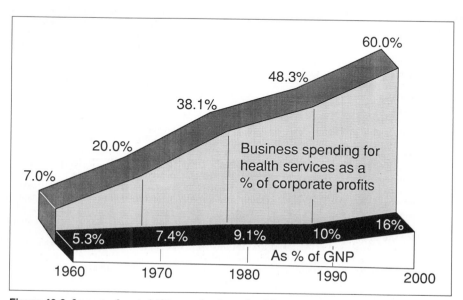

Figure 40-3. Impact of cost shifting on business health care costs. Source: Agency for Health Care Administration.

Disability Management

Costs related to the inability of employees to work have also been growing at a rapid rate. Disability costs include both medical payments and income outlays, the latter usually in the form of workers' compensation wages, short- and/or long-term disability payments, and disability pensions. These costs often account for 15 to 20% of a business's total health care expenditures, and there is evidence that they are growing as a percentage of that total [10] (Fig. 40-4). Whereas the medical payments for short- and long-term disability cases are included in personal illness costs, the health expenditures arising from workers' compensation are subject to state regulation and accounted for differently. The statutory nature of workers' compensation, the largest fraction of the disability dollar, leads to different incentives and different problems for business. The approaches to these challenges are discussed in Chaps. 34 and 39.

Future Considerations

Although it is clear that the US health care system will change in some way in the coming years, it is likely that employers will continue to be responsible for funding health insurance. Few believe today that the country will turn to a government-run model based on the Canadian system, funded by general taxes. More attention is being paid to the German model, which is an employer-based system that has managed to control its expenditures throughout the past two decades [11].

Even if price controls are to be adopted in a new system, business would still have short- and long-run financial stakes in health care. In the short run, it will take years to phase in a new system, and the financial exposure during the transition period will be as large, or larger, than it is currently. In the long run, even if costs only increase at the general inflation rate, business will be making an annual investment in health care that is quite substantial. Companies should pay as much attention to the value of this investment as they do their outlays to their other major suppliers.

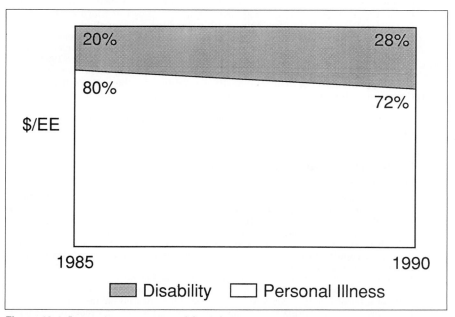

Figure 40-4. Increasing proportion of disability costs as percentage of total health care costs.

Business Strategies in Health Care Management

Employers have been actively trying to control their health costs for over 20 years. These efforts have encompassed three themes: restricting benefits, sharing cost with employees, and managing the delivery of health care [12]. The first wave of cost-containment efforts was run by traditional benefits managers, but by the early 1980s, an increasing number of large firms had carved out health care benefits, and had recruited experts or hired consultants from the health care industry to manage them.

Restricting Benefits and Self-Insurance

Many small firms have simply dropped their medical insurance benefits altogether because of the costs. Larger firms, often committed by collective bargaining to offering health care benefits, sought to decrease the scope of their health package. These businesses usually chose to be self-insured, meaning that they assumed the full risk for their employees' health costs, paying the actual cost of the medical encounters rather than an insurance premium. In a 1991 survey, 69% of companies had chosen this option [13]. The return for the risk in choosing self-insurance was twofold: (1) Under the federal ERISA statute, businesses could design their own benefit plan and be exempt from state mandates [14], and (2) no premium tax to the states was due. This has enabled businesses to restrict high-cost items such as treatment for infertility, open-ended payments for acquired immunodeficiency syndrome (AIDS), and long-term psychiatric treatment. These restrictions on benefits in the insured population have generated a great deal of concern nationally, and are believed to be a major contributor to the growing dissatisfaction with the American health care system.

Cost Sharing

Business has also increasingly shared the cost of medical benefits with employees. In the 1960s, "first-dollar" coverage policies were common in which employees had no financial responsibility for their health expenditures. In an effort to address this incentive for utilization (in insurance terminology, moral hazard), businesses began requiring employees to pay for a part of their medical expenses. Currently, three types of cost sharing exist: premiums, deductibles, and co-insurance. In a 1991 survey of 3323 employers, it was found that employees were paying on average 25 to 30% of their premiums (or of their total health expenditures in the case of self-insurance), the mean deductible was $475 for family coverage, and the median co-insurance rate was 20% [15]. Since 1987, when the Health Insurance Association of America began compiling statistics, employee cost sharing has increased at greater than the rate of medical inflation.

Managing the Delivery of Health Care

Utilization Review

Employers began using utilization review as a way of counteracting the incentives toward doing more in the health care system. Utilization review refers to the process in which services are reviewed by third parties in order to determine if they are medically appropriate and necessary. Payment for services is tied to this review, and only those services deemed necessary by the reviewer are authorized for payment. The most popular forms of utilization review are pre-admission certification and concurrent review of inpatient services. Both of these types of review seek to limit hospital days, as care delivered in this setting is the most expensive. Ironically, insurance plans of the 1960s had encouraged inpatient use by fully covering the costs of a hospital admission while requiring full or partial payment for outpatient procedures. Although this seems nonsensical in retrospect, the roots of this policy lie in the concept of insurance. Health insurance developed from the principles of classic indemnity insurance, examples of which are life or property and casualty insurance. The principle of classical insurance is that by pooling risk for unexpected and uncommon events, people could be financially protected from loss. Obviously, conditions such as myocardial infarctions and surgeries that require hospitalization fit the definition of uncommon occurrences. Other more common and predictable conditions, such as upper-respiratory infections and sprain/strains, did not, and they were not fully reimbursed.

However, by the late 1970s, it was evident that inpatient care was much more expensive than outpatient care, and that more procedures could safely be done in the outpatient setting, with considerable savings for the payer. By 1991, only 20% of the employers in the aforementioned survey did not use pre-admission certification [16]. Concurrent review, nearly as popular, addresses the issues of lengths of hospital stay for those conditions that require inpatient care. It was discovered that equal medical outcomes could be achieved with fewer hospital days, and utilization reviewers sought to concurrently evaluate cases, seeking justification for each hospital day used. Shorter stays have resulted from this approach. One dramatic example is the hospital stay for myocardial infarctions, which has decreased from 7 weeks in 1950 to 7 days in 1992.

Employers have used other forms of utilization review to monitor the delivery of their benefits. Case management is a form of review that attempts to manage the costliest cases early in their course. It is predicated on the fact that 10% of cases in a population can contribute to greater than 50% of the total costs. Mandatory second surgical opinion programs became popular in the 1980s, based on certain studies which indicated that unnecessary surgeries were a cause of rising health care costs [17].

The newest form of utilization review involves an intensified look at a specific area of high cost benefits, which are "carved out" from the health benefits package as a whole. This has been most commonly done with mental health and pharmacy services. Special utilization review firms have developed that only review this one aspect of benefits.

Managed Care

A way of changing the price incentives in the health care system is offered by health maintenance organizations (HMOs). In the classic staff-model HMO, premiums are prepaid on a capitated, or per-person, basis. This model combines the financing and the delivery of care in a single package, essentially shifting the economic risk to the providers of care. This means that the HMO needs to manage its care so that its actual expenditures are below its capitation. With doctors who are salaried and not fee-for-service, incentives are clearly for less costly care. This form of medical care lessens the need for utilization review, and if it does offer less costly care, obviates the need for benefit restriction and increasing cost sharing. As a result of legislation passed in 1973, the government required firms with greater than 25 employees (which offered health care benefits) to include an HMO as part of their benefit package.

Managed care organizations have expanded beyond staff-model HMOs in the past decade. Independent Practice Association (IPA)-model HMOs developed, in which individual doctors in private practice or free-standing physician groups formed organizations that contracted with a financing entity. This model lessens the link between the financing of care and the provision of care in that the doctors are usually paid on a discounted, fee-for-service basis. The financial risk that the physicians assume is in the form of a "withhold" of their payment, which is returned to the doctors only if certain budget targets are met. Because the "withholds" often represent only 10 to 15% of physician payment, their ability to change physician practice patterns is limited.

In response to the complaints of employees that HMOs restricted freedom of choice in selecting doctors, preferred provider organizations (PPOs) and point-of-service models have developed. In these models, selected networks of doctors and hospitals agree to accept discounts in prices and to cooperate with utilization review in exchange for the increase in patient volume that results from their being "preferred." Employees face a much lower copayment by choosing from the network, although they are free to choose any provider for a higher fee. The obvious problem with these plans is that the payment system is fee-for-service and not prepaid, so that the same incentives to increase volume and intensity of services that were found in the failing indemnity system exist here. Utilization may also be lacking.

Assessing Efforts at Cost Containment

The consensus among employers is that cost-containment efforts have not lived up to expectations [16]. Although it is not possible to estimate how much faster costs might have increased without the interventions described above, continuing double-digit increases at three to four times the CPI are considered unacceptable. Ironically, this sense of overall disappointment exists in the midst of individual, well-documented successes.

Employers view increased cost sharing with employees as a successful intervention. In a 1990 poll, close to 50% of employers viewed this as an effective way to control health care costs [13].

Certain types of utilization review have been documented to be cost saving. In the most comprehensive and methodologically sound study to date, Feldstein and associates [18] analyzed claims data on 222 groups of employees and dependents for the time period 1984 to 1985. The utilization review techniques used were pre-admission certification and concurrent review. Admissions were reduced by 12.3%, inpatient days by 8%, and total medical expenditures by 8.3%. The savings-to-cost ratio of utilization review was calculated at 8 : 1, even including the administrative costs of the review itself [18].

Other types of utilization review techniques have not been as successful. Although mandatory second surgical opinion programs were initially believed to be promising [17], the actual rates of avoided surgeries were less than 1% in the Medicare Program in 1991, prompting the Health Care Financing Administration to streamline the program to focus on a few selected procedures. Most utilization referral firms have adopted this streamlined approach. Although case management review is considered a successful intervention, no data are available to support this impression.

The biggest problem with utilization review is intrusion into the professional autonomy of the physician. Utilization review is usually done by nurses who have never seen the patient. And although the reviewers' medical necessity decisions are usually supported by some sort of practice guidelines or protocols, the uniqueness of the patient and the physician-patient bond cannot be factored into the decision. This kind of micromanagement is resented by physicians, and is not done in any other country besides the United States. Even health care managers who use it see it more as a necessary evil than as a desired intervention [19].

Managed care, particularly in the form of staff- and group-model HMOs, has had some success in modulating the increases in health costs. Early studies of HMOs showed that they did deliver less costly care, mainly by decreasing inpatient days [20]. However, despite one study to the contrary [21], suspicion has lingered that lower costs in HMOs have been a result of favorable selection (i.e., younger and healthier employees requiring less health care) and that the net savings for the entire workforce to the employer was unclear. However, the biggest problem with joining an HMO meant sacrificing freedom of choice in selecting doctors, and employees have not favored this. In 1991, less than 25% of medical care was delivered through staff-model HMOs.

A survey showed that in 1991 premium increases for HMOs were in the 10 to 15% range, compared to 15 to 20% for PPOs and 20 to 25% for indemnity plans [22]. Although these figures do represent a relative cost savings, increases of up to five times the CPI have not left employers satisfied. The 1991 National Executive Poll on health care costs sponsored by *Business and Health* magazine indicates that the percentage of employers who believe that HMOs and PPOs are effective in containing costs fell from around 30% in 1990 to 20% in 1991 [13]. Figure 40-5 shows the result of this *Business and Health* poll.

The prime reason why the first wave of cost-containment efforts was not more successful is that it did not adequately address the root causes of health care inflation. To the extent that benefit restrictions, cost sharing, and utilization review do not sufficiently alter the basic price insensitivity of the health care market, the underlying incentives for use and growth lead to attempts to circumvent the cost-containment efforts. Although employees have borne a progressively larger share of their health expenditures, they are still paying less than 20% of their total bill, which is below a critical value to change behavior. It also became obvious that providers can easily "game" the utilization review system, ranging from upcoding and unbundling services in billing to increasing the intensity of services for those cases that have been pre-approved. Common techniques used have been admitting

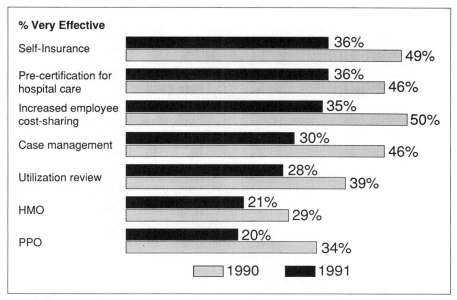

Figure 40-5. Effectiveness of health programs in containing costs. (From the 1991 national executive poll on health care costs and benefits. Reprinted from *Business and Health* September 1991. Pp. 62–68. © 1991, by Medical Economics Publishing, Inc., Montvale, N.J. All rights reserved.)

patients with mildly unstable conditions on an emergency basis, thereby bypassing precertification, and having hospitals reward doctors earning the highest revenue with purchases of new technology.

A second reason for the limited success was a result of another type of cost shifting that developed. This was the shift of inpatient costs to the outpatient setting. Schwartz and Mendelson [23] studied data from the American Hospital Association and the Health Care Financing Administration for the years 1981 to 1988 and found that outpatient utilization increased steadily over the time period, while inpatient days were being reduced at slower and slower rates. Their conclusion was that if the trend of decreasing reductions in inpatient days with increasing use of outpatient care continues, the net savings will be negligible [23].

A third cause of the relative failure of the initial cost-containment strategies was the realization that there was a profound gap in the information infrastructure of medicine. Health services researchers began studying patterns of medical care in the 1980s, and some surprising data emerged. Wennberg and associates [24] examined variation in medical practice between geographic areas, and found that for similar patients, coronary bypass surgery rates were twice as high in Boston, Massachusetts, as in New Haven, Connecticut. Although it was initially unclear which pattern of practice was "right," no benefit in clinical outcome was demonstrated for the higher intensity of services in Boston [24]. Similar findings of variations in practice patterns were found in New York State with respect to cesarean section rates [25]. On deeper examination, it was evident that no data existed to support one practice pattern over another.

Using guidelines for appropriateness of care, the Rand Corporation found that 17% of coronary angiographies and upper-gastrointestinal endoscopies, and 32% of carotid endarterectomies, were being done inappropriately [26]. Using a different set of criteria, researchers at the Lown Cardiovascular Center in Boston found that nearly 50% of coronary angiographies were unnecessary [27]. Although these studies have provoked considerable controversy in the medical field, it is clear that the actual outcomes of different interventions are not adequately understood.

The problems in medical practice patterns were not restricted to variation or overuse. As data became available that a great percentage of health care costs were being spent on potentially preventable diseases [28], it was also discovered that the health care system was not adequately addressing the issue of prevention [29]. Studies documented failures in the areas of both adequate treatment of hypertension and adequate immunization of children [30].

At the basis of the findings of practice variation and unnecessary services was the gap in medical information. Although the medical world had been involved in sophisticated basic science research since World War II, little of it had addressed the efficiency and outcomes of current treatments. It is estimated that less than a third of all the interventions in modern health care had ever been shown in scientific trials to help cure disease or preserve health [31]. According to David Eddy [32], a leader in the area of medical information: "The primary intellectual problem facing medicine today is that the information base is so poor. We simply do not know the consequences of a large proportion of medical activities. If we do not know the consequences of our activities, we cannot make intelligent choices."

As the data on the limits of cost containment were emerging, another line of inquiry began measuring satisfaction with the American health care system. It became evident that although employers were paying ever increasing amounts of money in what had become the most expensive health care system in the world, their employees were growing more dissatisfied with the system. Polls showed that in a 10-nation survey, Americans were the most dissatisfied with their health care system, with almost 90% feeling that either fundamental changes or a complete rebuilding of the system were necessary [33].

Not surprisingly, faced with evidence that expenditures on potentially preventable diseases were increasing, and that the services were frequently unnecessary, employers began to rethink their approach to cost containment. In surveys done with chief executive officers of the Fortune 500 companies, it was found that only 12.7% believed that they could control costs in the coming 2 years, and over 50% were dissatisfied with their current health strategies [16].

New Frontiers—Value Management

With the knowledge that efforts directed purely at cost containment were not sufficient, and that health expenditures were being used "unintelligently," employers became interested in moving from being "payers" to becoming "purchasers" [34]. Being a "purchaser" required that the value of expenditures is understood. The concept of value and quality in industry has undergone profound changes in the past 50 years as a result of the work of Juran, Shewart, and Deming in continuous quality improvement (CQI) and total quality management. One of the basic tenets of CQI is that variances in any process lead to variable quality rather than uniformly high quality. A corollary of this is that if variation is reduced, wasteful and unnecessary processes will have been identified and eliminated, and quality will be increased [35]. It became evident that the findings of variation in medical practice patterns made the health care field ripe for the applications of CQI. Purchasers of health care could be more confident of the value of their purchases if variation was reduced, and because reducing variations meant decreasing waste and increasing quality, it made sense to focus on quality improvement as the key to cost containment.

As employers have adopted the principles of CQI [35], their focus has been on three areas: increasing preventive interventions, involving the employee as a customer in the health care process, and working closely with suppliers to reduce variation in medical processes.

Prevention

A random survey of US worksites in 1985 revealed that 66% of businesses sampled had some health promotion activities. When firms with over 250 employees were isolated, greater than 80% had prevention programs [36]. These programs are usually designed to focus on cardiovascular risk factors, (i.e., smoking, nutrition, weight, exercise), the highest cost condition in the United States. Studies on the cost effectiveness of such programs have been mixed, with evidence that the more comprehensive and tightly designed programs will yield positive savings (see Chap. 32).

Employee as Customer

The continuous quality improvement model focuses on designing and strengthening processes that will meet the needs of the customer. Purchasers have increasingly demanded that their suppliers include satisfaction surveys in the package that is contracted. Surveys reveal that employees value freedom of choice, continuing relationships with their own doctors, and an increasing role in understanding and controlling their health care choices.

There is evidence that educating employees about self-care can decrease health care costs [37]. General Electric (GE) has piloted a program in which 24-hour free phone access is available to a group of employees who have any questions about health care. The phone line is staffed by experienced clinical nurses, who both educate employees and triage those problems not amenable to self-care to appropriate health care settings [19].

Relationships with Suppliers

As employers have moved to a purchaser model, their relationship with their suppliers has changed. Businesses no longer contract with insurance companies or managed care organizations and then simply leave the delivery of the benefits to these intermediaries. Employers are increasingly seeking a partnership rather than a vendor relationship. There is a perception among purchasers that because of the many stakeholders that managed care organizations must accommodate (i.e., providers, patients, and payers), their emphasis has been on pricing below indemnity insurance rather than on focusing on continuous improvement. This phenomenon of "shadow pricing" has led employers to commit resources to influence the processes of these managed care organizations.

In the CQI framework, purchasers are demanding to be treated like the customers of the intermediaries. One of the principles that is being insisted upon is that a process improvement approach be adopted both by the intermediaries and by the providers who are actually delivering the services. The belief is that the quality assurance model, which focuses on outliers, will not change the fundamental problems of the system. CQI techniques focus on mapping and improving processes in an effort to reduce variation.

Given that the weak medical evidence on which medical decisions are made is a prime factor in the variation in practice patterns, purchasers are insisting on outcome studies [38] and practice guidelines as a way of both improving the information base and optimizing what is already known. The ideal situation is believed to be one in which clinical and functional outcomes are understood for different medical interventions; decisions could then be made rationally about what benefits to reimburse. Purchasers are beginning to insist that their suppliers build data on these outcomes.

Developing practice guidelines or parameters is an attempt to organize the available medical evidence into clear recommendations. It is hypothesized that by having a guideline as a measuring stick variation can be reduced and quality improved. Efforts are currently under way by the US Government, through its Agency for Health Care Policy and Research (founded in 1989) and a plethora of speciality societies, managed care organizations, and insurers. The American Medical Association (AMA) has endorsed the concept of practice parameters, a change from its previous position of deriding them as "cookbook" medicine [39].

Opportunities for Occupational Physicians

As health care managers have begun their transition from frustrated payers to educated purchasers, and have sought to understand the processes of health delivery, they have found that physicians are crucial participants in this process. As stated by Charles Buck, Staff Executive for Health Care Management at GE [40]:

> Speaking as a nonphysician with responsibility for corporate-wide "value purchasing" activities, it is obvious that aggressive action on the part of the corporation and its employees, based on quality and value, requires substantial physician input. Are our insurance carriers using appropriate criteria to certify the necessity of procedures? Which of the many and various standards should we use? In selecting preferred networks, are we using the right criteria? What level of quality of care are we justified in claiming? More directly, which hospitals and physicians in a local area have the reputation for, and hopefully are, the highest in quality? Which physicians and hospitals pose problems? What should we do if our employees and their families are currently using "problem" providers? All of these issues arise in any aggressive pursuit of high value medical care on a day-to-day basis. Physician input is critical.

There are clear indications that physicians are moving to fill this role. Hospitals are increasingly placing physicians in charge of their organizations [41], and the American College of Physician Executives (ACPE), an organization of doctors involved in health care management, experienced 20% growth in membership between 1990 and 1992 [42]. However, the physicians moving to fill this role have largely not been occupational physicians. Less than 5% of the membership of the ACPE work for non–health care employers. As Buck goes on to say in the above article, if occupational physicians do not fill this needed role for employers, the physicians associated with the intermediaries, that is, the insurance companies or the managed care organizations, will. This leads to a basic question: Why has occupational medicine not moved to fill this role?

A primary reason has to do with the traditional scope of occupational medicine, which has focused on prevention and treatment of work-related illnesses and injuries. The code of ethical conduct adopted by the American College of Occupational Medicine in 1976 focuses exclusively on workplace-related issues of health and safety [43]. This focus arises at least in part out of the historical conflict between occupational medicine and the community of practicing physicians. Early in the twentieth century, the AMA demonstrated its concerns about the potential competition company-employed physicians represented by occasionally refusing them membership in the AMA. A distinct fear voiced by the AMA was that business might monopolize the medical community, thereby "corporatizing" the practice of medicine, and threaten the existence of private practice [5]. By restricting the definitions of occupational medicine to work-related problems only, conflict has been avoided and peaceful coexistence maintained. Although the American College of Occupational and Environmental Medicine (ACOEM) is slowly moving to broaden this scope, a recent report by the Medical Practice Committee of the College listed participation in planning, providing, and assessing the quality and cost of employee health benefits as only the seventh of eight possible elective components of an occupational health program [44].

Resulting from this traditional focus of occupational medicine, little attention has been paid to training in the discipline of health care management. Emphasis in occupational medicine in medical school and residency programs is on the traditional areas of toxicology, compliance requirements, and fitness-for-duty principles. Taking an active role in health care management requires a knowledge of health services research, economics, and issues of health delivery, little of which is offered in occupational medical training or residency programs.

A further explanation for occupational medicine's failure to take a lead role in health care management involves the potential ethical conflicts that could arise from deciding on benefit design and utilization issues. Occupational medicine has long struggled with the ethical dilemma of being between medicine and management. Walsh [45] has developed a model that accounts for the various functions and ethical conflicts of the occupational physician, which is shown in Fig. 40-6 (Table 40-2). According to this model, there are four distinct areas of occupational medical responsibility. In three of these areas, medical adjudication, environmental health, and health care services, ethical dilemmas abound. For example, in the medical adjudication role, a physician may have to determine an applicant's eligibility for a disability pension, where a negative determination can adversely impact the employee's social and financial status. This situation runs contrary to a physician's training to serve his or her patients solely in an advocacy role. This situation can arise in the environmental health sector and the health care service area as well, as in cases of employees with impairments who desire to work for financial reasons, but for whom continued work could jeopardize their health.

Although these conflicts are real and unavoidable, Walsh argues that occupational medicine has unnecessarily limited its scope by not expanding into a fourth area, that of strategy formulation. Particularly, as health care management has evolved from a pure cost-containment model to one of value management, decisions on quality of care may allow the occupational doctor to serve the interests of employees and employers simultaneously. Health promotion is one clear activity that achieves this. Involvement in issues such as benefits design and data analysis, however, can serve this purpose as well, as stated by Wood [46]:

> The corporate physician, in his or her role as protector of the health of workers as individuals and as a productive population, has the inherent interest and the expertise to make judgments about the clinical value of health care purchased for

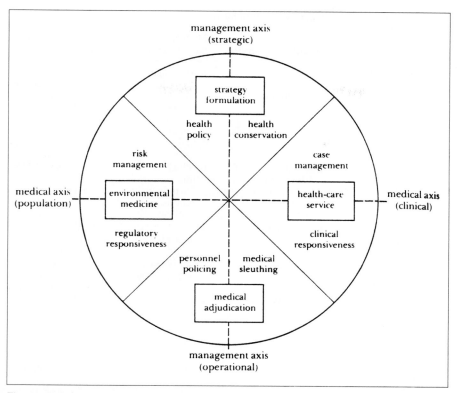

Figure 40-6. Sectors of corporate physician's role. (From D. C. Walsh, Employee assistance programs. *Milbank Quarterly.* 60:492, 1982.)

employees, and about the clinical validity of cost control measures, such as utilization review, that assess the appropriateness of the clinical process.

For these reasons the corporate physician has a responsibility to assert and insert himself or herself in the corporate health resource management process. One of the fundamental elements of this responsibility is that the physician be knowledgeable about the needs, the sources, the quality, the analysis, and the meaningful uses for data and the information and knowledge derived therefrom.

Although there may be potential conflict with practicing physicians over the issues of utilization review and managed care, there is evidence of a substantial difference in the attitude of the physician community in the late twentieth century as compared to the early twentieth century. The AMA has become involved in health care reform, and the American College of Physicians published a position paper in 1992 that offered solutions to the cost problem [47]. Ultimately, it is arguable that because someone on the purchaser side will be making benefit and utilization decisions, it is to the practicing doctor's advantage to have a fellow physician be influential in the decision-making process.

Models of Physician Involvement in Health Care Management

Existing classifications of the role of occupational physicians in health care management predate the rapid changes in health delivery in the 1980s [48]. Traditionally, occupational physicians have concerned themselves with issues of worksite health and safety, encompassing fitness for duty, toxicology, and prevention and

Table 40-2. Three major role sectors for corporate medicine

	Health care services	Medical adjudication	Environmental health
Historical roots	Emergency treatment, remote locations	Verification of eligibility and claims processing (workers' compensation and benefits associations)	Accident prevention and public health reforms
Functions	Early detection of illness, health conservation, case management	Medical interpretations for industrial relations applications	Risk assessment and management, organizational intelligence
Technique/ expertise	Clinical medicine	Medical administration	Epidemiology, biostatistics, toxicology
Conflicts	Organized medicine, regulators, employees, and public health sector vs. occupational medicine	Costs vs. health mission, line vs. staff	Worker vs. supervisor, in-house vs. outside physicians

Source: Adapted from D. C. Walsh. *Corporate Physicians.* New Haven: Yale University Press, 1987.

treatment of work-related injuries and illnesses. To the extent that employees are matched to their jobs, or injuries are prevented through safety programs, health care dollars are theoretically saved. The treatment of work-related conditions on site has theoretical cost savings, and may favorably impact workers' compensation costs [49]. However, other than treating episodic personal illness on a walk-in basis, for the most part occupational physicians have had little involvement in the management of non–work-related health costs, which represent over 70% of total employee health costs. According to Harris, on the infrequent occasions in which occupational doctors have been asked to participate in cost management, their focus has been on resisting any type of managed care and on preserving the right of the treating physician to have complete autonomy in practice style [53].

Although the published literature is limited, at least four distinct types of active involvement in health care management by occupational physicians can be classified in a contemporary model. These include (1) medical liaison, (2) medical treatment provider, (3) health management consultant, and (4) health management leader. The activities of any one occupational doctor do not necessarily fit into one classification and, indeed, may encompass two or three of the types.

Medical Liaison Model

In this model, occupational physician involvement in health care costs is through coordinating the activity of community providers with the worksite. This is the most common of the four models. The occupational physician takes the lead role in prevention of and convalescence from disease while the acute phase of medical treatment remains the responsibility of the community physicians. The occupational physician does have a role in ongoing care through referral of employees to the highest-quality, most cost-effective community doctors as well as through working with these providers on worksite issues. This triage role usually results from episodic treatment of employees on a walk-in basis.

Prevention and Health Promotion

The prevention of disease has long been within the scope of occupational medicine. Periodic health examinations of individuals are offered by most occupational health clinics, although the actual cost effectiveness of these examinations is unproven [50]. Over the past decade, full-scale health promotional programs have developed, which address the major risk factors of our times (smoking, nutrition, exercise, etc.). There is emerging evidence that specific types of these programs, and specific interventions within these programs, are saving health care dollars [52].

Employee assistance programs (EAP) serve as initial points of contact for employees with mental health or lifestyle problems. Usually run by trained, nonphysician counselors, these programs serve a triage function to appropriate outside providers. Given that mental health benefits have been the most rapidly rising area of health care benefits, the potential for cost savings by referral to cost-effective providers is substantial. More recently, EAP counselors are performing short-term treatment themselves. Certain programs have been found to have favorable cost-benefit ratios [53].

A third type of preventive activity is educating employees to be informed health care consumers. As described earlier in this chapter, one of the causes of health care cost increases is the lack of a functioning economic market, which requires informed consumers. Some corporate medical centers have been involved in this exercise, for which data exist that suggest a positive cost-benefit ratio [37].

Coordinating Chronic Disease

With respect to the treatment of personal illness, there is evidence that coordinating with primary care physicians on the treatment of hypertension has resulted in improved control of blood pressure at lower cost [54]. Although not proven, a similar program may be beneficial in other chronic conditions, such as diabetes and dyslipidemias.

Convalescence

The convalescence period has been a neglected area of potential cost savings. Utilization review focuses on inpatient treatment, and the optimum time for an employee to return to work has been understudied. When an employee is out of work, some form of income payment is usually generated, either as a short-term disability payment or as a workers' compensation weekly wage. Several companies have developed programs to monitor employees in this convalescence stage, either through contracting with external vendors or through in-house programs (R. S. Galvin; presented at ACOEM meeting, April 1990).

Chrysler has experienced savings with the Workability program, a software-based system developed and operated by Core Management, Inc. This system has established sophisticated disability durations for both occupational and nonoccupational injuries and illnesses, and provides guidelines for when employees can return to work. Between 1986 and 1989, Chrysler experienced a 9.1% decrease in the disability cost per employee for a total savings estimated at more than $16 million [55].

General Electric has developed the Convalescent Assistance to Recovering Employees (CARE) program, an in-house, nurse-run system that follows every employee with a medical absence of greater than 5 days. The program is based on employee advocacy; it coordinates benefits and case management, and facilitates return to work for all employees. Disability cost savings of 10% were measured in its pilot location (R. S. Galvin; presented at ACOEM meeting, April 1990).

Medical Treatment Model

Both free-standing occupational clinics and corporate medical departments have long provided episodic treatment of both work-related injuries and personal illness to employees. Indeed, the development of occupational medicine in the United States paralleled the growth of on-site clinics in the railroad industry. By 1910, when workers' compensation laws became established, it was estimated that there were over 6000 company doctors who specialized in surgery of railway workers [56].

As the health cost crisis has worsened, certain companies have expanded this on-site treatment model as a major strategy for containing costs [57]. This has been done for both personal illness and occupational disease.

Personal Illness

The attractions for providing medical care on site are many. For self-insured companies, whose costs are experience based, a visit to the on-site doctor avoids duplicate payment. It represents efficient use of a budgeted medical clinic and saves charges from community doctors. Equally attractive is the potential for optimizing the "gatekeeper" function. Health services research has indicated that physicians control 85 cents out of every health dollar spent, and that this expenditure is best managed by a primary care doctor who can treat most illnesses, and who can manage referrals to cost-effective specialists [58]. By having this gatekeeper be a salaried employee of the company, the expensive incentives of fee-for-service payment are diminished. A third possible source of cost savings is through controlling the pricing of expensive ancillary testing. As companies provide stress tests, endoscopies, and pharmaceuticals on site, significant price discounts are achieved.

There is the potential for other, more indirect savings. To the extent that an employee does not have to leave work to tend to his or her health needs, productivity increases. It is also likely that occupational physicians can better control medical absence through their understanding of job function and work restrictions. This can potentially save overtime, training, and replacement costs.

One of the most well-known proponents of the medical treatment model is the Gillette Company, based in Boston, Massachusetts. This company first offered full-scale on-site medical services to all employees in 1955. In a recent survey of six of its medical sites, all offered care for personal illness, and two provided full primary care, including afterhours coverage. The estimated annual saving is $800,000 based on a 1% decrease in absenteeism. The additional savings based on medical charges have not been published. The estimates were adjusted for a possible volume increase related to induced demand (W. E. Greer; presentation to the New England Occupational Medical Association, Fall 1992). Since the raw numbers from this estimate are not published, it is impossible to evaluate how the final sum was calculated. It is not clear if the total health dollars of the entire company were included, or how possible confounders contributing to decreased absenteeism were dealt with. It is clear that this program has been well received by both management and labor.

However, there are important potential problems with expanded on-site medical care. First, these clinics may attract minor illnesses and injuries, the cost of which is not significant. Second, to the extent that the clinic is used mostly by employees, the greater than 60% of total health care costs attributable to dependents is not impacted. Third, and most important, it is possible that having free treatment available may actually induce demand. A study by the Rand Corporation found that when compared to a system that required copayment, a free-care system led to 33% greater utilization of hospitalization and outpatient services [59]. The total medical expenditures were actually higher for the free-care group, without evidence of improvement in health status.

It is also possible that having on-site primary care treatment that exists parallel to the standard benefits plan may result in duplication of services and a problem with quality of care. When 24-hour coverage is not provided, the community doctor seeing the employee for the first time may end up ordering studies already performed through the worksite.

A second model of on-site treatment, which addresses some of these concerns, has been adopted by several companies that have used an outside vendor for their services. Both Goodyear Tire and Rubber Company, in 1985, and Nestlé, in 1992, have used Medicenter of Lawton, Oklahoma, to set up full-service clinics. Both of these companies address the limitations of employee-only treatment and free care by offering primary care to employees and dependents, which requires a copayment [60]. Neither company has published data relative to cost savings.

Southern California Edison (SCE) has constructed the most comprehensive program using the occupational physician in the medical treatment model [61]. The company has converted its numerous on-site clinics to be part of its managed care network. These sites are staffed by SCE-salaried primary care doctors, but the clinics are included in the company's PPO. Available to employees and dependents, there is a copayment for services identical to the fee charged at any community physician's office. This approach addresses many of the aforementioned problems of the medical treatment model: It provides full primary care services for employees and families as part of the company's overall benefit package.

Work-Related Conditions

The incentives for medical providers in the workers' compensation system are similar to those on the group health side. Although payment and financing are distinct, the fee-for-service system prevails. Since most workers' compensation injuries are out-patient-based problems, and by definition occur to employees only, the advantages of on-site treatment far outweigh the disadvantages, if the employee base is large enough.

Evidence exists that on-site physical therapy and work hardening can be cost effective. At one GE site, on-site physical therapy decreased lost workdays by 32% and overall costs by 37% for workers' compensation low back pain claims [49]. Although an increased number of low back claims were filed after the on-site pro-gram, the bulk of these did not involve lost time, and a net cost benefit was obtained. (For further discussion, see Chap. 39.)

Health Care Consultant Model

As health benefits managers have become more involved with the processes and outcomes of medical care, they have needed health care experts to serve as consul-tants. Although company occupational physicians would seem the most logical first choice, they have been mostly either uninterested or unable to help. However, there are examples of physicians becoming educated in health care management, and making valuable contributions.

Schneider [62] has described a situation at JP Morgan, Inc., in New York in which the corporate medical department has been included as part of a team headed by the human resources department that is responsible for health care benefit design. In addition to medical liaison and some medical treatment functions, the medical department provides advice relative to mental health benefits as well as to a second surgical opinion utilization review program.

At First National Bank of Chicago, the medical department and benefits depart-ment form a team that designs health care cost management strategies [63]. The team developed a database management system that integrates health risk appraisal data, medical claims data, and traditional occupational medical data. This innova-tive, integrated database is used to guide benefit decisions.

The most advanced example of the health care consultant model was pioneered at Northern Telecom, Inc., in Nashville in the mid-1980s. Analyzing health care costs and claims, the physician in charge of health and safety recommended a compre-hensive medical program, which was adopted by the company. The program included health promotion programs, on-site primary care, as well as a managed care strategy. The occupational physicians worked in a team with benefits and finance, but basi-cally were responsible for ongoing interpretation of health care cost and utilization data, on both personal illness and workers' compensation sides. Well-documented decreases occurred in risk factors, health care utilization, and health care costs [64].

Health Management Leader

This model places the business responsibility for health care management on the occupational physician. This least common of the four models adds the health man-agement function to the traditional responsibilities of the occupational medical role. The ultimate responsibility for costs, contracting, and benefit design comes under the medical director.

Although there has been theoretical support for occupational physicians assuming this role [43], few companies have chosen this path. The reasons have been alluded to earlier in this chapter and include reluctance on the part of both business and occupational medicine. However, there are compelling arguments for this role, the strongest of which is that physicians have a deeper understanding of the processes and incentives of the medical system by being part of it. Additionally, by having taken the Hippocratic oath, physicians are in the best position to develop a system that centers around the patient, rather than around administrative ease or cost savings. However, to the extent that physicians assume a leadership role, they are judged by the same criteria as any nonphysician. Expertise in finance, management, and strategic planning needs to coexist with the inherent understanding of medical processes.

Honeywell, Inc., created the position of Vice President for Health Management in the 1980s [65]. The physician who holds this position has the lead responsibility of developing health care strategies, and of contracting with various third-party administrators and managed care organizations. The corporate health care strategy has been cost control through quality management, defined as reimbursing only medical care that is based on the principles of medical necessity and medical appropriateness. This type of medical care is believed to be best delivered by networks of physicians organized into a managed care structure. The health management leader role at Honeywell is designed to highlight direct interaction with the provider groups as the mechanism to achieve the goals of quality and appropriateness. This interaction is obviously best done by a physician.

Using a similar model, General Electric appointed its New England medical director to become the regional health care manager in 1992. General Electric contracts with managed care organizations as third-party administrators to execute its self-insured benefit plan, taking an active partnership role with these organizations. The health care manager is responsible for these contracts and managing quality and cost trends with the health care organizations.

One company, Southern California Edison, has led the way with this approach [66]. Beginning in 1989, its medical director was put in charge of all health care and medical activities. The strategy has been to develop a managed care plan, Healthflex, of which Edison's 10 on-site occupational clinics are part. In addition, the company decided to bring all the administrative functions of the benefit plan in-house. This meant directing claims payment, provider and customer service, credentialing and utilization review by the medical department. Joint Commission on Accreditation of Healthcare Organizations (JCAHO) accreditation was secured for the health centers.

Summary

The role of the occupational physician in health care management has been expanding rapidly as rising health care costs have threatened US business competitiveness. Particularly as health services research has revealed practice pattern variation and unnecessary medical care, companies have moved from pure payers or buyers of care to informed purchasers. Given the paucity of clear guidelines in the highly technical health care field, physicians have played an increasingly important role in health care management.

This crisis among employers has led occupational physicians to move beyond their traditional roles as managers of worksite health and safety to assume more expanded roles as caregivers, consultants, or health care managers. Although there is still debate within the field of occupational medicine about the appropriateness of such an expanded role, both theoretical arguments and practical realities point to a tremendous opportunity for occupational physicians in these areas in future years.

References

1. Castro, J. Paging Dr. Clinton. *Time Magazine* January 18, 1993. Pp. 24–36.
2. Walsh, D. C. *Corporate Physicians: Between Medicine and Management.* New Haven: Yale University Press, 1987.
3. Iglehart, J. K. The American health care system—private insurance. *N. Engl. J. Med.* 326:1715, 1991.
4. Averbuch, R. *What Business Needs to Know About Health Care.* Massachusetts Business Roundtable, 1991.
5. Starr, P. *The Social Transformation of American Medicine.* New York: Basic Books, 1982.
6. Relman, A. S. The new medical-industrial complex. *N. Engl. J. Med.* 303:963, 1980.
7. Hemenway, D., et al. Physicians' responses to financial incentives: Evidence from a for-profit ambulatory care center. *N. Engl. J. Med.* 322:1059, 1990.
8. Greenfield, S., et al. Variations in resource utilization among medical specialties and systems of care: Results from the Medical Outcomes Study. *J.A.M.A.* 267:1624, 1992.

9. Williams, S. J., and Torreas, P. R. (eds.). *Introduction to Health Services*. Albany, NY: Delmar Publishers, 1988.
10. Robbins, F. The growing cost of disability. *Business and Health* Special Report, July 1993. Pp. 6–9.
11. Iglehart, J. K. Germany's health care system. Parts I and II. *N. Engl. J. Med.* 324:503, 1750, 1991.
12. Herzlinger, R., and Schwartz, J. How companies tackle health care costs. *Harvard Business Review* Part I, July, Aug.; pp. 69–81 and II, Sept., Oct.; pp. 108–120, 1985.
13. The 1991 national executive poll on health care costs and benefits. *Business and Health* September 1991. Pp. 62–68.
14. Mariner, W. K. Problems with employer-provided health insurance—the Employee Retirement Income Security Act and health care reform. *N. Engl. J. Med.* 327:1682, 1993.
15. Sullivan, C., et al. Employer-sponsored health insurance in 1991. *Health Affairs* 11:172, 1992.
16. Cantor, J. C., et al. Business leaders' views on American health care. *Health Affairs* 10:98, 1991.
17. Ruchlin, H. S., et al. The efficacy of second-opinion consultation programs: A cost-benefit perspective. *Med. Care* 20:3, 1982.
18. Feldstein, P. J., et al. Private cost containment: The effects of utilization review programs on health care use and expenditures. *N. Engl. J. Med.* 318:1310, 1988.
19. Darling, H. Employers and managed care: What are the early returns? *Health Affairs* 10:147, 1991.
20. Luft, H. S. How do health maintenance organizations achieve their savings? Rhetoric and evidence. *N. Engl. J. Med.* 298:1336, 1978.
21. Ware, J. E., et al. Comparison of health outcomes at a health maintenance organization with those of fee-for-service. *Lancet* 1:1017, 1986.
22. Schachner, M. Health plan premiums to increase 10 to 25%. *Business Insurance* 3:17, 1990.
23. Schwartz, W. B., and Mendelson, D. M. Hospital cost containment in the 1980s: Hard lessons learned and prospects for the 1990s. *N. Engl. J. Med.* 324:1037, 1991.
24. Wennberg, J. E., et al. Are hospital services rationed in New Haven or over-utilized in Boston? *Lancet* 1:1185, 1987.
25. Laditka, S., et al. GE goes after high medical costs. *Business and Health* 1:44, 1990.
26. Brook, R. H., et al. Predicting the appropriate use of carotid endarterectomy, upper gastrointestinal endoscopy, and coronary angiography. *N. Engl. J. Med.* 325:1173, 1990.
27. Graboys, T. B., et al. Results of a second opinion trial among patients recommended for coronary angiography. *J.A.M.A.* 268:2537, 1993.
28. Centers for Disease Control. Premature mortality in the United States: Public health issues in the use of years of potential life lost. *M.M.W.R.* 35 (Suppl. 25):15, 1986.
29. Lurie, N., et al. Preventive care: Do we practice what we preach? *Am. J. Public Health* 77:801, 1987.
30. Chassin, M. R. Practice guidelines: Best hope for quality improvement in the 1990's. *J.O.M.* 32:1199, 1990.
31. Berwick, D. M. Continuous improvement as an ideal in health care. *N. Engl. J. Med.* 320:53, 1989.
32. Eddy, D. *Decisions Without Information: The Intellectual Crisis in Medicine*. Harvard Community Health Plan Annual Report, 1989. Pp. 5–8 (Available through Harvard Community Health Plan, Inc., Ten Brookline Pl., West Boston, MA 02146.)
33. Blendon, R. J., et al. Satisfaction with health systems in ten nations. *Health Affairs* 9:185, 1990.
34. Patricelli, R. E. Employers as managers of risk, cost, and quality. *Health Affairs* 1:75, 1982.
35. Makens, P. K., and McEachern, J. E. Applications of industrial quality improvement in health care. *J.O.M.* 32:1177, 1990.
36. Fielding, J. F. Occupational health physician and prevention. *J.O.M.* 33:314, 1991.
37. Vickery, D. M., et al. Effect of self-care education program on medical visits. *J.A.M.A.* 250:2592, 1983.
38. Ellwood, P. Outcomes management: A technology of patient experience. *N. Engl. J. Med.* 318:1549, 1988.
39. Audet, A. M., et al. Medical practice guidelines: Current activities and future directions. *Ann. Intern. Med.* 113:709, 1990.

40. Buck, C. R. Assessing value in medical care for employees and dependents: An opportunity for occupational physicians. *J. Occup. Med.* 32:1165, 1990.
41. Nash, D. B. The physician-executive: Future challenges and opportunities. *Medical Interface* October 1, 1990. Pp. 45–48.
42. American College of Physician Executives. Internal publication, 1992.
43. American Occupational Medical Association. Code of ethical conduct for physicians providing occupational medical services. *J. Occup. Med.* January, 1994.
44. Occupational Medical Practice Committee of the American College of Occupational and Environmental Medicine. Scope of occupational and environmental health programs. *J.O.M.*: 34:436, 1992.
45. Walsh, D. C. "Is there a doctor in-house?" *Harvard Business Rev.*, 84:84, 1984.
46. Wood, L. W. A user's view of health care data management. *J.O.M.* 33:264, 1991.
47. Scott, H. D., and Shapiro, H. B.. Universal insurance for American health care. A proposal of the American College of Physicians. *Ann. Intern. Med.* 117:511, 1992.
48. Scholfield, et al. A Classification of Seven Corporate Health Clinics. In R. Egdahl et al. *Background Papers on Industry's Changing Role in Health Care Delivery.* New York: Springer-Verlag, 1977.
49. Galvin, R. S. Assuring Value in the Treatment of Low Back Pain. 1994 (in press).
50. Beck, H. D., et al. Assuring value in medical care for employees and dependents. *J.O.M.* 32:1161, 1990.
51. Galvin, R. S. The periodic health examination: Update and review. *The Occupational and Environmental Medicine Report,* May 1993.
52. Harris, J. S. The cost effectiveness of health promotion programs. *J.O.M.* 33:327, 1991.
53. Harris, J. S. Managing Health: What Employers Can Do About Health Care Costs. In J. Meyer and K. McLennon (eds.), *Background Papers on Health Care Cost.* Washington, DC: Committee for Economic Development, 1988
54. Foote, A., and Erfurt, J. Hypertension control: Formula for success. *Business Health* 1:13, 1984.
55. Carpenter, G. Disabilities management strategies: The Workability system. *Physical Medical and Rehab. State of the Art Rev.* Vol. 6; 2, June 1992.
56. Selleck, H. B., and Whitaker, A. H. *Occupational Health in America.* Detroit: Wayne State University Press, 1962.
57. Time for a fresh look at company doctors? *Wall Street Journal* June 12, 1990.
58. Franks, P., et al. Gatekeeping revisited—protecting patients from overtreatment. *N. Engl. J. Med.* 327:424, 1992.
59. Keeler, E. B., et al. How free care reduced hypertension in the health insurance experiment. *J.A.M.A.* 253:1926, 1985.
60. Bryant, M. "Comeback for the company doc?" *Business and Health* February 1991.
61. Gersel, J. Company-run clinics cutting health costs. An interview with Jacque Sokolove. *Business Insurance* March 5, 1990.
62. Schneider, W. J. A corporate medical department's role in medical benefits. *J.O.M.* 33:331, 1991.
63. Burton, W., et al. A computer-assisted health care cost management system. *J.O.M.* 33:268, 1991.
64. Dalton, B. A., and Harris, J. S. A comprehensive approach to corporate health management. *J.O.M.* 33:348, 1991.
65. Burns, J. M. The corporate physician as a health management leader. *J.O.M.* 33:335, 1991.
66. Schmitz, M., and Courtright, G. W. Case study: The corporate physician in a managed care environment. *J.O.M.* 33:351, 1991.

Further Information

Beck, H. D., Harris, J. S., and Wood, L. W. A strategy for employer health care value management. *J.O.M.* 33:386, 1991.
Summarizes the health care crisis and provides a framework for occupational physician involvement.

Briggs, D. Resource review. *J.O.M.* 32:1236, 1990.
Listing of journals and societies involved in the field of health care management.

Starr, P. *The Social Transformation of American Medicine.* New York: Basic Books, 1982.

Thorough sociologic and historical analysis of the role of medicine in American society. Provides an excellent guide for understanding the economic and social forces that shape medicine as an industry.

Starr, P. *The Logic of Health Care Reform: Transforming American Medicine for the Better.* The Grand Rounds Press, 1992.
A concise framework for the reshaping of the American health care system written by one of the architects of the White House Health Care Task Force. The likely future of employer involvement in the health care benefits arena is outlined in this short and well-written book.

Walsh, D. C. *Corporate Physicians: Between Medicine and Management.* New Haven: Yale University Press, 1987.
This book provides the most comprehensive look at the overall role of occupational physicians in industry. The ethical issues surrounding occupational medical involvement in health care benefit management are explored, with suggestions for resolutions of these issues.

Wood, L. W. Edited by J. S. Harris and H. D. Bock. *Managing Employee Health Care Costs: Assuring Quality and Value.* Boston: OEM Press, 1992.
This series of articles is compiled from two special editions of the Journal of Occupational Medicine *in 1990 and 1991 and a seminar at the Annual Meeting of the American College of Occupational Medicine in May 1991. It offers a state-of-the-art perspective on both the issues concerning employee health care costs and the involvement of specific companies and occupational physicians in addressing the cost and quality problems.*

Appendix to Chapter 40: Getting Involved

How does the physician get more involved in health care management? Increased involvement in health care management requires two conditions: opportunity and expertise. The opportunities in this area are abundant. As employers struggle with the increasingly sophisticated field of health care, their benefits departments have either contracted with health benefit consultants or added health care managers to their payroll. Few of these benefits professionals are physicians, and they are usually relieved to have a physician help them with issues of utilization review and medical management. The complaint heard among purchasers is not that there are too many occupational doctors involved, but that there are so few.

Expertise in health care management requires a knowledge of health services research and the economics of health care. The two physician organizations involved in health care management are the American College of Occupational and Environmental Medicine (ACOEM; 55 W. Seegers Rd., Arlington Heights, IL 60005-3922) and the American College of Physician Executives (ACPE; 4890 W. Kennedy Blvd., Suite 200, Tampa, FL 33609-2575). ACOEM has a Health Care Cost and Quality Management Committee that sponsors seminars at the semi-annual ACOEM meetings. The area of focus in the past decade has been on the value of group health and workers' compensation benefits. ACPE has a committee on corporate medical services, although the organization as a whole has historically been mostly focused on physicians working in the hospital and managed care industries. ACPE offers a three-part Physician Management Series, which presents a thorough introduction to health care management. However, although seminars and courses are useful, a masters-level program in health services administration, business, or public health is necessary to gain true expertise in the field.

Two publications focus on issues of health care management. *Business and Health* is a non–peer-reviewed journal that includes articles on the spectrum of health management issues. It is affiliated with the Washington Business Group on Health and is published monthly through Medical Economics Publishing (Five Paragon Dr., Montvale, NJ 07645-1742).

Health Affairs, an academic journal of health policy published quarterly, is peer reviewed and often referred to as the *New England Journal of Medicine* of the health policy field (Two Wisconsin Circle, Suite 500, Chevy Chase, MD 20815).

A third journal, *Physician Executive,* is peer reviewed and published monthly by ACPE, and has as its focus the issues of physicians as managers. Each issue usually includes one or two articles on health care management.

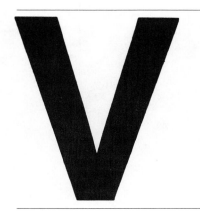

Environmental Medicine

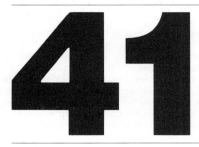

The Environment and Health

Tee L. Guidotti

Global ecologic change, including issues such as the greenhouse effect, stratospheric ozone depletion, interregional transport of pollution, and large-scale resource depletion, among others, has been much in the news. Increasingly, as occupational physicians are given responsibility for environmental affairs in major organizations, issues of ecologic changes arise that must be managed. In the past, these issues were related to public health and local effects of environmental pollution. In recent years, however, the scope of environmental issues has broadened considerably and forced the occupational physician to address serious issues beyond traditional medical and public health concerns. The purpose of this chapter is to provide the physician with sufficient background to follow the debate knowledgeably and to provide informed advice within the organization that he or she serves.

Some environmental problems, such as the human and medical wastes observed along the coastline of the northeastern United States a few years ago, represent extreme examples of traditional environmental and public health challenges. Other problems, such as chemical degradation of the ozone layer and the suspected "greenhouse effect" of global warming, are qualitatively different and on a scale far beyond our public health experience. The degradation of the environment has become a major global problem, outstripping its local public health dimensions and becoming a serious threat, perhaps even to human survival in the long run.

Many articles in the scientific literature have attempted to describe the most likely health outcomes of environmental degradation and have promoted action in response. Some have been particularly influential in drawing attention to the problem [1–6]. For example, the United Nations World Commission on Environment and Development described the dilemma of environmental degradation and development several years ago in the seminal "Brundtland Report," entitled *Our Common Future* (1987) [7], but this otherwise comprehensive treatise had little to say about health implications.

Dimensions of the Problem

The implications of environmental trends for weather, human habitation, and food supply suggest serious trouble ahead. On the other hand, the implications for human health are far from obvious and are likely to be indirect. Comparatively little attention has been paid so far to the possible effects of global environmental changes on human health and the adaptation required in health services. The descriptions of global and interregional ecologic changes described below are speculative, but are based on the informed judgment of a number of scientists, primarily authorities on geography, meteorology, and biology.

Atmospheric Changes

Climate Change and the Greenhouse Effect

The possible health consequences of global atmospheric changes have not been characterized in detail until recently. This section describes health effects based on the most likely climate changes predicted by the computer models presently in use, with an emphasis on North America. The exaggerated greenhouse effect and resultant "global warming" may result in changes in regional climate and weather patterns, and lead to health problems related to heat stress, natural weather disasters, changes in vector distribution, and consequently infectious disease endemicity.

Unreliable crop production, social disruptions leading to violent behavior, and stress on the health care system may also occur [5, 7, 8].

Climate, like the biologic phenomena more familiar to biomedical scientists, is affected by many factors. Some are deterministic, exerting an influence by direct action or in direct competition, but most are stochastic, and have the effect of increasing or reducing the probability of an event occurring. To use a medical analogy, understanding climate is like accounting for a multifactorial disease, such as heart disease or cancer: Seldom does a single factor explain everything; the interplay among risk factors is the most important aspect of the problem to appreciate. That is why there is no simple prediction as to what effect atmospheric changes will have on climate, except that there will *not* be a uniform, stable trend of rising temperature. "Global warming" is likely to produce *exaggerations* in existing weather trends and make extreme weather conditions more frequent. No one weather pattern, however, will predominate or envelop the planet. A major source of uncertainty is the lack of knowledge of cloud cover, which could be increased by ocean evaporation and cause paradoxical ground cooling [9].

The greenhouse effect contributes to stability of the world's temperature by allowing infrared radiation to reach the Earth's surface and by preventing the escape of radiant heat into space; this dual action maintains the biosphere within a temperature range conducive to life. If certain atmospheric gases trap too much infrared radiation, global temperature rises. A rapidly rising concentration of these so-called greenhouse gases is occurring in the troposphere (lower atmosphere). These gases include carbon dioxide (increasing at 0.4% per year), methane (increasing at about 1% per year), chlorofluorocarbons (increasing until recently at about 5% per year), oxides of nitrogen (increasing at 0.3% per year), ozone, and a miscellaneous group of others. This increase is mostly the result of industrial development, especially the use of internal combustion engines and coal-burning electric power generators. Methane also comes from agriculture and other sources, such as the decomposition of rotting vegetation. Of these gases carbon dioxide accounts for half of the greenhouse effect [9–13]. Carbon dioxide concentrations in the atmosphere today are thought to be the highest in 160,000 years, as judged from trapped bubbles in Antarctic glacier ice. Methane levels are also much increased in more recent ice core samples. A close association has been noted between carbon dioxide levels and estimated global average temperature throughout this period, as indicated by fossil biota and carbon isotope concentrations [12].

Carbon dioxide is absorbed by biota and is thereby removed from the atmosphere by natural processes and agriculture. The most significant "sinks" for carbon dioxide appear to be in the temperate zones of the Northern Hemisphere and in the Amazon rainforest. Destruction of the boreal and Amazonian forests might reduce the capacity of the biosphere to remove carbon dioxide and stabilize climate change [10, 12].

The accumulation of greenhouse gases appears to have raised average global temperature by an estimated one-half to one degree Celsius from 1880 to 1990, more rapidly in the last 10 years than in earlier periods. A warming trend is apparent since 1980. If an unusual ocean-driven "cold front" had not occurred in the summer of 1989, that year would have matched or exceeded 1988 as the warmest year ever recorded—0.23° warmer than the period 1951 to 1980. Rises of several degrees more are predicted in the coming century. In fact a global rise of between 3 and 4 degrees in the next 50 years is predicted by some experts. This increase may seem small, but on a global scale this average masks marked extremes that have substantial implications [9, 11].

This estimate in global temperature rise is supported by empiric evidence as well as by results of computer modeling conducted by American and British investigators. Called "general circulation models," these computer simulations are consistent in their predictions and vary primarily in their estimate of elapsed time required for the effects to appear [9, 12].

The net effect may be to restore the climatic regime that existed on Earth approximately 6000 years ago, but over a period of *dozens* rather than hundreds of years. These changes are unprecedented even considering the rapid changes at periods of transition at the end of the Ice Age. Unlike previous periods of rapid change in climate, humankind is now dependent on an intricate system of agriculture, trade, and communication that threatens to be disrupted. In addition, many modern cities are built in low-lying coastal areas, for historical reasons usually related to access and trade. As a result, these population centers face significant local threats due to global warming [13].

Regional predictions are more difficult than global predictions and are likely to be confounded by local factors. According to most models of future climate, the rise in average temperature is apt to be less at the equator and in high latitudes, and greatest in midlatitudes. Winters may be colder and the summers considerably warmer than at present.

Major cities of the world may have increased numbers of very hot days each year and a longer duration of "heat waves." The effect of this increase on mortality is likely to be diffuse, affecting all causes of death and not just cardiovascular disorders. An estimate of the likely effect of an increase in summer temperatures of only 2°C can be derived from a surveillance study of heat-related fatalities in the major cities in the state of Missouri from 1979 to 1987. In July 1980, a prolonged heat wave of this magnitude occurred; the temperature exceeded the normal daily maximum of 31°C for 21 days and exceeded 38°C on several occasions. Approximately 1 in every 4000 residents developed heat stroke and one in every 1400 developed a heat-related illness that was either fatal or required hospitalization. An excess of approximately 300 deaths from heat-related conditions was observed, somewhat under half due to heat stroke [14]. Violent behavior may tend to increase in frequency in hot weather, leading to the possibility of increased civil disturbance.

Global warming may disrupt ocean currents and establish anomalous flows of air, comparable to the trade winds and jet streams. As well as causing more prolonged droughts, global warming may increase the frequency of severe precipitation, especially in the tropics. The result may be to increase the frequency and severity of violent weather disturbances such as hurricanes, tornadoes, typhoons, floods, and blizzards. In 1988, North America experienced a major drought associated with the previous year's El Niño (a periodic midocean upwelling in the southeastern Pacific) and resulting displacement of the jet stream northward, diverting rain-carrying weather systems away from their usual region of precipitation. Whether this episode was influenced by a global warming trend is unclear. The conditions that were set up, however, appear to be very similar to those that would occur with increasing ocean temperatures [15].

A combination of effects from global warming could lead to food shortages [16]. The adverse effects on productivity of increased temperature and aridity on crop yields and growing ranges are likely to counteract growing yields predicted for many crops as a result of increased availability of carbon dioxide. Climate change may exert an unpredictable effect on the distribution of major pests and thus affect crop yields and food spoilage.

"Fossil" underground water (water stores not accumulated in modern times and not recharged by percolation from the surface), notably the artesian basin that lies under much of the southern United States, is being used faster than it is being replenished. The depletion of this water resource, in the absence of adequate precipitation to recharge underground aquifers, could create serious water shortages, a problem already present in some parts of the western United States.

Global warming may cause a rise of about a meter in sea level over the next 50 to 100 years. This change would threaten many coastal regions and low-lying wetlands. Sea level rise may slowly encroach on many coastal areas, including cities such as Vancouver, New Orleans, New York, Shanghai, Honolulu, Bangkok, Hong Kong, and London, and nations such as Bangladesh and large parts of the Netherlands. Exaggerated tides may threaten low-lying cities and coastal zones. Salt water intrusion into coastal aquifers may also compromise the fresh water supply of coastal cities [9].

The distribution of vegetation would change drastically in a short period of time, relative to the past rate of change on Earth, if global warming occurs on a massive scale. Climate change in the past has usually taken place over centuries, not decades. One likely consequence of this redistribution of temperature ranges is expansion in the geographic dispersion of insect vectors of human disease, including the anophelene and colicine mosquitoes. The arthropod-borne virus diseases, including viral hemorrhagic fevers such as yellow fever, dengue, and viral encephalitides, may extend beyond their current range. The tick-borne diseases, such as typhus and Lyme disease, may change their distribution because the range of the tick's mammalian host changes. Malaria may also extend its range, a phenomenon unlikely to be a problem in North America. Schistosomiasis, caused by a tropical and subtropical water-borne parasite that depends on a snail host, would likely spread as the range of its host expands, particularly with more damming to conserve water in arid regions. The endemic zones of diseases, which presently are limited to the tropics, may extend into temperate zones [17, 18].

Ozone Depletion and Ultraviolet Irradiation

In contrast to global warming, the public health consequences of depleted ozone in the stratosphere or upper atmosphere are more specific and more easily projected [19]. Stratospheric ozone depletion may increase exposure to ultraviolet (UV) radiation, which at the surface of the earth is most likely to result in damage to skin, eyes, and possibly the immune system.

Stratospheric ozone depletion is not to be confused with tropospheric ozone accumulation; ozone is an air pollutant in the lower troposphere and a greenhouse gas throughout the troposphere, but it is also a vital shield against potentially lethal UV-B irradiation in the stratosphere. Stratospheric ozone is regenerated by photolysis of oxygen and is minimally affected by migration of tropospheric ozone upward into the stratosphere.

Attenuation of UV radiation may occur from atmospheric dust, so that considerable variability occurs among locations. Ozone in the stratosphere absorbs ultraviolet radiation completely in the UV-C range (200–290 nm) and in a large portion of the UV-B range (290–320 nm). Intracellularly, UV absorption may cause breakage of covalent bonds in critical macromolecules and lead to carcinogenesis, accelerated aging, and cataracts [19–21]. Those at greatest risk for effects of UV exposure are people with fair skin who sunburn easily.

The stratospheric ozone layer was observed to be thinning over Antarctica about 12 years ago. Repeated observations have confirmed the attenuation and charted its progress. During 1956 to 1976, the first 20 years of observations from space, the ozone layer was stable; since then, it has declined in thickness over Antarctica from about 300 to between 125 and 200 Dobson units (units of concentration in a vertical atmospheric column under standard conditions). The cause of this depletion is the release into the atmosphere, and gradual diffusion into the stratosphere, of chemicals, particularly the chlorofluorocarbons (CFCs), that destroy ozone by catalytic action [20, 21].

Chlorofluorocarbons release chlorine by photolysis into the atmosphere; this free chlorine atom scavenges ozone and destroys it [22]. One CFC molecule may destroy as many as 10,000 ozone molecules. Release of CFCs into the atmosphere occurs through industrial activity, leaks, or the decommissioning of old refrigeration and air-conditioning units, as well as by use of aerosol cans that contain the compounds as propellants.

The human health effects of increased ultraviolet irradiation due to ozone depletion include higher risks of nonmelanoma skin cancer (particularly squamous cell carcinoma and actinic keratitis, a premalignant condition), malignant melanoma [23–30], cataract and retinal degeneration, and possibly impaired immunologic responses [29]. Relatively minor but cosmetically significant effects may include accelerated aging of skin [31] and perhaps increased frequency of pterygia [27], small wedge-shaped tissue webs on the whites of the eye. Although unlikely to result in serious health problems, these cosmetic effects may be just as significant in motivating action as the major health effects, which are discussed in greater detail below.

Substantial progress on curbing chlorofluorocarbon generation and release on a national level has already been made with the Montreal Protocol, an international treaty calling for reductions in CFC production and emissions. Given the long half-lives of the chlorofluorocarbons (75 years or more), however, the compounds already released are expected to continue their ozone-depleting reactions at significant levels well into the 22nd century.

The use of protective clothing, sunscreens, and eyeglasses, both tinted and clear, may significantly reduce exposure to ultraviolet light, as may changing fashions in sunbathing and outdoor recreation. These measures, taken by people to protect themselves, may not eliminate the risk. Commercial sunscreens may be effective against UV-induced sunburn if they have a high enough sun protection factor for the exposure period [32], but their effectiveness against UV-induced cancer is unproven [33]. Other measures, such as dark or reflective clothing, parasols, and hats, are unlikely to be accepted as permanent fashion statements by society. Increased shade will be more difficult to ensure in deforested rural areas or water-short communities.

Uncertainties remain regarding ozone depletion. Although stratospheric ozone levels are clearly and unambiguously reduced, measurements of UV-B irradiation at ground level do not show a consistent increase so far, although early suggestions of an increase have been noted in the Alps [34]. The first evidence of actual increases in surface UV-B radiation is expected to be seen in Australia and South America. Carbon dioxide accumulation and increased cloud cover, however, tend to offset the effects of ozone depletion, and thus introduce another set of variables that are poorly understood. Ozone depletion may not be the only factor to consider in projecting future UV-B radiation at ground level.

Acid Precipitation

In recent years, soil and water surveys in the Northern Hemisphere have shown increased acidity (or, more accurately, reduced acid neutralizing capacity) and presumably irreversible changes in pH in soils [35]. These changes are caused by increased production and airborne transport of acidifying emissions from industrial sources, principally sulfates and nitrates. Emissions of SO_2 and NO_2 combine with water vapor in the atmosphere to form sulfuric and nitric acids, respectively. The problem has been most severe and most heavily documented in Canada (largely as a result of emissions from the US Midwest) and Scandinavia (from Germany and Britain). The acidity has resulted in extensive changes in the biology of small bodies of water. Transregional transportation of pollution, as with acid deposition and the long-range transport of air toxics, may result in increased airways reactivity and asthma [36].

Acid precipitation is most detrimental to delicate aquatic ecosystems, marine biota, and some terrestrial species of plants and trees [37]. Although some adverse human health effects have been suggested, the associations are weak and inconsistent [38]. Most attention has been paid to airways reactivity [39, 40]. Some authors have speculated about the toxicologic implications if metals are leached into groundwater at excessive concentrations [41].

A major technical problem in developing control strategies for acid precipitation is the absence of a clear understanding of loading capacities, that is, the maximum emissions that an ecosystem can absorb before its capacity to neutralize, transform, or dilute the pollutant is exceeded.

Population

The detrimental effects of the population explosion are simple, but their implications for society are complex. The number of humans is increasing at a rate that has already outstripped our capacity to provide for them from the renewable resources of this planet, and this rate of increase is not declining sufficiently to ensure long-term economic and social stability.

At the time of Christ, the total world population was less than 300 million. It took well over 1500 years to approximately double to one-half billion in 1650. After only 200 more years, however, it had doubled again to 1 billion. By that time, the Industrial Revolution was in full swing, and after only another 80 years, the population had doubled again to 2 billion in 1930. It has only taken 45 years to more than double again to 5 billion, despite World War II, in which nearly 50 million people died. At the present rate, by the year 2025 about 8.4 billion people will inhabit the earth.

Our recent population growth is not the first population explosion humankind has experienced. In fact, this process has occurred at least twice before. The first population explosion occurred about 100,000 BC, when our ancestors learned how to organize into tribes, make stone tools, and hunt larger animals. The second surge appears to have occurred about 5000 BC, when humankind developed agriculture. In both of these prehistoric events, the big change came in the ability to produce food. With the coming of the Industrial Revolution, two changes occurred. Industry and more efficient agriculture allowed humankind to support a larger population. At the same time, improved public health and medical care both prolonged the average life span and increased the number of individuals who survived to bear children.

In each previous population explosion, the population eventually stabilized until the next fundamental change occurred in technology and society. In 1798, Thomas Malthus warned his fellow Englishmen that disaster was approaching. The human population, he said, increased by doubling with each successive generation, while food supply increased a plot at a time. Sooner or later, Malthus concluded, humankind would outstrip its food supply and the result would be starvation and a breakdown in social order. What kept the population from getting completely out of control, he believed, was the high death rate. This perspective was not popular in England at the height of the British Empire. While the British debated, however, famines in India, China, and Morocco afflicted over 100 million people, many of them British subjects.

Agricultural production has expanded enormously since then; essentially all the arable land in most parts of the world is under cultivation. The world has adopted the strategy of increasing the yield per acre by heavy fertilization and development of new crop strains. Even with the rapid spread of this "Green Revolution," however, world food production has been increasing only at about 4.5% per year overall and has actually been falling in Africa. By comparison, the world population is increasing by about 1.6% per year, which leaves a bare margin for improvement of chronic malnutrition in the underdeveloped world. This progress can be reversed at any time. In 1972, for example, the monsoons erased most of the progress India had made. In 1973, the US lost over 40% of its corn crop in the South to a fungus because the new high-yield strain was exceptionally susceptible. In the 1980s, overgrazing and overpopulation led to a terrible famine in sub-Saharan Africa. The Green Revolution is fragile and easily thwarted because it is expensive, requires education, depends on ideal weather, and puts farm laborers out of work in countries where there are no other jobs [42].

Since World War II, the basic technologies of industry, agriculture, and transportation have developed in such a way that they are drastically incompatible with natural environmental cycles and processes. The search for more profitable production and marketing has led to lopsided technology, successful at meeting narrowly defined economic goals but potentially harmful to the environment (e.g., the development of individualized, disposable packaging for consumer products). The effect on the environment of the average member of a developed society is enormously increased by the consumption and technological patterns in the society compared to those of the average resident of a developing country.

Thus, the impact of the US on the global environment is much greater than what might be expected on the basis of its population. The average American, for example, consumes a staggering amount of energy, raw materials, and food in his or her lifetime, about 6 to 10 times or more as much as the average Chinese, African, or Latin American. As the developing world matures economically, it is unrealistic to expect such a disproportionate imbalance in consumption of the world's resources to continue forever.

The US has a vast land area but its population centers draw their resources from far away. Los Angeles, for example, draws water from all over the state of California and from supplies that might be used by Arizona and Nevada. What is true for water is true for food, raw materials, arable land, and energy. It really does not make much difference whether people are concentrated in one place or scattered over the countryside. There is a limit to the population a region can support. Imported raw materials, energy, and food merely enlarge the region committed to sustaining a given population.

The situation is different in developing nations, where population has played a much more important role in impeding the achievement of a tolerable quality of life, similar to that of "developed" societies.

As nations become more affluent, the birth rate drops and population growth declines. The magnitude of the demographic transition, although initially larger than expected, has been insufficient to keep the world population under 5 billion. Even so, the demographic transition is based on the decisions of individuals who voluntarily limit their reproduction as the death rate declines and personal security increases. This phenomenon demonstrates how individual judgment may collectively result in a rational and productive direction for the society as a whole. The most promising avenues for population stabilization are planned national development, education of women, and reduction of infant mortality [5, 42].

Sustainable Development

Sustainable development is a concept critical to understanding solutions to large-scale ecologic degradation and resource depletion. Sustainable development involves establishing an economic structure that ideally consumes only as much as the natural environment produces and emits only as much as the natural environment can absorb. This goal is accomplished by reducing consumption and the scale of economic development as well as by recycling materials. The economic structure is "sustainable" in the sense that it can be "sustained" from one generation to another.

A sustainable economic structure will not be easily achieved, if at all. Movement toward such a system will likely raise controversies about economics and social organization. Issues of equity and community control over resources and decision-making will arise. The concept of sustainable development is closely linked, in the minds of many, with that of community empowerment and a host of associated issues related to social justice and cultural expression. There are other, less direct links that take the form of doctrines of ethical stewardship of resources.

Because of these ties with other, related issues, scientific information on the state of the global environment and the implications of large-scale ecologic change strike a deeply resonant chord in most people, even deeper than more abstract concern over survival. It is inevitable that there will be a temptation among many advocates to exaggerate scientific support for outcomes that are most dramatic or threatening and that force social change. It is equally inevitable that other vocal opponents will minimize the available evidence and distort scientific opinion in the opposite direction.

Implications for Physicians

Occupational and environmental physicians are, in many cases, assuming new roles in their organizations just at a time when these issues are coming onto the agenda of senior management. Sometimes the response to these issues is driven by a need to meet regulations. Many major corporations, however, are seeking ways to become "green," or environmentally sensitive, in their operations. This change in attitude is partly a response to public pressure; however, it is also a strategic way of positioning for survival in an era when ecologic issues are likely to affect public perception and, as a result, government activities. These organizations are likely to look to their medical director for guidance and answers to challenges on health issues associated with ecologic change. In many cases, they may delegate responsibility for environmental affairs to the medical department.

This responsibility places most physicians in a difficult situation. Little in medical training prepares the physician to deal with such vast and complicated issues in which the relationship to medicine is indirect. Likewise, the management of large-scale ecologic issues is far from the experience or expertise of all but a handful of physicians. The physician, however, will inevitably be called on to play a role because public concern about these issues is driven largely by their health implications.

References

1. Leaf, A. Potential health effects of global climatic and environmental changes. *N. Engl. J. Med.* 321:1577, 1989.
2. McCally, M., and Cassel, C. K. Medical responsibility and global environmental change. *Ann. Intern. Med.* 113:467, 1990.
3. Last, J. M., and Guidotti, T. L. Implications for human health of global ecological changes. *Public Health Rev.* 18:49, 1990/91.
4. Guidotti, T. L., and Last, J. M. Implications for human health of global atmospheric change. *Trans. R. Soc. Can.* Series 6, II:223, 1993.
5. Last, J. M. Global Environment, Health, and Health Services. In J. M. Last (ed.), Maxcy-Rosenau-Last Public Health, Norwalk, CT: Appleton and Lange, 1992.
6. Longstreth, J. Anticipated public health consequence of global climate change. *Environ. Health Perspect.* 96:139, 1991.
7. United Nations World Commission on Environment and Development. *Our Common Future.* Oxford and New York: Oxford University Press, 1987.
8. Suhrke, A. U. *Pressure Points: Environmental Degradation, Migration and Conflict.* Occupational Papers Series of the Project on Environmental Change and Acute Conflict, no. 3. Cambridge, MA: American Academy of Arts and Sciences, March 1993.

9. Mungall, C., and McLaren, D. (eds.). *Planet Under Stress: The Challenge of Global Change.* Toronto: Oxford University Press/Royal Society of Canada, 1990.

10. *Ozone Depletion, Greenhouse Gases, and Climate Change.* Washington, DC: National Academy Press, 1992.

11. Jones, P. D., and Wigley, T. M. L. Global warming trends. *Sci. Am.* 263:84, 1990.

12. Wuebbles, D., and Edmons, J. *A Primer on Greenhouse Gases.* Washington, DC: US Department of Energy, 1988.

13. Hansen, J., et al. Regional Greenhouse Climate Effects. In *Coping with Climate Change* (Proceedings of the Second North American Conference on Preparing for Climate Change, December 6–8, 1988). Washington, DC: Climate Institute, 1989.

14. Jones, T. S., et al. Morbidity and mortality associated with the July 1980 heat wave in St. Louis and Kansas City, Mo. *J.A.M.A.* 247:3327, 1982.

15. Trenberth, K. E., Branstator, G. W., and Arkin, P. A. Origins of the 1988 North American drought. *Science* 242:1640, 1988.

16. Daily, G. C., and Ehrlich, P. R. An exploratory model of the impact of rapid climate change on the world food situation. *Proc. R. Soc. Lond. [Biol]* 241:232, 1990.

17. Cook, G. C. Effect of global warming on the distribution of parasitic and other infectious diseases: A review. *J. Roy. Soc. Med.* 85:688, 1992.

18. Shope, R. Global climate change and infectious diseases. *Environ. Health Perspect.* 96:171, 1991.

19. Urbach, F. Potential health effects of climatic change: Effects of increased ultraviolet radiation on man. *Environ. Health Perspect.* 96:175, 1991.

20. Amron, D. M., and Moy, R. L. Stratospheric ozone depletion and its relationship to skin cancer. *J. Dermatol. Surg. Oncol.* 17:370, 1991.

21. Kripke, M. L., Pitcher, H., and Longstreth, J. D. Potential carcinogenic impacts of stratospheric ozone depletion. *J. Environ. Sci. Health* Part C, *Environ. Carcinogen Rev.* 7:53, 1989.

22. Lindley, D. CFCs cause part of global ozone decline. *Nature* 323:293, 1988.

23. Henriksen, T., et al. Ultraviolet radiation and skin cancer. Effect of an ozone layer depletion. *Photochem. Photobiol.* 51:578, 1990.

24. Vitasa, B. C., et al. Association of nonmelanoma skin cancer and actinic keratosis with cumulative solar ultraviolet exposure in Maryland watermen. *Cancer* 65:2811, 1990.

25. Longstreth, J. Cutaneous malignant melanoma and ultraviolet radiation: A review. *Cancer Metastasis Rev.* 7:321, 1988.

26. Olson, C. M. Increased outdoor recreation, diminished ozone layer pose ultraviolet radiation threat to eye. *J.A.M.A.* 261:1102, 1989.

27. Charman, W. N. Ocular hazards arising from depletion of the natural atmospheric ozone layer: A review. *Ophthalmic Physiol. Opt.* 10:333, 1990.

28. van Kuijk, F. J. G. M. Effects of ultraviolet light on the eye: Role of protective glasses. *Environ. Health Perspect.* 96:177, 1991.

29. Morison, W. L. Effects of ultraviolet radiation on the immune system in humans. *Photochem. Photobiol.* 50:515, 1989.

30. Kripke, M. L. Photoimmunology. *Photochem. Photobiol.* 52:919, 1990.

31. Dahlback, A., et al. Biological UV-doses and the effect of an ozone layer depletion. *Photochem. Photobiol.* 49:621, 1989.

32. Hendee, W. R. Harmful effects of ultraviolet radiation. *J.A.M.A.* 262:380, 1989.

33. Diffey, B. L., and Farr, P. M. Sunscreen protection against UVB, UVA, and blue light: An in vivo and in vitro comparison. *Br. J. Dermatol.* 124:258, 1991.

34. Blumthaler, M., and Ambach, W. Indication of increasing solar ultraviolet-B radiation flux in Alpine regions. *Science* 248:206, 1990.

35. Berden, M., et al. *Soil Acidification: Extent, Causes, and Consequences.* Publication no. 3292. Solna, Sweden: National Swedish Environment Protection Board, 1987.

36. Larson, T. V. The influence of chemical and physical forms of ambient air acids on airway doses. *Environ. Health Perspect.* 79:7, 1989.

37. Lioy, P. J., and Waldman, J. M. Acidic sulfate aerosols: Characterization and exposure. *Environ. Health Perspect.* 79:15, 1989.

38. Benarde, M. A. Health effects of acid rain: Are there any? *J. Roy. Soc. Health* 107:139, 1987.

39. Last, J. A. Global atmospheric change: Potential health effects of acid aerosol and oxidant gas mixtures. *Environ. Health Perspect.* 96:151, 1991.

40. Raizenne, M. E., et al. Acute lung function responses to ambient acid aerosols in children. *Environ. Health Perspect.* 79:179, 1989.

41. Goldstein, B., and Reed, D. J. Global atmospheric changes and research needs in environmental health science. *Environ. Health Perspect.* 96:193, 1991.
42. The environment and population growth: Decade for action. *Pop. Rep.* (Population Information Program, The Johns Hopkins University) Special Issue, Series M (20), May 1992.

Further Information

Chivian, E., et al. *Human Health and the Environment.* Boston: MIT Press, 1993.
New book, representing views of a group of experts associated with Physicians for Social Responsibility, an activist organization with a highly knowledgeable and insightful leadership.

Last, J. M. Global change: Ozone depletion, greenhouse warming, and public health. *Ann. Rev. Public Health* 14:115, 1993.
Good, concise introduction to basic issues.

Potential Health Effects of Climatic Change: Report of a WHO Task Group. Geneva: World Health Organization, 1990.
Highly authoritative, well referenced. Possibly the best short publication with which to begin.

WHO Commission on Health and Environment. *Our Planet, Our Health.* Geneva: World Health Organization, 1992.
Highly authoritative. Extends discussion from above reference and goes into some additional detail on indirect effects.

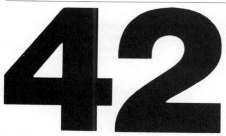

Environmental Medicine: The Regulatory Issues

William B. Bunn

Environmental protection policies and laws create an expansive set of regulations to control pollution and an excellent database on the types and quantities of pollutants, some of which may result in environmental illnesses. These statutory requirements and resulting exposure data generate an abundance of useful scientific information. Multiple reporting requirements under the Environmental Protection Agency (EPA) may arise when environmental illnesses are diagnosed [1–5].

The primary prevention of environmental exposure and disease is implemented by the combination of local, state, and federal regulations. In contrast to human risk–based occupational standards, many environmental regulations are oriented to minimize exposure by controlling emissions of *categories* of pollutants according to medium of exposure. However, environmental regulations are being carefully scrutinized to determine their impact on human health risk, an area of expertise for occupational and environmental physicians.

To comprehend the current approach to the prevention of environmental disease, one must understand the regulatory framework as well as the science that supports these rules. These prevention-based regulations serve as the bases for the control of hazardous exposure and, ultimately, prevention of disease. In fact, exposure control strategies must be recommended with clear knowledge of applicable regulations.

The Framework of Environmental Regulations

Before environmental regulations can be established, a bill must be passed by Congress and signed into law. This statute enables an appropriate agency, usually the EPA, to develop and promulgate regulations, which are first published in the *Federal Register* to solicit comment. These regulations become part of the Code of Federal Regulation (CFR) and serve as the legal framework for implementing environmental policy and reducing environmental exposures. If they are not followed, states or private individuals can bring suits in the civil courts to assure enforcement or to press for damages. A state may also seek criminal charges. Suits may be introduced in local, state, or federal courts. Case law, however, will help define the interpretation of the regulations promulgated in the instant jurisdiction.

Thus, both regulations and case law may be important in a particular case. In almost every environmental exposure/disease situation, multiple regulations may be involved [1, 2].

Chronology of Environmental Laws in the United States

Environmental regulations mirror public concern and its reflection of actual risk. As a result, regulations in the United States and other countries have been driven by a series of environmental issues, many of which arose from catastrophic situations. The EPA was established in 1970 by Congress one year after a major oil spill off the coast of California. The formation of EPA unified federal regulation of the environment under one federal agency. The EPA's charter included all media: air, water, and solid and hazardous waste (including liquid waste). The EPA began a sequential review and tightening of federal environmental protection regulation in the early 1970s [1, 2, 4].

The creation of the EPA was concurrent with other major legislative initiatives. For example, in January 1970, the National Environmental Policy Act (NEPA) was passed. This Act established a statement of national environmental policy that promoted concern for the environment by all federal agencies and established a Council of Environmental Quality (CEQ).

The Clean Air Act (CAA), passed in 1970 and amended in 1987 and 1990, is designed to prevent further air quality deterioration and to deal with ongoing emissions. Legislative regulation of water followed in 1972 with the Federal Water Pollution Control Act (Clean Water Act; CWA).

To summarize, in response to growing public concern, early congressional actions created a unified agency for environmental policy development and enforcement (EPA) and addressed the two major public issues with the Clean Air Act and Clean Water Act. These activities were followed by an expansion of federal authority into other areas of the environment.

Originally a recommendation of the CEQ founded under NEPA, the Toxic Substances Control Act (TSCA) was passed in 1976. TSCA responded to growing public concerns about the hazards of certain chemicals such as polychlorinated biphenyls (PCBs) and insecticides, such as kepone.

The Toxic Substances Control Act requires that scientific data be submitted to the EPA to evaluate the potential hazards of new or existing products. The EPA has the authority to interpret these data and regulate production, use, distribution, and disposal of the substance or product.

Also in 1976, the Resource Conservation and Recovery Act (RCRA) was passed to regulate the disposal of solid and liquid hazardous waste. It established the concept of "cradle to grave" management of hazardous waste. The passage of the TSCA and RCRA in the mid-1970s emphasized federal interest in comprehensively addressing environmental pollution and not simply cleaning up polluted air and water.

In 1980, the Comprehensive Environmental Response, Compensation and Liability Act (CERCLA) was passed. CERCLA addresses existing hazardous waste sites in the United States. Like other environmental regulations, it followed the national concern that focused on the health implications of a hazardous waste site in Love Canal, New York, and created a "superfund" to address the issue. CERCLA established retrospective responsibility and liability—unique for regulatory statutes. In 1986, CERCLA amendments, including another extension of the scope of environmental oversight with the Emergency Planning and Community Right to Know Act (EPCRA), were passed. In the aftermath of Bhopal, EPCRA requires industries to notify governmental authorities of the hazardous substances located on a site. For manufacturing sites, specific information must be submitted on the materials and the quantities used. These acts extended environmental protection retrospectively and incorporated the requirement to submit information to the public as well as to the EPA (see Chap. 48, Accessing Environmental Data).

Although this overview of major environmental actions does not cover the full scope of regulation or the subsequent amendments, it demonstrates a legislative pattern. First, a national policy was developed and an agency established for its enforcement. Second, the most obvious pollution problems of air and water were addressed. And third, acts were passed that established the comprehensive "cradle to grave" concept for pollution control. Later acts followed that addressed removal of existing hazardous waste and mandatory public communication.

Environmental Regulation and Its Interface With Environmental Medicine

There are a myriad of potential interfaces of environmental medicine with environmental regulations. The most important issues are: (1) recognition of the database for correlating an exposure to disease, (2) reporting requirements generated by environmental exposures, (3) knowledge of the regulatory system for environmental pollution, and (4) interventive strategies in environmentally induced disease or risk of disease [5, 6, 7] (Table 42-1).

Air Pollution Control

Air pollution control is accomplished primarily through the CAA, which addresses primary and hazardous pollutants. Primary pollutants include sulfur dioxide, par-

Table 42-1. Major US environmental regulatory statutes

Clean Air Act (42 USC §7401 et seq.)	Control and abate air pollution by regulating air emissions from stationary and mobile sources.
Clean Water Act (USC §1251 et seq.)	Restore and maintain the quality of the nation's surface waters by regulating the discharge of pollutants.
Resource Conservation and Recovery Act (RCRA) (42 USC §6901 et seq.)	Minimize threats to human health and the environment by regulating the treatment, storage, and disposal of waste, including releases to air, ground water, and land.
Toxic Substances Control Act (TSCA) (7 USC §136 et seq.)	Regulate the introduction of new and old chemical substances into the environment by requiring testing and reporting, and restricting use as necessary.
Comprehensive Environmental Response, Compensation and Liability Act (CERCLA) (42 USC §9601 et seq.)	Provide funding and enforcement authority for cleaning up thousands of hazardous waste sites and for responding to hazardous substance spills.
Emergency Planning and Community Right to Know Act (EPCRA) (Title III, Public Law 94-499)	Require state and local governments to develop plans for responding to emergency releases of environmentally hazardous substances, and require businesses to notify local emergency planning groups of the presence of such substances at facilities, to do emergency planning, and to report on inventories and releases.
Federal Insecticide, Fungicide and Rodenticide Act (FIFRA) (7 USC §136 et seq.)	Protect human health and the environment from hazards associated with pesticides and herbicides by requiring registration, testing, and reporting, and regulating distribution, sale, and use.
Safe Drinking Water Act (SDWA) (42 USC §300f et seq.)	Regulate public drinking water systems, set national standards for contaminants in drinking water, regulate underground injection wells, and protect sole source aquifers.

ticulate matter, ozone, carbon dioxide, nitrogen oxides, and lead. These substances are specifically regulated, whereas toxic emissions are regulated by the CAA through the National Emission Standards for Air Pollutants (NESHAPS). The control of emissions is accomplished by the establishment of National Ambient Air Quality Standards (NAAQS), which are implemented by the states through State Implementation Plans (SIPS). The CAA requires states to reduce emissions in conformance with the NAAQS. Specific requirements exist for newly constructed sources of pollution, new or modified sources in areas with better air quality, factories in nonattainment areas where air quality is poor, and chlorofluorocarbons (CFCs).

Site implementation of the CAA is based on obtaining a permit from the EPA to allow facility operation. The permit specifies the amount of pollutants that may be generated. It must be renewed and may require regular and specific monitoring for renewal (often, every 3 years). In the interim period, any excursions beyond permitted levels must be reported; EPA inspections and required testing (e.g., stack testing) may also be performed. The control of air pollution is usually achieved by scrubbers, incinerators, and filtering devices. Recently, more focus has been placed on process modification and pollution prevention. For example, the reduction of the use of hazardous substances is encouraged through the Superfund Amendments and Re-Authorization Act (SARA) Title III by reporting specific amounts of chemicals used and by the EPA's efforts to encourage voluntary reductions in emissions allowable by permit.

For the physician evaluating a person exposed to many chemicals, these regulations provide data on both the types and quantity of chemicals emitted into the air. In many situations, a calculation of the exposure that a person may receive from a "plume" from a stack may have already been performed and, thus, may be obtained from the industry or the EPA. Moreover, exceedences and unusual emissions must be reported under CAA and Emergency Right to Know provisions. These publicly available reports can provide excellent exposure data in evaluating an individual case or a cluster of cases [1–4].

Clean Water Standards

The federal CWA, originally titled the Federal Water Pollution Control Act, was passed in 1972 and refocused on toxic pollutants in 1977. The CWA has the following five major components: (1) a system of minimum national effluent guidelines, (2) water quality standards, (3) discharge permit programs, (4) provisions for special issues such as toxics, and (5) a grant program for publicly owned treatment works (POTWs). The most important change from previous regulations was the institution of an "end of the pipe" approach rather than state ambient water standards. Under this approach, industries must obtain a permit based on the National Pollutant Discharge Elimination Program (NPDES) or send waste water to a POTW, which must obtain a similar permit for the disposal of waste water. Either type of permit sets allowable limits of biologic and chemical constituents and specifies methods for measuring water quality to assure compliance. These specific requirements and measurements are available for regulatory or health risk analysis [1–4].

Storm water run-off is also regulated by the CWA. Although it is more difficult to know the exact chemical constituents of storm water, there are monitoring requirements in many industrial situations. Failures to meet discharge requirements for effluent or storm water must be reported to the EPA, normally at the state level. Records of all measurements will be available and reviewed in the event of an exceedence. The CWA also regulates spills of potentially hazardous substances. The programs developed are prevention oriented. Significant storage tank regulations also exist (see RCRA, below).

The Regulation of Storage and Disposal of Toxics: The Resource Conservation and Recovery Act

RCRA addresses the management of solid and liquid hazardous waste and is designed to minimize hazardous waste by regulation of its storage, treatment, and disposal. It establishes a "cradle to grave" approach for management. RCRA also addresses underground storage tanks (USTs), by establishing design, monitoring, reporting, and removal requirements.

RCRA requires each regulated industry to monitor all RCRA-listed chemicals from delivery to the facility until they are properly disposed. Chemical waste from specific industrial processes, with significant potential risk, are similarly regulated. The lists of regulated substances and processes are determined by risk assessment and rule-making procedures (see Chap. 50, Environmental Risk Assessment). Organic solvents, particularly chlorinated compounds and heavy metals, are among the most commonly listed substances requiring special disposal.

Regulations also apply to contaminated nonhazardous waste such as soil and to discarded products and waste chemicals. If a waste is not on a specific RCRA list, it is still regulated if it is ignitable, corrosive, reactive, or toxic. After determination that the substance is a "solid waste," the toxic characteristic is determined by specific testing techniques defined by the regulations and assessed against drinking water and other standards.

RCRA requires a regular inventory of all hazardous chemicals at a site in a "cradle to grave" process. That is, all use and discharge of a chemical at a plant must be accounted for from a public policy and individual health risk assessment perspective. This database provides excellent information to assess potential health risk.

The RCRA also regulates the transportation, storage, and disposal of hazardous wastes. Waste carriers must know the exact composition of the materials and the corresponding potential hazard of those materials. Disposal is regulated both in terms of process (e.g., incineration, burial) and the type and amount of chemical at each site. Recycling is encouraged by RCRA and is a growing area of regulation. Incentives for recycling solid and liquid hazardous waste have been instituted, along with special requirements to encourage purchase of products incorporating non-hazardous solid waste. RCRA has recently placed emphasis on biologic and medical wastes as well as chemical waste. The biologic waste control programs are not as developed as chemical programs but regulation is growing.

Superfund: Comprehensive Environmental Response Compensation and Liability Act

Congress enacted CERCLA (Superfund) in 1980 to supplement RCRA, which covers current hazardous waste disposal. CERCLA is designed to cover past hazardous waste activities. It also has reporting requirements for spills or other releases. In 1986, CERCLA was amended by SARA, which substantially expanded its scope.

CERCLA has broad authority over polluters and the substances regulated. For example, CERCLA jurisdiction is triggered by the release of any amount of a substance without threshold while other environmental statutes include a threshold before regulation.

CERCLA is also unique from the legal perspective. It is retrospective; that is, it applies to historic pollution, even if the disposal of the waste was legal or the waste was not considered hazardous at the time. Further, CERCLA is joint and several, in that any contributor to a waste site may be responsible for the entirety of the cost of the cleanup if other responsible parties cannot be found.

CERCLA may mandate cleanups of several types. Although the general mandate is for removal or remediation, or both, removal is rarely the total solution for large sites. Sites specifically regulated by CERCLA are maintained on the National Priority List (NPL). Of the tens of thousands of sites where there is the potential for EPA involvement, only a little over one thousand had been selected by 1990. Nonetheless, thousands of remediation plans have been submitted, reviewed by the EPA, and cleanup begun. The decision on the procedure for cleanup begins with a remedial investigation (RI) and feasibility study (FS) to characterize the site and the pollution. The RI stage addresses the contamination on the site and the FS notes the techniques for cleanup. The RI/FS package for a site is then submitted to EPA for a decision. The EPA's review and decision are published as a record of decision (ROD) and are available for public comment. The key issues for the ROD involve how clean the site should be and how far the contamination extends.

The decision on how clean the site should be is based on appropriate or relevant and appropriate requirements (ARAR). The ARAR are determined on a case-by-case basis and may be based on EPA regulations, a guidance document, or other applicable state/local regulations. Consideration is given to a number of other factors, including the health risks of removal and disposal of the contamination. The determinations made under CERCLA must take RCRA guidelines into consideration in the decision-making process for a waste site. The cost of the investigation and cleanup is commonly in the millions to hundreds of millions of dollars.

The costs will be borne not only by the owner of the waste site but also by every hauler of waste to the site or any manufacturer or company that transported hazardous materials to the site for disposal. The law requires contribution from each party up to the total cost of the remediation (e.g., joint and several liability). The EPA may also sue for damages to flora and fauna away from the remediation site, where applicable.

An important impact of CERCLA/Superfund has been in acquisitions and divestitures of property and businesses. In purchasing property or a business, the buyer assumes the environmental liability of the purchase. Since the environmental cleanup costs may be excessive, a major portion of due diligence investigations of potential purchases is an assessment of environmental liability (monetary/civil, administrative, and criminal). Due diligence teams will include a wide variety of health professionals to assess legal, monetary, and human health risks.

CERCLA also includes requirements for reporting of releases. If a certain quantity of any hazardous substance is released, immediate reporting is required to the National Response Center (NRC). There are stiff civil and criminal penalties for failures to report. Reporting does not include releases that are within the levels stated in the industry's permit. EPA has issued tables that will determine which substances require reporting when released and at what level (as expressed in the amount released during a 24-hour period).

The RI/FS/ROD site assessment and release reporting are excellent sources of data on potential environmental exposure. These reports are commonly used in tort actions to determine potential health risks. The information is also publicly available for use in evaluations of environmentally induced injury and illness. In addition, the parties responsible for exposures may be determined from EPA records and exposure information sought from that party for the chemical disposed or released. Information on toxicity developed by the manufacturers of the pollutants may also be obtained.

Superfund Amendments and Reauthorization Act: Emergency Planning and Community Right to Know Act

EPCRA is a free-standing provision of SARA. It is designed to make emergency planning entities aware of the presence of potentially hazardous substances through reporting requirements to state and local authorities. It also requires reporting of releases and inventories (i.e., utilization rates) of regulated substances. These reports are available to any interested persons and are commonly published by local and national media. This reporting of cumulative results is designed to encourage reduction in the use and disposal of potentially hazardous chemicals.

EPCRA has three subtitles. Subtitle A sets the framework for emergency planning and release notification. Subtitle B requires two types of reports of inventories of hazardous chemicals. The first section requires facilities to maintain and provide to local authorities data on listed hazardous substances. Material Safety Data Sheets (MSDS) must be prepared and provided to local authorities and the workforce in concordance with Occupational Safety and Health Administration (OSHA) regulations. Subtitle B also requires special reporting for certain larger manufacturers (SIC codes 20–39). These reports require reporting of the quantities of the listed substances at the facility (the chemicals are listed in the regulation as defined by risk assessment), how these substances are disposed of or treated, and how much of each chemical enters the environment by each medium. Subtitle C creates substantial civil, criminal, and administrative penalties for violations of the reporting requirements. Enforcement actions may be brought by citizens as well as by the state. Therefore, EPCRA requires the preparation and submission of substantial health risk information to local authorities and workers. These data will be available for assessment of potential environmentally related disease. In addition, quantification (by media) of releases is required. Results are available to the public.

The Toxic Substances Control Act

Before 1976, there were no federal regulations for testing of chemicals entering commerce and the environment. In the late 1960s and early 1970s, concerns arose about multiple chemical products, including organic mercury, PCBs, vinyl chloride, and kepone. In addition, NEPA and the CEQ had expressed an interest in preventing toxic pollution as well as setting standards for emission or remediation. TSCA addresses the need to fully evaluate the potential toxicity and environmental impact of existing and new chemicals. It also includes some specific regulations on PCBs and asbestos.

Premanufacture Notification

The heart of the TSCA is the requirement for premanufacture notification (PMN) of new substances introduced into commerce. A manufacturer (or importer) must notify the Office of Toxic Substances (OTS) 90 days before producing (or importing) a new chemical substance. For existing chemicals, the Act requires reporting of any significant adverse effects from animal or human studies or clinical cases that are not already known or reported.

Most companies approach the EPA well before the 90-day period preceding production. After notification, the EPA must publish in the *Federal Register* an item on the chemical, its intended use, its potential toxicity, and indicated testing. The

EPA must be satisfied that there is no "unreasonable risk to human health or the environment." If these requirements are not met, the EPA may either prohibit or limit production or distribution, or both, or require specific additional tests at the expense of the manufacturer.

To expedite the approval of testing of health effects, TSCA has issued testing guidelines [5]. There are specific exemptions for chemicals in the stages of research and development. To determine whether a chemical is "new," the TSCA has developed an inventory of existing chemicals (section 8b). The list was designed to cover all chemicals produced during a 3-year period, before the time of TSCA regulation. At that time, companies submitted chemicals to be placed on the list, which is updated by the EPA as chemicals are added to the inventory.

The Toxic Substances Control Act also regulates *new uses* of existing chemicals through significant new-use regulations (SNURs). Relevant issues as to whether existing chemicals come under the SNURs include changes in volume, type of exposure to humans or environment, duration of exposures, and life cycle of the chemical.

Reporting Requirements

In addition to the testing of new or existing chemicals, TSCA has a series of reporting requirements. First, under section 8b, an inventory of potentially toxic substances is compiled by the OTS. Section 8b also requires information from manufacturers that may lead to updating of the inventory. The inventory list is used in section 8 and other reporting requirements under the TSCA.

Section 8a requires submission of information on the listed chemical, the amount produced and distributed, and how it is manufactured. It applies to manufacturers, importers, and processors, although, as in most reporting requirements, exemptions are made for small quantities, research and development, and small industries. Section 8c is especially important for the occupational and environmental physician. This section requires recording and record maintenance for "significant adverse effects" alleged by any employee or user of the product/chemical. Employee allegations must be maintained for 30 years (nonemployee, 5 years). A significant adverse effect is described as "long-lasting irreversible damage to health or environment," but effects that indicate that such an ultimate effect could occur are also recordable. While all recorded allegations are not reportable unless requested, health effects are reportable (under section 8e) to the EPA if they meet the criteria of "substantial risk." If an effect is previously known, it is neither recordable nor reportable.

Section 8d requires submission to the EPA of all pertinent health and safety studies known to the manufacturer, importer, processor, or distributor on listed chemicals. Health and safety studies include those related to exposure (e.g., industrial hygiene studies) as well as toxicology and epidemiology. Unpublished studies are included; the requirement is retroactive for 10 years.

Section 8e requires submission of information "that reasonably supports the conclusion that such substance or mixture presents a substantial risk of injury to health or the environment." Reporting is required by manufacturers, processors, or distributors, but not by others receiving the information (e.g., testing laboratories). The EPA will often accept information that may not meet the "substantial risk" definition. Knowledge may be assumed to the corporation, including corporate management and officers, if anyone "capable of appreciating the information" obtains it. Civil fines may be substantial; criminal fines and sanctions also apply. If the finding has been previously reported or is a known effect, reporting is unnecessary. The reports must be received within 15 working days and will be available for public scrutiny.

Reporting responsibilities for TSCA 8c and 8e are significant. In fact, committees are commonly formed at the corporate level to evaluate 8c and 8e information and to determine the reportability and the wording of the report. These committees may include occupational and environmental physicians, industrial hygienists, toxicologists, operation managers, and environmental attorneys. Implementation of TSCA responsibilities may be coordinated through a product stewardship or member of the legal group, or both. Potential civil and criminal penalties, along with the public scrutiny of these reports, make the TSCA activities a highly sensitive area.

Furthermore, since occupational and environmental studies must be reported under the TSCA, an extensive database for the assessment of the potential toxicity of a chemical is available. In environmental medical cases, TSCA requirements are a source of reports regarding adverse health effects in people and in animals.

Testing Requirements and Regulation of Existing Chemicals

Premanufacture notification or reporting of potential health effects may prompt the need for additional testing under the TSCA. Testing requirements apply to situations in which more data are needed before a final decision may be made. Data may include those related to human exposures, potential toxicity, and/or environmental fate/impact. The cost of the testing is borne by the manufacturer.

If the data submitted are deemed not sufficient to meet the requirements of the Act, the TSCA has several alternatives. First, it can mandate additional testing before the chemical is sold. Second, the TSCA may limit the amount of a chemical produced, or prohibit or limit certain uses that increase exposures. Third, the TSCA may require specific warnings or labels, or extensive data on production or disposal of the substance. The TSCA also has the option of referring the issue to other regulatory bodies. For example, OSHA may be a more appropriate agency to review the material if only a workplace potential health hazard exists. Finally, if an "imminent and unreasonable risk" is present, the TSCA may actually ban the use of a chemical. The EPA has not chosen to use the total ban approach under section 7, but has focused on limitation of exposure by restriction of markets for such substances as CFCs and PCBs. Recently, regulations to phase out asbestos use were overturned by the courts.

The TSCA is of special importance for occupational and environmental physicians. Through the reporting of toxicologic and epidemiologic studies and "clinical adverse reactions," it mandates the establishment of a health risk database. It also includes several medical reporting requirements for manufacturers and importers. An awareness of these reports will be significant in any evaluation of environmentally based disease. The OTS, which administers TSCA, can be an extremely useful reference in assessing risks, especially when there is an ongoing scientific and regulatory debate concerning a chemical.

The Occupational and Environmental Physician's Role

Environmental statutes require the creation of a massive database that can be used by the occupational and environmental physician (OEP) in clinical cases, and in assessing the risks of working groups and the community. Access to the data will be as challenging as its interpretation and integration into the decision-making process. Access will be determined by the position of the OEP. For example, if the physician is employed by the industry generating the data, it is generally accessible. The data needed, however, should be carefully defined in a specific request to the corporate office or site environmental manager. A clear description of the intended use of the information is recommended. If the OEP needs data on a clinical case and is not employed by the industry, a request can be made through the employee or directly to management of the industry. Environmental record-keeping responsibilities are massive; as a result, a request for general data will not be acceptable. If the information is not made available, some of it may be accessed through environmental regulatory agencies. Local officials will usually be helpful; however, the physician may choose to call the regional EPA offices. Often, there is litigation and the records may be part of the discovery process. If special testing is needed and has not yet been performed, it may be requested from the industry or the EPA. Environmental testing services can be directly accessed. (The American Industrial Hygiene Association maintains a list of contractors specializing in environmental testing). (See Chap. 22.)

Just as industrial hygiene data may be difficult to access, environmental exposure data may present similar challenges, especially for physicians who evaluate workers as outpatients. If data access or interpretation is particularly difficult, subspecialists in environmental medicine can be contacted. Physicians in occupational and environmental residency training programs are an excellent resource when difficulties arise, since they commonly work with both industry and government and are often perceived as unbiased.

Summary

The system of environmental regulation in the United States can serve as a framework for understanding common environmental problems, as well as a reference source for the practice of environmental medicine. Regulations, well planned in the late 1960s, have matured over time. While most regulations have been oriented to exposure control rather than actual health risk, the data generated by these requirements are vital to assessing the potential relationship between exposure and disease.

Although environmental laws developed based on the medium, a comprehensive and preventive approach to environmental pollution is evolving. A new emphasis has been placed on risk assessment both for new regulations and for implementation of existing regulations. The ultimate product of this process is the assessment of risk to people. These assessments mirror the exposure/disease determination in a clinical case in a more formal fashion. The use of preventive approaches and human risk assessment makes the occupational and environmental physician a key participant in future regulations and their implementation.

In assessing a person with an illness potentially related to an environmental exposure, a determination of causation must include the most comprehensive exposure measurements available. Commonly, these measurements will be the product of regulatory requirements.

Whether data are requirements of permits or monitoring secondary to a release, they serve as a primary source of exposure information. In the occupational setting, personal monitoring data may be available. With environmental exposures, however, data require significant extrapolation and interpretation.

While the interpretation of data may be problematic, EPA officials and experts in occupational and environmental medicine can support these efforts. Although somewhat different from occupational health regulations, environmental statutes result in the generation of data that must be evaluated according to similar principles in exposure/disease/prevention assessments. Illness resulting from exposure to an environmental hazard is not different from that due to occupational exposure of similar concentration. The medical approach requires similar diligence to evaluate each piece of the clinical puzzle to formulate a diagnosis and treatment and to propose preventive strategies.

References

1. Arbuckle, J. G., et al. *Environmental Law Handbook*. Rockville, MD: Government Institutes, Inc., 1989.
2. Findley, R. W., and Farber, D. A. *Environmental Law*. St. Paul: West Publishing Co., 1988.
3. Rodgers, W. H. *Environmental Law*. St. Paul: West Publishing Co., 1984 (updates).
4. Anderson, F. R., and Mandelker, D. R. *Environmental Protection Law and Policy*. Boston: Little, Brown, 1988.
5. Conner, J. D., et al. *TSCA Handbook*. Rockville, MD: Government Institutes, Inc., 1989.
6. Tarcher, A. B. *Principles and Practice of Environmental Medicine*. New York: Plenum, 1992.
7. Sullivan, J. B., and Krieger, G. R. *Hazardous Materials Toxicology*. Baltimore: Williams & Wilkins, 1992.

Further Information

The environmental regulations and field of environmental laws are changing so rapidly that the most appropriate reading may be the *Federal Register* and a number of newsletters (e.g., *Environmental Reporter, EPA Today*) that will contain the more recent information. The texts listed above all contain good summary information, but details may not affect the current regulations. The *Environmental Law Handbook* is comprehensive and relatively easy to read, and the *TSCA Handbook* provides good detailed TSCA information.

Matthews, R. A., and Gray, P. L. *Superfund Claims and Litigation Manual*. New York: Executive Enterprises Publications Co., Inc., 1990.

43

Clinical Environmental Medicine

Alan M. Ducatman

Patients with significant exposures to hazardous materials or questions about exposures need not come from within workplaces. Occupational physicians possess a unique mix of skills including clinical care, epidemiology, and toxicology, which are essential for patients with environmental concerns. This chapter proposes to identify common environmental stressors from "beyond factory walls" and to suggest clinical and public health guidelines for occupational and environmental physicians. The several definitions suggested below describe environmental medicine, its clinical application, and its role as a public health discipline. A secondary purpose of the definition is to draw a distinction between the contents of this chapter and some of the misleading connotations carried by the word "environmental."

Environmental medicine can be considered to be "the study of effects upon human beings of external physical, chemical, and biologic factors in the general environment" [1]. *Clinical environmental medicine,* then, would be "the study of detectable human disease or adverse health outcomes from exposure to these environmental factors" [1]. The *discipline* of environmental medicine "combines clinical epidemiologic, and toxicologic approaches. It uniquely seeks to understand external causation and then to adopt policy, engineering, or human factor interventions to prevent or mitigate the caused outcomes" [1].

Clinicians who read these proposed definitions should be concerned by the absence of focus on usual pharmacologic or similar office-based interventions. The omission is deliberate. We can prevent environmental disease far more effectively and still more cost effectively than we can treat it. This generalization holds even for those few environmental diseases for which we have well-established and constantly improving treatment regimens, such as childhood lead poisoning. The prevention of lead poisoning features environmental hygiene primarily; pharmaceuticals are a tertiary intervention used in treatment.

Although the definitions state clearly that the diseases must be detectable, the distracting debate about clinical ecology/multiple chemical sensitivity forces one to reiterate several common scientific principles in the context of environmental health. Assignment of clinical or laboratory findings to environmental causes necessitates repeatability of those findings and clear epidemiologic linkage. Accuracy of diagnostic testing, in relation to exposures and efficacy of therapeutic interventions, needs to be tested by recognizable scientific means. Physicians who practice "clinical ecology" or who treat multiple chemical sensitivity must recall that neither environmental nor any other type of medicine is based on the application of "untested diagnostic and therapeutic regimens" [1]. Those who support new tests and procedures are obligated to prove effectiveness in appropriate scientific testing [1–6]. On the other hand, physicians alarmed by unsupported assertions need to recall that the patient's symptoms are real even when the science is suspect.

Table 43-1 lists office encounters common to environmental medicine, with attention to the scope of individual patient care. Table 43-2 lists community-based public health activities. Table 43-3 predicts future roles for physicians with clinical, epidemiologic, and toxicologic skills. Occupational and environmental physicians in training today will likely spend significant time performing the types of activities listed in the tables, perhaps as much as occupational physicians have devoted to workplace surveillance in the past.

The inclusion of issues such as childhood lead poisoning in Table 43-1 does not imply that occupational and environmental physicians should assume the primary therapeutic role of pediatricians when chelation therapy or other pharmacologic treatments are appropriate. (A few of my colleagues *do* have this role and probably wish that there were pediatricians in their area who were willing to take it from

Table 43-1. Examples of office encounters in environmental medicine*

Issue	Population
Lead exposure	Children, home renovators, hobbyists
Building-related complaints	Schoolchildren and their parents, home renovators, and tenants
Puzzling symptoms attributed to chemicals	See Multiple Chemical Sensitivity
Environmental cancer concerns	Residents near power lines, abandoned older (asbestos-containing) buildings, waste or incineration sites, areas with radon problems; residents with contaminated water
Reproductive concerns	See also, Lead, Hobbies, Environmental Cancer
Pulmonary disease (asthma, colds, bronchitis)	Residents near power plants or industries

*As in the rest of medicine, causation is a decision, not a certain implication of any encounter.

Table 43-2. Examples of community-based public health activities of environmental physicians*

Decisions	Activities
Siting an energy source for electric power generation	Predicted pulmonary increments for modeled ground-level emissions for fossil fuel sources
Siting and mode of waste disposal for a former chemical drum cleanup facility, with heavily contaminated soil, located upwind of one community and above the ground water of another	Consideration of neoplastic and reproductive hazards of ingestion
	Consideration of other potential outcomes for incidental emissions
	Description of epidemiologic nonatmospheric issues surrounding exposures, ranging from noise (coal trains/tracks) to electromagnetic fields (power lines)
Planning state programs for childhood lead exposure	Suggesting best areas for "trade-offs," based on existing community exposures
	Selecting best uses of scarce resources for population and environmental surveillance

*Examples taken from environmental questions facing several communities in 1992.

Table 43-3. Predicted future roles for occupational/environmental physicians

Product/work	Clients
Product labeling, Material Safety Data Sheet reviews	Corporations, labeling contractors
New product liability reviews	Corporate planners and attorneys, citizen groups, regulatory agencies
New product concepts, testing, and marketing	Corporations
Health policy decisions concerning public buildings, rights of way	Governments (all levels), citizen groups, public utilities
Health policy decisions concerning hazard abatement in and about private residences	Governments, public health agencies, citizen groups

them.) Rather, it means that occupational and environmental physicians will be relied on by patients for advice concerning sources of toxins, exposure prevention, and related public health interventions. These issues are ultimately more important.

Physician colleagues outside of occupational and environmental medicine have been slow to appreciate the importance of (and market potential for) public health counsel to communities, local governments, and industries in the give-and-take concerning air and water quality. Some of these are listed in Table 43-2. Our patients and even local government officials may be deeply dissatisfied with "risk assessment" as provided by current models. People on both sides of environmental issues perceive, with some justice, that elaborate mathematics of modern "risk assessments" obscure underlying assumptions and personal prejudices of risk assessors. A part of this chapter is intended to furnish physicians with a straightforward approach that can be provided by professionals already entrusted with community health (physicians) and presented in a way that patients can appreciate.

Office-Based Practice of Environmental Medicine

The physician who practices environmental medicine is likely to encounter patients with a variety of concerns about the potential health implications of exposure to environmental hazards. With advancing scientific knowledge of the health implications secondary to exposure, it is likely that physicians will continue to see more of these concerns. Some examples include lead paint and lead-contaminated soil or water; *asbestos* noted in the basement or attic; radon detected in the basement; formaldehyde detected in insulation or furnishings; organic chemicals including halogenated solvents detected in the water supply; pesticides sprayed inappropriately; and concerns raised about geographical proximity to a hazardous waste site, high tension wires, demolition, construction, or industrial point of source of emissions.

In the majority of these cases, the extent of the exposures are considerably less than in the traditional occupational setting. As a result, some of the diagnostic measures that are helpful in the occupational environment may not be appropriate for these settings. Nonetheless, the astute physician is urged to become familiar with techniques for accessing environmental data, especially those data that are available through federal and state agencies, as well as to become more sophisticated in the use of monitoring techniques to evaluate specific cause and effect relationships.

Lead Poisoning

Childhood lead poisoning and questions related to its prevention or mitigation represent an increasingly common office-based encounter. Referrals come from three sources. *Pediatricians* often feel uncomfortable with the public health and environmental aspects of lead poisoning. *Public health departments* (or public health nurse-run clinics) refer patients, families, or groups of affected patients. Most commonly, *families* self-refer when they face concerns about the future of affected children or available means of preventing ongoing exposures. Their tenacity in identifying a physician who recognizes the environmental decision-making aspects inherent to lead exposure is often impressive. The sophistication of referral questions and the physician's ability to arrange for appropriate public health interventions will vary remarkably from state to state. Some states (such as Massachusetts) have relatively sophisticated and legally mandated programs for family education, lead detection, and lead exposure abatement. Other states are only beginning to address this issue and have little or no infrastructure. In these states, testing of children or dwellings is hit-or-miss. There may be no trained and qualified home abatement personnel. There may be no established shelters or apartments to remove children from their source(s) of exposure. Dealing with absence of infrastructure is a challenge to office-based practice. Title X of the Affordable Housing Act (HR5334), signed into law on October 28, 1992, requires that states receiving any EPA grants also certify lead abatement contractors. The same law creates a source of funding for abatement work, although the adequacy of the funding pool is uncertain. Even if other states develop programs immediately, it will be some time before an infrastructure for prevention of childhood lead poisoning is available in many states.

Office referrals generally begin when childhood lead levels exceed 10 μg/100 ml of whole blood. This referral level from the Centers for Disease Control recommendations is based on a strong and steadily growing body of evidence that "low-level" lead intoxication causes significant intellectual deficit in the developing fetus and young child [7–11]. Clear decrements in performance can be measured at population exposure levels as low as 10 µg/100 ml.

For children whose lead exposure is recent, with a lead level between 10 and 20 µg/100 ml, no chelation treatment is warranted. (In some associated toxic torts, attorneys have tried to equate the absence of appropriate treatment with absence of harm. Whatever one feels about the value of toxic torts in this circumstance, physicians must avoid the obvious error of equating therapeutic risk/benefit ratios with the absence of adverse outcome.) Medications that help at this "low" level of recent exposure assure adequate iron and calcium stores. Inadequate iron stores potentiate several of the deleterious effects of lead. The critical public health intervention, which may exact considerable cost and social dislocation for families, assures that future lead encounters are minimized.

To accomplish this goal, physicians must impart several kinds of information to families. First, parents faced with social and economic dislocations may minimize the potential for serious harm to vulnerable children. One should clearly assert that continued risk of lead exposure is an important childhood health problem with real performance outcomes. Clinicians who provide this information must recognize the substantial emotional impact, with potential for associated parental guilt and grief. For clearly motivated parents, the potential for irreversible damage to their children does not need to be emphasized any more than is required to mobilize the family to accept and initiate needed public health measures.

In the overwhelming majority of childhood lead poisonings (or adult poisoning outside the workplace), the source of exposure is *lead paint*. Lead paint in obviously poor condition (peeling, chipping) is common but not required to cause toxic effects. Children without obvious pica frequently become lead intoxicated from paint. Home renovations or other sources of dust in air, in rugs, and in corners provide toddlers with invisible but adequate hand-mouth sources of lead poisoning. The most commonly implicated exposure areas of homes include windows (high lead levels, weathering, lots of friction), painted doorways (friction), porches (high lead levels, weathering), and even old radiators (exposed to blunt trauma). Any part of a home can be implicated, although older houses have higher lead levels. Even homes built after the lead paint prohibition of the late 1970s may have older paints applied within them. In fact, modern studies of "nonlead" paint may turn up surprising lead levels in some samples, particularly for outdoor and metal paints.

Soil is a secondary source of lead exposure. As a practical matter, young children have the most soil exposure near the home, often in the yard next to peeled outdoor paint. Paint from the home is the most important cause of accessible soil contamination. Play around parents' renovation jobs and childcare within other people's lead-contaminated homes represent similar risks for lead paint and soil exposure outside of the child's own home.

Water is a third and usually less important source. While municipal supplies, municipal plumbing, or personal wells are occasionally implicated, parents need to understand that most lead in drinking water comes from the solder contained in the last few feet of plumbing. (In cities where the EPA has discovered undesirable levels of lead in tap water, lead-*poisoned* children are still overwhelmingly characterized by their exposure to lead *paint*.) Another contributor to water-borne lead ingestion is boiling of babies' formula water. This activity may concentrate existing lead in water and lead from inappropriately constructed cookware. Still less common childhood ingestion sources include folk medicines and use of lead crystal for acid drinks. Unsuspected sources continue to be recognized. The most startling source in this author's experience was intoxication from an inappropriate lead-contaminated dye in pool cue chalk, a product made to be powdered indoors. Other environmental clinicians can provide equally strange tales of lead sources.

Residence near lead smelting operations is an important source in newly industrialized countries, where this industry is more common than in the United States. Inhalation (with secondary ingestion) exposures typify adult workplace rather than childhood home exposures in the United States. Workplace exposures also include paint. Bridge repair and junkyard workers, home renovators, and other construction workers face the same environmental risk as children.

The environmental clinician must recognize sources of exposure in order to provide families with a second, critical piece of information. Which of many possible steps should families take to prevent further childhood exposure? The easy "fixes" include removal of contaminated soil, cessation of the practice of boiling the water for baby's bottle (which may concentrate lead from water or utensil sources), and reconfiguring the last few feet of plumbing with nonleaded solder. Unfortunately, these easy measures are usually irrelevant to the underlying source of childhood lead poisoning. Environmental lead poisoning is overwhelmingly due to house paint, which is rarely just in one little area. Getting rid of the paint can be difficult and expensive, which leaves parents with unsatisfactory choices. They can more closely supervise their child in the same environment, although historically, this activity has had little impact on blood lead levels. A more proactive approach is to move from the offending environment. This advice is most attractive to renters, provided that alternative housing is available. The only medical requirement of "geographic removal protection" is that the new home is not another source of lead exposure.

An apparent compromise between these positions is to "abate" the lead in an existing home. This option is most attractive to parents who have invested life savings in their older home, with its ongoing renovation or maintenance requirements. They want to remain in the home and to do everything possible to protect their children within that environment. Simply cleaning up lead dust is not adequate abatement [9]. It is also necessary to physically remove (or, in some cases, cover) the old paint that provides the common source of the lead. As a public health measure, parents can be advised that abatement works well *if* it is done completely, *before* the family inhabits the dwelling, and by certified contractors with expert reputations. Abatement done as a reaction to already existing lead poisoning, on the other hand, can be disappointing. Abatements performed while the family still inhabits the house are a source of substantial additional risk, not safety. Abatements should not be performed in inhabited residences. Further, even when done very well and with the family safely in temporary quarters, abatements may not lower blood lead levels when the family returns, a disappointing experience to parents, who look for improvements when prevention of further increments may be all that is achievable.

Several interventions are recommended for children who have blood lead levels of 20 μg/100 ml or above [7]. Neurologic and neuropsychological evaluations are appropriate at the time lead intoxication is discovered, after environmental removal, and at intervals as the child progresses through the educational system. These studies are critical to understanding educational deficits associated with childhood lead toxicity. Grossly normal neurologic examinations, with visual and aural receptive processing problems on neuropsychological evaluation, accompanied by learning difficulties at school and sometimes coupled with subtle fine motor development problems are the most characteristic findings of "low-level" lead poisoning. Neuropsychological examinations are advantageously combined with frequent school evaluations, beginning in the preschool years. Deficits may become apparent by age 4 to 5 and be well characterized by age 7 to 8. Recognition of the need for special educational services can save families frustration. Educational performance of children whose disabilities would otherwise predict rapid failure in school systems can be enhanced by early and specialized interventions. Obtaining these services often requires firm insistence; the environmental physician can facilitate the process by explaining the nature of the problem to families and educators alike.

The threshold for chelation treatment of children (and adults) has been lowered dramatically in the past few years. Modern pharmacy textbooks still cite blood levels as high as 45 μg/100 ml whole blood as the threshold for treating childhood lead poisoning. Among pediatricians, neuropsychologists, and epidemiologists, there is an emerging consensus that treatments have substantial value for blood lead levels as low as 25 μg/100 ml [7, 8, 16]. No lower level threshold has been established for treatment effectiveness, and it is quite possible that treatments at still lower levels of lead exposure may be shown to have clinical advantages. Provocative chelation is often used to decide which children require chelation at "low" blood levels. Clinical trials randomized into treatment and nontreatment groups should further clarify threshold treatment levels in the next few years, likely at levels far lower than suggested by texts. Succimer (dimercaptosuccinic acid, a dimercaprol analogue) is gradually supplanting ethylenediaminetetraacetic acid (EDTA) as the chelating agent of choice. EDTA is a slightly but significantly better chelator in controlled clinical trials [11], but succimer is increasingly used because of lesser toxicity and ease of oral administration. Succimer may also mobilize mercury and arsenic, but it appears to mobilize essential trace metals far less than EDTA. Because succimer is the first successful oral lead chelating agent, clinicians must be alert to the public health inappropriateness of providing a pharmacologic therapy in circumstances in which the real issue is continued exposure. (Fear that easily available treatment may be substituted for prevention may be one of the reasons that succimer's entry into therapy of adult occupational exposures has been delayed.)

Succimer treatment generally begins in children one year or older, with 10 mg/kg every 8 hours for 5 days, followed by 10 mg/kg every 12 hours for an additional 2 weeks. Treatment beyond 3 weeks is not recommended, but repeated courses can be given after 2-week intervals. Succimer comes in 100-mg capsules. The capsule can be opened and the beads spread in food for children who are unable to swallow the capsule. Table 43-4 shows recommended pediatric doses [11]. While succimer should not be used in combination with any other chelation regimen, it can be used as outpatient follow-up to initial inpatient EDTA therapy. More severely intoxicated children can receive EDTA, 1.5 mg/m^2, for 5 days, with repeated courses at 5-day intervals if needed. Critical adverse side effects of EDTA include renal tubular and hepatocellular injury.

Usual lead treatment laboratory guidelines are applied to oral, intramuscular, and intravenous chelation treatments. Twenty-four hour urine collections are obtained for lead and creatinine clearance where possible. Renal functions are monitored before and during therapy. (Succimer may dialyze, but lead chelates do not.) Fluid intake must be maintained. Mild elevations of transaminases are seen in up to 10% of patients; "liver enzymes" should be obtained before and weekly during therapy. Use during pregnancy is a serious decision because of known teratogenicity and fetotoxicity in mice. Obstetricians, pediatricians, and pharmacologists should be part of the decision-making process if the aim is protection of the developing human. Nausea, vomiting, diarrhea, metallic taste, and, less often, rash are common side effects. Previous allergic reaction is a contraindication.

Since "rebound" (and reexposure) following cessation of any chelation therapy is common, the patient should be followed at frequent intervals after treatment. Formal performance measures are useful for assessing central nervous system (CNS) benefits in noninfant children and adults. Neuropsychological testing is a useful adjunct to therapy before and after treatment [7].

Renal damage, hearing loss, and hypertension are potential long-term effects of childhood lead poisoning. Appropriate testing should begin in childhood and occasional follow-ups are reasonable through young adulthood. A more complex research and social issue relates to the likelihood that childhood lead exposure causes chronic reproductive toxicity. One possibility, supported by preliminary population studies, is that children of lead-poisoned mothers have performance decrements independent of socioeconomic status or present lead levels. The exposure hypothesis relates to transplacental shift of maternal bone stores. No clinical advice pertains to this possibility for now, but clinicians should be alert that additional information may make this an educational intervention issue for children of exposed parents.

Clinically Based Risk Information, Including Biologic Monitoring for Environmental Exposures

Concerns with the health care system in general do not detract from the general faith in the judgment of *individual* clinicians. Clinicians who address questions about health outcomes of past or potential exposures are accorded enormous credibility. The local physician's opinion about an exposure or the cause of an outbreak

Table 43-4. Pediatric dose of succimer (100-mg capsules)

Weight (lb)	Dose (tid)*
18–35	100 mg
36–55	200 mg
56–75	300 mg
76–100	400 mg
> 100	500 mg

*Present recommendation is tid schedule for 5 days, followed by bid for 2 weeks [10].

is likely to be accorded more respect than the work of regulatory, public health, or research experts regardless of relative expertise. Occupational and environmental physicians are unique resources within communities because of their familiarity with environmental exposure-outcome data, including their availability, methods, quality, and potential weaknesses.

A responsibility of the clinician is to present exposure-outcome information in the same manner as clinical information (see Chap. 26). The information, including statistical uncertainty and the inability to draw definitive conclusions for some important questions, must be understood by patients. Risk assessment models typically fail the dual clinical requirement for simplicity and honesty. Their complex mathematics may also obscure hidden assumptions or inadequate data. One alternative is to "deconstruct" elaborate mathematical models into underlying exposure-outcome data. This approach requires familiarity with methodologic strategies, the data, and assumptions inherent in either the initial methods or subsequent models. Existing assessment models are still enormously useful since they often point out the complicating issues, and refer to many of the underlying peer-review studies. The key information in the model can be recapitulated by a literature search; review of primary references is essential whatever the starting point.

A situation that typically concerns communities involves the siting of a new facility, such as a factory, fossil fuel power generation station, highway, high-tension electric transmission wire, or a waste disposal incinerator. Questions also are raised about health effects from existing facilities and concerns about releases from abandoned sites. Air pollution is most commonly queried, but questions may also encompass drinking water pollution (waste sites) or asbestos exposure (abandoned buildings).

Investigation of a perceived disease outbreak, attributed to past or existing environmental conditions, is a third type of community-based clinical encounter. Investigation of disease "clustering" is common outside of workplaces, but far more likely to yield results in the work setting. Epidemiologists point out that most perceived disease clustering has no cause [12]. Before we dismiss the geographic/community "cluster," however, it is important to recall that "Epping jaundice," "Yu-Sho" and "Yu-Sheng" (in Pacific Rim communities from PCBs in rice oil), toxic oil syndrome, Parkinson-like symptoms from MPTP, eosinophilia myalgia, Lyme disease, and the immunodeficiency syndrome now ascribed to human immunodeficiency retrovirus were all recognized as community disease clusters [13]. Occupational and environmental physicians should be aware that most of what we know about environmental etiology was first noted as a perceived disease cluster.

Information needed by patients and community members depends on whether one starts with exposure(s) (from a facility, site, water supply) or outcome(s) (often a disease cluster). Both have clinical aspects, but we will confine the discussion to the more common situation—risk from identified exposures. The first obligation (Fig. 43-1) is to obtain exposure data. It is critically important that patients understand the source and accuracy of the data. Models, often used in the absence of measurements, are acceptable to patients only if exposures are so small that they cannot be measured accurately, or if future exposures are predicted based on past *measured* performance of the technology or facility in question. Otherwise models are relatively undesirable. The clinician should state clearly that exposure data are generated by others and that accuracy of (nonbiologic) exposure measurements is outside of physician control. It is acceptable to define a degree of confidence or skepticism concerning environmental exposure data collected (or modeled) by others, provided that the clinician is familiar with the techniques and technology involved.

For some exposures, *biologic monitoring* can be used to augment assessments of past exposures. Substances with long body half-lives are most accessible to biologic monitoring, particularly when partitioning is in equilibration with accessible body tissues (e.g., blood, urine, hair and nails). Concerns about lead exposure can be addressed in individuals or in populations routinely. The routine schedule for biologic monitoring of environmental lead in children is blood lead level measured at ages 1 and 2 for low-risk children, more frequently for children at high risk [7, 8] (Table 43-5). With slightly more effort, other heavy metals or polycyclic halogenated hydrocarbon exposures can be measured. These determinations provide valuable population and individual information in the event that the levels are elevated. Results are less helpful in individuals with normal or near normal levels. Concerns about temporal relationships of testing to exposure, competing sources of exposure (e.g.,

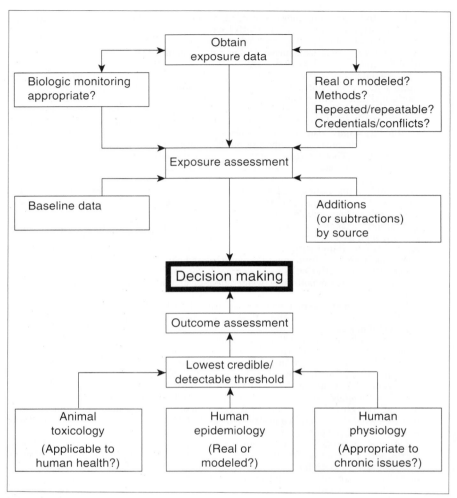

Figure 43-1. Risk assessment.

Table 43-5. Screening schedule for early detection of childhood lead exposure

Age	Low risk history	High risk history	Blood Pb ≥ 10 μg/100 ml
6 months		X	
1 year	X	X	
18 months		X	
2 years	X	X	
Every 3 months			X
Every 6 months		X	

Source: Adapted from Centers for Disease Control. *Preventing Lead Poisoning in Young Children.* US Department of Health and Human Services, 1991.

the seafood problem in arsenic surveillance), and inaccessibility of appropriate body compartment ("brown fat" in mercury exposure), present interpretation challenges.

In the introduction, problems of unproved diagnostic and therapeutic interventions were discussed. Patients continually bring to our offices evidence of unproved (not to mention illogical, unbelievable, and downright fraudulent) biologic monitoring results of environmental exposures. For example, office laboratories (frequently, but not always belonging to nonphysician providers) may claim to detect solvent levels *in* (not on) hair. Toxicologists acknowledge that solvent metabolism precludes any role for this type of diagnostic testing. Hair analysis of solvent exposure is without clinical benefit. The economic issue appears to be that the actual metabolism of solvents need not deter the enterprising laboratory. Similarly, the detection of solvents or solvent metabolites is achieved routinely in some laboratories *months, years,* or *decades* after exposure. The silliness of this enterprise deserves little discussion, except to note that some insurance mechanism must actually be paying.

A difficult issue is nonvalidated clinical uses of potentially legitimate research tests. The usual clinical scenario is a patient without physical findings who has been given a dreadful diagnosis, such as "chemical AIDS," based on unusual testing procedures. Most often abused are hapten-antibody tests (which can be valuable in the few laboratories that run blind controls), bizarre porphyrin metabolism tests run without blind controls, and even routine immunologic tests reported with unusually low thresholds for abnormal readings. The cost-effective approach is to repeat these tests at the appropriate university medical laboratory. The temptation to ignore the test leaves an open-ended question for the patient, who has no way of appreciating how infrequently these findings are validated. A present and future role of environmental clinicians will be identifying valid tests and defining appropriate clinical settings for their use. As health care payment systems evolve, tests ordered for environmental reasons will also come under cost-containment scrutiny. Valid public health testing procedures must be retained in payment mechanisms, a condition that will require the profession to describe testing algorithms.

Data from the exposure assessment should then be compared to the three types of outcome assessment information (Fig. 43-1); these are animal studies, human physiology studies, and human epidemiology studies. The affected population is most likely to need information concerning *the lowest credible exposure level that may produce measurable changes in human health*. In the case of cancer or reproductive outcomes (supposing the exposure to be a polycyclic polyhalogenated hydrocarbon, for example), lowest thresholds may be defined by animal studies that have uncertain applicability to human experience. In the case of respiratory risks such as asthma or bronchitis from air pollution, lowest thresholds may be defined by epidemiologic studies, which may in turn contain complex models and interesting assumptions. Traditional risk assessment models deal with the uncertainty by providing mathematical formulas whose margins encompass animal and human data, and then by presenting some central trend for discussion. It is no more effort and much more clinically honest to provide information concerning what we actually know about outcomes in minks, monkeys, and humans. (Minks are enormously more sensitive to reproductive hazards of PCBs than are humans, for example) [14]. With the underlying data, community decision-making may then be quite conservative, perhaps with a focus on minks rather than humans. Community policy-making is not without problems, but actual data shift the focus from angry revelations concerning "hidden" agendas to shared values about exposures and outcomes.

Summary of Clinical Issues

The scope of environmental practice is evolving rapidly [15], as is the impact of clinical research in environmental health [16]. Physicians are asked to integrate multidisciplinary regulatory, exposure, outcome, treatment, education, and decision-making information. They are thus involved directly in health evaluations (episodic or periodic), diagnosis and treatment, patient and community education, implementation of public health protection, and planned abatement of source stressors, exposure and outcome assessments (risk assessments), and, in an area of critical future need, disaster preparedness [17]. Each activity relates to existing or potential future exposures. For each activity, affected individuals and patients want and need to hear from their own physicians.

References

1. Ducatman, A. M., et al. What is environmental medicine? *J. Occup. Med.* 32:1130, 1990.
2. Committee on Environmental Hypersensitivities. *Report of the Ad Hoc Committee on Environmental Hypersensitivity Disorders.* Toronto, Ontario: Ministry of Health, 1985.
3. California Medical Association Scientific Task Force on Clinical Ecology. Clinical ecology—a critical appraisal. *West. J. Med.* 144:239, 1986.
4. American Academy of Allergy and Immunology. Position statement: Clinical ecology. *J. Allergy Clin. Immunol.* 78:269, 1986.
5. American College of Physicians. Position paper: Clinical ecology. *Ann. Intern. Med.* 111:168, 1989.
6. Coble, Y. D., et al. Clinical ecology: Council report. *J.A.M.A.* 268:3465, 1992.
7. Centers for Disease Control. *Preventing Lead Poisoning in Young Children.* US Department of Health and Human Services (USDHHS), 1991.
8. Agency for Toxic Substances and Disease Registry. *Case Studies in Environmental Medicine: Lead Toxicity.* USDHHS, 1990.
9. Weitzman, M., et al. Lead contaminated soil abatement and urban children's blood lead levels. *J.A.M.A.* 269:1647, 1993.
10. Ruff, H. A., et al. Declining blood lead levels and cognitive impairments in moderately lead poisoned children. *J.A.M.A.* 269:1641, 1993.
11. Olin, B. R., et al. (eds.). *Facts and Comparisons Drug Information.* St. Louis: Lippincott, December 1992 (updated monthly).
12. Anon. Nagging doubt, public opinion offers obstacles to ending "cluster" studies. Medical news and perspectives. *J.A.M.A.* 77:52, 1989.
13. Fleming, L. E., Ducatman, A. M., and Shalat, S. L. Disease clusters: A central and ongoing role in occupational health. *J. Occup. Med.* 33:818, 1991.
14. Ducatman, A. M., and Moyer T. P. The Role of the Clinical Laboratory in the Evaluation of the Polyhalogenated Polycyclic Toxins: DDT, PCBs, PBBs, Dibenzodioxins and Dibenzofurans. *Therapeutic Drug Monitoring,* Vol. 4. Washington, DC: American Association for Clinical Chemistry, June 1983. Pp. 1–18.
15. Perry, G. F., et al. Scope of occupational and environmental health programs and practice. *J. Occup. Med.* 34:436, 1992.
16. McCunney, R. J., Boswell, R., and Harzbecker, J. Environmental health in the journals. *Environ. Res.* 59:114, 1992.
17. Borak, J., Callan, M., and Abbott, W. *Hazardous Materials Exposure: Emergency Response and Patient Care.* Englewood Cliffs, NJ: Brady, 1992.

Further Information

Agency for Toxic Substances and Disease Registry. *Case Studies in Environmental Medicine: Lead Toxicity.* USDHHS/PHS/ATSDR, 1992 (revised).
This is the best available teaching tool concerning lead in children and adults for the busy physician.

Centers for Disease Control. *Preventing Lead Poisoning in Young Children.* USDHH/PHS/CDC, 1991.
This is the 4th revision of CDC's influential, basic recommendations for clinicians concerning childhood lead poisoning. It describes data available through 1990, which form the basis for the recommendations we follow. The goal is follow-up for all children with lead levels < 10 µg/100 ml; interventions begin at 15 µg/100 ml.

Cone, J. E., and Hodgson, M. J. (eds.) Problem buildings: Building associated illness and the sick building syndrome. *Occup. Med. State of the Art Rev.,*
This is a description of a variety of building issues that affect employed workers, school children, and others who spend time in institutional buildings.

Simon, G. E., et al. Immunologic, psychologic, and neuropsychologic factors in multiple chemical sensitivity. A controlled study. *Ann. Intern. Med.* 119:97, 1993.
The first designed, blinded study of multiple chemical sensitivity (MCS) demonstrates no immunologic response in MCS patients, and none of the previously attributed neuropsychological disorders. The authors also document, but do not discuss, some of the high-sensitivity/low predictive value immunologic testing that has plagued the MCS population.

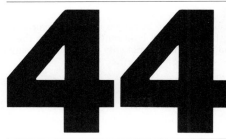

Indoor Air Pollution

Robert K. McLellan and
Robert J. McCunney

Indoor air pollution (IAP) did not begin with modern, energy-efficient office buildings. Open fire in primitive dwellings exposed our ancestors to a wide range of hazardous combustion products. People living in remote areas with the cleanest outdoor air imaginable still cook and heat indoors with poorly vented fires. These traditional practices potentially render the air in their drafty shelters more contaminated than contemporary, sealed office towers. Though high-level exposures to toxins such as combustion products occur in indoor settings, low-level exposures present the most important and most common challenge to the occupational health practitioner.

Historical Perspective

Complacency about the safety of indoor settings was shaken by a number of events beginning in the late 1970s. Newspaper headlines announced mysterious epidemics of health complaints in office buildings. Early investigators named the complaints the "tight building syndrome" because of their association with energy-conserving building construction and ventilation measures. Industrial hygienists often found low ventilation rates and contaminants considerably less than permissible exposure limits (PELs). In the absence of toxic exposure levels approaching PELs, some investigators ascribed office worker complaints to mass hysteria.

A series of widely publicized building-related incidents demonstrated the potential seriousness of indoor air exposures. In 1976, members of the American Legion convening in a Philadelphia hotel were struck by a pneumonia epidemic, resulting in 182 cases and 29 deaths [1]. Epidemiologic investigation linked the deaths to the contamination of a ventilation system with *Legionella pneumophila*. A fire in an office building in Binghamton, New York, resulted in widespread contamination of the interior with polychlorinated biphenyls released from electrical equipment. Concern about the health effects of indoor air was further piqued when an investigation of a radioactively contaminated nuclear power worker identified his home as an intense source of radon. After initial radon surveys revealed widespread residential contamination, the Surgeon General's office and the Environmental Protection Agency (EPA) released a joint statement in September 1988, recommending nearly universal radon testing of the residential environment [2].

As research progressed through the late 1980s, the federal government recognized IAP as a significant and expensive health concern. Investigators found that:

Poor indoor air quality (IAQ) was not simply a matter of comfort, but was associated with illness and death.
Many toxins were present at higher levels indoors than outdoors.
Changes in lifestyle over the last century had led average citizens of the United States to spend 90% of their lives indoors.
The most vulnerable segments of our population, the infirm, the very young, and the very old, were the most exposed.

These revelations led the EPA to place IAP among the top environmental priorities. From a business perspective, research on the impact of poor IAQ on productivity and illness may prove critically influential in decisions about facility construction and management [3].

Contemporary concerns for indoor air quality have prompted both the House and the Senate of the United States Congress to develop indoor air quality bills. At the time of this writing, this legislation has yet to be fully approved. Nevertheless, the public hearings associated with these proposed bills continue to focus the public's attention on the importance of indoor air quality, not only in promoting comfort, but also in preventing illness.

The Indoor Environment

Sources of IAP

Four sources contribute to IAP: external environment, building fabric, mechanical systems, and occupants.

External Sources
Without mechanical intervention, occupied buildings are usually under negative pressure with respect to the external environment. Temperature gradients, combustion devices, and wind contribute to this pressure differential, which allows contaminants to infiltrate a building. Not even the most aggressive attempts to seal a building can make it completely airtight.

Most modern, large office buildings are under positive pressure through the use of mechanical ventilation. Theoretically, positive pressure prevents passive infiltration; however, uneven pressurization may lead to passive infiltration in some areas of the building. More importantly, ventilation systems draw air into a building. The placement of outdoor intakes determines the cleanliness of the air entering the building. Investigations of problem buildings have often identified these intakes in polluted locations such as parking garages or in proximity to exhaust stacks.

Pollutants may also contaminate indoor air when carried indoors by water and natural gas pipelines. For example, well water may carry radon or a range of volatile organic chemicals (VOCs) that come out of solution when taps are turned on.

Building Fabric and Interior Furnishings
The building structure and interior furnishings may contribute to indoor air contamination through the emission of volatile components or physical degradation of products. A myriad of building products and finishes, ranging from urea formaldehyde foam insulation (UFFI) to composition board to new carpets to adhesives to paints, emit VOCs. The abrasion of products such as asbestos-containing floor coverings and pipe lagging can also pollute indoor air.

Building fabric and furnishings may be contaminated by floods, high humidity, smoking, and consumer chemical use. With appropriate moisture, room temperature, and the inevitable shower of organic debris from people and pets, absorbent materials like rugs or fiber glass ventilation duct liners serve as culture media for biologic contaminants such as dust mites and fungi. Physical agitation of these materials by vacuuming or human traffic can result in sprays of biologic aerosols. Absorbent materials may also serve as sinks for VOCs, pesticides, and other chemicals generated in the environment. These sinks will then slowly reemit the contaminants.

Mechanical Systems
Mechanical devices such as heating, ventilation, and air-conditioning systems (HVAC); humidifiers; dehumidifiers; wiring configurations; and lighting provide the operating infrastructure of a building. When not properly designed, operated, or maintained, HVAC systems may lead to excursions from accepted indoor comfort parameters such as temperature, humidity, or air velocity. They may also contribute to the distribution of hazardous contaminants. Humidifiers and cooling towers may contribute to biologic and particulate contamination of indoor air. Lighting characteristics such as flicker, spectral range, and luminance are important environmental influences. Wiring configurations and mechanicals also add vibration and electromagnetic fields.

Occupant-Generated Pollution
The habits, hobbies, business, and metabolism of buildings' occupants affect IAQ. Though increasingly restricted in public buildings, environmental tobacco smoke remains an important indoor pollutant. Personal products such as perfumes and deodorants can generate VOCs. In the office, copiers, laser printers, and fax machines may produce pollutants. Carbonless copy paper, marking pens, adhesives, cleaning

products, and pesticides contribute to the contaminant load. When buildings mix functions, office air may be polluted by adjoining laboratories or industries when their hazardous processes are improperly contained.

Characterizing Indoor Air

Broadly categorized, the key factors in IAQ are: biologic agents, combustion products, particulates, pesticides, radon, VOCs, and physical factors such as temperature, humidity, and air velocity (Table 44-1). Though the potency of contaminant sources is a key determinant of indoor pollutant concentrations, other variables are code-

Table 44-1. Common sources and types of indoor contaminants

Types	External	Building fabric	Mechanical systems	Occupant generated
Biologic	Local flora Animals Insects Microorganisms	Wet insulation Wet carpet Wet ceiling tiles	Cooling towers Condensate pans Humidifier Moisture in ductwork	Respiratory droplet
Combustion products	Combustion engines Incinerators Forest fires Residential and industrial heating devices		Poorly vented heating and cooking devices Malfunctioning heating and cooking devices	Tobacco smoke
Particulates	Wind-blown soil Industrial emissions Diesel emis- sions		Poorly vented heating and cooking devices Malfunctioning heating and cooking devices Humidifiers Degrading fiberglass ductwork	Tobacco smoke Remodeling Hobbies Cleaning
Pesticides	Aerial spraying Exterior exter- minations Tracked in on feet from ex- ternal appli- cation	Treated build- ing materials Paints	Contaminated ductwork HVAC biocides	Pest control activities
Radon	Soil gas Well water Natural gas	Stone, brick, cement block		
VOCs	Underground storage tanks Hazardous waste Industrial air pollution Tap water pol- lution	Composition board Adhesives Caulks Carpets Furnishing Paints	Office machines	Consumer prod- ucts Human metab- olism

terminants, including air exchange, ventilation mixing efficiency, building volume, and contaminant removal.

Biologic Aerosols

The metabolism and decay of large and microbial organisms produce gaseous pollution. Animals and humans shed hair, dander, epidermal scales, and allergens. Animal handling and changing of cage litter may result in exposures to saliva, urine, and feces. Animals nesting in ventilation systems can lead to wide dissemination of their products. Decaying carcasses of small animals lead to characteristic putrid odors.

Microbial contaminants include viruses, bacteria, protozoa, fungi, pollens, insect parts, and arachnid excrement. Humans transmit a variety of infectious diseases by respiratory droplet, some of which may be disseminated in indoor air.

Indoor microbial concentrations become more hazardous when amplified by variations in temperature, humidity, and nutrition. Hospitable microbial reservoirs include rugs, humidifiers, cooling towers, and condensate pans. Dissemination may occur through the actions of ventilation systems and machines, or agitation by occupant activities.

Combustion Products

Combustion generates gaseous and particulate products, some of which are prominent outdoor air pollutants: nitrogen oxides, sulfur dioxide, carbon monoxide, and respirable suspended particulates (RSP). Environmental tobacco smoke (ETS) alone adds more than 4000 compounds to indoor air. As many as 42 of these are known or suspected carcinogens [4].

Indoor exposures to combustion products vary seasonally and with the presence of smokers. In addition to fires, malfunctioning or unvented combustion devices in poorly ventilated areas can create short-term, hazardous excursions above Occupational Safety and Health Administration (OSHA) PELs. Uncommonly, carbon monoxide may reach intoxicating levels in work areas of buildings with parking garages.

Particulates

Indoor particulates are characterized by chemical composition and physical conformation. Gaseous air pollutants, such as radon daughters or formaldehyde, may adhere to suspended particulates and be inhaled.

Indoor levels of RSP may exceed National Ambient Air Quality Standards (NAAQS), although the building envelope typically excludes most outdoor particulates. Indoor sources are therefore the preeminent polluters. Tobacco smoke and unvented combustion devices are the most important generators of RSP; however, activities such as sanding, sweeping, construction, or unprofessional asbestos or lead abatement projects may generate short-term intense particulate exposures. Unfiltered ultrasonic humidifiers using tap water are capable of raising RSP above the NAAQS in a closed room.

Indoor exposure to asbestos has been intensely scrutinized. Chrysotile asbestos was used extensively in building materials until 1978, when most construction and insulation uses were banned. The EPA has estimated that 20% of public buildings (733,000) in the United States have some asbestos-containing materials [5]. This estimate excludes residential and school structures. Several studies indicate that steady-state indoor fiber counts are at least four orders of magnitude less than the current OSHA PEL of 0.2 fibers/cc. Further, the vast majority of indoor fibers tend to be the least toxic fiber—chrysotile—and less than 5 μ. On the other hand, poorly conducted asbestos abatement projects and activities that resuspend settled fibers, such as dry sweeping or vacuuming, can generate short-term exposures well over 100 fibers/cc [6]. As a result, current EPA policy recommends identification of indoor sources of asbestos, alerting persons potentially exposed about measures to minimize exposure, and in-place management. If asbestos-containing materials are at risk of being substantially disturbed through such actions as remodeling, full precautions are recommended, including asbestos removal.

The most important, preventable pediatric environmental disease is lead poisoning. According to the Agency for Toxic Substances and Disease Registry estimates, lead paint burdens 52% of all housing stock in the United States [7]. Ingestion of lead particulates from degrading paint remains the largest contributor to children's lead body burdens. Though many of these particulates are nonrespirable, remodeling efforts and unprofessional lead abatement projects that involve heating, scraping, and sanding can produce respirable lead particulates that become a hazard. (See

Chap. 43, Clinical Environmental Medicine, for a thorough discussion on childhood lead poisoning.)

Pesticides

Almost all indoor environments contain pesticides. Health effects may include acute systemic intoxication, irritating and immunopathic effects, and chronic effects such as neurobehavioral disorders and increased cancer risk. Although long-term concentrations are generally in the microgram range, reentering recently treated environments may result in exposures in the milligram range. As environmentally persistent products such as chlordane have been removed from the market because of long-term risks unacceptable to the EPA, they have often been replaced with more acutely toxic substances such as the carbamates and organophosphates.

Hundreds of chemicals classified as "inert ingredients" are included in pesticide formulations, many of which are of immediate toxicologic concern. Several are suspected carcinogens. Little toxicologic information is available to characterize the vast majority. A chemical banned for use as an active ingredient in pesticides may be used as an inert component.

Radon

Radon 222, an inert gas, is the by-product of the radioactive decay of uranium 238. With a half-life of 3.8 days, radon decays into several short-lived chemically reactive, and radioactive progeny: polonium 218, lead 214, bismuth 214, and polonium 214. The carcinogenic effects of radon are ascribed to these short-lived progeny, which, in contrast to radon, adhere to respiratory tissue.

Indoor radon levels combine with building factors such as ventilation rates to determine radon daughter concentrations. Though the technology exists to measure radon daughters directly, it is far cheaper to measure radon gas.

Radon exposures outdoors average less than 0.2 picocuries per liter (pCi/L). Indoor levels almost always are higher, averaging about 1.5 pCi/L in houses and ranging as high as 2700 pCi/L. By way of comparison, uranium miners' exposures are limited to less than 16 pCi/L today, with historic levels thought to be between 24 and 1380 pCi/L. The best estimates suggest that radon levels exceed 8 pCi/L in 1 to 3% of the basements (primarily) of homes in the United States [8].

The bulk of radon enters buildings as a soil gas, though other sources include tap water from private wells, building products, and, minimally, natural gas. As a soil gas, radon primarily affects the lower levels of a building; concentrations of radon tend to decrease in higher levels.

Volatile Organic Chemicals

A wide range of building products, furnishings, and consumer products emit volatile organic compounds. About two dozen of those substances are definite or probable human carcinogens. Peak exposures may exceed by 100 to 1000 times the ambient concentrations. Emission rates, however, typically drop dramatically within the first days to months of the installation. Many components of the indoor environment serve as sinks, which absorb, then reemit, VOCs under certain environmental conditions.

Volatile organic chemicals are usually detected at levels considerably lower than OSHA PELs. When the total weight of indoor VOCs is considered, however, levels can reach milligrams per cubic meter. The total exposure assessment methodology (TEAM) studies conducted by the EPA found that indoor air level of VOCs can be 2 to 10 times that of outdoor levels [9]. Using gas chromatography–mass spectrometry (GCMS), VOC emissions sources can be "fingerprinted" to identify specific contaminants.

Two VOCs have achieved particular notoriety. Formaldehyde is an omnipresent indoor contaminant emitted by myriad products and processes as well as inhabitants. Though regulations and litigation have resulted in decreased emissions from building products, indoor levels of formaldehyde may still exceed 0.2 ppm.

Although new carpets emit a myriad of VOCs, 4-phenylcyclohexene (4-PC) has been identified as the preeminent peak in GCMS analysis. Levels have been measured in the range of 0.3 to 40 ppb. Airborne concentrations exceeding 5 ppb are odiferous and easily noted. Levels of 4-PC greater than 1 ppb have been closely related to clusters of health complaints associated with the installation of new carpet, most famously at the EPA headquarters, although other factors, such as ventilation and maintenance, were involved [10]. Nonetheless, little is known about the toxicology of 4-PC. Carpet manufacturers have voluntarily agreed to take measures to reduce VOC emissions.

Physical Factors

Several physical attributes of the indoor environment influence human comfort and are associated with health complaints. Temperature, relative humidity, and air velocity are the key factors affecting thermal comfort. The American Society of Heating, Refrigeration, and Air-Conditioning Engineers (ASHRAE) publishes guidelines that define an acceptable level of thermal comfort that satisfies about 80% of the occupants of an interior space. Relative humidity and temperature also influence concentrations of pollutants. Increasing these parameters leads to higher rates of microbial growth, and emissions of some VOCs, such as formaldehyde. As relative humidity falls below 30%, mucous membranes become more susceptible to irritants. At low relative humidities, electrostatic fields increase.

Ergonomic analysis has identified optimal lighting characteristics for tasks ranging from living room conversation to work at a computer terminal [11]. Glare, reflections, flickers, contrasts, and spectral distribution of light are as important as luminance. Fluorescent lighting, in fact, has played a role in creating indoor smog through the photooxidation of VOCs and combustion products [12].

Rarely do indoor environments expose occupants to noise levels that induce hearing loss. On the other hand, ambient noise levels may interfere with normal conversation and concentration. Levels of noise below 40 dBA (A-weighted decibel) are considered comfortable. The average residence without music or appliances running has a noise level of about 30 dBa, whereas the average office has a level of about 50 dBA [11]. Proximity to vehicle traffic and jetports leads to noise exposures that are usually uncontrollable by building occupants. Community standards for ambient noise have been established by the EPA with reference to its annoying characteristics (see Chap. 16, Noise-Induced Hearing Loss).

The relevance of other physical factors such as negative ion deficiency or electromagnetic fields to environmental quality is controversial. Many indoor polluted environments have negative ion deficiencies when compared to settings such as waterfalls or ocean beachfronts. Nonetheless, no consensus exists regarding the role of negative and positive ion ratios in building-related health complaints. Some indoor environments have significantly increased levels of electromagnetic fields (EMF) generated by electrical transmission equipment, wiring configurations, video display terminals, and household appliances. Dosimetry reveals widely fluctuating exposures related to the operation of these devices. No consensus exists about the impact of these fields on human health.

The Problem Building

Buildings can be categorized by both the complaint rates of their occupants and environmental factors. By convention, *problem buildings* are buildings in which either greater than 20% of the occupants have building-related health complaints or specific environmental contaminants have been linked with building-related illnesses. A *crisis building* is one in which complaints and public concern have reached the point that normal activities have been severely disrupted. A building may be considered "at risk" if an audit reveals one or more environmental problems that are commonly associated with health problems. A *healthy building* refers to a structure that is designed, maintained, and operated to minimize environmental risk factors and maximize comfort, well-being, and productivity.

A considerable body of literature points to several building characteristics that increase the likelihood of occupant complaints [13]. A recent meta-analysis indicated that sealed, mechanically ventilated, humidified, and air-conditioned buildings are more likely to generate complaints than naturally ventilated buildings [14]. An extensive, systematic investigation of symptoms in relation to environment noted the following factors related to complaint rates: (1) the total weight and potential allergenic component of the floor dust, (2) the area of fleecy material (soft, absorbent fabric) per cubic meter of air, (3) the length of open shelving per cubic meter of air, (4) the number of work stations, and (5) the air temperature [15]. Users of photocopiers, carbonless copy paper, and video display terminals were more likely to have building-related complaints. Complaint rates are more closely related to the intensity of pollution sources than to ventilation rates [16].

Several organizations have generated guidelines for building design, commissioning, operation, and maintenance [17–19].

Health Effects of IAP: Acute Building-Related Illnesses

Adverse health effects from IAP have been broadly interpreted to include discomfort, irritation, and decreased productivity along with frank disease [20]. The health problems arising from IAP in nonindustrial environments are summarized by the term *building-associated illnesses,* which include building-related illnesses (BRI) and the sick building syndrome (SBS). BRI have a defined pathophysiology attributable to a specific building contaminant. In contrast, SBS describes a group of transient symptoms, affected by entering and leaving a particular building. Causes of SBS remain speculative and are probably multifactorial. Usually, the attack rate of BRI in a building is relatively low, but is commonly accompanied by an epidemic of SBS. The occupational physician is likely to be asked to address apparent building-related illnesses in terms of diagnosis as well as prevention and control. The nature of the symptoms and disease that have been noted before the occupational physician's involvement will have a major effect on the type of intervention as well as assessment that may need to be performed.

Hypersensitivity Diseases

ALLERGIES. About 25% of Americans have asthma or other allergic diseases. The most common diseases related to buildings are allergic syndromes affecting the eyes, upper airways, lungs, and occasionally skin. Symptoms are usually caused by exposure to biologic or chemical agents to which an individual has been sensitized. Though aeroallergens are ubiquitous, sensitizing or precipitating exposures may be linked to a specific building where exposure occurs at particularly high levels. After sensitization, trace amounts of the allergen may provoke episodes of illness in some individuals. The clinical presentation, skin testing, or the radioallergosorbent (RAST) test point to specific allergens, and provocative challenges confirm the diagnosis. Symptoms and peak flow diaries, pre- and postshift spirometry, and serial methacholine challenge tests can be used to implicate a specific environment's role in precipitating asthma. Both immediate and late-onset asthma are observed.

Uncommonly, allergic or pseudoallergic phenomena have been linked to indoor chemical contaminants. For example, a component of carbonless copy paper, alkylphenol novalac resin, has been found to be responsible for anaphylactoid reactions in a small number of users [21]. Challenge with the chemical re-creates the syndrome. Formaldehyde has been linked with allergic or pseudoallergic phenomena affecting the eyes, nose, skin, and lungs.

HYPERSENSITIVITY PNEUMONITIS. Hypersensitivity pneumonitis may result in fever, chest tightness, cough, shortness of breath, malaise, and myalgia. Laboratory findings may include restrictive patterns on pulmonary function tests, pulmonary infiltrates, leukocytosis, and elevated serum precipitins to biologic agents found in the building that is potentially implicated. Pulmonary diffusion capacity and pulmonary exercise tolerance tests are the most sensitive tests for the disease. T-lymphocyte–predominant alveolitis is noted on bronchial alveolar lavage, and lung biopsy usually reveals granulomatous changes. Precipitation of the illness by bronchial challenge with suspected antigens remains the gold standard for diagnosis, but the responsible antigen is often never identified. Smokers seem to be relatively protected from this disease and atopy is not a predisposing factor.

Symptoms and signs usually resolve spontaneously after the cessation of exposure to the offending agent. Because continued exposure to even a small amount of the responsible antigen can lead to a chronic, progressive interstitial lung disease, permanent removal from the precipitating environment may be necessary *even after remediation.* Though hypersensitivity pneumonitis usually affects only a small number of building occupants, the severity of this illness demands thorough environmental investigation and remediation.

HUMIDIFIER FEVER. Humidifier fever presents as a flu-like syndrome similar to hypersensitivity pneumonitis but without objective pulmonary findings or the risk for chronic sequelae. Symptoms usually begin within 4 to 8 hours and resolve spontaneously within 24 hours after cessation of exposure. In contrast to hypersensitivity pneumonitis, the attack rate is high—between 25 and 40%. Though biologic aerosols are the sine qua non of humidifier fever, the self-limited and benign nature of the illness has obstructed investigation of its pathophysiology. Many investigators believe that the illness may more closely resemble organic dust toxic syndromes caused by endotoxin than immunogenic antigens.

Infectious Diseases

After an incubation period of about 7 days, infection with the bacterium *L. pneumophila* causes a potentially fatal pneumonia and multisystem disease in a small percentage of exposed people. Historically, 15 to 20% of those infected die from the illness. Diagnosis is made by chest x-ray, isolation of the organism from body fluids, direct fluorescent antibody testing, and a significant increase in antibody titers. Treatment with erythromycin decreases morbidity and mortality.

Legionnaire's disease, uniquely transmitted by airborne droplet, occurs only sporadically in the community, despite the ubiquity of the *Legionella* organism. Infective aerosols have been traced to building reservoirs notable for the presence of water. Organisms may also originate from external sources such as excavation projects that liberate the organism from the soil.

Unlike Legionnaire's disease, Pontiac fever presents as a benign flu-like illness of fever, chills, headache, and myalgia, but no pulmonary involvement. Attack rates are high, sometimes nearing 100%. This illness is also caused by the *Legionella* organism. Though serologic testing demonstrates exposure, the organism has never been isolated from infected hosts. Why the same microbe can lead to two illnesses of very different severity and prognosis is not known.

In theory, epidemics of other respiratory illnesses that can be transmitted by aerosols may be linked to a building. Rare examples include histoplasmosis related to the disturbance of contaminated bird droppings concentrated near windows or air intakes. Opportunistic fungal pathogens, *Pseudomonas* and *Acinetobacter,* may contaminate therapeutic respiratory devices or humidifiers, but pose a risk only to immunocompromised hosts. A few airborne outbreaks of tuberculosis have been linked to poorly ventilated environments [22]. Some evidence, not yet conclusive, supports the theory that epidemics of common communicable viral respiratory diseases such as influenza, the common cold, measles, rubella, and chicken pox may be associated with airborne transmission in a building, due to inadequate ventilation. The multiplicity of opportunities for acquiring these illnesses in the community and by close personal contact makes linking an illness to a specific environment problematic.

Acute and Subacute Intoxications

Acute or subacute poisoning may occur from exposure to several chemicals, including carbon monoxide, heavy metals, pesticides, and volatile organics.

CARBON MONOXIDE. Though carbon monoxide poisoning rarely occurs in office settings, it is a leading cause of poisoning at home. About 1800 accidental deaths occur annually [23]. Many of these are caused by poorly vented or malfunctioning combustion devices. The number of fatalities may be considerably higher in people with preexisting cardiovascular disease, since carboxyhemoglobin levels in the 2 to 5% range can precipitate acute cardiovascular events. More insidiously, low-level carbon monoxide poisoning may present as a persistent flu-like syndrome. Reports have documented that between 2.8 and 23.6% of people presenting to an emergency room suffer from carbon monoxide poisoning [24].

HEAVY METALS. Though environmental lead poisoning is largely the result of lead paint, contaminated water ingestion, and lead-based pottery, poisoning may also occur by inhalation of dusts and fumes generated by the abrasion, heating, or burning of lead-painted surfaces. Hobbies such as glazing pottery, stained glass work, and making lead shot or fishing sinkers are particularly hazardous sources of airborne lead.

Acrodynia associated with exposure to a home recently painted with a latex paint containing phenyl mercury raised the concern of widespread exposures. Subsequently, an investigation identified elevated levels of mercury in other persons exposed to homes freshly painted with latex paint containing the preservative *phenylmercuric acetate* [25]. As a result, the EPA banned the manufacture of mercury compounds in all latex paints as of September 1991.

PESTICIDES. The banning of environmentally persistent pesticides such as chlordane has led to their substitution with shorter-acting products more acutely toxic to humans. Pesticides are the second most common cause of childhood poisoning in the US. At least 46.5% of accidental pesticide deaths between 1980 and 1985 occurred at home. Nonoccupational symptoms attributed to pesticides include sensitivity reactions, especially to pyrethrin products, which are antigenically similar to ragweed. The toxicology of many of the "inert" ingredients of pesticides is unknown.

Organic solvent carriers probably precipitate many of the acute symptoms attributed to pesticide use in buildings.

VOLATILE ORGANIC CHEMICALS. Exposure to VOCs, such as xylene, toluene, methylene chloride, and mineral spirits, may occur at levels exceeding OSHA PELs during remodeling efforts, with the use of solvent cleaning products or with hobbies such as furniture refinishing.

MYCOTOXICOSIS. Mycotoxicosis is a rare toxic response to some molds that produces fatigue, irritability, and myocarditis. A building-related outbreak was associated with *stachybotrys atra* [26].

Irritant Diseases

Rarely does a single indoor pollutant achieve sufficient levels to cause an acute, new-onset building-related illness such as conjunctivitis, rhinitis, pharyngitis, or reactive airway dysfunction syndrome (RADS). The mixture of chlorine and ammonia-based cleaners, however, and formaldehyde are examples. Poorly installed fibrous glass and carpet shampoo residues may provoke transient upper-respiratory and dermatologic irritant syndromes. More commonly, many airborne irritants are present at low levels and together aggravate preexisting allergic and respiratory diseases. The vapor and particulate mixture of ETS raises the risk of lower-respiratory infections and symptoms in children and irritates the eyes, nose, throat, and lower-respiratory tract of others. Though not firmly established, ETS can increase adult respiratory symptoms, and exacerbate asthma. Other combustion products, including particulates, sulfur dioxide, and nitrogen oxides, have been linked with respiratory illnesses in vulnerable populations.

Chronic Building-Related Diseases

Indoor pollutants have the potential for causing chronic diseases. Those of chief concern are cancer and neurobehavioral and pulmonary disorders.

Cancer

The presence of carcinogens in indoor air has prompted aggressive public health and regulatory actions. *Asbestos, benzene, radon, and ETS are all class A (EPA) carcinogens.* Though radon and ETS are of most concern, the risks of VOCs, pesticides, and, more recently, EMF have all been targeted.

Radon

The increased risk of lung cancer has been well demonstrated among uranium miners working underground with exposures to high concentrations of radon progeny. Most epidemiologic data suggest at least an additive if not a synergistic effect between smoking and radon. Extrapolating from the experience of uranium miners, various organizations have estimated that from 9000 to 16,000 excess lung cancer deaths annually are attributable to residential radon exposure [27]. Using EPA models, 50% of excess cancers occur at less than the mean residential level of 1.5 pCi/L due to radon. A recent case control study demonstrated that risks of lung cancer associated with residential radon exposure are consistent with estimates based on miner data [62].

ETS and Combustion Products

The International Agency for Research on Cancer, the EPA, the Surgeon General's office, and the National Research Council all consider ETS a human pulmonary carcinogen. OSHA may soon regulate ETS as an occupational carcinogen. Though the epidemiology has not yet been clarified, ETS probably interacts with other indoor carcinogenic pollutants such as radon.

Fossil fuel combustion also produces carcinogenic by-products, such as polynuclear aromatic hydrocarbons (PAH) that have been associated with cancer in coke oven and coal gas workers. Studies have revealed increased risks of nasopharyngeal cancer in populations in the developing world who heat and cook with poorly vented fires.

Particulates

Environmental Protection Agency risk estimates of cancer associated with indoor exposures to *asbestos* generated a massive regulatory and abatement effort in the 1980s. The estimates were based on the health experience of asbestos workers and their spouses along with assumptions about indoor exposures that have since been revised. In 1985, the EPA published lifetime estimated risks as high as $2.7 \times 10^{-3}/$ 0.01 fibers/cc of contracting cancer from asbestos [28]. At the time, the EPA calculated that school children were exposed to about 0.01 fibers/cc. Subsequent environmental hygiene surveys have demonstrated that typical indoor exposures are several orders of magnitude lower than occupational exposures except when asbestos-containing materials are disturbed. As a consequence, cancer risks from occupying buildings with asbestos are probably minimal [29].

Volatile Organic Chemicals and Pesticides

Individual risk estimates for the carcinogenic effects of VOCs and pesticides in indoor air have been generated [20]. These estimates have led to the withdrawal of several pesticides, such as chlordane, from commercial use and stricter regulation of some VOCs, such as formaldehyde and benzene. Six of the most prevalent and well-established carcinogenic VOCs may be responsible for 1000 to 5000 excess cancer cases annually [20].

Electromagnetic Fields

In the early 1980s, some reports raised concern that very low and extra low frequency EMF emanating from video display units were associated with reproductive effects. Since then, careful epidemiology, which for the first time included actual measurements of fields, refuted these concerns [30]. EMF has been associated with increasing risks of childhood leukemia and cancers in occupationally exposed workers. Great uncertainties remain regarding dose relationships of EMF to the studied health outcomes. Indeed, because of a lack of biologic plausibility, the question remains as to whether the association with EMF is confounded by other variables.

Neurobehavioral Disorders

Several indoor pollutants have the capability of causing chronic neurobehavioral disorders. These disorders include carbon monoxide, pesticide, and solvent encephalopathies resulting from high-dose acute intoxications. Whether chronic low-dose exposures to these agents as found in typical indoor settings can cause chronic encephalopathies remains controversial. Though the neurotoxicity of mercury is well understood, no one knows the extent to which mercury emitted from latex paints (phenylmercuric acetate) may have caused chronic neurologic disease.

Cognitive effects of lead have been identified at blood lead levels as low as 10 μg/ 100 ml [31]. Currently, in the US, between 3 and 4 million children younger than 6 years have blood lead levels over 15 μg/100 ml [31]. Though evidence is strong that these children have persistent measurable cognitive and behavioral problems with substantial social consequences, the biologic impact of lead burdens acquired in early childhood on neurobehavior in later adult life remains speculative.

Pulmonary Disorders

Several classes of indoor pollutants can cause chronic pulmonary disorders. Unremitting exposures to sensitizing chemical or biologic agents, such as mites, can lead to chronic asthma. Persistent exposures to immunogenic agents may also provoke hypersensitivity pneumonitis to progress to interstitial fibrosis. ETS has been well established to cause reduced lung development in children. Historically, para-occupational exposures to asbestos in family members of asbestos workers have been linked with pleural plaques, but typical indoor exposures to asbestos are not sufficient to cause fibrotic pulmonary diseases.

Sick Building Syndrome

Sick building syndrome is a constellation of nonspecific symptoms related to occupation of a specific building environment. Molhave [32] has grouped the symptoms into five classes, with the possibility that SBS may represent several pathophysiologic mechanisms: sensory irritation, neurologic or general health symptoms, skin irritation, nonspecific hypersensitivity reactions, and odor and taste problems. An individual typically suffers from SBS in the context of an epidemic of occupant complaints.

Though no specific environmental contaminants have been identified as causative agents of SBS, numerous hypotheses have been advanced. An early theory attributed high complaint rates to inadequate dilution of building contaminants with ventilation. Blind manipulations of ventilation have been shown to affect complaints in some buildings. Nonetheless, substantial evidence has accrued that inadequate ventilation is only one of the variables of importance in causing various health complaints between buildings. In fact, increasing ventilation rates in some buildings heighten dissatisfaction. Focus has therefore turned to categories and sources of pollution. One theory proposes that irritant and neurologic symptoms result from exposures to a large number of VOCs whose total weight (TVOC) reaches toxicologic significance. Though controlled laboratory evidence concerning the neurotoxic effects of low-level VOCs remains inconclusive, data clearly indicate dose-response relationships of mucous membrane irritation to VOC levels greater than 5 mg/m^3. Other credible theories implicate organic debris, endotoxin, respirable suspended particulates, and aberrant relative humidity. Causation is probably multifactorial.

Whatever their cause, nonspecific building-related health complaints are common. Systematic surveys of occupants of buildings in which environmental problems had not been previously identified consistently reveal complaint rates higher than 20%. At the extreme, a British study of 4373 office workers in 42 office buildings found that 80% of the workers had at least one work-related symptom [33].

Epidemiologic research has pointed to a role for individual and organizational psychosocial factors in building-associated nonspecific symptoms [34]. For example, women and those in clerical jobs report more symptoms than men and professional and managerial job categories. Organizational conflict and occupational stress have also been linked with higher complaint rates. Some investigators have interpreted these findings as sole explanations for SBS when building investigations have failed to reveal clear environmental etiologies. The importance of social dynamics, even in crisis buildings, should not be confused with mass psychogenic illness.

Mass Psychogenic Illness

Mass psychogenic illness (MPI) presents with symptoms compatible with hyperventilation, features not readily explained by organic mechanisms, a visual or verbal chain of transmission, and higher incidence in women [35]. Onset is usually explosive and new cases correlate with person-to-person transmission rather than a common source outbreak. Chronic building-related health complaints, though influenced by psychosocial dynamics, are unlikely to be caused by MPI. MPI should not be diagnosed merely because of an absence of an environmental explanation for occupant complaints.

Multiple Chemical Sensitivities

Practitioners interested in IAP will invariably encounter the clinical problem of multiple chemical sensitivities (MCS). Though controversy persists as to whether it represents a distinct diagnostic entity [36–41], MCS exists as a clinically recognizable syndrome [42]. Several working case definitions and plausible pathophysiologic mechanisms have been proposed [43–45].

Though the etiology of MCS has yet to be ascertained, many sufferers relate the onset and recurrent precipitation of their symptoms to exposures to IAP, particularly VOCs or pesticides.

Despite scientific uncertainties, the social trend has been to consider MCS as a bona fide handicap deserving of social security disability and reasonable accommodations under provisions of the Fair Housing Act and the Americans with Disabilities Act. Approaches to accommodating the individual reporting MCS have been reviewed elsewhere [46].

Clinical Evaluation of Building-Associated Illness

Building-associated illnesses resemble common clinical complaints and illnesses seen by primary care physicians. Only when armed with a high index of suspicion can the clinician identify the environmental contributors to these problems. Patients may present either with health complaints or anxiety about future health effects caused by building-related exposures.

Practitioners may reach one of five possible conclusions when evaluating patients with building-associated complaints: (1) The person has a disease caused by a *specific environmental agent;* for example, a child with neurobehavioral abnormalities has lead poisoning. (2) The person has a disease to which *multiple factors contribute,* including an indoor environment. A sample case could be lung cancer diagnosed in a smoker who has lived his life in a house contaminated with high levels of radon. (3) The individual may have a preexisting problem originally unrelated to a specific environment, such as asthma, that is *provoked* by indoor air exposures to low-level irritants. (4) A person is diagnosed with a problem, such as chronic fatigue syndrome, *that has no known environmental etiology.* (5) The individual is found to have a problem, such as systemic sclerosis, in which *environmental etiologies remain speculative.*

Healthy building occupants may also ask occupational physicians to evaluate future health risks associated with current exposures. Standard clinical toxicologic methods can be used with reference to published IAQ guidelines to communicate risks.

The *clinical evaluation* begins with an interview aimed at eliciting symptoms and the temporal sequence of those symptoms in relationship to specific environments and activities. The practitioner compares complaints to expected symptoms for particular building contaminants [11]. During the interview, the clinician should inquire about complaints of other building occupants. Individual and building population psychosocial dynamics should be explored. All underlying, known medical problems should be identified. Detailed occupational and environmental histories are essential [11, 18, 47]. Environmental data that have been collected by formal investigation should be reviewed.

Physical examination of patients with SBS complaints is usually unrevealing. Slit lamp examinations, however, reveal a preponderance of tear film instability and diminished foam in the inner canthus [48]. Results of examinations of patients with building-related illnesses (BRI), such as asthma, are characteristic of the illness itself.

Laboratory investigations are unhelpful in the assessment of SBS, but can be diagnostic with BRI.

The evaluation of hypersensitivity syndromes can be assisted with standard allergy tests, total and specific immunoglobulin E (IgE), and precipitating antibodies with specific reference to biologic agents identified in the suspect building. Standard reference laboratory hypersensitivity panels, however, may not include the offending agents. When critical for clinical or forensic purposes, samples from the building can be used to develop antigen preparations for in vitro tests and in vivo bronchial or nasal challenges. Positive antibody tests confirm exposure but do not by themselves establish etiology of complaints. Though helpful, appropriately timed chest radiography is not a sensitive tool in the diagnosis of hypersensitivity pneumonitis. Serial spirometry, peak flowmeters, and methacholine challenge are useful. Diffusion capacities are particularly sensitive in assessing hypersensitivity pneumonitis when timed to coincide with exposure to and avoidance of the suspected environment. Bronchial alveolar lavage and biopsy add confirmatory pathologic information when clinical diagnostic confusion persists about the possibility of hypersensitivity pneumonitis or bronchopulmonary aspergillosis.

The building-relatedness of upper-airway diseases and complaints, whether irritant or allergic in origin, is particularly difficult to confirm with laboratory tests. Timed with environmental challenges, clinical tools include rhinometry (a measure of nasal resistance), rhinoscopy, laryngoscopy, and computerized analysis of voice quality (available from many speech pathologists). Nasal smears or lavage help define the pathophysiology of rhinitis [49].

Occasionally, laboratory examination can be helpful in the evaluation of building-associated dermatologic complaints. Probably the most common example is fiberglass dermatitis. Scotch tape applied to actively pruritic skin before washing can be examined microscopically to identify certain types of fiberglass fibers.

An important clinical and legal responsibility of the physician is the decision about the relationship of a specific environment to an individual's symptoms. Medical diagnosis and appropriate therapeutic interventions may not be possible without an objective understanding of environmental exposures. As with all occupational and environmental illness, the most specific treatment of a building illness always begins with minimizing exposure to the offending agent(s). Even for illnesses with a suspected relationship to the environment, however, causative environmental agents may not be identified.

Litigation in the area of IAP is increasing rapidly. The range of these legal issues are reviewed elsewhere [50, 51].

Evaluation of Problem Buildings

Building evaluation protocols share a common theme. Investigations should be staged. Details of each of these phases for large and residential buildings have been reviewed elsewhere [52–54]. The most useful tools in the early phases of investigation are the senses and experience of the investigator. Detailed measurement of specific contaminants is seldom necessary. Sophisticated measurements should be performed only late in an investigation when attempting to confirm environmental or medical hypotheses. When assessments proceed beyond the initial phases, a multidisciplinary team including engineers, industrial hygienists, physicians, epidemiologists, and microbiologists becomes essential to a satisfactory outcome.

Analysis of the psychosocial dynamics of building complaints is best begun early in an investigation. Too often, psychosocial issues are invoked as an explanation for symptoms when environmental factors are not readily identified. The investigators' activities are likely to affect social dynamics. Confrontation can result when investigators and facility managers dichotomize environmental and psychological explanations. Organizational crisis may result, with decreased productivity and even evacuation, while occupants demand repeated investigations for "phantom" toxins. As part of a strategy to minimize opportunity for anxious speculation and distrust, building occupants should be kept informed of the progress and conclusions of the investigation. A task force that includes representatives of different job categories in a building serves this purpose well. The task force plays the equally important role of informing investigators and building managers about building occupant concerns and their hypotheses about causation.

The *first phase* of an investigation begins with the collection of general information about the building and occupant complaints. The use of semistructured questionnaires for the collection of data by interview and walk-around facilitates this process. In fact, protocols have been sufficiently refined so that many building managers are able to conduct the first phase of investigation and remediation without resorting to outside consultation. Occupants, facility managers, maintenance engineers, and custodial supervisors should be interviewed; appropriate representatives should accompany the investigator on the walk-around. Special attention should be focused on the HVAC system, extent of fleecy material, areas of moisture, smoking policies, occupant activities, remodeling efforts, maintenance procedures, cleaning products and practices, and occupant density. Measurements of temperature, relative humidity, and carbon dioxide are conveniently and cheaply included in this phase. Carbon dioxide concentrations are useful indicators of how effectively a space is ventilated for human occupation. Carbon dioxide levels above 800 ppm point to inadequate ventilation. On the other hand, carbon dioxide levels do not reflect the adequacy of the ventilation in dealing with nonphysiologic sources of contamination, such as ETS or VOCs [16].

This general environmental assessment in combination with a basic understanding of the epidemiology of building complaints often is sufficient to identify environmental risk factors worthy of intervention. If investigators identify individuals with suspected medical illness, especially pulmonary disorders, they should recommend medical evaluation.

The *second phase* of an investigation should proceed only with specific environmental or medical hypotheses in mind. In some cases, detailed epidemiology may be necessary to generate these hypotheses. Though seldom possible in practice, every attempt should be made to conduct such epidemiology with use of control buildings. Shotgun attempts to measure every possible pollutant should be avoided. One example of a specific hypothesis is a pattern of building-related headaches in people served by a ventilation system whose outdoor air intake is in a parking garage. This problem should lead to measurement of carbon monoxide levels. In another example, a history of extensive flooding of a carpet in an area of high complaints might lead to biologic sampling of the carpet and nearby air. The results of these environmental analyses would then be correlated with clinical data.

Industrial hygienists must be careful to use sampling methods appropriate for IAQ investigations [55, 56]. The sensitivity of industrial methods may not be appropriate. Timing of measurements will critically affect results. Climatic conditions, the operating state of HVAC systems, and building activities often affect contaminant levels. Establishing worst-case environmental scenarios is usually appropriate. For example, brief but intense showers of mold spores may be the event of interest in precipitating medical symptoms. This event may best be reproduced by actions such as banging a ventilation duct or jumping on a carpet. Research has also documented that personal breathing zone exposures may vary considerably from area samples in indoor settings. Biomonitoring for indoor contaminants has proved extremely useful in assessing exposure to such contaminants as ETS and carbon monoxide.

Seldom will contaminant levels exceed industrial guidelines, and many contaminants, particularly the bioaerosols, cannot be readily compared to a recommended limit. As a possible clue to the significance of a contaminant level, the investigator should compare concentrations measured in different locations in a building with outdoor concentrations. These contaminant variations may become meaningful when compared to the spatial distribution of health complaints in a building.

Particularly when environmental causation is elusive, biologic assays can be used to assess perceived pollution. Human panels have the greatest utility. A panel of people can be trained to reliably rate their dissatisfaction with air quality [57].

When an individual is affected and in the absence of recognized or readily corrected environmental hazards, medical removal is usually the action of choice. In other cases, environmental interventions may be recommended. Investigators should devise written and oral methods for notifying all building occupants about the study conclusions and action plans. Follow-up environmental and medical assessments of the impact of abatement should be made. In cases of SBS, building occupants and management must be informed that resolution of all building-related complaints is unlikely. Complaint rates are not likely to fall much below 20%.

Improving IAQ

Concerns about productivity, costs, and litigation have prompted concerted efforts from diverse business, professional, and governmental sectors to devise strategies for preventing IAQ problems. If building investigation protocols can be considered as tertiary prevention, then additional approaches may be categorized as secondary and primary prevention. Off-the-shelf IAQ guidelines now exist for those involved at every stage of a building's life cycle from its design to its commissioning, operation, maintenance, and remodeling [18, 19, 58, 59].

Secondary Prevention

Secondary prevention of poor IAQ involves the identification of environmental risk factors and occupant concerns before they become problems. Routine preventive maintenance schedules are advised, with particular focus on the HVAC system and known potential sources of IAP such as water-soaked carpeting. Facility managers should conduct periodic environmental audits using published check sheets. Some of these activities, such as asbestos and lead hazard identification, are mandated in certain buildings. Many states have laws about ETS in public buildings that require internal policies and monitoring. Radon levels should be measured according to current EPA recommendations.

Building managers are wise to devise a mechanism for soliciting and responding to occupant environmental concerns and comfort complaints. Notifying occupants about building audit activities is also recommended.

Primary Prevention

Steps to optimize IAQ can be taken in conjunction with other goals such as energy efficiency, structural integrity, safety, spatial utility, and aesthetics. Primary prevention begins with building and renovations design, for which guidelines have been published [18, 19, 58, 59].

Building, furnishing, and consumer product choices represent additional opportunities for minimizing IAP. As the result of regulatory actions, some of the most prevalent indoor contaminants, such as asbestos, lead paint, and chlordane, are not found in new buildings. Ironically, in each case their substitutes, man-made mineral fibers, mercury-contaminated latex paint, and organophosphate pesticides, have raised concerns of their own. Though desirable, substituting less hazardous products is unfortunately not always straightforward. Considerable controversy exists regarding the toxicity of many common building products and furnishings. Not only are there large gaps in basic toxicology for the thousands of chemicals used indoors, but other important questions remain. For example, products with highly volatile organic chemicals may have very high emission rates for the first week of installation that then dramatically fall off. Are these items more or less hazardous than products with lower rates but considerably longer periods of emission? Standardized methods for evaluating the emissions of building products and furnishings have been developed. Product choice schemes based on emission rates, known health effects, quantity used, and other considerations have been developed to assist construction and design managers in the midst of uncertainty [60].

Many administrative measures can also be taken to minimize IAP; these begin with the process of commissioning a building for its first use. Occupation should not occur until construction is finished and environmental controls are operating as designed. With the knowledge that new product emission rates are often high, some authorities have recommended that products be aged before installation or even that entire buildings be "baked" at increased ambient temperatures and ventilated at a high rate for a few days before occupation [61]. Renovations, maintenance activities, cleaning, exterminations, and other activities known to generate high levels of pollutants should be organized to minimize occupant exposures.

Finally, any comprehensive and successful attempt to manage air quality requires the training and education of all individuals managing the environment. Specific OSHA standards mandate this communication for specific hazards such as asbestos. Education of residential occupants has begun for lead, radon, asbestos, and a variety of other residential hazards through several governmental and voluntary agencies, but the education and practice of architects and construction contractors have lagged (see Chap. 37, Training and Communications).

Conclusion

Indoor air pollution has become a chief priority in the control of environmental threats to human health. Though our understanding of low-level air pollutants is hardly complete, known health effects range from discomfort, to illness, to death. Estimates of the associated economic impact are staggering. Those concerned with IAQ now have available considerable information to assist in the investigation, treatment, and prevention of building-associated illnesses.

References

1. Kreiss, K. The Epidemiology of Building-Related Complaints and Illness. In J. E. Cone and M. J. Hodgson (eds.), *Problem Buildings: Building-Associated Illness and the Sick Building Syndrome. Occup. Med. State of the Art Rev.* 4:575, 1989.
2. *New York Times,* September 11, 1988, p. 1.
3. Woods, J. E. Cost Avoidance and Productivity in Owning and Operating Buildings. In J. E. Cone and M. J. Hodgson (eds.), *Problem Buildings: Building-Associated Illness and the Sick Building Syndrome. Occup. Med. State of the Art Rev.* 4:753, 1989.
4. *Respiratory Health Effects of Passive Smoking: Lung Cancer and Other Disorders.* EPA/600/6-90/006F. Washington, DC: Office of Health and Environmental Assessment, Office of Research and Development, US Environmental Protection Agency, December 1992.
5. *EPA Study of Asbestos Containing Materials in Public Buildings—A Report to Congress.* Washington, DC: US Environmental Protection Agency, February 1988.

6. Balmes, J. R., DaPonte, A., and Cone, J. E. Asbestos Related Disease in Custodial and Building Maintenance Workers from a Large Municipal School District. In P. J. Landrigan and H. Kazemi (eds.), *The Third Wave of Asbestos Disease: Exposure to Asbestos in Place. Ann. N.Y. Acad. Sci.* 643:540, 1991.
7. *The Nature and Extent of Lead Poisoning in Children in the United States: A Report to Congress.* Agency for Toxic Substances and Disease Registry, Public Health Service, US Department of Health and Human Services, July 1988.
8. Nero, A. V., et al. Distribution of airborne radon-222 concentrations in U.S. homes. *Science* 234:992, 1986.
9. Wallace, L. A. Volatile Organic Chemicals. In J. M. Samet and J. D. Spengler (eds.), *Indoor Air Pollution—A Health Perspective.* Baltimore: The Johns Hopkins University Press, 1991. Pp. 252–272.
10. Sullivan, J. B., Van Ert, M., and Krieger, G. R. Indoor Air Quality and Human Health. In J. B. Sullivan, Jr., and G. R. Krieger, *Hazardous Materials Toxicology: Clinical Principles of Environmental Health.* Baltimore: Williams & Wilkins, 1992. P. 679.
11. *Introduction to Indoor Air Quality—A Self-Paced Learning Module.* EPA/400/3-91/002. US Environmental Protection Agency, United States Public Health Service, National Environmental Health Association, July 1991.
12. Sterling, E., and Sterling, T. The impact of different ventilation levels and fluorescent lighting types on building illness: An experimental study. *Can. J. Public Health* 74:385, 1983.
13. Kreiss, K. The sick building syndrome: Where is the epidemiologic basis? *Am. J. Public Health* 80:1172, 1990.
14. Mendell, M. J., and Smith, A. H. Consistent pattern of elevated symptoms in air conditioned office buildings: A reanalysis of epidemiologic studies. *Am. J. Public Health* 80:1193, 1990.
15. Kreiss, K. The Epidemiology of Building-Related Complaints and Illness. In J. E. Cone and M. J. Hodgson (eds.), *Problem Buildings: Building-Associated Illness and the Sick Building Syndrome. Occup. Med. State of the Art Rev.* 4:575, 1989.
16. Menzies, R., et al. *The effect of varying levels of outdoor air supply in the symptom of sick building syndrome. N. Engl. J. Med.* 328:821, 1993.
17. *Ventilation for Acceptable Indoor Air Quality.* ASHRAE Standard 62-1989.
18. *Building Air-Quality. A Guide for Building Owners and Facility Managers.* EPA/400/1-91/033, DHHS (NIOSH) Publications no. 91-114, December 1991.
19. Designing Healthy Buildings: Indoor Air Quality. Washington, DC: The American Institute of Architects, 1993.
20. *Introduction to Indoor Air Quality—A Reference Manual.* EPA/400/3-91/003. US Environmental Protection Agency, United States Public Health Service, National Environmental Health Association, July 1991.
21. Lamarte, F. P., Merchant, J. A., and Casale, T. B. Acute systemic reactions to carbonless copy paper associated with histamine release. *J.A.M.A.* 260:242, 1988.
22. Burge, H. A. Indoor Air and Infectious Disease. In J. E. Cone and M. J. Hodgson (eds.), *Problem Buildings: Building-Associated Illness and the Sick Building Syndrome. Occup. Med. State of the Art Rev.* 4:713, 1989.
23. Coultas, D. B., and Lambert, W. E. Carbon Monoxide. In J. M. Samet and J. D. Spengler (eds.), *Indoor Air Pollution—A Health Perspective.* Baltimore: The Johns Hopkins University Press, 1991. Pp. 187–208.
24. Heckerling, P. S., et al. Screening admissions from the emergency department for occult carbon monoxide poisoning. *Am. J. Emerg. Med.* 8:301, 1990.
25. Agocs, M. M., et al. Mercury exposure from interior latex paint. *N. Engl. J. Med.* 323:1096, 1990.
26. World Health Organization. *Indoor Air Quality: Biological Contaminants.* WHO Regional Publications, European Series no. 31, 1988.
27. Samet, J. M. Radon. In J. M. Samet and J. D. Spengler (eds.), *Indoor Air Pollution—A Health Perspective.* Baltimore: The Johns Hopkins University Press, 1991. Pp. 323–351.
28. US Environmental Protection Agency. *Airborne Asbestos Health Update.* EPA/600/8-84-003F. Research Triangle Park, NC: US EPA Office of Health and Environmental Assessment, 1985.
29. Spengler, J. D. Sources and Concentrations of Indoor Air Pollution. In J. M. Samet, and J. D. Spengler, *Indoor Air Pollution—A Health Perspective.* Baltimore: The Johns Hopkins University Press, 1991. Pp. 51–55.

30. Schnorr, T. M., et al. Video Display Terminals and the Risk of Spontaneous Abortion. *N. Engl. J. Med.* 324:727, 1991.
31. *Preventing Lead Poisoning in Young Children—A Statement by the Centers for Disease Control.* US Department of Health and Human Services, Public Health Service, Centers for Disease Control, October 1991.
32. Molhave, L. Controlled Experiments for Studies of the Sick Building Syndrome. In W. G. Tucker, et al. (eds.), *Sources of Indoor Air Contaminants: Characterizing Emissions and Health Impacts. Ann. N.Y. Acad. Sci.* 641:46, 1992.
33. Burge, S., et al. Sick building syndrome: A study of 4373 office workers. *Ann. Occup. Hyg.* 31:493, 1987.
34. Baker, D. B. Social and Organizational Factors in Office Building–Associated Illness. In J. E. Cone and M. J. Hodgson (eds.), *Problem Buildings: Building-Associated Illness and the Sick Building Syndrome. Occup. Med. State of the Art Rev.* 4:607, 1989.
35. Kreiss, K. The epidemiology of building-related complaints and illness. In J. E. Cone and M. J. Hodgson (eds.), *Problem Buildings: Building-Associated Illness and the Sick Building Syndrome. Occup. Med. State of the Art Rev.* 4:575, 1989.
36. Council on Scientific Affairs, American Medical Association. Clinical ecology. *J.A.M.A.* 268:3465, 1992.
37. American Academy of Allergy and Immunology. Position statements—clinical ecology. *J. Allergy Clin. Immunol.* 72:269, 1986.
38. American College of Physicians. Clinical ecology. *Ann. Intern. Med.* 111:168, 1989.
39. McLellan, R. K. *Clinical ecology. J.A.M.A.* 269:1634, 1993.
40. McLellan, R. K. *Multiple chemical sensitivities. J.A.M.A.* 265:2336, 1991.
41. McLellan, R. K. *Multiple chemical hypersensitivities. Ann. Intern. Med.* 111:953, 1989.
42. Cullen, M. (ed.). Workers with multiple chemical sensitivities. *Occup. Med. State of the Art Rev.* 2:655, 1987.
43. McLellan, R. K. A thoroughly modern malady. *Medical and Health Annual Encyclopedia Brittanica,* 1992. Pp. 353–358.
44. Rest, K. M. (ed.). Advancing the understanding of multiple chemical sensitivity. Proceedings of the Association of Occupational and Environmental Clinics (AOEC) Workshop on Multiple Chemical Sensitivity. *Toxicol. Industrial Health* 8:1, 1992.
45. Ashford, N. A., and Miller, C. S. *Chemical Exposures: Low Levels and High Stakes.* New York: Van Nostrand Reinhold, 1991.
46. McLellan, R. K. Responding to Chemical Sensitivity in the Workplace. *Indoor Air Quality Update* 4:8, December 1991.
47. Frank, A. L. *ATSDR Case Studies in Environmental Medicine. (26) Taking an Exposure History.* US Department of Health and Human Services, Public Health Service, Agency for Toxic Substances and Disease Registry, October 1992.
48. Kjaergaard S., Assessment of Eye Irritation in Humans. In W. G. Tucker, et al. (eds.), *Sources of Indoor Air Contaminants: Characterizing Emissions and Health Impacts. Ann. N.Y. Acad. Sci.* 641:187, 1992.
49. Koren, H. S., and Devlin, R. B. Human Upper Respiratory Tract Responses to Inhaled Pollutants with Emphasis on Nasal Lavage. In W. G. Tucker et al. (eds.), *Sources of Indoor Air Contaminants: Characterizing Emissions and Health Impacts. N.Y. Acad. Sci.* 641:215, 1992.
50. Kitsch, L. S. Legal Aspects of Indoor Air Pollution. In J. M. Samet and J. D. Spengler (eds.), *Indoor Air Pollution—A Health Perspective.* Baltimore: The Johns Hopkins University Press, 1991. Pp. 378–397.
51. Brennan, T. Untangling causation issues in law and medicine: Hazardous substance litigation. *Ann. Intern. Med.* 107:741, 1987.
52. Quinlan, P., et al. Protocol for the Comprehensive Evaluation of Building-Associated Illness. In J. E. Cone and M. J. Hodgson (eds.), *Problem Buildings: Building-Associated Illness and the Sick Building Syndrome. Occup. Med. State of the Art Rev.* 4:771, 1989.
53. National Institute for Occupational Safety and Health. *Guidance for Indoor Air Quality Investigations.* Cincinnati: Hazard Evaluation and Technical Assistance Branch, Division of Surveillance, Hazard Evaluations and Field Studies, NIOSH, 1987.
54. McLellan, R. K. *Assessing residential environmental hazards. Occup. Environ. Med. Rep.* 5:77, 1991.
55. Nagda, N. L., Rector, H. E., and Kountz, M. D. *Guidelines for Monitoring Indoor Air Quality.* New York: Hemisphere Publishing Corp., 1987.

56. American Conference of Governmental Industrial Hygienists. *Guidelines for the Assessment of Bioaerosols in the Indoor Environment.* Cincinnati, Ohio, 1989.

57. Odor evaluation as an investigative tool. *Indoor Air Quality Update* 4:10, July 1991.

58. Loftness, V., and Hartkopf, V. The Effects of Building Design and Use on Air Quality. In J. E. Cone and M. J. Hodgson (eds.), *Problem Buildings: Building-Associated Illness and the Sick Building Syndrome. Occup. Med. State of the Art Rev.* 4:643, 1989.

59. Indoor Air Quality Management Program. Anne Arundel County Public Schools, Annapolis, MD 21401.

60. Levin, H. Building Materials and Indoor Air Quality. In J. E. Cone and M. J. Hodgson (eds.), *Problem Buildings: Building-Associated Illness and the Sick Building Syndrome. Occup. Med. State of the Art Rev.* 4:667, 1989.

61. An office building bake-out: Methods and analysis. *Indoor Air Quality Update* 2:1, July 1989.

62. Pershagen, G., et al. Residential radon exposure and lung cancer in Sweden. *N. Engl. J. Med.* 330:159, 1994.

Further Information

Building Air-Quality. A Guide for Building Owners and Facility Managers. EPA 400/1-91/033, DHHS (NIOSH) Publication no. 91-114, December 1991.
An off-the-shelf, comprehensive guide for facility managers, maintenance personnel, and building investigators involved in preventing and correcting indoor air pollution problems.

Cone, J. E., and Hodgson, M. J. (eds.). *Problem Buildings: Building-Associated Illness and the Sick Building Syndrome. Occup. Med. State of the Art Rev.* 4:575–799, 1989.
A collection of articles concerning the source, control, and human and economic impact of indoor air pollution.

Gold, D. R. Indoor air pollution. *Clin. Chest Med.* 13:215, 1992.
A detailed summary of agents implicated in indoor air pollution, including practical guidelines for preventing exposure to common allergens, such as mites. (88 references)

Indoor Air Quality Update. Published monthly by Cutter Information Corp., 37 Broadway, Arlington, MA 02174-5539.
This is a monthly newsletter devoted to indoor air pollution and is filled with practical advice about the control of indoor air problems.

Samet, J. Environmental controls and lung disease. *Am. Rev. Respir. Dis.* 142:915, 1990.
A report on a workshop on environmental controls and lung disease. A comprehensive review of the taskforce of the American Thoracic Society, based on a 2-day workshop that addressed the major sources of indoor air pollution and their prevention.

Tucker W. G., et al. (eds.), *Sources of Indoor Air Contaminants: Characterizing Emissions and Health Impacts. Ann. N.Y. Acad. Sci.* 641:1–329, 1992.
This volume results from a conference of international experts on the frontier of characterizing indoor air contaminants and their acute effects on humans.

The Agency for Toxic Substances and Disease Registry

Frank L. Mitchell

In November 1990, the *Journal of Occupational Medicine* published a series of articles dealing with environmental medicine. The series was developed in preparation for a change in the name of the American College of Occupational Medicine to the American College of Occupational and *Environmental* Medicine. One of the papers defined environmental medicine ". . . to be the study of the effects upon human beings of external physical, chemical, and biologic factors in the general environment. *Clinical* environment medicine, then, would be the study of detectable human diseases or adverse health outcomes from exposure to these environmental factors" [1].

This chapter surveys environmental medicine, a relatively new medical discipline, and how it compares and contrasts with occupational medicine. While there are many similarities, there are also substantial differences. Environmental medicine is a broad field, covering essentially the entire population and their interactions with the environment and the contaminants it may contain. It considers how those interactions take place, and what effects they can produce. Those practicing environmental medicine will often be dealing with a patient, the patient's family, and the community of which they are a part. The physician will come to realize that environmental medicine is truly a public health practice.

Background

Before considering the medical evaluation of patients with environmentally related disease, the physician should have an understanding of how the materials affecting these patients became a part of the environment, how they can lead to adverse health effects in people, and how environmentally related illnesses have become widely recognized.

Industrialized countries produce large quantities of hazardous chemical substances. In the United States, about 60,000 to 70,000 chemicals are currently in commercial use, with another 1000 new ones being introduced yearly [2]. After production and use they become waste, which must be discarded. In the past, chemical wastes were often disposed of in landfills, waterways (rivers and lakes), through uncontrolled incineration, or by simply dumping onto the soil, an exercise that can contaminate both the earth and the groundwater supplies that lie beneath. This toxic legacy has caused harmful effects in humans and has the potential for more impact in the future.

The number of known hazardous waste sites in the United States is enormous. The Office of Technology Assessment [3] has reported that 255 to 275 million tons of hazardous waste are produced in the United States each year.

The Environmental Protection Agency (EPA) currently includes 33,000 sites in its inventory of known hazardous waste sites [2]. Of that number, about 1270 are on the National Priority List (NPL), which is a group of sites that the EPA considers its highest priority for remediation. The EPA has estimated that cleaning up the current NPL sites may cost more than $30 billion [2].

Facilities under the control of the federal government contain many thousands of additional hazardous waste sites that will also require clean-up. Some estimates predict that $150 billion may be necessary for the cleanup of these federal facilities alone [2].

In the late 1970s, the discoveries of toxic substances in residential communities such as Love Canal, New York; Times Beach, Missouri; and Elizabeth City, New

Jersey, captured the public's attention and led the US Congress to pass the Comprehensive Environmental Response, Compensation and Liability Act (CERCLA) of 1980. This Act became known as the "Superfund" Act because of its multibillion dollar size and its broad powers to deal with hazardous waste situations. The Act, which is financed through a trust fund made up of taxes on chemical producers, requires Congressional reauthorization every 5 years.

The Agency for Toxic Substances and Disease Registry

Although the Superfund Act is administered principally by the EPA, a new agency, the Agency for Toxic Substances and Disease Registry (ATSDR), was formed to help in understanding the human health impact of widespread environmental chemical contamination. The Superfund legislation created this relatively new federal agency to consider the harmful health effects that may be associated with hazardous waste.

The relationship between the EPA and ATSDR is, in some ways, similar to that of the Occupational Safety and Health Administration (OSHA) and the National Institute for Occupational Safety and Health (NIOSH), in that the regulatory and enforcement powers reside with the EPA. ATSDR's mission is "to prevent or mitigate adverse effects to both human health and the quality of life resulting from exposure to hazardous substances in the environment" [4].

The mandates for the Agency are many and varied. The most important, and the ATSDR response to each, are displayed in Table 45-1.

Role of ATSDR

A brief survey of how ATSDR works with a site and the surrounding community can help to illustrate issues that are common to many hazardous waste situations. Although all of the topics may not interest each physician, or be an issue at every site, several of them should be a part of any environmental health investigation and will be discussed in more detail.

A fundamental part of any evaluation is a survey of the health effects, real or potential, that may result from hazardous exposures. In ATSDR, this evaluation is called a *public health assessment* (PHA), and is defined as ". . . the evaluation of data and information on the release of hazardous substances into the environment in order to assess any current or future impact on public health" [5].

A formal health assessment is written only after ATSDR staff has assembled and reviewed detailed information about the area or site. The information necessary to develop a PHA is not the same for all sites, but in many cases, an extensive

Table 45-1. Legislative mandates and the ATSDR response

Legislative mandate	ATSDR response
Overall public health implications of a hazardous waste site	Public health assessment
Specific questions concerning a site	Health consultation
Toxicologic information of site contaminants	Toxicologic profile
Health surveillance of affected residents	Epidemiologic studies and registries
Educational and training materials	Case studies in environmental medicine, courses for physicians
Applied and substance-specific research	Sponsorship of intramural and academic research programs, conferences, etc.
Response to emergencies involving hazardous substances	24-Hour emergency response capability including on site, if required

investigation will be necessary before one can determine whether, and to what extent, people have or may have been exposed to hazardous substances. Examples of the information used in the typical PHA are listed in Table 45-2 [5].

A variation on the PHA is the *health consultation,* which is a less inclusive response to a request for information about health risks posed by a specific site, chemical release, or hazardous material. Health consultations often lead to specific actions. Water supplies, for example, may be restricted or replaced, environmental sampling may be initiated or intensified, access to the site may be restricted, or contaminated material may be removed or contained.

While it is impossible for an individual physician to carry out all these activities, an attempt should be made to acquire some understanding of the major points pertinent to each case. Without this knowledge, it is difficult to reach valid conclusions about the possibility of health effects resulting from exposure to the contaminated materials.

Many of the elements of the PHA are not unique, but one is: *the inclusion of community health concerns.* As a result, although scientific issues, such as the toxicology of the contaminants, are thoroughly investigated, efforts are made to blend that information with knowledge of the surrounding community to address a range of concerns about the site [5]. For example, while the specific contaminant may suggest that carcinogenesis is the major toxicologic issue, the results of the assessment may not be well accepted if the major concern is reproductive effects. Without an understanding of the worries of the area residents, and a willingness to address them, no health assessor, whether a governmental employee or an environmental physician, can expect to be well received, or even believed.

Thus, the physician who is attempting to deal with these environmental situations must, perhaps more than any other medical specialist, take on the *role of communicator.* To understand the feelings of the people potentially affected by the contamination, the practitioner must be as willing to work with community residents as with other experts in the field.

ATSDR is available for consultation by physicians working with environmentally related situations. The Agency is frequently consulted by the public on a wide variety of issues, and its staff can help in many ways. Each division also has physicians on its staff, and while they come from a number of medical specialties, they are all now involved in environmental medicine and are willing to discuss problems that the practicing physician may face. The questions most frequently asked tend to be toxicologic or they require referral assistance to environmentally experienced phy-

Table 45-2. Factors considered in a public health assessment

1. Setting
   Physical (landfill, spill, etc.)
   Geographic (natural and political)
   Historic (prior releases and actions)
   Operational (dates and process descriptions)
2. Environmental contamination
   Substances
   Concentrations in all relevant media
   Current and historical sampling data
3. Environmental pathways
   Groundwater
   Surface water
   Soil and sediment
   Air
   Biota
4. Health outcome data
   Community records
   Previous health studies
5. Community concerns
   Environmental and health complaints
   Previous actions by governmental units

sicians. Assistance with problems of risk communication and help in acquiring state and local information relating to specific sites are also commonly requested.

Consultation with ATSDR is available through its 10 regional offices or through its headquarters in Atlanta. The Agency can always be reached through its Emergency Response and Consultation Branch (ERCB) at 404-639-0615. This number is answered around-the-clock and serves as a conduit to the other parts of the Agency. A list of the ATSDR regional offices and the primary contacts in Atlanta are contained in the chapter appendix.

Evaluating Environmental Health Effects

The close relationship of occupational medicine to environmental medicine is reflected in the name change of the American College of Occupational and Environmental Medicine. Many physicians now practicing environmental medicine have had training in occupational medicine. This "cross-fertilization" and responsibility is logical, since one of the major issues in both fields is the interaction of humans with hazardous and toxic chemicals, adverse physical conditions, or radiation. The differences between occupational and environmental medicine, however, can be significant.

In cases of occupational exposure, the physician is usually able to make assumptions about the specific exposures encountered by the worker, the route of the exposure, and respective control measures. Thus, some characterization of the workplace is possible, and in conjunction with industrial hygiene expertise, conclusions can be formed concerning the source of the patient's complaints and how to reduce exposures to levels that will not cause further adverse effects. In the environmental setting, these procedures may be much more difficult to carry out. For example, a long-standing hazardous waste site may have an unknown number of contaminants. The exposure may be through the drinking water at levels that may be an order of magnitude lower than those seen in the workplace. Thus, the ability to measure or even estimate the dose the patient has received, or is receiving, is limited, and may be impossible. If the contaminant is volatile, for example, estimates of level of exposure from oral intake, skin penetration, or inhalation during showering must be made. Because the exposures may not occur at reasonably well-defined times and places, as in the workplace, the process of dose reconstruction can be difficult [6].

While the occupational physician is familiar with the working population, the environmental physician must consider all ages and sexes as well as a longer duration of exposure to lower concentrations of a hazard. The patient may also have preexisting illnesses, found in any sample of the general population. Environmental exposures tend to be continuous, without the daily or weekend cessation seen in the workplace. The only break from the environmental exposures, in fact, may be while the patient is at work.

Because typical environmental exposures are much smaller than occupational levels, the signs and symptoms may be considerably less than those traditionally expected of chemical exposures. They can be more typical of the litany of complaints handled every day in an average outpatient situation. In fact, there may be no signs of symptoms at all, merely a genuinely worried patient who is concerned about potential exposure to a nearby hazardous waste site. Common questions can range from, "What harmful effects could occur to the fetus of a 6-month-pregnant woman?" to "Is it safe to shower with well water contaminated by solvents?"

One issue common to both occupational and environmental medicine is the confounding effects of voluntary risks. If the patient is involved in hobbies or other pastimes having some exposure to toxic materials, problems can be created for the physician. This point needs emphasis because even though a question about hobbies is found on every history form, it is often not pursued to the degree it warrants [7]. A number of people have hobbies that involve significant exposures to a variety of very toxic materials, and if this is not explored while an environmental or occupational exposure situation is investigated, valuable information can be overlooked [7]. Examples are the amateur potter who works with metal-rich paints and glazes, the modeler who uses paints and several types of epoxy or cyanoacrylate adhesive systems, and the serious gardener who may have almost constant low-level exposure to various pesticides.

Diagnosis

The diagnostic process is further complicated by the fact that there are few laboratory tests that can be of any help. Biologic indicators of toxic exposure, adverse health effects, or susceptibility are termed "biologic markers," or "biomarkers." A biologic marker of *exposure,* for example, is an exogenous substance or its metabolites measured in a compartment of the body (e.g., blood lead); a biomarker of *effect* is a measurable alteration within an organism that can be recognized as an established or potential health impairment (e.g., changes in liver function tests following a solvent exposure); and a biomarker of *susceptibility* is an indicator of an individual's ability to respond to a xenobiotic challenge (e.g., genetic studies to determine the possibility of adverse responses) [8]. In most clinical situations, physicians rely primarily on the first two. However, since the chemical exposures are often at very low levels, there may not be measurable effects. Except for a few specific indicators, the diagnosis of environmentally related illness rests primarily on the patient's history and physical examination, and the characterization of the exposure.

The *history* is the fundamental tool for any environmental investigation, and it must include all of the patient's environments, occupational and otherwise. Not all patients, of course, will require an in-depth evaluation. However, all patients, particularly where the available evidence does not suggest a more plausible etiology, should be asked several broadly based questions that serve as a screen to determine whether further inquiry would be useful.

While most occupational physicians feel comfortable taking detailed occupational histories, they must, in an environmental situation, also concern themselves with the occupational histories of others with whom the patient may be in close contact. Particular attention should be paid to whether work clothes are brought home for laundering, and how they are cleaned.

Useful variations on the occupational history include the reverse of questions often asked. For example, does the problem get worse on weekends or vacations? Does it improve at work? Are there particular locations where it is worse?

To begin assessing the potential environmental source, inquire about recent home remodeling, new furniture or carpets, or new painting. What are the home construction materials, and how recently were they used? What is the type of heating used in the home, has it recently been changed, or is it in good repair? Are hazardous waste sites or other potential sources of environmental contaminants found in the community?

The physician should be careful not to assume that association is causation. There may be a number of potential sources of contamination, but unless a pathway to the patient can be confirmed and the known effects of the chemical reasonably associated with the patient's complaints at the reported level of exposure, the physician should continue searching for other, or additional, sources.

The *physical examination* should be thorough, remembering that early signs of environmental disease can be very subtle, and are often first seen in the organs most sensitive to contamination: the skin, the eyes, and the respiratory system. Unfortunately, complaints of these three areas are among the most common in any outpatient setting, and therefore the physical findings must be correlated with the information gained from the history.

Laboratory tests should be limited to those that are useful in any screening situation. Liver function tests, multichannel chemistries, and urinalysis may be very useful, but, again, the changes due to exposures to hazardous materials can be quite subtle. The physician must also consider false-positive results.

Reference Materials

Once the physician has gathered all the material from the patient and data about the possible contaminant, reference material will usually be needed. The lack of such information has been a major problem for practitioners of environmental medicine. With the increasing interest in this field, however, the situation is improving. ATSDR, for example, has developed and is producing informational publications aimed specifically at environmental situations. They include *Toxicological Profiles,* which are monographs on the health effects of specific hazardous substances, and *Case Studies in Environmental Medicine,* which are self-instructional exercises in environmental medicine that guide the practitioner through the diagnosis, treatment, and surveillance of persons exposed to a number of specific hazardous substances. Each case study includes a discussion of the substance and offers Continuing Medical Education credit after completion. These and other useful publications are listed under Further Information at the end of this chapter.

Electronic Databases

Electronic databases are the most rapidly growing source of information about environmental exposures. A number of databases are available to anyone with a personal computer and a modem. While their use has associated costs, there are several more economical databases available through the Toxicology Data Network (TOXNET) system of the National Library of Medicine (NLM). Generally, the most useful file is the Hazardous Substances Data Bank (HSDB), which contains toxicology information on over 4200 potentially hazardous chemicals. The HSDB also includes emergency handling procedures, environmental fate, regulatory information, and human exposure.

Another file of TOXNET is the Registry of Toxic Effects of Chemical Substances (RTECS). This file, which is maintained by NIOSH, contains data relating to irritation, carcinogenicity, mutagenicity, and reproductive effects on over 90,000 chemicals.

Information on any of the NLM systems, which are available 24 hours per day, 7 days per week, can be obtained from the NLM in Bethesda, Maryland. Examples of other electronic databases are listed under Further Information.

Assessment

After a careful evaluation of resource material and data relevant to the case, the physician can begin to consider diagnostic, therapeutic, and remedial actions that should be initiated. In the majority of cases, the environmental source of the patient's complaints can be determined and actions taken to diminish or eliminate the effects it may produce. This can involve removing the source, containing the source or its emissions, changing the ways hobbies are undertaken, or wearing personal protective equipment. In some cases, precautionary changes in lifestyles may be beneficial or even necessary.

Central to the treatment of environmentally related illnesses usually is removal of patients from the source of the contaminants affecting them. While other, more traditional medical care may be useful, the primary goal should be the elimination of pathways between the patient and the environmental contaminant.

A small percentage of patients may not respond to these procedures. Their history may include an initial chemical incident, perhaps a tight-building incident or pesticide exposure. Their symptoms, however, do not diminish with time, but in fact increase. After a variable period, they become symptomatic to a number of other chemicals. Their symptoms occur at levels of exposure that are common in everyday life and have no effect on others. For example, cosmetics, perfumes, cleaning materials, papers and inks, new construction, paint, and new clothing have been described as producing symptoms in this group of patients. They may have consulted a number of physicians due to a lack of improvement. Their condition has been labeled multiple chemical sensitivity (MCS) [9]. It is an affliction that has attracted considerable controversy and has been the subject of several national conferences [10, 11].

Summary

Environmental medicine, like the environment itself, is a broad and complex entity. While it has many points in common with occupational medicine, it is, in many other ways, unique. Occupational physicians who wish to enter the field have a large advantage over other specialists in that they understand the many varied, and sometimes contradictory, effects that chemicals can have on humans. Moreover, environmental exposures tend to be much less intense than those in the workplace, the effects can be very subtle, and diligent and often time-consuming investigations may be necessary to reach an understanding of the mechanisms in play. The rewards can be considerable, however, since they may affect an entire community and its quality of life.

References

1. Ducatman, A., et al. What is environmental medicine? (editorial). *J.O.M.* 32:1130, 1990.
2. Habicht, H. Plans, problems, and promises for the years ahead. *Hazardous Materials Control* Jan/Feb: 60, 1991.
3. Office of Technology Assessment. *Technologies and Management Strategies for Hazardous Waste Control.* Washington, DC: US Government Printing Office, 1983.
4. US Government Printing Office. *Fed. Register* 54:33617, August 15, 1989.
5. Agency for Toxic Substances and Disease Registry. *Public Health Assessment Guidance Manual.* Atlanta: ATSDR, March 1992.
6. Ram, N., Christman, R., and Cantor, K. Total Exposure to Volatile Organic Compounds in Potable Water. In N. Ram (ed.), *Significance and Treatment of Volatile Organic Compounds in Water Supplies.* Chelsea, MI: Lewis Publishers, 1990.
7. McCunney, R., Russo, P., and Doyle, J. Occupational illness in the arts. *Am. Fam. Physician* 36:145, 1987.
8. National Research Council. *Biologic Markers in Immunotoxicology.* Washington, DC: National Academy Press, 1992.
9. Cullen, M. The Worker with Multiple Chemical Sensitivities: An Overview. In M. Cullen (ed.), *Workers With Multiple Chemical Sensitivities. Occupational State of the Art Reviews.* Philadelphia: Hanley & Belfus, 1987.
10. National Research Council. *Multiple Chemical Sensitivities. Addendum to Biologic Markers in Immunotoxicology.* Washington, DC: National Academy Press, 1992.
11. Proceedings of the AOEC Workshop on Multiple Chemical Sensitivity. *Toxicology and Industrial Health* (special issue) 8:4, 1992.

Further Information

Books

ATSDR Public Health Assessment Guidance Manual. Chelsea, MI: Lewis Publishers, 1992.
This book was developed by ATSDR and is the most complete resource available for those wishing to know more about the investigation and management of a hazardous waste site.

ATSDR Toxicological Profiles, Case Studies in Environmental Medicine, and other publications.
Can be obtained on an as-available basis. For information and placement on mailing list, contact ATSDR, 1600 Clifton Rd., Atlanta, GA, 30333.

Borak, J., Callan, M., and Abbott, W. *Hazardous Materials Exposure.* Englewood Cliffs, NJ: Brady, 1991.
A book aimed primarily at the emergency medical services community that contains much worthwhile information on the handling and care of chemically exposed patients and the protection of the caregiver.

Sullivan, J., and Krieger, G. *Hazardous Materials Toxicology.* Baltimore: Williams & Wilkins, 1992.
A textbook that discusses the clinical principles of environmental health.

US Department of Transportation. *1992 Emergency Response Guidebook.* Washington, DC: US Government Printing Office, 1992.
A useful pocket-sized book containing chemical emergency response information.

Electronic Databases

CAMEO. National Oceanographic and Atmospheric Administration, Seattle, Washington.

A complete emergency planning and response package. Contains information from other governmental databases and tools for mapping community hazards, dispersion plumes, and right to know information.

CHEMTREC. Chemical Manufacturer's Association, Washington, DC.
Perhaps the most widely used database. Supplies basic information about most chemicals in use; can put caller into direct contact with the chemical's producer. Reached around the clock at 1-800-424-9300. MEDTREC is an extension of CHEMTREC that offers information to establish medical treatment protocols, communication on chemicals without known manufacturer, and training for poison control centers.

Hazardline. Occupational Medical Services, Secaucus, NJ.
Information on 70,000 chemicals, including physical and chemical properties, personal protective equipment, health exposure limits, lists of symptoms, and first-aid responses.

TOMES. Micromedix, Inc., Denver, CO.
Supplies medical treatment information, and hazardous materials handling information, and offers access to several governmental databases, as well as information gathered from a number of poison control centers.

Appendix to Chapter 45: ATSDR Contacts

Mailing address: ATSDR
                1600 Clifton Rd., E-28
                Atlanta, GA 30333

ATSDR Emergency Response and Consultation Branch: 404-639-0615

For current ATSDR regional office telephone numbers, contact the ATSDR Office of Regional Operations (404-639-0707).

Addresses of ATSDR regional offices:

Region I (CT, ME, MA, NH, RI, VT)
   Emergency Service Division ATSDR/Region I
   EPA Building
   60 Westview
   Lexington, MA 02173

Region II (NJ, NY, PR, VI)
   EPA Region II
   26 Federal Plaza
   New York, NY 10278

Region III (DE, DC, MD, PA, VA, WV)
   Hazardous Waste Mgt.
   Region III (3HW01)
   841 Chestnut Bldg.
   Philadelphia, PA 19107

Region IV (AL, FL, GA, KY, MS, NC)
   Waste Management Division
   EPA Region IV
   345 Courtland St. NE
   Atlanta, GA 30365

Region V (IL, IN, MI, MN, OH, WI)
   EPA Region V
   77 West Jackson Blvd.
   6th Floor—M/S HS-6J
   Chicago, IL 60604

Region VI (AR, LA, NM, OK, TX)
   Office of Health Response
   First Interstate Tower
   EPA Region VI (6H-E)
   1445 Ross Ave.
   Dallas, TX 75202

Region VII (IA, KS, MO, NE)
Waste Management Branch
EPA Region VII
726 Minnesota Ave.
Kansas City, KS 66101

Region VIII (CO, MT, ND, SD, UT, WY)
Region VIII 8HWM-FF
6th Floor—North Tower
999 18th St.
Denver, CO 80202

Region IX (AZ, CA, HI, NV, American Samoa, Guam, Marshall Islands)
ATSDR
75 Hawthorne St.
Rm. 09261, Mail Code H-1-2
San Francisco, CA 94105

Region X (AK, ID, OR, WA)
EPA Region X (M/S HW113)
1200 6th Ave.
Seattle, WA 98101

46 Environmental Medical Emergencies

Jonathan Borak

Emergency response planning is required at most worksites under a variety of federal and state regulations. Traditionally, occupational physicians have not been central to such planning. However, recent requirements contain specific medical components and involvement, and, as a result, occupational physicians are likely to be increasingly involved in the development and implementation of worksite emergency response plans. For that reason, physicians should be knowledgeable about the various emergency planning requirements that may affect those facilities at which they work or to which they provide medical services.

For the most part, worksite emergency planning requirements are found within the standards and regulations of the Occupational Safety and Health Administration (OSHA) and the Environmental Protection Agency (EPA). The focus and emphasis of those two agencies are fundamentally different. Because OSHA is primarily concerned with the health and safety of workers, its emergency focus is to protect employees, including emergency response personnel. By contrast, the EPA's concern is primarily protection of the "outside" world, that is, people, other living things, and the environment surrounding worksites.

Despite the differing perspectives of OSHA and the EPA, their actual emergency planning requirements overlap and cross-reference one another. As a result, it is of only limited usefulness to categorize requirements according to the issuing agency. Likewise, there is little practical benefit in distinguishing "worksite emergencies" from "environmental emergencies" because many incidents simultaneously involve both employees and the environment.

A more practical approach is to consider the regulatory requirements in light of the response functions and activities that are actually mandated in the event of an emergency. This chapter takes such an approach. Worksite emergency response requirements of relevance to occupational physicians are grouped and discussed according to the following five types of response functions and activities:

1. First aid and emergency medical care
2. Protection of emergency response personnel
3. Provision of emergency medical information
4. Medical surveillance
5. Coordination with community health care providers.

First Aid and Emergency Medical Care

The most basic requirement for worksite emergency planning is OSHA's requirement that there be ready access to first aid for all injured employees:

> In the absence of an infirmary, clinic, or hospital in near proximity to the workplace which is used for the treatment of all injured employees, a person or persons shall be adequately trained to render first aid. First aid supplies approved by the consulting physician shall be readily available. [29 CFR 1019.151(b)]

Although subject to interpretation, it is generally understood that "first aid" includes at least care for victims of trauma, response to corrosive and thermal injuries, and cardiopulmonary resuscitation (CPR). Many worksites meet this requirement by providing certification training to designated employees in first aid and CPR according to the guidelines of the American Red Cross or the National Safety Council.

The need for training and the number of individuals to be trained are determined in part by the proximity of the worksite to other sources of emergency care. As a rule of thumb, first aid and CPR must be available to employees within 5 minutes. Because even the most effective community emergency medical service (EMS) will often require longer than 5 minutes to respond to an emergency, most worksites must plan to provide first aid and CPR. In large facilities, it may be necessary to station trained individuals in multiple sites to assure an adequately prompt response to all employees.

The role of the consulting occupational physician in this setting is clear. At a minimum, that physician must approve the actual equipment and supplies used by first-aid providers. More logically, that physician would also oversee the actual training of emergency responders and assure that their training and number are adequate to meet OSHA requirements. In addition, special requirements for protection from bloodborne pathogens for first responders will necessitate medical oversight.

Similar but somewhat broader requirements are found in OSHA's Hazardous Waste Operations and Emergency Response Standard [29 CFR 1910.120], which deals with the health and safety of hazardous waste site workers and response personnel at hazardous materials emergencies. The EPA has issued identical rules [Worker Protection Standards for Hazardous Waste Operations and Emergency Response, 40 CFR 311], which apply to all workers and emergency response volunteers otherwise exempted from the OSHA standard.

OSHA and the EPA require that an emergency response plan be developed and implemented before the start of hazardous waste and emergency response operations at a facility: "The employer shall develop an emergency response plan for emergencies which shall address, as a minimum . . . Emergency medical treatment and first aid" [29 CFR 1910.120(1)]. These concerns relate to the effects of exposure to hazardous materials and the consequences of hazardous materials emergencies, but such concerns are broad and far reaching. The toxic effects of hazardous materials exposures can affect most of the body's organ systems. Thermal injuries and burns are common consequences of these incidents because nearly 65% of all hazardous materials are flammable. Explosions and trauma are also common outcomes. Accordingly, emergency response plans should include relatively comprehensive medical policies, protocols, and procedures for providing emergency care at the worksite under a variety of conditions.

Protection of Emergency Response Personnel

Emergency response personnel are exposed to greater variety and severity of health risks than are most other employees. For example, fire fighters regularly risk thermal injuries, toxic exposures, and trauma. Likewise, emergency medical technicians (EMT) and emergency physicians are at greater risk of bloodborne diseases than are most other health care workers. Employers are obliged by OSHA (and, in some cases, by the EPA) to provide acceptable levels of protection to those personnel. The occupational physician plays an important role in assuring that adequate protection is actually available to response personnel.

Use of respirators is one example. OSHA requires that self-contained breathing apparatus (SCBA) be provided to and used by members of industrial fire brigades [29 CFR 1910.156] and emergency personnel responding to hazardous materials releases [29 CFR 1910.120]. That latter requirement is also found in the EPA's Worker Protection Standards [40 CFR 311]. Employers must assure that response personnel are physically able to use the provided equipment, a process requiring the professional involvement of a physician:

> Persons should not be assigned to tasks requiring use of respirators unless it has been determined that they are physically able to perform the work and use the equipment. The local physician shall determine what health and physical conditions are pertinent. The respirator user's medical status should be reviewed periodically (for instance, annually). [29 CFR 1910.134(b)]

These requirements are commonly guided by consensus standards designed by organizations such as the National Fire Protection Association (see Appendix and Further Information section of this chapter).

Medical concerns also arise when emergency responders wear personal protective equipment (PPE), especially impervious clothing and encapsulating suits. By design, such PPE are impermeable to water and, therefore, the wearer quickly loses the temperature control benefits normally derived from sweating. The higher the ambient temperature and the longer the suits are worn, the greater is the risk of dehydration and heat stress. A protocol to monitor response personnel, including at least some measure of vital signs before donning of PPE and after PPE removal, should be developed, along with criteria for referral for medical evaluation.

A third example of protection for emergency response personnel is OSHA's Bloodborne Pathogens Standard [29 CFR 1910.1030]. That Standard requires employers to develop an exposure control plan, including training and the availability of hepatitis B vaccination for employees who, as a result of performing their duties, risk contact exposure of skin, eye, and mucous membranes or parenteral exposure to blood and other potentially infectious materials.

Employees who provide first aid are specifically included in this requirement. Training and vaccination must be provided in advance of exposure to employees who staff first-aid stations, health care workers, and those who are members of emergency response and public safety organizations. For employees who provide first aid only as a collateral duty to other routine work assignments, training must be provided in advance of exposure, but vaccination may be provided within 24 hours of exposure to blood or other infectious materials.

Provision of vaccinations and postexposure follow-up are medical functions for which the occupational physician should be responsible:

> The employer shall ensure that all medical evaluations and procedures including the hepatitis B vaccination series and postexposure evaluation and follow-up, including prophylaxis, are . . . Performed by or under the supervision of a licensed physician or by or under the supervision of another licensed health care professional. [29 CFR 1910.1030(f)]

Provision of Emergency Medical Information

Worksites at which hazardous substances are processed or stored should have detailed medical information available on the specific health effects of exposure to those substances. Facility emergency response plans should include protocols and procedures for medical treatment of exposure victims. Facility managers should be prepared to promptly provide detailed medical information, including treatment recommendations, to community response organizations in the event of a hazardous materials emergency. The quantity and type of information required exceed those commonly found on Material Safety Data Sheets.

The most explicit example of the need for such detailed information is the Emergency Notification requirement in Title III of EPA's Superfund Amendments and Reauthorization Act (Title III). That requirement applies to spills or releases of hazardous substance in excess of their "reporting quantities." ("Reporting quantity" is defined for "extremely hazardous substances" in Title III and for "hazardous substances" in the EPA's Comprehensive Environmental Response, Compensation and Liability Act, or CERCLA.)

In the event of such a spill or release exceeding the reporting quantity, the facility must immediately notify local and state emergency response officials of all local areas and states "likely to be affected by the release." Along with information identifying the released substance and the quantity released, the emergency notification must contain detailed medical information such as: "any known or anticipated acute or chronic health risks associated with the emergency and, where appropriate, advice regarding medical attention necessary for exposed individuals" [40 CFR 355.40(b)].

Initially, the required notification may be provided orally, but written notice must be given "as soon as practicable." Facilities that use or store quantities of hazardous substances should anticipate the possible need for such information and arrange for its preparation before, rather than following, emergencies. Occupational physicians should be involved in compiling and preparing the appropriate emergency medical information for those facilities at which they work or provide services.

Provision of emergency medical information is also required by OSHA [29 CFR 1910.120] and the EPA [40 CFR 311] in their parallel rules for hazardous waste and emergency response operations. Both agencies require emergency response plans that address "emergency medical treatment" of hazardous materials exposure victims. In turn, the emergency plans are an important component of employee training that is also required. Occupational physicians working at or consulting facilities that must comply with these regulations should be aware of the health-related information contained in those training programs. Physicians should also review and approve any emergency treatment protocols developed for implementation at the site and included in facility training programs.

Medical Surveillance

OSHA [29 CFR 1910.120] and the EPA [40 CFR 311] require employers to develop medical surveillance programs for emergency response personnel and other employees involved in hazardous materials emergencies. Members of "organized and designated HAZMAT teams" and others trained to the OSHA/EPA level of Hazardous Materials Specialist must receive baseline medical examinations, follow-up examinations at least every 12 to 24 months and at termination of employment, or reassignment if the previous examination was more than 6 months before. Medical consultation must also be provided to any emergency response personnel who "exhibit signs or symptoms which may have resulted" from exposure to hazardous substances during an emergency.

Medical examinations and consultations required by the regulations should include:

Medical and work history (or updated history if one is in the employee's file) with special emphasis on symptoms related to the handling of hazardous substances and health hazards, and to fitness for duty including the ability to wear any required PPE under conditions (i.e., temperature extremes) that may be expected at the worksite. The content of medical examinations or consultations . . . shall be determined by the attending physician. [29 CFR 1910.120(f)]

The employer must provide to the attending physician a copy of the relevant OSHA or EPA standard, a description of the employee's duties (that is, the emergency response duties of the individual), known or anticipated exposure levels, a description of the PPE available to the employee, and past medical history.

The physician must render a written opinion as to whether the employee has suffered a condition that increases the risk of "material impairment of the employee's health" from emergency response work or from use of respirators. It seems apparent that physicians cannot accomplish this specific task without an adequate understanding of the component roles and functions of the facility's emergency response program, the hazards and risks of the PPE available at an emergency, and the potential hazards to be encountered during emergencies at the facility.

Coordination with Community Health Care Providers

Important components of facility emergency response plans are explicit agreements between the facility and the surrounding community's emergency response organizations, including EMS organizations and hospitals. Such agreements are required under the EPA's Resource Conservation and Recovery Act (RCRA) [40 CFR 265 Subparta D], which mandates a contingency plan at facilities that generate, store, or process hazardous wastes. The facility contingency plan must contain actual letters of agreement signed by those organizations. If a community organization is unwilling to assist the facility, the facts of that refusal must be included in the plan.

Occupational physicians serve an important function by assisting the managers of industrial facilities to determine the community health care providers with which those facilities should develop agreements and by defining the parameters of those agreements. In communities with multiple hospitals, for example, it is often best to select and favor only one or a few for purposes of emergency planning and response.

The selection of such a hospital may reflect proximity to the facility, but other considerations should include the availability of specialized emergency care, such as trauma specialists, burn specialists, and toxicologists. In many communities, specific hospitals have been designated as providers of such specialty care (e.g., trauma centers, burn centers, poison control centers) and, where appropriate, those hospitals should be recognized and included as part of the emergency planning conducted at local industrial facilities.

It is important that occupational physicians correctly understand the abilities and limitations of the hospitals and EMS services that serve the facilities at which they work or to which they provide medical services. For example, many hospital emergency departments lack the equipment, knowledge, and experience to care for patients with toxic chemical exposures: In general, emergency physicians have only limited knowledge of industrial toxicology, and hospital emergency departments are not required by accrediting agencies (such as the Joint Commission) to maintain decontamination capabilities for victims of chemical or radiation exposures. Likewise, the strength of most poison control centers is medical toxicology (i.e., ingestion poisonings), not industrial toxicology, and most poison centers have only limited experience in responding to industrial emergencies. Training in industrial emergencies for poison control center employees has been proposed by the Chemical Manufacturer's Association, but has not been implemented. Facilities that manufacture or use large quantities of toxic chemicals should determine which local hospital is most capable of managing acute exposure victims and should develop agreements with that hospital to care for exposed workers. These items should be stated in the contingency plan.

There are also large differences among EMS services. Advanced services staffed with paramedics employ medications, endotracheal intubation, and cardiac monitoring, but basic services offer little more than first aid. Most EMS services, both advanced and basic, are not prepared to manage victims of toxic chemical exposures. Most EMT training courses devote little or no time to hazardous materials. Most EMS services lack decontamination protocols, carry no decontamination materials, and do not provide chemical protective equipment to their personnel. Although the National Fire Protection Association has established minimum competencies for EMS personnel responding to hazardous materials emergencies [NFPA Standard no. 473-92], that standard is voluntary and currently ignored by most services and states. OSHA has shown little enthusiasm for extending the protection of its Hazardous Waste Operations and Emergency Response Standard [29 CFR 1910.120] to EMS personnel.

Physicians should determine that local EMS services can provide the scope of emergency response support that might be required by the industrial facilities at which they work or to which they provide services. In many cases, those facilities can encourage and assist their EMS neighbors to develop necessary protocols and procedures. For example, industrial facilities using quantities of hydrofluoric acid should provide calcium gluconate gel to local EMS services along with appropriate training in its use for decontamination and burn care. Likewise, facilities that use or manufacture quantities of phenol should provide an appropriate skin cleanser such as polyethylene glycol 300 and training in its use.

Further Information

Borak, J., Callan, M., and Abbott, W. *Hazardous Materials Exposure: Emergency Response and Patient Care.* Englewood Cliffs, NJ: Prentice Hall, 1991.
A concise overview of planning issues for hazardous materials emergencies that can serve as a manual for OSHA-mandated training.

Dynes, R. R. *Community Emergency Planning: False Assumptions and Inappropriate Analogies.* Newark, DE: Disaster Research Center, University of Delaware, 1990.
A critical review of planning methodologies and models for community emergency planning.

Feldstein, B. D., et al. Disaster training for emergency physicians in the United States: A systems approach. *Ann. Emerg. Med.* 14:36, 1985.
A review of existing training systems for emergency physicians and a proposed approach to enhance capabilities for response to disasters of all sorts.

Leonard, R. B., and Teitelman, U. Manmade disasters. *Crit. Care Clin.* 7:293, 1991.
An overview and review of the toxicology of industrial disasters and war.

Leonard, R. B., et al. SARA (Superfund Amendments and Reauthorization Act) Title III: Implications for emergency physicians. *Ann. Emerg. Med.* 18:1212, 1989.

An overview of the SARA legislation with particular emphasis on those components of relevance to physicians and hospital emergency departments.

NFPA. *Competencies for EMS Personnel Responding to Hazardous Materials Incidents: NFPA Standard no. 473-92.* Quincy, MA: National Fire Protection Association, 1992.
Recommended training and performance standards for EMTs and paramedics involved in emergency medical response to victims of chemical exposure.

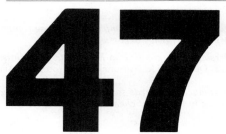

Emergency Response to Environmental Incidents

L. Kristian Arnold

The emergency response to environmental incidents combines the principles of occupational medicine (OM) and emergency medicine (EM). Considering the scope and purpose of this book, this chapter has been prepared from the knowledge bases of both disciplines with the intent of providing a practical resource for the occupational medicine practitioner. Since occupational medicine, like emergency medicine, is a relatively young field with many practitioners who do not have formal training, this chapter is focused on their needs, although it should also be a useful review for the specialist.

The field of environmental medicine continues to develop in scope. In fact, the definition of the environment has become increasingly global in relation to the activities of occupational medicine physicians. No longer does this term refer only to the physical and psychological milieu of the worker or to the confines of the property of the employer. As the geographic sphere of business responsibility has expanded, so have the responsibilities of the OM physician. This responsibility extends into the local and regional community, especially regarding adverse effects from "incidents" involving hazardous materials (HAZMATS). This additional role includes reducing liability, especially if operations involve handling of hazardous substances. Government agencies and community residents have filed successful suits against corporate officials, including criminal charges. This expanded scope and liability place the burden on the practitioner to assist in the development of safe operating policies and procedures, including emergency response plans, to minimize catastrophic events. With passage of the Superfund Amendments and Reauthorization Act (SARA) of 1986, among others, Congress established reporting and clean up requirements regarding accidental exposures to hazardous materials.

As the concept of the environment continues to expand, so do the lists of substances in the environment that represent a potential threat to human health and the ecosystem. At times, substances that are ordinarily considered benign may become a threat. For example, a tank car of cooking oil overturned and burst, spilling the oil into a local reservoir [1]. Secondary to such incidents, federal agencies with appropriate oversight may revise designated lists and measures regarding toxic materials. There are multiple listings of regulated hazardous substances and wastes that frequently cross-reference each other (Table 47-1).

Table 47-1. Listings of toxic and hazardous substances and wastes

Department of Transportation

Hazardous *substances*: 49 CFR 172.101 and appendices
Hazardous *wastes*: 49 CFR 171.8

Environmental Protection Agency

Characteristics of Hazardous *Waste*: 40 CFR 261.20-24
Lists of Hazardous *Wastes*: 40 CFR 261.30-33
Designation of Hazardous *Substances*: 40 CFR 302.4
Extremely Hazardous *Substances* and Their Threshold Planning Quantities:
    40 CFR 355, Appendix A and B

Occupational Safety and Health Administration

Hazardous *substances*: 29 CFR 1910.120.(a).(3).(A)-(D)
Toxic and hazardous *substances*: 29 CFR 1910, Subpart Z

Since the mid 1970s, emergency medical systems (EMS) throughout the United States have developed plans to cope with unexpected events that challenge routine capabilities of local and regional emergency response systems. These situations are known as mass casualty incidents (MCIs) and are classified into three categories (Table 47-2). Preparation for MCIs necessitates cooperation of multiple agencies from the local and regional levels, including treatment facilities. Only relatively recently has attention been turned to dealing with "disasters" that have as a *principle component* exposure to HAZMATS.

The potential for mishaps is underscored by the extent of hazardous materials in use. Government data gathered to support the Hazardous Materials Uniform Safety Act of 1990 indicated that around *4 billion tons* of regulated materials are transported annually and that approximately 500,000 movements of such materials occur daily [2]. Although these figures are enormous by any standard, relatively routine efforts such as moving a 55-gallon drum across a plant with a forklift are tabulated as well as driving a 10,000-gallon tank truck through a town. Since these figures are based on available data from before 1990, the actual number of activities involved in transporting substances is likely to be much greater. To regulate interstate transportation, the Department of Transportation (DOT) uses nine major classifications of regulated materials, including nearly 3000 individual substances [3] (Table 47-3). The final DOT category, "other regulated materials," contains many seemingly innocuous substances that represent hazards on the ecosystem level, as in the cooking oil incident cited earlier. The Chemical Transportation Emergency Center (CHEMTREC), a service of the Chemical Manufacturer's Association (CMA) that provides assistance in transportation incidents, received over 48,000 calls related to HAZMAT emergencies from 1986 through 1991 [4].

As governmental bodies enact stricter measures regarding the disposition of chemical wastes, the clandestine transport, storage, and dumping of such products are likely to increase. Transportation of hazardous materials has local as well as international implications. Border regions between countries with different levels of regulation present a particular problem. Children along the Rio Grande River, for example, have been known to get "high" by sniffing glowing green chunks of solidified solvents found along the river border [5]. In El Paso, Texas, an anonymous tip led to the discovery of four abandoned tractor-trailer rigs loaded with 175 55-gallon drums of polychlorinated biphenyls [5]. Although the clandestine transport of HAZMATS rarely involves the occupational physician, the expertise of the specialty may be valuable in an emergency release.

The more direct role of the OM practitioner (OMP) will involve developing and implementing HAZMAT "incident" response plans. OMPs are likely to also have

Table 47-2. Classification of mass casualty incidents

Level I	Manageable with resources available within the locality, with alterations in normal operations
Level II	Significant numbers of casualties that exceed normal medical response capability of local community
Level III	Medical disaster—overwhelms capabilities of local and regional resources, exceeds capacity of available multijurisdictional medical, mutual aid–state/federal support

Table 47-3. Department of Transportation regulated substances classification

Explosives
Gases
Flammable and combustible liquids
Flammable solids
Oxidizers and organic peroxides
Poisons
Radioactive materials
Corrosives
Other regulated materials

responsibility for monitoring and treating workers in the event of exposures. Incidents may involve no workers on site, a single worker or small group of workers, or an entire community/region.

A number of well-known catastrophes have occurred as a result of the release of hazardous materials. In December 1984, water entry into a storage tank containing methyl isocyanate (MIC) in Bhopal, India, resulted in release of a cloud of toxic gases. Controversy still exists as to whether the MIC or various reaction products such as hydrogen cyanide actually resulted in the deaths and injuries. Even the number of deaths directly related to the event remains uncertain; official government figures estimate about 1800 deaths, whereas other sources estimate between 2500 and 5000 deaths. Despite the mortality uncertainties, within 24 hours following the release, 90,000 people were evaluated by health care personnel. Due to uncertainty regarding the agent responsible for the toxic effects, most patients received only symptomatic management [6]. In this case, a complete lack of either a plant or regional response plan coupled with an inadequate understanding of the potential toxicity of the release resulted in the susceptible populations not being notified about precautionary measures.

In Springfield, Massachusetts, during a heavy rainstorm, water leaked through the ceiling of a warehouse onto fiber drums storing defective swimming pool chlorination crystals. The resultant heat released from the reaction ignited the paper drums and other warehouse materials, leading to a fire. A cloud of chlorine gas was released. That night, during another rainstorm, the same series of events occurred with a second release of chlorine gas! Approximately 25,000 people were evacuated from the surrounding area. Several firemen suffered inhalation injuries and skin damage but no civilian injuries occurred. Because the company failed to report the release to the National Response Center (NRC) and the local emergency planning committee (LEPC),[1] civil charges were brought by the federal government and the company was fined $89,840 in civil penalties. The Environmental Protection Agency (EPA) has delineated levels of penalties for failure to report releases. Failure to report may result in fines as much as *$25,000 per day* per incident. If found to have "knowingly and willfully" not complied with the reporting guidelines, guilty parties may be subject to a prison term of up to 2 years (5 years on repeat conviction) [7].

Frequently, such incidents have multiple components. For example, in February 1989, a runaway 48-car railroad train crashed into a three-unit engine in a rail yard on the outskirts of Helena, Montana, after going 12 miles downhill from the continental divide. On impact, a car filled with hydrogen peroxide exploded, which led to other explosions when derailed cars struck propane tanks placed along the track to fuel switch heaters. The resulting explosions caused extensive property damage and loss of electricity to 37,000 people, and 2000 people were evacuated at 4:30 AM amidst frigid temperatures ($-53°F$; $-85°$ with wind chill!). The fire was so intense that response personnel were unable to approach close enough to the tank cars to read any of the identifying placards.[2] In addition, there was significant concern about the potential for further danger from other railcars in the yard due to their proximity to the fire. Again, there was no loss of life or serious injury, a fortuitous outcome, since a major manufacturer in the area uses thousands of gallons of sulfuric acid daily with shipments arriving by rail. Hence, the possibility of the fire affecting tank cars loaded with sulfuric acid in the rail yard was also feared.

Although many incidents involve primarily one worker, events may contaminate other workers or rescue personnel. Hydrofluoric acid (HF), an etching agent used in the manufacture of computer chips, is highly corrosive and binds calcium. A worker was splashed with the agent on the upper body while working at a chip manufacturing plant in Massachusetts. Decontamination was an issue because of the risk of HF on the victim's clothing and in the surrounding area, affecting others. Unfortunately, the worker died within 4 hours of arrival at the hospital despite appropriate treatment by massive calcium infusion.

---

[1]Section 103 of CERCLA requires immediate reporting of releases of hazardous substances to the NRC. Section 304 of SARA Title III requires reporting in writing to the LEPC.
[2]Identification of contents of transportation vehicles is done through systems of placards and labels combined with the waybill carried on the carrier at the time of transport. The National Fire Protection Association has developed a system using a diamond divided into four smaller diamonds, with each field representing different characteristics (Fig. 47-1). The Department of Transportation has a system of specific labels and placards for different classes of HAZMATS. The United Nations has developed a system of numerical classification.

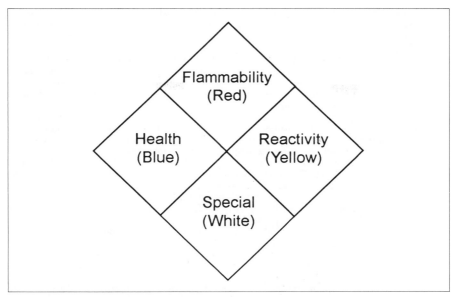

Figure 47-1. National Fire Protection Association 704 diamond. Each field except "special" has a number to indicate the relative degree of danger, with 1 indicating the least and 4 indicating the most dangerous. The "special" field has modification indicators, for example, OX = oxidizer. Copyright © 1990, National Fire Protection Association, Quincy, MA 02269. This warning system is intended to be interpreted and applied only by properly trained individuals to identify fire, health and reactivity hazards of chemicals. The user is referred to certain limited number of chemicals with recommended classifications in NFPA 49 and NFPA 325M which would be used as a guideline only. Whether the chemicals are classified by NFPA or not, anyone using the 704 system to classify chemicals does so at their own risk.

The above examples demonstrate some types of hazardous materials "incidents." In each situation, the occupational medicine physician has a significant contribution to make. It is essential, however, that the physician have a firm understanding of the toxicity of materials used at various sites to properly advise the planning for such emergencies. A well-developed and rehearsed *plan* is essential for responding appropriately to the types of incidents that may occur, including accidental exposures at a fixed site, or in the transportation and storage of hazardous materials.

Regulatory Authority

Since the mid 1970s, a number of federal statutes have been enacted that have direct relevance to the management of HAZMAT incidents. The most encompassing, in relation to employees at a worksite with potential exposure to HAZMATS, is SARA Title III [8]. SARA was enacted as an amendment to the Comprehensive Environmental Response, Compensation and Liability Act (CERCLA) of 1980, the original "Superfund Act" [9]. Title III is commonly known as the Emergency Planning and Community Right to Know Act (EPCRA). This legislation mandated the Occupational Safety and Health Administration (OSHA) to develop regulations regarding hazardous materials handling, which appears as OSHA's final rule for Hazardous Waste Operations and Emergency Response (HAZWOPER) [10]. The majority of the regulations in this section are directed at operations conducted at hazardous waste sites, particularly "Superfund sites."[3] Subsection (q) addresses non–

[3]These are federally designated sites, pursuant to CERCLA designation, that have been deemed to have particularly excessive amounts of designated toxic substances and hence are mandated to be cleaned to federally designated levels. A partial listing appears as the National Priority List of the EPA, published as Title 40 Code of Federal Regulations (CFR) 300, Appendix B.

waste sites; it covers *all* "emergency response operations for releases of, or substantial threats of releases of, hazardous substances without regard to the location of the hazard" [11]. The foundations for paragraph (q) are in section 303 of SARA Title III [12].

SARA Title III, section 311, requires filing Material Safety Data Sheets (MSDSs) or a chemical information list with the appropriate LEPC, the state emergency response commission (SERC), and the local fire department [13]. This section aids in planning for community response and promoting public awareness of hazardous materials present in the community.

Section 304 of SARA Title III (EPCRA) requires immediate reporting of accidental spills or releases of hazardous substances to a designated community emergency coordinator for the LEPC and to the SERC for any areas likely to be affected by the release. Additional reporting requirements can be found in several regulatory statutes, including the Resource Conservation and Recovery Act (RCRA), CERCLA, and the Clean Water Act. These requirements are codified by the EPA in Title 40 of the Code of Federal Regulations (Table 47-4). All releases, whether into water, air, or ground, are to be reported to the NRC per these EPA regulations.[4]

Regulation of transportation of HAZMATS is addressed largely through Public Law (PL) 101-615, entitled "Hazardous Material Transportation Uniform Safety Act of 1990." This law was passed as an amendment to the Hazardous Materials Transportation Act of 1975, since the original law did not address a number of issues such as precedence of jurisdiction and training of response personnel. The regulations generated by PL 101-615 appear in Volume 49 of the Code of Federal Regulations in various sections.

International standards vary greatly. At the time of this writing, the European Economic Community (EEC), for example, is trying to establish pan-European standards. This effort has led to heated political discussions. At this time, European standards are not as well codified as corresponding regulations in the US. Many Eastern European and developing countries have not yet addressed these issues.

The right to know sections of SARA Title III are a starting point for guidelines for the training of workers in handling hazardous materials. These same sections also address the filing of MSDSs and hazardous substance inventories with the LEPCs, to enable access to members of the community [14]. (As noted above, paragraph (q) of OSHA regulations 1910.120 addresses guidelines for workers involved in the emergency response to hazardous materials mishaps.) RCRA guidelines may also prevail.

Development of an Emergency Response Plan

Any facility or worksite that handles hazardous materials is required to develop an emergency response plan (ERP) consistent with the same regulations that govern

Table 47-4. Hazardous substance release reporting regulations[a]

Hazardous *waste*:[b]	
Generators	40 CFR 262.34(d) (5) (iv) (C)
Transport	40 CFR 263.30(c)
Treatment and storage disposal (TSD) facilities	40 CFR 264.56(d) (2)
TSD facilities	40 CFR 265.56(d) (2)
Hazardous *substances*:[c]	
Increase in continuous release	40 CFR 302.6
Noncontinuous release	40 CFR 302.6

[a]As codified by the Environmental Protection Agency.
[b]Mandated by the Solid Waste Disposal Act as amended by the Resource Conservation and Recovery Act of 1976, 42 USC 6901 et seq.
[c]As mandated by the Comprehensive Environmental Response, Compensation and Liability Act of 1980 and the Clean Water Act.

[4]The NRC is a division of the DOT and is managed by the Coast Guard. Its jurisdiction covers the 50 states, the Virgin Islands, Puerto Rico, Guam, and the Pacific Island Governments (Samoa and Northern Mariana). The telephone number for reporting is 1-800-424-8802.

reporting of releases as well as other EPA and OSHA regulations. The first decision to be made for any organization using hazardous materials is whether their own employees should participate in responses to releases, since OSHA regulations allow reliance on outside responders [15]. For small installations with good community support, the best course of action may be to simply have an OSHA-compliant emergency action plan in place [16].

Anticipation of Situations and Locations of Need

By conducting a facility survey of materials used and their respective processes, a *risk inventory* can be developed. As well as addressing means to avoid untoward events, this analysis will allow event-directed emergency response planning and the development of realistic drills.

To deal effectively with unexpected releases of HAZMATS, an ERP should take into account the following issues:

1. Exposures may affect the single worker or result in MCIs. A single worker exposure may escalate if not properly addressed.
2. Necessary contacts and information sources need to be outlined.
3. Guidelines should be prepared for grading the response (much like the concept of single- versus multi-alarm fire responses).

Many variations of the above may occur depending on the site's location, geography, number of personnel, and types of substances present. A number of basic concepts, however, are applicable in virtually any setting. As the plan is developed, though, the complexities become readily apparent. It is imperative that the authors of any plan pay particular attention to clarity and succinctness in the final version. OSHA delineates minimum elements for an ERP [17] (Table 47-5).

Determination of Scope of Plan

For companies that install their own response plans, the following should be addressed: (1) the type of events that will trigger an ERP, and the corresponding *level of response;* (2) the *responsibilities* of the emergency response team (ERT); (3) the relationship with *neighboring businesses* through mutual aid agreements; and (4) the role and *contact mechanisms* for local, state, and federal agencies. In determining the events that trigger a response, a thorough review of the toxicity of the materials of concern is critical (Table 47-6).

Emergency Response Team

Designating people or agencies who will respond to an incident as a team helps in planning for different levels of response. The ERT should specify *on-site* responders and *outside* agencies, such as fire, EMS, Coast Guard, and consultants. After defining off-site team members, agreements should be formalized *before* an incident. The composition of the ERT will vary according to the type and severity of an incident. ERTs for incidents involving hazardous substances are usually referred to as *HAZMAT teams,* the members of which all should have clearly defined roles. OSHA

Table 47-5. Minimum elements of an emergency response plan*

Pre-emergency planning
Personnel roles, lines of authority, and communications
Emergency recognition and prevention
Safe distances and places of refuge
Site security and control
Evacuation routes and procedures
Decontamination procedures that are not covered by the site safety and health
    plan
Emergency medical treatment and first aid
Emergency alerting and response procedures

*As proposed by the Occupational Safety and Health Administration [29 CFR 1910.120(1) (2)].

Table 47-6. Resources for information on toxicity and hazards[a]

Poison centers. Frequently do not have information on industrial or commercial toxic substances. MEDTREC service of the Chemical Manufacturer's Association[b] in cooperation with poison centers is preparing a reference base and training program that should improve this situation within a few years.

TOXNET. A service of the *National Library of Medicine.* Three reference sources:
  1. Hazardous Substances Data Bank
  2. Registry of Toxic Effects of Chemical Substances
  3. Chemical Carcinogenesis Research Information System

Sax, N. I., and Lewis, R. J. *Dangerous Properties of Industrial Materials.* New York: Van Nostrand Reinhold, 1989. *A comprehensive treatise.*

National Fire Protection Association.[b] Codes on a number of categories of substances, which include information on flammability, volatility, and explosivity.

[a]See also, references listed in Chaps. 25, Medical Surveillance, and 23, Toxicology.
[b]See Further Information at end of this chapter for address.

Table 47-7. Responder levels*

First-responder *awareness*	Know what hazardous substances are, how to recognize a release, how to notify the proper authorities
First-responder *operations*	Respond to a release to protect nearby persons, property, and environment through *defensive* actions, including basic decontamination
Hazardous materials *technician*	Respond for the purpose of actively trying to stop the leak
Hazardous materials *specialist*	Similar to technician but with more knowledge of various substances
On-scene *incident commander*	Able to take control of all the operations but would typically relinquish control to a fire department incident commander

*As defined by OSHA [29 CFR 1910.120(q) (6)].

defines four levels of responders and sets forth duty limitations and training guidelines for each level [18] (Table 47-7).

HAZMAT team members, starting at the technician level, must be familiarized with the proper use and care of personal protective equipment (PPE). The OM physician responsible for the medical aspects of the program must verify the physical capability of the person to use the designated type of PPE [19]. The term *PPE* is used primarily in the realm of protection of members of response teams. The term *chemical protective clothing (CPC)* is used more commonly in referring to protective garments for routine handling of chemicals. In selecting either PPE or CPC, the *substance* to which the garment will be exposed and the *duration of exposure* must be known. In conjunction with understanding the risk associated with *penetration* (bulk flow of liquid through material, seams, zippers, etc.) or *permeation* (passage through material on molecular level) of the material, one can critically evaluate various products.

Garments should be certified as having been tested in accordance with standardized methods. The American Society of Testing Materials (ASTM) methods, for example, are frequently used as standards for testing both penetration [20] and permeation [21]. The National Fire Protection Association (NFPA) also has standards for testing protective garments; those that meet their standards may carry a certification tag [22]. A number of OSHA regulations address standards for different components of protective garments (Table 47-8). The OSHA regulations often refer to both NFPA and American National Standards Institute (ANSI) statements on standards of protection (Table 47-8).

Table 47-8. Regulations and standards governing personal protective equipment

OSHA (29 CFR)

General	1910.132, 1910.1000,
(requirements for application,	subpart E, part 1926
selection, and use)	
Noise	1910.95
Eye and face	1910.133
Respiratory	1910.134
Head and foot	1910.135 and 1910.136
Electrical protection	1910.137

ANSI

General	Z37
Eye and face	Z87.1
Respiratory	Z88.2
Head	Z89.1
Footwear	Z41.1
Electrical	Z9.4

NFPA*

NFPA 1991	Standard on Vapor-Protective Suits for Hazardous Chemical Emergencies
NFPA 1992	Standard on Liquid Splash-Protective Suits for Chemical Emergencies
NFPA 1993	Standard on Support Function Protective Garments for Hazardous Chemical Operations

Key: ANSI = American National Standards Institute.
*Available from National Fire Protection Association (NFPA), One Batterymarch Park, Quincy, MA 02269.

Table 47-9. Personal protective equipment grades*

Level A	Totally encapsulating chemical-resistant suit
	Self-contained breathing apparatus (SCBA)
Level B	Splash protection with chemical-resistant clothing
	Positive-pressure, full–face-piece SCBA
Level C	Splash protection with chemical-resistant clothing
	Chemical-resistant, full–face-piece, air-purifying, cannister-type respirator
Level D	Standard work uniform with no special chemical-resistant properties and no respiratory protection

*These are partial descriptions to give an indication of the grades of protection. For a full description of required and optional gear at each level, refer to 29 CFR 1910.120, Appendix B, part A.

Personal protective equipment is classified into levels A, B, C, or D depending on the degree of protection afforded (Table 47-9). Table 47-10 outlines factors relevant to the choice of level of protection. Specialized equipment, despite being initially impervious to hazardous fluids and vapors, can be degraded such that the protective lifetime may be reduced to as short as several hours or less of continuous exposure. It is important to know the *composition of all components* of totally encapsulating suits used for maximum protection, as witnessed by the experience of Captain Gerald Grey of the San Francisco Fire Department. A totally encapsulating suit that he was wearing suffered severe damage to the faceplate due to exposure to anhydrous dimethylamine. Compatibility tables indicated that the suit, made of butyl rubber, was appropriate for the situation; however *the integrated faceplate,* made of polycarbonate, was not considered [23]. Tolerances of various PPE materials to potential hazards have been tabulated [24].

Employees required to use PPE must be evaluated regarding "fitness for . . . the

Table 47-10. Selection of level of PPE*

Level A	Maximum skin and respiratory protection from liquids, vapors, gases, and particulates; confined, poorly ventilated areas with unknown substances
Level B	Maximum respiratory protection; ambient $O_2 < 19.5\%$; lesser skin protection
Level C	Known substance and concentration meets specifications for air-purifying respirators; low skin toxicity
Level D	No anticipation of respiratory, skin, or mucous membrane toxicity

*29 CFR 1910.120, Appendix B, part B.

ability to wear any required PPE under conditions . . . that might be experienced at the worksite" [25]. These guidelines attempt to ensure that employees who need to use PPE are physically fit to wear the PPE in actual conditions. The most exacting of physical conditions in PPE are temperature extremes. Level A, which requires a totally encapsulating suit without ventilation, creates a potentially dangerous microclimate even at relatively cool ambient temperatures, especially if the wearer is engaged in heavy physical activity. Each worker required to use level A equipment needs to be evaluated for tolerance to heat stress. The NFPA has outlined a heat stress monitoring plan for persons using enclosed protective garments [26].

Levels of Response

A number of factors should be considered in delineating the level of response appropriate for categories of incidents, including: (1) level of *technical expertise* necessary to control the material(s) in question, (2) presence of *fire or explosion hazard,* and (3) potential *radius of risk,* that is, contained in a small room or over an entire city. Levels of response delineated for a site might be:

Individual or buddy system of worker teams
Divisional ERT
Facility ERT
Mutual aid ERT
"Outside" EMS/ERT

These levels could be activated in a sequential fashion or, based on information at the time of an incident, a higher level of response may be initiated. In all emergency situations involving HAZMATS, a buddy system is essential, wherein paired workers have protocols for checking the operations of each other and for providing immediate assistance to each other. As a part of the protocols for rendering assistance, *early notification of senior officials* is essential to enable them to summon medical assistance or activate a more comprehensive ERP.

Depending on the size and nature of the installation, the divisional and facility ERTs may be comprised of persons trained at the *HAZMAT technician* level. These personnel may be responsible for containing releases without endangering themselves or others while they await the outside team that is summoned for definitive action. Alternatively, the response teams of facilities such as large chemical manufacturing installations may be comprehensive and include their own fire control, medical, and decontamination capabilities. This situation is most common when the community response systems may not be politically or financially able to support such services, as, for example, in some foreign installations.

Activation of ERP

Much like any fire alarm system, the system for activation of the ERP must be treated with respect and yet not feared. Every employee should have the ability to activate the ERP and should not be discouraged to do so if he or she has an honest concern. A *protocol for internal verification* that is not so cumbersome as to delay necessary response should be in place. Although risk is involved simply in the response (for example, EMS and fire personnel driving at high speed to respond), it is preferable to respond in the early stages of an incident rather than after the situation has deteriorated.

Designation of Chain of Command

In the event of an incident, a clear *chain of command* is critical to prevent confusion. Authority needs to be designated at each level of response, including when authority will be relinquished to another designated incident commander (IC; for example, a shift foreman deferring command to a fire department official). The IC must coordinate the activities of uninjured workers remaining on site and ensure that volunteers without specific training and roles are not allowed to participate in any activities within restricted areas.

Decontamination

Decontamination of exposed personnel needs to be accomplished with strict adherence to guidelines that address four components:

1. *Location* of decontamination station, for example, at the site of the spill, within the "hot" zone, at the hospital; the site depends on the substances and injuries involved
2. *Removal of the substance* from contaminated personnel in a way that will not cause further harm to them
3. *Avoidance of exposure* of decontaminating personnel, who should be members of the ERT with specific decontamination training
4. *Containment* of offending agent in rinse solution, clothing, rescue material, and so forth.

It is often best to set up the decontamination zone in a "corridor" with progressive "stations" that move from fully contaminated to fully clean. Possible stations could include:

Initial shower/cleansing of exterior of PPE
Removal of PPE
Removal of any undergarments that may have been contaminated with leakage of the outer PPE
Personal shower/cleansing
Medical station for any immediate monitoring needs.

In addition to personnel, the entire site, *including equipment,* must be considered for decontamination. The emphasis in decontamination procedures should be on thoroughness rather than speed unless the victim(s) need emergency medical attention.

Decontamination procedures should always be performed at the most stringent levels appropriate for substances that may be present at the site. Procedures should be downgraded only when specific information regarding actual exposure becomes available. This point is particularly important for ERT members as they approach or enter the "hot zone." Although the means of decontamination is substance dependent, most hazardous substances do not react in a water-detergent environment and, hence, *water is an appropriate emergency starting point for liquid contaminants.* If the water reactivity of the contaminating substance is unclear or in the case of dry contaminants, removal of clothing and brushing or vacuuming the victims should be carried out initially. Chemical containing decontamination solutions should be used only when the offending agent is verified and an appropriate solution can be chosen.

Approaches for containment of decontamination waste range from using children's wading pools to collect flushing solutions to specially constructed trailers with self-contained air handling and waste water containers. More complete guidelines for decontamination exist in several of the resources listed under Further Information at the end of this chapter.

Containment of Incident

Containment should start at the first indication that a HAZMAT has been released; it may involve routine acts such as simply turning a switch or more complicated efforts such as dike-building. All workers should be acquainted with how to "shut down" the processes on which they are working. The emergency shutdown procedure should include instructions for stopping the flow of any reagents that are supplied to the process.

Once a response has been initiated, graded restricted zones should be established to prevent further injury and to allow containment and rescue operations to proceed unimpeded. Typically, three zones are designated: hot, warm, and cold, which are based on older plans designed for dealing with radioactive substances. Only "life-saving" treatment should occur in the "hot" area. In fact, only fully trained and properly attired HAZMAT specialists should enter the "hot" area, if at all. Additional zones can be designated if topography and weather conditions warrant them. Weather must be constantly monitored because changes, such as shifting wind direction, may require redesignation of safe areas as "hot." A *decontamination area* or areas should be designated as well.

Evacuation and Site Security

Like fire escape plans, hazardous materials evacuation plans should be established. Plans should be posted and reviewed as part of the right to know (RTK) orientation. Regional evacuation plans should be filed with the local government agency responsible for coordinating the responses of other services.

Plans for community evacuations must have contingencies for weather, explosions, and fires. Computers linked through modems to the National Weather Service for local and regional monitoring can assist in predicting evacuation needs. Computer programs are available that aid a sophisticated command center to make predictions regarding dispersion of any particular substance in light of local climate conditions.

Numerous factors are involved in securing the area of a release to allow for unimpeded rescue and containment activities as well as to prevent unnecessary exposure of personnel not on the HAZMAT team. Not least among the issues is *traffic control* and rerouting. Designation of perimeters and plans for patrolling and securing them may be necessary.

Systems of Outside Notification

Cooperation agreements with neighboring facilities and community and regional support systems should be drawn up with attention to a simplified notification process. A central agency, similar to an emergency services dispatch unit, can reduce confusion and chances of omitting a critical respondent. SARA Title III and RCRA require that facilities with designated quantities of extremely hazardous substances in excess of the EPA's threshold planning quantities must notify the LEPC with site/substance information [27].

Emergency notification procedures should include a checklist of information to be provided at the time of contacting respondents. *This checklist should be prominently posted next to each telephone that might be used for notification and include the following:*

Telephone number from which the call is coming
Name and location of the caller and facility/site
Time and location of the incident
Nature of incident (e.g., spill, explosion, confined space)
Material involved
Number of victims and extent of injuries
Condition and/or signs and symptoms of the victims
Name and phone number of safety officer responsible for the area of operations
    involved in the incident

If a community HAZMAT ERP does not exist, the responsible company will take the lead in establishing such a plan. A detailed discussion of *community HAZMAT ERPs* is beyond the scope of this chapter; however, excellent resources are described in Further Information. Planners should use a few resources to ensure that essential agencies are not omitted from the notification plan.

Site Communications

Effective communication among members of the ERT can be facilitated by using a *dedicated radio frequency* and by ensuring that all members of the team have radios. An analysis of a petroleum plant incident in Los Angeles in which hospital-based response teams participated indicated that some of the teams did not bring their HEAR[5] radios. Apparently, they felt there was too much feedback during drills due to the large number of radios operating on the same frequency [28]. A secondary system of communication should be in place, such as hand signals for crew members wearing PPE that have face masks. All members of the ERT should wear some form of external identification easily seen from a distance that is specific for their agency or division.

Role of Outside Agencies

The role of the municipal, county, state, federal, trade, and private consulting bodies that might be involved in an incident should be clearly defined. Many government agency roles will be obvious, but they should be stated in the ERP to avoid confusion and to reinforce their role and how they should be contacted.

Public Relations

A plan to notify and cooperate with local media to disseminate necessary information is essential. This plan should be conceived in a spirit of understanding the role of the media in both providing advice and information to those affected by the incident and to present a favorable image of the agencies and corporations involved in the response. The OM physician can be of valuable assistance in the public relations (PR) effort by assisting the director or by responding directly to the media. This latter effort can be a delicate responsibility that requires training, experience, and a savvy disposition. Some professional organizations, such as the CMA, provide this type of support for addressing the media in the event of a hazardous release.

At the scene, the PR director acts as the funnel and filter for transfer of information from the operations technicians to the media. The PR director may also be responsible for maintaining the incident log for use in debriefing. The PR director's role can be expanded to include creating links of acquaintance before any incidents occur. Previously established relationships with the media and community agencies will reduce adverse reactions and offer an opportunity for the company to present itself as responsible and prepared.

Debriefing

After an activation of the ERP, debriefings should occur at several levels. ERP planners/managers should confer with in-house personnel including workers on site at the location of the incident as well as members of the ERT. Evaluation of the events leading up to the incident, with attention to preventing similar series of events, should be the basic philosophy of the debriefings.

Actions of workers present at the time of the incident should be evaluated to enhance response performance and prevent additional personnel from becoming victims in future incidents. A study of a plant explosion in Norway, for example, revealed a number of correlates to "appropriate disaster response behavior" [29]. Among the correlates were *experience* in previous disasters, amount of *drilling,* and *previous maritime employment* (where there is a high attention to discipline regarding crisis situations as well as regular drills). Debriefings should be undertaken with partners in mutual aid agreements as well as local and regional public safety agencies. These debriefings should have a representative from, or at least share relevant conclusions and issues with, the LEPC.

All personnel who either were at direct or indirect risk during the incident should be offered the opportunity to participate in debriefings; these sessions should be structured like critical incident stress debriefing sessions (CISDS) performed by police, fire, and EMS agencies to mitigate the insidious psychological impact of major crises on affected personnel. Even off-duty personnel may be appropriate candidates

---

[5]*Hospital Emergency Administration Radio,* which operates on VHF frequencies and is prone to electrical static, known as feedback, if too many are operated in close proximity.

for CISDS-style debriefings, since they may manifest dysfunctional behavior patterns following a worksite disaster [30].

Finally, in regard to ERPs, the biggest factor in success is *repeated drilling*. A significant correlation between drilling experience and appropriate behavior in a stressful situation has been documented [29].

Role of the Occupational Physician

The Occupational Physician has an integral role in addressing emergencies surrounding hazardous materials. At the outset, the OM physician should be aware of potentially hazardous materials used in relation to the business for which he or she is working. Materials used on site for manufacturing, service, or maintenance should be addressed. If outside contractors come on site, the physician should be aware of the products they use that might affect employees. The physician should not rely solely on MSDSs for medical treatment guidelines, since the quality of these forms varies considerably. Once the physician is familiar with substances used, guidelines for safe handling and an ERP can be proposed in conjunction with the safety officer(s).

Depending on the degree of interest and expertise of the physician, involvement in ERP development may range from review and commentary of a plan to development of the plan itself. The OM physician should not limit attention to the individual business, but should be aware of potential ramifications of HAZMAT incidents on surrounding facilities and the local community. Thus, it is well within the purview of the OM physician to verify that the company has addressed regional problems, such as ground water contamination, that might arise in the event of a release. Meeting with local and regional EMS as well as EPA officials and participating in formation of mutual aid agreements will strengthen the OM physician's position in both planning and response phases. Corporate membership in LEPCs is encouraged and the OM physician would be an ideal candidate.

OSHA guidelines specify the role of the OM physician in relation to medical surveillance as well as pre- and postactivity assessments. In OSHA's regulations governing hazardous materials operations, virtually all workers who might be exposed to such materials are covered, whether they work at a waste site; a treatment and storage disposal (TSD) facility; manufacturer; transporter; or any other setting in which they might be exposed to hazardous materials [31]. For all of these employees, OSHA requires medical surveillance programs [32] (see Chap. 25, Medical Surveillance).

An occupational physician may perform required physical examinations or treat injured employees. Armed with information from the site survey and research on the effects of substances involved, the OM physician can either advise and treat directly or make informed choices of appropriate referrals.

Summary

At the time of this writing, most work on ERPs has been directed to larger operations such as petroleum and chemical manufacturing facilities as well as the bulk transportation industry. Relatively little has been done to assist smaller businesses and the service sector in this arena.

This chapter was written to aid the occupational health professional, whether physician, nurse, physician assistant, or safety officer, in dealing with appropriate response to hazardous materials releases. Since many of the courses offered by either government agencies or private organizations designed for familiarization and training last 2 to 5 days, this chapter should be considered as an introduction to the topic and a guide to further, more detailed resources.

References

1. Personal communication from DOT.
2. Hazardous Material Transportation Uniform Safety Act (1990), Public Law 101.615, section 2 ("Findings").
3. *Code of Federal Regulations,* Title 49, part 172, section 101 (commonly referred to as 49 CFR 172.101).

4. Chemical Transportation Emergency Center (CHEMTREC), Chemical Manufacturer's Association, 2501 M St., NW, Washington, DC 20037.
5. Tomsho, R. Environmental Posse Fights a Lonely War Along the Rio Grande. *The Wall Street Journal,* November 10, 1992.
6. Mehta, P. S., et al. Bhopal tragedy's health effects. *J.A.M.A.* 264:2781, 1990.
7. 40 CFR 355.50(a–c).
8. Enacted October 17, 1986, as Public Law 99-499 and published in v. 42 USC, sections 11001–11050. Relevant OSHA rulings are published in 29 CFR 1910.120.
9. Public Law 96-510.
10. 29 CFR 1910.120.
11. 29 CFR 1910.120.(a).(1).(v).
12. 42 USC 11003.
13. 42 USC 11021(a). EPA regulations covering this are in 40 CFR 370.
14. 40 CFR 370.
15. 29 CFR 1910.120 (1)(1)(ii).
16. 29 CFR 1910.38(a).
17. 29 CFR 1910.120(1)(2).
18. 29 CFR 1910.120.(q).(6).
19. 29 CFR 1910.120(f)(4)(i).
20. American Society for Testing and Materials, ASTM F739-91.
21. ASTM F903-90.
22. NFPA 1991. Standard on Vapor-Protective Suits for Hazardous Chemicals Emergencies; NFPA 1992, Standard on Liquid Splash-Protective Suits for Hazardous Chemical Emergencies; and NFPA 1993, Standard on Support Function Protective Garments for Hazardous Chemical Operations.
23. Grey, G. L. Supplement VII—Quick Reference Chemical Compatibility Chart for Protective Clothing. In M. F. Henry (ed.), *Hazardous Materials Response Handbook.* Quincy, MA: National Fire Protection Association, 1989. (This section, which includes an extensive listing based on a number of sources, does not appear in the latest [1992] edition.)
24. Johnson, J. S., and Anderson, K. J. *Chemical Protective Clothing, Product and Performance Information.* Akron: American Industrial Hygiene Association., 1990.
25. 29 CFR 1910.120(f)(4)(i).
26. Tokle, G. (ed.). Heat Stress Monitoring in Level C. *Hazardous Materials Response Handbook,* Quincy, MA: NFPA, 1992. Pp. 494–500.
27. 40 CFR 370.
28. Haynes, B. E., and Emmel, A. C., Role of a hospital team at an industrial explosion. Department of Emergency Medicine, Harbor/UCLA Medical Center, Torrance, California. *Am. J. Emerg. Med.* 6:260, 1988.
29. Weisaeth, L. A study of behavioral responses to an industrial disaster. Division of Disaster Psychiatry, Institute of Psychiatry, Gaustad. *Acta Psychiatr. Scand.* 355 (Suppl.):13, 1989.
30. Weisaeth, L., The stressors and the post-traumatic stress syndrome after an industrial disaster. Division of Disaster Psychiatry, Institute of Psychiatry, Gaustad. *Acta Psychiatr. Scand.* 355 (Suppl.):25, 1989.
31. 29 CFR 1910.120(a)(1)(i–iv).
32. 29 CFR 1910.120(f)(3–8).

Further Information

Agency for Toxic Substances and Disease Registry[6] This federal agency is a part of the Public Health Service. It was created by Superfund legislation in 1980 to "prevent or mitigate adverse human health effects and diminished quality of life resulting from exposure to hazardous substances in the environment." The agency provides a number of services, including training, research, and publications.

Managing Hazardous Materials Incidents, 1992
This is a three-volume series:

    I. *Emergency Medical Systems: A Planning Guide for the Management of Contaminated Patients.*

---

[6]See Chap. 45, The Agency for Toxic Substances and Disease Registry, for a comprehensive discussion of its role.

This volume addresses issues relevant to the prehospital setting and is primarily of concern to EMS personnel responding to an incident; however, much of the information would be helpful in organizing an on-site ERT.

II. *Hospital Emergency Departments: A Planning Guide for the Management of Contaminated Patients.*

This volume focuses on issues in dealing with hazardous materials incident victims in the emergency department setting. It is a good introduction to the topic and to relevant issues such as labeling and MSDSs. It would be a good resource for emergency departments that might serve a particular site.

III. *Medical Management Guidelines for Acute Chemical Exposure.*

This serves as a resource on the health effects of toxic substances and corresponding treatment protocols.

These publications are available on request through ATSDR, Emergency Response and Consultation Branch (E57), Division of Health Assessment and Consultation, 1600 Clifton Rd., NE, Atlanta, GA 30333 (404-639-6360).

American Society for Testing and Materials [1916 Race St., Philadelphia, PA 19103 (215-299-5400)] Standard testing procedures and other standards.

Chemical Manufacturer's Association, (2501 M St., NW, Washington, DC 20037)

Chemical Transportation Emergency Center (CHEMTREC) is a service provided by the CMA. With information from the placarding and waybill of a truck or train car, they may be able to contact the shipper/manufacturer to get further information regarding the exact contents. They are also able to give initial information on emergency response guidelines. Telephone: 1-800-424-9300.

MEDTREC is a service of the CMA designed to provide emergency medical treatment information for exposures to chemical substances. The service is available by calling the CHEMTREC number. The information provided is medically verified and peer reviewed for accuracy.

Community Awareness and Emergency Response Program Handbook. A handbook published by the Association, it goes through the process for developing emergency response plans for the chemical industry.

Decontamination Guideline Resources

Policy Guidance for Response to Hazardous Chemical Releases. US Dept. of Transportation (COMDTINST M16465.30), a US Coast Guard manual.

Hazardous Materials Response Handbook. National Fire Protection Association, One Battery Park, Quincy, MA 02269.

1990 Emergency Response Guidebook. DOT P5800.5. Washington, DC: US Department of Transportation, 1990.
This handbook lists chemicals by Chemical Abstracts (CAS) number for fast reference in the field. It also lists relevant telephone numbers for contacting in case of an incident. There is a table of initial isolation and protective action distances. The handbook is available directly from Department of Transportation, 400 7th St., SW, Washington, DC 20590.

Hazardous Materials Information Exchange (HMIX) An electronic bulletin board provided free of charge from the Federal Emergency Management Agency (FEMA). This service provides a database of information regarding training, resources, technical assistance, regulations, and emergency management. It *does not* function as assistance at the time of an emergency. For information on access, call: 1-800-752-6367 (outside Illinois) or 1-800-367-9592 (within Illinois).

The National Fire Protection Association (One Batterymarch Park, Quincy MA 02269)

Many federal standards cross-reference to publications of standards put forward by the NFPA. It will provide a catalogue on request. Several useful publications are the following:

Hazardous Materials Response Handbook.
This handbook includes the complete text of two helpful NFPA standards: Standard for Professional Competence of Responders to Hazardous Materials Incidents, NFPA 472, and Recommended Practice for responding to Hazardous Materials Incidents, NFPA 471. In addition there are eight supplements on topics ranging from a sample ERP *to guidelines for decontamination. This is a useful, practical reference.*

Hazardous Chemical Data, no. 49.

Properties of Flammable Liquids, Gases, and Volatile Solids, no. 325M.

Manual of Hazardous Chemical Reactions, no. 491M.

The National Library of Medicine (NLM)[7]

TOXNET system of three databases:

The Hazardous Substances Data Bank

Provides reviews on the toxicity, hazards, and regulatory status of over 4000 frequently used chemicals.

The Registry of Toxic Effects of Chemical Substances

The Chemical Carcinogenesis Research Information System.

All of these databases can be accessed using an inexpensive computer program available from the NLM called *Grateful Med* and a modem in any computer (Macintosh or IBM-compatible). Other computerized databases and technical support services are either a one-time purchase or subscription usually supplied on a compact disc, read-only memory (CD-ROM) format, which requires special software (generally provided by the vendor) and a special disc drive (not provided by the vendor).

For information regarding the services of the NLM, write: MEDLARS Management Section, National Library of Medicine, 8600 Rockville Pike, Bethesda, MD 20894; or Call: 1-800-638-8480 (outside Maryland) or 301-496-6193; or through INTERNET (gmhelp@gmedserv.nlm.nih.gov).

Sax, N. I., and Lewis, R. J. *Dangerous Properties of Industrial Materials.* New York: Van Nostrand Reinhold, 1989.

A comprehensive treatise that is an integral part of an office library for occupational/ environmental medicine.

United States Congress

Copies of any of the laws referred to in this chapter can be obtained by writing to House Document Room, US Capitol, Room H-226, Washington, DC 20515.

---

[7]See Chap. 27, Searching the Occupational Medical Literature, for a discussion of additional databases.

48

Accessing Environmental Data

David Mueller Gute

The etiologic contribution of the ambient environment to the development of human disease is a matter of controversy. This chapter does not enter into this debate, but suggests that there is increasing affirmation of the intricate relationship between the environment and human health. This chapter provides the reader with:

1. A consideration of available environmental information
2. A definition of and a means of *access* to environmental exposure databases
3. A delineation of *sources and the legal mandates* for the collection of such databases
4. Review of other types of environmental information available from government agencies
5. Possible applications of environmental exposure databases in the practice of clinical medicine

Ambient environmental information of relevance to the practicing clinician can take many forms. Information includes data collected as a result of statute, such as air pollution monitoring as mandated by the Clean Air Act to other burgeoning environmental exposure databases. Environmental information is collected by many levels of government: local, county, state, and federal, and even by private corporations. These data are also collected for different time periods and vastly different geographic units. Accessing environmental data systems may be of clinical interest, to improve diagnosis and treatment [1]. Another reason for accessing such data is to respond to patient queries on environmental health. Survey research indicates that the physician is highly regarded as a source of objective information on the environment by the public, but is usually untrained for addressing occupational/environmental health issues [2].

Physicians have been urged to become involved and knowledgeable about this content area because of "special responsibilities" owing to the advocacy role that they can fulfill as well as the role of agent to foster preventative actions by governments, corporations, and communities [3]. These relationships are likely to deepen as the intricate webs linking human health and the environment proliferate.

Environmental exposure databases were recently reviewed in a workshop hosted by the United States Environmental Protection Agency (EPA), the Agency for Toxic Substances and Disease Registry (ATSDR), and the National Center for Health Statistics (NCHS) [4]. This workshop was convened to consider the uses of environmental exposure databases collected at the federal level of government. In general, these databases report on *exposure* data, in contrast to the more clinically useful parameter of *dose*. It is of interest to note, however, that of the 67 federally sponsored data systems reviewed, 13 (approximately 20%) contained human tissue results.

Before reviewing available data, the manner in which databases are arrayed is described to consider which parameters are of potential clinical interest (Table 48-1). Selected comments on these parameters are also presented.

Information is presented on data sources available for the following environmental media: air, water, and soil, as well as hazardous waste. The chapter approaches these topical areas in a manner that will assist in medical practice.

Data Quality Issues

This chapter is based on the simple thesis that environmental information will benefit the practicing physician in the diagnosis, treatment, and prevention of disease. What separates data from information?

Table 48-1. Parameters of interest for environmental data

Parameter	Comments
Temporal period of data collection	Sufficient length of time to capture seasonal effects?
Collection *frequency*	Annual, monthly, daily
Smallest *unit* of geographic aggregation	City/town, census tract
Type of media	Soil, water, air

Table 48-2. Key questions in evaluating environmental data

1. How representative is the sample of the affected area?
2. Were standard laboratory methods used?
3. Were the samples handled, transported, and stored properly?
4. What were the quality assurance procedures?
5. How were the samples obtained?
6. What was the level of detection of the procedure? (What was the smallest amount of the substance that could be detected?)
7. If latency is a factor of interest, do retrospective exposure data exist?

Data are raw measurements concerning, for the purposes of this chapter, the ability to describe the concentration, distribution, and environmental fate of a given agent or contaminant. *Information,* on the other hand, represents data that are interpretable and useful to a decision maker for the purposes of coming to a conclusion. The products of any data system should be viewed through the lens of statistics.

Statistics are used to describe the natural world. The use of statistics revolves around key *parameters* of a given *population.* For instance, with sufficient resources, it is possible to measure the blood lead levels of all 6-year-old children in the United States. The mean value, or other measures of central tendency such as mode or median, would constitute a parameter of this population. The usual approach is to draw a sample of subjects from a population and then calculate statistics resulting from this sample. A key hurdle is the representativeness of the sample in reference to the underlying population from which it was drawn.

These basic points regarding data, including those from environmental media, consist of the following:

Validity: Do the data truly measure the desired attribute? Example: If you are measuring contaminant levels in a stream, are the sampling stations up- or downstream of a point source generator?

Accuracy: Is the method representative of the true value? That is, can the method adequately approach the true result?

Reliability: Can the method demonstrate *consistency* in the generation of values? For instance, a method may be highly reliable by generating consistent results in multiple tests. Reliability, however, should not be confused with accuracy. A technique can be very consistent, or reliable, without being accurate.

These are generic constraints in employing statistics to increase understanding of any problem. Practitioners in occupational and environmental medicine in particular are well aware of the vagaries that can plague indices of health, especially clinical laboratory results. A critical eye should also be cast with reference to environmental data. Cardinal concerns include questions to be used in conjunction with almost any of the databases discussed in this chapter (Table 48-2). The practitioner is urged to become a more sophisticated consumer of environmental data. This sophistication can result from familiarity with the sources of these data and from an intelligent appreciation of their use in the practice of medicine.

Types of Environmental Data

A variety of environmental data collection systems exist in the United States. (This chapter focuses on United States sources. This does not mean to imply that environmental health problems benefit from such insularity; rather, it is simply a decision predicated by available space.) Some of these systems exist because of regulatory requirements and fulfill either monitoring or surveillance requirements of statutes or regulations. These data may be collected at the federal or state level. It is important to keep in mind that many of these data systems are collected for *reasons other than human health concerns.*

The potential for human exposure to a specific contaminant is of primary clinical interest in that this information is central to diagnosis and treatment. A recent compilation of federal environmental exposure data systems reflects the profusion and variety of these sources [5]. This listing includes 67 data systems for data obtained from three distinct sources. These data can be generated from passive sensors located in an enclosed environment (e.g., radon sampling device), personal monitoring equipment actually worn by volunteers or workers (e.g., radiation badge), and biologic media for actual analysis (the quantitation of blood lead levels).

For a true picture of human exposure to emerge, the practitioner must address the cumulative nature of exposure from *multiple pathways,* including routes of exposure such as dermal, respiratory, and ingestion. Any such consideration must include the impact of food chain exposures, especially for substances readily stored (lead) or concentrated selectively in certain tissues, such as polychlorinated biphenyls (PCBs) in fat. Other factors to consider in relation to a patient's health include:

Magnitude of exposure: What is the effective concentration in biologic media? Measures of magnitude will be more likely expressed in a volume of environmental media such as air or water.

Duration of exposure: How long was the actual exposure? Acute or chronic exposure? A particular concern is whether sharp spikes in concentration for short periods may be relevant.

Frequency of exposure: How often does this exposure occur? Does it vary seasonally or temporally?

Data are also generated as a result of requirements of regulatory agencies and can be thought of as constituting three specific functions: monitoring, surveillance, and special studies tied to a geographic site. For instance, in the above-mentioned 67 data collection systems, 36 performed monitoring functions, 19 primarily supported regulatory activities, and 29 shaped research needs.

Monitoring data are routinely collected by federal, state, and sometimes local governments to measure environmental media (air, water, soil) for selected contaminants as specified either by statute (criteria pollutants as defined by the Clean Air Act) or special interest. Surveillance connotes a more encompassing and ambitious research plan for the visualization of a specific environmental agent (e.g., the National Health and Nutrition Examination Survey [NHANES] study, which characterizes, among other things, food chain exposure to selected environmental agents including lead). Special studies are performed for a variety of purposes, most notably in the area of hazardous waste, involving the cleanup and discovery process surrounding specific Superfund sites.

Agent-specific information concerning the toxicologic characteristics may be of use to practitioners in assessing the potential for health effects in a specific case. Two on-line data systems that can provide the practitioner with general information regarding an agent are the Toxicology Information (TOXLINE) and Toxicology Data Network (TOXNET). Both are supported by the MEDLARS management section of the National Library of Medicine. TOXLINE is composed of 16 subfiles, and TOXNET of 10 files, many of which could be of particular interest to the practitioner. Included among the subfiles of TOXNET are the following items:

Registry of Toxic Effects of Chemical Substances (RTECS) as maintained by the National Institute for Occupational Safety and Health. This file contains information on *agent-specific characteristics* including toxicity in both humans and animals and other characteristics of importance to clinicians.

Integrated Risk Management System (IRIS) from the EPA is an electronic on-line database of summary health risk assessment and regulatory information on chemical substances. The primary purpose of IRIS is to provide guidance risk values to EPA risk assessors and decision-makers for use in EPA risk assessments. IRIS is not an exhaustive toxicologic database, but rather presents a summary of information on hazard and dose-response assessments. As of April 1, 1993, IRIS contained 509 chemicals. This included 340 oral reference dose (RfD) and 78 inhalation reference concentration (RfC) summary sections, and 216 carcinogen assessments [6]. (See Chap. 23, Toxicology, for a review of relevant concepts.)

Toxic Release Inventory (TRI) represents a compilation of information on the release of toxic substances by manufacturing facilities. These data are available in an annual report as well as by accessing an EPA database via microcomputer telephone modem [7]. The federal statute that created TRI, the Emergency Planning and Community Right To Know Act of 1986, specifically required EPA to provide *public access* to this file *via an on-line format*. This law is one of the first instances in which the *mode of dissemination* of a database, in contrast to its content, was stipulated.

Commonly Asked Questions that Trigger Environmental Data Searches

Many analysts, in commenting on medical practice in the United States, note the rise in the public's interest in environmental health questions and the growing role of the physician in serving as an "expert" and opinion leader for answering such questions posed by patients [8]. Many of these questions are generated and fueled by patients' concerns surrounding news media coverage of environmental "pressure points." Examples include the possible health effects of a given agent, the environmental and health effects attributable to a hazardous waste site, the unknown consequences of a newly emerging technology (release of engineered microbes), or the possible health effects of mature technologies (electromagnetic fields).

Beyond helping patients interpret new events in environmental health, the practitioner must distill information of critical importance in the differential diagnosis and treatment of a patient. Such investigations can be enhanced with data concerning a hazardous agent. Inquiries may be started through data sources that contain agent-specific information. (Refer back to the toxicologic databases previously described.) In addition, the clinician must verify the exposure pathways in relation to a particular environmental agent. In performing such an analysis, the central tenets of exposure assessment (previously discussed) must be addressed.

Workers may be exposed to substances on the job that can affect their health. Transport of these same occupational agents to family members via the workers' clothes is widely acknowledged. Hobbies and recreational activities of workers must be critically evaluated for a comprehensive picture of all sources of potential exposure. In a similar manner, community residents may suffer complaints and health problems attributable to industrial facilities and/or hazardous waste sites or other facilities associated with solid waste streams, such as landfills, incinerators, and transfer stations.

The presentation of this type of complaint to the physician is an encounter of increasing frequency throughout the United States. Pivotal community environmental health cases in Times Beach, Missouri; Love Canal, New York; and Woburn, Massachusetts, among others, have forced local, state, and federal governments to develop and augment resources to address environmental disease. This transition has not been easy. Public health authorities have been upbraided for a variety of faults, including lack of compassion, deficiencies in the scope and focus of epidemiologic studies, and their general inability to include community representatives in the drafting and dissemination of community-based scientific protocols [9]. The questions posed to public health authorities regarding the linkages between site-specific contaminants and the relationship to somatic disease highlight some of the limits of epidemiology. These limits have been demonstrated in stark relief in celebrated cases and have resulted in thoughtful commentary concerning the feasibility of conducting such "reactive" epidemiology [10].

Agency Resources

Many federal and state agencies are responsible for the collection and dissemination of environmental data. This chapter focuses on the agencies listed here because of their singular importance to environmental health. (For more discussion of relevant regulatory agencies, see Chap. 3, The Role of Regulatory Agencies.)

Agency for Toxic Substances and Disease Registry

The ATSDR is a Health and Human Services Department agency created by the Comprehensive Environmental Response, Compensation and Liability Act of 1980 (CERCLA). Under CERCLA, commonly known as the Superfund Act, and the Superfund Amendments and Reauthorization Act of 1986, ATSDR's mission is to prevent or mitigate human health problems and diminished quality of life resulting from exposure to hazardous substances. ATSDR is also mandated to develop information and educational programs to help health professionals evaluate, diagnose, treat, and conduct surveillance on patients exposed to hazardous substances.

In 1984, amendments to the Resource Conservation and Recovery Act of 1976 (RCRA), which provides for the management of legitimate hazardous waste storage or destruction facilities, charged the ATSDR to conduct health assessments at these sites, when requested by the EPA, states, or individuals, and to assist the EPA in determining which substances should be regulated and the levels at which they may pose a threat to human health.

In 1986, amendments to CERCLA, known as the Superfund Amendments and Reauthorization Act of 1986 (SARA), broadened ATSDR's responsibilities in the areas of health assessments, toxicologic databases, information dissemination, and medical education.

Environmental Protection Agency

The EPA was formed in 1970 and acquired regulatory responsibility, under the Clean Air Act Amendments of 1970 and the Clean Water Act of 1972, to set national air and water standards for selected contaminants. As the EPA has developed and matured, it has placed greater reliance on the activity of its regional offices scattered throughout the country to maintain oversight. Added burdens imposed on the agency include the Toxic Substances Control Act of 1976 (TSCA) and CERCLA, or the Superfund Act (and its subsequent set of amendments, SARA). Superfund is grappling with an estimated 23,000 potential hazardous waste sites in the United States. The EPA has weathered severe criticism for the perceived lack of speed and responsiveness to the identification, control, and abatement of these sites. Given the complexity of achieving compliance and oversight of these statutes, many states (currently 41) have assumed delegated authority to enforce EPA mandates in these areas.

State Health and Environmental Departments

Because of the trend toward delegation, state-based resources in the form of state health and environmental agencies can represent useful resources for data, technical assistance, and information pertaining to the environment. State agencies are generally responsible for administering pollution control programs, and environmental monitoring programs for air and water, and, in conjunction with local officials, for the administration of an array of environmental protection activities.

Other Resources

Poison control centers, through the dispensing of critical clinical information for practitioners and patients alike have become well established in the medical landscape. The portion of inquiries that have some connection to the environment has continued to increase [11]. This reality, coupled with suggestions from organizations such as the Institute of Medicine that advocate "single access" sources of information for clinicians, has led certain poison control centers to move into the niche of supplying environmental health information. One of the first of these enhanced poison control centers has been established and staffed by the faculty of the Duke Medical School Division of Occupational and Environmental Health [12].

The physician may also rely on a personal computer and a modem to open new vistas of diverse environmental data. The profusion of on-line capability has expanded greatly and contains the familiar, such as MEDLINE, as well as the abstract and unfamiliar. Reviews of how to access, obtain, and utilize this technology are also improving [13].

Case Studies in Environmental Medicine

The following two cases attempt to provide the reader with concrete examples of how environmental data can be used by practitioners in ascertaining and evaluating putative environmental disease. The intent is to present practical advice as to how to approach two distinct classes of problems. The first case focuses on a particular disease and its relationship to a population at risk. The second case addresses not the disease endpoint as the critical focus, but rather pathways of exposure.

Case 1: Adult Diagnosed with Acute Leukemia

A 28-year old white man has been diagnosed with acute leukemia. His specific diagnosis is acute nonlymphocytic leukemia (ANLL), a category of leukemia that accounts for over 50% of all the leukemia in adults. The patient's family expresses the belief that other neighbors living nearby have recently been diagnosed with leukemia and other cancers. You are asked for your assessment of whether there is a possible environmental "factor" that may explain this situation. For an in-depth review of the etiology and epidemiology of the leukemia, the reader should consult Linet's book on this subject [14].

Your first steps should consist of the following. Respond to what your patient and his/her family are feeling and saying. It is critically important to listen and then give counsel. The astute clinician can represent the first line of intelligence with regard to the etiology of human carcinogens. One of the best examples of this occurrence is found in the association of vinyl chloride with angiosarcoma of the liver, which began in the practice of a single physician [15]. All too often, however, it will be hard to link the occurrence of community "clusters" of cancer with any specific etiologic agent.

In the case of leukemia, specifically ANLL, it would be prudent to review with the patient the known causes of this disease. The two most important causes are benzene exposure and ionizing radiation. Such exposures could come from a variety of sources, including both occupational and environmental sources, and, in the case of ionizing radiation, through medical therapy. In pursuing any evaluation of your patient's leukemia, it is important to seek information that carries with it the combined histopathologic and clinical classification scheme of the leukemia under study. Unfortunately, many epidemiologic studies simply lump all leukemias together, thus frustrating the attempt to improve on existing etiologic information for the major subtypes. A relatively new finding of some concern with reference to childhood leukemia is the proximity of cases to electromagnetic fields. These studies have found relative risks in the 0.8 to 2.0 range for this disease outcome. However, these studies are plagued by poor ascertainment of retrospective or historical exposure to the agent [16]. This lack of retrospective environmental data is a continuing problem for most investigations of occupational and environmental agents, and is a particular concern for health problems that exhibit long *latency*.

With regard to concerns about the existence of a community cluster or raised level of incidence in the immediate area, a number of possible sources of information are available. First, contact the local board of health or the state health department to inquire if a tumor or cancer registry exists. Statewide rates can be compared to those of the community of interest to yield some relative assessment of the magnitude of the problem. Ask for data that are at least aggregated over 3- to 5-year intervals, particularly for towns with small populations, so that the values for the area of interest are a little more stable. In addition, try to ascertain incidence instead of mortality. If the state health or county health agency does not maintain a registry, inquire at the regional tertiary cancer hospital and see if an institution-specific registry is maintained. The American Cancer Society maintains annual estimates of the number of cancer cases occurring in each state. These estimates are largely driven by mortality information but at least might be helpful in providing the family with some information.

The most important subject to pursue with the patient's family is a determination of the types of exposures that the patient may have suffered in his/her lifetime, either from occupational or environmental sources or from hobbies or crafts pursued by the individual. The goal of such an evaluation is to confront directly the fears that the disease resulted from some known agent that the patient could have avoided or have reduced exposure to if the information had been available. A structural problem to be discussed early in such a dialogue is that the science of epidemiology attempts to discern etiology for *groups* of people who exhibit certain characteristics. The generalizations gained from such analysis do not translate well into making statements about where *individual* cases of a particular disease arise.

Patients and families may want information about the number of cases of the cancer that have been found within the community. They may even supply you with lists of people who they have heard have been diagnosed with cancer. These lists should be passed on to the appropriate public health authority for verification and evaluation. Important parameters to check on such lists include the actual diagnosis, the date of diagnosis, and, if available, the length of residence in the neighborhood if the concern centers on a community risk of specific cancers. This level of detail is usually missing from community-generated lists, but is critical in order to support further epidemiologic evaluation. Such community-generated lists can suffer from a variety of problems including inaccurate information and various forms of information biases, which have been previously discussed in Chap. 24, Epidemiology and Biostatistics. .

Another factor to consider in any suspected environmental disease is the relative contribution of personal risk factors such as tobacco, drug, and alcohol use. In the case of ANLL, neither tobacco nor alcohol demonstrates consistent patterns as a major risk factor. In sum, listen to your patient and his/her family in their quest to understand "why" this disease happened. Be aware that your investigations may shed some light on etiology, but be prepared for the much more likely result that you will not be able to ascertain cause to the level of satisfaction of all concerned parties.

Case 2: Patient Concern Over Proximity to Superfund Hazardous Waste Site

A 34-year old woman presents to an occupational physician concerned about her proximity (1 mile) to a Superfund hazardous waste site and the possibility of air pollution and water pollution from this site influencing a variety of nonspecific symptoms that she is experiencing.

Given the nonspecific nature of the patient's symptoms, the first goal of your response should be to obtain information that describes what is known about the point source of interest. There are a variety of data sources that can be consulted. As a first step contact the local health authorities concerning the existence of a public health assessment of the Superfund site. The Superfund Amendments and Reauthorization Act of 1986 set a year deadline for the characterizing of sites after they are proposed for inclusion as a Superfund site and listing on the National Priorities List (NPL). Listing on the NPL qualifies the site for cleanup under CERCLA or Superfund authority. Sites that are not listed on the NPL are abated subject to state or private action. As of October 1990, about 1200 sites were on or proposed for the NPL. The EPA expects to add about 1000 sites to the list during the 1990s [17]. ATSDR has determined that hazardous substances had been released at 85% of the sites and that about 15% of these sites merited further public health investigation [18].

SARA requires that the public health assessments be based on such factors as the nature and extent of site contamination, the size and susceptibility of the community, and the effects of exposure. SARA sets out two goals for such assessments: deciding whether the exposure to a site's hazardous substances should be reduced and stating whether additional health studies should be conducted at the site. The law requires that ATSDR provide its health assessments to the EPA and to the states. ATSDR's role at Superfund sites is mostly advisory; the EPA is in charge of actual cleanup [17].

What are the likely pathways of exposure emanating from a hazardous waste site? There are three principal routes: airborne exposure, run-off to ground and surface waters, and dermal contact from community residents coming into direct contact with contaminated soils and agents. The routine monitoring of air concentrations of volatile agents on the site is usually not feasible. The study of this route, and others, is also plagued by the generally small number of exposed populations. The next route of exposure, water contamination, is not just confined to ingestion, but also should include airborne exposures from materials that can outgas during showering, bathing, or cooking, or can be absorbed through the skin.

The question of where water data can be obtained primarily turns on the source of the water. Private wells are generally tested at the initiative of the owner. Most regulatory agencies have been loath to accept responsibility for the regulation of this drinking water source. If the sources of drinking water are surface or ground, waters distributed as part of a municipal or regional system, quality can be obtained from the relevant water board or company. Most existing protocols in the United States are in place to guard against bacteriologic contamination and other threats that could affect gross water quality, such as turbidity and biologic oxygen (BOD). Special studies to characterize waterborne concentrations of hazardous materials such as lead have been implemented periodically by agencies such as the EPA or state environmental and health departments. The testing of residential water for organics, heavy metals, and other agents can usually be accomplished through commercial laboratories or in conjunction with special testing protocols provided by local authorities for residents. Some states are beginning to launch certification programs aimed at improving the accuracy and validity of data obtained from such commercial laboratories.

Under the federal Safe Drinking Water Act of 1974, the EPA is required to prepare and promulgate regulations and standards concerning public water supplies. Two different standards are required; they consist of the recommended maximum contaminant levels (RMCLs) and the maximum contaminant levels (MCLs). The RMCLs are not enforceable but exist for advisory purposes. In contrast the MCLs are enforceable; that is, an MCL, once exceeded, requires corrective action to be taken by the supplier to ensure compliance with the standard. Where no guidance exists from the EPA, states are left to their own devices in promulgating regulatory standards, particularly in the area of organic contaminants.

An associated problem is establishment of acceptable levels for soils through which ground water can percolate. Soil levels are also of concern in attempting to answer questions such as, "How clean is clean?" This question is regularly encountered in monitoring any abatement project. It poses the questions of what level of cleanliness to which a media should be returned before the site is returned to a more general pattern of use.

In general, the caveats that physicians are aware of in reference to the interpretation of clinical laboratory results hold for the interpretation of environmental data. Keep in mind some of the central questions that should inform your assessment of these data, as contained in Table 48-2.

A final possible route of exposure is through the medium of soil. Soil can obviously be ingested by young children, and serve as a means of uptake (along with airborne deposition), increasing the load on crops eaten for human consumption.

It is important to discuss with the patient all possible routes of exposure that exist in concern with the point source of interest. Often, if the possibility of exposure can be rigorously pursued, the level of fear and concern can either be substantiated or placed in an appropriate context. This is in contrast with Case 1, in which a specific health endpoint forms the basis of the investigation and dialogue between patient and physician. The presence of a Superfund site in a town can galvanize public concern. This public dimension of the problem will complicate an understanding of the levels of risk posed to your patient. Perception of risk from the perspective of your patient turns on issues with which you must be acquainted. These include the perceived benefit and attendant risks, the severity of the health endpoint associated with the risk, the certainty of the association, the ability of the individual to exercise some control of the risk, the newness of the risk, and whether the risk is limited to the individual or is also conferred on other family members or future generations, or both.

As in all professions, the skill of practitioners can only be improved by investing in training and education to enhance skills and competence. This chapter has attempted to lay out an overall framework for transforming data into the more clinically useful commodity of information. This transformation rests with the acumen and integrative abilities of the practitioner more than it does with a mastery of the hardware or software involved with the storage and dissemination of environmental data. There has been a palpable increase in the depth and the sophistication of continuing education and training programs directed at the physician community and targeting environmental health concerns. This change has ranged from the creation of environmental medicine residencies to a panoply of other formats and models [19]. Of greatest importance is that it is under way.

References

1. Goldman, R., and Peters, J. The occupational and environmental health history. *J.A.M.A.* 246:2831, 1981.
2. Levy, B. The teaching of occupational health in American medical schools: 5-year follow-up of an initial study. *Am. J. Public Health* 75:79, 1985.
3. McCally, M., and Cassel, C. K. Medical responsibility and global environmental change. *Ann. Intern. Med.* 113:467, 1990.
4. Sexton, K., et al. Estimating human exposures to environmental pollutants: Availability and utility of existing databases. *Arch. Environ. Health* 47:398, 1992.
5. US Environmental Protection Agency, National Center for Health Statistics, Agency for Toxic Substances and Disease Registry. *Inventory of Exposure-Related Data Systems Sponsored by Federal Agencies.* EPA/600/R-92/078, May 1992.
6. Anonymous. *Health and Environment Digest,* Freshwater Foundation 7:8, 1993.
7. US Environmental Protection Agency. *The Toxics Release Inventory: A National Perspective.* EPA/560/4-89-005. Washington, DC: US Government Printing Office, 1989.
8. Kilbourne, E. M., and Weiner, J. Occupational and environmental medicine: The internist's role. *Ann. Intern. Med.* 113:974, 1990.
9. Ozonoff, D., and Boden, L. I. Truth and consequences: Health agency responses to environmental health problems. *Science, Technology and Human Values* 12:70, 1987.
10. Anderson, H. A. Evolution of environmental epidemiologic risk assessment. *Environ. Health Perspect.* 62:389, 1985.
11. Litovitz, T. L., and White, J. D. Occupational and environmental illness and the poison center. *West. J. Med.* 152:178, 1990.
12. Darcey, D. J., Greenberg, G. N., and Jackson, G. W. Resource center for occupational and environmental medicine. *Ann. Intern. Med.* 114:607, 1991.
13. Alston, P. G. ENVIRONMENTONLINE: The greening of databases—Part 2. Scientific and technical databases. *DATABASE* October 1991. Pp. 34–52.
14. Linet, M. S. *The Leukemia-Epidemiologic Aspects.* New York: Oxford University Press, 1985.
15. US Department of Health and Human Services, Agency for Toxic Substances and Disease Registry. *Vinyl Chloride Toxicity. Case Studies in Environmental Medicine.* No. 2, 1990.
16. Tenforde, T. S. Health effects of low-frequency electric and magnetic fields. *Environmental Science and Technology* 27:56, 1992.
17. US General Accounting Office. *Superfund—Public Health Assessments Incomplete and of Questionable Value.* GAO/RCED-91-178. Washington, DC: US Government Printing Office, August 1991.
18. National Research Council. *Environmental Epidemiology. Public Health and Hazardous Waste.* Washington, DC: National Academy Press, 1991.
19. Byrns, G., Spahr, J., and Knapp, A. Emerging issues in health care: The role of the environmental health residency. *J. Environ. Health* July/August 1992. Pp. 31–35.

Further Information

Agency for Toxic Substances and Disease Registry, Division of Health Education, 1600 Clifton Rd., NE, Atlanta, GA 30333 (404-639-6205).
ATSDR offers continuing medical education credit for environmental case studies on toxic substances ranging from arsenic to vinyl chloride and provides medical management guidelines for acute chemical exposures. Many other physician-oriented educational activities are offered in cooperation with state health departments. Twenty-four-hour-a-day consultation for hazardous materials emergencies can be obtained through the emergency response and consultation program (404-639-0615).

Aldrich, T., and Griffith, J. *Environmental Epidemiology and Risk Assessment.* New York: Van Nostrand Reinhold, 1992.
The first comprehensive and systematic work that examines exposure to contamination

by hazardous materials in the ambient environment and that also examines the potential adverse effects on human health.

American Journal of Epidemiology 132 (Suppl. 1), 1990.
This entire issue reports on papers associated with the National Conference on Clustering of Health Events. This meeting was jointly sponsored by the Centers for Disease Control, the Agency for Toxic Substances and Disease Registry, and the Association of State and Territorial Health Officials. The issue describes state responses to hazardous waste sites, reports on protocols for the conducting of cluster studies, and provides details on appropriate analytic software, as well as the history of such inquiries. This discussion is for the practitioner who wants to be presented with both conceptual and applied information regarding environmental health surveillance as well as the conducting of cluster studies.

American Medical Association, Department of Preventive Medicine and Public Health, 515 North State St., Chicago, IL, 60610.
Reports on environmental topics as issued by the AMA Council on Scientific Affairs.

American Medical Association, Dr. Jerod Loeb, Assistant Vice President for Science and Technology (312-464-5456).
The AMA has prepared a brochure, entitled Why You Need to Learn More About Hazardous Substances. *The brochure explores the basics of SARA Title III "Right to Know" Amendments and delineates the roles played by the appropriate actors.*

Chivian, E., et al. (eds.). *Human Health and the Environment—A Doctor's Report.* Cambridge, MA: MIT Press, 1993.
This volume attempts to provide a comprehensive, yet brief, description of what is known medically about the effects of environmental degradation. It is intended to be accessible to a lay readership as well as to provide valuable and current references to practitioners. The volume also includes chapters concerning occupational health problems.

Environmental Issues in Primary Care. Wayzata, MN: Freshwater Foundation, 1991.
Provides an overview of the health effects of common environmental contaminants. The first four chapters review common contaminants found in water, air, and soil; Chap. 5 covers basic principles of risk assessment and communication. Chapter 6 addresses ways to incorporate questions about environmental and occupational exposures into a routine medical examination. A guide to federal, state, and published resources is also included. $20/copy.

Hazardous Substances and Public Health. Atlanta: ATSDR.
Bimonthly publication informing the audience of current developments at the Agency. Subscription information: Free *publication. Contact ATSDR, 1600 Clifton Rd., NE, Mailstop E33, Atlanta, GA 30333. Tel.: 404-639-6206. Fax: 404-639-6208.*

Health and Environment Digest.
A monthly publication of the Freshwater Foundation, a public nonprofit foundation whose mission is to help keep water usable for human consumption, industry, and recreation. The Digest *draws on the expertise of a network of representatives in 22 schools of public health, 50 state health departments, and over 75 research institutions, government agencies, state public health associations, and medical societies. The format of the* Digest *features a selected environmental topic of the month as prepared by guest expert authors. It also has an update section that provides brief, timely mentions of meetings, research, and educational opportunities as reported by the* Digest's *network of contributors. Subscription information: Government/public sector—$90; private sector—$115; $130 outside of the US and Canada. Spring Hill Center, 725 County Rd. 6, Wayzata, MN 55391 (612-449-0092).*

Institute of Medicine, Division of Health Promotion and Disease Prevention. *Meeting Physicians' Needs for Medical Information on Occupations and Environments.* Report of a Study by the Committee on Enhancing the Practice of Occupational and Environmental Medicine, Subcommittee on Information Systems. Washington, DC: National Academy Press, 1990.
A short and concise statement by a diverse multidisciplinary committee on the status and future prospects for the improvement of health information available to occupational/environmental health clinicians.

IRIS User Support, ECAO/EPA (MS-190), 26 West Martin Luther King Dr., Cincinnati, OH 45268. Tel.: 513-569-7916; Fax: 513-569-7916.

Kids and the Environment, California Public Health Foundation, 318A, 2001 Addison St., Suite 210, Berkeley, CA 94704 (501-540-2386).
Health care providers working with children traditionally receive no training in pediatric environmental health. In response to their need for information, the California Public Health Foundation, working with the California Department of Health Services, and Children's Hospital of Oakland under funding from a co-operative agreement with the ATSDR have developed a curriculum on environmental health and children.

National Research Council. *Environmental Epidemiology—Public Health and Hazardous Wastes.* Washington: DC: National Academy Press, 1991.
This report provides an in-depth discussion of the intersection between human health and the distribution of hazardous wastes in the United States. It also attempts to identify research gaps in our present level of knowledge concerning this relationship.

Physicians for Social Responsibility, 1000 16th St., NW, Suite 810, Washington, DC 20036 (202-785-3777).
This 25,000 member organization has recently expanded its campaign against the proliferation of nuclear weapons to include environmental issues. A national conference, Human Health and the Environment, was held in Cambridge, Massachusetts, on October 10–11, 1992.

Appendix to Chapter 48: Other Inventories of Environmental or Health Databases

Abramowitz, J. N., Baker, D. S., and Turnstall, D. B. *Guide of Key Environmental Statistics in the U.S. Government.* Washington, D.C.: World Resources Institute, 1990.

Directory of Exposure-Related Data Bases. Task Force on Environmental Cancer and Heart and Lung Disease, 1981.

Frisch, J. D., Shaw, G. M., and Harris, J. A. Epidemiologic research using existing databases of environmental measures. *Arch. Environmen. Health* 45:303, 1990.

Information Resources Directory. Environmental Protection Agency, Office of Information and Resources Management, 1989.

National Center for Health Statistics, US Department of Health and Human Services. *Environmental Health: A Plan for Collecting and Coordinating Statistical and Epidemiologic Data.* DHSS Publication no. (PHS) 80-1248. Washington, DC: US Government Printing Office, 1980.

National Center for Health Statistics, US Department of Health and Human Services. *Environmental Health: A Study of the Issues in Locating, Assessing and Treating Individuals Exposed to Hazardous Substances.* DHHS Publication no. (PHS) 81-1275. Washington, DC: US Government Printing Office, 1981.

The Potential for Linking Environmental and Health Data. Washington, DC: National Governors' Association, 1989.

Some Publicly Available Sources of Computerized Information on Environmental Health and Toxicology. US Public Health Service, Centers for Disease Control, Center for Environmental Health and Injury Control, February 1988.

US Department of Health and Human Services. *HHS Data Inventories.* Washington, DC: US Government Printing Office, Various years of issue.

49

The Environmental Audit

Ridgway M. Hall, Jr., and
William B. Bunn

The environmental audit serves an increasingly important role in the United States and internationally. It is conducted by companies that seek to identify and correct current and potential environmental problems. The audit process reduces the risk of legal liability for current activities and identifies future environmental issues, with attention to cost-effective strategic planning.

The term *environmental audit* is used to describe a process that includes the gathering of information on the activities at a facility that may impact the environment or human health, especially any activities subject to legal or regulatory requirements. Examples of the information obtained include releases to the air and water, hazardous and solid waste management and disposal practices, compliance with permit requirements, and numerous other activities that are regulated at the federal, state, and local level. The data are then measured against the regulatory requirements to determine a facility's "compliance profile."

Typically, areas of noncompliance are noted, as well as activities that, though not illegal, could expose the company to liability. At the conclusion of this process, an action plan is developed, which sets forth all findings that need a response, states the proposed action, and includes a timetable for completion with a designation of responsibility.

The audit may be conducted by experts within the organization or from other institutions. The qualifications of auditors will vary, depending on the situation. Environmental engineers, environmental attorneys, process engineers, industrial hygienists, and other occupational and environmental professionals may serve as auditors or as part of the audit team. The key areas of expertise are an understanding of pertinent regulations and the ability to carefully analyze the manufacturing process, from the raw materials to the final product.

The document produced by an environmental audit is usually comprehensive and contains substantial information on processes and programs as well as a list of observations for management consideration.

The Role of the Environmental Audit

The most important role of the environmental audit is to ensure regulatory compliance and prevent violations, fines, public relations problems, and even criminal charges. Fines begin at up to $25,000 per day for civil violations. In addition, corporations and corporate officers may be fined up to $50,000 per day for criminal charges and face jail sentences under certain circumstances. Further, civil suits may then be filed by any person who claims personal injury or property damage. Although a regulatory violation is a significant part of the evidence for any litigation, liability can be imposed even absent a violation. Compliance with a permit or regulation may not be an adequate defense to a common-law "toxic tort" if business activities are held accountable for injuries.

The risks of fines and litigation are not the only financial reasons for establishing environmental audit programs. Cost-effective planning that anticipates changing regulations or enforcement practices will result in timely use of capital investments. Moreover, the capital requirements that are used in pollution control may increase efficiency and product quality. Insurance can be purchased to cover certain damages if they are anticipated. In addition, environmental audits may identify strategies for waste minimization that will decrease disposal costs. In evaluating potential environmental diseases or clusters or in assessing potential risk, the environmental audit can provide a wealth of information to the occupational physician. A properly conducted environmental audit can serve as an excellent overview of the regulatory compliance issues. It will also help assess the potential health risks of the facility's operations to the workforce and surrounding community.

The Timing of the Environmental Audit

There are several occasions on which environmental audits should be conducted: (1) as an ongoing review of environmental programs—regular review (e.g., 1–3 years) is commonly scheduled by major industries; (2) at the time of the decision to invest in new or upgraded existing facilities; (3) during acquisition and divestitures; and (4) in anticipation of an external audit.

The Legal Basis

The environmental audit will address federal, state, and local regulations and be separated into different foci. For example, clean water and effluent issues can be structurally separated from clean air considerations. Superfund responsibilities may involve visits to nonproducing or disposal sites away from the actual manufacturing facilities. Audits commonly address Occupational Safety and Health Administration (OSHA) regulations as well, particularly in areas of overlap with environmental statutes. Environmental audits also focus on legal issues, which are not regulatory, such as the risk of toxic torts or for insurance purposes.

Conducting the Audit

The audit itself is divided into several steps. The first step is information gathering, which usually precedes the actual visit to the site. This step involves an extensive questionnaire on the environmental programs at the site. A request for copies of substantial numbers of documents may accompany the questionnaire. For example, plant layouts and flow diagrams, process and product information, permits and applications, notifications, monitoring reports, spill control plans, emergency response plans, training programs, shipping manifests, manuals, inspectional reports, complaints or legal proceedings, and product safety data are usually reviewed [1]. Permits and documentation of discussions with regulatory agencies are of particular interest. Applicable federal, state, and local laws and regulations are reviewed before the visit.

At the site visit, information gathering focuses on facility inspections using checklists. Site inspection focuses on emissions sources, such as effluent pipes and stacks, storage areas for all wastes, and processing areas. Specific checklists are usually developed for major areas (e.g., air, water, hazardous waste) or may simply address areas of focused concern, such as spill control [1]. These are keyed to the applicable legal requirements. The site review focuses on the entire process from the raw materials to the final product. The physical layout of the operating facility, industrial processes, sampling and analysis program, waste and by-products assessments, disposal practices, and environmental releases are reviewed. Actual samples of soil, air, or water are taken when indicated. The ultimate objective of this activity is to develop a "compliance profile"—in short, a picture of the extent to which a plant is or is not in compliance with regulatory requirements. Areas not in compliance or areas of potential liability are noted.

Interviews with plant personnel are an essential part of the on-site audit process; they also may be conducted with regional Environmental Protection Agency (EPA) or state agency personnel. People responsible for site environmental compliance are usually interviewed in the initial stages. Senior management, however, should also be addressed early in the site inspection process. People who know the manufacturing process and its problems, along with operations and maintenance workers, can provide valuable insights for understanding potential environmental risks.

At the conclusion of the site visit, an exit interview is usually held to discuss the auditors' impressions. Significant problems will be highlighted; however, many observations will require further analyses, especially if sampling is necessary or local regulations are involved.

A report is then prepared that may be "privileged" through a rather complex legal process or may be submitted without privilege [2]. The report may be extensive and run into hundreds of pages. An executive summary along with a succinct list of observations should be expected. The purpose of the audit report is to identify areas of noncompliance, recommend cost-effective corrective measures, and describe items that could become violations in the future. The audit report, usually targeted to a specific audience, such as site or corporate management, discusses both strengths and weaknesses of different programs and makes specific observations.

While not technically part of the audit, a staged follow-up action plan is developed by most companies. This plan addresses each finding of apparent noncompliance or other problems, and will set forth the steps to correct the problems, with an anticipated time line for carrying them out. Action plans are prioritized, reflecting the seriousness of the observations. Notes of the auditors and other materials used to prepare the audit report are usually maintained for a varying period of time depending on company policies. The action plan is often entered into a spreadsheet computer database to enhance data management.

For example, environmental audits might reveal patterns of increasing air (or water) emissions such as volatile organic compound (VOCs) that will exceed permit requirements in the future (1–2 years). This finding prompts consideration of at least three options: a new permit or variance, new emissions equipment—often incinerators, or a process change. Since in most industrial areas, permitted emissions are decreasing, the choice is narrowed to expensive new pollution abatement equipment (often tens to hundreds of millions of dollars) or a process change. A process change requires significant lead time. A change to an aqueous-based rather than solvent-based process that eliminates use of VOCs requires not only research to assure that the process works but also the development of new equipment since components will be different (aqueous systems cause rusting). Finally, because the product will not be identical, a marketing strategy must be developed and piloted. Only with the clear direction of an audit finding and a well-developed action plan is the lead time commonly available to make an effective process change and product transition.

Because the environmental audit details regulatory issues facing a facility, it will serve as a general indicator of potential health risk, to the extent that compliance reflects protection of the workforce and community. In fact, a thorough audit will reveal whether exceedances from recommended or required guidelines have occurred and when. Thus, if a person has an illness that may be related to an environmental or workplace exposure, the review of the audit may indicate a correlation with a specific release and exposure. Although a release may not be reported, the audit should define current and potential exposures. The latter issue is of particular concern in the context of the EPA's Toxic Release Inventory reporting requirements. An audit and the organization's response to the corresponding observations help demonstrate a commitment to health safety and environmental programs.

The Role of the Occupational and Environmental Physician

Occupational and environmental medicine (OEM) physicians may be a part of the environmental audit team, review the audit report, or be informed users of it. The OEM physician has a unique understanding of the relationship between human health and environmental exposure. Although the audit commonly focuses on regulatory compliance, protection of human health is the ultimate goal of regulations. In fact, many regulations essentially require an assessment of health risk. As a result, the OEM physician may increasingly become a part of the audit team and participate in report preparation.

A second role for the OEM physician is to review the audit. This activity may focus on the accuracy of the observations and conclusions, especially the implications of the audit on the health of the workforce or community, or both, and the need for preventive actions. Although the audit does not usually include an initial action plan, a plan is commonly generated for each major observation noted in the audit. Implementing and integrating the substance of this plan with ongoing health programs is an important activity that may require the knowledge of an OEM physician. For example, particularly in acquisition audits, representative sampling of soils and final products will be conducted. The product may be contaminated with substances that may present a health risk for the product or require hazard labeling under OSHA's Hazard Communication Standard. The OEM physician's multidisciplinary skills are valuable in interpreting audit results. For example, many raw products from mines often contain crystalline silica or some form of asbestos. When the substance is used in consumer products, in particular food or beverages, a clear assessment of both public health risk and labeling and other regulatory requirements is critical. The recognition of route of exposure for crystalline silica (inhalation versus ingestion) and the potential difference in toxicity (and significant difference in regulation) of cleavage fragment tremolite asbestos are risk-determining issues that require a knowledge of pathophysiology and toxicology as well as regulatory requirements. In both instances, the future of the company or product may turn on the OEM physician's appropriate interpretation and communication of audit results.

A third interface of the OEM physician with environmental auditing is to use the data, especially exposure sampling findings, modeling results, and risk assessment reports. This information may prove useful in evaluating a clinical case or an illness among groups of individuals, or in communicating risk to members of the community. Reliable data should be preferentially used, especially those that document exposure, concentration, biologic dose, and potential health effect.

Although the environmental audit may seem specific to regulatory compliance, it provides an important role for the occupational and environmental physician, who can benefit from using the results and participating in the audit process.

References

1. Hall, R. M., and Case, D. R. *All About Environmental Auditing,* (2nd ed.). Washington, DC: Federal Publications Inc., 1992.
2. Arbuckle, J. G., et al. *Environmental Law Handbook.* Rockville, MD, Government Institutes, 1989.

Further Information

Association of Groundwater Scientists and Engineers (a division of the National Groundwater Association). *Guidance to Environmental Site Assessments.* September 1992.
Explains and discusses the numerous tasks involved in conducting an environmental site assessment, including working checklists and suggestions for the content of an environmental audit report.

Herz, M. Environmental auditing and environmental management: The implicit and explicit federal regulatory mandate. *Cardozo Law Rev.* 12:1241, 1991.

Multimedia Compliance Audit Procedures. US Environmental Protection Agency, Office of Enforcement and Compliance Monitoring, March 1989.
The EPA's manual for facility inspectors who conduct inspections or compliance audits of industrial facilities for compliance with applicable environmental laws and regulations; includes the EPA's inspection checklists.

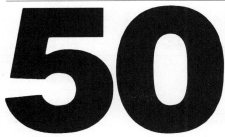

Environmental Risk Assessment

Roger O. McClellan and
William B. Bunn

The clinical approach to environmental illness is described in Chap. 43. Although there is always a spectrum of approaches to evaluating any disease, low-level exposures that may produce chronic diseases, particularly neoplasms, are often managed through the process of qualitative or quantitative risk assessment. This approach is particularly desirable where large numbers of individuals may be exposed, the exposures vary, and clinical, biologic, or physiologic markers are unavailable or not practical. Risk assessments are also used for policy decisions at local, state, and federal levels, and in multiple regulatory settings, such as air and water permitting, Superfund cleanup, and Toxic Substances Control Act (TSCA) decision-making. Although risk assessment mirrors clinical analysis of an environmental medicine clinical case, it is of necessity a more formal process because public policy is often formulated based on the results.

Qualitative risk assessment is commonly performed by "authoritative bodies," including the International Agency for Research on Cancer (IARC), American Conference of Governmental Industry Hygienists (ACGIH), Environmental Protection Agency (EPA), National Toxicology Program (NTP), and other agencies. These organizations weigh available evidence and categorize carcinogens or "safe levels" for exposure to toxicants.

Quantitative risk assessments are typically developed for carcinogens. For example, lifetime exposures estimated to lead to one cancer in 100,000 individuals is a customary approach; mathematical models are incorporated and analysis is performed by governmental agencies such as the EPA to prioritize risk reduction strategies. Quantitative analysis involves substantial "default assumptions" (to be described) in the absence of specific scientific knowledge so that all factors are addressed in a mathematical model. In Chap. 26, risk assessment is addressed in the clinical setting using a "general approach," and an example is given. Since environmental regulation is driven by specific and quantitative assessments, a more detailed review of risk analysis in the environmental setting is important.

The Risk Assessment Process

The basis of risk assessment and management is the proper interpretation of the biologic research available. (See Fig. 50-1 from the National Academy of Science/National Research Council [NAS/NRC] paradigm.) The end product is a listing of identified hazards for support in clinical decision-making, regulations, and determination of acceptable levels for those substances in the various media (air, water, soil).

The risk assessment process, as codified by the National Academy of Sciences (NAS), involves four steps. The first, *hazard identification,* is qualitative; that is, it assesses the toxicant's potential for causing health effects. The second, *exposure-dose-response assessment,* establishes a quantitative relationship between exposure and response. Both of these steps use human data if available. In the absence of comprehensive human data (which is usually the case), information from studies with laboratory animals, cells, and/or tissues from animals and people must be used. *Exposure assessment,* the third step, may use actual measurements or, more frequently, results obtained by modeling. The fourth and final step, *risk characterization,* involves integration of results from steps 2 and 3 to assess risk for the specific exposure scenario under consideration (Fig. 50-1) [1].

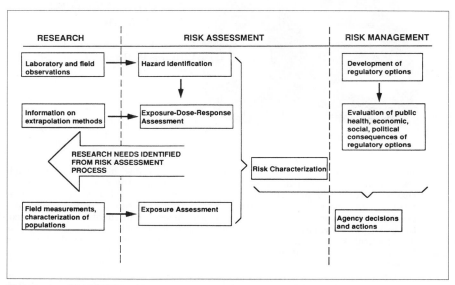

Figure 50-1. NAS/NRC risk assessment/management paradigm [1].

Approaches to Acquiring Information

In many situations, a defined benchmark dose from the EPA or other agencies may be appropriate for the determination of risk. However, if the case has public health or occupational impact or involves regulatory or policy-making considerations, more formal integration of all available toxicity and exposure data may be indicated. State-of-the-art risk assessments are not common in the nonoccupational/environmental clinical situation, and, thus, it may be advisable to consult experts in the risk assessment process. Further, the contribution of people with knowledge of human and animal biology/pathobiology may be necessary to aid the physician in appreciating the complexities and subtleties of the analysis.

For the establishment of National Ambient Air Quality Standards (NAAQS), information from multiple sources is used in the risk assessment process and in setting standards. Each approach has advantages and disadvantages, as is discussed briefly below [2].

Clinical and epidemiologic studies are especially useful in that the data are obtained on people. Clinical studies with exposures carried out under carefully controlled laboratory conditions allow the test atmosphere to be precisely defined and the exposure concentration and duration of exposure to be experimentally controlled. A drawback in such studies is the extent to which the range of exposure conditions must be limited to those that the clinician feels confident will not produce irreversible effects; to study higher exposure conditions would be unethical. A wide range of procedures can be used to evaluate biologic changes related to the exposure conditions. The resulting data can be readily evaluated to qualitatively or quantitatively define exposure-response relationships.

It is possible to study people under natural exposure conditions rather than to use carefully controlled conditions of the laboratory. In these studies, comparisons may be made between responses evaluated under low and high pollutant conditions. The exposure gradients and the quality of the exposure characterization are likely to be best for short-term (days) rather than long-term (months) observations. Although usually conducted in the field, a broad range of procedures can be conducted to evaluate the functional status of the individuals being studied. The results of such studies can be evaluated to provide a semiquantitative or, perhaps in some cases, a quantitative relationship between exposure and response. The relevance of the exposure is not open to debate, since it occurred naturally.

Epidemiologic studies, beyond their advantage of directly studying humans, also have the advantage of involving real-world conditions. However, a related major difficulty is that the exposure conditions are not controlled—one must study the exposure conditions provided. The range of procedures that can be used to evaluate the health status of individuals and changes related to exposure are substantial and range from symptom questionnaires to sophisticated pulmonary function evaluations to mortality records. Because the exposure conditions in the epidemiologic studies may not be precisely defined, especially for long periods of observation, the exposure-response relationship tends to be more qualitative than quantitative. It is especially difficult to establish even semiquantitative relationships between exposure and response for chronic diseases, such as emphysema and bronchitis, when the outcome is presumably related to years of exposure.

Laboratory animal studies, like controlled human exposure studies, have the advantage of using carefully defined conditions matched to the experimental needs. Moreover, the range of procedures used to evaluate the "dose of pollutant" received by the experimental subjects can include invasive procedures as well as end-of-life observations that could not be used with people. The study of intact mammals is advantageous in that all of the body functions are subject to the complex integrated physiology that occurs in people. Because exposure conditions and evaluation procedures can be rigorously controlled, it is possible to develop quantitative assessments of exposure-response relationships. Approaches to the conduct of animal bioassays with inhaled or ingested chemicals, however, must be carefully scrutinized. Standard protocols are commonly used. Laboratory animal studies have the major disadvantage of requiring extrapolation of results to people. However, we are rapidly approaching the point where such extrapolations can be facilitated by using species characteristics in the process.

In vitro studies that use cells and tissues from people and laboratory animals represent the ultimate "reductionist" approach of defining pollutant effects. They have the advantage in that exposure conditions can be precisely controlled and a wide range of procedures of varying complexity can be used to evaluate responses. Observations can be made at a level of detail that cannot be readily made in laboratory animals or people. For example, the influence of pollutants on the production and release of specific cellular mediators from defined cell populations can be assessed. The disadvantage is that the observations must be extrapolated to the intact mammal, which has a complex array of feedback mechanisms that modulate interactions.

In the final analysis, a risk assessment for a substance, such as an air pollutant, should be based on available data regardless of the methods used to acquire them. Maximum use should be made of human data, with results from other systems employed to complement and extend the value of the human data, frequently by giving insight into the mechanisms that may be operative in people. In the absence of human data, priorities should be given to data obtained in controlled studies of laboratory animals, preferably those that include life span assessments. If concern exists for the material as an air pollutant with inhalation as the primary route of entry to people, then it is appropriate to conduct laboratory animal studies using inhalation exposures. This approach obviates the need for making extrapolations between routes of exposure, such as from oral intake to inhalation intake. Studies with isolated cells or tissues can be used as "screening" systems to identify and rank potential toxicants and give insight into mechanisms of action. Finally, in the absence of data from biologic systems, insight into the potential toxicity of new materials can be gained from evaluating structure-activity relationships for the new material relative to materials that have been extensively studied in biologic systems [3, 4].

Approaches to Conducting Risk Assessment

The use of formal qualitative and quantitative risk assessment in occupational and environmental cases will vary depending on the situation. Authoritative determinations of the IARC, EPA, NTP, Occupational Safety and Health Administration (OSHA), and others must be given significant weight in determining if the exposure can cause the disease. Although newer literature may be available, it will very likely not be accepted until it has been subjected to the scrutiny of world experts and been endorsed by regulatory agencies. In each case, a consensus opinion of authoritative bodies is preferred. Most agencies, however, identify and characterize hazards on a generic basis; that is, they assess the chemical to determine if there is any evidence in the literature that a hazard, such as cancer, has been identified. The fact that the preponderance of the literature has not found the adverse effect or that exposure levels associated with the effect do not exist in occupational or environmental situations, is *not* considered. The clinician, however, must evaluate the context of the exposure, estimate the dose to the target organ, and correlate exposure with disease. Quantitative risk assessments may support clinical judgment in evaluating cases, but these determinations are best used as part of communicating risk to individuals or groups. Regardless of a physician's preference to avoid numeric estimates, quantitative determinations and regulatory definitions of safe or acceptable levels may be useful in assessing a clinical case. Since quantitative analyses are designed not to *understate* risks, these risk assessments may also serve to reassure individual clinicians of their judgment in settings with multiple and complex factors.

A range of approaches to conducting risk assessments, and especially exposure-dose-response assessments, has evolved for both noncancer health endpoints and cancer. Because of differences in the approaches for the two endpoints, they are discussed separately.

Noncancer "Endpoints"

The approach used by the ACGIH and EPA for noncancer endpoints makes use of "safety factors" (or "uncertainty factors," the term used most recently by the EPA in establishing reference doses for noncancer endpoints) (Table 50-1). In both cases, the starting point is the use of human data, if available. Otherwise laboratory animal data must be used. A series of safety factors are employed to extrapolate from levels of observed effect or absence of effect to levels of exposure that may be viewed as acceptable limits. This acceptable level of exposure is believed to provide a margin of safety below a threshold at which no effect has been found [5, 6].

The EPA uses a similar but less rigorously quantitative approach in assessing exposure-response relationships for "criteria pollutants" (sulfur dioxide, particulate matter, ozone, carbon dioxide, nitrogen oxides, and lead). With criteria pollutants, such as ozone, a substantial amount of human exposure-response data is available, especially for short-term exposures. With significant human data available on short-term exposures, the primary extrapolation is from levels of observable effects to lower levels of exposure. This extrapolation involves the critical issue of determining an "ample margin of safety" that may lead to differences of opinion regarding the methods used to assure the protection of the public or sensitive individuals [7].

Cancer

Authoritative risk assessments for cancer were initially directed to whether a compound was a carcinogen, based on evidence from epidemiologic studies. Later, the assessment was broadened to include consideration of results from animal experimentation. This change gave rise to formalized criteria for evaluating the carcinogenic risks to humans such as those used by the IARC. In 1969, IARC initiated a program to evaluate the carcinogenic risk of chemicals to humans and produce monographs on individual chemicals. This program has had substantial impact on cancer risk assessment because the IARC *Monographs* are widely viewed as authoritative and serve as the basis for action by other groups, including state and federal regulatory agencies as well as other countries [8].

The IARC conducts a formalized risk assessment that leads to a qualitative classification of a compound's carcinogenic potential. It provides an excellent model of a formal risk assessment/hazard identification process. The IARC approach uses international working groups of experts with contributions from the IARC staff to carry out five tasks: (1) ascertain that all appropriate references have been collected, (2) select the data relevant for the evaluation on the basis of scientific merit, (3) prepare accurate summaries of the data to enable the reader to follow the reasoning of the working group, (4) evaluate the results of experimental and epidemiologic studies, and (5) make an overall evaluation of the carcinogenic potential of the agent to humans [8].

In the *Monographs,* the term *carcinogen* denotes an agent that is capable of increasing the incidence of malignant neoplasms. Traditionally, the IARC has eval-

Table 50-1. Use of uncertainty factors in deriving reference dose

	Standard uncertainty factor
H—Human to sensitive human	Use a 10-fold factor when extrapolating from valid experimental results from studies using prolonged exposure to average healthy humans. This factor is intended to account for the variation in sensitivity among the members of the human population.
A—Animal to human	Use a 10-fold factor when extrapolating from valid results of long-term studies on experimental animals when results of studies of human exposure are not available or are inadequate. This factor is intended to account for the uncertainty in extrapolating animal data to the case of average healthy humans.
S—Subchronic to chronic	Use up to a 10-fold factor when extrapolating from less than chronic exposure results on experimental animals or humans when there are no useful long-term human data. This factor is intended to account for the uncertainty in extrapolating from less than chronic NOAELs to chronic NOAELs.
L—LOAEL to NOAEL	Use up to a 10-fold factor when deriving an RfC from an LOAEL, instead of an NOAEL. This factor is intended to account for the uncertainty in extrapolating from LOAELs to NOAELs.
D—Incomplete to complete data	Use up to a 10-fold factor when extrapolating from valid results in experimental animals when the data are "incomplete." This factor is intended to account for the inability of any single animal study to adequately address all possible adverse outcomes in humans.

Modifying factor

Use professional judgment to determine another uncertainty factor (MF) that is ≤ 10. The magnitude of the MF depends on the professional assessment of scientific uncertainties of the study and database not explicitly treated above, e.g., the number of animals tested. The default value for the MF is 1.

LOAEL = lowest observed adverse effect level; NOAEL = no observable effect level; RfC = reference concentration.
Source: Jarabek, A. M., et al. The U.S. Environmental Protection Agency's inhalation RFD methodology: risk assessment for air toxics. *Toxicol. Ind. Health* 6:279, 1990.

uated the evidence for carcinogenicity independent of the underlying mechanism(s) involved. In 1991, it convened a group of experts to consider how mechanistic data could be used in the classification process. This group suggested a greater use of mechanistic data including information relevant to extrapolation between laboratory animals and humans.

The evaluation process considers three types of data: human carcinogenicity data, experimental carcinogenicity data, and supporting evidence of carcinogenicity. Definitive evidence of human carcinogenicity can only be obtained from epidemiologic or clinical studies. The epidemiologic evidence is classified into four categories: (1) Sufficient evidence of carcinogenicity is used when a causal relationship has been established between exposure to the agent and human cancer. (2) Limited evidence of carcinogenicity is used when a positive association between exposure to an agent and human cancer is considered to be credible, but change, bias, or confounding could not be ruled out with reasonable confidence. (3) Inadequate evidence of carcinogenicity is used when available studies are of insufficient quality, consistency, or statistical power to permit a conclusion regarding the presence or absence of a causal association. (4) Evidence suggesting lack of carcinogenicity is used when there are several adequate studies covering the full range of doses to which humans are known to be exposed, which are mutually consistent in showing no positive association between exposure and any studied cancer at any observed level of exposure.

The IARC evaluation process gives substantial weight to carcinogenicity data from laboratory animals. In the first 11 *Monograph* volumes, 44 agents were identified for which there is sufficient or limited evidence of carcinogenicity to humans. It should be noted that all agents have been adequately tested experimentally and produced cancer in at least one laboratory animal species. The IARC concluded that "in the absence of adequate data in humans, it is biologically plausible and prudent to regard agents for which there is sufficient evidence of carcinogenicity in experimental animals as if they presented a carcinogenic risk to humans."

Thus, the IARC classifies the strength of the evidence of carcinogenicity in experimental animals in a fashion analogous to that used for the human data. In the past, the IARC has not commented on the extent of their carcinogenic potency or on the mechanisms involved. Based on the recommendations of the 1991 Working Group on Use of Mechanistic Data, it is anticipated that these data will be fully evaluated and commented on in the future. This approach should be especially useful in classifying agents that may cause species-specific effects such as those associated with alpha (2u) globulin–mediated renal toxicity and neoplasia in the male rat.

The evidence of carcinogenicity is classified into four categories: (1) Sufficient evidence of carcinogenicity is used when a working group considers that a *causal* relationship has been established between the agent and an increased incidence of malignant neoplasms or an appropriate combination of benign and malignant neoplasms in two or more species of animals or in two or more independent studies in one species carried out at different times, in different laboratories, or under different protocols. A single study in one species might be considered under exceptional circumstances to provide sufficient evidence when malignant neoplasms occur to an unusual degree with regard to incidence, site, type of tumor, or age at onset. (2) Limited evidence of carcinogenicity is used when the data suggest a carcinogenic effect but are limited for making a definitive evaluation. (3) Inadequate evidence of carcinogenicity is used when studies cannot be interpreted as showing either the presence or absence of a carcinogenic effect because of major qualitative or quantitative limitations. (4) Evidence suggesting lack of carcinogenicity is used when adequate studies involving at least two species are available that show that, within the limits of the tests used, the agent is not carcinogenic (Table 50-2) (see Appendix D). Such a conclusion is inevitably limited to the species, tumors, and doses of exposure studied.

Supporting evidence for the classification includes a range of information, such as structure-activity correlations, toxicologic information, and data on kinetics, metab-

Table 50-2. IARC cancer classification

Group 1: The agent is carcinogenic to humans. This category is used only when there is sufficient evidence of carcinogenicity in humans.

Group 2: This category is used for a range of agents, from those for which the human evidence of carcinogenicity is almost sufficient to those for which no human data are available but for which there is experimental evidence of carcinogenicity.

Group 2A: The agent is probably carcinogenic to humans. The category is typically used when there is limited evidence of carcinogenicity in humans and sufficient evidence of carcinogenicity in experimental animals.

Group 2B: The agent is possibly carcinogenic to humans. This category is typically used when there is limited evidence in humans in the absence of sufficient evidence in experimental animals or when there is sufficient evidence of carcinogenicity in experimental animals in the face of inadequate evidence or no data in humans.

Group 3: The agent is not classifiable as to carcinogenicity in humans. This category is used when agents do not fall into any other group.

Group 4: The agent is probably not carcinogenic to humans. This category is typically used for agents for which there is evidence suggesting lack of carcinogenicity in humans together with evidence suggesting lack of carcinogenicity in experimental animals.

---

olism, and genotoxicity. Data from laboratory animals, humans, and lower levels of biologic organization such as tissues and cells are included. In short, any information that may provide a clue as to the cancer-causing potential of an agent will be reviewed and presented.

Finally, all relevant data are integrated and the agent categorized on the basis of the *strength of the evidence* derived from humans, animals, and other studies [8].

The IARC categorization scheme does not address the potency of carcinogens, which poses constraints on the utility of IARC classification for use beyond hazard identification. In short, a carcinogen is a carcinogen irrespective of potency. This "lumping" of carcinogens regardless of potency can be misleading to the nonspecialist including policy makers and the public. Another group of the World Health Organization, the International Programme for Chemical Safety (IPCS), addresses potency through an assessment of actual occupational and environmental risk. The IPCS reviews substances studied by IARC and produces documents that go farther than identification of potential risk. Unfortunately, IPCS documents do not receive the same attention as IARC documents, and they are not incorporated in policy making even though they parallel IARC documents [2, 4, 6–8].

In 1986, the EPA issued guidelines for cancer risk assessment to codify the agency's practices, which built on a policy document prepared by the United States Office of Science and Technology Policy on chemical carcinogens. The 1986 EPA guidelines use an approach similar to that of IARC in categorizing agents based on the weight of the evidence of carcinogenicity, except ending up with an alpha rather than a numeric notation for the categories (Table 50-3). The classification of environmental

Table 50-3. EPA and IARC carcinogenicity groupings

EPA group	IARC group	Evaluation		Evidence in humans	Evidence in animals
	1	Carcinogenic to humans		Sufficient	
A		Human carcinogen		Sufficient	
	2A	Probably carcinogenic to humans		Limited	Sufficient
B1		Probable human carcinogen		Limited	Sufficient
B2		Probable human carcinogen		Inadequate	Sufficient
	2B	Possibly carcinogenic to humans			Absence of sufficient evidence
			or	Inadequate	Sufficient
			or	Inadequate	Limited
C		Possible human carcinogen		Absent	Limited
	3	Not classifiable as to carcinogenicity to humans		No data	No data
D		Not classified as to human carcinogenicity		Inadequate	Inadequate
			or	No data	No data
	4	Probably not carcinogenic to humans		Evidence in humans and animals suggests lack of carcinogenicity	
E		Evidence of noncarcinogenicity for humans		No evidence of carcinogenicity in at least two adequate animal tests in different species or in both adequate epidemiologic and animal studies.	

tobacco smoke as a class A carcinogen is a notable example. It is expected that in 1994 the EPA will propose revised guidelines for cancer risk assessment. For quantitative risk assessment, regulatory agencies commonly use a multistage model that is *linear* at low doses to determine risk, and then use the upper confidence limit of that model to provide a greater level of certainty. From these calculations, a lifetime risk acceptable to the agency must be met [9–11].

In the quantitative analysis of carcinogens, the 1986 EPA guidelines go beyond the IARC approach in offering guidance for developing quantitative estimates of carcinogen potency, that is, cancer risk per unit exposure. Because the information base for individual chemicals varies markedly and is rarely complete, the guidelines include a number of "default" options that are used in the assessment process unless compelling scientific data exist. Some of the key "default" assumptions are: (1) humans are as sensitive as the most sensitive laboratory animal species, strain, or sex evaluated; (2) chemicals act like radiation at low doses in inducing cancer with a linearized multistage model appropriate for estimating dose-response relationships below the range of experimental observations; (3) the biology of humans and laboratory animals, including the rate of metabolism of chemicals, is a function of body surface area; (4) a given unit of intake of chemical has the same effect irrespective of the intake time or duration; and (5) laboratory animals are a surrogate for humans in assessing cancer risks, with positive cancer bioassay results in laboratory animals taken as evidence of the chemical's potential to cause cancer in people. All of the default assumptions have been vigorously debated as to their validity [2].

Similar analytic processes are used by other authoritative and regulatory bodies. The NTP conducts a similar although less formal assessment and categorization. [6–8].

The Occupational and Environmental Physician

The results of qualitative and quantitative risk assessments performed by governmental or authoritative bodies or by the occupational and environmental medicine (OEM) physician should be an integral part of the evaluation of a disease potentially related to the environment. Risk identification processes (such as performed by the IARC) and the listing of potentially hazardous agents will help the OEM physician determine if a potential association between exposure and disease is plausible. Quantitation of the risk at specific exposure levels allows a more refined evaluation and can be used to communicate information to individuals or groups.

Risk assessments specific to an exposure situation may also be available. For example, an important determination is the potential risk from a site where hazardous wastes have been improperly disposed, a potential Superfund site. The risk is initially defined during the remedial investigation feasibility (RI/FS) study of the site. The assessed risk will be quantitated and the quantitation will determine priority. If the priority is high, the site may become a part of the National Priority List (NPL) established by the EPA, and cleanup mandated. In addition to the initial risk assessment of the site, each NPL site will also be evaluated by the Agency for Toxic Substances and Disease Registry (ATSDR). These assessments are available for public use. The data from the RI/FS and ATSDR studies and detailed risk assessments can be very useful in answering questions raised by individual cases or by community groups. While generic dispersion models and default values must be examined, it is important that OEM physicians use all the data available in each exposure/disease situation.

In addition to utilizing risk assessments in clinical practice, the physician knowledgeable in occupational and environmental medicine can play a valuable role in evaluating and refining default options associated with risk assessment. There may be physiologic reasons that humans are not equivalent to rodents when studies report excesses of cancer that are sex and strain specific. One may also offer judgment as to whether a threshold or linearized multistage model should be applied, particularly as exposure levels approximate background levels. The problems of extrapolating results from maximum tolerated doses in animals (which by definition overcome defense mechanisms) to low doses in humans must be scrutinized carefully. For example, the metabolism of humans is not always similar to that of animals and exposure levels are not equivalent between species.

Specific knowledge of the actual occupational and environmental exposure situation may be most important. The extent to which the agent is respirable must be considered in evaluating exposure to fibers and particles. The likelihood of a particular route of exposure actually occurring as well as the comparative level of occupational or environmental exposure is of crucial importance in determining the actual human risk.

Further, the OEM physician has a role both in standard-setting process through risk assessment and interpreting the standards based on knowledge of the specific situation. When regulations are proposed, it is not always possible to analyze each integral element of the risk assessment process. Key questions should be posed and default assumptions and risk characterizations challenged, when appropriate, by OEM physicians. Risk assessments based on regulatory guidelines always need to be considered as candidates for refinement based on specific knowledge.

In summary, risk assessment, qualitative and quantitative, can be instrumental in environmental medicine. This approach must be carefully integrated with clinical assessments. Furthermore, the clinician should take an active part in the determination of risk assessment when appropriate and in the examination of qualitative or quantitative risk assessments that are used in formulating regulatory policies or enforcement proceedings.

References

1. National Academy of Sciences/National Research Council. *Risk Assessment in the Federal Government: Managing the Process.* Washington, DC: National Academy Press, 1983.
2. McClellan, R. O., Medinsky, M. A., and d'A. Heck, H. J. Developing Risk Assessments for Airborne Materials. In D. E. Gardner et al. (eds.), *Toxicology of the Lung.* (2nd ed.). New York: Raven Press, 1993. Pp. 603–651.
3. Hooper, L. D., Oehme, F. W., and Krieger, G. R., Risk Assessment for Toxic Hazards. In J. B. Sullivan and G. R. Krieger (eds.), *Hazardous Materials Toxicology.* Baltimore: Williams & Wilkins, 1991. Pp. 65–75.
4. Scala, R. A. Risk Assessment. In M. O. Amdur, J. Doull, and C. Klaassen (eds.), *Toxicology.* New York: Pergamon Press, Pp. 985–995, 1991.
5. American Conference of Governmental Industrial Hygienists. *Threshold Limit Values and Biological Exposure Indices for 1991, 1992.* Cincinnati: ACGIH, 1991.
6. Shouf, C. R. Current assessment practices for noncancer end points. *Environ. Health Perspect.* 94:111, 1991.
7. United States Environmental Protection Agency. Guidelines for carcinogenic risk assessment. *Fed. Register* 51:33992, 1986.
8. International Agency for Research on Cancer (IARC). Diesel and gasoline engine exhausts and some nitroarenes. *IARC Monogr. Eval. Carcinog. Risk Chem. Hum.* 46:87, 1989.
9. Office of Science and Technology Policy (OSTP). *Chemical Carcinogens: A Review of the Science and its Associated Principles,* 1985.
10. Jarabek, A. M., et al. The U.S. Environmental Protection Agency's inhalation RFD methodology: risk assessment for air toxics. *Toxicol. Ind. Health* 6:279, 1990.
11. Environmental Protection Agency. *Respiratory Health Effects of Passive Smoking: Lung Cancer and Other Disorders.* Washington, DC: Office of Health and Environmental Assessment, Office of Research and Development, US EPA, December 1992.

Further Information

Andersen, M. E. Quantitative risk assessment and occupational carcinogens. *Appl. Ind. Hyg.* 3:267, 1989.

Anderson, E. L. Quantitative Approaches in Use in the United States to Assess Cancer Risk. In V. B. Vouk et al. (eds.), *Methods for Estimating Risk of Chemical Injury: Human and Non-Human Biota and Ecosystems.* New York: Wiley, 1985.

Barnes, D. G., and Dourson, M. Reference dose (RfD): description and use in health risk assessments. *Reg. Toxicol. Pharmacol.* 8:471, 1988.

Breslow, N. E., and Day, N. E. *Statistical Methods in Cancer Research: The Analysis of Case Control Studies.* Lyon, France: International Agency for Research on Cancer, 1980. Part 1.

Breslow, N. E., and Day, N. E. *Statistical Methods in Cancer Research: The Design and Analysis of Cohort Studies.* Lyon, France: International Agency for Research on Cancer, 1987. Part 2.

Brown, H. S., West, C. R., and Bishop, D. R. Chemical health effects assessment methodology for airborne contaminants. *Risk Anal.* 7:389, 1987.

Flamm, W. G. Risk assessment policy in the United States. *Prog. Clin. Biol. Res.* 208:141, 1986.

Grant, L. D., and Jordan, B. C. *Basis for Primary Air Quality Criteria and Standards.* United States Environmental Protection Agency. Environmental Criteria and Assessment Office, Research Triangle Park, NC, Springfield National Technical Information Service, NTISPB88-180070, 1988.

Harkema, J. R., et al. Effects of ambient level of ozone on primate nasal epithelial mucosubstances: Quantitative histochemistry. *Am. J. Pathol.* 127:90, 1987.

Lippmann, M. Effective strategies for population studies as acute air pollution health effects. *Environ. Health Perspect.* 81:115, 1989.

National Academy of Sciences/National Research Council. *Human Exposure Assessment for Airborne Pollutants: Advances and Opportunities.* Washington, DC: National Academy Press, 1990.

Office of Science and Technology Policy (OSTP). *Chemical Carcinogens: A Review of the Science and its Associated Principles,* 1985.

United States Environmental Protection Agency. Interim procedures and guidelines for health risk and economic impact assessments of suspect carcinogens. *Fed. Register* 41:21402, 1976

United States Environmental Protection Agency. Guidelines for the health assessment of suspect developmental toxicants. *Fed. Register* 54:9386, 1989.

United States Environmental Protection Agency. *Alpha Globulin Association with Chemically Induced Renal Toxicity and Neoplasia in the Male Rat.* Washington, DC: EPA/625-3-91/019P, 1991.

United States Environmental Protection Agency. *Interim Methods for Development of Inhalation Reference Concentrations.* EPA/600/8 90/006A, 1990.

United States Environmental Protection Agency. *National Air Quality and Emissions Trends Report, 1990.* Research Triangle Park, NC: EPA 150/4 91-023, 1991.

Vianio, H., et al. Working group on mechanisms of carcinogenesis and evaluation of carcinogenic risks. *Cancer Res.* 52:2357, 1991.

Vocci, F., and Farber, T. Extrapolation of animal toxicity data to man. *Reg. Toxicol. Pharmacol.* 8:389, 1988.

Wilbourn, J., et al. Response of experimental animals to human carcinogens: An analysis based upon the IARC Monograph Programme. *Carcinogenesis* 7:1853, 1986.

Appendixes

Appendixes

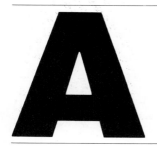

Health Effects of Common Substances

Howard Frumkin, Robert J. McCunney, and Cheryl Barbanel

This appendix presents chemical substances that may be encountered in the workplace or the environment, and their respective hazards. The type of work where exposure may occur, the route of exposure, and the range of symptoms that may result from exposure are noted. Guides to diagnosis and medical monitoring are indicated, where appropriate. Readers are advised to consult primary materials for a more comprehensive description of the context of the exposure associated with the health effect described.

Fundamental principles involved in assessing potential occupational or environmental illness should be applied in using this information. The appendix is designed to serve as guide and rapid reference, not as comprehensive source of every acknowledged health effect associated with a hazard. A selected list of references is included after the table.

This table has evolved from original material in Levy and Wegman's book *Occupational Health and Safety* and has been further expanded and reorganized in alphabetical order to facilitate use. Thirty new entries were added to the list from the first edition, which included information on approximately fifty substances. This expanded version includes special notations for those materials for which specific OSHA standards exist. Classifications of the International Agency for Research on Cancer (IARC) are noted for human and animal carcinogens. See Appendix D for a comprehensive summary of IARC classifications.

Health Effects of Common Substances

Agent	Exposure	Route of entry	System(s) affected	Primary manifestation(s)	Aids in diagnosis[a]	Remarks
Acetonitrile (methyl cyanide)	Laboratory and industrial solvent, synthetic	Inhalation, skin absorption, ingestion	Pulmonary CNS Eye	Asphyxiation Malaise, stupor, weakness, nausea, headache Irritation	Blood cyanide and thiocyanate	Most common chemical causing health-related incidents to date in biotechnology research
Acrylamide	Used in soil waterproofing during mining and tunneling operations, in polymers, sizing for paper and fabrics, dyes, adhesives, waste treatment, and ore processing	Inhalation, percutaneous absorption, ingestion	CNS Skin	Fatigue, dizziness, confusion, peripheral neuropathy, ataxia, dysarthria, excessive sweating Irritation of skin and mucous membranes, exfoliation	No biologic monitoring method to routine screening is available	IARC 2B
Acrylonitrile*	Plastics, synthetic fibers, adhesive chemical intermediates, fumigant	Inhalation of vapors, percutaneous absorption	Cellular metabolism Skin	Asphyxiation, eye irritation, headache, nausea, dizziness, weakness Dermatitis, vesicular	Blood cyanide and thiocyanate	Associated with brain tumors, lung and bowel cancer; IARC 2A
Aldrin. *See* Chlorinated hydrocarbons						
Ammonia	Refrigeration; petroleum refining; mfg. of nitrogen-containing chemicals, synthetic fibers, dyes, and optics	Inhalation of gas	Upper respiratory tract	Upper respiratory irritation		Also irritant of eyes and moist skin[b]

Substance	Source of exposure	Route	System	Clinical effects	Monitoring	Comments
Antimony	Exposure maximal during mining and smelting; used in the semiconductor industry, battery grids, type castings, bearings and cable sheaths, munitions, glass, pottery, paints, and lacquers, rubber, solder	Inhalation of dust and fumes, percutaneous contact	Pulmonary; Gastrointestinal; Skin; Cardiac	Irritation, pneumoconiosis; Nausea, vomiting, bloody diarrhea; Dermatitis, pustular; Arrhythmia	Urinary antimony	Suspected carcinogen (lung, bladder) IARC 2B
Arsenic*	Alloyed with lead and copper for hardness; mfg. of pigments, glass, pharmaceuticals; by-product in copper smelting; insecticides; fungicides; rodenticides; tanning	Inhalation and ingestion of dust and fumes	Neuromuscular; Gastrointestinal; Skin; Pulmonary	Peripheral neuropathy, sensory motor; Nausea and vomiting, diarrhea, constipation; Dermatitis, finger and toenail striations, skin cancer, nasal septum perforation; Lung cancer	Arsenic in urine	Urinary arsenic levels affected by amount of seafood consumed; IARC 1
Arsine	Accidental by-product of reaction of arsenic with acid; Semiconductor manufacturing	Inhalation of gas	Hematopoietic	Intravascular hemolysis: hemoglobinuria, jaundice, oliguria or anuria	Arsenic in urine	
Asphyxiant gases (simple): nitrogen, hydrogen, methane, and others	Enclosed spaces in a variety of industrial settings	Inhalation of gas	CNS	Anoxia	O_2 in environment	No specific toxic effect; act by displacing O_2

(continued)

Agent	Exposure	Route of entry	System(s) affected	Primary manifestation(s)	Aids in diagnosis[a]	Remarks
Benzene	Mfg. of organic chemicals, detergents, pesticides, solvents, paint removers; used as a solvent Gasoline	Inhalation of vapor; slight percutaneous absorption	CNS Hemato-poietic Skin	CNS depression Leukemia, aplastic anemia Dermatitis	Urinary phenol	About 3% of commercial gasoline is benzene; IARC 1
Benzidine*	Manufacturing of dyes and pigments; hardener for rubber	Inhalation, percutaneous absorption	Eyes, nose, respiratory CNS Skin Hematologic	Irritation Giddiness, headache, nausea, staggering gait, fatigue Dermatitis Bone marrow suppression	Urine benzidine	Associated with bladder tumors in humans; IARC 1
Beryllium	Hardening agent in metal alloys; special use in nuclear energy production	Inhalation of fumes or dust	Pulmonary (and other organs)	Granulomatosis and fibrosis	Beryllium in urine (acute) Beryllium in tissue (chronic) Chest x-ray Lymphoblast transformation test	Pulmonary changes virtually indistinguishable from sarcoid on chest x-ray; IARC 1
Bipyridyls: paraquat, diquat		Inhalation, ingestion, percutaneous absorption	Pulmonary	Rapid massive fibrosis, only following paraquat ingestion		An interesting toxin in that the major toxicity, pulmonary fibrosis, apparently occurs only after ingestion

Substance	Uses/Sources	Routes	Target organs	Health effects	Monitoring	Comments
1,3-Butadiene	Used in the production of rubber and other polymers	Inhalation, percutaneous absorption	Eyes, nose, throat; CNS; Skin	Irritation, cough; Depression, drowsiness; Frostbite	Hemoglobin adduct of 1,3-butadiene	Probable carcinogen, IARC 2A; possible reproductive hazard
Cadmium*	Electroplating; solder for aluminum; metal alloys; process engraving; nickel-cadmium batteries	Inhalation or ingestion of fumes or dust	Pulmonary; Renal	Pulmonary edema (acute); Emphysema (chronic); Nephrosis	β-2 microglobulin (urinary); Urinary protein; Pulmonary function test (PFT)	May be a pulmonary carcinogen; IARC 1
Carbamates: carbaryl (Sevin) and others		Inhalation, ingestion, percutaneous absorption	Neuromuscular	Same as organophosphates	Plasma cholinesterase; urinary 1-naphthol (index of exposure)	Treatment of carbamate poisoning is the same as that of organophosphate poisoning except that 2-PAM is contraindicated
Carbon Dioxide	By-product of ammonia production, lime-kiln operations, and fermentation; used in carbonated beverages, propellant in aerosols, dry ice for refrigeration, fires, indoor environment	Inhalation, dermal contact	Pulmonary; Skin; CVS; Eye	Asphyxiation, dyspnea, restlessness, convulsions; Frostbite; Elevated blood pressure and heart rate; May cause retinal damage	Levels > 800 ppm suggest inadequate ventilation	In environments with inadequate ventilation, elevations can occur; background levels usually less than 300 ppm

(continued)

Agent	Exposure	Route of entry	System(s) affected	Primary manifestation(s)	Aids in diagnosis[a]	Remarks
Carbon disulfide	Solvent for lipids, sulfur, halogens, rubber, phosphorus, oils, waxes, and resins; mfg. of organic chemicals, paints, fuels, explosives, viscose rayon	Inhalation of vapor, percutaneous absorption of liquid or vapor	CNS PNS Renal Cardiovascular Skin Reproductive	Parkinsonism, psychosis, suicide Peripheral neuropathies Chronic nephritic and nephrotic syndromes Acceleration or worsening of atherosclerosis; hypertension Irritation; dermatitis Menorrhagia and metrorrhagia	Iodine-azide reaction with urine (nonspecific since other bivalent sulfur compounds give a positive test); CS_2 in expired air, blood, and urine	A solvent with unusual multisystem effects, especially noted for its cardiovascular, renal, and nervous system actions
Carbon monoxide	Incomplete combustion in foundries, coke ovens, refineries, furnaces, etc.	Inhalation of gas	Blood (hemoglobin)	Headache, dizziness, double vision	Carboxyhemoglobin	A major cause of accidental death; chronic manifestations have included parkinsonism
Carbon tetrachloride	Solvent for oils, fats, resins, lacquers, varnishes, etc.; used as a degreasing and cleaning agent	Inhalation of vapor	Hepatic Renal CNS Skin	Toxic hepatitis Oliguria or anuria CNS depression Dermatitis	Expired air and blood levels	Carbon tetrachloride is the prototype for a wide variety of solvents that cause hepatic and/or renal damage. This solvent, like trichloroethylene, acts synergistically with ethanol. Rarely used in commerce today, since many substitutes are available.

Substance	Uses/Sources	Route	Affected system	Clinical effects	Laboratory tests	Comments
Cellusolve. *See* Ethylene glycol ethers						
Chlordecone. *See* Chlorinated hydrocarbons						
Chlorinated hydrocarbons; chlordane, DDT, heptachlor, chlordecone (Kepone), aldrin, dieldrin, uridine		Ingestion, inhalation, percutaneous absorption	CNS	Stimulation or depression	Urinary organic chlorine, or *p*-chlorophenyl acetic acid; specific blood levels have been measured	The chlorinated hydrocarbons may accumulate in body lipid stores in large amounts.
Chlorine	Paper and textile bleaching; water disinfection; chemical mfg.; metal fluxing; detinning and dezincing iron	Inhalation of gas	Middle respiratory tract	Tracheobronchitis, pulmonary edema (delayed), pneumonitis	CXR, PFTs	Chlorine combines with body moisture to form acids, which irritate tissues from nose to alveoli
Chlorofluorocarbons	Aerosol propellants, refrigerants, intermediate process product	Inhalation, percutaneous absorption	Cardiac; Pulmonary; CNS; Skin	Arrhythmias, palpitations, dizziness; Irritation, cough; Anesthesia, nausea, vomiting, loss of consciousness; Dermatitis		CFCs are of relatively low toxicity unless used in very high concentrations; Control of these compounds has resulted in improvement in the ozone layer over Antarctica

(continued)

Agent	Exposure	Route of entry	System(s) affected	Primary manifestation(s)	Aids in diagnosis[a]	Remarks
Chloroform	Mfg. of fluorocarbons for refrigerants, aerosol propellants, plastics, purifying antibiotics, solvents, photographic processing, and dry cleaning	Inhalation	CNS Liver Renal Cardiovascular	CNS depressant, anesthetic Hepatomegaly, hepatitis Nephropathy, ATN Arrhythmias	Blood or breath chloroform	IARC 2B; Acute exposure may result in delayed hepatotoxicity within 2–5 days
Chloromethyl ethers*	Used in the manufacture of ion exchange resins, bactericides, pesticides, dispersing agents, water repellents, and solvents for industrial polymerization	Inhalation, percutaneous absorption	Eyes, Skin Pulmonary	Irritation of mucous membranes, corneal damage Cough, wheeze, and edema; respiratory tract cancer		Bis(chloromethyl) ether is associated with lung cancer in humans and in animal studies; IARC 1
Chromium	In stainless and heat resistant steel and alloy steel; metal plating; chemical and pigment mfg.; photography	Percutaneous absorption, inhalation, ingestion	Pulmonary Skin	Lung cancer Dermatitis, skin ulcers, nasal septum perforation	Target organ manifestations	
Cobalt	Used in steel and tungsten carbide tools, paint pigments, therapeutic agents	Inhalation of dust and fumes	Pulmonary Skin	Cough, pulmonary fibrosis ("hard metal disease") Allergic dermatitis	Urine cobalt level	Accumulates in the serum of uremic patients. Associated with cardiomyopathy when it was used as an additive in beer.

Substance	Uses/Source	Route of Exposure	Organ/System	Health Effects	Biological Monitoring	Comments
Cyanides	Metallurgy, electroplating	Inhalation of vapor, percutaneous absorption, ingestion	Cellular metabolic enzymes (especially cytochrome oxidase)	Enzyme inhibition with metabolic asphyxia and death	SCN^- in urine or blood	Emergency procedure includes amylnitrate; "cyanide kit" may be helpful
DDT. *See* Chlorinated hydrocarbons						
Dibromochloropropane	Nematocide	Inhalation, percutaneous absorption	CNS Eyes, nose, throat Reproductive Pulmonary	Nausea, drowsiness Irritation Azoospermia		Banned in US, except in Hawaiian pineapples; IARC 2B
p-Dichlorobenzene*	Used as a deodorant, disinfectant, and insecticide	Inhalation of vapors or particulates	Eye and nose, skin Pulmonary Liver Renal	Irritation, profuse rhinitis Irritation Necrosis, anorexia, nausea, jaundice Renal tubular damage	2,5-dichlorophenol in urine	IARC 2B; liver and kidney tumors in animals
Dieldrin. *See* Chlorinated hydrocarbons						
Dimethyl-formamide	Laboratory and industrial solvent	Inhalation, percutaneous absorption, ingestion	Liver Skin CVS	Hepatomegaly, hepatonecrosis, nausea, vomiting, anorexia Facial flushing, dermatitis Elevated blood pressure	Methylformamide in urine within 4 hours of exposure	Ingestion of alcohol during or after exposure can result in a disulfram-like reaction

(continued)

Agent	Exposure	Route of entry	System(s) affected	Primary manifestation(s)	Aids in diagnosis[a]	Remarks
Dioxane	Used as a solvent for a variety of materials, including cellulose acetate, dyes, fats, greases, resins, polyvinyl polymers, varnishes, and waxes	Inhalation of vapor, percutaneous absorption of liquid	CNS Renal Liver	Drowsiness, dizziness, anorexia, headaches, nausea, vomiting, coma Nephritis Chemical hepatitis		Dioxane has caused a variety of neoplasms in animals. *Dioxane should not be confused with "dioxin"* (2,3,7,8-trichlorodibenzo-*p*-dioxin), a contaminant of the chlorphenoxy herbicide, 2,4,5-T (2,4,5-trichlorophenoxyacetic acid) and a known teratogen.
Ethylbenzene	Solvent, fuel additive, chemical intermediate in the production of styrene	Inhalation, percutaneous absorption	Eyes and nose, skin CNS	Irritation, lacrimation CNS depression, dizziness	Mandelic acid in the urine	
Ethylene oxide*	Chemical intermediate, sterilization	Inhalation	Liver	Hepatotoxic Spontaneous abortions		IARC 2A

Substance	Sources/Uses	Route of Exposure	System	Effects	Monitoring	Comments
Ethylene glycol ethers Ethylene glycol monoethyl ether (cellosolve) Ethylene glycol monoethyl ether acetate (cellosolve acetate) Methyl- and butyl-substituted compounds such as ethylene glycol monomethyl ether (methyl cellosolve)	The ethers are used as solvents for resins, paints, lacquers, varnishes, gum, perfume, dyes, and inks; the acetate derivatives are widely used solvents and ingredients of lacquers, enamels, and adhesives. Exposure occurs in dry cleaning, plastic, ink, and lacquer manufacturing, and textile dying, among other places Semiconductor industry	Inhalation of vapor, percutaneous absorption of liquid	CNS Renal Liver Hematopoietic Reproductive	Fatigue, lethargy, nausea, headaches, anorexia, tremor (due to encephalopathy) Renal failure (following acute ingestion) Chemical hepatitis Pancytopenia In animals, reduced fertility and spontaneous abortions		Some glycol ethers have been associated with reproductive hazards in the semiconductor industry Effects associated with ethylene glycol monomethyl ether (methyl cellosolve)
Fluorine	Uranium processing; mfg. of fluorine-containing chemicals; oxidizer in rocket fuel systems	Inhalation of gas	Middle respiratory tract	Laryngeal spasm, bronchospasm, pulmonary edema	CXR, PFTs, urinary fluoride levels	Potent irritant of eyes, mucous membranes, and skin; IARC 3
Fluorocarbons	Refrigeration, degreasing, polymer intermediates	Inhalation	CNS	Mild CNS depression		Many commercial types in use; please check for specific toxicity in other sources; IARC 3

(continued)

Agent	Exposure	Route of entry	System(s) affected	Primary manifestation(s)	Aids in diagnosis[a]	Remarks
Formaldehyde*	Chemical industry, consumer products—wallboard, carpeting	Inhalation	Skin Pulmonary	Irritation Asthma	Urinary formic acid level	Levels between 0.1 and 1.0 ppm can cause upper respiratory irritation in some people; IARC 2A
Hexachlorobenzene	Used as a fungicide in control of smut diseases in seed wheat	Ingestion	Skin Joints Liver	Blistering epidermolysis of the face and hands, hypertrichosis, cutaneous porphyria Interphalangeal joint swelling Weight loss, hepatomegaly	Hexachlorobenzene in whole blood, plasma, or fat biopsy; Urinary porphyrin levels may be elevated following high exposures	Immunosuppressive; Withdrawn from the market in 1959; IARC 2B
n-Hexane	Solvents, adhesives, component of naphtha	Percutaneous, inhalation	PNS	Distal neuropathy	Urinary 2,5,-hexanedione	
Hydrochloric acid	Chemical mfg.; electroplating; tanning; metal pickling; petroleum extraction; in rubber, photographic, and textile industries	Inhalation of gas or mist	Upper respiratory tract Skin	Upper respiratory irritation Irritation		Strong irritant of eyes, mucous membranes, and skin; IARC 3
Hydrofluoric acid	Chemical and plastic mfg.; catalyst in petroleum refining; aqueous solution for frosting, etching, and polishing glass Semiconductor industry	Inhalation of gas or mist	Upper respiratory tract Skin Eye	Upper respiratory irritation Dermal ulceration Corneal ulceration	Serum calcium levels and resting EKG may be helpful	In solution, causes severe and painful burns of skin. Prompt treatment essential Calcium gluconate gel is an effective antidote

Substance	Source/Use	Route	Organ system	Health effect	Monitoring	Comments
Hydrogen. *See* Asphyxiant gases						
Hydrogen sulfide	Used in mfg. of sulfur-containing chemicals: by-product of petroleum product use; decay of organic matter	Inhalation of gas	CNS	Respiratory center paralysis, hypoventilation	PaO$_2$	
			Pulmonary	Respiratory tract irritation		
Isocyanates TDI (toluene diisocyanate) MDI (methylene diisocyanate) Hexamethylene diisocyanate and others	Polyurethane manufacture; resin binding systems in foundries; coating materials for wires, certain types of paint	Inhalation of vapor	Predominantly lower respiratory tract	Asthmatic reaction and accelerated loss of pulmonary function	CXR, PFTs	Isocyanates are both respiratory tract "sensitizers" and irritants in the conventional sense.
Isopropanol	Industrial and laboratory chemical	Accidental ingestion	Eyes, nose throat	Irritation	Isopropanol in breath or blood	IARC 3; Isopropanol manufacture (strong-acid process) IARC 1
			Skin	Dry cracking skin		
			CNS	Drowsiness, dizziness, muscle weakness		
			CVS	Hypotension, bradycardia		
			Renal	Acute renal failure		
			Hematologic	Hemolytic anemia		

(continued)

Agent	Exposure	Route of entry	System(s) affected	Primary manifestation(s)	Aids in diagnosis[a]	Remarks
Ketones Acetone Methyl ethyl ketone (MEK) Methyl n-propyl ketone (MPK) Methyl n-butyl ketone (MBK) Methyl isobutyl ketone (MIBK)	A wide variety of uses as solvents and intermediates in chemical mfg.	Inhalation of vapor, percutaneous absorption of liquid	CNS PNS Skin	Acute CNS depression Chronic CNS depression MBK has been linked with peripheral neuropathy Dermatitis	Neuropsychiatric testing Acetone in blood, urine, expired air (used as an index of exposure, not for diagnosis) Urinary levels for MEK may be helpful	The ketone family demonstrates how a pattern of toxic responses (i.e., CNS narcosis) may feature exceptions (i.e., MBK peripheral neuropathy).
Lead*	Storage batteries; mfg. of paint, enamel, ink, glass, rubber, ceramics; chemical industry	Ingestion of dust, inhalation of dust or fumes	Hematologic Renal Gastrointestinal Neuromuscular CNS Reproductive	Anemia Neuropathy Abdominal pain ("colic") Palsy ("wrist drop") Encephalopathy, behavioral abnormalities Spontaneous abortions	Blood lead Urinary ALA Zinc protoporphyrin (ZZP); free erythrocyte protoporphyrin (FEP)	Lead toxicity, unlike that of mercury, is believed to be reversible, with the exception of late renal and some CNS effects; Organic, IARC 3; Inorganic, IARC 2B
Lindane	Organochlorine insecticide for agriculture and control of body lice	Inhalation, percutaneous absorption, ingestion	Eyes, Nose, Throat CNS Hematologic	Irritation Clonic convulsions, emotional changes, mental confusion Anemia, aplastic anemia	Blood lindane	

Malthione. *See* Organophosphates						
Manganese	Used in the mfg. of steel, welding rods, batteries, ceramics, ink, glass, refractory materials, mining and preservatives	Inhalation, ingestion	Respiratory CNS	Metal fume fever Headache, restlessness, insomnia, mental confusion, irritability, extrapyramidal symptoms, speech and hearing impairment	Urinary manganese	
Mercury (Hg) Elemental	Electronic equipment; paint, metal and textile production; catalyst in chemical mfg.; pharmaceutical production	Inhalation of vapor; slight percutaneous absorption	Pulmonary CNS	Acute pneumonitis Neuropsychiatric changes (erethism); tremor	Urinary Hg	Mercury illustrates several principles. The chemical form has profound effect on its toxicology, as is the case for many metals. Effects of Hg highly variable. Though inorganic
Inorganic		Some inhalation and GI and percutaneous absorption	Pulmonary Renal CNS Skin	Acute pneumonitis Proteinuria Variable Dermatitis	Urinary Hg	
Organic	Agricultural and industrial poisons	Efficient GI ab-			Blood and urine Hg,	

(continued)

Agent	Exposure	Route of entry	System(s) affected	Primary manifestation(s)	Aids in diagnosis[a]	Remarks
Mercury (Hg) Organic (cont.)		sorption, percutaneous absorption, and inhalation	CNS	Sensorimotor changes, visual field constriction, tremor	but ? sensitivity	Hg poisoning is primarily renal, elemental and organic Hg poisoning are primarily neurologic. These responses are difficult to quantify, so dose-response data are generally unavailable. Classic tetrad of gingivitis, sialorrhea, irritability, and tremor is associated with both elemental and inorganic Hg poisoning; the four signs not generally seen together. Many effects of Hg toxicity, especially those in CNS, are irreversible; IARC 3

Substance	Source/Use	Route of Exposure	Target	Clinical Effects	Laboratory	Comments
Methane. *See* Asphyxiant gases						
Methanol	Formaldeyhyde production; used in paints, varnishes, cements, inks, dyes	Inhalation of vapor, percutaneous absorption of liquid	Acid-base Ocular	Metabolic acidosis Optic nerve damage and blindness	Urinary formic acid; methanol in blood and urine; acidosis	Methanol acts through its metabolites formaldehyde and formic acid. Notable is its specific nerve toxicity IARC 3
Methyl bromide	Fumigant of soil and stored food, methylating agent	Inhalation, percutaneous absorption	CNS Respiratory Skin	Vertigo, coma, tremor, weakness, organic brain damage, peripheral neuropathy, visual disturbances Pulmonary edema Erythema, edema, vesiculation	Serum bromide	
Methylene chloride	Solvent, refrigerant, propellant	Percutaneous	Skin	Irritation	In vivo metabolism leads to formation of carboxyhemoglobin	
Nickel	Corrosion-resistant alloys; electroplating; catalyst production; nickel-cadmium batteries	Inhalation of dust or fumes	Skin Pulmonary	Contact dermatitis ("nickel itch") Paranasal sinus cancer Asthma		
Nickel carbonyl	Intermediate in nickel refining; catalyst in petroleum, plastic, rubber industries	Inhalation of vapor, percutaneous absorption of liquid	Pulmonary	Severe irritation, pneumonitis Paranasal sinus cancer	Urinary nickel (acute)	
Nitrogen. *See* Asphyxiant gases						

(continued)

Agent	Exposure	Route of entry	System(s) affected	Primary manifestation(s)	Aids in diagnosis[a]	Remarks
Nitrogen oxides	Mfg. of acids, nitrogen-containing chemicals, explosives, etc.; by-product of many industrial processes	Inhalation of gas	Lower respiratory tract	Pulmonary irritation, bronchiolitis fibrosa obliterans ("silo filler's disease"), mixed obstructive-restrictive changes	CXR, PFTs	Common components of automobile exhaust. Major contributor to acid rain formation ($NO_x + H_2O \rightarrow HNO_3$).
Nitrosamines	Used in rubber industry; as a solvent, organic accelerator, retardant, antioxidant; used in leather tanning, synthetic cutting fluid, and as a meat preservative; present in cigarette smoke	Inhalation, percutaneous absorption, ingestion	Liver Pulmonary, renal	Nausea, vomiting, diarrhea, abdominal pain, jaundice, hepatic necrosis Dysfunction	No specific medical surveillance is recommended	Probable human carcinogen; N-Nitrosodiethylamin, N-Nitrosodimethylamine; IARC 2A

Substance	Source/Use	Route of entry	Target organ	Effects/Symptoms	Diagnostic tests	Comments/Treatment
Organophosphates: malathion, parathion, and others	Inhalation, ingestion, percutaneous absorption	Neuro-muscular	Cholinesterase inhibition, cholinergic symptoms: nausea and vomiting, salivation, diarrhea, headache, sweating, meiosis, muscle fasciculations, seizures, unconsciousness, death	Refractoriness to atropine; plasma or red cell cholinesterase	As with many acute toxins, rapid treatment of organophosphate toxicity is imperative. Thus, diagnosis is often made based on history and a high index of suspicion rather than on biochemical tests. Treatment is atropine, to block cholinergic effects and 2-PAM (2-pyridine-aldoxine methiodide) to reactivate cholinesterase.
Ozone	Inert-gas-shielded arc welding; food, water, and air purification; food and textile bleaching; emitted around high-voltage electrical equipment	Inhalation of gas	Lower respiratory tract	Delayed pulmonary edema (generally 6–8 hr following exposure)	CXR, PFTs	Ozone has a free radical structure and can produce experimental chromosome aberrations; it may thus have carcinogenic potential.
Paraquat	Herbicide	Inhalation, percutaneous absorption, ingestion	Skin, nose, eye / Pulmonary / Liver / Gastrointestinal	Dermatitis, fingernail damage, epistaxis, eye damage / Fibrotic lung changes, dyspnea / Jaundice / Epigastric pain, vomiting	Urinary paraquat	

(continued)

Agent	Exposure	Route of entry	System(s) affected	Primary manifestation(s)	Aids in diagnosis[a]	Remarks
Parathion. *See* Organophosphates						
Pentachlorophenol	Wood preservative, contact herbicide, disinfectant, mildew retardant	Inhalation of vapors from treated wood, percutaneous absorption, ingestion	Eye, nose, throat	Irritation, sneezing	Pentachlorophenol in plasma and urine	Most commercial use in the U.S. has been suspended due to its carcinogenic potential; IARC 2B
			Pulmonary	Dyspnea, cough		
			CNS	Headache, dizziness, fever		
			Gastrointestinal	Anorexia, nausea, vomiting, weight loss		
Perchloroethylene (tetrachloroethylene)	Dry cleaning; chemical intermediate, degreaser	Inhalation, percutaneous	Skin	Irritation	Breath analysis	IARC 2B
			Liver			
			CNS	Acute and chronic CNS depression (see Toluene)		
Phenol	Cleaning agent, paint stripper, disinfectant, chemical intermediate for epoxy resins and drugs	Inhalation of vapors, percutaneous absorption	CNS	CNS depressant, anesthetic	Phenol in urine	IARC 3
			Skin	Potent irritant, corrosive		
			Liver	Necrosis, cytotoxic, abdominal pain		
			Renal	Acute renal failure		
Phosgene	Mfg. and/or burning of isocyanates, and mfg. of dyes and other organic chemicals; in metallurgy for ore separation; burning near trichloroethylene	Inhalation of gas	Lower respiratory tract	Delayed pulmonary edema (delay seldom longer than 12 hours)	CXR, PFTs	Effects can be life-threatening.

Substance	Sources/Uses	Route of exposure	System affected	Signs/symptoms	Monitoring	Comments
Polychlorinated biphenyls (PCBs)	Transformers, electrical equipment	Skin, inhalation of vapors	In animals, *liver* dysfunction; Skin	Chloracne	Serum PCB level	
Polycyclic aromatic hydrocarbons	Incomplete combustion of coke, coal tar and pitch, used in asphalt and oil plastics, dye industry, aluminum smelting electrodes, and present in cigarette smoke	Inhalation, percutaneous absorption, ingestion	Skin; Gastrointestinal; Hematopoietic; Pulmonary	Photodermatitis, conjunctivitis; Nausea, diaphoresis, vomiting; Hemolytic anemia, lymphoma; Chronic bronchitis	Direct measurement of all PAHs is not clinically useful; Benzo[a]pyrene is measured to indicate the presence of PAHs; Serum antibodies to PAH-DNA adducts can be measured; In laboratory animals, measurement of urinary levels of 1-hydroxy pyrene have been associated with exposure to PAH compounds	Epidemiologic studies indicate that workers exposed to PAHs may be at increased risk of cancer at many sites including scrotal, skin, lung, GI, laryngeal and pharyngeal
Sevin. *See* Carbamates						
Stoddard solvent	Degreasing, paint thinning	Inhalation of vapor, percutaneous absorption of liquid	Skin; CNS	Dryness and scaling from defatting; dermatitis; Dizziness, coma, collapse (at high levels)		A mixture of primarily aliphatic hydrocarbons, with some benzene derivatives and naphthenes
Styrene	Chemical intermediate, solvent used in the mfg. of plastics	Inhalation, percutaneous absorption	CNS; Liver; Eyes, skin	CNS depression, fatigue, unsteady gait, headache; Hepatotoxic, nausea; Irritation of mucous membranes, dermatitis	Urinary mandelic acid and phenylglyoxylic acid, blood styrene	May cause adverse reproductive effects; IARC 2B

(continued)

Agent	Exposure	Route of entry	System(s) affected	Primary manifestation(s)	Aids in diagnosis[a]	Remarks
Sulfur dioxide	Mfg. of sulfur-containing chemicals; as a food and textile bleach; tanning; metal casting	Inhalation of gas, direct contact of gas or liquid phase on skin or mucosa	Middle respiratory tract	Bronchospasm (pulmonary edema or chemical pneumonitis in high dose)	CXR, PFTs[c]	Strong irritant of eyes, mucous membranes, and skin; Combined with moisture, leads to acid rain (H_2SO_4); IARC 3
Toluene	Organic chemical mfg.; solvent; fuel component	Inhalation of vapor, percutaneous absorption of liquid	CNS Skin	Acute CNS depression Irritation, dermatitis Chronic CNS depression	Urinary hippuric acid Neuropsychiatric testing	Toluene lacks the leukemogenic effect of benzene, but commercial toluene is often contaminated with benzene.
1,1,1-Trichloroethane	Degreaser, propellant	Inhalation, percutaneous	Skin Liver CNS	Irritation Acute and chronic CNS depression (see Toluene)	Breath analysis	
Trichloroethylene (TCE)	Solvent in metal degreasing, dry cleaning, food extraction; ingredient of paints, adhesives, varnishes, inks	Inhalation, percutaneous absorption	CNS PNS Skin Cardiovascular	CNS depression Peripheral and cranial neuropathy Irritation, dermatitis Arrhythmias	Breath analysis for TCE Urinary trichloroacetic acid	TCE is involved in an important pharmacologic interaction. Within hours of ingesting alcoholic beverages, TCE workers experience flushing of the face, neck, shoulders, and back. Alcohol may also potentiate the CNS effects of TCE. The probable mechanism is competition for metabolic enzymes.

Substance	Uses	Route	Organ systems	Health effects	Biological monitoring	Comments
Trimellitic anhydride	Used as a curing agent for alkyl and epoxy resins, polymers, polyesters, vinyl chloride plasticizer, paints and pigments	Inhalation of dust or fumes, percutaneous absorption, ingestion	Pulmonary / Immunologic / Skin	Pulmonary edema, hemorrhage / Sensitization, asthma, rhinitis / Irritation of the mucous membranes	Serum antibodies to TMA	Causes late respiratory distress syndrome
Uranium	Processing of uranium ore for nuclear fuel	Inhalation	Pulmonary / Immune system / Renal	Irritation, lung damage, lung cancer / Lymph node damage, bone marrow suppression / Albuminuria, hematuria	Urinary uranium	IARC 1 (radon and its decay products)
Uridine. *See* Chlorinated hydrocarbons						
Vanadium pentoxide	Dyes, paints, insecticides, alloying agent in hard steel	Inhalation of dust and fumes	Pulmonary / Skin, eyes, mucous membranes	Cough, wheezing, dyspnea, pneumonitis / Irritation, green tongue	Urine vandium concentrations	Favorable prognosis with removal
Vinyl chloride*	Intermediate in the synthesis of polyvinyl chloride resins for plastic piping, floor coverings, upholstery, appliances, and packaging	Inhalation	Pulmonary / CNS / Liver / Skin	Respiratory tract irritation / Lethargy, headache / Hepatosplenomegaly, angiosarcoma / Acrocyanosis, Raynaud's phenomenon, skin thickening	Breath analysis for vinyl chloride, or urine thiodiglycolic acid	May cause adverse reproductive effects; IARC 1

(continued)

Agent	Exposure	Route of entry	System(s) affected	Primary manifestation(s)	Aids in diagnosis[a]	Remarks
Xylene	A wide variety of uses as a solvent; an ingredient of paints, lacquers, varnishes, inks, dyes, adhesives, cements; an intermediate in chemical mfg.	Inhalation of vapor; slight percutaneous absorption of liquid	Pulmonary	Irritation, pneumonitis, acute pulmonary edema (at high doses)	Methylhippuric acid in urine, xylene in expired air, xylene in blood.	
			Eyes, nose, throat	Irritation		
			CNS	Acute CNS depression Chronic CNS depression	Neuropsychiatric testing	
Zinc oxide	Welding by-product; rubber mfg.	Inhalation of dust or fumes that are freshly generated		"Metal fume fever," (fever, chills, and other symptoms)	Urinary zinc (useful as an indicator of exposure, not for acute diagnosis)	A self-limiting syndrome of 24–48 hours, with apparently no sequelae.

*OSHA standards apply to this chemical or class.
[a]Occupational and medical histories are, in most instances, the most important aids in diagnosis.
[b]The less water-soluble the gas, the deeper and more delayed its irritant effect.
[c]PFTs are useful aids in diagnosis of irritant effects if the patient is subacutely or chronically ill.
Source: Adapted from H. Frumkin. Some Illustrative Toxins and Their Effects. In B. S. Levy and D. H. Wegman (eds.), *Occupational Health*. Boston: Little, Brown, 1983. Revised by R. J. McCunney.

References for Appendix A

Amdur M., Doull J., and Klaassen C., (ed.). *Casarett and Doull's Toxicology: The Basic Science of Poisons*. New York: McGraw-Hill, 1991.

Baselt R. *Biological Monitoring Methods for Industrial Chemicals* (2nd ed.). Littleton, Ma.: PSG, 1988.

Clayton G., and Clayton F. (eds.). *Patty's Industrial Hygiene and Toxicology: Toxicology* (4th ed.). New York: Wiley, 1991–1994.

Ellenhorn M., and Barceloux D. *Medical Toxicology: Diagnosis and Treatment of Human Poisoning*. New York: Elsevier, 1988.

Frumkin H., Health Effects of Common Substances. In Levy B. S., and Wegman D., (eds.). *Occupational Health and Safety,* Boston: Little, Brown, 1983.

Hathaway G., et al. *Proctor and Hughes' Chemical Hazards in the Workplace* (3rd ed.). New York: Van Nostrand Reinhold, 1991.

NIOSH. *NIOSH Pocket Guide to Chemical Hazards*. Cincinnati, Ohio: NIOSH, 1990. DHHS (NIOSH) Publication No. 90–117.

Que Hee S. *Biological Monitoring: An Interpretive Approach*. New York: Van Nostrand Reinhold, 1993.

Sullivan, J., and Krieger G. *Hazardous Materials Toxicology: Clinical Principles of Environmental Health*. Baltimore: Williams & Wilkins, 1992.

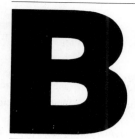

Government and Regulatory Agencies

Nancy English

The Occupational Safety and Health Administration (OSHA), part of the Department of Labor, is charged with enforcing workplace health and safety standards. This federal agency also has responsibility for establishing safe exposure limits and other protective measures required of various workplaces. Although OSHA plays a fundamental role in the enforcement of workplace health standards, the agency can also be instrumental in providing consultative support to business and industry. For more information contact:

Occupational Safety and Health Administration (OSHA)
Headquarters Office
US Department of Labor
3rd and Constitution Ave., NW
Washington, DC 20210

There are 10 regional OSHA offices where information, advice, and lists of currently available publications can be obtained. These offices can answer questions and can direct inquiries to appropriate local offices or specialized OSHA services. States may administer their own plans if these plans are at least as effective as federal requirements and the state plans are approved by OSHA. Currently, 25 states have state plans. Check with your regional office for more information.

Region I (CT, ME, MA, NH, RI, VT)
133 Portland St., 1st Floor
Boston, MA 02114
617-565-7164

Connecticut
Federal Office Bldg.
450 Main St.
Hartford, CT 06103
203-240-3152

Maine
US Federal Bldg.
40 Western Ave., Rm. 121
Augusta, ME 04330
207-622-8417

Massachusetts
1145 Main St., Rm. 108
Springfield, MA 01103
413-785-0123

639 Granite St., 4th Floor
Braintree, MA 02184
617-565-6924

New Hampshire
Federal Bldg., Rm. 334
55 Pleasant St.
Concord, NH 03301
603-225-1629

Rhode Island
380 Westminster Mall
Rm. 243
Providence, RI 02903
401-528-4669

Region II (NJ, NY, PR, VI)
201 Varick St., Rm. 670
New York, NY 10014
212-337-2378

New Jersey
Plaza 35, Suite 205
1030 Saint Georges Ave.
Avenel, NJ 07001
201-750-3270

2 E. Blackwell St.
Dover, NJ 07801
201-361-4050

500 Rte. 17 South, 2nd Floor
Hasbrouck Heights, NJ 07604
201-288-1700

Marlton Executive Park
701 Rte. 73, South Bldg. 2
Marlton, NJ 08053
609-757-5181

New York
Leo W. O'Brien Federal Bldg.
Clinton Ave. and N. Pearl St.
Rm. 132
Albany, NY 12207
518-472-6085

42-40 Bell Blvd., 5th Floor
Bayside, NY 11361
718-279-9060

5360 Genesee St.
Bowmansville, NY 14026
716-684-3891

90 Church St., Rm. 1407
New York, NY 10007
212-264-9840

100 S. Clinton St., Rm. 1267
Syracuse, NY 13260
315-423-5188

990 Westbury Rd.
Westbury, NY 11590
516-334-3344

Puerto Rico
US Courthouse and FOB
Carlos Chardon St., Rm. 559
Hato Rey, PR 00918
809-766-5457

Region III (DC, DE, MD, PA, VA, WV)
Gateway Bldg., Suite 1200
3535 Market St.
Philadelphia, PA 19104
215-596-1201

Maryland
Federal Bldg., Rm. 1110
Charles Ctr., 31 Hopkins Plaza
Baltimore, MD 21201
301-962-2840

Pennsylvania
850 N. 5th St.
Allentown, PA 18102
215-776-4220

Rothrock Bldg., Rm. 408
121 West 10th St.
Erie, PA 16501
814-453-4351

Progress Plaza
49 N. Progress St.
Harrisburg, PA 17109
717-782-3902

US Custom House, Rm. 242
Second and Chestnut St.
Philadelphia, PA 19106
215-597-4955

1000 Liberty Ave., Rm. 2236
Pittsburgh, PA 15222
412-644-2903

Penn Pl., Rm. 2005
20 N. Pennsylvania Ave.
Wilkes-Barre, PA 18701
717-826-6538

West Virginia
550 Eagan St., Rm. 206
Charleston, WV 25301
304-347-5937

Region IV (AL, FL, GA, KY, MS, NC, SC, TN)
Peachtree St., NE, Suite 587
Atlanta, GA 30367
404-347-3573

Alabama
2047 Canyon Rd., Todd Mall
Birmingham, AL 35216
205-731-1534

Florida
299 East Broward Blvd., Rm. 302
Fort Lauderdale, FL 33301
305-527-7292

3100 University Blvd. South
Jacksonville, FL 32216
904-791-2895

700 Twiggs St., Rm. 624
Tampa, FL 33602
813-228-2821

Georgia
Bldg. 7, Suite 110
La Vista Perimeter Office Park
Tucker, GA 30084
404-331-4767/0353

Kentucky
John C. Watts Federal Bldg., Rm. 108
330 W. Broadway
Frankfort, KY 40601
502-227-7024

Mississippi
Federal Bldg., Suite 1445
110 West Capitol St.
Jackson, MS 39269
601-965-4606

North Carolina
Century Station, Rm. 104
300 Fayetteville Street Mall
Raleigh, NC 27601
919-856-4770

South Carolina
1835 Assembly St., Rm. 1468
Columbia, SC 29201
803-765-5904

Tennessee
2002 Richard Jones Rd., Suite C-205
Nashville, TN 37215-2809
615-736-5313

Region V (IL, IN, MI, MN, OH, WI)
230 S. Dearborn St., Rm. 3244
Chicago, IL 60604
312-353-2220

Illinois
1600 167th St., Suite 12
Calumet City, IL 60409
312-891-3800

2360 E. Devon Ave., Suite 1010
Des Plaines, IL 60018
312-803-4800

344 Smoke Tree Business Park
North Aurora, IL 60542
312-869-8700

2001 W. Willow Knolls Rd.
Suite 101
Peoria, IL 61614-1223
309-671-7033

Indiana
46 East Ohio St., Rm. 423
Indianapolis, IN 46204
317-269-7290

Michigan
300 E. Michigan Ave., Rm. 305
Lansing, MI 48993
517-377-1892

Minnesota
110 South 4th St., Rm. 425
Minneapolis, MN 55401
612-348-1994

Ohio
Federal Office Bldg., Rm. 4028
550 Main St.
Cincinnati, OH 45202
513-684-3784

Federal Office Bldg., Rm. 899
1240 East Ninth St.
Cleveland, OH 44199
216-522-3818

Federal Office Bldg., Rm. 620
200 N. High St.
Columbus, OH 43215
614-469-5582

Federal Office Bldg., Rm. 734
234 N. Summit St.
Toledo, OH 43604
419-259-7542

Wisconsin
2618 North Ballard Rd.
Appleton, WI 54915
414-734-4521

2934 Fish Hatchery Rd.
Suite 225
Madison, WI 53713
608-264-5388

Suite 1180
310 W. Wisconsin Ave.
Milwaukee, WI 53203
414-291-3315

Region VI (AR, LA, NM, OK, TX)
525 Griffin St., Rm. 602
Dallas, TX
214-767-4731

Arkansas
Savers Bldg., Suite 828
320 West Capitol Ave.
Little Rock, AR 72201
501-378-6291

Louisiana
2156 Wooddale Blvd.
Hoover Annex, Suite 200
Baton Rouge, LA 70806
504-389-0474

New Mexico
320 Central Ave., SW
Suite 13
Albuquerque, NM 87102
505-776-3411

Oklahoma
420 West Main Pl., Suite 725
Oklahoma City, OK 73102
405-231-5351

Texas
611 E. 6th Street, Rm. 303
Austin, TX 78701
512-482-5783

Government Plaza, Rm. 300
400 Mann St.
Corpus Christi, TX 78401
512-888-3257

North Star 2 Bldg., Suite 430
8713 Airport Freeway
Fort Worth, TX 76180-7604
817-885-7025

2320 La Branch St., Rm. 1103
Houston, TX 77004
713-750-1727

1425 W. Pioneer Dr.
Irving, TX 75061
214-767-5347

Federal Bldg., Rm. 421
1205 Texas Ave.
Lubbock, TX 79401
806-743-7681

Region VII (IA, KS, MO, NE)
911 Walnut St.
Kansas City, MO 64106
816-426-5861

Kansas
216 N. Waco, Suite B
Wichita, KS 67202
316-269-6644

Missouri
911 Walnut St., Rm. 2202
Kansas City, MO 64106
816-426-2756

4300 Goodfellow Blvd., Bldg. 105E
St. Louis, MO 63120
314-263-2749

Nebraska
Overland-Wolf Bldg., Rm. 100
6910 Pacific St.
Omaha, NE 68106
402-221-3182

Region VIII (CO, MT, ND, SD, UT, WY)
Federal Bldg., Rm. 1576
1961 Stout St.
Denver, CO 80294
303-844-3061

Colorado
1244 Speer Blvd.
Colonnade Ctr., Suite 360
Denver, CO 80204
303-844-5285

Montana
19 N. 25th St.
Billings, MT 59101
406-657-6649

North Dakota
Federal Bldg., Rm. 348
PO Box 2439
Bismarck, ND 58501
701-250-4521

Utah
1781 South 300 West
Salt Lake City, UT 84115
801-524-5080

Region IX (AZ, CA, HI, NV, American Samoa, Guam, Trust Territories of the Pacific)
71 Stevenson St., Rm. 415
San Francisco, CA 94105
415-744-6670

Arizona
3221 N. 16th St., Suite 100
Phoenix, AZ
602-640-2007

California
71 Stevenson St., Suite 415
San Francisco, CA 94105
415-744-6670

Hawaii
300 Ala Moana Blvd., Suite 5122
Honolulu, HI 96850
808-541-2685

Nevada
1413 N. Carson Blvd., 1st Floor
Carson City, NV 98701
702-885-6963

Region X (AK, ID, OR, WA)
1111 Third Ave., Suite 715
Seattle, WA 98174
206-442-5930

Alaska
Federal Bldg., USCH Rm. 211
222 West 7th Ave., #29
Anchorage, AK 99513-7571
907-271-5152

Idaho
Suite 134
3050 N. Lake Harbor Lane
Boise, ID 83903
208-334-1867

Oregon
1220 SW Third Ave., Rm. 640
Portland, OR 97204
503-326-2251

Washington
121 70th Ave., NE
Bellevue, WA 98004
206-442-7520

The National Institute for Occupational Safety and Health (NIOSH) was established by the Occupational Safety and Health Act of 1970, which made NIOSH responsible for conducting research to make the nation's workplaces healthier and safer. NIOSH was within the US Public Health Service until 1973, when it became part of the Centers for Disease Control.

NIOSH may require employers to measure and report employee exposure to potentially hazardous materials and to provide medical examinations and tests to determine the incidence of occupational illness among employees. NIOSH is required by law to respond to urgent requests for assistance from employers, employees, and their representatives where imminent hazards are suspected. To identify hazards, NIOSH is authorized to conduct workplace inspections.

NIOSH conducts laboratory and epidemiologic research, publishes its findings, and makes recommendations for improved working conditions to regulatory agencies such as OSHA and the Mine Safety and Health Administration. NIOSH has completed and published many surveys and studies on hazards in the workplace, as well as recommendations for limits on certain workplace exposures. For more information or to obtain a list of publications contact:

Department of Health and Human Services
Public Health Service
Centers for Disease Control
National Institute for Occupational Safety and Health
Robert A. Taft Laboratories
4676 Columbia Pkwy.
Cincinnati, OH 45226

NIOSH technical information resources can be accessed at 1-800-35-NIOSH.

NIOSH offers many services that may be requested by both employers and employees: (reference CDD/NIOSH).

NIOSH maintains extensive databases of occupational safety and health information from around the world. Databases: 513-533-8326.

NIOSH supports educational resource centers at 14 US universities to help assure an adequate supply of trained occupational safety and health professionals. Educational Resource Centers: 513-533-8241.

NIOSH sponsors extramural research in priority areas and coordinates this with its intramural and contract research and that of other HHS and US departments. Extramural Grants: 404-639-3343.

NIOSH identifies risk factors for work-related fatalities and injuries through its Fatal Accident Circumstances and Epidemiology project. Fatal Accident Investigations: 304-291-4575.

Employers, employees, or their representatives who suspect a health problem in the workplace can request a NIOSH Health Hazard Evaluation (HHE) to assess the problem. Health Hazard Evaluation: 1-800-35-NIOSH.

NIOSH administers periodic chest x-rays to coal miners to facilitate early detection of coalworker's pneumoconiosis. Miners' x-rays: 304-291-4301.

NIOSH publishes and distributes a variety of publications related to occupational safety and health. Publications: 513-533-8287.

NIOSH tests and certifies respirators to assure their compliance with federal requirements. Respirators: 304-291-4331.

NIOSH has offices in four locations:

NIOSH Headquarters
Bldg. 1, Rm. 3007
Centers for Disease Control
1600 Clifton Rd.
Atlanta, Georgia 30333
404-639-3061

NIOSH Washington Office
200 Independence Ave., SW
Washington, DC 20201
202-472-7134

Appalachian Laboratories
944 Chestnut Ridge Rd.
Morgantown, WV 26505-2888
Division of Respiratory Disease Studies: 304-291-4474
Division of Safety Research: 304-284-5100

Cincinnati Laboratories
4676 Columbia Pkwy.
Cincinnati, OH 45226-1998
Division of Biomedical and Behavioral Science: 513-533-8465
Division of Standards Development and Technology Transfer: 513-533-8302
Division of Training and Manpower Development: 513-533-8221

Division of Physical Sciences and Engineering: 513-841-4321
Division of Surveillance, Hazard Evaluation and Field Studies: 513-841-4428

The US Environmental Protection Agency (EPA), created in 1970, administers nine
comprehensive environmental protection laws: the Clean Air Act (CAA); the Clean
Water Act (CWA); the Safe Drinking Water Act (SDWA); the Comprehensive Environmental Response, Compensation and Liability Act (CERCLA or Superfund)
amended by the Superfund Amendments and Reauthorization Act (SARA); the Resource Conservation and Recovery Act (RCRA); the Federal Insecticide, Fungicide
and Rodenticide Act (FIFRA); the Toxic Substances Control Act (TSCA); the Marine
Protection Research and Sanctuaries Act (MPRSA); and the Uranium Mill Tailings
Radiation Control Act (UMTRCA). The EPA is responsible for implementing these
federal laws and for conducting research relevant to environmental concerns.

The EPA has 10 regional offices from which information and publications can be
obtained.

Region 1 (CT, ME, MA, NH, RI, VT)
JFK Federal Bldg.
Boston, MA 02203
617-565-3420

> **Connecticut**
> Federal Office Bldg.
> 450 Main St.
> Hartford, CT 06103
> 203-240-3152
>
> **Maine**
> US Federal Bldg.
> 40 Western Ave., Rm. 121
> Augusta, ME 04330
> 207-622-8417
>
> **Massachusetts**
> JFK Federal Bldg.
> Boston, MA 02203
> 617-565-3420
>
> **New Hampshire**
> Federal Bldg., Rm. 334
> 55 Pleasant St.
> Concord, NH 03301
> 603-225-1629
>
> **Rhode Island**
> 380 Westminster Mall
> Rm. 243
> Providence, RI 02903
> 401-528-4669

Region 2 (NJ, NY, PR, VI)
Jacob K. Javits Federal Bldg. 26
Federal Plaza
New York, NY 10278
212-264-2515

> **New Jersey**
> Plaza 35, Suite 205
> 1030 Saint Georges Ave.
> Avenel, NJ 07001
> 201-750-3270

2 E. Blackwell St.
Dover, NJ 07801
201-361-4050

500 Rte. 17 South, 2nd Floor
Hasbrouck Heights, NJ 07604
201-288-1700

Marlton Executive Park
701 Rte. 73, South Bldg. 2
Marlton, NJ 08053
609-757-5181

New York
Leo W. O'Brien Federal Bldg.
Clinton Ave. and N. Pearl St.
Rm. 132
Albany, NY 12207
518-472-6085

42-40 Bell Blvd., 5th Floor
Bayside, NY 11361
718-279-9060

5360 Genesee St.
Bowmansville, NY 14026
716-684-3891

90 Church St., Rm. 1407
New York, NY 10007
212-264-9840

100 S. Clinton St., Rm. 1267
Syracuse, NY 13260
315-423-5188

990 Westbury Rd.
Westbury, NY 11590
516-334-3344

Puerto Rico
US Courthouse and FOB
Carlos Chardon St., Rm. 559
Hato Rey, PR 00918
809-766-5457

Region 3 (DC, DE, MD, PA, VA, WV)
841 Chestnut St.
Philadelphia, PA 19107
215-597-9370

Maryland
Federal Bldg., Rm. 1110
Charles Ctr., 31 Hopkins Plaza
Baltimore, MD 21201
301-962-2840

Pennsylvania
850 N. 5th St.
Allentown, PA 18102
215-776-4220

Rothrock Bldg., Rm. 408
121 West 10th St.
Erie, PA 16501
814-453-4351

Progress Plaza
49 N. Progress St.
Harrisburg, PA 17109
717-782-3902

US Custom House, Rm. 242
Second and Chestnut St.
Philadelphia, PA 19106
215-597-4955

1000 Liberty Ave., Rm. 2236
Pittsburgh, PA 15222
412-644-2903

Penn Pl., Rm. 2005
20 N. Pennsylvania Ave.
Wilkes-Barre, PA 18701
717-826-6538

West Virginia
550 Eagan St., Rm. 206
Charleston, WV 25301
304-347-5937

Region 4 (AL, FL, GA, KY, MS, NC, SC, TN)
345 Courtland St., NE
Atlanta, GA 30365
404-347-3004

Alabama
2047 Canyon Rd., Todd Mall
Birmingham, AL 35216
205-731-1534

Florida
299 East Broward Blvd., Rm. 302
Fort Lauderdale, FL 33301
305-527-7292

3100 University Blvd. South
Jacksonville, FL 32216
904-791-2895

700 Twiggs St., Rm. 624
Tampa, FL 33602
813-228-2821

Georgia
Bldg. 7, Suite 110
La Vista Perimeter Office Park
Tucker, GA 30084
404-331-4767/0353

Kentucky
John C. Watts Federal Bldg., Rm. 108
330 W. Broadway
Frankfort, KY 40601
502-227-7024

Mississippi
Federal Bldg., Suite 1445
110 West Capitol St.
Jackson, MS 39269
601-965-4606

North Carolina
Century Station, Rm. 104
300 Fayetteville Street Mall
Raleigh, NC 27601
919-856-4770

South Carolina
1835 Assembly St., Rm. 1468
Columbia, SC 29201
803-765-5904

Tennessee
2002 Richard Jones Rd., Suite C-205
Nashville, TN 37215-2809
615-736-5313

Region 5 (IL, IN, MI, MN, OH, WI)
230 S. Dearborn St.
Chicago, IL 60604
312-353-2072

Illinois
1600 167th St., Suite 12
Calumet City, IL 60409
312-891-3800

2360 E. Devon Ave., Suite 1010
Des Plaines, IL 60018
312-803-4800

344 Smoke Tree Business Park
North Aurora, IL 60542
312-869-8700

2001 W. Willow Knolls Rd.
Suite 101
Peoria, IL 61614-1223
309-671-7033

Indiana
46 E. Ohio St., Rm. 423
Indianapolis, IN 46204
317-269-7290

Michigan
300 E. Michigan Ave., Rm. 305
Lansing, MI 48993
517-377-1892

Minnesota
110 South 4th St., Rm. 425
Minneapolis, MN 55401
612-348-1994

Ohio
Federal Office Bldg., Rm. 4028
550 Main St.
Cincinnati, OH 45202
513-684-3784

Federal Office Bldg., Rm. 899
1240 East Ninth St.
Cleveland, OH 44199
216-522-3818

Federal Office Bldg., Rm. 620
200 N. High St.
Columbus, OH 43215
614-469-5582

Federal Office Bldg., Rm. 734
234 N. Summit St.
Toledo, OH 43604
419-259-7542

Wisconsin
2618 North Ballard Rd.
Appleton, WI 54915
414-734-4521

2934 Fish Hatchery Rd.
Suite 225
Madison, WI 53713
608-264-5388

Suite 1180
310 W. Wisconsin Ave.
Milwaukee, WI 53203
414-291-3315

Region 6 (AR, LA, NM, OK, TX)
1445 Ross Ave., Suite 1200
Dallas, TX 75202
214-655-2200

Arkansas
Savers Bldg., Suite 828
320 West Capitol Ave.
Little Rock, AR 72201
501-378-6291

Louisiana
2156 Wooddale Blvd.
Hoover Annex, Suite 200
Baton Rouge, LA 70806
504-389-0474

New Mexico
320 Central Ave., SW
Suite 13
Albuquerque, NM 87102
505-776-3411

Oklahoma
420 West Main Pl., Suite 725
Oklahoma City, OK 73102
405-231-5351

Texas
611 E. 6th Street, Rm. 303
Austin, TX 78701
512-482-5783

Government Plaza, Rm. 300
400 Mann St.
Corpus Christi, TX 78401
512-888-3257

North Star 2 Bldg., Suite 430
8713 Airport Freeway
Fort Worth, TX 76180-7604
817-885-7025

2320 La Branch St., Rm. 1103
Houston, TX 77004
713-750-1727

1425 W. Pioneer Dr.
Irving, TX 75061
214-767-5347

Federal Bldg., Rm. 421
1205 Texas Ave.
Lubbock, TX 79401
806-743-7681

Region 7 (IA, KS, MO, NE)
726 Minnesota Ave.
Kansas City, KS 66101
913-551-7003

Kansas
216 N. Waco, Suite B
Wichita, KS 67202
316-269-6644

Missouri
911 Walnut St., Rm. 2202
Kansas City, MO 64106
816-426-2756

4300 Goodfellow Blvd., Bldg. 105E
St. Louis, MO 63120
314-263-2749

Nebraska
Overland-Wolf Bldg., Rm. 100
6910 Pacific St.
Omaha, NE 68106
402-221-3182

Region 8 (CO, MT, ND, SD, UT, WY)
999 18th St., Suite 500
Denver, CO 80202
303-293-1692

Colorado
1244 Speer Blvd.
Colonnade Ctr., Suite 360
Denver, CO 80204
303-844-5285

Montana
19 N. 25th St.
Billings, MT 59101
406-657-6649

North Dakota
Federal Bldg., Rm. 348
PO Box 2439
Bismarck, ND 58501
701-250-4521

Utah
1781 South 300 West
Salt Lake City, UT 84115
801-524-5080

Region 9 (AZ, CA, HI, NV, American Samoa, Guam, Northern Mariana Islands)
1235 Mission St.
San Francisco, CA 94103
415-556-5145

Arizona
3221 N. 16th St., Suite 100
Phoenix, AZ
602-640-2007

California
71 Stevenson St., Suite 415
San Francisco, CA 94105
415-744-6670

Hawaii
300 Ala Moana Blvd., Suite 5122
Honolulu, HI 96850
808-541-2685

Nevada
1413 N. Carson Blvd., 1st Floor
Carson City, NV 98701
702-885-6963

Region 10 (AK, ID, OR, WA)
1200 Sixth Ave.
Seattle, WA 98101
206-442-1465

Alaska
Federal Bldg., USCH Rm. 211
222 West 7th Ave., #29
Anchorage, AK 99513-7571
907-271-5152

Idaho
Suite 134
3050 N. Lake Harbor Lane
Boise, ID 83903
208-334-1867

Oregon
1220 SW Third Ave., Rm. 640
Portland, OR 97204
503-326-2251

Washington
121 70th Ave., NE
Bellevue, WA 98004
206-442-7520

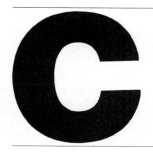

A History of the American College of Occupational and Environmental Medicine and the Growth of a Specialty

Jean Spencer Felton

Not only in antiquity but in our own times also laws have been passed in well-ordered cities to secure good conditions for the workers; so it is only right that the art of medicine should contribute its portion for the benefit and relief of those for whom the law has shown such foresight; indeed we ought to show peculiar zeal, though so far we have neglected to do so, in taking precautions for their safety, so that as far as possible they may work at their chosen calling without loss of health.

Bernardino Ramazzini (1713)

Although physicians in the United States were knowledgeable about the existence of work-related illness and injury in the late nineteenth century, it was only at the century's turn that comprehensive texts began to appear in this country, with the emphasis on the trauma sustained by the worker [1–5]. While there were practitioners in the field of the then-termed "industrial medicine," there was no formal organization for such physicians. Departments had been established at certain universities in the early years and a few clinics for the study of occupational diseases were established, but were short lived [6]. There was no activity in the United States at that time that matched the publications, dedicated hospitals, or morbidity studies emanating from European sources. A summation of the current status was well stated at an international conference in Brussels by a member of the Belgian Labor Department, who said, "It is well known that there is no industrial hygiene in the United States. *Ça n'existe pas*" [7].

The Birth of a Society

With the initial passage of liability laws and the subsequent enactment of workers' compensation legislation, there was an awakening in several industries of the need for better standards in the burgeoning field of medical care for injured employees. With the creation of the National Safety Council in 1912, the health and safety movement began to grow and programs headed by physicians were found in such corporate entities as the Norton Grinding Company of Worcester, Massachusetts; the Cincinnati Milling Machine Company; People's Gas Company of Chicago; General Motors Corporation, Ford Motor Company; E. I. du Pont de Nemours and Company of Wilmington, Delaware; and Sears, Roebuck and Company of Chicago.

In an early conversation between Drs. Harry E. Mock of Sears and Andrew M. Harvey of the Crane Company, the thought of an association of physicians serving industry emerged. Eventually, in Detroit on June 12, 1916, the American Association of Industrial Physicians and Surgeons (AAIPS) was organized with over 100 members [6]. The stated objective of the Association was to ". . . foster the study and discussion of the problems peculiar to the practice of industrial medicine and surgery; to develop methods adapted to the conservation of health among workmen in the industries; to promote a more general understanding of the purposes and results of the medical care of employees; and to unite into one organization members of the medical profession specializing in industrial medicine and surgery for their mutual advancement in the practice of their profession" [6]. While the scope of the field has enlarged into research, education, and the involvement of bodies of workers outside of industry, the founding tenets still have validity.

Apart from the changes undergone by the specialty over the ensuing decades, interesting socioeconomic observations may be made about the founding of AAIPS.

The dues were set at $2.00 per annum and the initial banquet held at the Cadillac Hotel carried a charge of $2.00 with no provision for the inclusion of cigars [6].

The mix of the officers elected at the initial gathering foretells, in a sense, the various affiliations of the membership to follow over the years. The president was Dr. Joseph W. Schereschewsky of the relatively new Office of Industrial Hygiene of the Public Health Service, seen today as the National Institute for Occupational Safety and Health (NIOSH). In the position of vice president was Dr. Robert T. Legge from the University of California, Berkeley. Dr. Francis D. Patterson served as second vice president; he was a member of the Pennsylvania Department of Labor. Dr. Harry E. Mock was elected secretary-treasurer and, as indicated earlier, was from industry [6].

Members of AAIPS became active during World War I, becoming involved with both the introduction of placement physical examinations and the identification, and possibly the control, of occupational health hazards. In 1917, Dr. Alice Hamilton published a list of 2432 cases of work-related poisonings, of which 1389 were caused by nitrous fumes, as were 28 of 58 deaths. Second in number were 660 relating to trinitrotoluene (TNT), of which 13 were deaths [7].

The Boost by War

Little in the way of growth was seen in occupational medicine following the conclusion of World War I. Some research was conducted in academe and the beginnings of epidemiologic studies were seen in some of the states' official agencies.

The period between the wars had seen the elimination of phosphorus as a hazard in the match industry [8] and the substitution of other carroting agents for mercury in the making of felt hats [9]. Also, the causation of osteogenic sarcoma among radium dial painters was identified [10].

That there was growing recognition of the value of a medical service in industry was seen in the creation of the Knudsen Award in 1938, named after the General Motors president, that was to be given annually to "the industrial physician making the most outstanding contribution to industrial medicine" [6]. The presentation of the award at the annual meeting of AAIPS and its successors has highlighted the honors ceremonies conducted during the American Occupational Health Conference.

In the early 1930s, an episode of great proportion was seen in the boring of the Hawk's Nest Tunnel through a vein of silica near the town of Gauley Bridge, West Virginia. The tunnel was cut in order to bring water from a river to a hydroelectric power plant. The engineering activity was undertaken during the early years of the depression and workers came from all over the United States for the employment opportunity. About 5000 men worked on the project and 50 to 60% saw some service underground. There were three times as many blacks as whites in the labor force. Within 5 years following completion of the tunnel, over 700 deaths resulted from acute or chronic silicosis or other pneumoconioses [11]. The toll of lives led to a congressional investigation in 1936 and the recognition of silicosis—despite negative thought among industrial health professionals—as a definite occupational disease entity. Several conferences followed and research efforts were begun. In the words of the epidemiologist who put the data together, "Not all was in vain, however. By the end of 1937, forty-six states had enacted laws covering workers afflicted with silicosis. Where the federal government had failed, the states, through the workers' compensation system, had recognized silicosis as the prototypical occupational disease" [11].

That industrial medicine had finally reached a point of recognition was seen in the creation of the Council on Industrial Health by the American Medical Association (AMA) in late 1937. The Council continued to act until 1960, when its functions were absorbed by other segments of the AMA. The designation of the Council, a standing committee of the AMA, was based on the objective of studying further work-related disease so that uniform workers' compensation laws might result [6]. For many years, members of AAIPS served on the Council.

It was the technology of World War II and the demand for workers, however, that led to the medical staffings of the large war production plants. Physicians in uniform were assigned posts in armed services facilities, for the installations had taken on all of the characteristics of heavily staffed industries, and programs in occupational medicine were needed. In late 1942, it was determined that the Army alone owned and operated more than 160 plants, with an employee population of approximately 400,000 [12.]

The first general directive concerning the Army industrial medical program was promulgated in early 1943, calling for the establishment of such programs in all Army-owned and operated plants, arsenals, depots, and ports of embarkation [13]. Many of the young medical officers serving at military facilities remained in occupational medicine after the war and were added to the membership of AAIPS.

Almost in parallel with this augmentation of worker care was the development of the Manhattan District Project with its various subprojects, all of which had as their objective the production of an atomic bomb that, it was hoped, would end World War II. As the effects of exposure to ionizing radiation were not known fully and since many of the workers had little idea of the materials with which they were in contact, there was ". . . a need for physicians who were competent not only to distinguish the illnesses due to special hazards but who were also capable of seeing that all types of cases were treated properly" [14]. During the developmental phase and until war's end, the physicians assigned industrial medical responsibilities were oncologists or radiologists, but in early 1946 they were replaced by practitioners experienced in the organization of plant programs.

Certification and Education

During these early years, many elder statesmen of AAIPS tried to obtain board certification for its members, but repeatedly the concept was rejected due to a lack of appropriate training in the specialty, if, indeed, it was one. One of the last remaining objections to the proposal was the absence of a period of hospital training, which was deemed essential by the AMA for the establishment of a board. It was believed at the time, and later proved to be true, that a year of in-plant training would be the equivalent of a hospital year, the latter not being a feasible site for a practicum in a specialty practiced at worksites. It was finally accepted that occupational medicine could be a subspecialty of the American Board of Preventive Medicine and, in June 1955, after a long and diligent effort, board certification became a reality. Of some 325 names that were submitted for initial diplomate status, 100 were chosen to form a "grandfather group" [6].

Board certification has subsequently been sought by graduates of the various residency training programs that followed. By 1993, 1867 physicians had been certified by the American Board of Preventive Medicine in the subspecialty of occupational medicine. In 1992, 169 applications were filed by prospective examinees; in 1991, 195 applied, and in 1990, 166 sought examination, an increase over the 131 applicants of 1989. In 1992, 62% of those physicians applying passed the examination [15].

To substantiate board status, training programs were needed. Although "the first intensified course in industrial medicine" was offered by the Department of Industrial Hygiene of the University of Pittsburgh School of Medicine in 1938 in cooperation with the Allegheny County Medical Society [16], the longer in-residence programs were yet to be developed.

In 1950, for the first time, at a University of Pittsburgh convocation, the degree of Doctor of Industrial Medicine was conferred on three graduates who had completed the special course established by Dr. T. Lyle Hazlett. In the same year, the new graduate school of public health was created at the University of Pittsburgh, headed by the eminent Dr. Thomas Parran, former Surgeon General of the US Public Health Service, and the degrees to be granted became the Master and Doctor of Public Health, the degrees currently being granted at several approved graduate schools [6]. Since 1984, graduates may be admitted to the board examination only after completing accredited training in preventive medicine, with no equivalency pathways available. The specialty examination today comprises material on the workplace, the worker, occupational medical services, occupational medical practice, clinical occupational medicine, industrial toxicology, physical hazards, and biologic hazards. All graduates must have completed courses for the core examination, including administration, biostatistics, clinical (medicine), epidemiology, behavioral (science), and environmental (science) [17].

The special requirements for residency education in preventive medicine and its subspecialties are laid down by the Accreditation Council for Graduate Medical Education (ACGME). The Council is sponsored jointly by the American Board of

Medical Specialties, the American Hospital Association, the American Medical Association, the Association of American Medical Colleges, and the Council of Medical Specialty Societies. The ACGME is responsible for the evaluation and accreditation of programs in graduate medical education in keeping with established standards and mechanisms that are designed to ensure that acceptable graduate medical education is provided. Various residency review committees meet periodically to determine compliance of a residency program with both general and special requirements, and representatives of the occupational medical organization have served as the specialty society members [18, 19].

Presently, there are 37 accredited residency programs in occupational medicine, based in schools of medicine, schools of public health, hospitals, and specialized health agencies, or in combinations of such organizations [20]. Periodic reviews of the programs offered assure currency of the programs and compliance with established requirements.

In Step with the Times

While AAIPS was gaining members slowly, it was realized that the designation "AAIPS" was cumbersome and not necessarily representative of its constituency. While remnants of surgical practice remained in day-to-day clinic sessions, the focus of practice was more on medicine, particularly preventive medicine. In April 1951, the name of the organization became the Industrial Medical Association. That this designation was not to remain permanently was seen because of the various work populations being covered by occupational health services. The term "industrial" had a connotation of corporate America, with its large manufacturing plants and thousands of employees. However, many occupations in the United States were not found in such installations though they presented health hazards unique to their work. Such groups as servicemen, students, beauticians, farmers, aircraft pilots, and retail sales personnel did not work in industry, as such, yet required the same kind of preventive health programs offered to corporate workers.

With this realization, in 1974, the Industrial Medical Association became the American Occupational Medical Association, the new name implying that its members were concerned with the health of persons in *all* occupations, irrespective of size, service, end product, or locale of the operation or activity.

Other thought began to germinate with the ensuing years. In 1946, the American Academy of Occupational Medicine had been founded, its membership comprising full-time physicians in occupational medicine. Annual meetings were held and the program content was always scientifically solid. However, with the passage of the years, it was believed that some consolidation was needed, so that in late 1988, the American College of Occupational Medicine was created, combining the Academy and the Association, and thus avoiding immediate identification of either component body in the new name.

This newest designation was short lived, for attention was being given to the extension of occupational medicine to include environmental health as an area of activity [21, 22]. In keeping with this expansion of the professional's concern, a new name was given to the organization in 1992—the American College of Occupational and Environmental Medicine (ACOEM). That the latest title was truly representative of the College's interests has been seen in subsequent supportive writings [23, 24], and the change now requires the College "to move forward and broaden its educational offerings, its scientific reporting, and its societal influence into the discipline of environmental medicine" [25].

College Activities

The American College of Occupational and Environmental Medicine consists of over 6500 physicians worldwide. The College's organizational structure consists of an executive committee as well as a board of directors, whose function is to set policy, oversee committee activities and other related functions, and generally act in the best interest of the membership. Members of the board are elected to 3-year terms. Each year, approximately five new board members assume office. The executive committee consists of elected officers, such as the president, president elect, and first and second vice president, as well as the secretary, treasurer, and executive director.

In addition to the national organization, ACOEM consists of 29 chapters in the United States. Each chapter has a range of members and is entitled to one representative in the House of Delegates per each 100 members of the chapter. Like the national organization, the local chapters function primarily in an educational and professional role by promoting scientific meetings and professional exchanges.

The majority of College activities are carried out by respective committees, which are overseen by councils. Numerous areas of professional practice in occupational medicine are addressed, including epidemiology, toxicology, publishing, and external affairs. In addition, a government affairs committee attempts to keep the membership alerted to various regulatory and legislative activities that may affect the practice of occupational medicine. The college owns and publishes the *Journal of Occupational Medicine,* the editor of which, although a member of ACOEM, functions independently of the organization with respect to editorial prerogative. The College's main activity is to sponsor two educational conferences a year. The Spring meeting is the largest professional meeting in the world of occupational health professionals and annually attracts over 6000 physicians, nurses, and various exhibitors. The College also publishes a monthly newsletter, sponsors standing courses in occupational medicine, and coordinates a basic curriculum in occupational medicine for those physicians new to the field. In the fall of 1993, a core curriculum in environmental medicine was introduced.

Within the past few years, the College has been successful in acquiring its own headquarters in Arlington Heights, north of Chicago. The College's activities are administrated by a variety of staff at the corporate headquarters, who assist in meeting planning and development and operational aspects of the College, and also help to promote interchange with other medical disciplines.

A survey of the membership of ACOEM was conducted in March 1993. Approximately 70% of over 1500 people who completed a questionnaire practice full time in occupational medicine. The survey rate, which comprised 27% of those who received the ACOEM monthly report, indicated that half of those responding had been practicing occupational medicine for fewer than 10 years, and that only 30% were board certified. Topics in ergonomics and toxicology, especially risk assessment and occupational cancer, were highlighted as areas that were worthy of the College's formal attention.

The American College of Occupational and Environmental Medicine is open to physicians and doctors of osteopathic medicine worldwide. Members of the College are invited to participate in a variety of committees and educational and professional challenges assumed by the organization.

The College and Education

Education is one objective of ACOEM and was seen early on, when in 1961 the first intensive refresher courses were offered as preliminary to the American Industrial Health Conference. Included were "Cardiology in Industry," "Treatment of Radiation Injuries," "Dermatology in Industry," and "Hearing Conservation in Industry." Such courses have increased in number and precede the annual conference.

As a related organization, the Samuel Bacon Research and Education Fund Board, now the Bacon Foundation, was founded in 1976 "to promote educational, scientific and charitable work of ACOEM by accepting, holding, administering and investing such funds and property . . . as may . . . be given it; disburse . . . the income and principal . . . in the form of grants; promote and develop educational activities related to advanced training in occupational medicine, and promote and support scientific research in occupational medicine" [26]. The Foundation is active and continues to receive and disburse funds. Royalties from the sale of this text benefit the Foundation.

The Occupational Health Institute was created in 1945 as a trust for educational purposes in connection with occupational medical research and education. While it functioned for several years, supporting certain courses and publishing activities, it ceased to exist in recent years as its functions were absorbed by ACOEM.

Education took another form in the association of AAIPS with the journal *Industrial Medicine* (later *Industrial Medicine and Surgery*), first published in 1932. Apart from the *Journal of Industrial Hygiene,* initiated in 1919, there was no periodical devoted to the specialty. While it represented AAIPS and its successor designations, it was not truly the "official" publication of the Association. In 1959, Volume 1,

Number 1 of the *Journal of Occupational Medicine* appeared, under the dedicated editorship of Dr. Adolph G. Kammer. The *Journal* is the official publication of ACOEM and is currently edited by Dr. Paul W. Brandt-Rauf of Columbia University. Frequently, special issues are published that explore subjects in depth, for example, "Conference on Medical Screening and Biological Monitoring for the Effects of Exposure in the Workplace," which appeared in two parts, consuming 1126 pages [27]. The *Journal* carries such departments as the Occupational Medicine Forum (answers to subscribers' questions), Selected Reviews from the Literature, Original Articles, Letters to the Editor, Committee Reports, Book Reviews, General Information for Authors, and People and Events, among others.

It is the publication of Committee Reports that brings guidelines to the readership in the practice of occupational medicine. The Reports are approved by ACOEM's board of directors and represent a knowledgeable consensus regarding an issue at hand. Examples of such conclusive opinions are seen in "Scope of Occupational and Environmental Health Programs and Practice" [28] and "ACOEM Position Statement on Residential Radon Exposure" [29].

In 1978, the position of Director of Education was created at the ACOEM headquarters office to stimulate and oversee the College's educational activities.

Occupational Medicine in the 1990s

The annual conferences have continued to reflect the changing concerns of the specialty. While recent clinical studies and research in toxicology share a primary post of interest with epidemiology at the workplace, program management, economics, ergonomics, health care, substance abuse, counseling, stress, and musculoskeletal problems continue to capture the attention of writers and investigators. Other organizations maintain their interest in the expansion of occupational medicine into their own specialty areas, such as the Institute of Medicine [30], the American Medical Association [31], and the American College of Physicians [32]. A publishing house, established in 1987, OEM (Occupational and Environmental Medicine) Health Information, based in Beverly, Massachusetts, is the only publisher whose products are devoted to a single specialty—occupational and environmental medicine—and that carries some 300 related monographs in stock.

Graduates of the training programs are turning more to academic posts and consultant practices as industry continues to downsize. NIOSH and the Occupational Safety and Health Administration (OSHA) fluctuate in strength and effectiveness in keeping with the philosophic tenor of the administration in power. Legislative dicta such as the Occupational Safety and Health Act; the Federal Toxic Substances Control Act (TSCA); the Federal Mine Safety and Health Act (FMSHA); the Comprehensive Environmental Response, Compensation and Liability Act of 1980 (CERCLA-Superfund); and the Americans with Disabilities Act (ADA) will continue to demand the attention of ACOEM members. Occupational safety and health is number 10 among 22 priority areas of the year 2000 national health objectives and Public Health Service lead agencies [33], and remains a concern of the Centers for Disease Control and Prevention, designated as the lead agency. Although all residency posts at various universities are not filled, federal funding has become stronger and the numbers of graduates and programs increase in comparison with related specialties [34]. The 29 component societies of ACOEM continue to gain new members.

It is anticipated that ACOEM will return to a physician director in the years ahead, will begin to produce annual reports, and will develop upscale educational modalities whose use will carry continuing medical education credits.

The future bodes well for ongoing growth, for, as stated in a mid-1993 report, "The field of occupational and environmental medicine is not static. The demand for trained occupational and environmental physicians in private industry, education, and governmental agencies far exceeds the supply, and the need continues to grow" [35]. To paraphrase *Occupational Health in America*'s closing statement, "[I]t is safe to say that whatever the triumphs of chemical therapy, whatever miracles are wrought in the war on ailments that scourge society and whatever feats man may perform in the conquest of space, organized occupational medicine, and the American College of Occupational and Environmental Medicine with its 6000 members, will play a vital role in their accomplishment" [6].

History of the ACOEM **755**

References

1. Eastman, C. *Work-Accidents and the Law.* New York: Russell Sage Foundation, Charities Publication Committee, 1910.
2. Thompson, W. G. *The Occupational Diseases: Their Causation, Symptoms, Treatment, and Prevention.* New York: D. Appleton, 1914.
3. Price, G. M. *The Modern Factory: Safety, Sanitation, and Welfare.* New York: Wiley, 1914.
4. Kober, G. M., and Hanson, W. C. (eds.). *Diseases of Occupation and Vocational Hygiene.* Philadelphia: P. Blakiston's Son, 1916.
5. Mock, H. E. *Industrial Medicine and Surgery.* Philadelphia: Saunders, 1920.
6. Selleck, H. B. and Whittaker, A. H. *Occupational Health in America.* Detroit: Wayne State University Press, 1962.
7. Cited in Hamilton, A. *Exploring the Dangerous Trades.* Boston: Little, Brown, 1943.
8. Felton, J. S. Phosphorus necrosis—a classical occupational disease. *Am. J. Indust. Med.* 3:77, 1982.
9. Goldwater, L. J. *Mercury—A History of Quicksilver.* Baltimore: York Press, 1972. P. 270.
10. Sharpe, W. D. The New Jersey radium dial painters: A classic in occupational carcinogenesis. *Bull. Hist. Med.* 52:560, 1978.
11. Cherniak, M. *The Hawk's Nest Incident—America's Worst Industrial Disaster.* New Haven: Yale University Press, 1986.
12. Medical Department, United States Army. *Preventive Medicine in World War II.* Volume IX, Special Fields. Washington, DC, 1969, P. 110.
13. *Industrial Medical Program of the United States Army,* War Department Circular no. 59, February 24, 1943.
14. Stone, R. S. (ed.). *Industrial Medicine on the Plutonium Project.* New York: McGraw-Hill, 1951. P. 20.
15. Hyland, C. Personal communication.
16. Hazlett, T. L., and Hummel, W. W. *Industrial Medicine in Western Pennsylvania 1850–1950.* Pittsburgh: University of Pittsburgh Press, 1957. P. 174.
17. The American Board of Preventive Medicine, Inc. *Study Guide Materials, Exam Content Outlines.* Schiller Park, IL: The Board, 1993. Pp. 1–4, 9–14.
18. *Manual of Structure and Functions for Graduate Medical Education Review Committees.* Chicago: Accreditation Council for Graduate Medical Education, 1993.
19. *An Orientation to Residency Review Committees.* Chicago: Accreditation Council for Graduate Medical Education, 1993.
20. *Residency Programs Verification List—Specialty: Preventive Medicine: Occupational [Medicine].* Chicago: Accreditation Council for Graduate Medical Education, 1993.
21. Goldstein, B. D., and Gockfeld, M. Role of the physician in environmental medicine. *Med. Clin. North Am.* 74:245, 1990.
22. American College of Physicians. Occupational and environmental medicine: The internist's role. *Ann. Intern. Med.* 113:975, 1990.
23. Ducatman, A. M. Occupational physicians and environmental medicine. *J. Occup. Med.* 35:251, 1993.
24. Goldstein, B. D. Global issues in environmental medicine. *J. Occup. Med.* 35:260, 1993.
25. De Hart, R. L. Accepting the environmental medicine challenge. *J. Occup. Med.* 35:265, 1993.
26. *ACOEM Executive Manual,* July 1992. P. F-11.
27. Halperin, W. F., Schulte, P. A, and Greathouse, D. G. (eds.). Conference on Medical Screening and Biological Monitoring for the Effects of Exposure in the Workplace. *J. Occup. Med.* 28:543, Part I, 1986; 28:913, Part II, 1986.
28. Occupational Medical Practice Committee, ACOEM. Scope of occupational and environmental health programs and practice. *J. Occup. Med.* 34:436, 1992.
29. Ad Hoc Committee on Residential Radon, ACOEM. ACOEM position statement on residential radon exposure. *J. Occup. Med.* 34:1028, 1992.
30. *Addressing the Physician Shortage in Occupational and Environmental Medicine. Report of a Study by the Institute of Medicine.* Washington, DC: National Academy of Sciences, 1991.
31. American Medical Association Council on Long Range Planning and Development. *The Future of Family Practice.* Chicago: American Medical Association, 1988.

32. American College of Physicians. *Role of Internist in Occupational Medicine.* Philadelphia: The College, 1984.
33. Healthy People 2000: National health promotion, disease prevention objectives of the year 2000. *J.A.M.A.* 264:2057, 1990.
34. Stoll, D. A. Personal communication, June 10, 1993.
35. Publications Committee of the American College of Occupational and Environmental Medicine (ACOEM). Careers in occupational and environmental medicine. *J. Occup. Med.* 35:628, 1993.

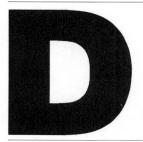

Lists of Carcinogens Rated by the International Agency for Research on Cancer (IARC)

In the first 58 volumes of *Monographs,* over 700 agents (chemicals, groups of chemicals, complex mixtures, occupational exposures, and cultured habits) have been evaluated.

In the following lists, the agents are classified as to their carcinogenic risk to humans in accordance with the procedures adopted as standard IARC practice:

Group 1—The agent (mixture) is carcinogenic to humans. The exposure circumstance entails exposures that are carcinogenic to humans.
Group 2
    Group 2A—The agent (mixture) is probably carcinogenic to humans.
    The exposure circumstance entails exposures that are probably carcinogenic to humans.
    Group 2B—The agent (mixture) is possibly carcinogenic to humans.
    The exposure circumstance entails exposures that are possibly carcinogenic to humans.
Group 3—The agent (mixture or exposure circumstance) is not classifiable as to its carcinogenicity to humans.
Group 4—The agent (mixture) is probably not carcinogenic to humans.

These lists should be read only in conjunction with the IARC Preamble and the IARC User's Guide and it is strongly recommended to refer also to the individual monographs concerning the agents in which you may be interested (see also the cumulative index given in each volume of *IARC Monographs*). This booklet will be updated periodically.

Each monograph consists of a brief description, where appropriate, of the potential exposure to the agent, by providing data on chemical and physical properties, methods of analysis, methods and volumes of production, use, and occurrence. Then, the relevant epidemiologic studies are summarized. Subsequent sections cover evidence for carcinogenicity obtained in experimental animals, and a brief description of other relevant data, such as toxicity and genetic effects. The Agency makes every effort to ensure that the factual material presented is reported without bias, and it is meticulously checked for accuracy.

The *Monographs* are used widely by research scientists, public health authorities, and national and international regulatory authorities. These users apply the information contained in the mongraphs in different ways, but it is hoped that none use the overall evaluations of carcinogenicity in isolation from the body of scientific evidence on which they are based.

Overall Evaluations of Carcinogenicity to Humans
IARC Monographs Volumes 1–58 (768)

Group 1—Carcinogenic to Humans (60)
Agents and Groups of Agents
Aflatoxins [1402-68-2] (1993)[1]
4-Aminobiphenyl [92-67-1]

Source: Reprinted from World Health Organization International Agency for Research on Cancer. *IARC Monographs on the Evaluation of Carcinogenic Risks to Humans: Lists of IARC Evaluations.* Lyon, France: IARC, May 1993.
[1]Year in parentheses: Year in which the evaluation was published subsequent to the Supplement

Group 1 (continued)
Arsenic [7440-38-2] and arsenic compounds[2]
Asbestos [1332-21-4]
Azathioprine [446-86-6]
Benzene [71-43-2]
Benzidine [92-87-5]
Beryllium [7440-41-7] and beryllium compounds (1993)
N,N-Bis(2-chloroethyl)-2-naphthylamine (Chlornaphazine) [494-03-1]
Bis(chloromethyl)ether [542-88-1] and chloromethyl methyl ether [107-30-2] (technical grade)
1,4-Butanediol dimethanesulfonate (Myleran) [55-98-1]
Cadmium [7440-43-9] and cadmium compounds (1993)
Chlorambucil [305-03-3]
1-(2-Chloroethyl)-3-(4-methylcyclohexyl)-1-nitrosourea (methyl-CCNU) [13909-09-6]
Chromium [VI] compounds (1990)
Cyclosporin [79217-60-0] (1990)
Cyclophosphamide [50-18-0] [6055-19-2]
Diethylstilbestrol [56-53-1]
Erionite [66733-21-9]
Estrogen replacement therapy
Estrogens, nonsteroidal[2]
Estrogens, steroidal[2]
Melphalan [148-82-3]
8-Methoxypsoralen (methoxsalen) [298-81-7] plus ultraviolet radiation
MOPP and other combined chemotherapy including alkylating agents
Mustard gas (sulfur mustard) [505-60-2]
2-Naphthylamine [91-59-8]
Nickel compounds (1990)
Oral contraceptives, combined[3]
Oral contraceptives, sequential
Radon [10043-92-2] and its decay products (1988)
Solar radiation (1992)
Talc containing asbestiform fibers
Thiotepa [52-24-4] (1990)
Treosulfan [299-75-2]
Vinyl chloride [75-01-4]

Mixtures
Alcoholic beverages (1988)
Analgesic mixtures containing phenacetin
Betel quid with tobacco
Coal tar pitches [65996-93-2]
Coal tars [8007-45-2]
Mineral oils, untreated and mildly treated
Salted fish (Chinese-style) (1993)
Shale oils [68308-34-9]
Soots
Tobacco products, smokeless
Tobacco smoke

Exposure Circumstances
Aluminum production
Auramine, manufacture of
Boot and shoe manufacture and repair
Coal gasification
Coke production
Furniture and cabinetmaking

7 Working Group for agents, mixtures, or exposure circumstances considered in Volumes 43–58 of the *Monographs*. Numbers in brackets refer to the chemical's CAS number.
[2]This evaluation applies to the group of chemicals as a whole and not necessarily to all individual chemicals within the group.
[3]There is also conclusive evidence that these agents have a protective effect against cancers of the ovary and endometrium.

Hematite mining (underground) with exposure to radon
Iron and steel founding
Isopropanol manufacture (strong-acid process)
Magenta, manufacture of (1993)
Painter (occupational exposure as a) (1989)
Rubber industry
Strong-inorganic-acid mists containing sulfuric acid (occupational exposure to) (1992)

Group 2A—Probably Carcinogenic to Humans (51)

Agents and Groups of Agents
Acrylonitrile [107-13-1]
Adriamycin[4] [23214-92-8]
Androgenic (anabolic) steroids
Azacitidine[4] [320-67-2] (1990)
Benz[*a*]anthracene[4] [56-55-3]
Benzidine-based dyes[4]
Benzo[*a*]pyrene[4] [50-32-8]
Bischloroethyl nitrosourea (BCNU) [154-93-8]
1,3-Butadiene [106-99-0] (1992)
Captafol[4] [2425-06-1] (1991)
Chloramphenicol[4] [56-75-7] (1990)
1-(2-Chloroethyl)-3-cyclohexyl-1-nitrosourea[4] (CCNU) [13010-47-4]
para-Chloro-*ortho*-toluidine [95-69-2] and its strong acid salts (1990)
Chlorozotocin[4] [54749-90-5] (1990)
Cisplatin[4] [15663-27-1]
Dibenz[*a,h*]anthracene[4] [53-70-3]
Diethyl sulfate [64-67-5] (1992)
Dimethylcarbamoyl chloride[4] [79-44-7]
Dimethyl sulfate[4] [77-78-1]
Epichlorohydrin[4] [106-89-8]
Ethylene dibromide[4] [106-93-4]
Ethylene oxide [75-21-8]
N-Ethyl-*N*-nitrosourea[4] [759-73-9]
Formaldehyde [50-00-0])
IQ[4] (2-Amino-3-methylimidazo[4,5-*f*]quinoline) [76180-96-6] (1993)
5-Methoxypsoralen[4] [484-20-8]
4,4′-Methylene bis(2-chloroaniline) (MOCA) [101-14-4] (1993)
N-Methyl-*N*′-nitro-*N*-nitrosoguanidine[4] (MNNG) [70-25-7]
N-Methyl-*N*-nitrosourea[4] [684-93-5]
Nitrogen mustard [51-75-2]
N-Nitrosodiethylamine[4] [55-18-5]
N-Nitrosodimethylamine[4] [62-75-9]
Phenacetin [62-44-2]
Procarbazine hydrochloride[4] [366-70-1]
Propylene oxide[4] [75-56-9]
Silica [14808-60-7], crystalline
Styrene oxide[4] [96-09-3]
Tris(2,3-dibromopropyl)phosphate[4] [126-72-7]
Ultraviolet radiation A (1992)
Ultraviolet radiation B (1992)
Ultraviolet radiation C (1992)
Vinyl bromide[4] [593-60-2]

Mixtures
Creosotes [8001-58-9]
Diesel engine exhaust (1989)
Hot mate (1991)

[4]Overall evaluation upgraded from 2B to 2A with supporting evidence from other relevant data.

Group 2A (continued)
Nonarsenical insecticides (occupational exposures in spraying and application of) (1991)
Polychlorinated biphenyls [1336-36-3]

Exposure Circumstances
Art glass, glass containers, and pressed ware (manufacture of) (1993)
Hairdresser or barber (occupational exposure as a) (1993)
Petroleum refining (occupational exposures in) (1989)
Sunlamps and sunbeds (use of) (1992)

Group 2B—Possibly Carcinogenic to Humans (206)

Agents and Groups of Agents
A-α-C (2-Amino-9H-pyrido[2,3-b]indole) [26148-68-5]
Acetaldehyde [75-07-0]
Acetamide [60-35-5]
Acrylamide [79-06-1]
AF-2 [2-(2-Furyl)-3-(5-nitro-2-furyl)acrylamide] [3688-53-7]
Aflatoxin M1 [6795-23-9] (1993)
para-Aminoazobenzene [60-09-3]
ortho-Aminoazotoluene [97-56-3]
2-Amino-5-(5-nitro-2-furyl)-1,3,4-thiadiazole [712-68-5]
Amitrole [61-82-5]
ortho-Anisidine [90-04-0]
Antimony trioxide [1309-64-4] (1989)
Aramite [140-57-8]
Atrazine[5] [1912-24-9] (1991)
Auramine [492-80-8] (technical-grade)
Azaserine [115-02-6]
Benzo[b]fluoranthene [205-99-2]
Benzo[j]fluoranthene [205-82-3]
Benzo[k]fluoranthene [207-08-9]
Benzyl violet 4B [1694-09-3]
Bleomycins[5] [11056-06-7]
Bracken fern
Bromodichloromethane [75-27-4] (1991)
Butylated hydroxyanisole (BHA) [25013-16-5]
β-Butyrolactone [3068-88-0]
Caffeic acid [331-39-5] (1993)
Carbon-black extracts
Carbon tetrachloride [56-23-5]
Ceramic fibers
Chlordane [57-74-9] (1991)
Chlordecone (Kepone) [143-50-0]
Chlorendic acid [115-28-6] (1990)
α-Chlorinated toluenes
para-Chloroaniline [106-47-8] (1993)
Chloroform [67-66-3]
Chlorophenols
Chlorophenoxy herbicides
4-Chloro-*ortho*-phenylenediamine [95-83-0]
CI Acid Red no. 114 [6459-94-5] (1993)
CI Basic Red no. 9 [569-61-9] (1993)
CI Direct Blue no. 15 [2429-74-5] (1993)
Citrus Red no. 2 [6358-53-8]
Cobalt [7440-48-4] and cobalt compounds (1991)
para-Cresidine [120-71-8]
Cycasin [14901-08-7]
Dacarbazine [4342-03-4]
Dantron (Chrysazin; 1,8-dihydroxyanthraquinone) [117-10-2] (1990)

---

[5]Overall evaluation upgraded from 3 to 2B with supporting evidence from other relevant data.

Daunomycin [20830-81-3]
DDT [p,p'-DDT, 50-29-3] (1991)
N,N'-Diacetylbenzidine [613-35-4]
2,4-Diaminoanisole [615-05-4]
4,4'-Diaminodiphenyl ether [101-80-4]
2,4-Diaminotoluene [95-80-7]
Dibenz[*a,h*]acridine [226-36-8]
Dibenz[*a,j*]acridine [224-42-0]
7*H*-Dibenzo[*c,g*]carbazole [194-59-2]
Dibenzo[*a,e*]pyrene [192-65-4]
Dibenzo[*a,h*]pyrene [189-64-0]
Dibenzo[*a,i*]pyrene [189-55-9]
Dibenzo[*a,l*]pyrene [191-30-0]
1,2-Dibromo-3-chloropropane [96-12-8]
para-Dichlorobenzene [106-46-7]
3,3'-Dichlorobenzidine [91-94-1]
3,3'-Dichloro-4,4'-diaminodiphenyl ether [28434-86-8]
1,2-Dichloroethane [107-06-2]
Dichloromethane [75-09-2]
1,3-Dichloropropene [542-75-6] (technical-grade)
Dichlorvos [62-73-7] (1991)
Diepoxybutane [1464-53-5]
Di(2-ethylhexyl)phthalate [117-81-7]
1,2-Diethylhydrazine [1615-80-1]
Diglycidyl resorcinol ether [101-90-6]
Dihydrosafrole [94-58-6]
Diisopropyl sulfate [2973-10-6] (1992)
3,3'-Dimethoxybenzidine (*ortho*-Dianisidine) [119-90-4]
para-Dimethylaminoazobenzene [60-11-7]
trans-2-[(Dimethylamino)methylimino]-5-[2-(5-nitro-2-furyl)-vinyl]-1,3,4-oxadiazole
   [25962-77-0]
2,6-Dimethylaniline (2,6-xylidine) [87-62-7] (1993)
3,3'-Dimethylbenzidine (*ortho*-Tolidine [119-90-4]
Dimethylformamide [68-12-2] (1989)
1,1-Dimethylhydrazine [57-14-7]
1,2-Dimethylhydrazine [540-73-8]
1,6-Dinitropyrene [42397-64-8] (1989)
1,8-Dinitropyrene [42397-65-9] (1989)
1,4-Dioxane [123-91-1]
Disperse Blue no. 1 [2475-45-8] (1990)
Ethyl acrylate [140-88-5]
Ethylene thiourea [96-45-7]
Ethyl methanesulfonate [62-50-0]
2-(2-Formylhydrazino)-4-(5-nitro-2-furyl)thiazole [3570-75-0]
Glasswool (1988)
Glu-P-1 (2-Amino-6-methyldipyrido[1,2-*a*:3',2'-*d*]imidazole) [67730-11-4]
Glu-P-2 (2-Aminodipyrido[1,2-*a*:3',2'-*d*]imidazole) [67730-10-3]
Glycidaldehyde [765-34-4]
Griseofulvin [126-07-8]
HC Blue no. 1 [2784-94-3] (1993)
Heptachlor [76-44-8] (1991)
Hexachlorobenzene [118-74-1]
Hexachlorocyclohexanes
Hexamethylphosphoramide [680-31-9]
Hydrazine [302-01-2]
Indeno[1,2,3-*cd*]pyrene [193-39-5]
Iron-dextran complex [9004-66-4]
Lasiocarpine [303-34-4]
Lead [7439-92-1] and lead compounds, inorganic
Magenta [632-99-5] (containing CI Basic Red no. 9) (1993)
MeA-α-C (2-Amino-3-methyl-9*H*-pyrido[2,3-*b*]indole) [68006-83-7]
Medroxyprogesterone acetate [71-58-9]
MeIQ (2-Amino-3,4-dimethylimidazo[4,5-*f*]quinoline) [77094-11-2] (1993)
MeIQx (2-Amino-3,8-dimethylimidazo[4,5-*f*]quinoxaline) [77500-04-0] (1993)

Group 2B (continued)
Merphalan [531-76-0]
2-Methylaziridine [75-55-8]
Methylazoxymethanol acetate [592-62-1]
5-Methylchrysene [3697-24-3]
4,4'-Methylene bis(2-methylaniline) [838-88-0]
4,4'-Methyleneadianiline [101-77-9]
Methylmercury compounds (1993)
Methyl methanesulfonate [66-27-3]
2-Methyl-1-nitroanthraquinone [129-15-7] (uncertain purity)
N-Methyl-*N*-nitrosourethane [615-53-2]
Methylthiouracil [56-04-2]
Metronidazole [443-48-1]
Mirex [2385-85-5]
Mitomycin C [50-07-7]
Monocrotaline [315-22-0]
5-(morpholinomethyl)-3-[(5-nitrofurfurylidene)amino]-2-oxazolidinone [3795-88-8]
Nafenopin [3771-19-5]
Nickel, metallic [7440-02-0] (1990)
Niridazole [61-57-4]
Nitrilotriacetic acid [139-13-9] and its salts (1990)
5-Nitroacenaphthene [602-87-9]
6-Nitrochrysene [7496-02-8] (1989)
Nitrofen [1836-75-5] (technical-grade)
2-Nitrofluorene [607-57-8] (1989)
1-[(5-Nitrofurfurylidene)amino]-2-imidazolidinone [555-84-0]
N-[4-(5-Nitro-2-furyl)-2-thiazolyl]acetamide [531-82-8]
Nitrogen mustard *N*-oxide [126-85-2]
2-Nitropropane [79-46-9]
1-Nitropyrene [5522-43-0] (1989)
4-Nitropyrene [57835-92-4] (1989)
N-Nitrosodi-*n*-butylamine [924-16-3]
N-Nitrosodiethanolamine [1116-54-7]
N-Nitrosodi-*n*-propylamine [621-64-7]
3-(*N*-Nitrosomethylamino)propionitrile [60153-49-3]
4-(*N*-Nitrosomethylamino)-1-(3-pyridyl)-1-butanone (NNK) [64091-91-4]
N-Nitrosomethylethylamine [10595-95-6]
N-Nitrosomethylvinylamine [4549-40-0]
N-Nitrosomorpholine [59-89-2]
N'-Nitrosonornicotine [16543-55-8]
N-Nitrosopiperidine [100-75-4]
N-Nitrosopyrrolidine [930-55-2]
N-Nitrososarcosine [13256-22-9]
Ochratoxin A [303-47-9] (1993)
Oil Orange SS [2646-17-5]
Panfuran S (containing dihydroxymethylfuratrizine [794-93-4])
Pentachlorophenol [87-86-5] (1991)
Phenazopyridine hydrochloride [136-40-3]
Phenobarbital [50-06-6]
Phenoxybenzamine hydrochloride [63-92-3]
Phenyl glycidyl ether [122-60-1] (1989)
Phenytoin [57-41-0]
PhIP (2-Amino-1-methyl-6-phenylimidazo[4,5-*b*]pyridine) [105650-23-5] (1993)
Ponceau MX [3761-53-3]
Ponceau 3R [3564-09-8]
Potassium bromate [7758-01-2]
Progestins
1,3-Propane sultone [1120-71-4]
β-Propiolactone [57-57-8]
Propylthiouracil [51-52-5]
Rockwool (1988)
Saccharin [81-07-2]
Safrole [94-59-7]
Slagwool (1988)

Sodium *ortho*-phenylphenate [132-27-4]
Sterigmatocystin [10048-13-2]
Streptozotocin [18883-66-4]
Styrene[5] [100-42-5]
Sulfallate [95-06-7]
2,3,7,8-Tetrachlorodibenzo-*para*-dioxin (TCDD) [1746-01-6]
Tetrachloroethylene [127-18-4]
Thioacetamide [62-55-5]
4,4'-Thiodianiline [139-65-1]
Thiourea [62-56-6]
Toluene diisocyanates [26471-62-5]
ortho-Toluidine [95-53-4]
Trichlormethine (Trimustine hydrochloride) [817-09-4] (1990)
Trp-P-1 (3-Amino-1,4-dimethyl-5*H*-pyrido[4,3-*b*]indole) [62450-06-0]
Trp-P-2 (3-Amino-1-methyl-5*H*-pyrido[4,3-*b*]indole) [62450-07-1]
Trypan blue [72-57-1]
Uracil mustard [66-75-1]
Urethane [51-79-6]

Mixtures
Bitumens [8052-42-4], extracts of steam-refined and air-refined
Carrageenan [9000-07-1], degraded
Chlorinated paraffins of average carbon chain length C_{12} and average degree of
    chlorination approximately 60% (1990)
Coffee (urinary bladder)[6] (1991)
Diesel fuel, marine[5] (1989)
Engine exhaust, gasoline (1989)
Fuel oils, residual (heavy) (1989)
Gasoline[5] (1989)
Pickled vegetables (traditional in Asia) (1993)
Polybrominated biphenyls [Firemaster BP-6, 59536-65-1]
Toxaphene (polychlorinated camphenes) [8001-35-2]
Toxins derived from *Fusarium moniliforme* (1993)
Welding fumes (1990)

Exposure Circumstances
Carpentry and joinery
Textile manufacturing industry (work in) (1990)

Group 3—Unclassifiable as to Carcinogenicity to Humans (450)

Agents and Groups of Agents
Acridine orange [494-38-2]
Acriflavinium chloride [8018-07-3]
Acrolein [107-02-8]
Acrylic acid [79-10-7]
Acrylic fibers
Acrylonitrile-butadiene-styrene copolymers
Actinomycin D [50-76-0]
Agaritine [2757-90-6]
Aldicarb [116-06-3] (1991)
Aldrin [309-00-2]
Allyl chloride [107-05-1]
Allyl isothiocyanate [57-06-7]
Allyl isovalerate [2835-39-4]
Amaranth [915-67-3]
5-Aminoacenaphthene [4657-93-6]
2-Aminoanthraquinone [117-79-3]
para-Aminobenzoic acid [150-13-0]
1-Amino-2-methylanthraquinone [82-28-0]
2-Amino-4-nitrophenol [99-57-0] (1993)

---

[6]There is some evidence of an inverse relationship between coffee drinking and cancer of the large bowel; coffee drinking could not be classified as to its carcinogenicity to other organs.

Group 3 (continued)
2-Amino-5-nitrophenol [121-88-0] (1993)
4-Amino-2-nitrophenol [119-34-6]
2-Amino-5-nitrothiazole [121-66-4]
11-Aminoundecanoic acid [2432-99-7]
Ampicillin [69-53-4] (1990)
Anesthetics, volatile
Angelicin [523-50-2] plus ultraviolet A radiation
Aniline [62-53-3]
para-Anisidine [104-94-9]
Anthanthrene [191-26-4]
Anthracene [120-12-7]
Anthranilic acid [118-92-3]
Antimony trisulfide [1345-04-6] (1989)
Apholate [52-46-0]
Attapulgite [12174-11-7]
Aurothioglucose [12192-57-3]
Aziridine [151-56-4]
2-(1-Aziridinyl)ethanol [1072-52-2]
Aziridyl benzoquinone [800-24-8]
Azobenzene [103-33-3]
Benz[*a*]acridine [225-11-6]
Benz[*c*]acridine [225-51-4]
Benzo[*ghi*]fluoranthene [203-12-3]
Benzo[*a*]fluorene [238-84-6]
Benzo[*b*]fluorene [243-17-4]
Benzo[*c*]fluorene [205-12-9]
Benzo[*ghi*]perylene [191-24-2]
Benzo[*c*]phenanthrene [195-19-7]
Benzo[*e*]pyrene [192-97-2]
para-Benzoquinone dioxime [105-11-3]
Benzoyl chloride [98-88-4]
Benzoyl peroxide [94-36-0]
Benzyl acetate [140-11-4]
Bis(1-aziridinyl)morpholinophosphine sulfide [2168-68-5]
Bis(2-chloroethyl)ether [111-44-4]
1,2-Bis(chloromethoxy)ethane [13483-18-6]
1,4-Bis(chloromethoxymethyl)benzene [56894-91-8]
Bis(2-chloro-1-methylethyl)ether [108-60-1]
Bis(2,3-epoxycyclopentyl)ether [2386-90-5] (1989)
Bisphenol A diglycidyl ether [1675-54-3] (1989)
Bisulfites (1992)
Blue VRS [129-17-9]
Brilliant Blue FCF, disodium salt [3844-45-9]
Bromochloroacetonitrile [83463-62-1] (1991)
Bromoethane [74-96-4] (1991)
Bromoform [75-25-2] (1991)
n-Butyl acrylate [141-32-2]
Butylated hydroxytoluene (BHT) [128-37-0]
Butyl benzyl phthalate [85-68-7]
γ-Butyrolactone [96-48-0]
Caffeine [58-08-2] (1991)
Cantharidin [56-25-7]
Captan [133-06-2]
Carbaryl [63-25-2]
Carbazole [86-74-8]
3-Carbethoxypsoralen [20073-24-9]
Carbon blacks [1333-86-4]
Carmoisine [3567-69-9]
Carrageenan [9000-07-1], native
Catechol [120-80-9]
Chlordimeform [6164-98-3]
Chlorinated dibenzodioxins (other than TCDD)
Chlorinated drinking water (1991)

Chloroacetonitrile [107-14-2] (1991)
Chlorobenzilate [510-15-6]
Chlorodibromomethane [124-48-1] (1991)
Chlorodifluoromethane [75-45-6]
Chloroethane [75-00-3] (1991)
Chlorofluoromethane [593-70-4]
4-Chloro-*meta*-phenylenediamine [5131-60-2]
Chloroprene [126-99-8]
Chloropropham [101-21-3]
Chloroquine [54-05-7]
Chlorothalonil [1897-45-6]
2-Chloro-1,1,1-trifluoroethane [75-88-7]
Cholesterol [57-88-5]
Chromium [III] compounds (1990)
Chromium [7440-47-3], metallic (1990)
Chrysene [218-01-9]
Chrysoidine [532-82-1]
CI Acid Orange 3 [6373-74-6] (1993)
Cimetidine [51481-61-9] (1990)
Cinnamyl anthranilate [87-29-6]
CI Pigment Red no. 3 [2425-85-6] (1993)
Citrinin [518-75-2]
Clofibrate [637-07-0]
Clomiphene citrate [50-41-9]
Copper 8-hydroxyquinoline [10380-28-6]
Coronene [191-07-1]
Coumarin [91-64-5]
meta-Cresidine [102-50-1]
Cyclamates [sodium cyclamate, 139-05-9]
Cyclochlorotine [12663-46-6]
Cyclohexanone [108-94-1] (1989)
Cyclopenta[*cd*]pyrene [27208-37-3]
D & C Red no. 9 [5160-02-1] (1993)
Dapsone [80-08-0]
Decabromodiphenyl oxide [1163-19-5] (1990)
Deltamethrin [52918-65-5] (1991)
Diacetylaminoazotoluene [83-63-6]
Diallate [2303-16-4]
1,2-Diamino-4-nitrobenzene [99-56-9]
1,4-Diamino-2-nitrobenzene [5307-14-2] (1993)
2,5-Diaminotoluene [95-70-5]
Diazepam [439-14-5]
Diazomethane [334-88-3]
Dibenz[*a,c*]anthracene [215-58-7]
Dibenz[*a,j*]anthracene [224-41-9]
Dibenzo[*a,e*]fluoranthene [5385-75-1]
Dibenzo[*h,rst*]pentaphene [192-47-2]
Dibromoacetonitrile [3252-43-5] (1991)
Dichloroacetonitrile [3018-12-0] (1991)
Dichloroacetylene [7572-29-4]
ortho-Dichlorobenzene [95-50-1]
trans-1,4-Dichlorobutene [110-57-6]
2,6-Dichloro-*para*-phenylenediamine [609-20-1]
1,2-Dichloropropane [78-87-5]
Dicofol [115-32-2]
Dieldrin [60-57-1]
Di(2-ethylhexyl)adipate [103-23-1]
Dihydroxymethylfuratrizine [794-93-4]
Dimethoxane [828-00-2]
3,3'-Dimethoxybenzidine-4,4'-diisocyanate [91-93-0]
para-Dimethylaminoazobenzenediazo sodium sulfonate [140-56-7]
4,4'-Dimethylangelicin [22975-76-4] plus ultraviolet A radiation
4,5'-Dimethylangelicin [4063-41-6] plus ultraviolet A radiation
N,*N*-Dimethylaniline [121-69-7] (1993)

Group 3 (continued)
Dimethyl hydrogen phosphite [868-85-9] (1990)
1,4-Dimethylphenanthrene [22349-59-3]
3,7-Dinitrofluoranthene [105735-71-5]
3,9-Dinitrofluoranthene [22506-53-2]
1,3-Dinitropyrene [75321-20-9] (1989)
Dinitrosopentamethylenetetramine [101-25-7]
2,4'-Diphenyldiamine [492-17-1]
Disperse Yellow no. 3 [2832-40-8] (1990)
Disulfiram [97-77-8]
Dithranol [1143-38-0]
Dulcin [150-69-6]
Endrin [72-20-8]
Eosin [15086-94-9]
1,2-Epoxybutane [106-88-7] (1989)
1-Epoxyethyl-3,4-epoxycyclohexane [106-87-6]
3,4-Epoxy-6-methylcyclohexylmethyl-3,4-epoxy-6-methylcyclohexane carboxylate
    [141-37-7]
cis-9,10-Epoxystearic acid [2443-39-2]
Estradiol mustard [22966-79-6]
Estrogen-progestin replacement therapy
Ethionamide [536-33-4]
Ethylene [74-85-1]
Ethylene sulfide [420-12-2]
Ethyl selenac [5456-28-0]
Ethyl tellurac [20941-65-5]
Eugenol [97-53-0]
Evans blue [314-13-6]
Fast Green FCF [2353-45-9]
Fenvalerate [51630-58-1] (1991)
Ferbam [14484-64-1]
Ferric oxide [1309-37-1]
Fluometuron [2164-17-2]
Fluoranthene [206-44-0]
Fluorene [86-73-7]
Fluorescent lighting (1992)
Fluorides (inorganic, used in drinking water)
5-Fluorouracil [51-21-8]
Furazolidone [67-45-8]
Furosemide (Frusemide) [54-31-9] (1990)
Glass filaments (1988)
Glycidyl oleate [5431-33-4]
Glycidyl stearate [7460-84-6]
Guinea Green B [4680-78-8]
Gyromitrin [16568-02-8]
HC Blue no. 2 [33229-34-4] (1993)
HC Red no. 3 [2871-01-4] (1993)
HC Yellow no. 4 [59820-43-8] (1993)
Hematite [1317-60-8]
Hexachlorobutadiene [87-68-3]
Hexachloroethane [67-72-1]
Hexachlorophene [70-30-4]
Hycanthone mesylate [23255-93-8]
Hydralazine [86-54-4]
Hydrochloric acid [7647-01-0] (1992)
Hydrochlorothiazide [58-93-5] (1990)
Hydrogen peroxide [7722-84-1]
Hydroquinone [123-31-9]
4-Hydroxyazobenzene [1689-82-3]
8-Hydroxyquinoline [148-24-3]
Hydroxysenkirkine [26782-43-4]
Hypochlorite salts (1991)
Iron-dextrin complex [9004-51-7]
Iron sorbitol-citric acid complex [1338-16-5]

Isatidine [15503-86-3]
Isonicotinic acid hydrazide (isoniazid) [54-85-3]
Isophosphamide [3778-73-2]
Isopropanol [67-63-0]
Isopropyl oils
Isosafrole [120-58-1]
Jacobine [6870-67-3]
Kaempferol [520-18-3]
Lauroyl peroxide [105-74-8]
Lead, organo [75-74-1], [78-00-2]
Light Green SF [5141-20-8]
d-Limonene [5989-27-5] (1993)
Luteoskyrin [21884-44-6]
Malathion [121-75-5]
Maleic hydrazide [123-33-1]
Malonaldehyde [542-78-9]
Maneb [12427-38-2]
Mannomustine dihydrochloride [551-74-6]
Medphalan [13045-94-8]
Melamine [108-78-1]
6-Mercaptopurine [50-44-2]
Mercury [7439-97-6] and inorganic mercury compounds (1993)
Metabisulfites (1992)
Methotrexate [59-05-2]
Methoxychlor [72-43-5]
Methyl acrylate [96-33-3]
5-Methylangelicin [73459-03-7] plus ultraviolet A radiation
Methyl bromide [74-83-9]
Methyl carbamate [598-55-0]
Methyl chloride [74-87-3]
1-Methylchrysene [3351-28-8]
2-Methylchrysene [3351-32-4]
3-Methylchrysene [3351-31-3]
4-Methylchrysene [3351-30-2]
6-Methylchrysene [1705-85-7]
N-Methyl-N,4-dinitrosoaniline [99-80-9]
4,4'-Methylenebis(N,N-dimethyl)benzenamine [101-61-1]
4,4'-Methylenediphenyl diisocyanate [101-68-8]
2-Methylfluoranthene [33543-31-6]
3-Methylfluoranthene [1706-01-0]
Methylglyoxal [78-98-8] (1991)
Methyl iodide [74-88-4]
Methyl methacrylate [80-62-6]
Methyl parathion [298-00-0]
1-Methylphenanthrene [832-69-9]
7-Methylpyrido[3,4-c]psoralen [85878-62-2]
Methyl red [493-52-7]
Methyl selenac [144-34-3]
Modacrylic fibers
Monuron [150-68-5] (1991)
Morpholine [110-91-8] (1989)
1,5-Naphthalenediamine [2243-62-1]
1,5-Naphthalene diisocyanate [3173-72-6]
1-Naphthylamine [134-32-7]
1-Naphthylthiourea (ANTU) [86-88-4]
Nithiazide [139-94-6]
5-Nitro-*ortho*-anisidine [99-59-2]
9-Nitroanthracene [602-60-8]
7-Nitrobenz[*a*]anthracene [20268-51-3] (1989)
6-Nitrobenzo[*a*]pyrene [63041-90-7] (1989)
4-Nitrobiphenyl [92-93-3]
3-Nitrofluoranthene [892-21-7]
Nitrofural (nitrofurazone) [59-87-0] (1990)
Nitrofurantoin [67-20-9] (1990)

Group 3 (continued)
1-Nitronaphthalene [86-57-7] (1989)
2-Nitronaphthalene [581-89-5] (1989)
3-Nitroperylene [20589-63-3] (1989)
2-Nitropyrene [789-07-1] (1989)
N'-Nitrosoanabasine [37620-20-5]
N'-Nitrosoanatabine [71267-22-6]
N-Nitrosodiphenylamine [86-30-6]
para-Nitrosodiphenylamine [156-10-5]
N-Nitrosofolic acid [29291-35-8]
N-Nitrosoguvacine [55557-01-2]
N-Nitrosoguvacoline [55557-02-3]
N-Nitrosohydroxyproline [30310-80-6]
3-(*N*-Nitrosomethylamino)propionaldehyde [85502-23-4]
4-(*N*-Nitrosomethylamino)-4-(3-pyridyl)-1-butanal (NNA) [64091-90-3]
N-Nitrosoproline [7519-36-0]
5-Nitro-*ortho*-toluidine [99-55-8] (1990)
Nitrovin [804-36-4]
Nylon 6 [25038-54-4]
Orange I [523-44-4]
Orange G [1936-15-8]
Oxazepam [604-75-1]
Oxyphenbutazone [129-20-4]
Paracetamol (acetaminophen) [103-90-2] (1990)
Parasorbic acid [10048-32-5]
Parathion [56-38-2]
Patulin [149-29-1]
Penicillic acid [90-65-3]
Pentachloroethane [76-01-7]
Permethrin [52645-53-1] (1991)
Perylene [198-55-0]
Petasitenine [60102-37-6]
Phenanthrene [85-01-8]
Phenelzine sulfate [156-51-4]
Phenicarbazide [103-03-7]
Phenol [108-95-2] (1989)
Phenylbutazone [50-33-9]
meta-Phenylenediamine [108-45-2]
para-Phenylenediamine [106-50-3]
N-Phenyl-2-naphthylamine [135-88-6]
ortho-Phenylphenol [90-43-7]
Picloram [1918-02-1] (1991)
Piperonyl butoxide [51-03-6]
Polyacrylic acid [9003-01-4]
Polychloroprene [9010-98-4]
Polyethylene [9002-88-4]
Polymethylene polyphenyl isocyanate [9016-87-9]
Polymethyl methacrylate [9011-14-7]
Polypropylene [9003-07-0]
Polystyrene [9003-53-6]
Polytetrafluoroethylene [9002-84-0]
Polyurethane foams [9009-54-5]
Polyvinyl acetate [9003-20-7]
Polyvinyl alcohol [9002-89-5]
Polyvinyl chloride [9002-86-2]
Polyvinyl pyrrolidone [9003-39-8]
Ponceau SX [4548-53-2]
Potassium bis(2-hydroxyethyl)dithiocarbamate [23746-34-1]
Prednimustine [29069-24-7] (1990)
Prednisone [53-03-2]
Proflavine salts
Pronetalol hydrochloride [51-02-5]
Propham [122-42-9]
n-Propyl carbamate [627-12-3]

Propylene [115-07-1]
Ptaquiloside [87625-62-5]
Pyrene [129-00-0]
Pyrido[3,4-*c*]psoralen [85878-62-2]
Pyrimethamine [58-14-0]
Quercetin [117-39-5]
para-Quinone [106-51-4]
Quintozene (pentachloronitrobenzene) [82-68-8]
Reserpine [50-55-5]
Resorcinol [108-46-3]
Retrorsine [480-54-6]
Rhodamine B [81-88-9]
Rhodamine 6G [989-38-8]
Riddelline [23246-96-0]
Rifampicin [13292-46-1]
Rugulosin [23537-16-8]
Saccharated iron oxide [8047-67-4]
Scarlet Red [85-83-6]
Selenium [7782-49-2] and selenium compounds
Semicarbazide hydrochloride [563-41-7]
Seneciphylline [480-81-9]
Senkirkine [2318-18-5]
Sepiolite [15501-74-3]
Shikimic acid [138-59-0]
Silica [7631-86-9], amorphous
Simazine [122-34-9] (1991)
Sodium chlorite [7758-19-2] (1991)
Sodium diethyldithiocarbamate [148-18-5]
Spironolactone [52-01-7]
Styrene-acrylonitrile copolymers [9003-54-7]
Styrene-butadiene copolymers [9003-55-8]
Succinic anhydride [108-30-5]
Sudan I [842-07-9]
Sudan II [3118-97-6]
Sudan III [85-86-9]
Sudan Brown RR [6416-57-5]
Sudan Red 7B [6368-72-5]
Sulfafurazole (sulfisoxazole) [127-69-5]
Sulfamethoxazole [723-46-6]
Sulfites (1992)
Sulfur dioxide [7446-09-5] (1992)
Sunset Yellow FCF [2783-94-0]
Symphytine [22571-95-5]
Talc [14807-96-6], not containing asbestiform fibers
Tannic acid [1401-55-4] and tannins
2,2′,5,5′-Tetrachlorobenzidine [15721-02-5]
1,1,1,2-Tetrachloroethane [630-20-6]
1,1,2,2-Tetrachloroethane [79-34-5]
Tetrachlorvinphos [22248-79-9]
Tetrafluoroethylene [116-14-3]
Tetrakis(hydroxymethyl)phosphonium salts (1990)
Theobromine [83-67-0] (1991)
Theophylline [58-55-9] (1991)
Thiouracil [141-90-2]
Thiram [137-26-8] (1991)
Titanium dioxide [13463-67-7] (1989)
Toluene [108-88-3] (1989)
Toxins derived from *Fusarium graminearum, F. culmorum,* and *F. crookwellense*
    (1993)
Toxins derived from *Fusarium sporotrichioides* (1993)
Trichlorfon [52-68-6]
Trichloroacetonitrile [545-06-2] (1991)
1,1,1-Trichloroethane [71-55-6]
1,1,2-Trichloroethane [79-00-5] (1991)

Group 3 (continued)
Trichloroethylene [79-01-6]
Triethylene glycol diglydicyl ether [1954-28-5]
Trifluralin [1582-09-8] (1991)
4,4',6-Trimethylangelicin [90370-29-9] plus ultraviolet A radiation
2,4,5-Trimethylaniline [137-17-7]
2,4,6-Trimethylaniline [88-05-1]
4,5',8-Trimethylpsoralen [3902-71-4]
Triphenylene [217-59-4]
Tris(aziridinyl)-*para*-benzoquinone (Triaziquone) [68-76-8]
Tris(1-aziridinyl)phosphine oxide [545-55-1]
2,4,6-Tris(1-aziridinyl)-*s*-triazine [51-18-3]
Tris(2-chloroethyl)phosphate [115-96-8] (1990)
1,2,3-Tris(chloromethoxy)propane [38571-73-2]
Tris(2-methyl-1-aziridinyl)phosphine oxide [57-39-6]
Vat Yellow no. 4 [128-66-5] (1990)
Vinblastine sulfate [143-67-9]
Vincristine sulfate [2068-78-2]
Vinyl acetate [108-05-4]
Vinyl chloride-vinyl acetate copolymers [9003-22-9]
4-Vinylcyclohexene [100-40-3]
Vinyl fluoride [75-02-5]
Vinylidene chloride [75-35-4]
Vinylidene chloride-vinyl chloride copolymers [9011-06-7]
Vinylidene fluoride [75-38-7]
N-Vinyl-2-pyrrolidone [88-12-0]
Wollastonite [13983-17-0]
Xylene [1330-20-7] (1989)
2,4-Xylidine [95-68-1]
2,5-Xylidine [95-78-3]
Yellow AB [85-84-7]
Yellow OB [131-79-3]
Zectran [315-18-4]
Zineb [12122-67-7]
Ziram [137-30-4] (1991)

Mixtures
Betel quid, without tobacco
Bitumens [8052-42-4], steam-refined, cracking-residue, and air-refined
Crude oil [8002-05-9] (1989)
Diesel fuels, distillate (light) (1989)
Fuel oils, distillate (light) (1989)
Jet fuel (1989)
Maté (1990)
Mineral oils, highly refined
Petroleum solvents (1989)
Tea (1991)
Terpene polychlorinates (Strobane) [8001-50-1]

Exposure Circumstances
Flat-glass and specialty glass (manufacture of) (1993)
Hair coloring products (personal use of) (1993)
Leather goods manufacture
Leather tanning and processing
Lumber and sawmill industries (including logging)
Paint manufacture (occupational exposure in) (1989)
Pulp and paper manufacture

Group 4—Probably Not Carcinogenic to Humans

Caprolactam [105-60-2]

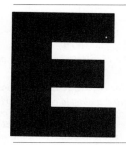

References in Occupational and Environmental Medicine

Joseph Harzbecker, Jr.

This Appendix is a comprehensive overview of the specialized literature that may be of value in the practice of occupational medicine. It includes a large amount of information related to indices, abstracts, encyclopedias, legal sources, and statistics, among others. A familiarity with these sources will serve as a background from which to launch the search.

1. Specialized Reference Sources in Toxicology and Occupational/Environmental Medicine

Reference sources are used primarily for consulting factual information, and fall into two categories: compendiums that furnish information and bibliographic aids that indicate the location of additional items. This section covers sources specific to occupational health and toxicology.

1.1. Indices

Indices allow access to journal article citations, reviews, reports, dissertations, proceedings, and government documents by author, agency, or subject. Some indices include title access. The typical index is divided by author and subject.

1.1.1. *American Statistics Index (ASI)*. Washington, DC: Congressional Information Service.

ASI remains one of the strongest comprehensive indices for American statistical information. It identifies, catalogues, announces, describes, indexes, and publishes on microfiche statistics published by the United States government.

1.1.2. Bower, C. E., and Rhoads, M. L. (eds.). *EPA Indices: A Key to US Environmental Protection Agency Reports and Superintendent of Documents and NTIS Numbers*. Phoenix: Oryx Press, 1983.

This is a listing of EPA reports before 1982. It provides SuDoc number (government document classification) for each publication listed.

1.1.3. *Government Reports and Announcements Index*. Springfield, VA: National Technical Information Service.

Technical reports from the US government. Toxicology literature may be located in section 6, Biological and Medical Science.

1.1.4. *Hospital Literature Index*. Chicago: American Hospital Association with the National Library of Medicine.

Journal articles from hospital management, Medicare, Medicaid, malpractice, occupational health services, and others. Subject access through Medical Subject Headings.

1.1.5. *Index to Health Information*. Bethesda, MD: Congressional Information Service.

Statistical data from international, state, and federal organizations, commercial publishers, associations, universities, and independent research organizations. Serves very much like the ASI. Data taken from approximately 2000 issuing sources.

1.1.6. *Index Medicus*. Bethesda, MD: National Library of Medicine.

The premier index for international biomedical information. MeSH used for subject indexing and access. Contains review literature. Clinical medicine subset published in the abridged Index Medicus. *Covers more than 4000 journal titles.*

1.1.7. *MEDOC*. Salt Lake City: Spencer S. Eccles Health Sciences Library.

US government publications in the medical and health sciences. Contains some toxicology and occupational health information. Using the MeSH, monographs, pamphlets, and series are indexed.

1.1.8. *Science Citation Index*. Philadelphia: Institute for Scientific Information.

The Citation Index *can be used to determine who has cited a classic research article. For example, if you have a paper written by McCunney on trichlorethylene, you could use this index, through a preliminary scan of the indices, to determine other authors who cited the work. Divided into source, permuterm (subject), and citation index sections. "International interdisciplinary index to the literature of science, medicine, agriculture, toxicology, and the behavioral sciences."*

1.2.   Abstracts

These abstract sources are indices to journal literature. In addition to bibliographic citations (author, title, and journal name), an abstract is appended to each citation. The following list of sources contains information relevant to occupational medicine and toxicology.

1.2.1. *Biological Abstracts* (*BA* and *Biological Abstracts/RRM*). Philadelphia: Biosciences Information Services.

A large biological abstracting service that contains author, biosystematic, generic, and subject indices. A toxicology section is divided into antidotes and preventive toxicology, environmental and industrial, foods, food residues and additives, and preservatives; and general, pharmacologic, and veterinary toxicology. BA focuses on serial articles, while RRM includes reports, meetings, and reviews.

1.2.2. *Chemical Abstracts*. Columbus, OH: Chemical Abstracts Service.

The premier resource for journal article literature in chemistry and related fields. Contains abstracts to articles and numerous complex indices. More than 14,000 scientific and technical journals are covered. Patents are included.

1.2.3. *Excerpta Medica*. Amsterdam: Excerpta Medica Foundation.

Information is divided into 46 sections. Section 35 covers occupational health and industrial medicine, while section 52 covers toxicology. Subject vocabulary is arranged in the EMTREE system. EMTREE is similar to the NLM MeSH.

1.2.4. *Pollution Abstracts*. Bethesda, MD: CSA.

International technical literature on many aspects of environmental pollution.

1.2.5. *Toxicology Abstracts*. Bethesda, MD: CSA.

Monitors over 5000 primary journals and other source materials. Toxicology is divided into food additives, toiletries, metals, toxins, social poisons, and others.

1.3.   Encyclopedias

Encyclopedias contain concise articles, with bibliographic references on particular subjects. Some encyclopedias include information provided by societies, associations, or other groups to define their function, activity, and purpose. Directories contain names and addresses of organizations and identify key personnel.

1.3.1. Burek, D. M. (ed.). *Encyclopedia of Associations*. Detroit: Gale.

"A guide to over 22,000 national and international organizations." Contains relevant information from a wide range of associations, societies, and organizations.

1.3.2. Batten, D. (ed.). *Encyclopedia of Governmental Advisory Organizations*. Detroit: Gale.

Reference guide to over 6000 permanent, continuing, or ad hoc US presidential, public, and congressional interagency advisory committees and other government taskforces and commissions. A valuable reference tool in focusing on the activities of government advisory organizations.

1.3.3. *Encyclopaedia of Occupational Health and Safety*. Geneva: International Labour Office, 1983.

Alphabetical list of relevant subjects from "accident" to "zoonoses." Coverage of chemical and physical data, exposure limits, unit of measurement, abbreviations, and bibliographic references. More than 1150 articles and 600 bibliographic references.

1.3.4.   *International Directory of Occupational Safety and Health Institutions.* Geneva: International Labour Office, 1990.

Listing of research and national scientific institutes, national safety councils, and social security institutions from 92 countries.

2.   Legal Resources and Related Government Publications for the Occupational Health Practitioner

2.1.   Code of Federal Regulations. Washington, DC: Office of the Federal Register, National Archives and Records Service, General Services Administration.

Annually published, the Code of Federal Regulations (CFR) consists of the Final Rules published in the Federal Register *(see below). These Final Rules are codified and added to the CFR. The most relevant titles for health: Title 21, Food and Drugs; Title 40, Protection of the Environment; Title 25, Public Welfare; Title 29, Labor (which contains Occupational Safety and Health Administration [OSHA] standards).*

2.2.   *Federal Register.* Washington, DC: Office of the Federal Register, National Archives and Records Service, General Services Administration.

Federal Register *publishes proposed rules to elicit response from the public, background information, and Final Rules. Subject access is very tedious. Includes presidential proclamations.*

2.3.   *Occupational Safety and Health Cases.* Washington, DC: Bureau of National Affairs.

Full text of Occupational Safety and Health Review Commission decisions. Published since 1974.

2.4.   Rothstein, M. A. *Occupational Safety and Health Law.* St. Paul, MN: West Publishing Co., 1990.

Handbook of law and legislation regarding this subject in the United States.

2.5.   *Occupational Safety and Health Reporter.* Washington, DC: Bureau of National Affairs.

Up-to-date information on legislation and regulations; weekly coverage of governmental actions related to occupational safety and health. Published since 1971.

2.6.   *Shepard's Federal Occupational Safety and Health Citations.* Colorado Springs, CO: Shepard's/McGraw-Hill.

Contains subsequent case histories. Lists citations to law reviews and other secondary sources. Provides parallel citations to other legal reporters. Includes OSHA citations.

2.7.   United States Code. Washington, DC: US Government Printing Office.

Every 6 years a new US Code is published, codified by topic, which includes by title the public laws appearing in the Statutes at Large. Title 42 covers The Public Health and Welfare; Title 29, Labor; Title 21, Food and Drugs. United States Statutes at Large contains the slip laws of each session of Congress.

3.   Sources Used to Locate Occupational Health Statistics

3.1.   National Center for Health Statistics. *Health United States.* Washington, DC: US Government Printing Office.

In-depth profiles of specific health subjects from both public and private sources. Published annually.

3.2.   *MMWR: Morbidity and Mortality Weekly Report.* Atlanta: Centers for Disease Control (CDC).

3.3.   *Annual Summary MMWR: Morbidity and Mortality Weekly Report.* Atlanta: CDC.

3.4.   Surveillance Summaries. Atlanta: CDC.

These three sources comprise the MMWR *Information Series.* MMWR *includes cases of specified notifiable diseases (for particular week covered, and cumulated for the year), notifiable diseases of low frequency (cumulated for the year only), cases of specified notifiable diseases (for week covered and the week of the preceding year by geographic region), and deaths for all causes (week only) in 121 US cities.* Annual Summary *is published in the last issue in each volume and covers the previous year. It does not contain an index. See* ASI *(1.1.1),* Index Medicus *(1.1.6), or* MEDLINE *for index access. Surveillance Summaries are published quarterly and contain annual data on conditions monitored in the surveillance programs of the CDC.*

3.5.   *Statistical Reference Index.* Bethesda, MD: Congressional Information Service.

This covers the same six objectives as the ASI (1.1.1). Coverage of US government agency statistics, social trends, business, industry, and economics. In 1989, approximately 2070 titles were indexed and abstracted, including 1450 annual or recurring reports.

3.6.   US Bureau of the Census. *Statistical Abstract of the United States.* Washington, DC: US Government Printing Office.

This serves as both a primary and secondary source for an extensive range of national data. It remains a good first choice in searching for statistical data. It contains over 1600 tables and charts on business, economics, politics, and health.

3.7.   Vital and Health Statistics Series. Hyattsville, MD: National Center for Health Statistics.

The "Rainbow" series (named for the various colors of its sections) contains 23 sections on vital and health statistics. Best used in conjunction with the ASI (1.1.1).

3.8.   *World Statistics Annual.* Geneva: World Health Organization.

Three volumes: Vital Statistics and Causes of Death, Infectious Disease: Cases and Deaths, *and* Health Personnel and Hospital Establishments.

3.9.   Milton, J. S., and Tsokos, J. O. *Statistical Methods in the Biological and Health Sciences.* New York: McGraw-Hill, 1983.

This book is meant to serve as a first course in statistical methods for students of health and biological sciences.

3.10.   Colton, T. *Statistics in Medicine.* Boston: Little, Brown, 1974.

Covers the principles of statistics for the "present or future practicing physician."

3.11.   Darnay, A. J. *Statistical Record of the Environment.* Detroit: Gale, 1992.

". . . a comprehensive presentation of statistical materials drawn from governmental and private sources." SRE is divided into 10 chapters that present environmental statistics, which begin with the media (overview) and are followed by others that present specific aspects of environmental concern. Over 800 tables, many with illustrated maps or graphs.

3.12.   Guides to the Statistics Sources

Useful information found in reference sources published by librarians. In addition to the source in this section, please refer to those listed in 3.

3.12.1.   Weise, F. *Health Statistics: A Guide to Information Sources.* Health Affairs Information Guide Series, Vol. 4. Detroit: Gale, 1980.

An excellent annotated bibliography with complete coverage of statistics reported by local, state, and federal governments. A valuable guide to the structure of the compilation process of the US government.

4.   Recommended Readings in Epidemiology

4.1.   Hennekens, C. H., and Buring, J. E. *Epidemiology in Medicine.* Boston: Little, Brown, 1988.

The chief objective is to enable readers to interpret and apply the principles of epidemiology to their own needs. Divided into four sections: basic concepts of epidemiology, discussions of various study designs, issues and analyses in interpretation of data, and examples of application of epidemiologic principles and methods to disease control within screening programs.

4.2.   Lilienfeld, A. M., and Lilienfeld, D. E. *Foundations of Epidemiology.* New York: Oxford University Press, 1980.

This text has wide applications for students of medicine, dentistry, allied health, nursing, public health, veterinary science, and environmental health. It presents concepts and methods of epidemiology as applied to various disease problems.

4.3.   Bernier, R. H., and Mason V. M. *EPISOURCE: A Guide to Resources in Epidemiology.* Roswell, GA: The Epidemiology Monitor, 1991.

The growth of the field of epidemiology in the 1980s prompted the authors to write this comprehensive directory of materials and resources available.

4.4. Last, J. M. *A Dictionary of Epidemiology.* New York: Oxford University Press, 1988.

This dictionary ". . . is an attempt to bring some order to the occasionally chaotic nomenclature of epidemiology." Bibliography included.

5. Guides and Manuals

5.1. *Major Hazard Control: A Practical Manual.* Geneva: International Labour Office, 1990.

This manual covers the design, planning, operation, and safety of plants. Specifically emphasizes the roles of authorities, employees, and management.

5.2. Grad, F. O. *The Public Health Law Manual.* Washington, DC: American Public Health Association, 1990.

Legal aspects of the public health field. Written for public health professionals who enforce, administer, and provide health services.

5.3. Office of the Federal Register, National Archives and Records Administration. *The United States Government Manual.* Washington, DC: US Government Printing Office.

Annual official handbook of the US federal government. Comprehensive information on the agencies of the legislative, judicial, and executive branches.

6. Handbooks

Handbooks are practical guides to a field, with tables, formulas, or other pertinent information.

6.1. Sunshine, I. *CRC Handbook Series in Analytical Toxicology.* Boca Raton, FL: CRC, 1979.

"In addition to collating the physical and chemical properties of drugs and chemical hazards, summaries of published methods for their detection in biological specimens are presented."

6.2. Kaye, S. *Handbook of Emergency Toxicology.* Springfield, IL: Thomas, 1988.

General facts and some detail to assist the clinician in making reliable, rapid diagnoses of poisoning. Additional information on crack, nitrogen dioxide, and fish poisoning (ciguatera).

6.3. Plunkett, E. R. *Handbook of Industrial Toxicology.* New York: Chemical Publishing Co., 1987.

A quick-reference, practical guide for those employed in protecting the health of the worker. The Threshold Limit Values (TLV) are based on current American Conference of Governmental Industrial Hygienists (ACGIH) recommendations.

6.4. Sittig, M. *Handbook of Toxic and Hazardous Chemicals and Carcinogens.* Park Ridge, NJ: Noyes Publications, 1991.

Presents concise chemical, safety, and health information on over 800 toxic and hazardous chemicals. Written for those who work with these chemicals or have direct contact with third-party exposure. Extensive coverage of EPA hazardous wastes, substances, NIOSH information profiles, and carcinogens identified by the US National Toxicology Program.

6.5. Weiss, G. (ed.). *Hazardous Chemicals Data Book.* Park Ridge, NJ: Noyes Data Corporation, 1980.

The Chemical Hazard Response Information System (CHRIS) was designed to provide information to those who transport hazardous chemicals through waterways. Compilation of 1350 hazardous chemicals.

6.6. Proctor, N. H., Hughes, J. P., and Fischman, M. L. *Chemical Hazards of the Workplace.* Philadelphia: Lippincott, 1988.

Provides authoritative, critical information on some 438 chemicals likely to be encountered in the workplace. This includes all of the 386 chemicals identified in the NIOSH/OSHA Standards Completion Project.

7. Important Bibliographic Databases that Relate to Occupational Health and Toxicology

7.1. MEDLARS

The Medical Literature and Analysis Retrieval System (MEDLARS) family of databases is the product of the National Library of Medicine. It consists of more than 20 database files, including specific ones that are presented here. MEDLARS began in the mid-1960s. It is an evolving system.

7.2. MEDLINE

This heavily used biomedical database may be accessed through many formats; it covers more than 4000 journals from around the world. Indexing is based on MeSH. Citations contained in Index to Dental Literature, International Nursing Index, *and* Index Medicus *are found in MEDLINE. Coverage begins with 1966 and continues to the present. Over 250,000 records are added each year.*

7.3. CANCERLIT

A MEDLINE companion file that overlaps with MEDLINE, but includes material from symposia, proceedings, and abstracts not published in standard journal literature. Includes abstracts that appeared in Carcinogenesis Abstracts *from 1963 to 1969 and in* Cancer Therapy Abstracts *from 1967 to 1979.*

7.4. CANCERPROJ

Listing of cancer research throughout the United States.

7.5. TOXLINE and TOXLIT

TOXLINE and TOXLIT are comprehensive bibliographic databases for toxicologic, occupational medicine, pharmacologic, biochemical, and physiologic effects. When the files are combined, one has access to approximately 3 million citations. TOXLINE coverage begins with 1965 and continues to the present. TOXLIT contains citations that require royalty charges, while TOXLINE does not. Since this coverage may vary among database vendors, it is imperative to understand what you are getting. Both databases are composed of files from secondary sources. These are identified as "subfiles." Each subfile has its own internal standards. All have been included here, and are as follows:

TOXBIB: Citations from MEDLINE. This is the "toxicity bibliography." Indexing based on MeSH. Citations from MEDLINE that have the subheadings adverse effects, poisoning, or toxicity.

BIOSIS: Toxicologic aspects of environmental health. Former name: Health Effects of Environmental Pollutants (HEEP). Coverage from 1970 to present. Expanded in 1985 to include occupational health, air, soil, water pollution, and waste disposal. Compiled by the Biosciences Information Service.

CA: Contains specific sections of Chemical Abstracts Service on toxicology from 1965.

IPA: Coverage of specific sections of the American Society of Hospital Pharmacists' *International Pharmaceutical Abstracts* from 1970 to the present. Toxicologic aspects of pharmaceuticals.

EMIC: Mutation literature from the Environmental Mutagen Information Center file at the Oak Ridge National Laboratory, 1965 to the present.

ETIC: Birth defects (teratology) literature from the Environmental Teratology Information Center file, 1950 to the present.

NTIS: National Technical Information Service, Toxicology Document and Data Depository, October 1979 to the present. Lists citations from the *Government Reports and Announcements Index* (1.1.3) on toxicology.

NIOSH: National Institute for Occupational Safety and Health coverage of selected NIOSH publications. Approximately 150 journals on occupational safety and health information since 1984.

PESTAB: Coverage from 1966 through 1981 of the EPA's *Pesticides Abstracts*. Effects of pesticides on humans and epidemiology.

EPIDEM: Produced by the Food and Drug Administration's (FDA's) Center for Food Safety, the Epidemiology Information System File dates back to the 1940s. Special coverage of natural toxicants.

CIS: Coverage since 1981 of toxicology-related material from the International Labour Office (ILO) database.

CRISP: Toxicology research projects selected from the National Institute of Health's (NIH's) CRISP system. Information on projects and research grants supported by the Public Health Service, or conducted "intramurally" by the NIH and the National Institute of Mental Health.

TSCATS: Health and safety studies on chemicals submitted by industry to the EPA's office of Toxic Substances under the Toxic Substances Control Act (TSCA).

ANEUPL: The aneuploidy file from the Environmental Mutagen Information Center Special Collection. These citations are related to abnormal chromosome number ". . . induced by physical, chemical, or biological agents."

HMTC: Information on the management of hazardous materials (transportation, storage, and disposal) from the Hazardous Materials Technical Center.

PPBIB: Poisonous Plants Bibliography. Citations from this subfile are from 1976 and earlier. Coverage of the toxicology of poisonous plants.

FEDRIP: This subfile consists of project reports on toxicology and related areas, derived from the NTIS database of the same name. Emphasis on research in progress. FEDRIP stands for Federal Research in Progress.

DART: Developmental and Reproductive Toxicology. Literature on chemical, physical, and biologic agents that may cause birth defects. Approximately 60% of DART is contained in MEDLINE. DART is a continuation of the ETIC subfile and contains citations published since 1989.

7.6. The TOXNET System

TOXNET (Toxicology Data Network) is a computerized system of files on toxicology, hazardous chemicals, and related areas. Managed by the National Library of Medicine's (NLM's) Division of Specialized Information Services through its Toxicology Information Program, TOXNET possesses an "integrated approach" to building and updating records, with a sophisticated retrieval module. The following is a complete list of TOXNET files:

HSDB: The Hazardous Substances Data Bank is factual information on over 4300 potentially hazardous chemicals. HSDB contains information on exposure potential, emergency medicine, and regulatory requirements. The file undergoes peer review by expert toxicologists and scientists.

RTECS: The Registry of Toxic Effects of Chemical Substances (11.5) contains data on more than 106,000 chemicals. The file is built and maintained by NIOSH.

CCRIS: The National Cancer Institute sponsors the Chemical Carcinogenesis Research Information system (CCRIS), which contains over 2500 records on mutagenicity, tumor studies, and carcinogenicity.

IRIS: The EPA sponsors the Integrated Risk Information System (IRIS). Health risk and regulatory information is provided on 500 chemicals. Also contains EPA Health Advisories issued by their Office of Drinking Water.

GENE-TOX: Another EPA file that contains genetic toxicology (mutagenicity) data on over 3000 chemicals. This is a review system of the "open scientific" literature. A "multi-phase" effort to "review and evaluate" existing literature and assay systems available in this field of toxicology.

EMIC/EMICBACK: Two files created by the Oak Ridge National Laboratory's Environmental Mutagen, Carcinogen, and Teratogen Information Program. Bibliographic databases on the chemical, biologic, and physical agents tested for genotoxic activity.

DART/ETICBACK: Developmental and Reproductive Toxicology/Environmental Teratology Information Center backfile. Bibliographic file on teratology and developmental toxicology. Produced jointly by the EPA and the National Institute of Environmental Health Sciences.

DBIR: Directory of Biotechnology Information Resources. This guide to biotechnology resources includes on-line databases, networks, and publications.

TRI: The Toxic Release Inventory was mandated by the Emergency Planning and Community Right to Know Act. Contains data on the estimated releases of toxic chemicals to the environment. Also includes information on chemical waste sites.

TRIFACTS: Toxic Chemical Release Inventory Facts. A new component of TOXNET. Written in lay language, this file grew out of the New Jersey State Hazardous Substances Fact Sheets.

7.7. Additional Databases

A large number of bibliographic databases exist through various commercial vendors besides the US government. A partial list is included in this section.

7.7.1. BIOBUSINESS

This file is created by the BIOSIS group in Philadelphia and provides current and retrospective information to business executives and product and marketing professionals. It has been included here because it covers various medical subjects, such as pesticides, occupational health, toxicology, and pharmaceuticals. 1985 to present; over 200,000 records.

7.7.2. BIOSIS PREVIEWS

This contains the on-line equivalent of the Biological Abstracts, Biological Abstracts/ RRM, *and* BioResearch Index *(1.2.1). Covers approximately 275,000 accounts of original research each year from almost 9000 primary journals and monographs. An extensive, comprehensive database. 1969 to present.*

7.7.3. CA SEARCH

Chemical Abstracts *coverage goes back to–1967. This is the on-line equivalent of the index by the same name (1.2.2)*

7.7.4. CHEMTOX ONLINE

Comprehensive coverage of over 6400 regulated toxic and hazardous substances. Includes physical, chemical, and toxicological properties; health, safety, and risk management. Total integration of toxicity data including carcinogenicity status.

7.7.5. CIN

Chemical Industry Notes *indexes over 80 important international journals and newspapers that reflect events in the industry. Produced by Chemical Abstracts Service and the American Chemical Society. 1974 to the present; over 800,000 records.*

7.7.6. CRGS

Chemical Regulations and Guidelines System *is produced by CRC systems in Fairfax, Florida. It is an index to US federal regulatory material relating to the control of chemical substances. Also included: federal guidelines, statutes, and promulgated regulations. CRGS follows the regulatory cycle, including main document and revisions found in the* Federal Register. *Regulations in effect since 1982.*

7.7.7. CSNB

Chemical Safety Newsbase *is produced by the Royal Society of Chemistry and covers workplace hazards encountered in industry and laboratories. This on-line equivalent of the* Chemical Hazards in Industry *and* Laboratory Hazards Bulletin *has been in existence since 1981.*

7.7.8. EMBASE

This on-line version of the Excerpta Medica *(1.2.3) begins in 1974. The file contains over 4 million records and an additional 100,000 annual records that do not appear in printed journals.*

7.7.9. ENVIROLINE

A comprehensive international database of environmental information covering more than 5000 primary and secondary sources, including rulings in the Federal Register *and* Official Gazette *of the US Patent and Trademark Office. Coverage since 1971 with more than 140,000 records.*

7.7.10. HAZARDLINE

Provides safety and handling information on 3000 hazardous substances. Information taken from court decisions, monographs, and periodicals.

7.7.11. MSDS-CCOHS Database

Produced by the Canadian Centre for Occupational Health and Safety, available through Chemical Abstracts/STN. This is the "largest publicly available collection" of Material Safety Data Sheets. Information on 70,000 records.

7.7.12. NTIS

The National Technical Information Service covers a wide range of subjects. Includes government-sponsored research, development, and engineering. Over 240 US government agencies covered. Interdisciplinary database from 1964 to the present. More than one million records.

7.7.13. NIOSH

The NIOSH database covers citations from more than 400 journals and 70,000 monographs and technical reports since 1973. A pertinent source for occupational health, hazards, and safety literature. More than 160,000 records.

7.8. Aids for Searching Common Database Files

Included here are popular, time-tested aids to searching common databases, such as MEDLINE. It is important to consult these aids to conduct your own searches.

7.8.1. *MEDLINE: A Basic Guide to Searching.* Chicago: MLA, 1985

Strong overview of the MEDLINE search mechanics, indexing practices, and other important aspects of searching. The differences between searching MEDLINE on three systems is compared.

7.8.2. Basics of Searching MEDLINE: A Guide for the Health Professional. MEDLARS Management Section, Bibliographic Services Division, Library Operations, National Library of Medicine, 1986.

Self-instructional guide to the concepts and skills required in searching MEDLINE.

7.8.3. The NLM Technical Bulletin. US Department of Health and Human Services, Public Health Service, National Institutes of Health, National Library of Medicine.

The bulletin covers the changes in each MEDLARS database. If you search MEDLARS files, it is worth reading this publication each month.

7.8.4. Medical Subject Headings—Annotated Alphabetic List. US Department of Health and Human Services, Public Health Service, National Institutes of Health, National Library of Medicine.

The list of medical subject headings (MeSH), which is updated annually and described as the "bible" of MEDLARS. Subjects are arranged in alphabetical order with scope notes and alphanumeric codes for the Tree Structures (7.8.6)

7.8.5. Medical Subject Headings—Permuted Headings.

This serves as a thesaurus for the MeSH headings. Subjects are listed by each significant word in the MeSH heading.

7.8.6. Medical Subject Headings—Tree Structures.

The Tree Structures is a subject-arranged listing of terms from the annotated list. Subjects are grouped into 15 broad categories that are hierarchically arranged; hence the "tree structure."

7.8.7. MEDLEARN. US Department of Health and Human Services, Public Health Service, National Institutes of Health, National Library of Medicine.

A computer tutorial program for learning MEDLINE searching.

7.8.8. TOXLEARN. US Department of Health and Human Services, Public Health Service, National Institutes of Health, National Library of Medicine.

A computer tutorial program for searching TOXLINE.

7.8.9. List of Journals Indexed in Index Medicus. US Department of Health and Human Services, Public Health Service, National Institutes of Health, National Library of Medicine.

An annual publication of current titles included in Index Medicus. Includes NLM standard abbreviations, titles added in the previous year, arrangement by subject, and country of origin. 3030 titles listed in 1992.

7.8.10. List of Serials Indexed for On-line Users. US Department of Health and Human Services, Public Health Service, National Institutes of Health, National Library of Medicine.

Annual list of complete bibliographic information for over 7000 serials indexed in the Hospital Literature Index, International Nursing Index, Index Medicus, and International Dental Index. Includes standard NLM abbreviations. Special list indicators for population studies, biotechnology, dentistry, nursing, health planning.

7.8.11. Kelner, L. W. *Searching the MEDLARS Database: A Practical Guide for Profilers.* Latham, NY: Bibliographic Retrieval Services, 1981.

Describes MEDLARS as a system and how to search it, concentrating on areas that are most troublesome.

7.9. Guides to Databases

Many databases exist throughout the world. These constantly change, and it is often difficult to keep up with these changes. Some of the following sources represent a sample list of reference books that catalogue the availability of databases.

7.9.1. Barg, J. C. (ed.). *Directory of On-line Databases*. Detroit: Gale.

Over 4000 on-line bibliographic and nonbibliographic databases are included. Coverage of statistical, alphanumeric, textual numeric, and full-text databases.

7.9.2. Zarozny, S. (ed.). *Federal Database Finder*. Chevy Chase, MD: Information USA, 1987.

Coverage of approximately 4200 databases and datafiles available to the public. Many of these are available at no charge.

8. Guides to the Health Sciences Literature

Many of these guides are indispensable in locating the correct sources for information. The purpose of these books is to overview a particular discipline and often to provide lists of reference books with or without annotations.

8.1. Chih-Chen, C. *Health Information Sources*. Cambridge, MA: MIT Press, 1981.

A broad, comprehensive treatment of information sources within the health sciences. Covers titles from 1975 to April 1980.

8.2. Chitty, M. G., and Schatz, N. *Federal Information Sources in Health and Medicine*. New York: Greenwood Press, 1988.

Since much toxicology and occupational health information pertains to government activity, this book is an important guide to the literature. Annotations of up to 1200 government publications; 100 databases from 90 federal agencies, institutes, and information centers. Toxicology is covered in Chap. 43, occupational health in Chap. 37.

8.3. *Occupational Safety and Health: A Sourcebook* New York: Garland, 1985.

Annotated bibliographic guide to approximately 500 English-language publications, including audiovisuals, statistical sources, and reference works published between 1970 and 1984. Includes the text of the 1970 Occupational Safety and Health Act.

8.4. Roper, F. W., and Boorkman, J. A. *Introduction to Reference Sources in the Health Sciences*. Chicago: MLA, 1984.

Selected annotated list of medical library reference, bibliographic, and information sources used on a regular basis. A useful and popular reference.

8.5. Wexler, P. *Information Resources in Toxicology*. New York: Elsevier, 1988.

An essential, comprehensive guide to national as well as international toxicology resources. The book of choice in locating toxicology resources.

8.6. Deck, K. S., and Bonzo, S. E. *Some Publicly Available Sources of Computerized Information on Environmental Health and Toxicology*. Atlanta: US Department of Health and Human Services, Public Health Service, Centers for Disease Control, Center for Environmental Health and Injury Control, Information Resources Management Group, 1991.

Another important guide to toxicology information resources.

9. Style Manuals

If you are preparing research for publication, you will need to consult some style manuals. If used correctly, these sources will enable you to organize material and save precious time.

9.1. *The Chicago Manual of Style* (14th ed.). Chicago: University of Chicago Press, 1994.

Readable, well organized, a great source of guidance in the preparation of manuscripts and other bibliographic formats.

9.2. *Manual of Style* (8th ed.). Chicago: American Medical Association, 1989.

This manual assists in the preparation of manuscripts. It defines the types of articles, and covers legal and ethical considerations, style, grammar, measurements, terminology, and other technical information.

9.3.　Schwanger, E. *Medical English Usage and Abusage.* Phoenix: Oryx Press, 1991. *A concise, relevant guide for the medical writer.*

10.　General List of Occupational Medicine and Toxicology Monographs

A short list of monographs is provided as a starting point for research in this area. Some are "reference" books (books consulted for factual information).

10.1.　Amdur, M. O., Doull, J., and Klaassen, C. D. (eds.). *Cassarett and Doull's Toxicology.* New York: Pergamon, 1991.

10.2.　Sax, N. I., and Lewis, R. J., Jr. *Dangerous Properties of Industrial Materials.* New York: Van Nostrand Reinhold, 1989.

10.3.　*Hamilton and Hardy's Industrial Toxicology.* Littleton, MA: John Wright PSG Publications, Inc., 1985.

10.4.　Williams, P. L., and Burson, J. L. (ed.). *Industrial Toxicology. Safety and Health Applications in the Workplace.* New York: Van Nostrand Reinhold, 1985.

10.5.　*Occupational Exposure to Airborne Toxic Substances.* Geneva: International Labour Office, 1991.

10.6.　Waldron, H. A. *Occupational Health Practice.* Boston: Butterworth, 1989.

10.7.　Waldron, H. A., and Harrington, J. M. (eds.). *Occupational Hygiene: An Introductory Text.* Oxford: Blackwell, 1980.

10.8.　Morgan, W. K. C., and Seaton, A. *Occupational Lung Diseases.* Philadelphia: Saunders, 1984.

10.9.　Parkes, W. R. *Occupational Lung Disorders.* London: Butterworth, 1982.

10.10.　Clayton, G. D., and Clayton, F. E. (eds.). *Patty's Industrial Hygiene and Toxicology.* New York: Wiley, 1991.

10.11.　Verschueren, K. *Handbook of Environmental Data on Organic Chemicals.* New York: Van Nostrand Reinhold, 1983.

10.12.　Viccellio, P. *Handbook of Medical Toxicology.* Boston: Little, Brown, 1993.

10.13.　Foden, C. *Hazardous Materials.* Boca Raton, FL: CRC, 1991.

10.14.　Lawrence, K. (ed.). *National Toxicology Programs.* Philadelphia: Lea & Febiger, 1992.

10.15.　Smith, R. P. *Primer of Environmental Toxicology.* Philadelphia: Lea & Febiger, 1992.

10.16.　Rom, W. N. *Environmental and Occupational Medicine.* Boston: Little, Brown, 1992.

10.17.　Zenz, C. *Occupational Medicine.* St. Louis: Mosby–Year Book, 1993.

10.18.　Levy, B. S., and Wegman, D. H. *Occupational Health: Recognizing and Preventing Work-Related Disease.* Boston: Little, Brown, 1988.

10.19.　Koren, H. *Handbook of Environmental Health and Safety: Principles and Practices.* Chelsea, MI: Lewis, 1991.

10.20.　Tarcher, A. B. *Principles and Practice of Environmental Medicine.* New York: Plenum, 1992.

11.　Additional Reference Sources

These sources belong in a general reference collection for the occupational health specialist.

11.1. Curry, A. S. *Advances in Forensic and Clinical Toxicology.* Cleveland: CRC, 1972.

This is an overview of the literature on substances such as carbon monoxide, cannabis, LSD, barbiturates, lead, and mercury.

11.2. Lewis, R. J., Sr. *Hazardous Chemicals Desk Reference.* New York: Van Nostrand Reinhold, 1991.

Includes safe storage and handling of chemicals, respirators, protective chemical clothing, fire protection, first aid, abbreviations, (CAS) and RTECS numbers, hazard ratings, molecular properties, OSHA air standards, American Conference of Governmental Industrial Hygienists Threshold Limit Values, German Research Society's values, US DOT classifications, and the Toxic and Hazard Review.

11.3. *The Merck Index.* Rahway, NJ: Merck & Co., 1989

Comprehensive encyclopedia of chemicals, drugs, and biologic substances.

11.4. *Merck Manual of Diagnosis and Therapy.* Rahway, NJ: Merck & Co., 1992.

Reference guide for a broad range of medical disorders. Discussions of factors related to rational diagnostic reasoning and therapy.

11.5. Registry of Toxic Effects of Chemical Substances (RTECS). Cincinnati: NIOSH.

Arrangement by chemical substance. Purpose: to identify all known toxic substances in the environment and to codify toxic doses. When available, the following are provided: CAS registry number, molecular weight and formula, toxic dose data, US and NIOSH documents citing standards for handling these substances.

11.6. Report of the Task Group on Reference Man. Report no. 23, International Commission on Radiographical Protection. New York: Pergamon, 1977.

Report originally prepared to assist in radiation studies. The compilers focused attention on human characteristics "which are known to be important or which are likely to be significant for estimation of dose from sources of radiation within or outside the body . . ."

11.7. Ellenhorn, M., and Barceloux, D. G. *Medical Toxicology.* New York: Elsevier, 1988.

A general approach to the poisoned patient, therapeutic drugs, drugs of abuse, chemical products, and natural toxins.

12. Translations and Translation Services

Although English has become the international language of communication, you may find materials that require translation. Here is a sample list of directories and services.

12.1. Congrat-Butlar, Stefan. *Translation and Translators: An International Directory and Guide.* New York: Bowker, 1979.

12.2. National Technical Information Service. Office of International Affairs. *Directory of Japanese Technical Resources.* Springfield, VA: NTIS, 1987–

A result of the Japanese Technical Literature Act of 1986. Entries give bibliographic information. Subject terms and availability information.

12.3 American Translator's Association. *Translation Services Directory.* Arlington, VA: ATA, 1985–

12.4 University Microfilms International, Inc. Ann Arbor, MI.

Contact UMI for more information: 1-800-521-3042; 313-761-4700.

12.5 World Translation Index. Delft, Netherlands: International Translations Centre, 1978–

Former title: World Transindex. *Subject listings with author and source index.*

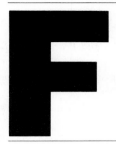

Recommended Library for Occupational and Environmental Physicians

Occupational Medicine: General

Core

Encyclopedia of Occupational Health and Safety (3rd ed.). International Labor Office, 1983.

McCunney, R. J. (ed.). *A Practical Approach to Occupational and Environmental Medicine* (2nd ed.). Boston: Little, Brown, 1994.

Rosenstock, L., and Cullen, M. R. (eds.). *Clinical Occupational Medicine.* Philadelphia: Saunders, 1986.

Advanced

Jong, E. C. *The Travel and Tropical Medicine Manual.* Philadelphia: Saunders, 1987.

LaDou, J. (ed.). *Occupational Medicine.* E. Norwalk, CT: Appleton & Lange, 1990.

Last, J. M., and Wallace, R. B. (eds.). *Maxcy-Rosenau-Last Public Health and Preventive Medicine* (13th ed.). E. Norwalk, CT: Appleton & Lange, 1991.

Levy, B. S., and Wegman, D. H. (eds.). *Occupational Health: Recognizing and Preventing Work-Related Diseases* (3rd ed.). Boston: Little, Brown, 1994.

Raffle, P. A. B., et al. (eds.). *Hunter's Diseases of Occupations* (8th ed.). Boston: Little, Brown, 1988.

Rom, W. N. (ed.). *Environmental and Occupational Medicine* (2nd ed.). Boston: Little, Brown, 1992.

Rose, S. R. *International Travel Health Guide.* Northampton, MA: Travel Medicine Inc, 1992.

Wolfe, M. S. Travel medicine. *Med. Clin. North Am.* 76:1261, 1992.

Zenz, C. *Occupational Medicine: Principles and Practical Applications* (3rd ed.). St. Louis: Mosby, 1994.

Environmental Medicine: General

Core

ATSDR Case Studies in Environmental Medicine. US Public Health Service, Agency for Toxic Substances and Disease Registry.

ATSDR Toxicologic Profiles. US Public Health Service, Agency for Toxic Substances and Disease Registry.

Tarcher, A. B. (ed.). *Principles and Practice of Environmental Medicine.* New York: Plenum, 1992.

Advanced

Brooks, S. M., et al. *Environmental Medicine: Principles and Practices.* St. Louis: Mosby, 1994.

Cone, J., and Hodgson, M. Problem buildings: Building-associated illness and the sick building syndrome. *Occup. Med. State of the Art Rev.,* 4:575, 1989.

Holland, C. D., and Sielken, R. L. *Quantitative Cancer Modeling and Risk Assessment.* Englewood Cliffs, NJ: Prentice Hall, 1993.

Samet, J. M., and Spengler, J. D. *Indoor Air Pollution: A Health Perspective.* Baltimore: Johns Hopkins Press, 1991.

US Environmental Protection Agency. *Building Air Quality.* Office of Air and Radiation, US Department of Health and Human Services, US Government Printing Office, 1991.

Epidemiology and Biostatistics

Core

Friedman, G. D. *Primer of Epidemiology* (3rd ed.). New York: McGraw-Hill, 1987.

Morton, R. F., Hebel, J. R., and McCarter, R. J. *A Study Guide to Epidemiology and Biostatistics* (3rd ed.). Rockville, MD: Aspen Publishing, 1990.

Advanced

Ahlbom, A., and Norrell, S. *Introduction to Modern Epidemiology* (2nd ed.). Newton, MA: Epidemiology Resources Inc, 1990.

Checkoway, H., Pearce, N. E., and Crawford-Brown, D. J. *Research Methods in Occupational Epidemiology.* New York: Oxford University Press, 1989.

Hennekens, C. H., Buring, J. E., and Mayrent, S. L. *Epidemiology in Medicine.* Boston: Little, Brown, 1988.

Karvonen, M., and Mikheev, M. I. *Epidemiology of Occupational Health.* WHO Regional Publications, 1986.

Kleinbaum, D. G., Kupper, L. L., and Morganstern, H. *Epidemiologic Research.* New York: Van Nostrand Reinhold, 1982.

Last, J. M. *A Dictionary of Epidemiology* (2nd ed.). New York: Oxford University Press, 1988.

Monson, R. R. *Occupational Epidemiology* (2nd ed.). Boca Raton, FL: CRC Press, 1990.

Rothman, K. J. *Modern Epidemiology.* Boston: Little, Brown, 1986.

Health Promotion and Screening

Core

Eddy, D. M. (ed.). *Common Screening Tests.* Philadelphia: American College of Physicians, 1991.

Scofield, M. E. Worksite health promotion. *Occup. Med. State of the Art Rev.* 5:653, 1990.

US Preventive Services Task Force. *Guide to Clinical Preventive Services: An Assessment of the Effectiveness of 169 Interventions.* Baltimore: Williams & Wilkins, 1989.

Advanced

O'Donnell, M. P., and Ainsworth, T. E. *Health Promotion in the Workplace*. Albany, NY: Delmar Publishers, 1992.

Toxicology

Core

Ellenhorn, M. J., and Barceloux, D. G. *Medical Toxicology: Diagnosis and Treatment of Human Poisoning*. Philadelphia: Elsevier Science Publishers, 1988.

Hathaway, G. J., et al. *Proctor and Hughes' Chemical Hazards of the Workplace* (3rd ed.). New York: Van Nostrand Reinhold, 1991.

Lauwerys, R. R., and Hoet, P. *Industrial Chemical Exposure: Guidelines for Biologic Monitoring* (2nd ed.). Chelsea, MI: Lewis Publishers, 1993.

Sullivan, J. B., and Krieger, G. R., (eds.). *Hazardous Material Toxicology*. Baltimore: Williams & Wilkins, 1992.

Advanced

Amdur, M. O., Doull, J., and Klaassen, C. D. (eds.). *Casarett and Doull's Toxicology: The Basic Sciences of Poisons* (4th ed.). New York: McGraw-Hill, 1991.

Finkel, A. J. *Hamilton and Hardy's Industrial Toxicology* (4th ed.). St. Louis: Mosby, 1982. (*This book is currently out of print. It can be obtained through local medical libraries.*)

Goldfrank, L. R., et al. (eds.). *Goldfrank's Toxicologic Emergencies* (4th ed.). E. Norwalk, CT: Appleton & Lange, 1990.

Gosselin, R. E., Smith, R. P., and Hodge, H. C. *Clinical Toxicology of Commercial Products* (5th ed.). Baltimore: Williams & Wilkins, 1984.

Haddad, L. M., and Winchester, J. F. *Clinical Management of Poisoning and Drug Overdose* (2nd ed.). Philadelphia: Saunders, 1990.

Lewis, R. J. *Sax's Dangerous Properties of Industrial Materials* (8th ed.). New York: Van Nostrand Reinhold, 1992.

Hazardous Chemicals Desk Reference (3rd ed.). Lewis, R. J. New York: Van Nostrand Reinhold, 1993.

Clayton, G. D., and Clayton, F. E. (eds.). *Patty's Industrial Hygiene and Toxicology* 3rd Rev Ed.: Vol. I, A & B; Vol. II, A–F, 1993–1994. Vol. III, A & B. 4th Ed.: Cralley, L. J., and Cralley L. V. (eds.). 1992–1994. New York: Wiley.

Williams, P. L., and Burson, J. L. (eds.). *Industrial Toxicology: Safety and Health Applications in the Workplace.*New York: Van Nostrand Reinhold, 1985.

Ergonomics and Musculoskeletal Medicine

Core

Grandjeans, E. *Fitting the Task to the Man* (4th ed.). Philadelphia: Taylor & Francis, 1988.

Hadler, N. M. *Occupational Musculoskeletal Disorders*. New York: Raven Press, 1993.

Moore, J. S., and Garg, A. Ergonomics: Low back pain, carpal tunnel syndrome, and upper extremity disorders in the workplace. *Occup. Med. State of the Art Rev.* 7:593, 1992.

Putz-Anderson, V. *Cumulative Trauma Disorders: A Manual for Musculoskeletal Diseases of the Upper Limbs*. Philadelphia: Taylor & Francis, 1988.

Advanced

Chaffin, D. B., and Andersson, G. B. J. Occupational Biomechanics (2nd ed.). New York: Wiley, 1991.

Eastman Kodak Co. *Ergonomic Design for People at Work*. Vols. I and II. New York: Van Nostrand Reinhold, 1986.

Iserhagen, S. J. *Work Injury: Management and Prevention*. Rockville, MD: Aspen Publishers, 1988.

Pope, M. H., et al. *Occupational Low Back Pain*. St. Louis: Mosby, 1991.

Steinberg, G. G., Akins, C. M., and Baron, D. T. *Ramamurti's Orthopedics and Primary Care* (2nd ed.). Baltimore: Williams & Wilkins, 1992.

Clinical Occupational and Environmental Medicine

Dermatology

Core
Adams, R. M. *Occupational Skin Disease* (2nd ed.). Philadelphia: Saunders, 1990.

Maibach, H. I. *Occupational and Industrial Dermatology*. St. Louis: Mosby, 1987. (*This book is currently out of print. It can be obtained through local medical libraries.*)

Advanced
Marks, J. G., and DeLeo, V. A. *Contact and Occupational Dermatology*. St. Louis: Mosby, 1992.

Ear, Nose, and Throat

Core
Sataloff, R. T., and Sataloff, J. *Occupational Hearing Loss* (2nd ed.). New York: Marcel Dekker, 1993.

Respiratory Medicine

Core
Parkes, R. *Occupational Lung Disorders* (3rd ed.). New York: Butterworth-Heinemann, 1994.

Advanced
Bardana, E. J., Montanaro, A., and O'Hallaren, M. T. Occupational asthma. St. Louis: Mosby-Year Book, 1992.

Beckett, W. S., and Basson, K. Occupational lung disease. *Occup. Med. State of the Art Rev.* 7:189, Apr 1992.

Bernstein, I. L., et al. *Asthma in the Workplace*. New York: Marcel Dekker, 1993.

Harber, P., and Balmes, J. R. Prevention of pulmonary disease. *Occup. Med. State of the Art Rev.* 6: 1991.

Occupational Lung Diseases. International Labor Office, 1991.

Industrial Hygiene

Core

Plog, B. A. Fundamentals of Industrial Hygiene (3rd ed.). National Safety Council, 1988.

Threshold Limit Values and Biological Exposure Indices for 1993–1994. American Conference of Governmental Industrial Hygienists, 1993.

Advanced

Documentation of the Threshold Limit Values and Biological Exposure Indices (6th ed.). American Conference of Governmental Industrial Hygienists, 1991.

Administration

Core

American Medical Association: Guide to the Evaluation of Permanent Impairment (4th ed.). American Medical Association, 1993.

Guidotti, T. L., Cowell, J. W. F., and Jamieson, G. G. *Occupational Health Services: A Practical Approach*. American Medical Association, 1989.

Reed, P. *The Medical Disability Advisor* (2nd ed.). Horsham, PA: LRP Publications, 1994.

Swotinsky, R. B. *The Medical Review Officers Guide to Drug Testing*. New York: Van Nostrand Reinhold, 1992.

Advanced

DiBenedetto, D. V., Harris, J. S., and McCunney, R. J. *OEM Occupational Health and Safety Manual*. OEM Health Information Inc., 1992, updated 1993.

Edwards, F. C. *Fitness for Work: The Medical Aspects*. New York: Oxford University Press, 1988.

Equal Employment Opportunity Commission. *A Technical Assistance Manual on the Employment Provision of the Americans with Disabilities Act*. Washington, DC: US Government Printing Office, 1992.

Felton, J. S. *Occupational Medical Management: A Guide to the Organization and Operation of In-Plant Occupational Health Services*. Boston: Little, Brown, 1989.

Moser, R. *Effective Management of Occupational and Environmental Health and Safety Programs: A Practical Guide*. Boston: OEM Health Information Inc., 1992.

The Recommended Library for Occupational and Environmental Physicians was compiled by the Publications Committee of the American College of Occupational and Environmental Medicine (ACOEM). Questions regarding the Library should be directed to the ACOEM Publications Department, 55 W. Seegers Road, Arlington Heights, IL 60005.

Source: Reprinted with permission from the *Journal of Occupational Medicine* Vol. 36(7), July 1994.

Index

Index

system of outside notification in, 676
team in, 671–674
protection of response personnel in, 661–662
provision of medical information in, 662–663
regulatory authority in, 669–670
role of occupational physician in, 678
Emergency response plan, 670–677. *See also*
Emergency response
Emergency response team, 671–674
protection of, 661–662
responder levels on, 672
EMF. *See* Electromagnetic fields
EMG. *See* Electromyography
Emotional disabilities, 71–72
Emotional factors in physical symptoms, 272–274
Emphysema, 153
Employee
assessment of, 467. *See also* Health promotion
Americans with Disabilities Act and, 64
assistance programs for. *See* Employee assistance programs
as customer of health care services, 590–591
drug testing of. *See* Drug testing
emergency plans for, 538
emergency protection for, 661–662
employment examinations for, 66–68
exposure of. *See* Exposure
handling hazardous chemicals, 544. *See also* Chemical, hazardous
in industry with high noise levels, 232
international travel of, 548. *See also* International occupational health
matching job with, in primary prevention programs, 48–50
Material Safety Data Sheets for, 542
medical records of, 39
medical surveillance of, 366–367
reproductive hazards for. *See* Reproductive hazards
right-to-know law and, 541
training of, in primary prevention programs, 50
Employee assistance programs, 52, 265–267
economics of, 497
evaluation of, 475
occupational health information system and, 526
occupational physician in, 595
in worksite health promotion, 471
Employer
in accommodation of workplace for applicants or employees, 492–493
economic benefits for, 491. *See also* Economics
health care spending of, 583
insurance coverage by, 581–582, 583
EMS. *See* Emergency Medical Service
EMTs. *See* Emergency Medical Technicians
Enamels in dermatoses, 261, 262
Encephalopathy, 217
clinical evaluation of, 221–223
international travel and, 552
from solvents, 642
Energy expenditure, 205–207
of job, 412–413
model for, 413
Engineering controls
in medical center occupational health, 429
in skin disorder prevention, 255
for sterilants, 436
Enteric pathogens, 432
Entrapment neuropathy, 294–295. *See also* Cumulative trauma disorders
Environment. *See also* Environmental medicine
in accreditation, 136

Agency for Toxic Substances and Disease Registry and, 654
as cause of medical problem, 304–305
contamination of, 306. *See also* Exposure
emergency response to. *See* Emergency response
in history taking in occupational illness, 303
tobacco smoke in
in building-related diseases, 641
as indoor air pollutant, 636
Environmental audit, 693–696
conducting, 694–695
legal basis for, 694
physician in, 695–696
role of, 693–694
timing of, 694
Environmental data, 682–692. *See also* Data; Databases
agency resources for, 685–686, 690–692
agent-specific information in, 684
case studies and, 686–690
commonly asked questions triggering searches in, 685
key questions in evaluating, 683
parameters of interest for, 683
types of, 683–685
Environmental Epidemiology and Risk Assessment, 690–691
Environmental exposure. *See* Exposure
Environmental health. *See also* Environmental medicine
Agency for Toxic Substances and Disease Registry and, 654
corporate medicine in, 594
programs for, 5
Environmental Issues in Primary Care, 691
Environmental medicine. *See also* Environment
accessing data in. *See* Environmental data
acid precipitation and, 609
Agency for Toxic Substances and Disease Registry in, 651–659. *See also* Agency for Toxic Substances and Disease Registry
atmospheric changes and, 605–610
audit in, 693–696
climate change and, 605–608
clinical, 623–632
biologic monitoring for exposures in, 628–631
community-based public health activities in, 624
lead poisoning in, 625–628
office-based practice in, 625–631
office encounters in, 624
risk information in, 628–631
databases for. *See* Databases
defined, 623
dimensions of problems in, 605–611
emergencies in, 660–681. *See also* Emergency response
greenhouse effect and, 605–608
ozone depletion and, 608–609
population growth and, 609–610
regulatory issues in, 614–622
air pollution control, 615–617
chronology of laws on, 614–615
clean water, 617
Comprehensive Environmental Response Compensation and Liability Act and, 618–619
Emergency Planning and Community Right to Know Act and, 619
framework of, 614
interface of, 615, 616
physician and, 621
Resource Conservation and Recovery Act and, 617–618
storage and disposal of toxics and, 617–618
Superfund Amendments and Reauthorization Act and, 619

economics of, 500
environmental, 697–706
  acquiring information in, 698–699
  cancer in, 700–703, 704
  conducting, 699–703
  NAS/NRC paradigm for, 698
  noncancer "endpoints" in, 700
  occupational and environmental physician in, 703–705
  process of, 697, 698
  qualitative or quantitative, 697, 699
methods and terminology in, 379–381
principles of, 381
terminology of, 379–381
Risk characterization in assessment, 697
Risk factors
  for coronary heart disease, 199
  for low back injuries, 166–167
  medical surveillance of, 361
  premature deaths and, 502
  prevalence of, in employed populations, 502
  relative risk of death and, 501
  in worksite health promotion, 466–467
Risk spreading in workers' compensation, 571
RMCLs. See Recommended contaminant levels
RNA. See Ribonucleic acid
Rocky mountain spotted fever, 313
ROD. See Record of decision
Roemer's law, 583–584
Rohmert curve, 399
Roland Disability Questionnaire, 95
ROS. See Review of systems
Rotator cuff tears, 179
RSP. See Respirable suspended particulates
RTECS. See Registry of Toxic Effects of Chemical Substances
Rubber
  in dermatoses, 260, 261, 262, 263, 264
  in gloves. See Gloves
Rubella, 312
  immunizations for, 508, 509
  international travel and, 551
  in medical center occupational health, 430, 433
RWL. See Recommended Weight Limit

Safe Drinking Water Act, 616, 689
Safety
  in environmental risk assessments, 700
  in hazardous chemical management, 539–540
  health information system and, 527
  international health and, 559
  legal issues in, 26–31
Salicylate with bismuth, 557–558
Salmonella, 342, 432
Sample size in epidemiology, 350
Santa Ana Form Board Test, 219
SARA. See Superfund Amendments and Reauthorization Act
SBS. See Sick building syndrome
Scabies, 433
SCBA. See Self-contained breathing apparatus
Scheduling of appointments, 525
Schizoid personality, 276
Schizophrenia, 275
Schizotypal personality, 276
Schools of public health, 513–514
Science Technology and the Constitution, 383
Screening
  economics of, 500
  for lead exposure, 630
  software for, 528
  of traveler upon return, 557–558
  in worksite health promotion, 468–469
Scrotum, malignant neoplasm of, 315
SDWA. See Safe Drinking Water Act

Search strategies in occupational medical literature, 387–391
Seat belts, 501, 502
Second-generation mini-computer systems, 521
Second opinions, 503
Secondary prevention program, 50, 52–54
  in occupational health nursing, 82
Secondary sources of medical literature, 384
Selenium, 463
Self-Assessment Manual, 134
Self-care, economics of, 499, 503
Self-contained breathing apparatus, 661
Self-insurance in cost containment, 586, 588
Seminars, 513–514
Sensitization, testing for, 340. See also Chemical, sensitivity to
Sensorineural hearing loss, 245
Sensory conduction
  measurement of, 216
  in peripheral neuropathies, 224, 225
Sensory nerve action potentials, 224
Sentinel health events, 305, 482–483
Sentinel health events-occupational, 366
Sentinel physicians, 366
Sequoiosis, 318
Server based computer networking, 533–534
Sevin. See Carbaryl
SHE. See Sentinel health events
SHE-O. See Sentinel health events-occupational
Shellfish, 158
Shift work, 271–272
Shingles, 430, 433
Shortage of physicians, 510
Shoulder disorders, 178–179, 296
SIC Codes for manufacturing groups. See Standard Industrial Classification Codes for manufacturing groups
Sick building syndrome, 642–643
Sickness Impact Profile, 95
Significant new-use regulations, 619–620
Significant threshold shift, 238, 240–241, 242, 243, 244
Silica, 151, 154. See also Silicosis
Silicosis, 151–152, 319
  history of deaths from, 750
  nodule in, 152
  physical examination in, 146
Silicotuberculosis, 311
SIP. See Sickness Impact Profile
Skeletal fluorosis, 320
Skin disorders, 248–264. See also Dermatitis
  absorption of toxin in, 335–336
  administrative controls and, 256
  after international travel, 557
  causes of, 249
  clinical expressions of, 250
  engineering controls and, 255
  environmental causes of, 304
  evaluation of, 248–250
  hazardous materials in, 57
  history and physical examination in, 250–254
  patch testing in, 255
  prevention of
    closed systems in, 255
    exposure, 255–256
    materials selection in, 255
    personal protective measures for, 255–256
    ventilation in, 255
  risks specific to occupation in, 260–264
  significance of, 248–264
  site of, 251, 252
  toxic agents and, 334
  toxin effects in, 543
  treatment of, 256–258
    resulting in or prolonging disorder, 250–253
  worksite evaluation of, 254–255
Skin testing, 280–281